GENERAL ULTRASOUND

GENERAL ULTRASOUND

EDITED BY

Carol A. Mittelstaedt, M.D.

Professor of Radiology and Obstetrics and Gynecology
Department of Radiology
University of North Carolina at Chapel Hill School of Medicine
Director, Abdominal Imaging Section
Department of Radiology
University of North Carolina Hospitals
Chapel Hill, North Carolina

CHURCHILL LIVINGSTONE
New York, Edinburgh, London, Melbourne, Tokyo

Library of Congress Cataloging-in-Publication Data

General ultrasound / edited by Carol A. Mittelstaedt.
    p. cm.
  Includes bibliographical references and index.
  ISBN 0-443-08735-0
  1. Diagnosis, Ultrasonic. I. Mittelstaedt, Carol A.
  [DNLM: 1. Ultrasonography. WB 289 G326]
RC78.7.U4G46 1992
616.07'543—dc20
DNLM/DLC
for Library of Congress   92-25436
                          CIP

Distributed in the United Kingdom by Churchill Livingstone, Robert Stevenson House, 1–3 Baxter's Place, Leith Walk, Edinburgh EH1 3AF, and by associated companies, branches, and representatives throughout the world.

Accurate indications, adverse reactions, and dosage schedules for drugs are provided in this book, but it is possible that they may change. The reader is urged to review the package information data of the manufacturers of the medications mentioned.

The Publishers have made every effort to trace the copyright holders for borrowed material. If they have inadvertently overlooked any, they will be pleased to make the necessary arrangements at the first opportunity.

Acquisitions Editor: *Nancy Mullins*
Copy Editor: *Bridgett Dickinson*
Production Designer: *Patricia McFadden*
Production Supervisor: *Sharon Tuder*

Printed in the United States of America

First published in 1992   7 6 5 4 3 2 1

CONTRIBUTORS

Carol B. Benson, M.D.
Associate Professor, Department of Radiology, Harvard Medical School; Co-Director, Division of Ultrasound, Department of Radiology, Brigham and Women's Hospital, Boston, Massachusetts

Barbara A. Carroll, M.D.
Professor, Department of Radiology, Duke University School of Medicine; Chief, Division of Diagnostic Ultrasound, Department of Radiology, Duke University Medical Center, Durham, North Carolina

Peter M. Doubilet, M.D, Ph.D.
Associate Professor, Department of Radiology, Harvard Medical School; Co-Director, Division of Ultrasound, Department of Radiology, Brigham and Women's Hospital, Boston, Massachusetts

Bruno D. Fornage, M.D.
Professor, Department of Radiology, University of Texas Medical School at Houston; Chief, Section of Ultrasound, Department of Diagnostic Radiology, The University of Texas M.D. Anderson Cancer Center, Houston, Texas

Gretchen A. W. Gooding, M.D.
Professor and Vice Chairman, Department of Radiology, University of California, San Francisco, School of Medicine; Chief, Department of Radiology, San Francisco Veterans Administration Medical Center, San Francisco, California

Edward G. Grant, M.D.
Professor of Radiology and Vice-Chairman, Department of Radiology, University of California, Los Angeles, UCLA School of Medicine, Los Angeles, California; Chairman, Department of Radiology, Veterans Administration Medical Center, West Los Angeles, California

D. Bradley Koslin, M.D.
Director, Section of Ultrasonography, Department of Radiology, Baylor University Medical Center, Dallas, Texas

John P. McGahan, M.D.

Professor, Department of Radiology, University of California, Davis, School of Medicine, Davis, California; Director, Division of Abdominal Imaging and Ultrasound, Department of Radiology, University of California, Davis, Medical Center, Sacramento, California

Carol A. Mittelstaedt, M.D.

Professor of Radiology and Obstetrics and Gynecology, Department of Radiology, University of North Carolina at Chapel Hill School of Medicine; Director, Abdominal Imaging Section, Department of Radiology, University of North Carolina Hospitals, Chapel Hill, North Carolina

Susan A. Mulligan, M.D.

Diagnositic Radiologist, Radiology Associates of Birmingham, P.C., Birmingham, Alabama

Steve H. Parker, M.D.

Staff Radiologist, Radiology Imaging Associates, P.C., The Centrum, Englewood, Colorado

Etta D. Pisano, M.D.

Assistant Professor, Department of Radiology, University of North Carolina at Chapel Hill School of Medicine; Chief, Breast Imaging Section, Department of Radiology, University of North Carolina Hospitals, Chapel Hill, North Carolina

David Thickman, M.D.

Clinical Associate Professor, Department of Radiology, University of Colorado School of Medicine; Staff Radiologist, Radiology Imaging Associates, P.C., Porter Hospital, Denver, Colorado

Lawrence M. Vincent, M.D.

Ultrasound Specialist, Bellevue, Incorporated, P.S., Bellevue, Washington

PREFACE

There have been many advances in the field of ultrasound since the publication of *Abdominal Ultrasound* in 1987. Not only has there been further improvement in the ultrasound image quality (with the most noted changes in small parts scanning), but there has also been expansion of many of the known applications (kidney, lower urinary tract, penis, scrotum, gastrointestinal tract, and interventional). In addition, there has been the development of newer applications, such as endocavitary ultrasound (transrectal, endovaginal, endoscopic, endovascular), as well as dramatic changes in Doppler ultrasound, such as color Doppler evaluation of transplants, impotence, vascular disorders, and tumors. *General Ultrasound* is designed to keep pace with these advances and to cover all areas of ultrasound, with the exception of obstetrics and gynecology (which is a broad enough topic in itself).

General Ultrasound represents a culmination of the information published by sonographers and sonologists worldwide, from my own experience, and from my contributors' experience. A comprehensive and authoritative textbook would not have been possible without the assistance of a number of experts in the field of ultrasound. This text is intended to be a comprehensive reference of general ultrasound topics for use by practicing physicians, residents, medical students, and sonographers.

Each chapter is organized with a preliminary discussion of sonographic technique and pertinent normal anatomy followed by a review of abnormalities. The areas covered include musculoskeletal and breast, neck (including Doppler), abdominal (liver, biliary, pancreas, gastrointestinal tract, peritoneal, and abdominal wall), retroperitoneum (vascular, general retroperitoneal, kidney [native and transplant], and lower urinary tract), male pelvis (penis, scrotum, and prostate), peripheral vascular evaluation, and interventional abdominal ultrasound. In each chapter, where appropriate, a discussion of ultrasound's diagnostic accuracy and a comparison of ultrasound and other imaging techniques are included.

I hope *General Ultrasound* will benefit both the radiologist and sonographer as a reference and textbook.

Carol A. Mittelstaedt, M.D.

ACKNOWLEDGMENTS

This text represents the culmination of numerous individuals' efforts. A comprehensive and authoritative textbook would not have been possible without the efforts of the contributing authors who kindly provided chapters in their areas of expertise. The high-quality images are the product of many talented sonographers at the contributing authors' institutions, at the University of North Carolina Hospitals, and at numerous institutions worldwide. Many thanks to these people, as well as to those who have kindly contributed scans, so it was possible to completely illustrate this text.

Credit for photography goes to the contributing authors' photographers and, especially, to Robert Strain of the University of North Carolina for my chapters and for Chapters 2, 3, 9, and 19. A special note of gratitude goes out to the contributors' secretaries with particular appreciation to my secretary, Tracy Hall, for extraordinary and tireless efforts.

I would like to thank Joseph K. T. Lee, M.D., Chairman of the Department of Radiology at the University of North Carolina, for his support in this endeavor. Finally, a word of gratitude to Churchill Livingstone for the production of this first-class text, with particular praise to Bridgett Dickinson, Senior Copy Editor, and to Nancy Mullins, Senior Editor, for their tireless dedication and advice throughout this entire project.

Carol A. Mittelstaedt, M.D.

CONTENTS

Color plates follow page 370.

1

Musculoskeletal Evaluation

Bruno D. Fornage

High-resolution sonography is an ideal modality for imaging superficial soft tissues such as muscles, tendons, joints, and other subcutaneous tissues, particularly in the extremities. In the past decade, musculoskeletal imaging has been revolutionized in the United States by the advent of magnetic resonance imaging (MRI), which has become the preferred imaging modality of many clinicians, in great part because the images more closely resemble anatomic sections and because the technique is less operator-dependent than sonography is. However, in many situations, ultrasound can provide similar information at a much lower cost. In addition, with the development of very high frequency (20-MHz) transducers, sonography has recently made possible cross-sectional imaging of the skin and subcutaneous tissues.

Because traumatic and inflammatory disorders of muscles and tendons, which account for most pathologic conditions of the extremities, are associated with athletic as well as occupational activities, cooperation between radiologists and specialists in sports medicine has played a significant role in the development of musculoskeletal ultrasound. Vascular sonography of the extremities, which has undergone tremendous advancement with the refinement of Doppler sonographic techniques, is covered in Chapter 18.

TECHNIQUE

Equipment

The use of real-time scanners makes sonographic examination fast and complete, leaving no blind area between the scans. Because of their wider field of view and better resolution in the near field, flat linear-array electronic transducers are more appropriate than mechanical or phased-array sector scanners for the evaluation of superficial structures.[1] Because the parallel lines of sight of the former are grossly perpendicular to the interfaces encountered, the amplitude of echoes is optimal, whereas the diverging beam of sector transducers is responsible for beam-scattering artifacts that leave only a narrow central portion of the scan unaffected. Whereas 7.5- or 10-MHz probes are needed for the evaluation of very superficial soft tissues such as tendons, distal extremities, and subcutaneous tissues, examination of deep muscles of the extremities is usually performed with a 5-MHz probe. On occasion, a 3.5-MHz probe, which provides scans as wide as 7 or 8 cm along with sufficient penetration, may be needed to visualize a deeply located structure in a patient with a well-developed musculature or excessive subcutaneous fat deposition or to encompass a long anatomic segment or lesion. As the nominal frequency of the transducer increases, the depth of the field of view decreases, as usually does its width, so that scans obtained with most 7.5- or 10-MHz linear-array transducers are about 3 or 4 cm wide. However, most real-time units equipped with linear-array transducers can display two and sometimes three adjacent scans on the video monitor (split-screen mode). This permits visualization and measurement of structures or lesions whose size exceeds the width of the probe, although extreme care must be taken when juxtaposing the contiguous scans on the screen. Although long criticized for their suboptimal image quality, some small portable ultrasound units now provide acceptable gray-scale images of sufficient diagnostic quality when equipped with 5.0- or

7.5-MHz transducers. Scanners dedicated to the examination of the skin are now commercially available; the mechanically activated transducer has a frequency of 20 or 30 MHz and is housed in a water-filled chamber.[2]

Examination

The use of a standoff pad allows visualization of the skin and the most superficial structures. Standoff pads are made of anechoic gel-like material such as the mixture of oil and viscoelastic polymer initially used in flotation rest pads designed to prevent decubitus ulcers (Kitecko; 3-M, St. Paul, MN).[3] The standoff pad is placed on the skin after liberal application of couplant. Its suppleness allows optimal contact between a flat linear-array transducer and the skin in areas with uneven surfaces. When a standoff pad is used, it is necessary to verify continuously that the beam is perpendicular to the interfaces examined to ensure optimal reflection. Because the pad adds to the beam pathway, only thin pads should be used with high-frequency transducers.

The combination of longitudinal and transverse scans is mandatory for three-dimensional localization of lesions and calculation of their volume. A scan of the symmetric area in the contralateral extremity or region can serve as a reference of normal anatomy. However, it must be kept in mind that some pathologic conditions, such as tendinitis in the lower extremities, may occur bilaterally.

Sonography is the only real-time cross-sectional imaging modality, and the operator should take advantage of this capability by examining mobile structures such as muscles and tendons first with the patient at rest and then during active or passive maneuvers that mobilize the involved structure.[1] Sonography also allows palpation under real-time ("sonoscopic") monitoring, enabling a sonographic study to be focused on palpable abnormalities and, conversely, palpation to be directed to sonographically equivocal areas.

Doppler Studies

With high-sensitivity color Doppler equipment, vessels can be identified in normal muscles and increased flow during exercise can be demonstrated. Hypervascularization associated with inflammatory processes rang-

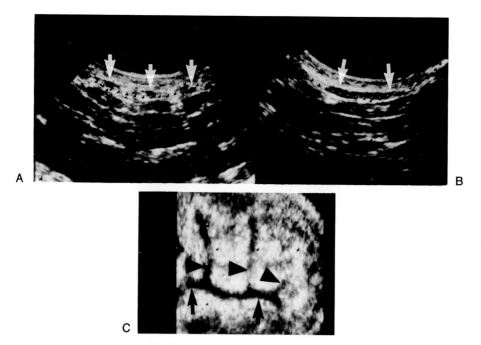

Fig. 1-1. Three-dimensional ultrasound images of the palm of the hand using a special 7.5-MHz sector transducer and built-in reconstruction software (Combison 330, Kretztechnik, Austria). **(A)** Transverse scan showing the three common palmar digital arteries (arrows). **(B)** Sagittal scan showing a common palmar digital artery (arrows). **(C)** Reconstructed "concave" coronal scan showing the palmar arch (arrows) and the origin of the three common palmar digital arteries (arrowheads).

ing from tendinitis to abscess can be depicted by color Doppler examination. Malignant soft tissue tumors are usually hypervascularized; color Doppler imaging can help determine the relationship between a tumor and neighboring vessels, although it cannot replace angiography for preoperative assessment.

Ultrasound-Guided Biopsy

Real-time sonography is ideal for guiding needle biopsy of soft tissue lesions. Fluid collections are aspirated with fine (20- to 25-gauge) needles, although the presence of thick material such as pus may require the use of a larger needle. If an expert cytopathologist is available, many solid masses can be diagnosed by ultrasound-guided fine-needle aspiration. If this is not the case or if the mass is hard to aspirate (fibrous), it is advantageous to use automatic biopsy devices (Biopty gun) and large (18- to 14-gauge) Tru-Cut-type needles, which have a very high tissue recovery rate.[2]

Intraoperative Sonography

Sonography is the only cross-sectional imaging modality that can be used in the operating theater. Intraoperative ultrasound has proved to be instrumental in localizing nonpalpable tumors and foreign bodies.

Three-Dimensional Sonography

Ultrasound scanners that automatically scan a volume, store the received echoes, and display reconstructed coronal scans and even three-dimensional views, in addition to standard longitudinal and transverse sections, have recently appeared on the market, and significant research and development are under way. Although the concept is appealing, it is difficult to predict the impact of such reconstructed images on the sonographic examination of soft tissues (Fig. 1-1).

Other Ultrasound Techniques

In ultrasound transmission imaging, images are obtained from beams that are transmitted, not reflected. The transmitted beams are refocused on an array of receiving transducers to create a video signal. Images are planar projections comparable to plain radiographs.[4]

Acoustic holography was developed in the late 1960s[5]: Ultrasonic holograms are obtained by mixing a coherent reference beam with beams that have propagated through the object, the whole being decoded by various techniques, including illumination by a laser light source; appropriate focusing produces images at various selected planes within the object.

Although they hold promise for imaging soft tissues, these two techniques have not yet reached the level of clinical usefulness.

SKELETAL MUSCLES

NORMAL ANATOMY

The echopattern is similar for all normal skeletal muscles. On longitudinal scans, the connective tissue that surrounds the bundles of fibers, or perimysium, gives rise to parallel echogenic striae, which project over a hypoechoic background representing the bulk of the muscle fibers per se (Fig. 1-2A). On transverse scans, the cross-sectional perimysium appears as scattered dot echoes (Fig. 1-2B). The intermuscular fasciae are brightly echogenic. During contraction, the thickness of the body of the muscle increases, the echogenic striae become more oblique, and the background becomes even more hypoechoic than at rest.[1,2] Color Doppler examination can demonstrate intramuscular blood flow

in vessels too small to be depicted on B-mode images (Plate 1-1).

Artifacts and Pitfalls

When included entirely within the scan plane, prominent flat intramuscular septa may appear on longitudinal scans as misleading echogenic areas. The pitfall can be correctly identified on transverse scans[1] (Fig. 1-3). Large intramuscular veins such as those seen in the soleus muscle may mimic areas of fiber discontinuity.

Trauma Abnormalities

Trauma is the prevailing cause of pathologic conditions involving muscles.

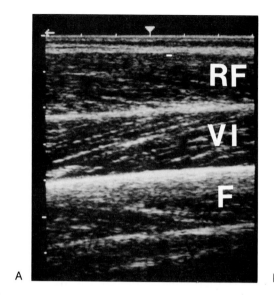
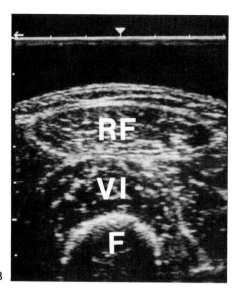

Fig. 1-2. Normal skeletal muscle. **(A)** Longitudinal scan of the anterior aspect of the thigh showing the rectus femoris *(RF)* and vastus intermedius *(VI)* muscles with the typically striated, echogenic perimysium over a markedly hypoechoic background. *(F, femur.)* **(B)** Transverse scan of the same region showing the perimysium with a dotted and reticular pattern. *(F, femur; RF, rectus femoris; VI, vastus intermedius.)*

Acute Injuries

Contusions resulting from direct trauma may cause a moderately echogenic hemorrhage that infiltrates the muscle without a frank discontinuity of muscular fibers[6] (Fig. 1-4). Recent intramuscular hematomas are often ill-defined, and the enlargement of the injured muscle compared with the contralateral muscle may be the sole sign of an intramuscular hematoma.[7] Special reference must be made to muscular hematomas of the calf, which may mimic thrombophlebitis[8] and cause posterior compartment syndrome.[9] Diagnosis of spontaneous intra-

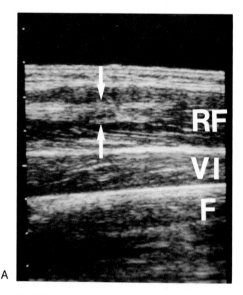
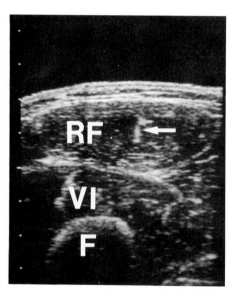

Fig. 1-3. Pitfall related to an intramuscular septum. **(A)** Sagittal scan of the anterior thigh showing a hyperechoic area (arrows) in the rectus femoris *(RF)* muscle. *(F, femur; VI, vastus intermedius.)* **(B)** Transverse scan of the same region showing the sagittally oriented intramuscular septum (arrow) responsible for the echogenic area seen on the sagittal scan. *(F, femur; RF, rectus femoris; VI, vastus intermedius.)* (From Fornage,[2] with permission; © 1991 by BD Fornage.)

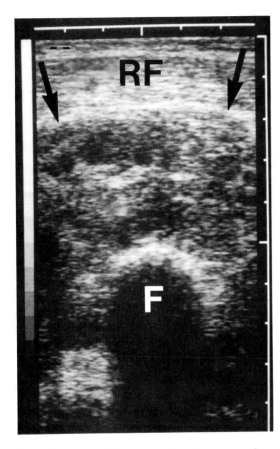

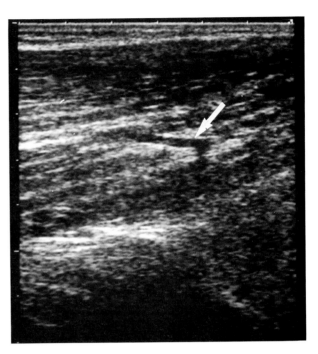

Fig. 1-5. Partial rupture of the short head of the biceps femoris muscle. Longitudinal scan of the posterior thigh showing the discontinuity with a minimal amount of hemorrhage (arrow).

Fig. 1-4. Hematoma following a direct trauma to the vastus intermedius muscle. Transverse scan showing a large nonhomogeneous hematoma involving the entire vastus intermedius (arrows) and laminating the rectus femoris *(RF)* muscle anteriorly. *(F,* femur.) (From Fornage,[2] with permission; © 1991 by BD Fornage.)

muscular hematomas in hemophiliacs has also benefited from ultrasound.[7,10,11]

Frank muscular ruptures are characterized by a discontinuity in muscular fibers (direct sign) and an associated hematoma (indirect sign) (Fig. 1-5). The "clapper-in-the-bell" sign is the visualization of a retracted ruptured muscle surrounded by hematoma[6,12] (Fig. 1-6). The sonographic appearance of a muscular hematoma varies over time. Ill-defined areas of increased echogenicity seen within a few hours of hemorrhage may mask a partial underlying rupture, so a repeat examination 2 or 3 days later may be indicated. During the following weeks, the liquefying hematoma appears as an anechoic collection, which may contain echogenic fibrinous strands or debris (Fig. 1-7) and whose size progressively decreases on follow-up examinations.[13]

Occasionally, trauma results in the detachment of fibers from the epimysium and an associated hematoma

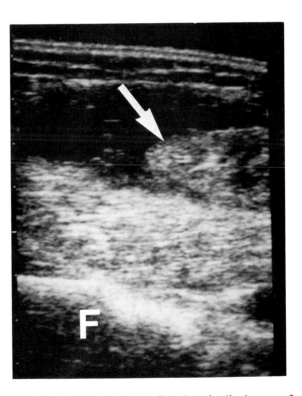

Fig. 1-6. Clapper-in-the-bell sign. Longitudinal scan of a large rupture of the biceps femoris muscle showing the retracted lower fragment (arrow) surrounded by the sonolucent hematoma. *(F,* femur.)

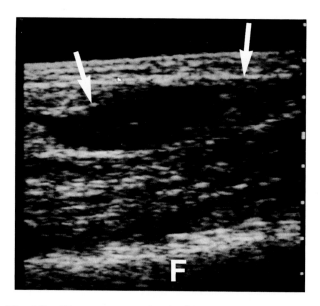

Fig. 1-7. Hematoma associated with a rupture of the long head of the biceps femoris muscle. Longitudinal scan of the posterior thigh showing the collection (arrows) with internal fibrinous strands. (*F*, femur.)

(Fig. 1-8). Such an injury is common in the distal portion of the gastrocnemius medialis muscle.

Muscle hernias through a ruptured or weakened aponeurosis are readily diagnosed by real-time sonography, which confirms the alteration of the shape of the muscle during contraction (Fig. 1-9).

Chronic Injuries

Intramuscular fibrous scars, a complication of neglected or recurrent ruptures,[12] appear as focal, stellate, echogenic areas, often abutting the epimysium (Fig. 1-10). The mere presence of a scar predisposes the muscle to recurrent rupture. In such a case, the preexisting chronic lesions limit the accuracy of ultrasound in the diagnosis of superimposed acute traumatic changes.

Sonography can demonstrate the rare cystic transformation of a hematoma associated with a muscle rupture. Ossification of muscular hematomas (post-traumatic myositis ossificans) gives rise to characteristic bright foci with acoustic shadowing[12,14] (Fig. 1-11). Heterotopic ossification can also develop after orthopaedic surgery, such as total hip arthroplasty.

Tumors

The major indication for sonography has long been the differentiation of cystic from solid palpable masses. However, with state-of-the-art equipment, sonography can now be used to detect nonpalpable masses, such as local tumor recurrences.

Lipomas and hemangiomas are the most common benign tumors of the muscles. Lipomas may be well-circumscribed or ill-defined. The presence of areas of increased echogenicity should suggest a fatty tumor (Fig. 1-12), although lipomas may also be diffusely hypoechoic[15,16] (Fig. 1-13). Angiomas can be ill-defined and

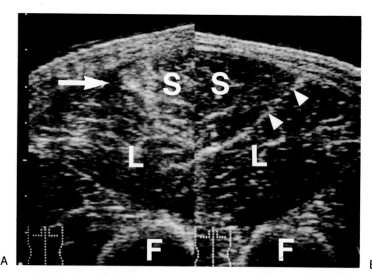

Fig. 1-8. Small partial detachment of the short head of the biceps femoris muscle from the epimysium. **(A)** Transverse scan of the left posterior thigh showing the disruption of the epimysium between the short *(S)* and long *(L)* heads of the biceps femoris *(F)* muscle. Note the presence of a minimal hematoma (arrow) and the increased echogenicity of the retracted short head. (*F*, femur.) **(B)** Comparative contralateral scan showing the well-defined echogenic epimysium between the two heads of the biceps femoris (arrowheads). (*L*, long head of biceps femoris; *S*, short head of biceps femoris; *F*, femur.)

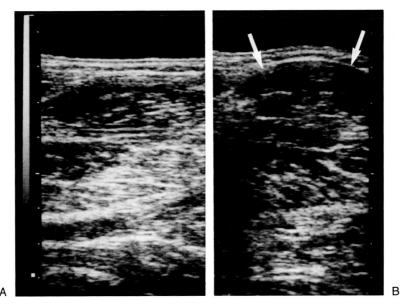

Fig. 1-9. Hernia of the semitendinosus muscle. **(A)** Longitudinal scan of the posterior thigh at rest. **(B)** Scan obtained during contraction showing that the palpable mass in the lower thigh corresponds to the herniated semitendinosus (arrows) muscle, whose echotexture remains grossly normal.

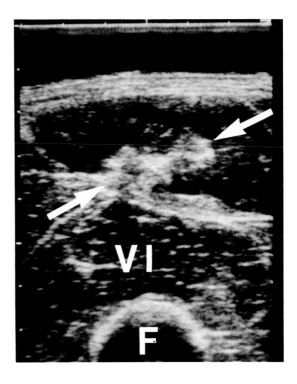

Fig. 1-10. Fibrous scar in the rectus femoris muscle resulting from a neglected partial rupture. Transverse scan of the quadriceps muscle showing a stellate echogenic area (arrows) abutting the epimysium of the rectus femoris. (*F*, femur; *VI*, vastus intermedius.)

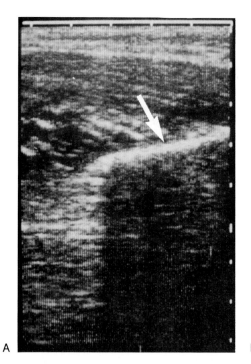

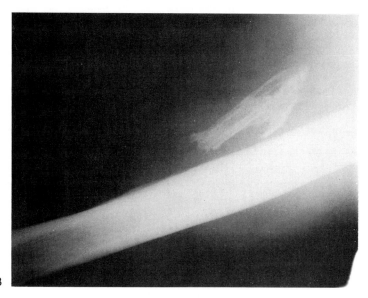

Fig. 1-11. Traumatic myositis ossificans following a rupture of the adductor longus muscle. **(A)** Longitudinal scan of the inner thigh showing linear echoes (arrow) with acoustic shadowing, suggesting the presence of calcified material. **(B)** Low-kilovoltage radiograph confirming the post-traumatic heterotopic ossification. (From Fornage et al,[12] with permission.)

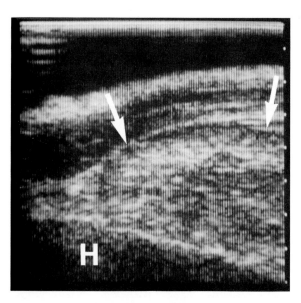

Fig. 1-12. Lipoma of the brachialis anterior muscle. Longitudinal scan of the arm showing a well-encapsulated echogenic mass (arrows). (*H*, humerus.)

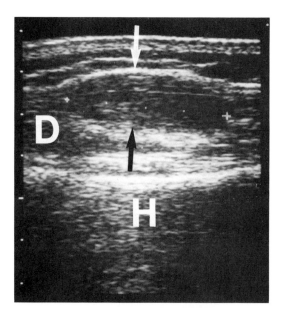

Fig. 1-13. Lipoma of the deltoid muscle. Coronal scan of the shoulder showing a nonencapsulated hypoechoic mass (arrows) in the deltoid muscle. (*D*, deltoid; *H*, humerus.) (From Fornage,[2] with permission; © 1991 by BD Fornage.)

can also have a wide spectrum of echogenicity[17] (Figs. 1-14 and 1-15). The diagnosis of angioma should be suggested in the presence of hyperechoic foci representing calcified thrombi (phleboliths) or if the size of the tumor increases after exercise; Doppler studies help in assessing the hemodynamic status of these lesions (Fig. 1-15). Angiolipomas are often echogenic because of their high fat content, and they may exhibit an infiltrating pattern.[2] Among the rarer benign tumors, intramuscular myxomas are characterized by well-defined margins and a markedly hypoechoic, sometimes pseudocystic appearance[2] (Fig. 1-16).

Sarcomas are the most common malignant primary tumors of muscles. They generally appear as hypoechoic masses (Fig. 1-17). Although it would be hazardous to infer a particular histopathologic type from the sonographic appearance, the following associations should be kept in mind: calcifications can be seen within synovial sarcomas; extensive intratumoral necrosis is often associated with rhabdomyosarcomas (Fig. 1-17); lymphomas are often markedly hypoechoic; and the presence of echogenic components should suggest a well-differentiated liposarcoma. In experienced hands, sonography is the most accurate and cost-effective technique for guiding needle biopsy of superficial soft tissue tumors. The use of automatic biopsy systems such as the Biopty gun has made obtaining large-core specimens easier and less painful.

Intramuscular metastases also appear as hypoechoic masses (Fig. 1-18). The presence of calcifications should raise the possibility of a metastatic gastrointestinal carcinoma.

Because the volume of a given tumor is easily calculated by the prolate ellipsoid volume formula from the three greatest diameters measured on two perpendicular scans, sonography is a convenient tool with which to monitor and quantify the response of a malignant tumor to conservative therapy. In such cases, tumor volume reduction may be accompanied by changes in echotexture such as those due to necrosis (Fig. 1-19). More importantly, sonography has shown a very high sensitivity in the early detection of nonpalpable tumor recurrence after surgical excision of a soft tissue sarcoma (Fig. 1-20), with an accuracy similar to that of MRI.[18] It is therefore legitimate in such cases to use high-resolution sonography as a first-line modality for follow-up. When a nonpalpable recurrence has been detected, ultrasound can be used to guide the confirmatory fine-needle aspiration and eventually to localize the tumor preoperatively (or intraoperatively).

Infection

On sonograms, muscular abscesses appear as hypoechoic or complex masses with echogenic debris and occasionally gas bubbles responsible for ring-down artifacts or shadowing (Fig. 1-21), although areas of increased echogenicity can also be seen in patients with pyomyositis.[19,20] The diagnosis is established through ultrasound-guided needle aspiration, and sonography can be used to monitor the percutaneous drainage.[19,21,22] The relationship between the abscess and adjacent bones should be carefully studied to rule out osteomyelitis.

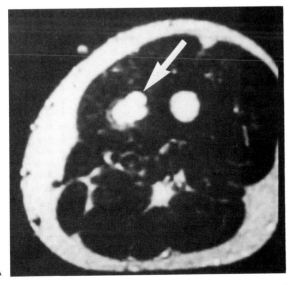
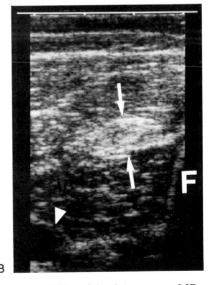

Fig. 1-14. Nonpalpable angioma of the left vastus medialis muscle. **(A)** T_2-weighted transverse MR scan showing a rounded area of increased signal intensity (arrow). **(B)** Transverse sonogram showing the hyperechoic angioma (arrows). (arrowhead, superficial femoral artery; F, femur.)

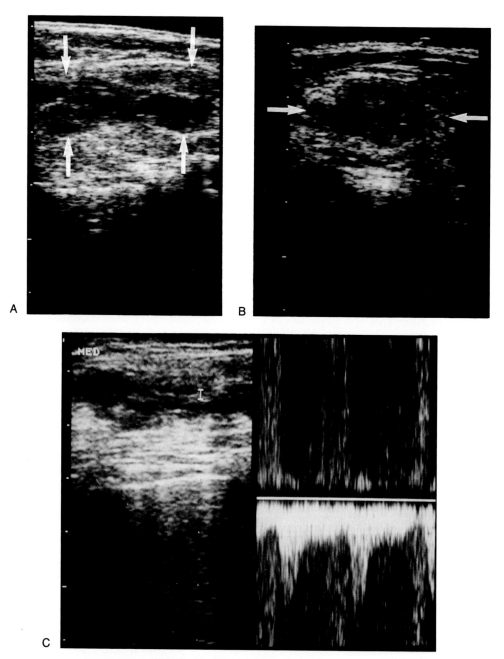

Fig. 1-15. Intramuscular angioma of the lower posterior thigh. **(A)** Longitudinal and **(B)** transverse scans of the inner hamstring muscles showing an ill-defined hypoechoic mass (arrows) with a few internal anechoic areas representing blood lakes. **(C)** Duplex sonogram identifying arterial Doppler signals within the mass.

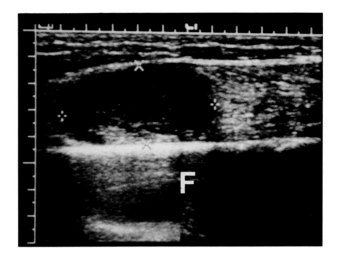

Fig. 1-16. Intramuscular myxoma of the thigh. Coronal scan of the lateral aspect of the thigh showing a well-defined, markedly hypoechoic mass (calipers) in the vastus intermedius muscle, adjacent to the femur *(F)*. Note the distal sound enhancement.

Miscellaneous

Rhabdomyolysis

Rhabdomyolysis, the necrosis of muscle fibers, may develop whenever the muscular fibers suffer from ischemia. The most common causes include crush syndrome, drug toxicity, illegal drug abuse, and, in athletes, exhaustion as observed in marathon runners. Sonography shows that in the acute phase, the smooth architecture of the muscle is replaced with nonhomogeneous patchy areas of decreased echogenicity (Fig. 1-22). Later, the areas may become more hypoechoic[23,24] and may even be transformed into fluid-filled collections.[25] Recently, MRI has been reported to be more accurate than sonography or computed tomography (CT).[26]

Nontraumatic Myositis Ossificans

Nontraumatic heterotopic ossification is associated with a number of neurologic disorders, including spinal cord injuries, closed head injuries, encephalitis, multiple sclerosis, and poliomyelitis, but it can also develop apparently de novo in a normal individual. Initially, there is local swelling, warmth, redness, and limitation of the range of motion of the affected segment. The differential diagnosis includes hematoma, deep venous thrombosis, cellulitis or abscess, and tumor. Early in the process, ultrasound demonstrates a nonspecific hypoechoic area,[27] while color Doppler imaging confirms the hypervascularity of the lesion. Within 3 or 4 weeks, deposition of echogenic calcific material at the periphery of the lesion can be seen on sonograms, first without and then

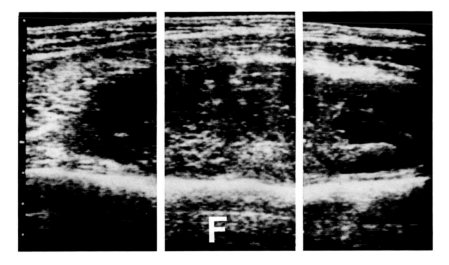

Fig. 1-17. Rhabdomyosarcoma of the thigh. Montage of three contiguous longitudinal scans of the thigh showing a nonhomogeneous mass located in the vastus intermedius muscle. Note the areas of necrosis. (*F,* femur.)

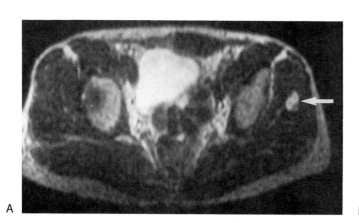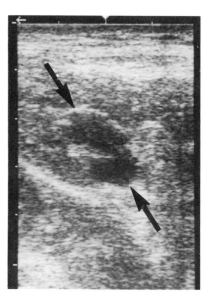

Fig. 1-18. Nonpalpable metastatic melanoma in the buttock. (**A**) T_2-weighted MR scan showing a hyperintense focus (arrow) in the left buttock. Surgical exploration guided by MRI failed to retrieve the tumor. (**B**) Sonogram clearly identifying the hypoechoic tumor (arrows), which was confirmed by ultrasound-guided fine-needle aspiration and then excised under intraoperative ultrasound guidance. (From Fornage,[2] with permission; © 1991 by BD Fornage.)

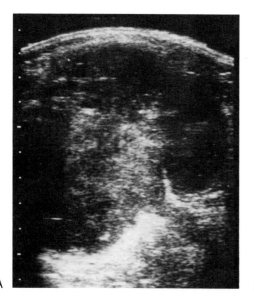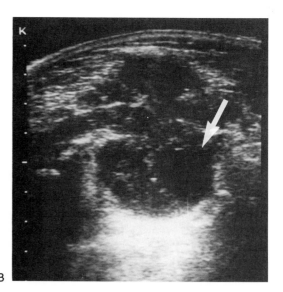

Fig. 1-19. Ultrasound evaluation of response to treatment of an undifferentiated sarcoma of the gluteus maximus muscle. (**A**) Initial longitudinal scan of the buttock showing the bulky tumor. (**B**) Scan obtained after two courses of chemotherapy showing significant shrinkage of the tumor, which contains a fluid-filled necrotic area (arrow). (From Fornage,[2] with permission; © 1991 by BD Fornage.)

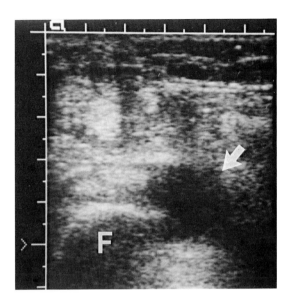

Fig. 1-20. Nonpalpable recurrent malignant fibrous histiocytoma of the thigh. Transverse sonogram showing a 2-cm hypoechoic mass (arrow) adjacent to the femur *(F).* Note the altered texture of the anterior thigh as a result of postoperative changes. (From Fornage,[2] with permission; © 1991 by BD Fornage.)

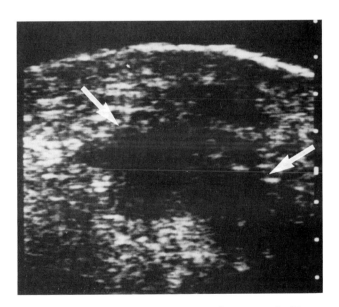

Fig. 1-21. Abscess of the gluteus maximus muscle. Transverse scan showing an ill-defined complex mass (arrows).

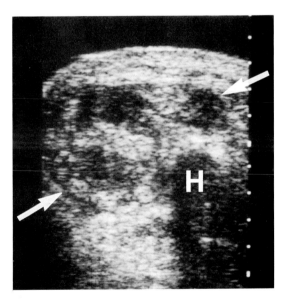

Fig. 1-22. Rhabdomyolysis of the triceps brachii muscle. Transverse scan of the posterior aspect of the arm showing the swollen muscle, which has a nonhomogeneous texture (arrows). (*H,* humerus.)

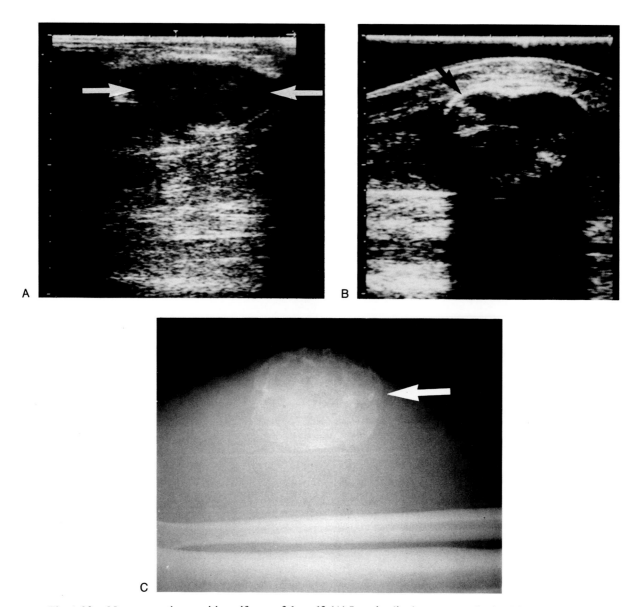

Fig. 1-23.   Nontraumatic myositis ossificans of the calf. **(A)** Longitudinal sonogram obtained 2 weeks after the onset of clinical symptoms showing an ovoid, hypoechoic lesion (arrows). **(B)** Longitudinal sonogram obtained 7 weeks later showing a well-defined peripheral calcific ring (arrows). Note the presence of internal calcified material and the marked acoustic shadow. **(C)** Lateral radiograph of the leg showing a well-circumscribed calcified mass in the calf (arrow). (From Fornage and Eftekhari,[27] with permission.)

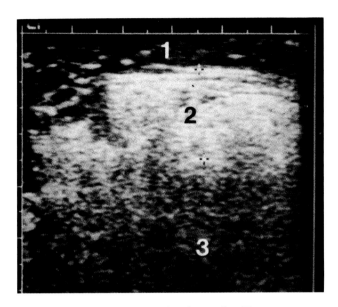

Fig. 1-24. Duchenne muscular dystrophy. Transverse scan of the thigh showing hyperechoic quadriceps *(2)* with marked sound attenuation. The femur shaft *(3)* is completely obscured. (*1*, subcutaneous fat.) (From Fischer et al,[29] with permission.)

with shadowing[27,28] (Fig. 1-23). The typical rim ossification pattern, confirmed by plain radiography or CT, differentiates the condition from an osteogenic soft tissue sarcoma, whose calcifications are coarser and located more centrally.

Neuromuscular Diseases

The common denominator in muscular dystrophies is a marked increase in the echogenicity of the affected muscles, owing to replacement of muscle fibers by connective tissue and fat (Fig. 1-24). A possibly distinctive "moth-eaten" pattern has been described in neuropathies.[29] Sonography is useful for measuring the muscle/soft tissue ratio, and recently, quantification of abnormal muscle echotexture by measurement of the density of perimysial reflections has been attempted.[30] However, because CT and MRI provide global and symmetric scans of the limbs and better reproducibility than sonography, these modalities are preferred for evaluation and follow-up of patients with neuromuscular diseases.

TENDONS, LIGAMENTS, AND JOINTS

TENDONS AND LIGAMENTS

Normal Anatomy

Tendons and ligaments consist of dense, fibrous connective tissue with longitudinally oriented collagen fibers. Tendons are surrounded by the peritenon, from which emanate internal echogenic septa separating the bundles of fibers. Blood supply is poor. In the absence of mechanical constraint, tendons lie in a loose connective tissue, the paratenon. Where it is needed, additional mechanical protection is provided by synovial sheaths and, in specific areas, by fibrous bands or retinacula. Synovial bursae containing a minute amount of synovial fluid facilitate the play of certain tendons.

All normal tendons are echogenic and exhibit the same fibrillar echotexture, best demonstrated on longitudinal sonograms[1,31] (Fig. 1-25A). On transverse sections, most tendons are oval to round (Fig. 1-25B). With the use of a very high frequency (20-MHz) transducer, a subtle hypoechoic underlining can be seen around the superficial tendons that lie in synovial sheaths (e.g., the flexor tendons of the fingers) (Fig. 1-26). Large synovial bursae appear as flattened, hypoechoic structures adja-

cent to the tendons and are rarely more than 2 to 3 mm thick.

The most significant artifact in tendon sonography is the false hypoechogenicity that results from the slightest obliquity of the ultrasound beam in relation to the tendon fibers[32] (Fig. 1-27). This artifact, which can be seen on both longitudinal and transverse sections, may obscure minute textural abnormalities and mimic tendinitis (see below).

Abnormalities

Trauma

Complete tendon ruptures are usually diagnosed by physical examination. However, ultrasound can be helpful when physical examination has been delayed and is hampered by inflammatory changes. On sonograms, a variable space filled with hypoechoic blood or granulomatous tissue separates the two fragments[31] (Fig. 1-28). When a tendon has been torn from its bony insertion, avulsed bone fragments may appear as hyperechoic foci with acoustic shadowing.[33]

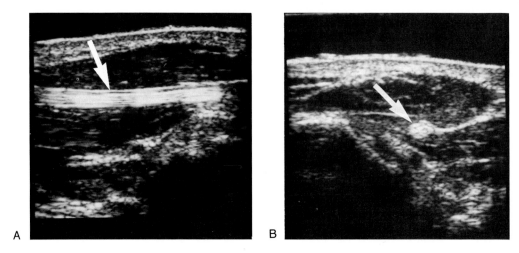

Fig. 1-25. Normal tendon. **(A)** Longitudinal sonogram of the tendon of the flexor pollicis longus in the thenar area showing the markedly hyperechoic tendon and its fibrillar texture (arrow). **(B)** Transverse sonogram showing the echogenic, rounded cross-section of the same tendon (arrow).

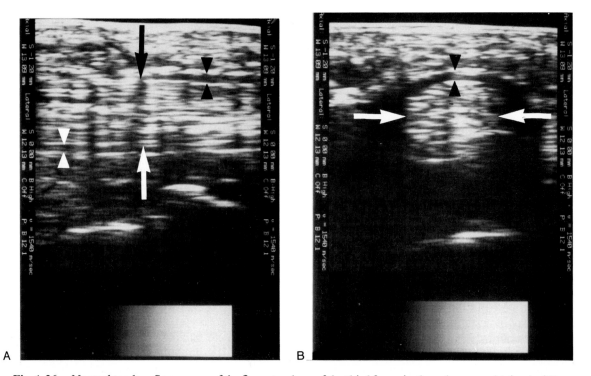

Fig. 1-26. Normal tendon. Sonograms of the flexor tendons of the third finger in the palm were obtained with a 20-MHz scanner. **(A)** Longitudinal sonogram showing the echogenic superficial and deep flexor tendons (arrows). (arrowheads, 0.3-mm-thick fluid-filled synovial sheath around the two tendons.) **(B)** Transverse sonogram confirming the subtle anechoic rim (arrowheads) around the echogenic tendons (arrows).

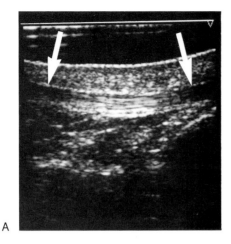
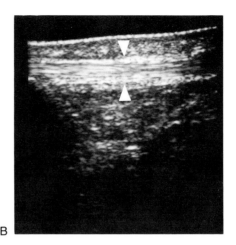

A   B

Fig. 1-27. False hypoechogenicity of the patellar tendon resulting from the slight obliquity of the beam in relation to the tendon fibers. **(A)** Longitudinal sonogram obtained with the knee extended and the quadriceps muscle relaxed. The tendon is concave anteriorly, and on each side of the scan the obliquity of the fibers in relation to the beam of the flat linear-array transducer results in scattering of the beam and decreased echogenicity (arrows). **(B)** Sonogram along the same orientation with the quadriceps contracted. The tendon (arrowheads) has been straightened, and the artifact has been cleared.

Sonography is more useful in the diagnosis of partial tendon ruptures, which are often misdiagnosed clinically. They appear on sonograms as hypoechoic focal defects within the echogenic, fibrillar echotexture[31,33] (Fig. 1-29). Early detection of partial tendon ruptures allows for timely surgery and improved functional outcome. Conversely, because of its high negative predictive value, a normal sonogram can prevent unnecessary surgery.

Inflammatory Conditions

Sonography can be used to diagnose and monitor tendinitis, tenosynovitis, and bursitis. In acute tendinitis, the tendon is swollen, its echogenicity is decreased, and its contours are blurred[31,33] (Fig. 1-30). Intratendinous calcifications can develop in chronic tendinitis; they appear on sonograms as hyperechoic foci with or without acoustic shadowing and/or comet tail artifact, depend-

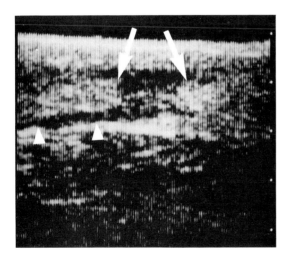

Fig. 1-28. Complete tendon rupture. Longitudinal sonogram of the Achilles tendon showing the two completely separated fragments (arrows). Note the anechoic hematoma surrounding the tendon (arrowheads).

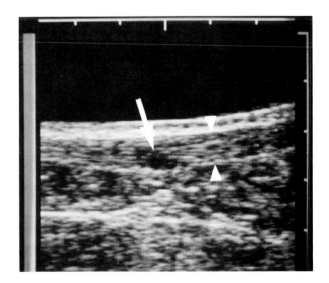

Fig. 1-29. Partial tendon rupture. Longitudinal sonogram of the Achilles tendon (arrowheads) showing the focal discontinuity of the fibers (arrow).

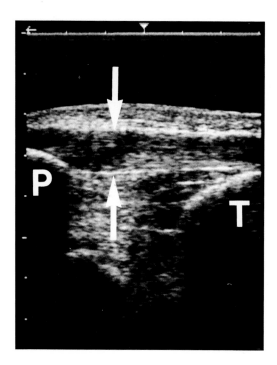

Fig. 1-30. Patellar tendinitis. Longitudinal sonogram of the patellar tendon showing thickening, decreased echogenicity, and blurred margins of the tendon (arrows). (*P*, patella; *T*, tibia.)

ing on their size and reflectivity.

In acute tenosynovitis, ultrasound demonstrates the presence of fluid in the synovial sheath[31,33,34] (Fig. 1-31). Echogenic debris can be seen in infected effusions.[35] In addition to the presence of fluid in the sheath, chronic tenosynovitis is often associated with a hypoechoic thickening of the synovium.[33]

In bursitis, sonograms show an enlarged, fluid-filled bursa with ill-defined margins. The subdeltoid, olecranal, patellar, and calcaneal bursae are most frequently involved. Calcifications can develop in chronic calcified bursitis.[2]

Postoperative Patterns

After surgery, tendons remain thickened and nonhomogeneously hypoechoic for an extended period, so it may not be possible to differentiate between such a postoperative pattern and a recurrent tendinitis or partial rupture[31,33] (Fig. 1-32).

Miscellaneous

Ganglion cysts are typically located in the hand and wrist. Xanthomas in patients with hypercholesterolemia and intratendinous rheumatoid nodules are hypoechoic, whereas gouty tophi are echogenic and cast a shadow.[36]

Neoplasms that develop from tendons or their sheaths are rare. The most common benign type is the giant cell tumor, the localized form of pigmented villonodular synovitis, which appears hypoechoic and relatively well circumscribed. Synovial sarcomas may develop from a tendon sheath, although at the time of diagnosis the site of origin is rarely identified.

JOINTS

Sonography is undisputedly superior to other imaging modalities in diagnosing fluid collections and should be the first-line imaging modality for the diagnosis of joint effusions and synovial cysts.

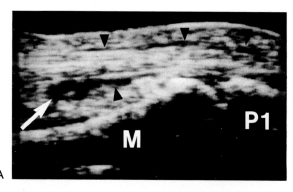
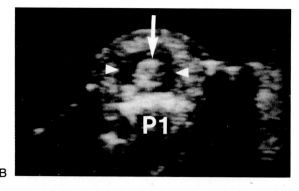

Fig. 1-31. Acute tenosynovitis of the flexor tendons of the second finger. **(A)** Longitudinal sonogram of the palm showing a small amount of fluid in the sheath (arrowheads) pooling in the proximal cul-de-sac (arrow). (*M*, metacarpal; *P1*, first phalanx.) **(B)** Transverse sonogram at the level of the first phalanx *(P1)* showing the normal tendons (arrow) surrounded by the fluid collection (arrowheads). (From Fornage,[2] with permission; © 1991 by BD Fornage.)

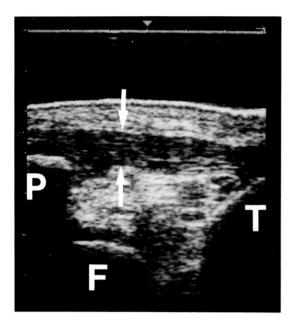

Fig. 1-32. Postoperative tendon. Longitudinal sonogram of the patellar tendon 1 year after surgical treatment of tendinitis showing persistent thickening, decreased echogenicity, and irregular margins of the tendon (arrows). (*F*, femur; *P*, patella; *T*, tibia.)

Normal Anatomy

The proximal surface of cortical bone is outlined as a brightly reflective line, whereas the articular cartilage appears as a thin anechoic rim, about 1 to 2 mm thick. The joint capsule is rarely identified, and periarticular ligaments usually cannot be distinguished from the surrounding fat. In neonates, the nonossified cartilaginous epiphyses are hypoechoic, and sonography can demonstrate the ossification centers as hyperechoic foci with acoustic shadowing.

Abnormalities

Effusions

Joint effusions are readily diagnosed as anechoic intra-articular fluid collections distending the joint cavity. Septic effusions may contain debris, whereas recent hemarthrosis may show an echogenic, sedimented layer of erythrocytes, which may change with the patient's position. Sonography is ideal for guiding aspiration of small effusions (e.g., in the hips of children).

Synovial Proliferations

In proliferative diseases of the synovium, such as pigmented villonodular synovitis or rheumatoid arthritis, high-frequency ultrasound can depict the hypoechoic, thickened synovium, particularly when it is outlined by an effusion.

SHOULDER

Ultrasound examination of the shoulder is performed primarily to evaluate the rotator cuff and the biceps tendon.

Technique

Ultrasound examination of the rotator cuff is difficult and requires considerable experience because of the complex anatomy of the shoulder and the numerous beam propagation-related artifacts. Because of the convexity of the cuff, sector transducers should not be used. Flat linear-array transducers of 7.5 MHz are satisfactory. Since the slightest obliquity of the beam results in a false hypoechogenicity of the cuff, the operator should maintain the position of the transducer so that the region of interest in the cuff lies as perpendicular to the beam (i.e., parallel to the footprint of the probe) as possible.[32]

The examination is performed bilaterally with the patient sitting, the elbows flexed to 90 degrees, and the

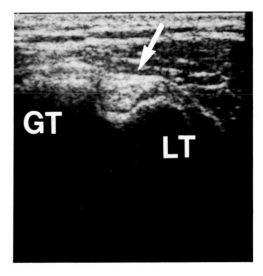

Fig. 1-33. Normal anatomy of the shoulder on ultrasound. Transverse scan of the biceps tendon showing the hyperechoic tendon (arrow) in the bicipital groove. (*LT*, lesser tuberosity of humerus; *GT*, greater tuberosity.)

hands resting on the thighs. Identification of the biceps tendon on transverse scans of the bicipital groove is the first step of the examination (Fig. 1-33). Each component of the cuff is then examined along two perpendicular planes, which are grossly coronal and sagittal. Special attention should be paid to the distal supraspinatus tendon, including the "critical zone," where most rotator cuff tears occur. Standard scans should be complemented by a dynamic examination of the shoulder during passive maneuvers of abduction and adduction.[37] Hyperextended internal rotation of the arm (with the patient's arm behind the back), another useful technique, allows visualization of a longer segment of the supraspinatus.[38] Plain films of the shoulder should be available at the time of the examination to avoid such pitfalls as tendon calcifications.

Normal Anatomy

The rotator cuff is composed, from front to back, of the tendons of the subscapularis, supraspinatus, infraspinatus, and teres minor muscles. Key anatomic landmarks include the deltoid muscle, with the characteristic texture of skeletal muscle; the underlying subdeltoid bursa, whose collapsed walls appear as an echogenic interface less than 2 mm thick between the deltoid and the cuff; the bony surface of the humeral head; and the biceps tendon, which courses between the subscapularis and the supraspinatus tendons. When it is properly scanned, the rotator cuff displays the typical fibrillar echogenicity of tendons (Fig. 1-34). All components of

the tendinous cuff have the same echopattern. The thickness of the cuff ranges from 6 mm posteriorly to 9 mm anteriorly and is similar on both sides of the body. The bony surface of the humeral head is smooth and regular, except for the bicipital groove.

Abnormalities

Rotator Cuff Tears

The incidence of rotator cuff tears increases with age, as the cuff deteriorates. Pain and arm weakness are the usual symptoms. The unequivocal ultrasound criterion for a complete tear is nonvisualization of the avulsed rotator cuff retracted under the acromial process (Fig. 1-35). This is often accompanied by a joint effusion, best demonstrated around the biceps tendon, or by an intrabursal effusion.[37] Focal thinning of the cuff is frequently found in the critical zone of the supraspinatus. Focal discontinuity appearing as a fluid-filled defect within the substance of the cuff is another useful sign of rupture (Fig. 1-36). The presence of foci of increased echogenicity in the cuff, thought to represent granulation tissue, is the least reliable sign of rotator cuff tear and should be considered only when a frank asymmetry is found between the shoulders.[39]

The technical difficulty and operator dependence of rotator cuff sonography are reflected in the significant variation in the reported accuracy of this method in diagnosing tears. Although early reports claimed that the accuracy of ultrasound was close or even superior to that

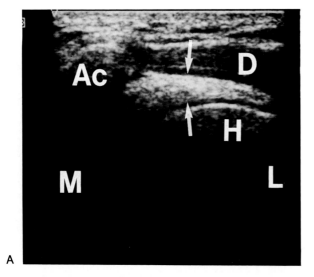
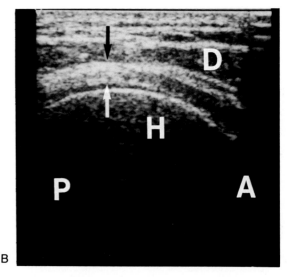

Fig. 1-34. Normal rotator cuff. **(A)** Longitudinal scan showing the tapering echogenic cuff (arrows) underneath the deltoid muscle *(D)* and covering the humeral head *(H)*. The proximal cuff is obscured by the shadow from the acromion *(Ac)*. (*L*, lateral; *M*, medial.) **(B)** Transverse scan of the cuff (arrows). Note the artifactual hypoechogenicity of the cuff anteriorly. (*A*, anterior; *D*, deltoid muscle; *H*, humerus; *P*, posterior.)

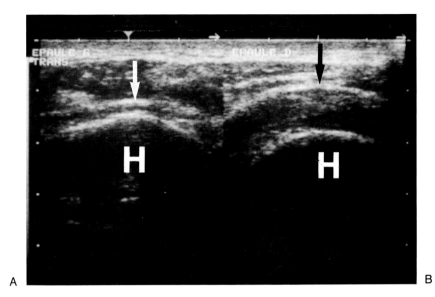

Fig. 1-35. Complete rupture of the rotator cuff. **(A)** Transverse scan shows the absence of a cuff (arrow). **(B)** Transverse scan of the normal contralateral cuff (arrow) is shown for comparison. (*H*, humerus.)

of arthrography,[40,41] recent studies have indicated a sensitivity for ultrasound of only about 60 percent.[42–44] Sonography is reasonably accurate in the diagnosis of the normal rotator cuff and complete tears but is less reliable in the diagnosis of partial tears. Arthrography should be performed in patients with normal sonograms when there is a strong clinical suspicion of a tear or when conservative therapy has failed. In patients with a positive sonogram, arthrography may still be necessary for a more objective preoperative assessment of the tear. Because of its relatively low cost, sonography can be used as

a screening tool in patients with shoulder pain, particularly the elderly. However, its role may have to be reevaluated as MRI continues to be improved.

Significant changes in cuff appearance as well as in anatomic landmarks occur postoperatively and must be carefully evaluated when diagnosing a recurrent tear. The cuff is usually thinner and more echogenic than normal, and changes in the humeral head contour are noticed in cases of tendon reimplantation. Nevertheless, satisfactory results have been reported in the diagnosis of recurrent tears.[45,46]

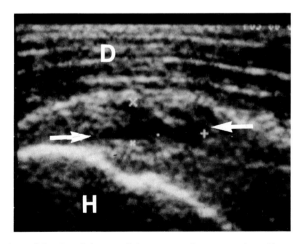

Fig. 1-36. Partial tear of the supraspinatus tendon. Coronal scan of the shoulder showing the ill-defined discontinuity of the fibers (arrows). (*D*, deltoid muscle; *H*, humerus.) (Courtesy of P. Farin, M.D.)

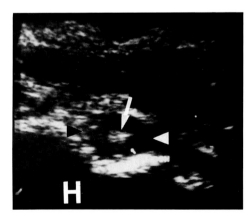

Fig. 1-37. Fluid collection in the biceps tendon sheath associated with a rotator cuff tear. Transverse scan of the bicipital groove showing the anechoic fluid (arrowheads) around the tendon (arrow). (*H*, humerus.) (From Fornage,[2] with permission; © 1991 by BD Fornage.)

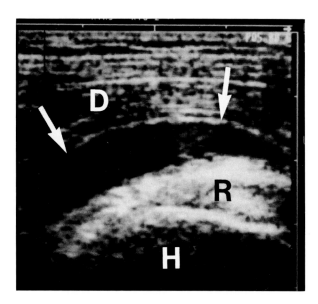

Fig. 1-38. Impingement syndrome. Longitudinal scan showing the fluid-distended subdeltoid bursa (arrows). (*D*, deltoid muscle; *H*, humerus; *R*, rotator cuff.) (Courtesy of P. Farin, M.D.)

Biceps Tendon

Visualization of the echogenic biceps tendon in the bicipital groove is an important landmark in sonography of the rotator cuff.[47] Nonvisualization of the tendon in-

dicates a complete rupture or dislocation.[48] The possibility of an artifactual "empty groove" resulting from an improperly angled scan plane must be excluded in all cases. In tendinitis, the tendon is thickened and hypoechoic. Fluid around the tendon in the bicipital groove is seen in tenosynovitis and joint effusions (Fig. 1-37). It is associated with about 10 percent of rotator cuff tears and should therefore trigger a meticulous search for such a lesion.[47]

Other Applications

Fluid accumulation in the subdeltoid bursa can be demonstrated by sonography. This condition has been reported to be common in patients with impingement syndrome[37] (Fig. 1-38), but can also occur in patients with rheumatoid arthritis, gout, and pyogenic infections. Calcifications within the cuff can also be visualized on sonograms as bright foci often associated with shadowing (Fig. 1-39).

Sonography can demonstrate pathologic changes of the acromioclavicular joint, including osteoarthritis and dislocation. More interesting is its ability to detect subtle fractures of the greater tuberosity, which may not be well seen on initial plain radiographs. Such a fracture appears as an abrupt discontinuity of the smooth echogenic bony contour.[49,50]

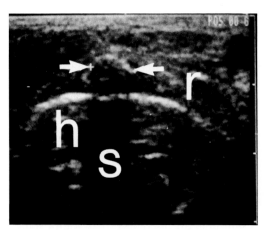

A

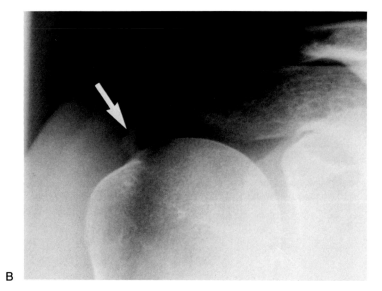

B

Fig. 1-39. Calcification of the rotator cuff. **(A)** Sonogram showing a curved linear echo with an acoustic shadow (arrows). (*h*, humerus; *r*, rotator cuff; *s*, shadow.) **(B)** Radiograph confirming the calcification (arrow). (Courtesy of P. Farin, M.D.)

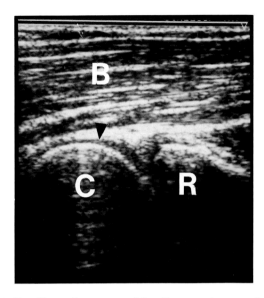

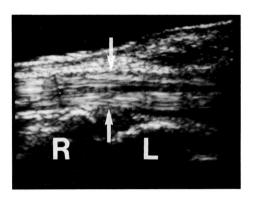

Fig. 1-42. Normal anatomy of the wrist on ultrasound. Longitudinal scan showing the echogenic superficial and deep flexor tendons of the third finger (arrows) coursing over the distal extremity of the radius *(R)* and the lunate *(L).*

Fig. 1-40. Normal anatomy of the elbow on ultrasound. Sagittal scan of the anterior aspect of the extended elbow showing the capitulum *(C)* and the radial head *(R).* Note the thin articular cartilage (arrowhead). (*B,* brachioradialis.)

ELBOW

Normal Anatomy

In children, the cartilaginous epiphyses are hypoechoic with minute scattered bright dots. As ossification centers develop, their echogenicity increases and shad-

owing becomes apparent.[51] In adults, sonography delineates the bony contours (Fig. 1-40) and can demonstrate the major tendons, including those of the biceps and triceps muscles (Fig. 1-41), as well as the common flexor and common extensor tendons, which insert on the medial and lateral epicondyles of the humerus, respectively.[31] Vessels are easily identified by color Doppler imaging, and the radial and ulnar nerves can be visualized using high-frequency transducers.[2]

Abnormalities

Trauma causes most pathologic conditions involving the elbow. In children, sonography has the advantage of allowing direct visualization of the epiphyses and their displacement. As with any other joint, sonography is useful in demonstrating joint effusions in the elbow. Although very rare, synovial cysts may develop from the elbow, particularly in patients with rheumatoid arthritis, and can be diagnosed on sonograms. Ultrasound has also been used in the diagnosis of epicondylitis, with the demonstration of a thickened, hypoechoic tendon, which sometimes contains calcifications.

HAND AND WRIST

When examining the hand and wrist, a thin standoff pad is often needed to ensure proper contact between the flat transducer and the skin. Dynamic examination is instrumental in identifying the tendons.[52]

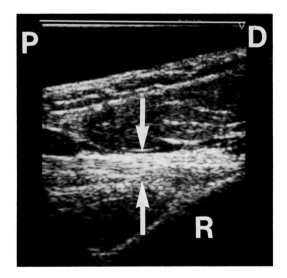

Fig. 1-41. Normal anatomy of the elbow on ultrasound. Sagittal scan of the anterior aspect of the elbow showing the echogenic biceps tendon (arrows) inserting on the radial tuberosity. (*D,* distal; *P,* proximal; *R,* radius.)

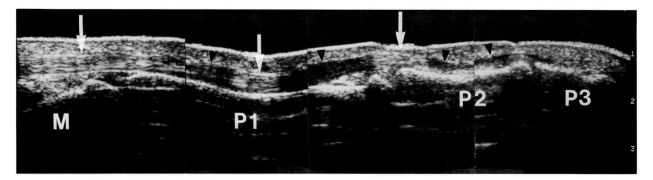

Fig. 1-43. Normal anatomy of the fingers on ultrasound. Montage of longitudinal scans of the third finger showing the superficial and deep flexor tendons coursing along the phalanges. Tendons exhibit normal echogenicity only in the segments in which they are parallel to the linear-array transducer (arrows) and are falsely hypoechoic in any segment in which they are not strictly perpendicular to the beam (arrowheads). (*M*, third metacarpal; *P1*, first phalanx; *P2*, second phalanx; *P3*, third phalanx.)

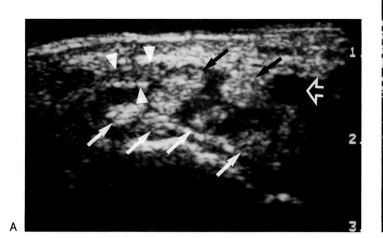
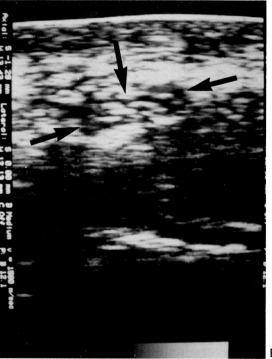

Fig. 1-44. Normal median nerve in the wrist. **(A)** Transverse scan of the wrist at 10 MHz showing the echogenic cross-sections of the flexor tendons of the fingers (arrows) in the ulnar bursa. (arrowheads, echogenic median nerve; open arrow, ulnar artery.) **(B)** Transverse scan obtained at 20 MHz showing the fascicular texture of the nerve more clearly (arrows).

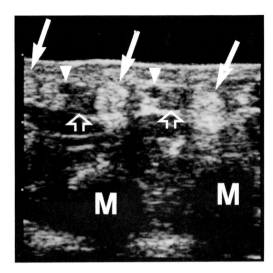

Fig. 1-45. Normal anatomy of the hand on ultrasound. Transverse scan of the palm showing the echogenic round cross-sections of the deep and superficial tendons of the second, third, and fourth fingers (arrows). (open arrows, adjacent hypoechoic lumbrical muscles; arrowheads, common palmar digital arteries; *M*, metacarpal bone.)

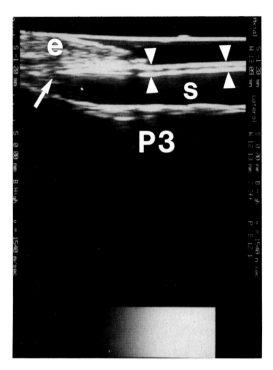

Fig. 1-46. Normal anatomy of the fingers on ultrasound. Longitudinal scan of the dorsal aspect of the tip of the third finger showing the proximal nail, which is 0.3 mm thick (arrowheads), and the nail root with the nail matrix (arrow). (*e*, eponychium; *P3*, third phalanx; *s*, subungual space.)

Normal Anatomy

Longitudinal scans of the normal wrist demonstrate the bony contours of the radius, the ulna, and the carpal bones. The flexor tendons of the fingers are demonstrated in the volar aspects of the wrist and the hand as brightly echogenic structures with a fibrillar echotexture (Fig. 1-42). In the fingers, the flexor tendons follow the curvature of the bony phalanges, and their echogenicity may be artificially decreased in the segments in which the fibers are not perpendicular to the beam[1] (Fig. 1-43). At the dorsum of the wrist, hand, and fingers, extensor tendons of the fingers also display the typical echopattern of tendons.

Transverse scans of the carpal tunnel show the echogenic cross-sections of the flexor tendons in the radial and ulnar bursae. The median nerve lies anterior to the tendons, beneath the palmar carpal ligament[1] (Fig. 1-44). In the palm, the cross-sections of the echogenic superficial and deep flexor tendons of the fingers are seen adjacent to the hypoechoic lumbrical muscles (Fig. 1-45). The hypoechoic interosseous muscles and hyperechoic metacarpal bones are seen posteriorly.

The nails and the subungual spaces, which represent a common site for glomus tumors, can be evaluated by high-frequency transducers (Fig. 1-46). The superficial palmar arch and the common digital arteries in the palm and the digital arteries in the fingers are routinely seen with color Doppler imaging (Plate 1-2).

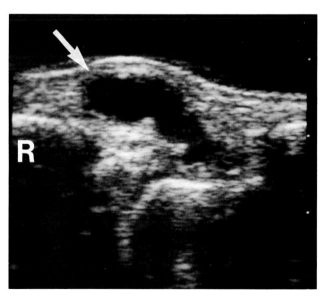

Fig. 1-47. Ganglion cyst of the wrist. Longitudinal scan of the dorsal aspect of the wrist showing the lobulated anechoic cyst (arrow) originating from the wrist joint. (*R*, radius.) (From Fornage,[2] with permission; © 1991 by BD Fornage.)

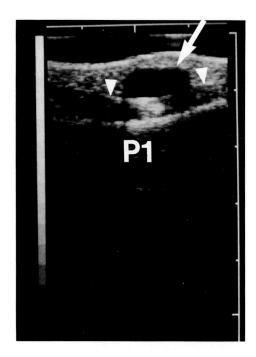

Fig. 1-48. Ganglion cyst of a finger. Longitudinal scan of the volar aspect of the first phalanx showing the anechoic cyst (arrow) anterior to the flexor tendons (arrowheads). (*P1*, first phalanx.)

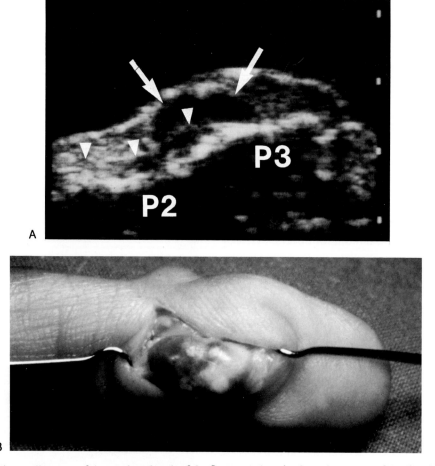

Fig. 1-49. Giant cell tumor of the tendon sheath of the flexor tendons in the volar aspect of the tip of the second finger. **(A)** Longitudinal scan showing a lobulated hypoechoic mass (arrows) lying just anterior to the distal flexor tendons (arrowheads) and the distal interphalangeal joint. (*P2*, second phalanx; *P3*, third phalanx.) (Fig. A from Fornage et al,[53] with permission.) **(B)** Intraoperative view of the tumor.

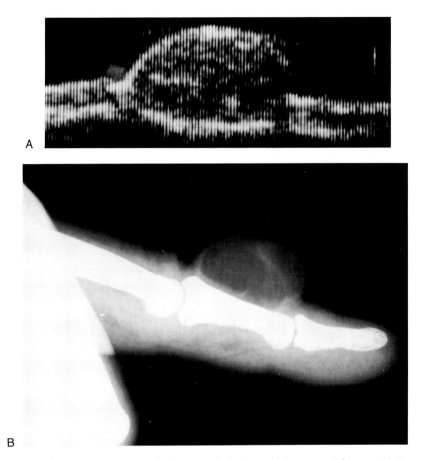

Fig. 1-50. Lipoma of the dorsal aspect of the second phalanx of the second finger. **(A)** Longitudinal scan showing a moderately echogenic mass dorsal to the second bony phalanx. **(B)** Low-kilovoltage radiograph showing the radiolucent lipoma. (From Fornage et al,[53] with permission.)

Abnormalities

Soft Tissue Masses

Ganglion cysts usually develop from the wrist joint with which they communicate and are also found adjacent to tendon sheaths[53,54] (Figs. 1-47 and 1-48). They are usually sonolucent, but internal low-level echoes can be found in chronic or inflammatory cysts.[52] Artifactual echoes from volume averaging (slice thickness artifact) may fill in minute cysts.

The vast majority of soft tissue tumors in the hand are benign. Most commonly found are giant cell tumors, fibrous histiocytomas, angiomas, lipomas, and nerve sheath tumors. Sonography confirms the solid nature of such a mass, allows precise measurement, and shows the relationship of the tumor to adjacent structures, notably the tendons (Fig. 1-49). Except for some lipomas that are echogenic (Fig. 1-50), soft tissue neoplasms of the hand appear as nonspecific hypoechoic masses.[53] Epidermoid

(inclusion) cysts may contain hyperechoic keratin plugs mimicking calcifications or foreign bodies (Fig. 1-51).

Ultrasound has been used successfully in the diagnosis and preoperative localization of glomus tumors of the hand. Glomus tumors are small (less than 1 cm), usually nonpalpable tumors that are characterized clinically by exquisite tenderness and temperature sensitivity. They

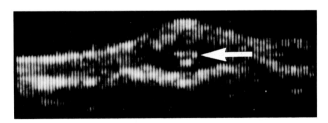

Fig. 1-51. Epidermoid (inclusion) cyst of the dorsal aspect of the second finger. Longitudinal scan showing a hypoechoic mass with echogenic foci representing keratin plugs (arrow).

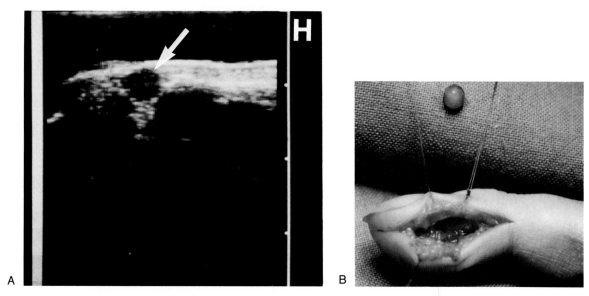

Fig. 1-52. Glomus tumor of the tip of the fifth finger. **(A)** Coronal scan showing a well-defined, rounded, hypoechoic mass (arrow) lying in the concavity of the third bony phalanx. (*H*, toward patient's head.) **(B)** Intraoperative view showing the excised 5-mm tumor. (From Fornage and Rifkin,[52] with permission.)

are often localized in the tips of digits, typically in the subungual space. On sonograms, glomus tumors are markedly hypoechoic to sonolucent[55] (Fig. 1-52).

Inflammatory Changes

In tenosynovitis, sonography accurately demonstrates even small amounts of fluid (Fig. 1-31), thickening of the synovial sheath, or both.[34,35] In patients with rheumatoid tenosynovitis, ultrasound shows the markedly hypoechoic pannus involving the sheath (Fig. 1-53) and may demonstrate tendon ruptures.[52,56]

In Dupuytren's contracture (palmar fibromatosis), sonography shows an ill-defined hypoechoic mass in the subcutaneous tissues of the palm, associated with skin retraction, usually beginning over the course of the flexor tendons of the fourth or fifth finger (Fig. 1-54). Initially, the flexor tendons are not involved by the slow-progressing inflammatory process, as confirmed by real-time ultrasound.

Carpal Tunnel Syndrome

In patients with carpal tunnel syndrome, sonography can detect a nonpalpable causal abnormality, such as a deeply located ganglion cyst, lipoma, or tenosynovitis.[57] When the median nerve is markedly inflamed, it appears swollen and hypoechoic on sonograms[2] (Fig. 1-55). However, in most cases, the nerve is more clearly depicted on MRI.

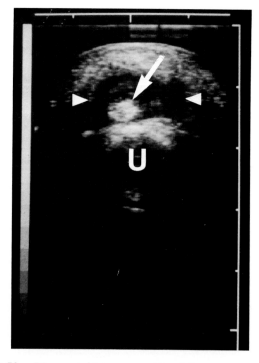

Fig. 1-53. Rheumatoid tenosynovitis of the extensor carpi ulnaris tendon. Transverse scan of the wrist showing the echogenic, slightly irregular cross-section of the tendon (arrow) surrounded by the ill-defined hypoechoic pannus (arrowheads). (*U*, ulna.)

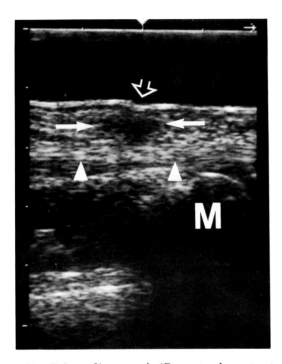

Fig. 1-54. Palmar fibromatosis (Dupuytren's contracture). Longitudinal scan of the palm through the flexor tendons of the fourth finger showing a poorly defined hypoechoic area in the subcutaneous tissues (arrows). Note the retraction of the overlying skin (open arrow). The play of the flexor tendons (arrowheads) was not impaired, as confirmed by the real-time study. (*M*, head of the fourth metacarpal.)

Foreign Bodies

Sonography is very helpful in the diagnosis and three-dimensional localization of foreign bodies, which are most commonly found in the distal extremities (see below).

PEDIATRIC HIP

Sonography of the hip has recently become popular in neonates and infants for the diagnosis of congenital dislocation of the hip[58-65] and in children for the diagnosis of hip effusions.[66-73]

Technique

Whatever the technique used, it is crucial that the infant be relaxed at the time of ultrasound examination. Several techniques of hip examination have been described. Harcke and others have recommended the lateral approach (i.e., scanning the supine patient from the lateral aspect of the hip) and emphasized the dynamic assessment of the hip's position and stability, in particular during the Barlow and Ortolani maneuvers.[60-62] Harcke et al use three basic scans: the transverse view with the hip in the neutral position, the transverse view with the hip flexed, and the coronal view with the hip flexed. On the other hand, as advocated by Graf,[59] most

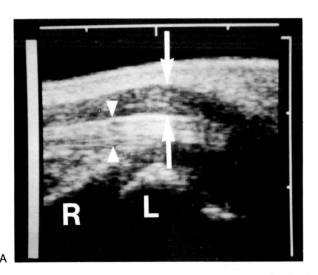

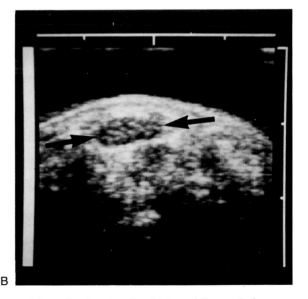

A B

Fig. 1-55. Carpal tunnel syndrome. **(A)** Longitudinal scan of the wrist showing the thickened, hypoechoic median nerve (arrows) anterior to the echogenic flexor tendons of the second finger (arrowheads). (*R*, radius; *L*, lunate.) **(B)** Transverse scan showing the enlarged nerve (arrows). (From Fornage,[2] with permission; © 1991 by BD Fornage.)

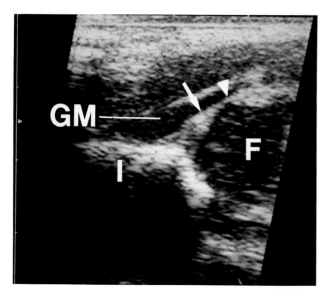

Fig. 1-56. Normal neonatal hip. Coronal scan of the right hip in a 3-day-old neonate showing the hypoechoic cartilaginous femoral head with a characteristic fine stippled pattern, resting against the bony acetabulum. Note the echogenic tip of the labrum (arrow) and the thin echogenic capsule (arrowhead). (*F*, femoral head; *GM*, gluteus minimus muscle; *I*, iliac line.) (Courtesy of V. Tran-Minh, M.D.)

European authorities have relied on the coronal view obtained with the hip in the neutral position and the measurement of two angles, the α angle between the iliac bone baseline and the bony acetabular roof and the β angle between the iliac bone baseline and the cartilaginous acetabular roof.[59,63]

Normal Anatomy

Anatomic landmarks include the hypoechoic triradiate or Y-shaped cartilage, the echogenic iliac line on coronal views, the labrum and its echogenic tip, the rounded hypoechoic femoral head with its ossification center appearing within a few months of life, and the echogenic hip joint capsule. Ultrasound examination reveals the positional relationship between the acetabulum and the hypoechoic femoral head (Fig. 1-56). On the coronal/neutral view, the iliac bone baseline passes grossly through the center of the femoral head and the α and β angles are grossly equal. The α angle is about 50 degrees at birth and reaches 60 degrees at the age of 3 months. The size of the ossification center of the femoral head can be appreciated on sonograms; after the age of 1 year, ultrasound examination of the hip is prevented by the associated shadow.[74]

Abnormalities

Congenital Dislocation and/or Dysplasia

In subluxation or dislocation, the femoral head is usually displaced posteriorly, superiorly, and laterally (Fig. 1-57). The ultrasound diagnosis of congenital disloca-

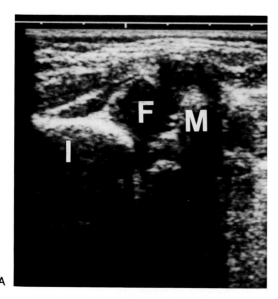

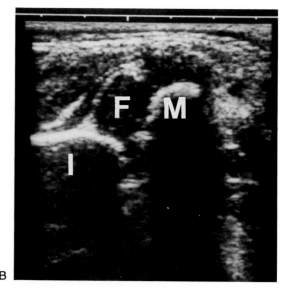

Fig. 1-57. Congenital dislocation of the hip in a 4-day-old neonate. **(A)** Coronal scan in the neutral position showing the superolateral displacement of the femoral head *(F)*. (*I*, iliac line; *M*, femoral metaphysis.) **(B)** Coronal scan obtained during adduction showing greater displacement of the femoral head *(F)*. (*I*, iliac line; *M*, femoral metaphysis.) (Courtesy of V. Tran-Minh, M.D.)

tion of the hip is straightforward, and sonography has proved to be more sensitive than physical examination in the detection and diagnosis of this condition.[65] Hip laxity, although common before the age of 1 month, should be monitored. For practical reasons, sonographic screening cannot be recommended for every newborn; currently, the technique is used to evaluate infants with abnormal or suspicious physical findings and those at risk.[64] For these purposes, sonography has virtually replaced standard radiography.

Ultrasound is a useful tool for observation of borderline cases and for monitoring the efficacy of therapy, particularly with the Pavlik harness.[75]

Other Pediatric Applications

In children with hip pain, sonography is instrumental in diagnosing hip joint effusions. Transverse oblique scans along the axis of the femoral neck are obtained from an anterior approach with the patient supine and the hip in the neutral position. The normal capsule is concave anteriorly, and the distance between the capsule and the anterior aspect of the femoral neck ranges from 2 to 5 mm (mean, 2.5 mm) in children without abnormalities. A distance greater than 6 mm is suggestive of an effusion, as is a difference between the hips of 3 mm or greater[72] (Fig. 1-58). A bulging capsule is a reliable sign of effusion. The hypoechoic psoas muscle should not be confused with an effusion. In a series of 111 children with acute hip pain, sonography diagnosed an effusion in 71 percent compared with only 15 percent for radiography, and sonography has therefore been proposed as the first-line examination technique for children up to 8 years of age with an irritable hip.[73] Common conditions associated with a hip effusion include transient synovitis, traumatic synovitis, Legg-Calvé-Perthes disease, septic

arthritis, and osteomyelitis. When needle aspiration of the fluid is required, ultrasound provides safe and accurate guidance.

Although sonography occasionally permits visualization of the femoral head fragmentation in Legg-Calvé-Perthes disease or a step at the level of the epiphyseal plate in a patient with slipped femoral capital epiphysis, its role in the diagnosis of these conditions is anecdotal and radiography remains the standard technique for diagnosis.

Various techniques for the measurement of femoral torsion by using static or real-time ultrasound equipment have been described, with emphasis placed on the low cost and wide availability of the equipment and on the lack of irradiation.[76,77] However, the reliability of sonography in this application has been controversial, and the gold standard remains CT (or MRI).[78]

ADULT HIP

Sonography can be used in the adult to diagnose hip joint effusion and guide needle aspiration. This has proved particularly helpful in patients with a suspected infection of a hip prosthesis.[79] In patients with acute lower abdominal pain and symptoms referable to the groin and thigh, ultrasound examination of the hip may reveal an unsuspected effusion.[80]

The iliopectineal bursa lies anterior to the hip joint space, lateral to the femoral vessels. It can increase in volume, usually in the cephalocaudal direction, resulting in a sausage-shaped fluid-filled collection (Fig. 1-59). Large synovial cysts arising from this bursa may extend into the pelvis.[81]

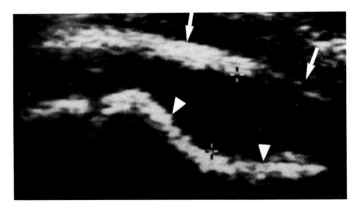

Fig. 1-58. Hip effusion in a child with transient synovitis. Scan obtained along the axis of the femoral neck showing the fluid effusion. The distance between the concave femoral neck (arrowheads) and the bulging capsule (arrows) is 1.1 cm (calipers). (From Alexander et al,[72] with permission.)

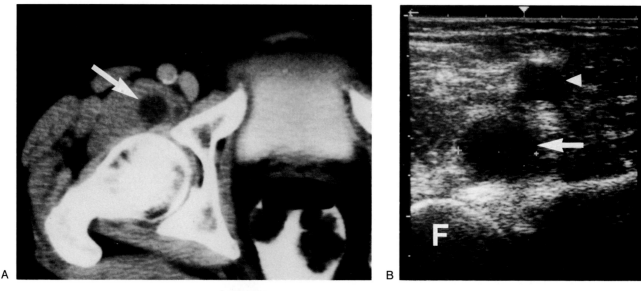

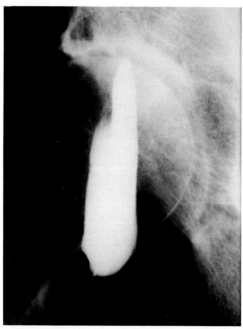

Fig. 1-59.   Enlarged iliopectineal bursa. **(A)** CT scan showing a hypodense rounded structure anterior to the right hip joint (arrow). **(B)** Transverse sonogram demonstrating the fluid-filled bursa (arrow) immediately anterior to the joint capsule. (arrowhead, femoral artery; *F*, femoral head.) **(C)** Ultrasound-guided bursography fails to demonstrate a communication between the opacified bursa and the joint space. (From Fornage,[2] with permission; © 1991 by BD Fornage.)

KNEE

The best uses of ultrasound examination of the knee are the evaluation of the extensor tendons, the diagnosis of a mass in the popliteal fossa, and the confirmation of a joint effusion.

Normal Anatomy

The quadriceps tendon inserts on the base of the patella, and the patellar tendon is a flat band that extends from the patella to the tibial tuberosity. The two tendons are connected by prepatellar fibers. Because both tendons may be concave anteriorly when the knee is extended and at rest, the best longitudinal scans are obtained during contraction of the quadriceps muscle, which straightens the tendons, thereby clearing any area of false hypoechogenicity and showing the normal, echogenic, fibrillar texture of tendons[31] (Figs. 1-27 and 1-60). With the use of high-frequency transducers, prepatellar tendon fibers are visualized, as are the thin subcutaneous prepatellar and infrapatellar bursae and the slightly larger deep (subtendinous) infrapatellar bursa (Fig. 1-61). On transverse sections, the quadriceps tendon is oval, whereas the patellar tendon has a meniscus shape with a convex anterior and flat posterior surface[1] (Fig. 1-62). At its midpoint, the patellar tendon is about 4 to 5 mm thick and about 20 to 25 mm wide.[31]

Abnormalities

Quadriceps and Patellar Tendons

Complete ruptures of the quadriceps or patellar tendons are usually recognized by physical examination, but partial ruptures are less easily diagnosed. Although direct trauma can occur — including perforation during arthroscopy — most tears of the quadriceps or patellar tendons are caused by excessive tension on the tendon. In partial ruptures, sonography demonstrates a focal defect within the tendon along with some swelling; there is minimal or no associated hematoma. Partial detachment of the patellar tendon from the apex of the patella gives rise to a characteristic midline hematoma[33] (Fig. 1-63).

Tendinitis is characterized by a thickened, hypoechoic tendon, sometimes with blurred margins[31,82,83] (Fig. 1-30). Focal areas of decreased echogenicity may mimic partial tears. Doppler studies can reveal increased vascularity (Fig. 1-64). Intratendinous calcifications are associated with chronic tendinitis. Sonography is highly sensitive in the detection of minute tendon calcifications, but their shape and size are better appreciated on low-kilovoltage radiographs or xerograms.[84]

Following surgery, ultrasound demonstrates a thickened tendon (Fig. 1-32) and can depict sutures or reinforcement material such as polydioxanone sulfate bands.[31]

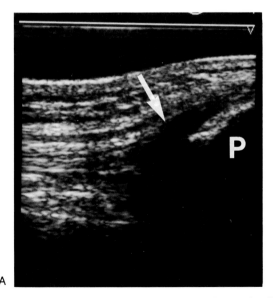
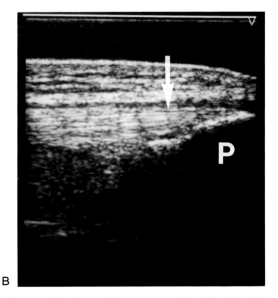

A   B

Fig. 1-60. Normal quadriceps tendon. **(A)** Longitudinal scan with the quadriceps at rest. The distal tendon (arrow) is falsely hypoechoic because of the obliquity of the fibers to the beam. (*P*, patella.) **(B)** Scan obtained during contraction of the quadriceps showing the straightened, brightly echogenic tendon (arrow). (*P*, patella.)

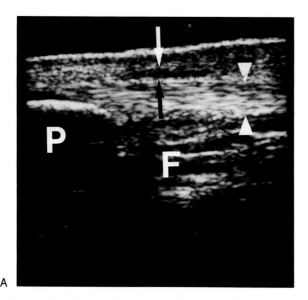 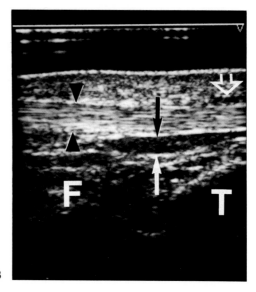

Fig. 1-61. Normal bursae associated with the patellar tendon. **(A)** Longitudinal scan of the upper tendon showing prepatellar bursa (arrows). (arrowheads, patellar tendon; *P*, patella; *F*, fat pad of knee.) **(B)** Longitudinal scan of the lower tendon showing the deep (subtendinous) (arrows) and subcutaneous (open arrow) infrapatellar bursae. (arrowheads, patellar tendon; *F*, fat pad of the knee; *T*, tibia.)

Popliteal Masses

The most common masses in the popliteal fossa are cysts and aneurysms of the popliteal artery, both of which are readily diagnosed by sonography. Popliteal cysts result from distention of the gastrocnemiosemimembranosus bursa, which may communicate with the

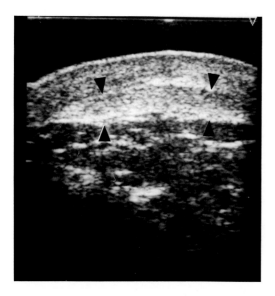

Fig. 1-62. Transverse scan of the upper patellar tendon (arrowheads) showing the typical meniscus shape with a convex anterior and flat posterior surface.

knee joint. A predisposing factor is increased intra-articular pressure from capsular sclerosis or synovial hypertrophy, as observed in rheumatoid and other arthritides. Small popliteal cysts may be asymptomatic, whereas large cysts cause pain and impair knee function. Large cysts extending into the calf, ruptured cysts, and infected cysts can all produce a swollen painful limb, mimicking thrombophlebitis.

Sonograms of a popliteal cyst demonstrate a fluid-filled collection[85-87] (Fig. 1-65). Early cysts have a tendency to wrap around the origin of the medial gastrocnemius muscle, and such a cyst may appear on longitudinal scans through the muscle as a biloculated effusion, with the anterior part being smaller. Transverse scans confirm that both areas represent parts of the same cyst (Fig. 1-66). Internal echoes representing fibrinous strands or debris and synovial thickening can be seen in inflammatory cysts. The advantage of sonography over arthrography is the visualization of noncommunicating cysts and of cysts that are poorly opacified because of their thick contents. However, in patients with rheumatoid arthritis, cysts may be completely filled with pannus and may therefore mimic solid masses (Fig. 1-67). Osteochondromatosis with hyperechoic loose bodies in a popliteal cyst has also been reported.[88] Sonograms of a ruptured cyst show the residual cyst, which has decreased in size, and the presence of fluid dissecting along the calf[87] (Fig. 1-68). However, when the examination is delayed, the diagnosis may be missed if most of the leaking fluid has

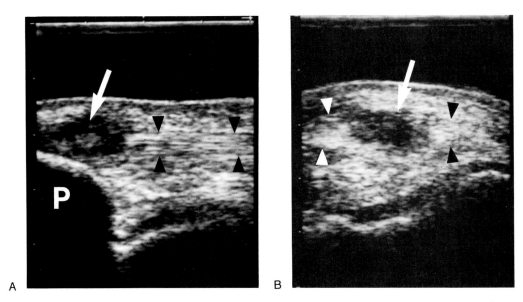

Fig. 1-63. Partial detachment of the patellar tendon from the patellar apex. **(A)** Longitudinal scan of the upper tendon showing the focal discontinuity and the hematoma (arrow). (arrowheads, normal tendon; *P*, patella.) **(B)** Transverse scan confirming that the tear is limited to the center (arrow) and that the lateral aspects of the tendon are not involved (arrowheads).

already been resorbed, because only an ill-defined hypoechoic area will remain at the previous site of the cyst. In patients with systemic predisposing factors such as rheumatoid arthritis, it is recommended that the contralateral fossa be examined for an early nonpalpable cyst.

Sonography and color Doppler imaging are effective means of diagnosing aneurysms of the popliteal artery.[89,90] Uncomplicated aneurysms are anechoic structures located centrally within the upper or mid-fossa, and longitudinal scans can document their continuity with the normal popliteal artery. Unlike angiography, ultrasound can demonstrate totally thrombosed aneurysms, which usually contain some echogenic material. Because aneurysms of the popliteal artery often occur

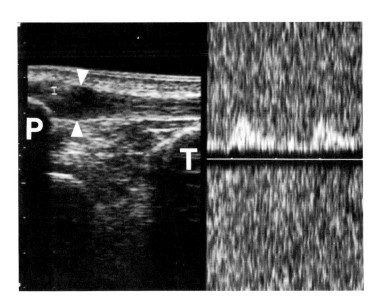

Fig. 1-64. Patellar tendinitis. Longitudinal duplex sonogram showing increased vascularity in the thickened, hypoechoic upper half of the tendon (arrowheads). (*P*, patella; *T*, tibia.)

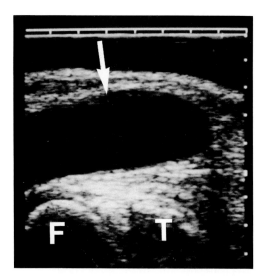

Fig. 1-65. Typical popliteal cyst. Longitudinal scan of the popliteal fossa showing a well-defined, ovoid fluid collection (arrow) lying posterior to the origin of the gastrocnemius medialis muscle. (*F*, femur; *T*, tibia.)

bilaterally, it is good practice to scan the contralateral fossa.

Tumors that can develop in the popliteal fossa include lipomas and nerve sheath tumors, soft tissue sarcomas, and, infrequently, lymph node metastases.[2,90] On rare occasions, sonography performed to evaluate a "firm soft tissue mass" will reveal an osteochondroma.[2]

Joint Effusions and Synovial Abnormalities

Sonography can confirm the presence of small effusions in the knee joint, which generally collect in the suprapatellar bursa when the knee is extended.[91] If needed, aspiration can be performed under ultrasound guidance.

In various proliferative diseases of the synovium, including osteochondromatosis, pigmented villonodular synovitis, and rheumatoid arthritis, sonography can be used to visualize and measure the thickened synovium[92,93] (Fig. 1-69). Synovial thickening can also be demonstrated in hemophiliac patients with iterated blood effusions. The anecdotal demonstration of synovial plicae of the knee by sonography has been reported.[94]

Miscellaneous

Encouraging results have been reported in the evaluation of Osgood-Schlatter disease by sonography.[95] Initially, the anechoic cartilage of the ossification center of the tibial tubercle is swollen and the overlying soft tissues are moderately thickened. As the disease progresses, the fragmented ossification center can be seen as multiple hyperechoic foci, the distal patellar tendon becomes thickened and hypoechoic, and fluid accumulates in the deep infrapatellar bursa. More studies are needed to define the role of sonography in the evaluation of this con-

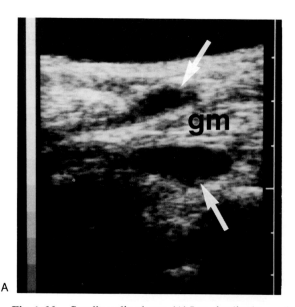
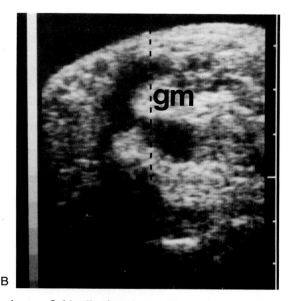

Fig. 1-66. Small popliteal cyst. **(A)** Longitudinal scan showing two fluid collections (arrows) located posteriorly and anteriorly to the gastrocnemius medialis muscle *(gm)*. **(B)** Transverse scan showing that both collections are parts of the same cyst, which wraps medially around the origin of the gastrocnemius medialis muscle *(gm)*. (dotted line, orientation of the scan plane in Fig. A.) (From Fornage,[2] with permission; © 1991 by BD Fornage.)

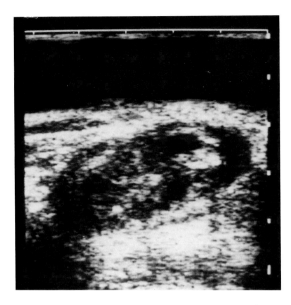

Fig. 1-67. Popliteal cyst in a patient with rheumatoid arthritis. Longitudinal scan showing a popliteal cyst filled with echogenic material.

for evaluating the knee menisci, except for the rare meniscal cysts[100] (Fig. 1-71).

Portions of the articular cartilage of the distal femur can be visualized by sonography. The normal cartilage of the weight-bearing portion of the femoral condyles is 1.2 to 2 mm thick.[101] In patients with arthritis and osteoarthritis, the cartilage is thinned and irregular.[101,102] It is doubtful, however, that this application of sonography will be used routinely.

Normal collateral ligaments of the knee are difficult to identify on sonograms. Despite encouraging results in demonstrating intra-articular hemorrhage, widening of the joint space under stress, and discontinuity of the torn ligament in recent trauma,[103] the feasibility of this application on a routine basis is doubtful. Cruciate ligaments of the knee cannot be satisfactorily imaged by sonography. MRI is the imaging modality of choice for menisci, articular cartilage, and collateral and cruciate ligaments of the knee.

ANKLE

Sonography of the ankle is performed primarily to evaluate the Achilles tendon.

Normal Anatomy

The Achilles tendon is formed by the fusion of the aponeuroses of the soleus and both gastrocnemius muscles. It inserts on the posterior surface of the calcaneus.

dition. Larsen-Johansson disease, a rarer condition with similar ultrasound findings, involves the accessory ossification center of the patella.

Menisci of the knee are echogenic, with a homogeneous echopattern[96,97] (Fig. 1-70). However, their visualization is incomplete and inconstant. Despite initial reports claiming promising results in the diagnosis of meniscal tears,[98,99] sonography is not a reliable modality

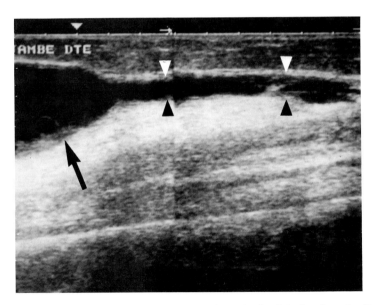

Fig. 1-68. Ruptured popliteal cyst mimicking deep venous thrombosis of the leg. Longitudinal scan of the calf showing the popliteal cyst (arrow) and the leaking fluid dissecting along the calf (arrowheads). (From Fornage,[2] with permission; © 1991 by BD Fornage.)

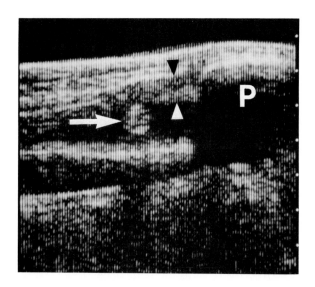

Fig. 1-69. Osteochondromatosis of the knee. Longitudinal scan of the knee showing the fluid-distended suprapatellar bursa with a thickened synovium (arrowheads) and a cartilage body (arrow). (*P*, patella.)

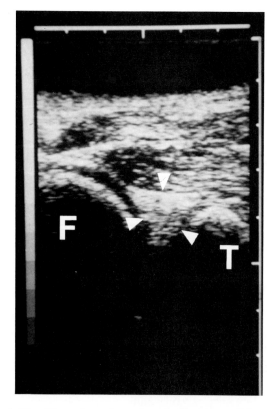

Fig. 1-70. Normal meniscus. Longitudinal scan of the posterior aspect of the knee showing the posterior horn of the lateral meniscus as a triangular echogenic structure (arrowheads). (*F*, femur; *T*, tibia.)

The patient is scanned in the prone position with the foot hanging over the edge of the table so that a dynamic examination with plantar flexion and dorsiflexion can be performed. Because of the subcutaneous location of the tendon, a thin standoff pad is required for the best images.

On longitudinal scans, in the absence of technique-related artifacts, the normal Achilles tendon is echogenic with well-defined margins and a characteristic fibrillar texture[1,31,104-107] (Fig. 1-72). Anterior to the distal half of the tendon lies the fatty Kager's triangle, whose overall echogenicity is variable. The hypoechoic subtendinous calcaneal bursa is sometimes seen in the angle formed by the tendon and the calcaneous (Fig. 1-72). At the insertion on the calcaneus, the fibers may have an oblique course anteriorly. The false hypoechogenicity that results should not be confused with the subcutaneous calcaneal bursa, which is not normally seen.

On transverse sonograms, the tendon is grossly elliptical and is thinner medially. Because the tendon plane is oriented obliquely, there is a risk of overestimating the thickness of the tendon on strictly sagittal scans of the leg, so measurements should be made on transverse scans[1] (Fig. 1-73). At 2 to 3 cm above its insertion, the Achilles tendon is 5 to 7 mm thick and 12 to 15 mm wide.[104]

Abnormalities

Achilles Tendon

A complete tear appears as a total disruption of the tendon. The variable gap between the retracted fragments is filled with hematoma or granulomatous tissue, depending on the chronicity of the tear (Fig. 1-28). In large ruptures, the hematoma may surround the tendon over a long distance.[33] In patients with a partial tear of the tendon, sonography shows a focal discontinuity within the otherwise echogenic substance of the tendon, sometimes associated with a focal swelling[104,107,108] (Fig. 1-29).

In Achilles tendinitis, the tendon is hypoechoic and thickened, with extensive nonhomogeneity.[104,107] In peritendinitis, the grossly intact central tendon is surrounded by the hypoechoic, diffusely thickened peritenon, whose margins are blurred (Fig. 1-74). Calcifications may develop in chronic Achilles tendinitis, particularly in the case of enthesitis.

Tendon thickening and decreased echogenicity are also found in patients with systemic inflammatory diseases such as rheumatoid arthritis, ankylosing spondylitis, lupus erythematosus, Reiter syndrome, psoriasis, or

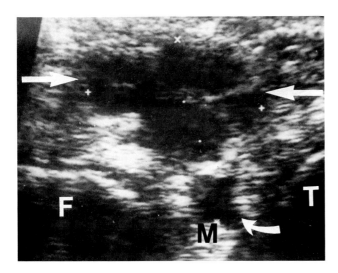

Fig. 1-71. Meniscal cyst. Longitudinal scan showing a septated cystic mass (arrows) with an intrameniscal component (curved arrow). (*F*, femur; *M*, meniscus; *T*, tibia.) (Courtesy of P. Peetrons, M.D.)

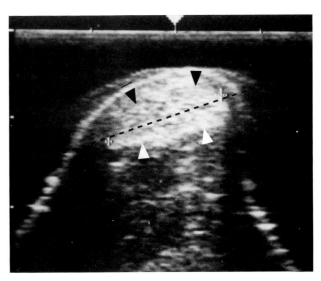

Fig. 1-73. Normal Achilles tendon. Transverse scan showing the hyperechoic tendon (arrowheads). Note the obliquity of the tendon plane (dotted line). The tendon measures 14 × 5 mm.

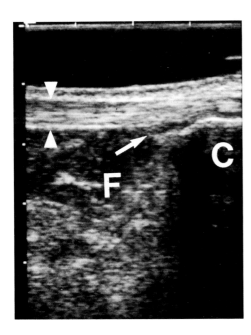

Fig. 1-72. Normal Achilles tendon. Longitudinal scan showing the well-defined echogenic tendon (arrowheads). Note the small subtendinous calcaneal bursa (arrow). (*C*, calcaneus; *F*, fatty Kager's triangle.)

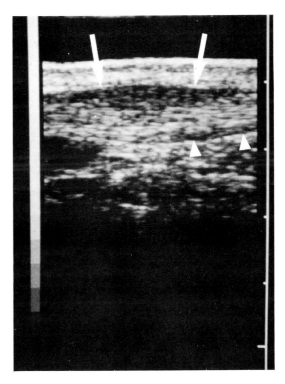

Fig. 1-74. Achilles peritendinitis. Longitudinal scan showing the thickened hypoechoic peritenon (arrows) responsible for the posterior bulge. There is also minor involvement of the peritenon anteriorly (arrowheads).

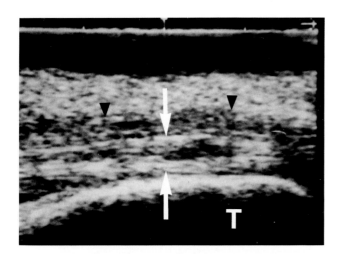

Fig. 1-75. Partial rupture of the posterior tibial tendon. Longitudinal scan showing the frayed tendon (arrows). Note the thickened sheath (arrowheads). (*T*, medial malleolus.)

gout. Retrocalcaneobursitis, which can be isolated or associated with tendinitis, appears sonographically as an enlarged anechoic bursa, sometimes with ill-defined contours.[107,109]

In patients with familial hypercholesterolemia, Achilles tendon thickening may be diffuse or focal, as in xanthomas, with an average reported thickness of 13 mm.[110,111] Sonography can be used to monitor the effects of pharmacotherapy on tendon size.

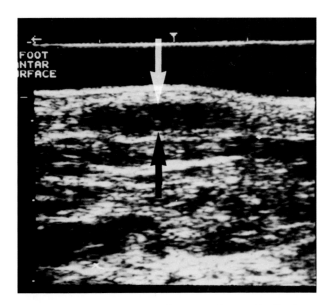

Fig. 1-76. Recurrent plantar fibromatosis. Longitudinal scan of the sole showing an ill-defined elongated hypoechoic mass in the subcutaneous tissue (arrows).

Sonography is highly accurate in detecting morphologic abnormalities of the Achilles tendon. When scanning artifacts have been carefully excluded, all disturbances of the homogeneous tendon structure indicate lesions. However, the tendon may appear normal in some patients with "functional" achillodynia (i.e., pain due to overstress of the dorsal muscle apparatus of the leg). Usually this pain resolves within a few weeks or months.[107]

Postoperatively, tendons are thickened and irregular, and echogenic suture material can be demonstrated.[104,112]

Other Tendons of the Ankle

Other tendons of the ankle that can be evaluated by sonography include those of the peroneus longus and brevis muscles laterally; the tibialis posterior muscle medially; and the tibialis anterior, extensor hallucis longus, and extensor digitorum longus muscles anteriorly. All these tendons are wrapped in synovial sheaths. Because of their curvature, it is difficult to display more than 2 to 3 cm of any of them at a time. Sonography has proved useful in the diagnosis of rupture and tenosynovitis of the tendons of the posterior tibial and peroneus muscles, which occur more frequently in patients with rheumatoid arthritis[33,113,114] (Fig. 1-75).

FOOT

Indications for ultrasound of the soft tissues of the foot are similar to those for ultrasound of the hand. Many pathologic conditions that affect the soft tissues of the hand can also be found in the foot; these include synovial cysts, benign solid tumors (e.g., lipomas, nerve sheath tumors, and glomus tumors), inflammatory changes (e.g., tenosynovitis, arthritis), and trauma (e.g., hematomas, foreign bodies).[52] A special mention must be given to Morton's neuroma, a fibrotic pseudotumor arising from the interdigital plantar nerves and located near the heads of the metatarsal bones. On sonograms, the small lesion (7 mm on average) is hypoechoic and well-defined.[115] Plantar fibromatosis, like palmar fibromatosis, appears sonographically as an ill-defined, elongated, hypoechoic mass in the subcutaneous tissue, superficial to the echogenic plantar fascia[116] (Fig. 1-76). The differential diagnosis for this poorly circumscribed lesion includes desmoid tumor and sarcoma. Sonography can also be used in the assessment of plantar fasciitis[117] (Fig. 1-77).

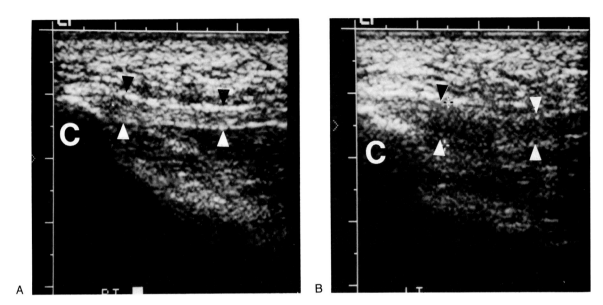

Fig. 1-77. Plantar fasciitis. **(A)** Sagittal scan of the contralateral heel showing the normal echogenic plantar fascia, which is about 4 mm thick (arrowheads). (*C*, calcaneus.) **(B)** Sagittal scan of the affected heel showing the markedly thickened, hypoechoic fascia with poorly defined margins (arrowheads). (*C*, calcaneus.)

Accurate and reproducible results have been obtained with sonography in the measurement of heel pad thickness, which is increased under various conditions, including acromegaly and treatment with phenytoin.[118]

Other studies have shown a significant decrease in the thickness of the heel and of the sole over the first and second metatarsals in diabetic patients with foot ulcers.[119]

BONES

Because bones interrupt the propagation of the beam, bone imaging by sonography has long been disregarded. However, this long-neglected application of diagnostic ultrasound is being revived today. Studies are needed to define indications for bone sonography in routine practice.

NORMAL ANATOMY

The proximal surface of the bony cortex appears on sonograms as a smooth, densely reflective line[1,2] (Fig. 1-40). The articular cartilage is a thin, anechoic rim. In children, nonossified hyaline cartilage is seen as a markedly hypoechoic area with scattered low-level dot echoes (Fig. 1-56). Ossification centers appear on sonograms earlier than on radiographs as areas of increased echogenicity and eventually cause shadowing.[74] Sonography

is routinely used to measure the femur length in utero and has been used by some authors, with variable results, to measure the degree of femoral torsion.[76,78]

ABNORMALITIES

Deformity or destruction of the bony cortex can be depicted by sonography, within the resolution limits of the available ultrasound equipment.

Trauma

Subperiosteal hematomas appear as meniscus-shaped hypoechoic areas bulging under the thin, echogenic periosteum. On occasion, bone fractures in adults have been detected by sonography as a discontinuity of the smooth cortical line[2,49,50] (Fig. 1-78). Ultrasound examination

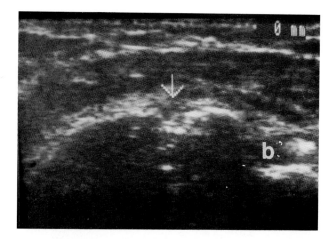

Fig. 1-78. Unsuspected fracture of the humeral head detected by sonography. Axial scan of the humeral head showing a compression defect (arrow) lateral to the bicipital groove *(b)*. (From Hammond,[49] with permission.)

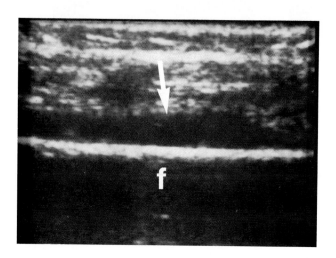

Fig. 1-79. Osteomyelitis of the fibula in a 13-year-old child. Longitudinal scan of the calf showing a fluid collection (arrow) in contact with the fibula *(f)*. (From Abiri et al,[124] with permission.)

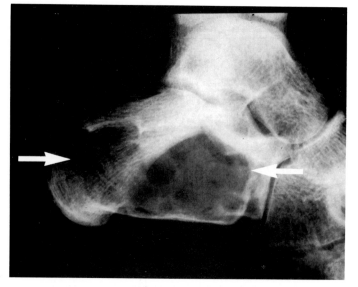

A

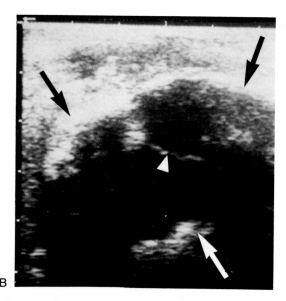

B

Fig. 1-80. Calcaneal bone cyst. **(A)** Lateral radiograph of the foot showing the radiolucent lesion (arrows) occupying most of the calcaneus. **(B)** Transverse sonogram of the lateral aspect of the hindfoot obtained with a 5.0-MHz transducer showing the cystic lesion (arrows) in the calcaneus. Note the internal septum (arrowhead). (From Fornage et al,[127] with permission.)

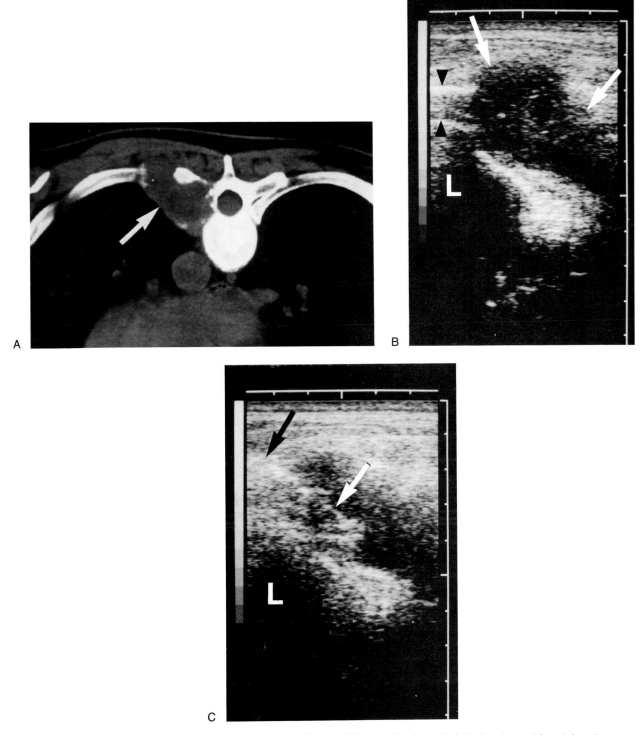

Fig. 1-81. Malignant fibrous histiocytoma of a rib. **(A)** CT scan showing a lytic lesion (arrow) involving the proximal rib and invading the vertebral body. **(B)** Transverse sonogram of the left paravertebral region showing the hypoechoic malignant tumor (arrows), which has destroyed the proximal rib. (arrowheads, rib; *L*, lung.) **(C)** Transverse sonogram obtained during real-time ultrasound-guided percutaneous biopsy showing the obliquely inserted Tru-Cut needle (arrows). (*L*, lung.)

should include the underlying or adjacent bones as well as the soft tissues, particularly in areas (such as the humeral head) that are difficult to evaluate radiographically.[49,50] Of significant interest is the potential of sonography to diagnose fractures and dislocations involving nonossified epiphyses in neonates and children.[120,121]

Recently, sonography has been used in the operating room to monitor the closed reduction of femoral fractures, thereby reducing significantly the duration of fluoroscopic exposure.[122] Sonography can also demonstrate bone formation at the fracture site many weeks before its appearance on radiographs, and it has been used successfully to monitor bone production at the distraction site in Ilizarov limb-lengthening procedures.[123]

Through the specific reverberation artifacts associated with metallic bodies, ultrasound can identify bone fixation devices and localize them in three dimensions.[2]

Osteomyelitis

In the proper clinical setting, the ultrasound demonstration of a fluid collection abutting the bone is a reliable sign of osteomyelitis[124] (Fig. 1-79). Occasionally, sonography can visualize a detached sequestrum as a brightly echogenic structure with an acoustic shadow, lying at a variable distance from the bone.

Tumors

Sonography can identify bone tumors that deform or destroy the superficial cortex.[125] Bone lesions that have markedly thinned the cortex also can be detected by sonography[126,127] (Fig. 1-80). Osteochondromas are readily visualized, and their hypoechoic cartilaginous cap demonstrated.[128] In malignant tumors, the focal cortex destruction may unmask part of the tumor, which is usually hypoechoic (Fig. 1-81). Tumor infiltration into the adjacent soft tissues can also be delineated. Ultrasound guidance can be used with safety and accuracy for needle biopsy of bone tumors that are visible on sonograms[127] (Fig. 1-81).

NERVES

It is only recently that normal peripheral nerves have been clearly identified by high-frequency ultrasound.[1,129]

NORMAL ANATOMY

Sonographically, normal nerves appear as hyperechoic tubular structures. On longitudinal scans, the echotexture is fibrillar, similar to that of tendons (Fig. 1-82A). On transverse scans, nerves exhibit a rounded or oval cross-section with a coarsely dotted pattern[1,129] (Fig. 1-82B). The false hypoechogenicity artifact resulting from obliquity of the ultrasound beam, described above for tendons, applies to nerves as well. Because a falsely hypoechoic normal nerve mimics a diseased nerve, the scanning technique should be adjusted so that all nerves are displayed perpendicular to the beam (i.e., parallel to the footprint of the transducer on longitudinal scan). As with tendons, the echogenic nerve trunks are best visualized when they are surrounded by hypoechoic muscles.

In the upper extremity, sonography can identify the median nerve in the forearm and carpal tunnel (Figs. 1-44 and 1-82), the radial nerve in the arm and at the elbow, and the ulnar nerve at the elbow and in the forearm. In the lower extremity, the sciatic nerve is visible in the posterior thigh (Fig. 1-83) and the tibial and popliteal nerves can be seen in the popliteal fossa.

ABNORMALITIES

Tumors

Benign nerve sheath tumors of the peripheral nerves include schwannomas (or neurilemmomas) and neurofibromas. On sonograms, both types of tumors are hypoechoic.[129-134] Often, high-frequency sonography can demonstrate the junction between the hypoechoic tumor and the normal echogenic nerve, thus confirming the diagnosis of nerve tumor[135] (Figs. 1-84 and 1-85). Schwannomas tend to be rounded or oval, well circumscribed, and eccentric in relation to the nerve axis, with internal cystic cavities and good sound-through transmission, sometimes mimicking a cyst (Fig. 1-84); neurofibromas, on the other hand, are often elongated along the nerve axis and lobulated. In reality, there is consider-

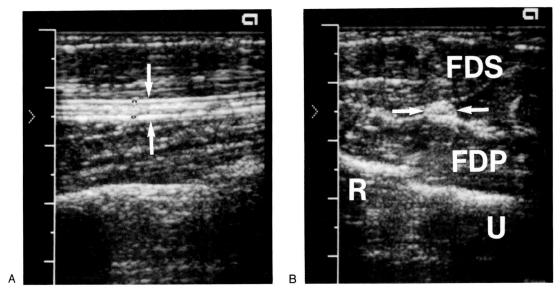

Fig. 1-82. Normal median nerve in the forearm. **(A)** Longitudinal scan showing the hyperechoic median nerve (arrows) with typical fascicular texture. **(B)** Transverse scan showing the rounded cross-section of the nerve (arrows). (*FDP,* flexor digitorum profundus muscle; *FDS,* flexor digitorum superficialis muscle; *R,* radius; *U,* ulna.)

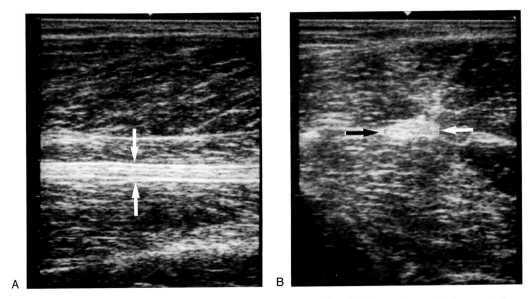

Fig. 1-83. Normal sciatic nerve in the posterior thigh. **(A)** Longitudinal scan shows the hyperechoic nerve (arrows). **(B)** Transverse scan showing the oval cross-section of the nerve (arrows).

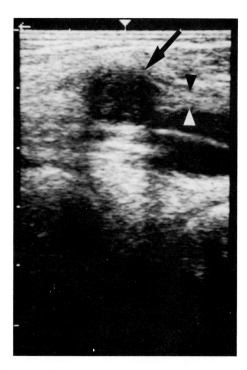

Fig. 1-84. Benign schwannoma of the tibial nerve. Longitudinal scan of the popliteal fossa showing a 1.3-cm pseudocystic mass (arrow) adjacent to the popliteal vessels. (arrowheads, normal nerve.)

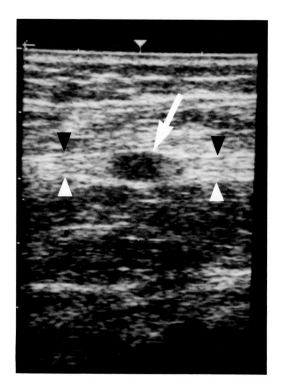

Fig. 1-86. Minute schwannoma of the sciatic nerve. Longitudinal scan of the buttock showing the echogenic nerve (arrowheads) with a small (9 × 5 mm) hypoechoic mass (arrow).

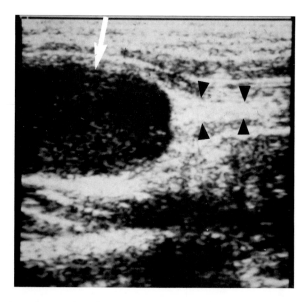

Fig. 1-85. Neurofibroma of the radial nerve. Longitudinal scan of the anterior aspect of the elbow showing an ovoid hypoechoic mass (arrow). Note the junction with the normal echogenic distal nerve (arrowheads).

able overlap between the ultrasound appearance of schwannomas and neurofibromas.

Malignant schwannoma (or neurofibrosarcoma) is the most frequent malignant nerve tumor, accounting for about 10 percent of all soft tissue sarcomas. The sciatic nerve and the brachial plexus are frequently involved. Sonographically, tumors are ill-defined and hypoechoic. Intratumoral necrosis or hemorrhage may result in a nonhomogeneous texture. As for other soft tissue sarcomas, sonography is expected to play a significant role in the early detection of local tumor recurrence following surgical excision.

High-frequency sonography is highly sensitive in the detection of nerve sheath tumors of the extremities (Fig. 1-86). Even though a given nerve is not distinctly visualized along its entire course, continuous scanning along its expected course allows detection of even minute hypoechoic nerve sheath tumors.

Ultrasound-guided needle biopsy of nerve sheath tumors has occasionally been attempted.[2] The insertion of the needle into the tumor, particularly in neurofibromas, may trigger a lightning pain, which forces interruption of the procedure but indirectly confirms the neural origin of the tumor.

Miscellaneous

The inflamed nerve in peripheral neuritis cases appears thickened and hypoechoic.[129] In leprosy, ultrasound visualization of markedly thickened nerves and abscess formation has been reported.[136] Although sonography can demonstrate a thickened, hypoechoic irritated median nerve in patients with carpal tunnel syndrome[2,57] (Fig. 1-55), MRI depicts the structure of the wrist more consistently and more clearly.

Traumatic neuromas develop after nerve injuries such as a cutting section and appear on sonograms as ill-defined, hypoechoic areas.[129] Morton's neuroma is discussed above in the section on the foot.

SUBCUTANEOUS TISSUES

Highly detailed images of the subcutaneous tissues are now available with the use of transducers with frequencies of 7.5 MHz or higher.

NORMAL ANATOMY

The subcutaneous tissues are composed mainly of subcutaneous fat, which is hypoechoic and shows linear echoes representing strands of connective tissue. Sonography has been used to measure the thickness of subcutaneous tissues in healthy individuals and in those with various pathologic conditions.[118,119,137-140] Subcutaneous veins can be seen if the pressure on the transducer is kept minimal to maintain their patency. Sonography has been used to guide venipuncture when venous access by palpation is difficult (e.g., for venography in patients with leg edema).[141]

ABNORMALITIES

Tumors

High-frequency sonography is highly sensitive in the visualization of subcutaneous tumors. Exceptions include poorly defined and isoechoic lipomas and angio-

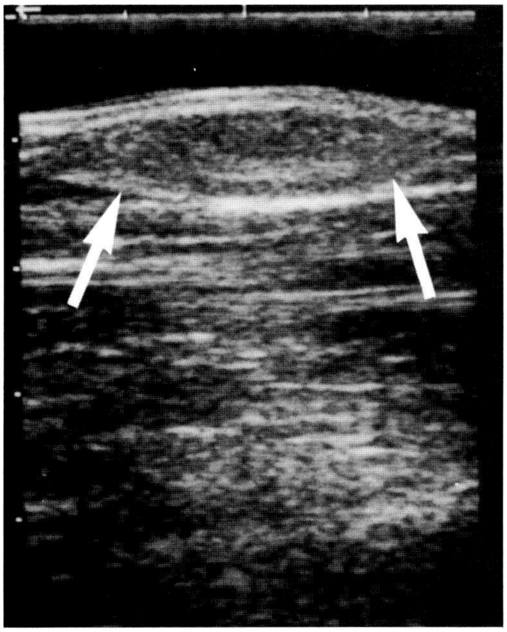

Fig. 1-87. Subcutaneous lipoma of the forearm. Longitudinal scan showing a lenticular, echogenic mass (arrows).

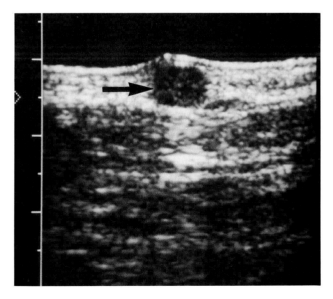

Fig. 1-88. Subcutaneous schwannoma. Sonogram showing a rounded, hypoechoic (8 × 6 mm) mass (arrow).

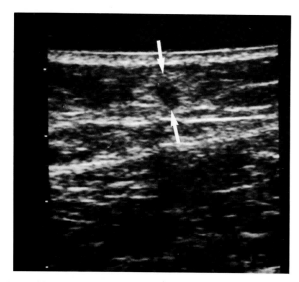

Fig. 1-89. Nonpalpable metastatic melanoma (5 × 3 mm) (arrows) in the subcutaneous fat. Note the irregularity of the margins and the greatest axis perpendicular to the general orientation of the tissue planes.

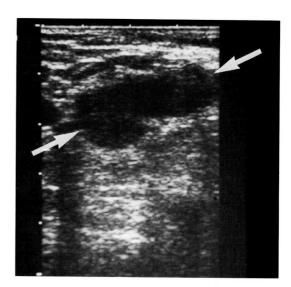

Fig. 1-91. Reactive benign hyperplastic axillary lymph node in a patient with breast carcinoma. Sonogram showing the diffusely enlarged, hypoechoic node (arrows).

mas, which may require palpation under real-time sonoscopy for identification. Lipomas often contain hyperechoic areas and are markedly elongated, with their greatest diameter being parallel to the skin[16] (Fig. 1-87). Hemangiomas are mostly hypoechoic and may contain hyperechoic phleboliths. Most other subcutane-

ous tumors are hypoechoic (Fig. 1-88), and a reliable diagnosis of their nature cannot be made from their ultrasound appearance alone.[142]

High-frequency sonography is a powerful tool for the detection of recurrent soft tissue sarcomas.[18] Sonography has also been used for follow-up after excision of a

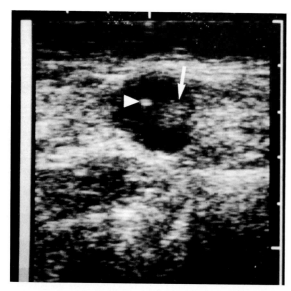

Fig. 1-90. Metastatic axillary lymph node in a patient with breast carcinoma. Sonogram showing the grossly rounded, enlarged node with irregular margins and an eccentric residual fatty hilus (arrow). (arrowhead, tip of needle during the fine-needle aspiration biopsy.)

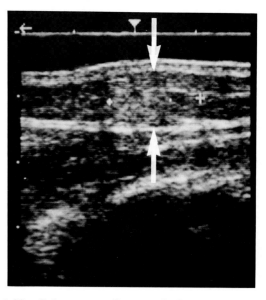

Fig. 1-92. Subcutaneous fat necrosis. Sonogram showing an ill-defined area of increased echogenicity (arrows) in the subcutaneous fat.

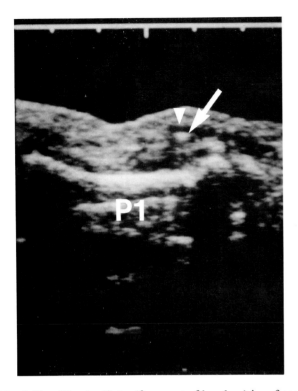

primary cutaneous malignant melanoma; for this application, the operator should screen wide areas around the scar and include the regional node-bearing areas. Nonpalpable recurrences or in-transit metastases as small as a few millimeters can be detected (Fig. 1-89). An advantage of real-time sonography over other cross-sectional imaging techniques is its dramatic accuracy in guiding fine-needle aspiration biopsy of tiny lesions, thus confirming early recurrence within minutes.[143] Other primary cancers, notably of the breast, lung, and colon, can also disseminate in the subcutaneous tissues.

Nonpalpable metastatic lymph nodes can be detected by sonography.[144,145] Nodes that are significantly enlarged, focally deformed, or rounded; that have sharp margins; or that show distal sound enhancement or a thinned, distorted, or absent echogenic hilus are more likely to harbor metastatic deposits[146-148] (Fig. 1-90). However, inflammatory (reactive) lymph nodes may also be significantly enlarged and markedly hypoechoic (Fig. 1-91). The internal texture may not be a reliable criterion for differentiating benign from malignant nodes.[148] In a patient with a history of cancer, fine-needle aspiration of an enlarged node may be needed to rule out a metastasis.[149] Increased vascularity, as demonstrated by color Doppler imaging, is found in both malignant and inflammatory lymphadenopathy (Plate 1-3), but the flow distribution within the node in relation to the internal configuration of the node may become a useful indicator as the resolution and sensitivity of color Doppler equipment increase.[150]

Fig. 1-93. Wood splinter (fragment of bamboo) in a finger. Sonogram of the volar aspect of the finger showing the echogenic foreign body (arrow) anterior to the flexor tendons. Note the subtle, hypoechoic surrounding inflammation (arrowhead). (*P1*, first phalanx.) (From Fornage,[2] with permission; © 1991 by BD Fornage.)

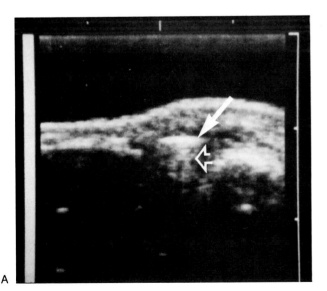

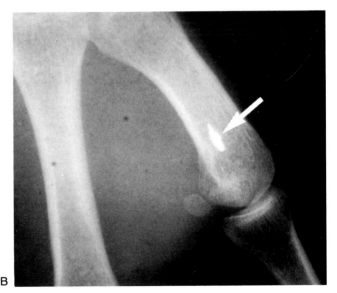

A   B

Fig. 1-94. Metallic foreign body in the thumb. **(A)** Sonogram showing the bright reflector (arrow) and the associated comet tail artifact (open arrow). **(B)** Radiograph showing the metal fragment (arrow). (From Fornage,[2] with permission; © 1991 by BD Fornage.)

Inflammation

Sonography can differentiate between an abscess and diffuse cellulitis.[151] Fat necrosis appears as a nonhomogeneous, focal or diffuse area of moderately increased echogenicity (Fig. 1-92). Panniculitis, which occurs in patients with systemic diseases such as scleroderma or lupus erythematosus and can also be induced by trauma, has a similar appearance.

Foreign Bodies

Retained foreign bodies, usually fragments of wood, glass, or metal from penetrating injuries of soft tissues, are most commonly seen in the distal extremities. The advantage of sonography over plain radiography is its capability to visualize low-density, radiotransparent bodies such as wood splinters[52,152–158] (Fig. 1-93). Foreign bodies appear as echogenic foci associated with acoustic shadowing and/or comet tail artifact, or neither, depending on their nature. The comet tail artifact is strongly suggestive of a metallic body[59] (Fig. 1-94). Inflammatory changes around the foreign body appear as an ill-defined hypoechoic area.[52,152] Although radiographic techniques (including CT) demonstrate the shape and size of radiopaque foreign bodies much better, sonography has the advantage of providing accurate preoperative (and, if needed, intraoperative) three-dimensional localization, thereby limiting the surgeon's incision and possible damage to the adjacent tissues.[157,159,160]

SKIN

Sonography of the skin is rarely performed by radiologists. However, this application of diagnostic sonography is gaining popularity among dermatologists.

TECHNIQUE

Although skin lesions of sufficient size can be evaluated with the 7.5- or 10-MHz transducers available in radiology departments, B-mode ultrasound evaluation of lesions confined to the skin is best performed by using commercially available dedicated scanners operating at 20 MHz, which provide an axial and lateral resolution of approximately 80 and 200 μm, respectively[2] (Fig. 1-95). Doppler imaging of skin lesions has been successfully performed using high-frequency (10-MHz), continuous-wave equipment[161]; larger lesions can be evaluated by duplex ultrasound or color Doppler, available on 7.5- or 10-MHz transducers.

NORMAL ANATOMY

At 7.5 or 10 MHz, the skin appears as a regular layer of tissue with medium echogenicity and variable thickness, depending on the region examined.[162] The epidermis and dermis cannot be differentiated, and skin appendages are not seen. At 20 MHz, the echogenic dermis is sharply contrasted from the hypoechoic subcutaneous fat, but the thin epidermal layer still cannot be distinguished from the dermis. Hair follicles are visible as obliquely oriented linear or rounded hypoechoic structures, depending on whether they are scanned longitudinally or transversely[135] (Fig. 1-96). Higher frequencies (up to 40 MHz) are needed to clearly identify the epidermis from the dermis.[163] In the sun-exposed skin of elderly patients, a hypoechoic band thought to result from an age-related deficit in collagen bundles is often noted in the superficial dermis. This hypoechoic band is also noted in the skin of neonates; in this case it is probably related to collagen network immaturity. Depending on the location, the thickness of normal adult skin as measured by sonography ranges from 1.4 to 4.8 mm; the skin is thicker in men than in women.[162]

ABNORMALITIES

Nodular Lesions

Epidermoid cysts appear on sonograms as well-circumscribed, anechoic or hypoechoic lesions. Not infrequently, the typical distal sound enhancement is lacking, possibly because of the lipidic or keratinic content.

Virtually all skin tumors are hypoechoic and are therefore well demarcated from the echogenic dermis. Crusts and ulcerations cast acoustic shadows, which preclude a satisfactory study. Common benign tumors of the skin include nevi (Fig. 1-97), seborrheic keratosis, dermatofibromas (Fig. 1-98), and hemangiomas.

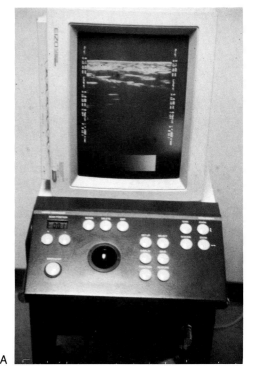
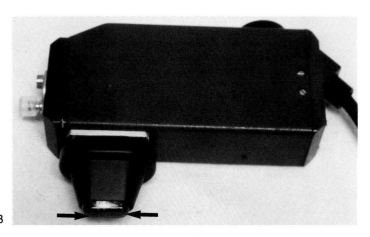

Fig. 1-95. Dedicated ultrasound scanner for the examination of the skin (Dermascan, Brymill, Vernon, CT). (A) View of the console. (B) View of the 20-MHz hand-held real-time transducer. Arrows point to the narrow footprint of the water bath.

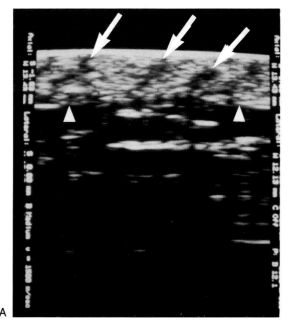
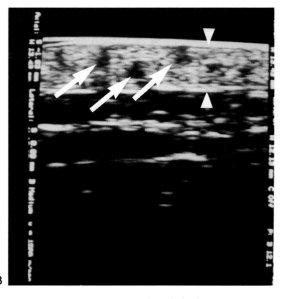

Fig. 1-96. Normal skin. (A) Scan performed at 20 MHz showing the oblique hypoechoic hair follicles (arrows). (arrowheads, deep margin of the dermis.) (B) The scan plane has been rotated 90 degrees. The cross-sections of the hair follicles appear as rounded hypoechoic structures (arrows). (arrowheads, skin.)

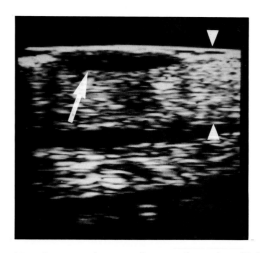

Fig. 1-97. Compound nevus. Scan performed at 20 MHz showing a well-defined, elongated, markedly hypoechoic lesion (arrow) located in the superficial dermis. (arrowheads, skin.)

At 20 MHz, these lesions are usually markedly hypoechoic and well defined, although hemangiomas and dermatofibromas may exhibit irregular margins.

Primary malignant melanomas are markedly hypoechoic, and deep-margin irregularity is noted with large tumors. Because of the overlap in the ultrasound appearance of benign and malignant skin tumors, sonography is not expected to contribute significantly to differentiating benign from malignant lesions, although Doppler studies have confirmed the increased vascularity of malignant skin tumors, particularly melanomas[161] (Fig. 1-99). Tumor thickness, which has a significant prognostic value in melanoma, can be directly measured on sonograms,[164] and software for three-dimensional visualization and volume measurement has recently become available. Of the other primary malignant skin tumors, including basal cell carcinoma, squamous cell carcinoma, and Kaposi sarcoma, none can be differentiated from melanoma on the basis of the ultrasound appearance alone.

Inflammation

Sonography is useful in the evaluation of various inflammatory conditions of the skin. In patients with skin edema, the thickness of the skin may exceed 1 cm. The skin becomes generally hypoechoic, and there is poor demarcation between the skin and subcutaneous tissues. Color Doppler examination can demonstrate increased vascularity.

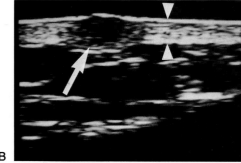

Fig. 1-98. Dermatofibroma. **(A)** Scan performed at 10 MHz barely identifying the lesion (arrow). **(B)** Scan performed at 20 MHz showing the lesion clearly (arrow). Note the irregular contours. (arrowheads, skin.)

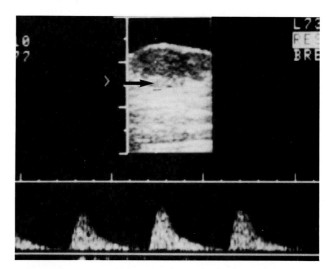

Fig. 1-99. Duplex sonography of a large malignant melanoma. The Doppler gate is placed at the deep surface of the tumor (arrow). Increased vascularity of the tumor is demonstrated.

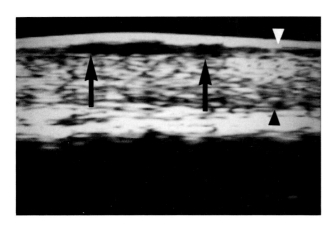

Fig. 1-100. Psoriasis. Sonogram of the skin at 20 MHz showing a characteristic superficial hypoechoic band (arrows), which represents acanthosis and lymphocytic infiltration into the papillary dermis. (arrowheads, skin.)

Skin thickness measurements by sonography have been used in the evaluation and follow-up of patients with scleroderma, a thickening and hardening of the skin, which occurs as a localized or systemic disease.[165,166] In patients with psoriasis, high-frequency sonography shows a characteristic superficial hypoechoic band representing a combination of acanthosis and lymphocytic infiltration into the papillary dermis (Fig. 1-100). In these patients, ultrasound is a potential tool with which to monitor objectively the effects of therapy.

Other possible future applications of skin sonography include monitoring of wound healing and testing of pharmaceutical agents and cosmetic products.

SUMMARY

In the United States, musculoskeletal sonography has remained in the shadow of MRI. However, the role of sonography should be reappraised, especially at a time when the health care system is being reviewed in the light of drastic attempts to contain costs. For the evaluation of soft tissues, sonography is valuable in confirming morphologic abnormalities, with a high negative predictive value; determining the cystic or solid nature of a mass; guiding percutaneous needle biopsy or drainage; localizing nonpalpable lesions pre- or intraoperatively; and monitoring lesions that are treated conservatively.

Limitations of musculoskeletal ultrasound include the reduced width of view of the scans, difficulties in reproducing scans on serial examinations, inability of clinicians to read sonograms, and inability to "see through" bones and to portray certain structures in areas of complex anatomy. Sonography cannot be used for staging malignant tumors or evaluating muscular dystrophies, which are indications for MRI or CT. However, in many situations involving soft tissues, sonography should be the first-line examination technique, with MRI being used only as a problem-solving tool.

REFERENCES

1. Fornage BD: Ultrasonography of Muscles and Tendons. Examination Technique and Atlas of Normal Anatomy of the Extremities. Springer-Verlag, New York, 1988
2. Fornage BD: Echographie des Membres. (Ultrasound of the Extremities.) Vigot, Paris, 1991
3. Fornage BD, Touche DH, Rifkin MD: Small parts real-time sonography: a new "water-path." J Ultrasound Med 1984;3:355
4. Hentz VR, Marich KW, Dev P: Preliminary study of the upper limb with the use of ultrasound transmission imaging. J Hand Surg 1984;9:188
5. Weiss L, Holyoke ED: Detection of tumors in soft tissues by ultrasonic holography. Surg Gynecol Obstet 1969;128:953
6. Fornage BD: Sports injuries: ultrasound imaging. In Golding SJ, Wilson DJ (eds): Imaging in Musculoskeletal Disease, Oxford University Press, Oxford, (in press)

7. Aspelin P, Pettersson H, Sigurjonsson S, Nilsson IM: Ultrasonographic examinations of muscle hematomas in hemophiliacs. Acta Radiol Diagn 1984;25:513
8. Giyanani VL, Grozinger KT, Gerlock AJ et al: Calf hematoma mimicking thrombophlebitis: sonographic and computed tomographic appearance. Radiology 1985;154:779
9. Auerbach DN, Bowen AD III: Sonography of leg in posterior compartment syndrome. AJR 1981;136:407
10. Kumari S, Fulco JD, Karayalcin G, Lipton R: Gray scale ultrasound: evaluation of iliopsoas hematomas in hemophiliacs. AJR 1979;133:103
11. Graif M, Martinovitz U, Strauss S et al: Sonographic localization of hematomas in hemophilic patients with positive iliopsoas sign. AJR 1987;148:121
12. Fornage BD, Touche DH, Segal P, Rifkin MD: Ultrasonography in the evaluation of muscular trauma. J Ultrasound Med 1983;2:549

13. Wicks JD, Silver TM, Bree RL: Gray scale features of hematomas: an ultrasonic spectrum. AJR 1978;131:977

14. Kramer FL, Kurtz AB, Rubin C, Goldberg BB: Ultrasound appearance of myositis ossificans. Skeletal Radiol 1979;4:19

15. Behan M, Kazam E: The echographic characteristics of fatty tissues and tumors. Radiology 1978;129:143

16. Fornage B, Tassin G: Sonographic appearances of superficial soft-tissue lipomas. J Clin Ultrasound 1991; 19:215

17. Derchi LE, Balconi G, De Flaviis L et al: Sonographic appearances of hemangiomas of skeletal muscle. J Ultrasound Med 1989;8:263

18. Choi H, Varma DGK, Fornage BD et al: Soft-tissue sarcoma: MR imaging vs sonography for detection of local recurrence after surgery. AJR 1991;157:353

19. Yousefzadeh DK, Schumann EM, Mulligan GM et al: The role of imaging modalities in diagnosis and management of pyomyositis. Skeletal Radiol 1982;8:285

20. Quillin SP, McAlister WH: Rapidly progressive pyomyositis. Diagnosis by repeat sonography. J Ultrasound Med 1991;10:181

21. Van Sonnenberg E, Wittich GR, Casola G et al: Sonography of thigh abscess: detection, diagnosis, and drainage. AJR 1987;149:769

22. Christensen RA, Van Sonnenberg E, Casola G, Wittich GR: Interventional ultrasound in the musculoskeletal system. Radiol Clin North Am 1988;26:145

23. Fornage BD, Nerot C: Sonographic diagnosis of rhabdomyolysis. J Clin Ultrasound 1986;14:389

24. Vukanovic S, Hauser H, Curati WL: Myonecrosis induced by drug overdose: pathogenesis, clinical aspects, and radiological manifestations. Eur J Radiol 1983;3:314

25. Kaplan GN: Ultrasonic appearance of rhabdomyolysis. AJR 1980;134:375

26. Lamminen AE, Hekali PE, Tiula E et al: Acute rhabdomyolysis: evaluation with magnetic resonance imaging compared with computed tomography and ultrasonography. Br J Radiol 1989;62:326

27. Fornage BD, Eftekhari F: Sonographic diagnosis of myositis ossificans. J Ultrasound Med 1989;8:463

28. Peck RJ, Metreweli C: Early myositis ossificans: a new echographic sign. Clin Radiol 1988;39:586

29. Fischer AQ, Carpenter DW, Hartlage PL et al: Muscle imaging in neuromuscular disease using computerized real-time sonography. Muscle Nerve 1988;2:270

30. Dock W, Happak W, Grabenwoger F et al: Neuromuscular diseases: evaluation with high-frequency sonography. Radiology 1990;177:825

31. Fornage BD, Rifkin MD: Ultrasound examination of tendons. Radiol Clin North Am 1988;26:87

32. Fornage BD: The hypoechoic normal tendon: a pitfall. J Ultrasound Med 1987;6:19

33. Fornage BD: The tendons. p. 627. In Rumack CM, Wilson SR, Charboneau JW (eds): Diagnostic Ultrasound. Vol. 1. Mosby-Year Book, St. Louis, 1991

34. Gooding GAW: Tenosynovitis of the wrist. A sonographic demonstration. J Ultrasound Med 1988;7:225

35. Jeffrey RB Jr, Laing FC, Schechter WP et al: Acute sup-purative tenosynovitis of the hand: diagnosis with US. Radiology 1987;162:741

36. Tiliakos N, Morales AR, Wilson CH Jr: Use of ultrasound in identifying tophaceous versus rheumatoid nodules (letter). Arthritis Rheum 1982;25:478

37. Farin PU, Jaroma H, Harju A, Soimalkallio S: Shoulder impingement syndrome: sonographic evaluation. Radiology 1990;176:845

38. Crass JR, Craig EV, Feinberg SB: The hyperextended internal rotation view in rotator cuff sonography. J Clin Ultrasound 1987;15:416

39. Middleton WD: Status of rotator cuff sonography. Radiology 1989;173:307

40. Crass JR, Craig EV, Thompson RC, Feinberg SB: Ultrasonography of the rotator cuff: surgical correlation. J Clin Ultrasound 1984;12:487

41. Middleton WD, Reinus WR, Totty WG et al: Ultrasonographic evaluation of the rotator cuff and biceps tendon. J Bone Jt Surg 1986;68-A:440

42. Brandt TD, Cardone BW, Grant TH et al: Rotator cuff sonography: a reassessment. Radiology 1989;173:323

43. Burk DL Jr, Karasick D, Kurtz AB et al: Rotator cuff tears: prospective comparison of MR imaging with arthrography, sonography, and surgery. AJR 1989;153:87

44. Miller CL, Karasick D, Kurtz AB, Fenlin JM: Limited sensitivity of ultrasound for detection of rotator cuff tears. Skeletal Radiol 1989;18:179

45. Crass JR, Craig EV, Feinberg SB: Sonography of the postoperative rotator cuff. AJR 1986;146:561

46. Mack LA, Nyberg DA, Matsen FA III et al: Sonography of the postoperative shoulder. AJR 1988;150:1089

47. Middleton WD, Reinus WR, Totty WG et al: US of the biceps tendon apparatus. Radiology 1985;157:211

48. Conrad MR, Nelms BA: Empty bicipital groove due to rupture and retraction of the biceps tendon. J Ultrasound Med 1990;9:231

49. Hammond I: Unsuspected humeral head fracture diagnosed by ultrasound (letter). J Ultrasound Med 1990;10:422

50. Patten RM, Mack LA, Wang KY, Lingel J: Nondisplaced fractures of the greater tuberosity of the humerus: sonographic detection. Radiology 1992;182:201

51. Barr LL, Babcock DS: Sonography of the normal elbow. AJR 1991;157:793

52. Fornage BD, Rifkin MD: Ultrasound examination of the hand and foot. Radiol Clin North Am 1988;26:109

53. Fornage BD, Schernberg FL, Rifkin MD: Ultrasound examination of the hand. Radiology 1985;55:785

54. De Flaviis L, Nessi R, Del Bo P et al: High-resolution ultrasonography of wrist ganglia. J Clin Ultrasound 1987;15:17

55. Fornage BD: Glomus tumors in the fingers: diagnosis with US. Radiology 1988;167:183

56. Fornage BD: Soft tissue changes in the hand in rheumatoid arthritis: evaluation with US. Radiology 1989; 173:735

57. Buchberger W, Schon G, Strasser K, Jungwirth W: High-resolution ultrasonography of the carpal tunnel. J Ultrasound Med 1991;10:531

58. Novick G, Ghelman B, Schneider M: Sonography of the neonatal and infant hip. AJR 1983;141:639
59. Graf R: Classification of hip joint dysplasia by means of sonography. Arch Orthop Traum Surg 1984;102:248
60. Harcke HT, Clarke NMP, Lee MS et al: Examination of the infant hip with real-time ultrasonography. J Ultrasound Med 1984;3:131
61. Clarke NMP, Harcke HT, McHugh P et al: Real-time ultrasound in the diagnosis of congenital dislocation and dysplasia of the hip. J Bone Jt Surg 1985;67-B:406
62. Boal DB, Schwentker DP: The infant hip: assessment with real-time ultrasound. Radiology 1985;157:667
63. Zieger M, Hilpert S, Schulz RD: Ultrasound of the infant hip. Part 1. Basic principles. Pediatr Radiol 1986;16:483
64. Clarke NMP, Clegg J, Al-Chalabi AN: Ultrasound screening of hips at risk for CDH. J Bone Jt Surg 1989;71-B:9
65. Tonnis D, Storch K, Ulbrich H: Results of newborn screening for CDH with and without sonography and correlation of risk factors. J Pediatr Orthop 1990;10:145
66. Wilson DJ, Green DJ, MacLarnon JC: Arthrosonography of the painful hip. Clin Radiol 1984;35:17
67. Adam R, Hendry GMA, Moss J et al: Arthrosonography of the irritable hip in childhood: a review of 1 year's experience. Br J Radiol 1986;59:205
68. Egund N, Wingstrand H, Forsberg L et al: Computed tomography and ultrasonography for diagnosis of hip joint effusion in children. Acta Orthop Scand 1986;57:211
69. Berman L, Catterall A, Meire H: Ultrasound of the hip: a review of the applications of a new technique. Br J Radiol 1986;59:13
70. Marchal GJ, Van Holsbeeck MT, Raes M: Transient synovitis of the hip in children: role of ultrasound. Radiology 1987;162:825
71. Harcke HT, Grissom LE, Finkelstein MS: Evaluation of the musculoskeletal system with sonography. AJR 1988;150:1253
72. Alexander JE, Seibert JJ, Glasier CM et al: High-resolution hip ultrasound in the limping child. J Clin Ultrasound 1989;17:19
73. Bickerstaff DR, Neal LM, Booth AJ et al: Ultrasound examination of the irritable hip. J Bone Jt Surg 1990;72-B:549
74. Harcke HT, Lee MS, Sinning L: Ossification center of the infant hip: sonographic and radiographic correlation. AJR 1986;147:317
75. Grissom LE, Harcke HT, Kumar SJ et al: Ultrasound evaluation of hip position in the Pavlik harness. J Ultrasound Med 1988;7:1
76. Moulton A, Upadhyay SS: A direct method of measuring femoral anteversion using ultrasound. J Bone Jt Surg 1982;64-B:469
77. Upadhyay SS, O'Neil T, Burwell RG et al: A new method using ultrasound for measuring femoral anteversion (torsion): technique and reliability. Br J Radiol 1987;60:519
78. Lausten GS, Jorgensen F, Boesen J: Measurement of anteversion of the femoral neck: ultrasound and computer-ised tomography compared. J Bone Jt Surg 1989;71-B:237
79. Komppa GH, Northern JR, Haas DK et al: Ultrasound guidance for needle aspiration of the hip in patients with painful hip prosthesis. J Clin Ultrasound 1985;13:433
80. Graif M, Strauss S, Heim M, Itzchak Y: Sonography of the hip joint as part of the evaluation of acute lower abdominal pain. J Clin Ultrasound 1988;16:99
81. Janus C, Hermann G: Enlargement of the iliopsoas bursa: unusual cause of cystic mass on pelvic sonogram. J Clin Ultrasound 1982;10:133
82. Fornage BD, Rifkin MD, Touche DH, Segal PM: Sonography of the patellar tendon: preliminary observations. AJR 1984;143:179
83. Mourad K, King J, Guggiana P: Computed tomography and ultrasound imaging of jumper's knee. Patellar tendinitis. Clin Radiol 1988;39:162
84. Fornage B, Touche D, Deshayes JL, Segal P: Diagnostic des calcifications du tendon rotulien. Comparaison écho-radiographique. J Radiol 1984;65:355
85. McDonald DG, Leopold GR: Ultrasound B-scanning in the differentiation of Baker's cyst and thrombophlebitis. Br J Radiol 1972;45:729
86. Moore CP, Sarti DA, Louie JS: Ultrasonographic demonstration of popliteal cysts in rheumatoid arthritis. A noninvasive technique. Arthritis Rheum 1975;18:577
87. Gompels BM, Darlington LG: Evaluation of popliteal cysts and painful calves with ultrasonography: comparison with arthrography. Ann Rheum Dis 1982;41:355
88. Moss GD, Dishuk W: Ultrasound diagnosis of osteochondromatosis of the popliteal fossa. J Clin Ultrasound 1984;12:232
89. Silver TM, Washburn RL, Stanley JC, Gross WS: Gray scale ultrasound evaluation of popliteal artery aneurysms. AJR 1977;129:1003
90. Pathria MN, Zlatkin M, Sartoris DJ et al: Ultrasonography of the popliteal fossa and lower extremities. Radiol Clin North Am 1988;26:77
91. Richardson ML, Selby B, Montana MA, Mack LA: Ultrasonography of the knee. Radiol Clin North Am 1988;26:63
92. Kaufman RA, Towbin RB, Babcock DS, Crawford AH: Arthrosonography in the diagnosis of pigmented villonodular synovitis. AJR 1982;139:396
93. Cooperberg PL, Tsang I, Truelove L, Knickerbocker WJ: Gray scale ultrasound in the evaluation of rheumatoid arthritis of the knee. Radiology 1978;126:759
94. Derks WHJ, De Hooge P, Van Linge B: Ultrasonographic detection of the patellar plica in the knee. J Clin Ultrasound 1986;14:355
95. De Flaviis L, Nessi R, Scaglione P et al: Ultrasonic diagnosis of Osgood-Schlatter and Sinding-Larsen-Johansson diseases of the knee. Skeletal Radiol 1989;18:193
96. Dragonat P, Claussen C: Sonographische Meniskusdarstellungen. ROFO 1980;133:185
97. Selby B, Richardson ML, Montana MA et al: High resolution sonography of the menisci of the knee. Invest Radiol 1986;21:332

98. Selby B, Richardson ML, Nelson BD et al: Sonography in the detection of meniscal injuries of the knee: evaluation in cadavers. AJR 1987;149:549

99. Sohn C, Gerngross H, Bähren W, Danz B: Meniskussonographie. Alternative zur invasiven Meniskusdiagnostik? Dtsch Med Wochenschr 1987;112:581

100. Peetrons P, Allaer D, Jeanmart L: Cysts of the semilunar cartilages of the knee: a new approach by ultrasound imaging. A study of six cases and review of the literature. J Ultrasound Med 1990;9:333

101. Aisen AM, McCune WJ, MacGuire A et al: Sonographic evaluation of the cartilage of the knee. Radiology 1984;153:781

102. McCune WJ, Dedrick DK, Aisen AM, MacGuire A: Sonographic evaluation of osteoarthritic femoral condylar cartilage. Correlation with operative findings. Clin Orthop 1990;254:230

103. De Flaviis L, Nessi R, Leonardi M, Ulivi M: Dynamic ultrasonography of capsulo-ligamentous knee joint traumas. J Clin Ultrasound 1988;16:487

104. Fornage BD: Achilles tendon: US examination. Radiology 1986;159:759

105. Blei CL, Nirschl RP, Grant EG: Achilles tendon: US diagnosis of pathologic conditions. Radiology 1986;159:765

106. Mathieson JR, Connell DG, Cooperberg PL, Lloyd-Smith DR: Sonography of the Achilles tendon and adjacent bursae. AJR 1988;151:127

107. Kainberger FM, Engel A, Barton P et al: Injury of the Achilles tendon: diagnosis with sonography. AJR 1990;155:1031

108. Leekam RN, Salsberg BB, Bogoch E, Shankar L: Sonographic diagnosis of partial Achilles tendon rupture and healing. J Ultrasound Med 1986;5:115

109. Gerster JC, Anderegg A: Ultrasound imaging of Achilles tendon (letter). J Rheumatol 1988;15:382

110. Steinmetz A, Schmitt W, Schuler P et al: Ultrasonography of Achilles tendons in primary hypercholesterolemia. Comparison with computed tomography. Atherosclerosis 1988;74:231

111. Yuzawa K, Yamakawa K, Tohno E et al: An ultrasonographic method for detection of Achilles tendon xanthomas in familial hypercholesterolemia. Atherosclerosis 1989;75:211

112. Maffulli N, Dymond NP, Regine R: Surgical repair of ruptured Achilles tendon in sportsmen and sedentary patients: a longitudinal ultrasound assessment. Int J Sports Med 1990;11:78

113. Downey DJ, Simkin PA, Mack LA et al: Tibialis posterior tendon rupture: a cause of rheumatoid flat foot. Arthritis Rheum 1988;31:441

114. Stephenson CA, Seibert JJ, McAndrew MP et al: Sonographic diagnosis of tenosynovitis of the posterior tibial tendon. J Clin Ultrasound 1990;18:114

115. Redd RA, Peters VJ, Emery SF et al: Morton neuroma: sonographic evaluation. Radiology 1989;171:415

116. Reed M, Gooding GAW, Kerley SM et al: Sonography of plantar fibromatosis. J Clin Ultrasound 1991;19:578

117. Gibbon WW: Plantar fasciitis: US imaging (letter). Radiology 1992;182:285

118. Gooding GAW, Stess RM, Graf PM, Grunfeld C: Heel pad thickness: determination by high-resolution ultrasonography. J Ultrasound Med 1985;4:173

119. Gooding GAW, Stess LM, Graf PM et al: Sonography of the sole of the foot. Evidence for loss of foot pad thickness in diabetes and its relationship to ulceration of the foot. Invest Radiol 1986;21:45

120. Graif M, Stahl-Kent V, Ben-Ami T et al: Sonographic detection of occult bone fractures. Pediatr Radiol 1988;18:383

121. Broker FHL, Burbach T: Ultrasonic diagnosis of separation of the proximal humeral epiphysis in the newborn. J Bone Jt Surg 1990;72-A:187

122. Mahaisavariya B, Suibnugarn C, Mairiang E et al: Ultrasound for closed femoral nailing. J Clin Ultrasound 1991;19:393

123. Young JWR, Kostrubiak IS, Resnik CS, Paley D: Sonographic evaluation of bone production at the distraction site in Ilizarov limb-lengthening procedures. AJR 1990;154:125

124. Abiri MM, Kirpekar M, Ablow RC: Osteomyelitis: detection with US. Radiology 1988;169:795

125. Kratochwil A, Zweymüller K: Ultrasonic examination in orthopedic surgery. p. 343. In Kazner E, de Vlieger M, Muller HR, McCready VR (eds): Ultrasonics in Medicine. Excerpta Medica, Amsterdam, 1975

126. Mukuno DH, Lee TG, Watanabe AS, McIff EB: Aneurysmal bone cyst presenting as a pelvic mass on sonographic examination. J Ultrasound Med 1986;5:215

127. Fornage BD, Richli WR, Chuapetcharasopon C: Calcaneal bone cyst: sonographic findings and ultrasound-guided aspiration biopsy. J Clin Ultrasound 1991;19:360

128. Longo JM, Rodriguez-Cabello J, Bilbao JI et al: Popliteal vein thrombosis and popliteal artery compression complicating fibular osteochondroma: ultrasound diagnosis. J Clin Ultrasound 1990;18:507

129. Fornage BD: Peripheral nerves of the extremities: imaging with US. Radiology 1988;167:179

130. Chinn DH, Filly RA, Callen PW: Unusual ultrasonographic appearance of a solid schwannoma. J Clin Ultrasound 1982;10:243

131. Reuter KL, Raptopoulos V, DeGirolami U, Akins CM: Ultrasonography of a plexiform neurofibroma of the popliteal fossa. J Ultrasound Med 1982;1:209

132. Hoddick WK, Callen PW, Filly RA et al: Ultrasound evaluation of benign sciatic nerve sheath tumor. J Ultrasound Med 1984;3:505

133. Hughes DG, Wilson DJ: Ultrasound appearances of peripheral nerve tumors. Br J Radiol 1986;59:1041

134. Cantos-Melian B, Arriaza-Loureda R, Aisa-Varela P: Tibialis posterior nerve schwannoma mimicking Achilles tendinitis: ultrasonographic diagnosis. J Clin Ultrasound 1990;18:671

135. Fornage BD: Current status of musculoskeletal sonography. Appl Radiol 1991;20:29

136. Fornage BD, Nerot C: Sonographic diagnosis of tuberculoid leprosy. J Ultrasound Med 1987;6:105

137. Heckmatt JZ, Pier N, Dubowitz V: Measurement of quadriceps muscle thickness and subcutaneous tissue thickness in normal children by real-time ultrasound imaging. J Clin Ultrasound 1988;16:171

138. Koskelo EK, Kivisaari LM, Saarinen UM, Siimes MA: Quantitation of muscles and fat by ultrasonography: a useful method in the assessment of malnutrition in children. Acta Paediatr Scand 1991;80:682

139. Vincent LM: Ultrasound of soft tissue abnormalities of the extremities. Radiol Clin North Am 1988;26:131

140. van Holsbeeck M, Introcaso JH (eds): Sonography of the dermis, hypodermis, periosteum, and bone. p. 207. In Musculoskeletal Ultrasound. Mosby-Year Book, St. Louis, 1991

141. Johns CM, Sumkin JH: US-guided venipuncture for venography in the edematous leg. Radiology 1991;180:573

142. Nessi R, Betti R, Bencini PL et al: Ultrasonography of nodular and infiltrative lesions of the skin and subcutaneous tissues. J Clin Ultrasound 1990;18:103

143. Fornage BD, Lorigan J: Sonographic detection and fine-needle aspiration biopsy of nonpalpable recurrent or metastatic melanoma in subcutaneous tissues. J Ultrasound Med 1989;8:421

144. Bruneton JN, Normand F, Balu-Maestro C et al: Lymphomatous superficial lymph nodes: US detection. Radiology 1987;165:233

145. Pamilo M, Soiva M, Lavast E: Real-time ultrasound, axillary mammography, and clinical examination in the detection of axillary lymph node metastases in breast cancer patients. J Ultrasound Med 1989;8:115

146. Sakai F, Kiyono K, Sone S et al: Ultrasonic evaluation of cervical metastatic lymphadenopathy. J Ultrasound Med 1988;7:305

147. Tohnosu N, Onoda S, Isono K: Ultrasonographic evaluation of cervical lymph node metastases in esophageal cancer with special reference to the relationship between the short to long axis ratio (S/L) and the cancer content. J Clin Ultrasound 1989;17:101

148. Shozushima M, Suzuki M, Nakasima T et al: Ultrasound diagnosis of lymph node metastasis in head and neck cancer. Dentomaxillofacial Radiol 1990;19:165

149. Van den Brekel MWM, Castelijns JA, Stel HV et al: Occult metastatic neck disease: detection with US and US-guided fine-needle aspiration cytology. Radiology 1991;180:457

150. Mitchell DG, Merton DA, Liu J-B, Goldberg BB: Superficial masses with color Doppler imaging. J Clin Ultrasound 1991;19:555

151. Sandler MA, Alpern MB, Madrazo BL, Gitschlag KF: Inflammatory lesions of the groin: ultrasonic evaluation. Radiology 1984;151:747

152. Fornage BD, Schernberg FL: Sonographic diagnosis of foreign bodies of the distal extremities. AJR 1986;147:567

153. Little CM, Parker MG, Callowich MC, Sartori JC: The ultrasonic detection of soft tissue foreign bodies. Invest Radiol 1986;21:275

154. Gooding GAW, Hardiman T, Sumers M et al: Sonography of the hand and foot in foreign body detection. J Ultrasound Med 1987;6:441

155. Torfing KF, Teisen HG, Skjodt T: Computed tomography, ultrasonography and plain radiography in the detection of foreign bodies in pork muscle tissue. ROFO 1988;149:60

156. Wilson DJ: Ultrasonic imaging of soft tissues. Clin Radiol 1989;40:341

157. Banerjee B, Das RK: Sonographic detection of foreign bodies of the extremities. Br J Radiol 1991;64:107

158. Kaplan PA, Matamoros A Jr, Anderson JC: Sonography of the musculoskeletal system. AJR 1990;155:237

159. Fornage BD: Preoperative sonographic localization of a migrated transosseous stabilizing wire in the hand. J Ultrasound Med 1987;6:471

160. Fornage BD, Schernberg FL: Sonographic preoperative localization of a foreign body in the hand. J Ultrasound Med 1987;6:217

161. Srivastava A, Hughes BR, Hughes LE, Woodcock JP: Doppler ultrasound as an adjunct to the differential diagnosis of pigmented skin lesions. Br J Surg 1986;73:790

162. Fornage BD, Deshayes JL: Ultrasound of the normal skin. J Clin Ultrasound 1986;14:619

163. Murakami S, Miki Y: Human skin histology using high-resolution echography. J Clin Ultrasound 1989;17:77

164. Shafir R, Itzchak Y, Heyman Z et al: Preoperative ultrasonic measurements of the thickness of cutaneous malignant melanoma. J Ultrasound Med 1984;3:205

165. Cole GW, Handler SJ, Burnett K: The ultrasonic evaluation of skin thickness in scleredema. J Clin Ultrasound 1981;9:501

166. Myers SL, Cohen JS, Sheets PW, Bies JR: B-Mode ultrasound evaluation of skin thickness in progressive systemic sclerosis. J Rheumatol 1986;13:577

2

Breast

Etta D. Pisano

Ultrasound is an important tool in the evaluation of breast abnormalities, both for diagnostic imaging and for intervention. This chapter details how and in what clinical context breast ultrasound should be performed. In addition, the ultrasonic appearance of normal breast anatomy and pathologic lesions are described. Finally, instruction on how to perform intraventional procedures using breast ultrasound is provided.

TECHNIQUE

Instrumentation

There are two types of ultrasound units currently being used for breast imaging: high-frequency auto-mated whole breast scanners and high-frequency hand-held units with an offset pad or built-in fluid offset. A recent survey of 319 radiologists showed that of those doing breast ultrasound, 93 percent used handheld units.[1] Both types of units are equally good at identifying cystic and solid masses in the breast.[2] Each type of unit has its advantages. Automated units produce tomographic images of the entire breast, and a technologist alone can perform the examination for later review by a radiologist. These units also allow for more exact localization of lesions, which is especially useful when multiple abnormalities exist in the same breast. In addition, automated units are designed to allow the sonographer to adjust the focal zone independently for each breast.[3,4] However, handheld units are generally cheaper, take up

less space, and do not require a trained technologist for operation. The examination time is considerably shorter than for automatic units.[5] In addition, handheld instrument allow the operator to have a better appreciation of inhomogeneities and discontinuities in breast echotexture and the presence of tissue fixation.[6]

The optimal transducer for breast imaging allows visualization of fine detail while providing adequate depth of penetration for the lesion being evaluated. Generally, 7.5-MHz transducers are necessary to allow a high enough resolution to distinguish between small masses and surrounding breast parenchyma and fat.[3,7] Depth of focus should be 3 cm or less.[8] For lesions that lie deep within the breast, a lower frequency transducer might be necessary. In one series of 89 patients, the depth of penetration of higher frequency transducers was thought to limit the examination in only 16 percent of the cases examined, which was considered a mild limitation only.[3] The patient can be positioned so that the area of interest lies close enough to the transducer to allow usage of the higher resolution (high-frequency) transducers. New transducers that allow the operator to vary either the central frequency output of the transducer, or the band path of the receiver improve image contrast. They may also improve detection of breast masses and allow depiction of greater internal architectural detail[9] (Fig. 2-1).

Ultrasound Technique

Breast ultrasound is quite technically dependent. Many artifacts can interfere with the depiction of the true cystic or solid nature of breast masses.

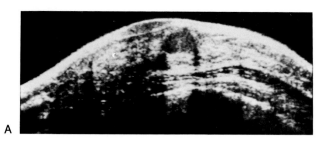

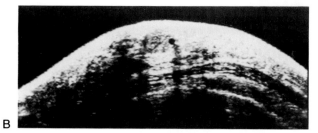

Fig. 2-1. Tunable transducer. These transverse sonograms of a breast mass of a 45-year-old woman reveal the potential usefulness of a tunable transducer. **(A)** Obtained using a 7.5-MHz transducer, pulsed to yield a center frequency of 8.0 MHz, with a standard receiver. **(B)** Obtained using a 10-MHz transducer, pulsed to yield a center frequency of 11 MHz, with the tunable receiver set for a narrow band-pass. A small cyst on the margin of the lesion becomes visible with the tunable transducer. Biopsy revealed a fibroadenoma. (From Kelly-Fry et al,[9] with permission.)

When a handheld unit is used, the patient is first examined in the supine position with the ipsilateral arm under the head and the contralateral arm down by the patient's side.[10] For the inner quadrants, the patient lies flat (Fig. 2-2), and for the outer quadrants, the patient lies in the contralateral oblique position (Fig. 2-3). This can be facilitated by placing a wedge beneath the patient. If the area of interest is not adequately visualized with these positions, the patient is rolled until the area lies within the transducer's focal zone. This may even require upright positioning (Fig. 2-4). The examination is adequate if the underlying pectoral muscles and ribs are visualized.[3,10]

The area of interest in the breast is surveyed with slow sweeping motions in both the transverse and longitudinal planes. Planes must overlap to allow small lesions to be visualized.[6] Pressure must be light and even and good skin contact must be maintained. To examine deeper areas of the breast, greater compression may be used.[6] For phased array and linear transducers, an offset pad should be used to avoid near field reverberation artifacts.[8] Some higher frequency transducers have built-in fluid offsets. A directed examination of specific abnormality takes an average of 5 to 15 minutes.[11-13] For a survey of the whole breast, examination with a handheld unit takes approximately 30 minutes.[5]

For most automated examinations, the patient lies prone with her breasts suspended, one at a time, in a water tank (Figs. 2-5 to 2-7). Transverse whole breast images are first obtained at 2-mm intervals to allow small lesions to be detected.[5,14] Section thickness at the transducer focus increases as the transducer frequency decreases. Areas with equivocal findings or mammogra-

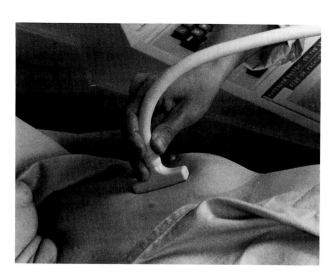

Fig. 2-2. Supine scanning technique. If the lesion lies within 1 to 2 cm of the skin surface, a fluid offset should be utilized.

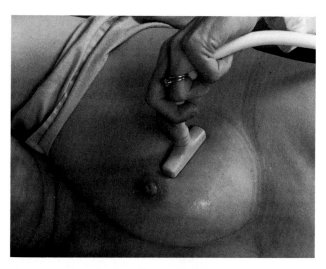

Fig. 2-3. Technique for lateral lesions. Note that the patient is in the opposite decubitus position with her arm resting on her head and neck. If the lesion lies within 1 to 2 cm of the skin surface, a fluid offset should be utilized.

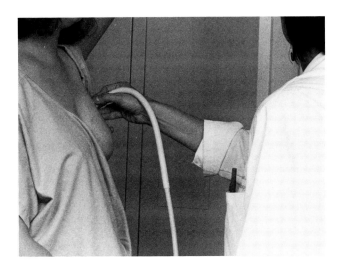

Fig. 2-4. Upright position scanning technique. If a lesion cannot be visualized using the supine or decubitus positions, scanning with the patient in the upright position might be useful.

phic or palpable abnormalities are rescanned at 1 mm intervals in the region of interest with compression applied. A complete examination takes 30 to 40 minutes.[5] This test has been well accepted by patients and referring physicians.[15] Currently the only commercially available automatic breast scanner is the Labsonics dedicated water-path breast unit (Labsonics, Inc., Mooresville, In-

diana),[16] which allows for supine scanning of a limited selected area of the breast. It uses a water bag that not only couples the sound and applies pressure to the breast, but also allows for delicate control of the angle of incidence of the sound beam, which allows the operator to minimize refraction and beam defocusing[3] (Fig. 2-8).

As described by Bassett and Kimme-Smith,[8] there are many artifacts that can interfere with proper breast ultrasonography. Breast tissue is heterogeneous owing to multiple impedance mismatches at tissue interfaces, which causes extensive defraction and beam defocusing.[4] As mentioned previously, a standoff pad or built-in fluid offset must be used to best visualize the near field. If this is not done, artifactual filling in of cysts with low-level echoes will occur (Fig. 2-9). Optimal visualization of the far field is also difficult owing to the divergence of the beam. This causes impaired lateral resolution, which blurs the margins of large masses, fills in shadows behind small masses, and impairs visualization of small masses.[8] This can be solved by repositioning the patient and scanning from a different surface, or by applying greater compression at the same surface.[7] The power and time-gain-compensation (TGC) curve must be appropriately set so that detailed evaluation of masses is possible. The power, or voltage applied to the transducer, should be set as low as possible to allow for penetration of the breast all the way to the chest wall without losing anatomic detail. If the power is too great, the image will be excessively bright without the gray levels necessary to see detail[8]

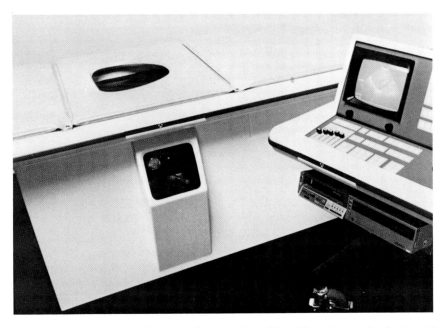

Fig. 2-5. Ausonics system I water path breast ultrasound machine. Note the opening in the table. The patient lies prone with one breast suspended through this hole into a water bath. (Courtesy of Ausonics Corporation.)

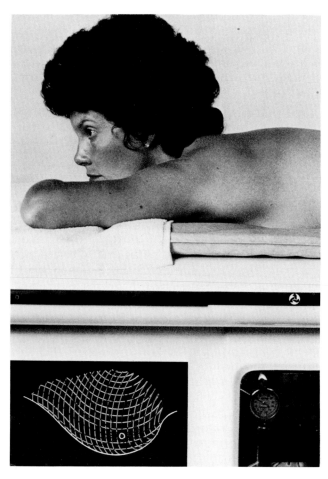

Fig. 2-6.   Correct patient position for Ausonics water path breast ultrasound. (Courtesy of Ausonics Corporation.)

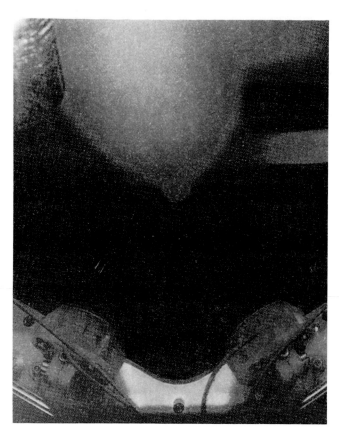

Fig. 2-7.   Breast position for Ausonics water path breast ultrasound. The patient's breast is suspended within the water bath for whole breast ultrasound using the Ausonics system I unit. This unit has four 4.5-MHz transducers (located on the lower corners of the photograph). (Courtesy of Ausonics Corporation.)

(Figs. 2-10 and 2-11). The TGC curve must be adjusted for each patient depending on breast density and size. Denser breasts generally require steeper curves since they attenuate more of the beam than do fatty breasts. The curve must not be too steep, however, or detailed anatomy will not be visualized in the deeper portions of the breast.[8]

NORMAL ANATOMY

The breast is composed of parenchyma and supporting structures. The parenchyma consists of the functioning elements, namely the milk-secreting acini and ducts; the supporting structures consist of fat and connective tissue. In a premenopausal, nonpregnant, nonlactating patient, each breast contains 15 to 25 lobes. Each lobe is drained by a separate lactiferous duct that dilates into a lactiferous sinus just deep to the nipple. Each lobule contains the milk-producing acini and secretory ducts,

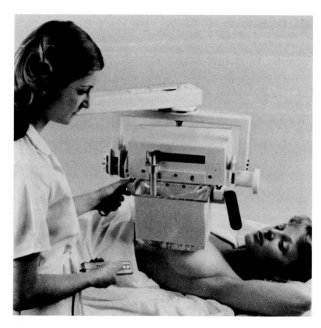

Fig. 2-8.   Labsonics unit. The Labsonics dedicated water path breast unit. (Courtesy of Labsonics, Inc., Morresville, IN.)

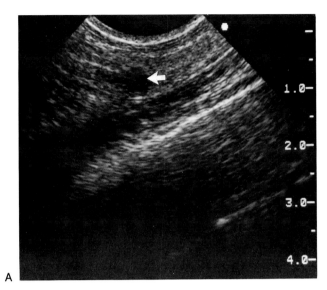
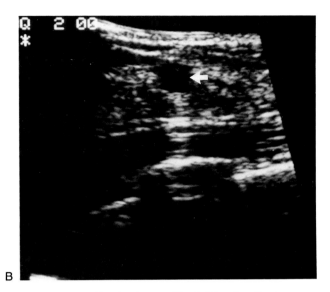

Fig. 2-9. Importance of using a fluid offset for near field lesion. **(A)** No offset has been utilized. The visualized hypoechoic mass (arrow) is somewhat ill defined and contains some internal echoes. Only minimal enhanced through transmission is seen. **(B)** With the fluid offset, the same mass (arrow) is now obviously a simple cyst. (Courtesy of Lawrence W. Bassett, M.D., UCLA School of Medicine.)

which are poorly developed in nonpregnant, nonlactating women.[17]

Four distinct areas of variable thickness may be seen on the well-performed sonogram of the breast: the skin and nipple, subcutaneous layer, mammary layer, and the retromammary layer[8] (Fig. 2-12). The skin is seen as a brightly echogenic line that is 0.5 to 2 mm thick. If high resolution equipment is used, it can be seen as two distinct lines with a hypoechoic central region. The nipple and surrounding areola cause extensive shadowing owing to their connective tissue composition[8] (Figs. 2-13 to 2-15). Subareolar ducts can often be visualized[8] (Fig. 2-16).

The next most superficial layer, the subcutaneous tissue, is composed of fat and connective tissue. The fat is divided into distinct groups of fat cells by connective tissue septa or Cooper's ligaments. These distinct structures are called fat lobules. The fat has relatively low acoustic impedance compared with the surrounding Cooper's ligament. Thus, one sees hypoechoic areas surrounded by brighter echoes,[17] which creates multiple pseudomasses. By examining these structures in two planes, they usually can be seen to be elongated on one image[8] (Fig. 2-17).

The next layer down from the transducer is the mammary layer, which contains parenchymal elements plus some fat and connective tissue. This layer is quite variable from patient to patient and is partially dependent on the woman's age and hormonal status.[18] For women with a lot of breast parenchyma (dense breasts by mammography), this region can appear very echogenic (Fig.

2-18). For women with atrophic parenchyma (completely fatty breasts on mammography), this area cannot be distinguished as a separate region. It appears continuous with subcutaneous and retromammary fat and contains hypoechoic areas interrupted by brightly echogenic connective tissue septa (Fig. 2-19). For women with intermediate amounts of breast parenchyma (mixed density breasts on mammography), the two patterns are mixed on the sonogram with brightly echogenic parenchyma mixed with hypoechoic fat lobules separated by echogenic connective tissue septa (Fig. 2-20).

The deepest layer on a breast sonogram is the retromammary layer, which consists of fat and connective tissue arranged in the same pattern as they are in the subcutaneous layer.[17] This layer is usually thinner than the subcutaneous layer and contains smaller fat lobules.[8] The ribs and pectoral muscle are visible deep to this layer.[19]

Pregnancy causes the proliferation of the parenchymal elements within the breast, which causes an enlargement and increase in echogenicity of the mammary layer with a concomitant reduction in size of the subcutaneous and retromammary layers[17] (Fig. 2-21).

INDICATIONS FOR BREAST SONOGRAPHY

Since it was first described by Wild and Neal in 1952,[20] breast ultrasound has been utilized in a variety of circumstances. This topic has been the subject of consider-

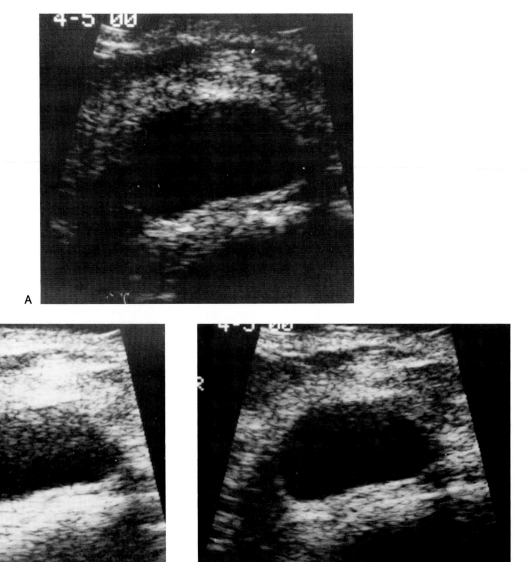

Fig. 2-10. Importance of appropriate power and scale setting. **(A)** Simple cyst at low power with a linear scale. **(B)** Same cyst at high power with a linear scale. **(C)** Same cyst at high power with a logarithmic scale. The appearance varies markedly depending on the settings selected. (Courtesy of Lawrence W. Bassett, M.D., UCLA School of Medicine.)

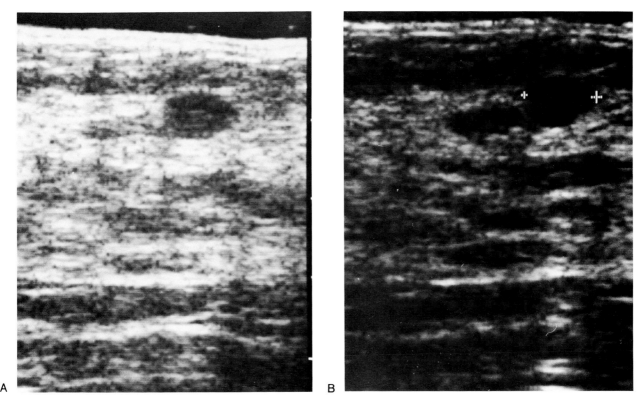

Fig. 2-11. Importance of appropriate power (gain). **(A)** Cyst with the gain adjusted inappropriately high. It contains internal echoes. Enhanced through transmission is not evident. **(B)** Same cyst (calipers) with the gain set appropriately. All of the features of a cyst are now apparent.

able controversy over the last 40 years. With the publication in the mid-1970s of a well-publicized article criticizing screening mammography because of its carcinogenic potential,[21] tremendous attention was placed on sonography as a screening modality for breast cancer. Early articles suggested that the ultrasonographic appearance of cancer was distinct from that of benign lesions. Unfortunately, this has not been confirmed by later work. As discussed below in detail, there is a great deal of overlap between the appearance of benign and malignant masses.[13,24-26] Furthermore, to be useful for screening, a modality should be reasonably sensitive. Unfortunately, with present technology, ultrasound cannot reliably detect mammographically apparent microcalcifications, which are frequently the only indicator of an intraductal cancer. In one series, only 6 percent of such lesions were detected.[27] Furthermore, there are only few anecdotal reports of ultrasound detection of mammographically occult nonpalpable cancers.[10,14,15,28] Kopans et al[29] reported no evidence for malignancy at 3 to 4 years follow-up on 255 positive ultrasound examinations with negative physical examination and mammography. Sickles et al[27] compared sonography with

high-quality mammography and found that mammography detected more cancers than ultrasound (97 versus 58 percent) and was better than ultrasound at detecting nonpalpable (96 versus 30 percent) and node-negative cancers (95 versus 48 percent). Similar results have been reported by others.[15,30] Given these facts, the consensus among experts is that ultrasound should not be used for screening for breast cancer.[2,5,11-13, 16,18,29,31-33] Some experts have advocated ultrasound screening only for asymptomatic patients with dense breasts on mammography.[14,15,34] This is not supported by a review of 796 examinations performed for this purpose in which only one malignancy was found.[35]

The major use of ultrasound is in determining whether a mass is cystic or solid once it is detected by mammography and/or physical examination.[2,5,6,13-16,32,36,37] In fact, if strict criteria to divide cystic and solid lesions are observed (see below), the accuracy of ultrasound approaches 100 percent.[13,15,37] Sonography can thus spare a large number of women unnecessary biopsies[37] since cysts represent approximately 25 percent of palpable and mammographically apparent masses.[13,27] There is a simple test for confirming that an abnormality detected on

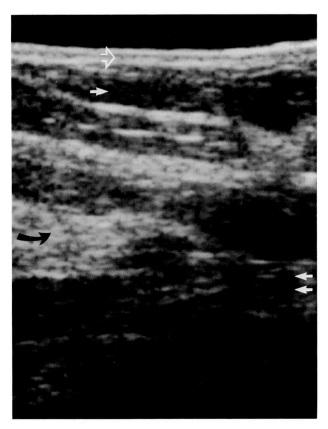

Fig. 2-12. Normal breast anatomy. The skin is visible most superficially as a double echogenic line (open arrow). The next most superficial layer is the subcutaneous fat. Unlike fat elsewhere in the body, fat in the breast is hypoechoic (arrow). The next layer is the breast glandular tissue, which appears echogenic (curved arrow). The deepest layer is the retromammary fat, which is also hypoechoic (double arrows). These layers vary in thickness depending on the composition of the individual patient's breasts (see Figs. 2-18 to 2-20). Note the use of the fluid offset in order to visualize the superficial layers optimally.

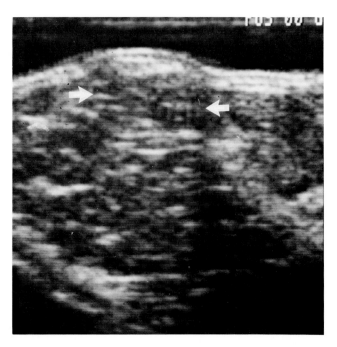

Fig. 2-13. Normal nipple and areola. Note the shadowing occurring at the edges of the areola (arrows), which is a normal finding and should not be confused with pathology. Obviously if a lesion lies deep to this region, one must angle around the areolar shadowing to get an adequate image of it. Again note the use of the fluid offset in order to best visualize the superficial structures.

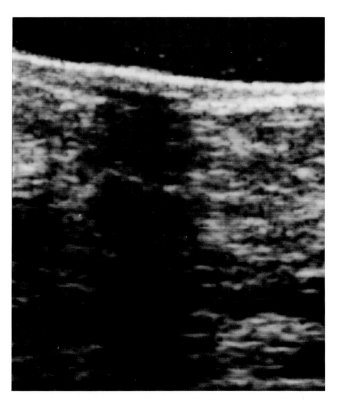

Fig. 2-14. Dense areolar shadowing. Sometimes areolar shadowing can be quite dense, as in this sonogram. Again, this is a normal finding.

ultrasound corresponds to a mammographic finding. After the ultrasound examination is completed, a metallic marker is placed over the area that has been examined and the mammogram is repeated with the marker in place.[10] This step is usually not necessary in most cases.

There is more controversy regarding whether ultrasound has a place in the management of palpable lesions.[38-40] Some authors advocate using this modality only after aspiration has been unsuccessful since an extra imaging procedure merely adds to the expense and time of diagnosis, and most palpable cysts can be readily aspirated.[6,41] However, other experts believe ultrasound is useful in this setting since many patients would prefer to avoid the anxiety and discomfort caused by cyst aspiration, a procedure that can be deferred after definitive sonographic diagnosis of a cyst.[5,36] Furthermore, some

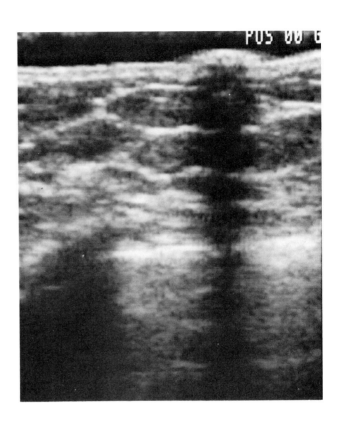

Fig. 2-15. Shadowing from a skin lesion. This sonogram demonstrates a dense shadow caused by a skin mole. Careful correlation with skin lesions must be made in order not to confuse these types of findings with breast parenchymal pathology.

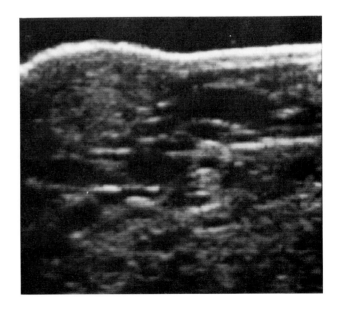

Fig. 2-16. Lactiferous sinuses. This image was obtained of a lactating woman as she experienced "let-down." The anechoic tubular structures just deep to the nipple represent the lactiferous sinuses and large terminal ducts.

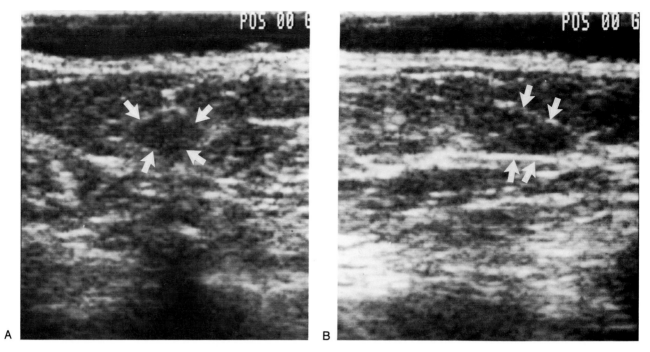

Fig. 2-17. Fat lobule. **(A)** Fat lobules can appear mass-like in one sonographic projection because they are surrounded by echogenic lines representing the fibrous support structure of the breast, Cooper's ligaments (arrows). These can be easily distinguished from masses by turning the transducer and evaluating them in the opposite plane. **(B)** Fat lobules will elongate (arrows). Masses will retain a rounded configuration.

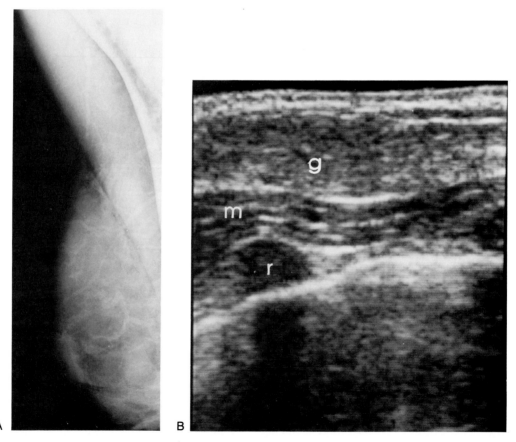

Fig. 2-18. Dense breast. **(A)** This patient's breasts are very dense. They contain a large amount of somewhat homogeneous fibroglandular tissue without much intervening fat. **(B)** Sonogram of the same breast as in Fig. A contains homogeneous glandular tissue *(g)*. There are no definite subcutaneous or retromammary fatty layers. The two hypoechoic layers deep to the breast tissue represent pectoralis muscles *(m)*. The deep shadowing structure is a rib *(r)*.

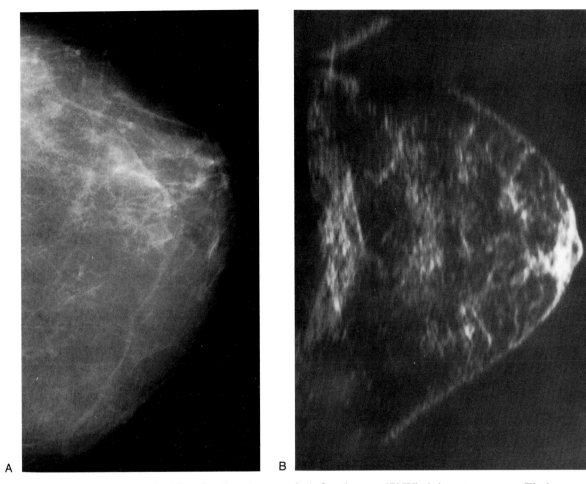

A   B

Fig 2-19. Fatty breast. **(A)** This patient has almost entirely fatty breasts. **(B)** Whole breast sonogram. The breast is almost entirely hypoechoic with no definite glandular layer visualized. The bright lines interrupting the hypoechoic fat represent the supporting structures of the breast, Cooper's ligaments.

patients have palpable lesions that lie in the periphery of the breast but cannot be visualized on two mammographic views despite compulsive technique.[42] This is especially true in patients who have undergone augmentation mammoplasty even if the Eklund view[43] is used.[44] Therefore, ultrasound can be used in this setting to prove the palpable abnormality is a cyst to avoid further evaluation and excess radiation exposure to the patient.[11,31–33,45] Likewise, some masses are too large to evaluate well with mammography and can be imaged successfully with this technique.[46]

The use of ultrasound to evaluate an asymmetric density that was detected on mammography for an occult underlying mass is not well supported.[31,47] Of three patients reported on by Bassett et al,[5] who were evaluated for this reason, ultrasound did not elucidate a cause for the asymmetric tissue. Jackson[31] reports similar results. Some experts do advocate using ultrasound for this purpose, however.[32,36]

Some advocate using ultrasound to evaluate patients with multiple nonpalpable masses.[5,11,17,34,48] However, this is a tedious and sometimes confusing examination that can cause many false-positive evaluations and unnecessary biopsies. Such breasts are probably best managed by short-term mammographic follow-up unless one mass is clinically or radiographically distinct.[45,49]

Ultrasound should be the first examination performed on pregnant women[12] and on any woman younger than 30 to 35 years old with a palpable mass.[15,16,36,50,51] Mammography is less sensitive in such patients because they almost always have dense breasts. In addition, the risk of cancer is low and the risk of radiation carcinogenesis is relatively higher (though it is still low) in young patients.[5] If the palpable mass is shown to be cystic by ultrasound, no further imaging or intervention is required. If a solid mass or no mass is seen, a single view oblique mammogram can be performed to look for other signs of malignancy.[17,31]

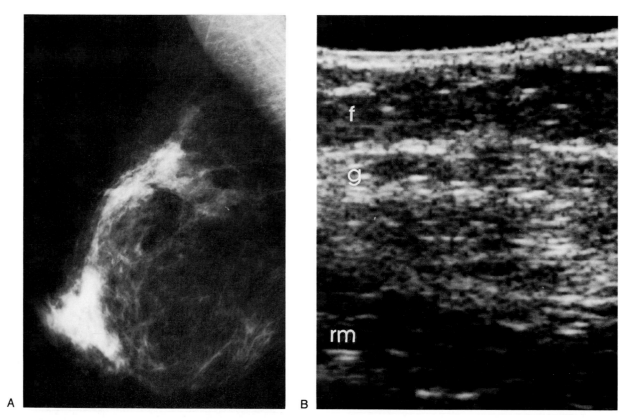

A   B

Fig. 2-20. Mixed density breast. **(A)** This patient has mixed density breasts. Note the definite presence of subcutaneous fat, glandular layer, and retromammary fat. **(B)** The corresponding sonogram reveals the presence of all three layers of tissue as expected from the mammogram. Just below the skin is the hypoechoic subcutaneous fat *(f)*. Beneath the subcutaneous fat is the echogenic glandular layer *(g)*. The deepest layer is the hypoechoic retromammary fat *(rm)*. Note that the resolution within the deepest layer is not as good as it is within the two more superficial layers. Deep lesions can easily be missed. If one is suspected clinically or owing to mammographic findings, the patient's breast tissue should be rolled so that the transducer lies as close to the lesion as possible.

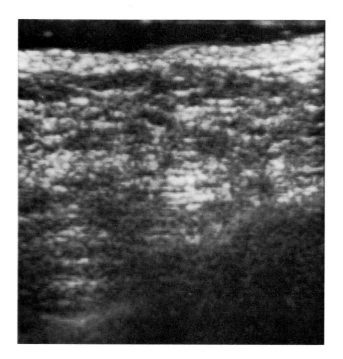

Fig. 2-21. Pregnant patient's breast. There are homogeneous echoes extending from the skin to the chest wall. This is secondary to hypertrophy of the fibroglandular elements. A pregnant woman's breasts have almost no fat. The subcutaneous and retromammary layers get crowded out by breast glandular elements.

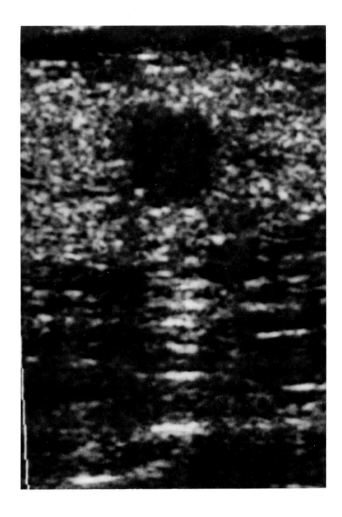

Fig. 2-22. Breast abscess. This irregular hypoechoic mass with some enhanced through transmission proved to contain pus when it was aspirated using ultrasound guidance. This abscess occurred most likely through hematogenous spread of organisms from this patient's skin lesions. (Courtesy of Ellen B. Mendelson, M.D., Breast Diagnostic Imaging Center, Western Pennsylvania Hospital.)

Fig. 2-23. Normal submuscular breast implant. The implant contents are anechoic. The surface itself is fairly smooth. In real-time, no surface discontinuities should be visualized. (Courtesy of Judy Destouet, M.D., Mallinckrodt Institute of Radiology.)

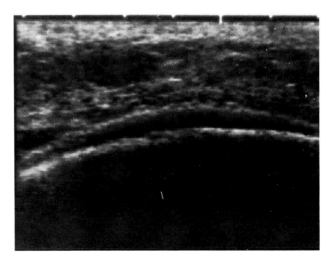

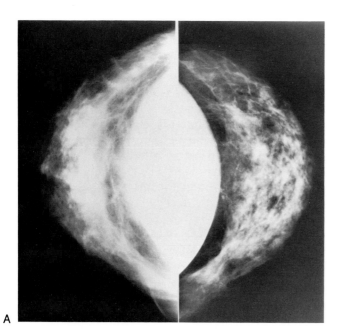
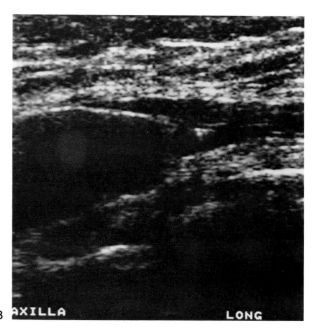

A   B

Fig. 2-24. Leaking breast implant. **(A)** The Eklund position craniocaudal view of this patient's mammogram reveals asymmetric denser breast tissue on the left. This correlated with physical examination findings consistent with inflammatory carcinoma. **(B)** The sonogram of the left implant shows echoes within the implant and a discontinuity of its surface that was consistently visualized on real-time examination, which proved to be a leaking implant. The leaking caused an inflammatory response in the surrounding tissues that simulated inflammatory carcinoma. (From Mendelson,[56] with permission.)

Ultrasound is sometimes used in the evaluation of localized breast pain or tenderness in the hope of finding a nonpalpable and mammographically occult cyst that might be causing the patient's discomfort.[36] For patients with clinical evidence of infection, ultrasound can aid in surgical management by identifying frank abscess cavities that require open drainage[31] (Fig. 2-22).

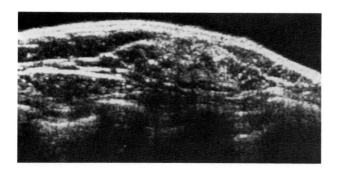

Fig. 2-25. Simple gynecomastia. No masses are evident. The echogenic focus behind the nipple represents this 45-year-old man's breast tissue. The remainder of his breast enlargement is due to fat deposition. (Courtesy of Valerie P. Jackson, M.D., Indiana University Medical Center.)

Ultrasound also has a role in localizing lesions seen on only one mammographic projection,[33,36] guiding fluid aspiration or fine needle aspiration of nonpalpable cystic or solid masses,[52-54] and guiding wire placement prior to open surgical biopsy.[52] (See Interventional Ultrasound for techniques for these procedures.)

For patients with breast implants, who present with hardening of the prosthesis or pain and tenderness, ultrasound can help delineate the cause of their symptoms. Specifically, this examination has been used to search for adjacent abscess, implant displacement, leakage, and fibrous capsule formation.[55] Leakage is likely when there is disruption in the bright echo corresponding to the implant surface[56] (Figs. 2-23 and 2-24). Fibrous capsule formation is suggested when the implant shape is distorted.[55]

Men with gynecomastia have also been evaluated using ultrasound.[57,58] Simple gynecomastia appears as a small retroareolar hypoechoic area. As more breast tissue develops, it can appear more hyperechoic and encompass a larger area[57] (Fig. 2-25). In a review of sonograms of 41 men with this problem, Jackson and Gilmor[59] have found that, just as with female patients, there is a large overlap between the appearance of gynecomastia and malignant lesions. The one malignancy found in the group studied was quite subtle.[59] Therefore, the most appropriate place for ultrasound in the workup of abnormalities in the male breast is as an adjunct to mammographic imaging (Figs. 2-26 and 2-27).

There may be some role for breast ultrasound in the staging of breast cancers. One series evaluated 60 consecutive breast cancer patients with clinical examination, axillary ultrasound, and node dissection. Ultrasound detected 72.7 percent of the axillary nodal metastases found at surgery compared with a detection rate of only 45.4 percent for physical examination.[60] A similar study of 140 breast cancer patients revealed a sensitivity of 66 percent for ultrasound compared with a sensitivity of only 42 percent for physical examination.[61] Ultrasound has also been shown to be more sensitive than axillary mammography for staging breast cancer (72.7 versus 38.9 percent).[62] This technique is probably not useful or necessary in patients who will undergo node dissection anyway. However, for patients with cancer treated only by irradiation, insufficient dissec-

tions, or with large tumors not amenable to surgery, ultrasound might provide invaluable information about clinical status and prognosis.[60] The technique, as described by Pamilo et al[62] used a 5-MHz linear probe focused in the near field. The examination was considered positive for adenopathy if a rounded hypoechoic lesion greater than 5 mm in size was visualized in the axilla. The pectoral muscles, muscles of the proximal humerus, subclavian axillary artery and vein were visualized in all examinations[62] (Figs. 2-28 and 2-29).

More recent work by Tsunoda et al[63] suggests that intraductal spread of malignancy might also be detectable by ultrasound. They correlated preoperative sonograms with pathologic findings after mastectomy. In their series of four patients, hypoechoic tubular structures adjacent to a primary tumor appeared to correlate with ducts containing malignancy at surgery[63] (Fig. 2-30). If this is confirmed by other authors, it may have significant impact on preoperative evaluation of patients.

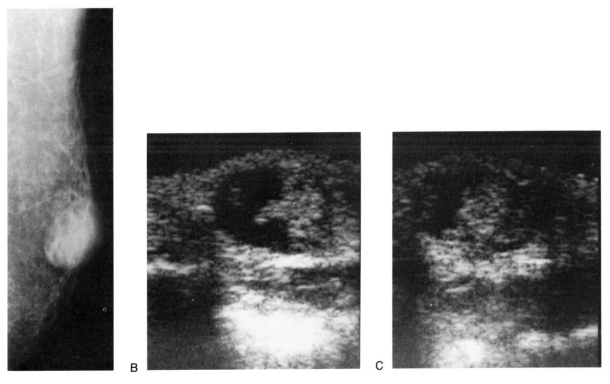

Fig. 2-26. Carcinoma of the male breast. An elderly man presented with a palpable breast mass. **(A)** Mammogram. The mass is moderately well defined on most borders with some suggestion of irregularity and even spiculation along the superior aspect. **(B & C)** Scans of the patient's mass. Most of the lesion is cystic but there is a large papillary outpouching into the cyst lumen along one wall. This lesion proved to be intracystic papillary carcinoma. Fortunately the patient's nodes were negative at the time of surgery.

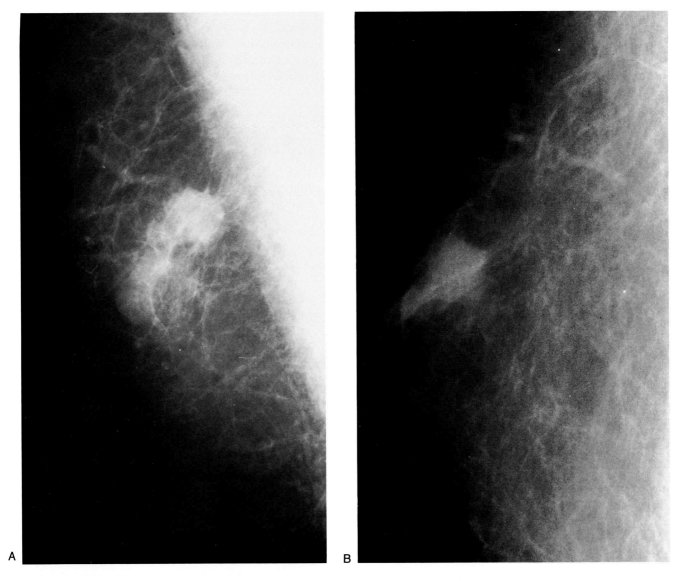

Fig. 2-27. Carcinoma of the male breast. This patient is a 69-year-old white man who decided to have his right bloody nipple discharge investigated after his sister was diagnosed with breast cancer. **(A & B)** Mammogram. There is an obvious partially ill-defined, partially spiculated mass in the right subareolar region. *(Figure continues.)*

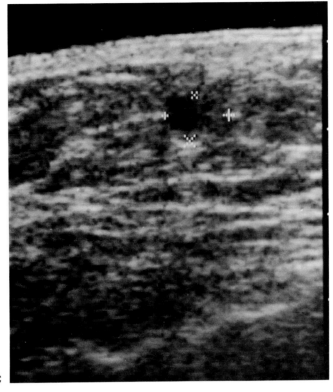

C

Fig. 2-27 *(Continued).* **(C)** Sonogram of this region (calipers) reveals an ill-defined hypoechoic focus without enhanced through transmission. Biopsy of this lesion revealed invasive ductal carcinoma. The patient had positive nodes at the time of surgery.

ULTRASONIC FEATURES OF BREAST LESIONS

Cysts

Cysts represent 25 percent of palpable and/or mammographically detected masses.[13,37] In one series evaluating 1,500 women with ultrasound, mammography, and physical examination, ultrasound found all 241 cysts detected by mammography and all 254 cysts detected by physical examination, plus an additional 362 cysts detected by neither of the other two modalities—an accuracy of 100 percent.[37] Other series have reported accuracies ranging from 96 to 98 percent.[13,15] Cysts as small as 2 mm can be reliably detected with good technique.[15]

Fig. 2-28. Axillary ultrasound. Lymph notes *(N)* involved with breast cancer are seen from the ipsilateral breast. The axillary artery *(A)* and vein *(V)* are also visualized. (Courtesy of Jean-Noel Bruneton, Centre Antoine-Lacassagne, Nice, France.)

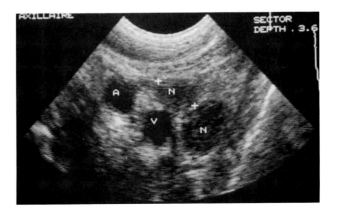

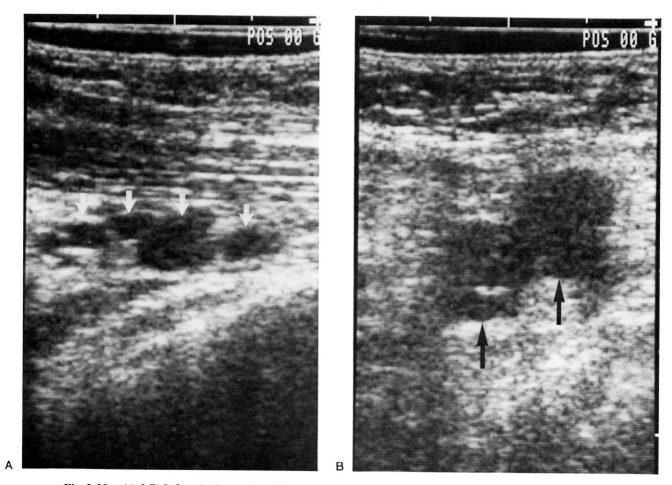

Fig. 2-29. (A & B) Infected adenopathy. This patient with AIDS had palpable, painful axillary masses (arrows). These sonograms reveal them to be enlarged axillary nodes. Ultrasound-guided aspiration of the largest node yielded frankly purulent material. Cultures were negative, probably because the patient had been on broad spectrum antibiotics prior to aspiration.

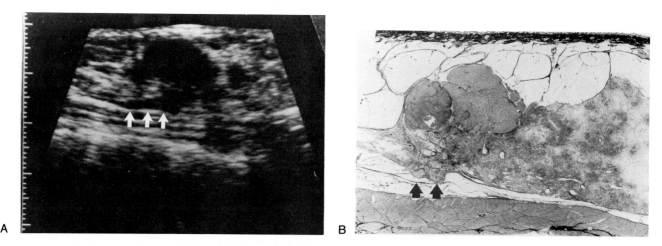

Fig. 2-30. Sonographic depiction of ductal invasion. **(A)** A large carcinoma with invasion into an adjacent duct is seen. The duct appears as a tubular structure protruding from the deep aspect of the lesion (arrows). **(B)** Histologic correlate with the sonogram. The arrows label the involved duct. This tumor had penetrated the basement membrane of this duct. (From Tsunoda et al,[63] with permission.)

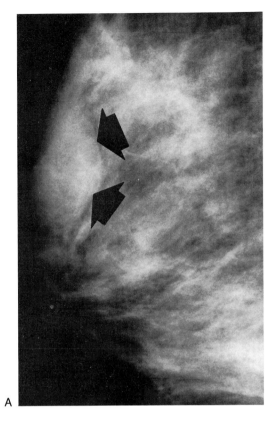

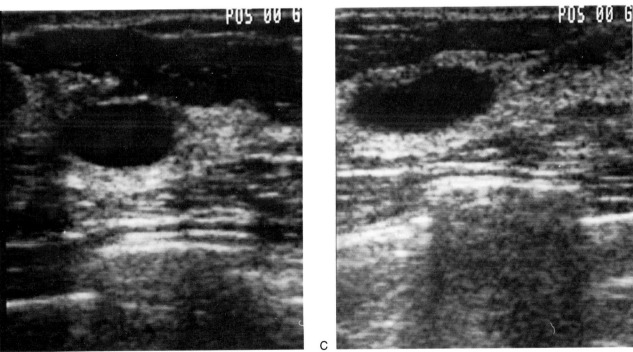

Fig. 2-31. Typical nonpalpable cyst. **(A)** A perimenopausal patient presented for screening mammography. A moderately well-defined mass (arrows) is seen with some borders obscured by adjacent parenchyma. **(B & C)** Sonograms of this mass. All of the features typical of a cyst are visualized: (1) oval shape, (2) smooth sharp back wall, (3) no internal echoes, and (4) enhanced through transmission. Note that the refractive shadows at the edge of the mass are normal findings and do not make the diagnosis of a cyst less likely. In Fig. C, the mass is seen to change shape, becoming more flattened, with minimal additional compression.

One series, however, did report four cancers originally mistaken for cysts,[5] which illustrates the need for adherence to strict criteria in the classification of any mass as a cyst before aspiration is deferred. A mass should only be classified as a simple cyst if it (1) is round or oval, (2) has smooth back and front walls without any mural projections, (3) demonstrates back wall enhancement and through transmission, and (4) is anechoic[64] (Fig. 2-31A & B and Fig. 2-32). If any of these features are lacking, a mass should be considered ultrasonographically indeterminate or solid.[16,31] Another feature, which, if present, confirms the diagnosis of a cyst, is compressibility of the lesion[10] (Fig. 2-31C).

Proving that a lesion is cystic can be somewhat difficult, however (Fig. 2-33). In one series, 25 percent of proven cysts did not demonstrate through transmission on all images.[13] This probably relates to the position of the mass relative to the transducer's focal zone. In addition, echoes at the edge of cysts can be caused by a refraction from the cyst capsule and not by attenuation.[5,65] As mentioned previously, location in the near field and excessive power settings can also "fill in" cysts with internal echoes (Figs. 2-5 and 2-6). To assure maximum accuracy in the diagnosis of a cyst, the examination should be performed before needle aspiration to assure that internal echoes are not created by intracystic hemorrhage.

Solid Masses

Malignant Lesions

For all solid masses detected by ultrasound, carcinoma cannot be excluded by the sonographic appearance, despite early reports to the contrary. Originally, it was thought that solid benign masses have well-defined margins and homogeneous internal echoes without distal shadowing. Malignant masses were said to have irregular margins with heterogeneous internal echoes and distal shadowing.[22,23,66] In a study of 41 malignant masses, Harper et al,[67] found irregular margins in 88 percent, inhomogeneous internal echoes in 70 percent, and distal attenuation in 97 percent of the lesions studied. Kobayashi[22] found distal attenuation in 83 percent of malignancies studied. Thus, if these findings are present, the risk of malignancy is high (Figs. 2-34 and 2-35); however, their absence does not preclude a diagnosis of carcinoma. In a review of the ultrasonic appearance of 130 known breast cancers, Kopans et al,[24] found that only 35 percent demonstrated acoustic shadowing and only 16 percent appeared as hypoechoic masses with ill-defined margins. On the other hand, 25 percent appeared as well-defined hypoechoic masses and 12 percent had enhanced through transmission[24] (Figs. 2-36 to 2-40).

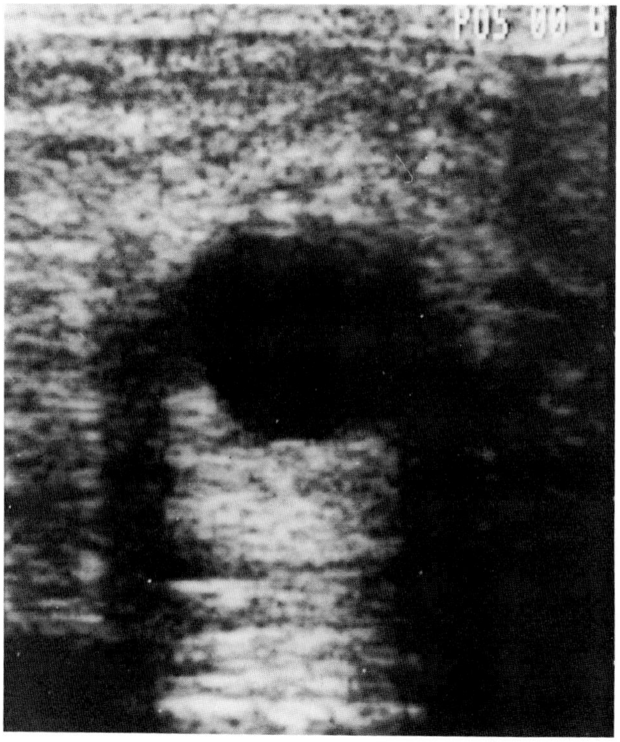

Fig. 2-32. Typical palpable cyst. This perimenopausal patient presented with a readily palpable mass. Again the typical features of a cyst are present. This cyst is rounder and contains a small amount of reverberation echo in its anterior portion. Again note the extensive refractive edge shadows.

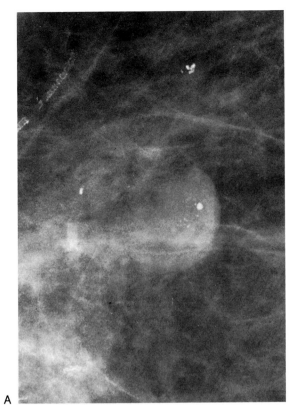

A

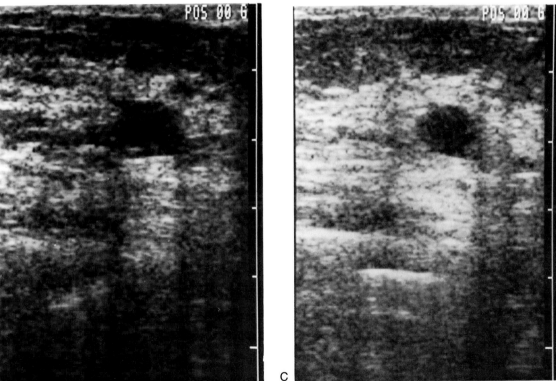

B   C

Fig. 2-33. Atypical cyst. This 68-year-old woman presented with the 1-cm mass found on routine screening mammography. (A) Magnification of the routine craniocaudal view reveals predominately well-defined borders and some round somewhat amorphous calcifications. (B & C) Sonograms of lesion. While some of the features of a cyst are present (enhanced through transmission and round shape), the lesion is not completely anechoic and does not have completely sharp borders, especially in Fig. C. The patient underwent needle localization. During this procedure, the lesion was punctured and a few milliliters of greenish black fluid drained out of the needle. Subsequent mammogram showed no residual mammographic density. This case illustrates how debris within a cyst can cause it to appear atypical on sonography. Such atypical lesions require either needle aspiration to confirm their cystic nature or very close mammographic, sonographic, and clinical follow-up.

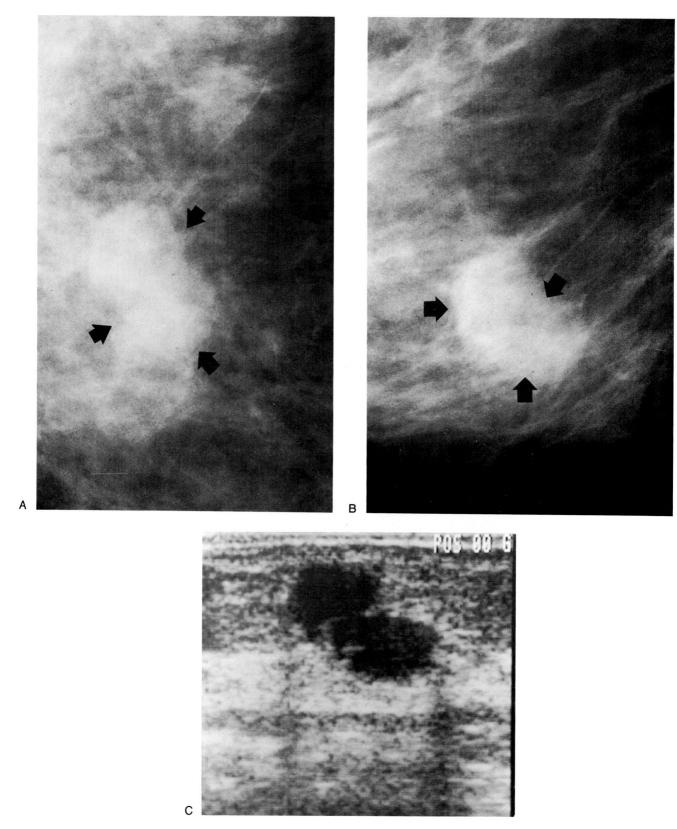

Fig. 2-34. Hypoechoic cancer. **(A & B)** This perimenopausal patient presented for baseline screening mammography with an ill-defined mass (arrows). **(C)** The accompanying sonogram reveals the mass to be irregular and lobulated. Although it is hypoechoic, there are some internal echoes. There is no enhanced through transmission. Again, there are refractive echoes at the borders of the mass. This lesion proved to be infiltrating ductal carcinoma.

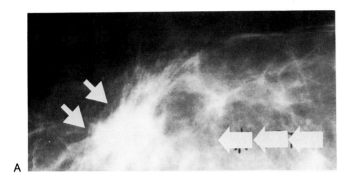

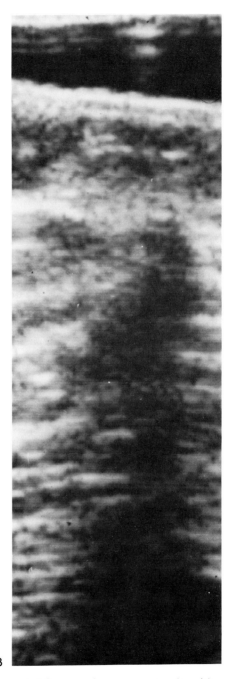

Fig. 2-35. Shadowing carcinoma. **(A)** This middle-aged woman presented for screening mammography with this new spiculated mass (arrows) in the right subareolar region. **(B)** Sonogram of this lesion reveals only a shadowing focus with no definite mass. This lesion proved to be tubular carcinoma.

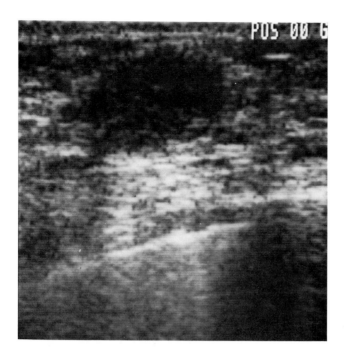

Fig. 2-36.   Carcinoma with through transmission. This carcinoma is ill defined, hypoechoic, and demonstrates enhanced through transmission.

One ultrasonic feature that has recently shown promise in helping to distinguish benign from malignant masses is the ratio of tumor transverse diameter or length (L) to anteroposterior (AP) diameter. In one series, this ratio was measured in 100 pathologically proven fibroadenomas and 28 invasive carcinomas. Eighty-six percent of the fibroadenomas had an L/AP ratio of greater than 1.4. None of the cancers did.[68] A similar result was obtained by Nishimura et al[69] who analyzed 30 benign and 68 malignant masses.[69]

Other features that have been described as useful in distinguishing benign from malignant lesions are the presence of secondary signs of malignancy, namely architectural distortion, skin thickening, or retraction and increased echogenicity of the subcutaneous fat.[14] None of these signs is specific for malignancy and there have been no studies documenting the utility of a search for them with ultrasound in distinguishing benign from malignant masses.

Duplex sonography and color Doppler have been advocated by some authors as useful adjuncts in distinguishing benign from malignant solid masses. One series examining 38 lesions showed 100 percent sensitivity: the 12 lesions with positive duplex ultrasound signals proved to be infiltrating ductal carcinoma, while the 26 lesions with no signal proved to be benign.[70] Since this study did not use consecutive patients, a selection bias might have occurred. Other studies have shown 69 to 95 percent sensitivity in the diagnosis of cancer with these techniques, with cancers demonstrating increased color

signal or higher peak systolic frequencies than the contralateral mirror image breast region.[71-73] Unfortunately, this is a tedious examination[73] and methods to quantify vascularity are somewhat cumbersome and crude at present.[72] Scoutt et al,[74] consider a duplex signal to be suggestive of malignancy if the peak systolic frequency in the region of the lesion exceeds by 2 KHz the peak systolic frequency in the opposite breast in a mirror image location and if the end diastolic frequency in the region of the lesion exceeds by 0.8 KHz the end diastolic frequency in the opposite breast in a mirror image location. They use a 10-MHz continuous wave pencil probe and angle the probe so that the peak systolic shifts are recorded[74] (Fig. 2-41 and Plate 2-1). Additional research must be performed on these techniques before they can be considered useful in the workup of solid breast masses.

There have been some studies correlating ultrasonic features with tumors of particular histopathologic type. One series reviewed 80 infiltrating ductal carcinomas. The most common ultrasonographic features of this lesion were irregular contour (72 percent), weak internal echoes (74 percent), intermediate anterior boundary echoes (56 percent), and weak to absent posterior boundary echoes (55 percent). Sixty percent showed great distal attenuation.[75] The nine lobular cancers described by the same group showed irregular markings (100 percent), weak internal echoes (89 percent), and great distal attenuation (78 percent).[75] Distal attenuation correlated well with the amount of fibrous tissue

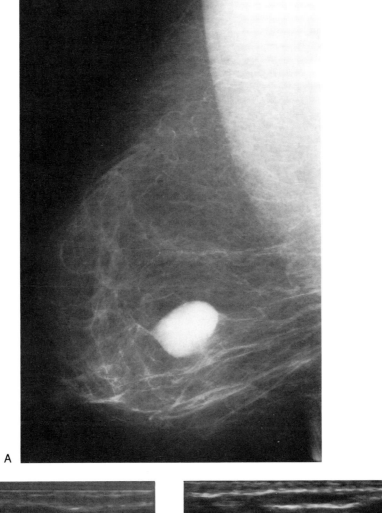

A

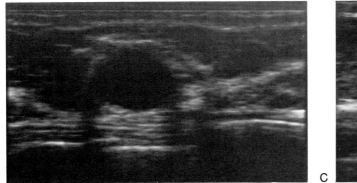

B

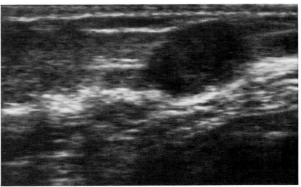

C

Fig. 2-37. Cystic or solid? **(A)** An 89-year-old woman presented with a predominately well-defined mass on her mammogram. **(B)** Initial sonogram revealed a round, well-defined anechoic mass with enhanced through transmission. The preliminary diagnosis of a cyst was made. **(C)** After adjustment of the gain settings so that more detail is visible within the surrounding breast parenchyma, the mass is now obviously solid with internal echoes and ill-defined borders. This mass proved to be infiltrating adenoid cystic carcinoma. This case illustrates the importance of proper technical settings in the evaluation of any breast mass. (Courtesy of Daniel Sullivan, M.D., Duke University School of Medicine.)

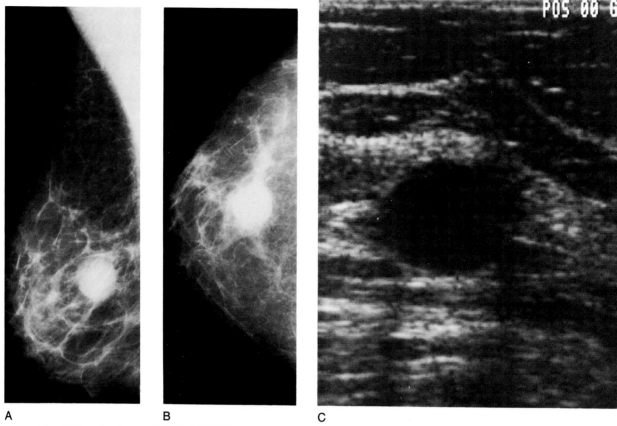

A   B   C

Fig. 2-38.   Cystic or solid? **(A & B)** This postmenopausal patient on estrogen presented for screening mammography with this new mass. It is predominately well-defined, although it is somewhat obscured by adjacent breast parenchyma. **(C)** This lesion is seen to be round, anechoic, and well-defined with mildly enhanced through transmission. However, again the gain settings are lower than they should be. This mass proved to be solid on aspiration. Surgery revealed a very homogeneous infiltrating ductal carcinoma. This case illustrates a pitfall of breast sonography. Solid masses that are homogeneous without tissue interfaces to create internal echoes mimic cysts.

relative to epithelial tissue in the infiltrating ductal and lobular carcinomas studied.[75]

In a review of 24 pathologically proven medullary carcinomas, 25 percent appeared as well-defined hypoechoic masses. While there was inhomogeneity of echotexture in this group of patients, all lesions demonstrated enhanced through transmission.[76] A recent review of three invasive papillary carcinomas showed all three lesions to be hypoechoic with good through transmission of sound.[77] Cole-Beuglet et al[75] found intermediate to great attenuation in the papillary carcinomas that they studied.[75] Obviously, for most cell types, the number of cases studied is so small that definitive statements about ultrasonic features cannot be made.

Cystosarcoma phylloides is a rare breast tumor with low-grade malignant potential. When this lesion has a benign clinical course, it is also called a giant fibroadenoma. Of 21 cases reported in the literature,[12,14,49,68,78-80] the most common appearance (seen in 8 cases) is a smooth, well-defined round mass, with inhomogeneous internal echoes. The echotexture was homogeneous in another eight cases; and posterior enhancement has been noted in six cases. Two lesions had fluid-filled clefts (Fig. 2-42). There are no particular distinguishing ultrasonographic features to determine whether one of these tumors has undergone malignant transformation.[14,78]

Lymphoma of the breast appears the same as this tumor does elsewhere in the body: a large lobulated, well-defined, hypoechoic mass.[12]

Metastases to the breasts are variable in appearance. Most frequently, they appear as smooth, well-defined masses with homogeneous low-level faint internal

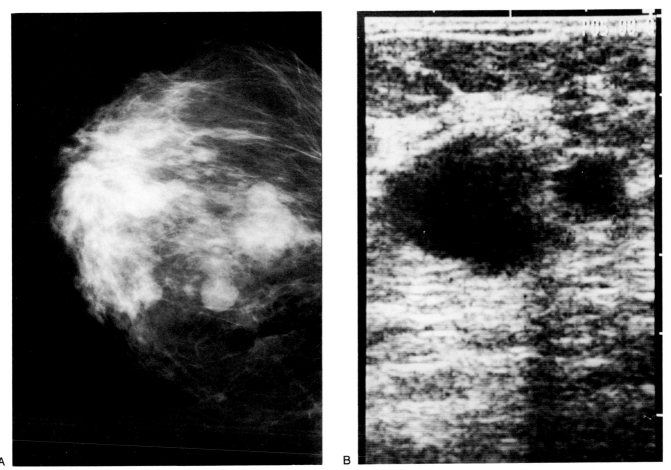

A

B

Fig. 2-39. Multifocal carcinoma presenting with atypical cysts. A 42-year-old woman had recently undergone right mastectomy for infiltrating ductal carcinoma. **(A)** Mammography of the left breast revealed multiple rounded well-defined masses. Because several of these had increased in size since the previous examination, sonography was performed to evaluate the lesions that had changed. **(B)** Sonogram of the largest mass revealed it to be hypoechoic, lobulated, and somewhat irregular in contour. No definite enhanced through transmission was demonstrated. Other visualized masses that had grown since the prior mammogram had a similar appearance. Fine needle aspiration cytology of all of the enlarging masses were highly suspicious for malignancy. Subsequent biopsies revealed multifocal infiltrating ductal carcinoma. This case illustrates the importance of ultrasound in evaluating masses that are not very suspicious on mammography. The most likely diagnosis in a patient of this age with this mammographic appearance is multiple cysts. The ultrasound revealed the lesions to be atypical for cysts, thus prompting further workup.

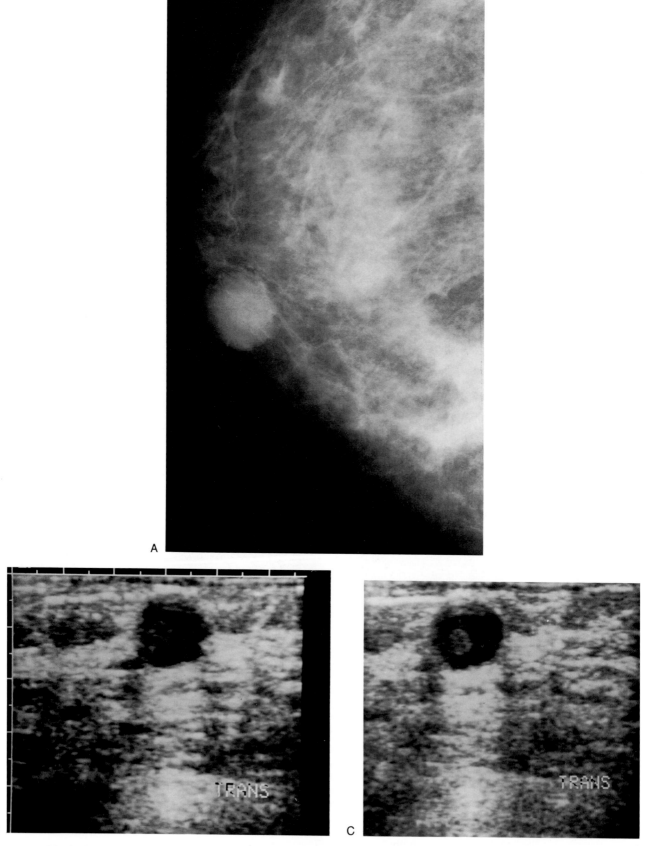

Fig. 2-40. Intracystic carcinoma. **(A)** The patient presented with a well-defined mass on her mammogram. **(B & C)** Sonography reveals the mass to be somewhat irregular but predominately smooth and round. There is some enhanced through transmission. There is a solid mass projecting from the wall of this mass into the lumen of the cystic component. Biopsy revealed an intracystic papillary carcinoma. If this lesion had been scanned incompletely, this small tumor might have been missed within this predominately cystic mass. (Courtesy of J. Stittmatter, M.D., Gainesville, GA.)

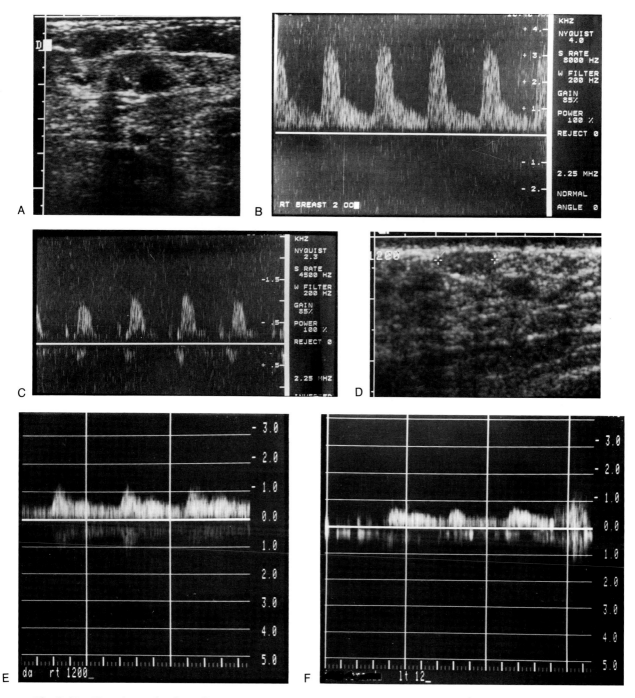

Fig. 2-41. Doppler evaluation of breast masses. **(A)** The ill-defined inhomogeneous mass shown proved to be infiltrating ductal carcinoma on biopsy. **(B)** Continuous-wave Doppler signal from the region of the tumor. **(C)** Continuous-wave Doppler signal from the opposite breast in a mirror image location. By Scoutt's criteria, this is an examination that is suggestive of malignancy. The peak systole and end diastole frequencies for the tumor side are greater than the normal side by the required amounts. **(D)** A somewhat isoechoic, moderately well-defined mass is demonstrated with slightly enhanced through transmission (calipers). **(E)** Continuous-wave signal from the side of the tumor. **(F)** Signal from the opposite side. This lesion is not suspicious by the Doppler criteria described in the text. It proved to be a fibroadenoma. *(Figure continues.)*

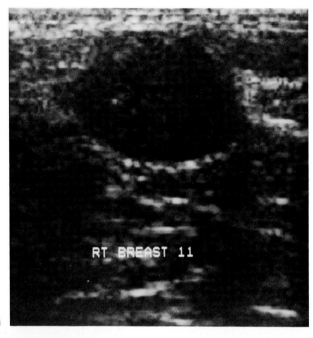

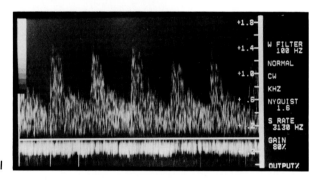

Fig. 2-41 *(Continued).* **(G)** Hypoechoic mostly well-defined mass with some enhanced through transmission. **(H)** The continuous-wave signal from the lesion is shown. **(I)** The signal from the contralateral breast is shown. While this lesion easily meets criteria suggesting malignancy, this proved to be a false-positive examination since biopsy demonstrated only a fibroadenoma. (See also Plate 2-1.) (Courtesy of Leslie Scoutt, M.D., Yale University School of Medicine.)

echoes.[81,82] Multiple lesions within the same patient have been described as being all the same in appearance in four cases[81] and different in one case[82] (Fig. 2-43).

Angiosarcoma of the breast is an extremely rare and highly malignant lesion. Case reports of this entity are rare. Of 10 lesions described in the literature, 4 were well-defined multilobular large masses with mixed echotexture. The hypoechoic areas apparently corresponded to regions of necrosis and hemorrhage.[83] Three lesions with homogeneous echotexture have been recently reported on. All three occurred in the same patient, who had undergone radiation therapy and wedge resection

for infiltrating ductal carcinoma. These tumors were not necrotic on pathologic examination.[84]

Benign Lesions

The most common benign solid breast mass is the fibroadenoma.[27] There have been several series delineating the ultrasonographic appearance of this mass.

Clinically or mammographically apparent fibroadenomata are often difficult to detect on ultrasound, particularly when they lie in the midst of a fatty region of the breast.[26] Typically, 60 to 84 percent of fibroadenomata

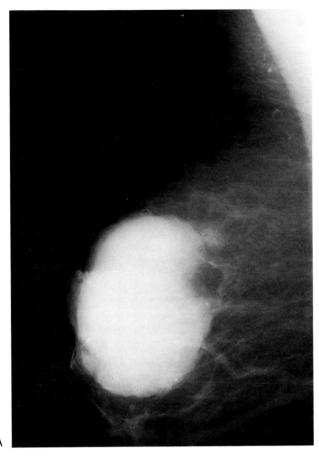

A

Fig. 2-42. Cystosarcoma phylloides. **(A)** This 71-year-old woman reported that she palpated this large, somewhat lobulated well-defined mass only in the month prior to this mammogram. *(Figure continues.)*

detected can be imaged by ultrasound.[25,26,85] Of those detected, the classic ultrasonic appearance is a smooth round hypoechoic mass with homogeneous echoes and either unchanged or enhanced distal echoes (Figs. 2-44 and 2-45). One large series reviewing the sonograms of 62 fibroadenomata revealed that only 19 percent had these classic features. The other 81 percent all had at least one atypical feature.[26] Various series have shown that 25 to 58 percent of fibroadenomata have irregular borders.[26,68,85] Fifteen to thirty-one percent have lobulated margins,[26,68,85] 4 to 11 percent were hyperechoic or had intermediate echoes,[68,85] and 11 to 52 percent were inhomogeneous.[26,67,68,85] Distal shadowing was seen in 9 to 33 percent of the cases studied.[26,67,68,85] Acoustic shadowing may relate to the presence of calcifications within the lesion, but in one series, this was thought to be the cause of shadowing in only six of the nine lesions in which it was demonstrated.[68] Thus, the ultrasonic ap-

pearance of this tumor is quite variable (Figs. 2-46 and 2-47).

The breast hamartoma, also known as the lipofibroadenoma or fibroadenolipoma, is a rare lesion. A recent review of the ultrasound features of 10 hamartomas reveal that the most frequent appearance of this lesion, seen in four cases, was a moderately well-circumscribed hypoechoic mass with posterior shadowing. The other six hamartomata showed variable ultrasonic appearances: three were of mixed echogenicity with shadowing and/or enhanced distal acoustic properties, two were isoechoic and thus poorly demonstrated, and one was hyperechoic with distal shadowing[86] (Figs. 2-48 and 2-49). Mendelson[10] reports that the hamartomata she examined were well-defined masses with increased or mixed echogenicity and posterior shadowing.

Galactoceles are uncommon breast lesions that occur in lactating women. Pathologically they are milk-filled

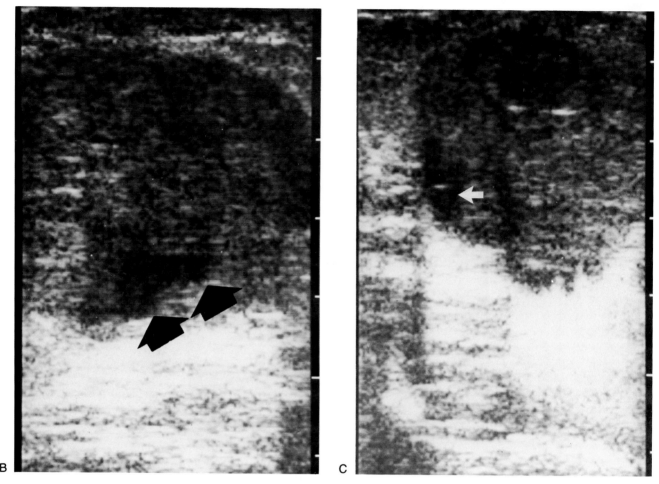

Fig. 2-42 *(Continued).*   **(B & C)** Sonography revealed a large, lobulated, predominately well-defined homogeneous mass with enhanced through transmission. There are some hypoechoic areas (arrows) within the mass corresponding pathologically to fluid-filled clefts within this large cystosarcoma phylloides.

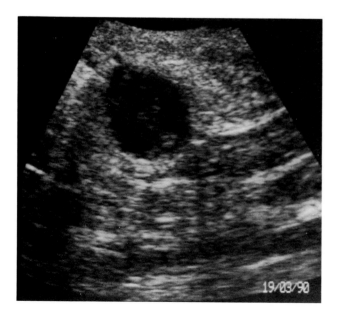

Fig. 2-43.   Breast metastasis. This hypoechoic, well-defined mass with some minimally enhanced through transmission proved to be malignant melanoma metastatic to the breast. (Courtesy of Lorenzo E. Derchi, M.D., Universita di Genova, Italy.)

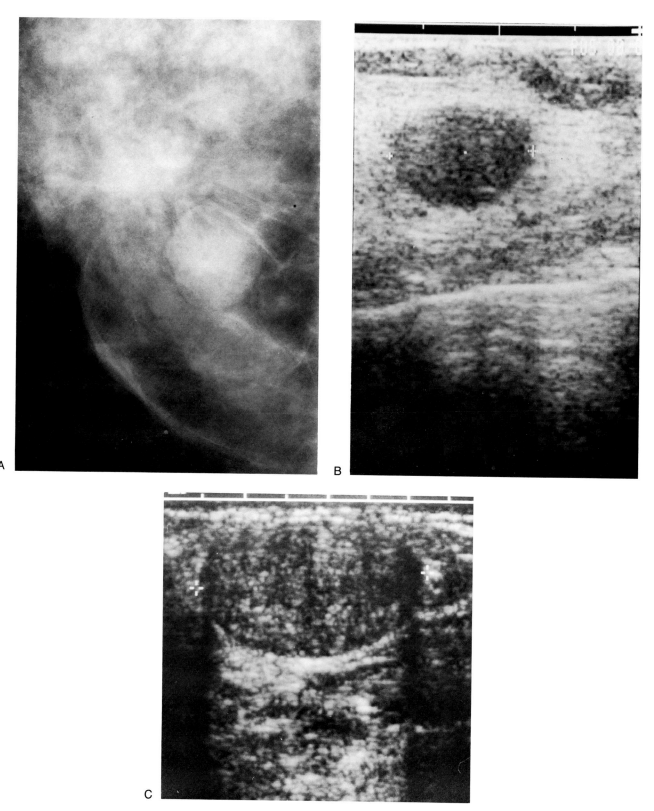

Fig. 2-44. "Typical" fibroadenomas. **(A)** A 45-year-old woman presented for screening mammography with a well-defined mass. There is some associated architectural distortion due to a prior unsuccessful attempt to biopsy this mass. **(B)** Accompanying sonogram reveals a homogeneous well-defined hypoechoic mass (calipers) without enhanced through transmission, which proved to be a fibroadenoma. **(C)** Another "typical" fibroadenoma (calipers). It is an oval homogeneous, hypoechoic mass with enhanced distal echoes. (Fig. C courtesy of Leslie Scoutt, M.D., Yale University School of Medicine.)

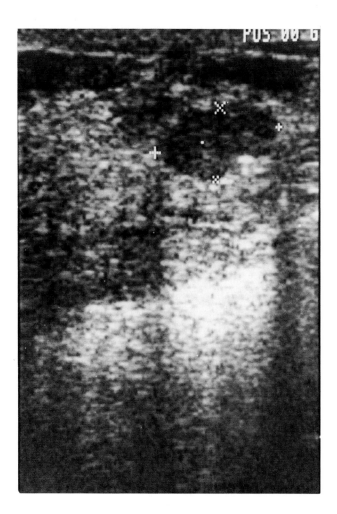

Fig. 2-45. Lobulated but otherwise typical fibroadenoma. This fibroadenoma is also hypoechoic and well-defined, but it is lobulated and demonstrates enhanced through transmission as well (calipers).

cysts. The two cases reported by Heywang et al[25] had different appearances. One was a well-circumscribed hypoechoic mass with an internal septum and no posterior enhancement (Fig. 2-50). This lack of enhancement may be secondary to the high fat content of the contained milk with a large discrepancy in attenuation between galactocele and surrounding tissue. The only other galactocele described was evident only as a shadowing structure inhibiting delineation of the internal detail of the mass[25] (Fig. 2-51). Galactoceles may also appear as echogenic masses[87] (Fig. 2-52).

Lipomas, which occur most often in elderly women, are completely fatty masses on mammography demarcated by a thin capsule. On ultrasound, they appear as well-defined masses with medium level echoes, more echogenic than the usual fat lobules seen on mammography[10] (Fig. 2-53).

Intraductal papillomas, which may be visualized as irregularities of the walls of dilated ducts, also occur as papillary out pouchings within cysts (Fig. 2-39). One report of three cases of juvenile papillomatosis of the breast revealed these rare types of lesions to be ill-defined, inhomogeneous masses, with small rounded hypoechoic areas noted mainly in the periphery of the lesion[88] (Fig. 2-54).

The diagnosis of breast abscess or hematoma is often apparent from clinical history. These usually appear as hypoechoic ill-defined masses with some internal echoes, thick walls, and septations[13,25,45,88] (Fig. 2-55). As a hematoma matures, it more closely resembles a simple cyst[89] (Fig. 2-56).

The sonographic appearance of fat necrosis, which can appear as an ill-defined hypoechoic mass with or without acoustic shadowing, architectural distortion, and skin retraction[10,14,25] (Figs. 2-57 and 2-58), is quite varied and may be indistinguishable from carcinoma.

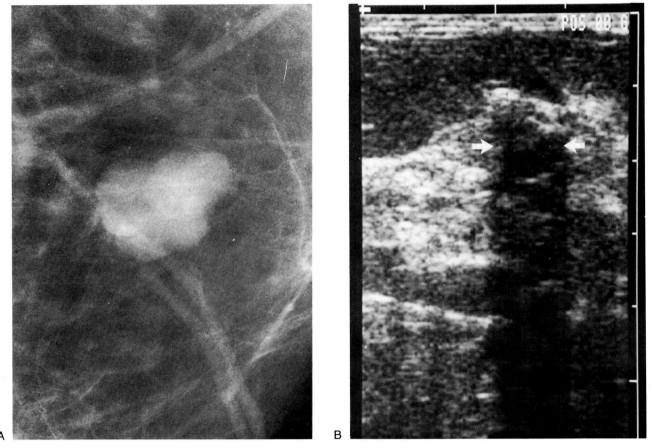

A   B

Fig. 2-46. Atypical fibroadenoma. (A) This lobulated moderately well-defined mass was found on baseline screening mammogram of a perimenopausal woman. (B) Poorly defined hypoechoic mass (arrows) is shown with dense distal shadowing. This lesion also proved to be a fibroadenoma and demonstrates the variability of the sonographic appearance of this common benign tumor.

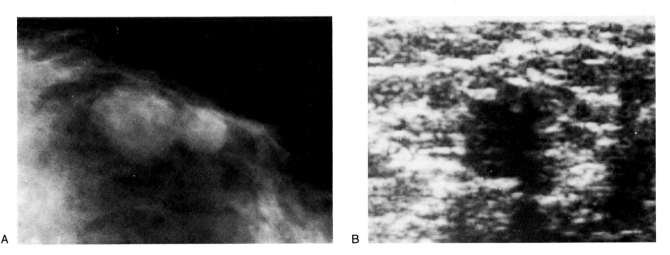

A   B

Fig. 2-47. Atypical fibroadenoma. (A) This perimenopausal woman presented with this moderately ill-defined lobulated 1.5-cm mass on screening mammography, which was not palpable. (B) Sonogram of this lesion. Despite its good definition on mammography, this lesion appears very poorly defined on ultrasound evaluation. This lesion also proved to be a fibroadenoma.

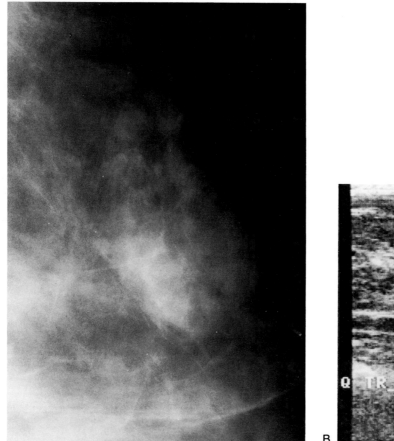

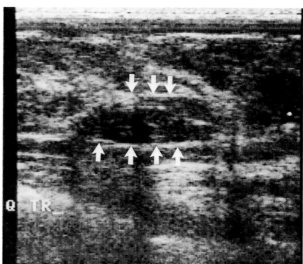

A   B

Fig. 2-48.   Hamartoma. **(A)** Typical radiographic appearance of a hamartoma: a well-defined mass with mixed fat and soft tissue density. **(B)** Slightly hypoechoic mass (arrows) that almost blends into the background breast parenchyma. Its borders are difficult to define and there is both enhanced through transmission and distal shadowing. (Courtesy of Dorit Adler, M.D., University of Michigan.)

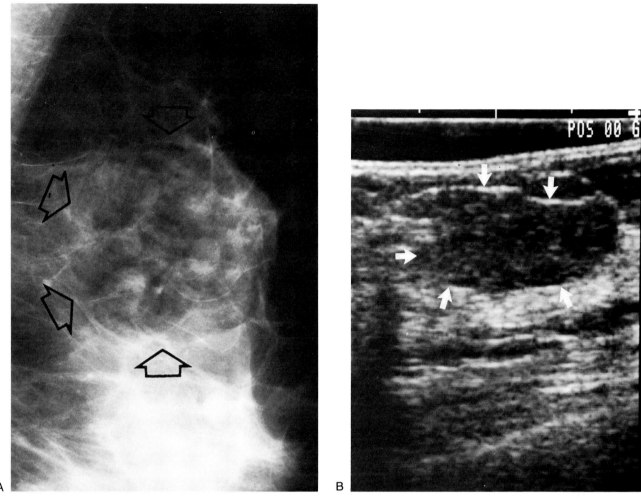

Fig. 2-49. Hamartoma. **(A)** This mammogram was performed because of a palpable mass. This represents a typical breast hamartoma (arrows). **(B)** Sonogram reveals a predominately hypoechoic, somewhat heterogeneous mass (arrows) that is slightly better defined than the hamartoma shown in Fig. 2-48B. Neither enhanced through transmission nor distal shadowing was demonstrated.

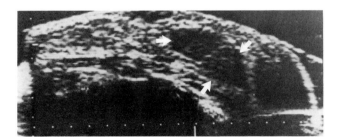

Fig. 2-50. Galactocele. A well-defined hypoechoic mass with an internal septum (arrows) is shown. (From Heywang et al,[25] with permission.)

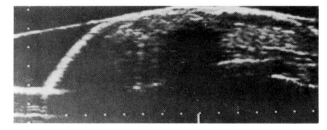

Fig. 2-51. Galactocele. An ill-defined shadowing structure is demonstrated. (From Heywang et al,[25] with permission.)

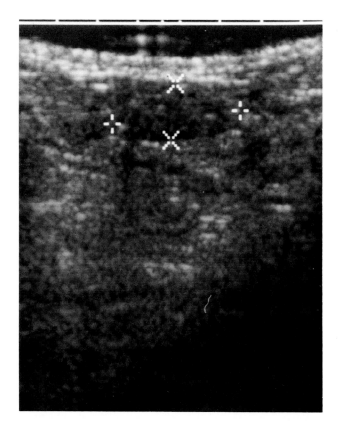

Fig. 2-52. Galactocele. An ill-defined mass is seen that is partially isoechoic with surrounding breast parenchyma (calipers).

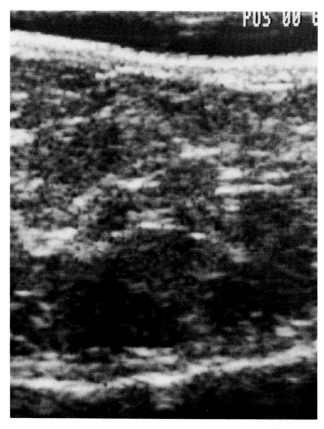

Fig. 2-53. Large lipoma. This lipoma was so large that its border extended beyond the field of view and occupies virtually the entire image. Note the more typical hypoechoic breast fat located in the deeper parts of the image.

INTERVENTIONAL ULTRASOUND

Ultrasound has been utilized to localize nonpalpable masses prior to cyst aspiration,[52,90] fine needle aspiration cytology sampling of solid masses,[91-93] and for localization of occult lesions prior to open biopsy.[52,94,95]

The first step in all of these procedures involves placing a needle tip within the area of interest. The breast is prepped and draped and the transducer is draped as with any aseptic procedure. The area of interest is scanned with a 5- to 7.5-MHz transducer. The skin may be anesthetized, although many experts believe that this step is unnecessary. The needle is placed with direct real-time visualization with or without the aid of a needle guide on the transducer. Direct visualization precludes the need for exact measurement of depth prior to the procedure. Alternatively, the skin site directly overlying the lesion can be marked with a pen or shadowing object prior to skin preparation. Depth of the lesion is then measured from recorded images. As the needle is placed, it is often

useful to have the breast immobilized by an assistant with the skin overlying the lesion held taut. A needle stop can be placed on the needle prior to insertion to ensure that the required depth is not exceeded. With this technique, lesions as small as 8 mm have been sampled (Fig. 2-59).

Generally, a 19- to 23-gauge needle is used. The larger gauge needles are necessary for good, fine needle aspirates for cytologic interpretation. Cyst aspiration or core biopsies require smaller gauge needles. The length of the needle can vary depending on the depth of the lesion. Most lesions can be reached with a 100 mm long needle, although some will require needles up to 400 mm in length. The type of needle is not that important. A simple spinal needle will suffice to obtain cytologies. Franceen or Chiba needles are appropriate choices. Needle manufacturers are currently producing needles with rough edges to enhance ultrasonographic visualization. A needle adapted to accept a hookwire is desirable for localization prior to open biopsy.[96]

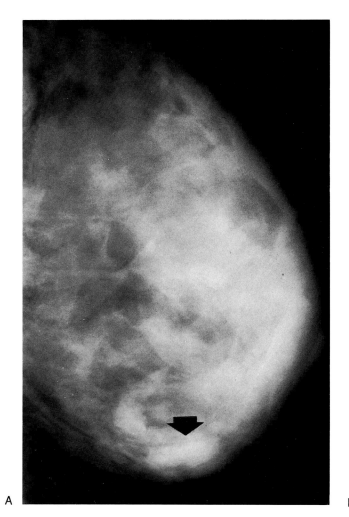

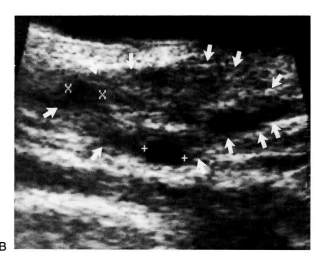

A   B

Fig. 2-54. Juvenile papilloma. **(A)** This 32-year-old woman presented with a palpable mass, visualized as a poorly defined mass on this mammogram (arrow). **(B)** Accompanying sonogram reveals an ill-defined inhomogeneous mass (arrows) containing several hypoechoic areas. This proved to be a large juvenile papilloma on biopsy. (From Kersschot et al,[88] with permission.)

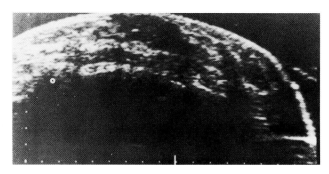

Fig. 2-55. Hematoma. This hypoechoic irregular mass represents a post-traumatic hematoma. (From Heywang et al,[25] with permission.)

Once the needle tip is correctly positioned as confirmed on subsequent ultrasonographic images (Fig. 2-60), fine needle aspiration cytology or cyst aspiration is accomplished by placing suction on the needle by means of a 20-ml syringe or a biopsy gun. For cyst drainage, the needle tip is placed in the far portion of the cyst and is withdrawn gradually. The breast can be squeezed to facilitate complete emptying of cyst contents. Follow-up mammography should be performed afterward to confirm that no residual suspicious density is in the region of the drained cyst. Some authors advocate air insufflation of cyst cavities to prevent the reaccumulation of fluid.[97] In one series of 434 cysts thus treated, 97 percent did not

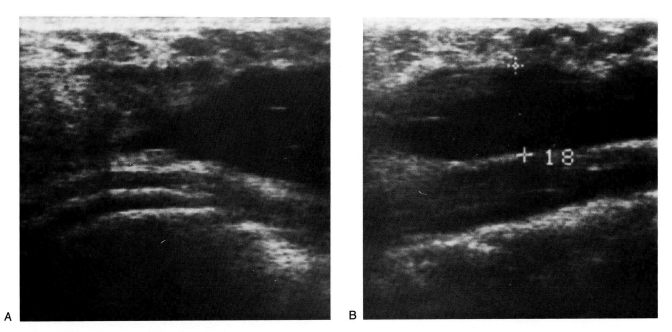

Fig. 2-56. (A & B) Hematoma. This patient developed a large painful left chest wall mass after a chest wall expander had been placed after subcutaneous mastectomy and before reconstructive surgery. Ultrasound reveals a large somewhat irregular hypoechoic mass that proved to be a hematoma. (Courtesy of Judy Destouet, M.D., Mallinckrodt Institute of Radiology.)

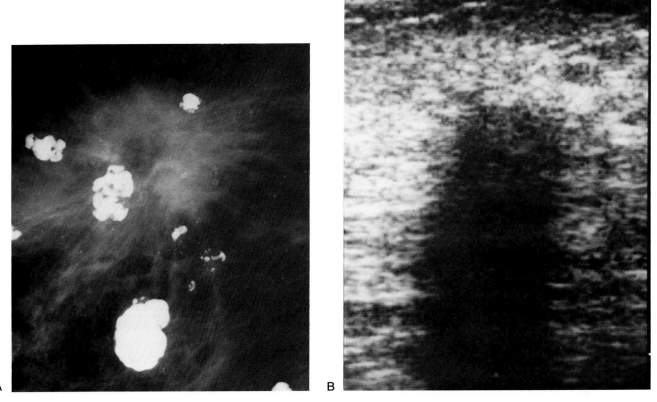

Fig. 2-57. Fat necrosis. This patient had undergone prior biopsy for benign disease. **(A)** The area of architectural distortion and coarse calcifications adjacent to several large degenerating calcified fibroadenomas had been stable for many years and probably represents a focal area of fat necrosis. **(B)** Sonogram of this area revealed a dense shadowing area without a definite mass. The fibroadenomas not shown in this picture were visualized as separate echogenic structures with dense shadowing.

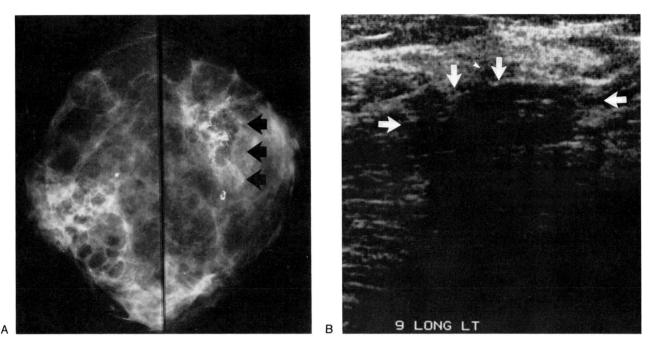

A   B   9 LONG LT

Fig. 2-58. Fat necrosis. **(A)** Mammogram demonstrating the typical appearance of fat necrosis (arrows). **(B)** Inhomogeneous, hypoechoic area (arrows) with acoustic shadowing that corresponds to this area. Some of the small echogenic foci may represent calcifications. (Courtesy of Ellen Mendelson, M.D., Breast Diagnostic Imaging Center, Western Pennsylvania Hospital.)

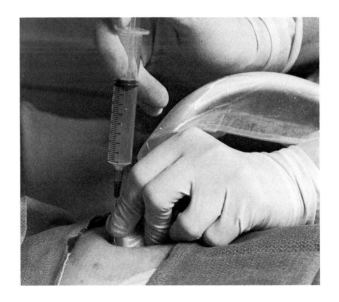

Fig. 2-59. Technique for localizing a lesion using sonographic guidance. The lesion is aligned with an edge of the transducer. This allows for the introduction of the needle in a path directly parallel to the edge of the transducer. While the needle is not visualized in its entire course using this method, the depth of the lesion will be known and it can thus be inserted to the exact depth appropriate for cytologic sampling or cyst aspiration. Alternative methods involve using a needle guide or triangulation, as with ultrasound-guided aspiration of any other organ in the body.

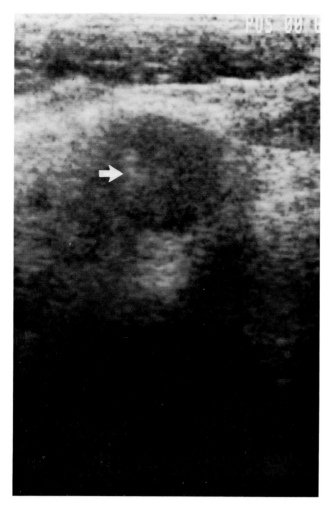

Fig. 2-60. Needle tip within a lesion. A 21-gauge needle tip within this hypoechoic breast mass (arrow) is demonstrated. Cytologic evaluation of this mass was diagnostic for fibroadenoma.

recur after pneumocystography. Other experts have not been able to replicate these results (D.B. Kopans, personal communication). There is considerable debate regarding whether cyst fluid should be evaluated after it is withdrawn. At my institution if it is clear or translucent blue, it is discarded; if it is bloody or blood-tinged, it is sent for cytologic evaluation.

For fine needle aspiration cytology, approximately 7 ml of suction must be placed on the needle as it is moved about vigorously in the mass in an up-and-down motion along the long axis of the needle with concomitant rotational motion of the needle shaft. As the needle is withdrawn from the lesion, suction is released. The specimen is immediately placed on glass slides and fixed. Any delay in this step may severely damage the acquired specimen. It is helpful to have a skilled cytologist available to immediately analyze the specimen to determine whether an adequate sample has been obtained. Up to three attempts are made before a lesion is judged to be unamenable to cytologic sampling. This occurs in approximately 3 to 20 percent of lesions sampled.[92,93,98] If a definitive diagnosis of malignancy is obtained, the patient can proceed to therapy. If only a suspicion of malignancy is raised, or if sampling is inadequate, open biopsy can be performed. But, "negative" cytologies do not necessarily exclude malignancy. The false-negative rate has varied from 0 to 12 percent of cases studied.[91-93] If a negative cytology is obtained, either open biopsy[91] or repeat mammography after an appropriate interval along with careful clinical follow-up[93] can be performed.

If localization of the mass is desired prior to open biopsy, a spring hookwire is introduced into the mass in the same way that this is done for mammographically guided localizations.[96]

Once the needle is withdrawn after any of these procedures, it is wise to compress the breast to prevent hematoma formation. These procedures are generally painless and well tolerated by the patient.[91]

SUMMARY

As can be seen, properly performed breast ultrasound is a useful and important procedure in certain limited contexts, most importantly in the evaluation of clinically occult masses to determine whether the lesion is cystic or solid. With practice, it can also be used to facilitate several diagnostic and therapeutic procedures involving the breast.

REFERENCES

1. Bassett LW, Diamond JJ, Gold RH: Survey of mammography practices. AJR 1987;149:1149
2. Kimme-Smith C, Bassett LW, Gold RH: High-frequency breast ultrasound: hand-held versus automated units, examination for palpable mass versus screening. J Ultrasound Med 1988;7:77
3. Jackson VP, Kelly-Fry E, Rothschild PA et al: Automated breast sonography using a 7.5 MHz PVDF transducer: preliminary clinical evaluation. Work in Progress. Radiology 1986;159:679–684
4. Kossoff G, Jellins J. The physics of breast echography. Semin US CT MR 1982;111:5
5. Bassett LW, Kimme-Smith C, Sutherland LK et al: Automated and hand-held breast ultrasound: effect on patient management. Radiology 1987;162:103
6. Rubin E, Miller VE, Berland LL et al: Hand-held real-time breast sonography. AJR 1985;144:623
7. Dempsey PJ: The importance of resolution in clinical application of breast sonography. Ultrasound Med Biol, suppl. 1, 1988;14:S43

8. Bassett LW, Kimme-Smith C: Breast sonography: technique, equipment, and normal anatomy. Semin US CT MR 1989;10:82

9. Kelly-Fry E, Morris ST, Jackson VP et al: Variation of transducer frequency output and receiver bandpass characteristics for improved detection and image characterization of solid breast masses. Ultrasound Med Biol, suppl. 1, 1988;14:143

10. Mendelson EB: Breast sonography p. 31. In Syllabus for the Categorical Course in Breast Imaging. American College of Radiology, Reston, VA, 1990

11. Smallwood JA, Guyer P, Dewberry K et al: The accuracy of ultrasound in the diagnosis of breast disease. Ann R Coll Surg Engl 1986;68:19

12. Guyer PB, Dewbury KC, Warwick D et al: Direct contact B-scan ultrasound in the diagnosis of solid breast masses. Clin Radiol 1986;37:451

13. Hilton SW, Leopold GR, Olson LK, Willson SA: Real-time breast sonography: application in 300 consecutive patients. AJR 1986;147:479

14. McSweeney MB, Murphy CH: Whole-breast sonography. Radiol Clin North Am 1985;23:157

15. Egan RL, Egan KL: Detection of breast carcinoma: comparison of automated water-path whole breast sonography, mammography, and physical examination. AJR 1984;143:493

16. Bassett LW, Kimme-Smith C: Breast sonography. AJR 1991;156:449

17. Schneck CD, Lehman DA: Sonographic anatomy of the breasts. Semin US CT MR 1982;3:13

18. Bloomberg TJ, Chivers RC, Price JL: Real-time ultrasonic characteristics of the breast. Clin Radiol 1984;35:21

19. Kaizer L, Fishell EK, Hunt JW et al: Ultrasonographically defined parenchymal patterns of the breast: relationship to mammographic patterns and other risk factors for breast cancer. Br J Radiol 1988;61:118

20. Wild JJ, Neal D: The use of high frequency ultrasonic waves for detecting changes of texture in the living tissue. Lancet 1952;1:655

21. Bailar JC: Mammography: a contrary view. Ann Intern Med 1976;83:77

22. Kobayashi T: Diagnostic ultrasound in breast cancer: analysis of retrotumerous echo patterns correlated with sonic attenuation by cancerous connective tissue. JCU 1979;7:471

23. Kobayashi T, Takatani O, Hattori N, Kimura K: Differential diagnosis of breast tumors: the sensitivity graded method of ultrasonotomography and clinical evaluation of its diagnostic accuracy. Cancer 1974;33:940

24. Kopans DB, Meyer JE, Steinbock RT: Breast cancer: the appearance as delineated by whole breast water-path ultrasound scanning. JCU 1982;10:313

25. Heywang SH, Lipsit ER, Glassman LM, Thomas MA: Specificity of ultrasonography in the diagnosis of benign breast masses. J Ultrasound Med 1984;3:453

26. Jackson VP, Rothschild PA, Kreipke DL et al: The spectrum of sonographic findings of fibroadenoma of the breast. Invest Radiol 1986; 21:34

27. Sickles EA, Filly RA, Callen PW: Breast cancer detection with sonography and mammography: comparison using state-of-the-art equipment. AJR 1983;140:843

28. Egan RL, Egan KL: Automated water-path full-breast sonography: correlation with histology of 176 solid lesions. AJR 1984;143:499

29. Kopans DB, Meyer JE, Lindfors KK: Whole breast US imaging: four-year follow-up. Radiology 1985;157:505

30. Cole-Beuglet C, Goldberg BB, Kurtz AB et al: Ultrasound mammography: a comparison with radiographic mammography. Radiology 1981;139:693

31. Jackson VP: The role of ultrasound in breast imaging. Radiology 1990;177:305

32. Pera A, Freimanis AK: The choice of radiologic procedures in the diagnosis of breast disease. Obstet Gynecol Clin North Am 1987;14:635

33. Kopans DB: Nonmammographic breast imaging techniques: current status and future developments. Radiol Clin North Am 1987;25:961

34. Walsh P, Baddeley MB, Timms H, Furnival MB: An assessment of ultrasound mammography as an additional investigation for the diagnosis of breast disease. Br J Radiol 1985;58:115

35. Rothschild P, Kimme-Smith C, Bassett LW, Gold RH: Ultrasound breast examinations of asymptomatic patients with normal but radiodense mammograms. Ultrasound Med Biol 1988;14:113

36. Feig S: The role of ultrasound in a breast imaging center. Semin US CT MR 1989;10:90

37. Sickles EA, Filly RA, Callen PW: Benign breast lesions: ultrasound detection and diagnosis. Radiology 1984;151:467

38. Harper AP, Kelly-Fry E: Ultrasound visualization of the breast in symptomatic patients. Radiology 1980;137:465

39. Jellins J, Reeve TS, Croll J, Kossof G: Results of breast echographic examination in Sydney, Australia. Semin US CT MR 1982;3:58

40. VanDam PA, VanGoethem MLA, Kersschot E et al: Palpable solid breast masses: retrospective single and multimodality evaluation of 201 lesions. Radiology 1988;166:435

41. Kopans DB, Meyer JE, Sadowsky N: Breast imaging. N Engl J Med 1984;310:960

42. Guyer PB, Dewbury KC: Ultrasound of the breast in the symptomatic and x-ray dense breast. Clin Radiol 1985;36:69

43. Eklund GW, Busby RC, Miller SH, Job JS: Improved imaging of the augmented breast. AJR 1988;151:469

44. Leibman AJ, Kruse B: Breast cancer: mammographic and sonographic findings after augmentation mammoplasty. Radiology 1990;174:195

45. Pisano ED, McLelland R: Mammographic analysis of breast masses. p. 17. In Syllabus for the Categorical Course in Breast Imaging, American College of Radiology, Reston, VA, 1990

46. Guyer PB: The use of ultrasound in benign breast disorders. World J Surg 1989;13:692

47. Kopans DB, Swann CA, White G et al: Asymmetric breast tissue. Radiology 1989;171:639

48. Lee ME, Hashimoto B, Carter L: Role of direct contact,

real-time breast ultrasound: one-year's experience. Ultrasound Med Biol 1988;14:109

49. Dempsey PJ, Moskowitz M: Is there a role for breast sonography? Clin Diagn Ultrasound 1987;20:17

50. Frazier TG, Murphy JT, Furlong A: The selected use of ultrasound mammography to improve diagnostic accuracy in carcinoma of the breast. J Surg Oncol 1985;29:231

51. Ysrael M, Bassett LW, Gold RH, Ysrael C: Effect of mammography and breast sonography in women under 35 years. Radiology 1989;173:231

52. Kopans DB, Meyer JE, Lindfors KK, Buchianeri SS: Breast sonography to guide cyst aspiration and wire localization of occult solid lesions. AJR 1984;143:489

53. Fornage BD, Faroux MJ, Simatos A: Breast masses: US-guided fine-needle aspiration biopsy. Radiology 1987; 162:409

54. D'Orsi CJ, Mendelson EB: Interventional breast ultrasonography. Semin US CT MR 1989;10:132

55. Cole-Beuglet C, Schwartz G, Kurtz AB et al: Ultrasound mammography for the augmented breast. Radiology 1983;146:737

56. Mendelson EB: Imaging the post-surgical breast. Semin US CT MR 1989;10:154

57. Wigley KD, Thomas JL, Bernardino ME, Rosenbaum JL: Sonography of gynecomastia. AJR 1981;136:927

58. Cole-Beuglet C, Schwartz GF, Kurtz AB et al: Ultrasound mammography for male breast enlargement. J Ultrasound Med 1982;1:301

59. Jackson VP, Gilmor RL: Male breast carcinoma and gynecomastia: comparison of mammography with sonography. Radiology 1983;149:533

60. Bruneton JN, Caramella E, Hiry M et al: Axillary lymph note metastases in breast cancer: preoperative detection with ultrasound. Radiology 1986;158:325

61. Tate JJT, Lewis V, Archer T et al: Ultrasound detection of axillary lymph node metastases in breast cancer. Euro J Surg Oncol 1989;15:139

62. Pamilo M, Soiva M, Lavast E: Real-time ultrasound, axillary mammography, and clinical examination in the detection of axillary lymph node metastases in breast cancer patients. J Ultrasound Med 1989;8:115

63. Tsunoda HS, Ueno E, Tohno E, Akesada M: Echogram of ductal spreading of breast carcinoma. Jpn J Med Ultrasonics 1990;17:44

64. Jellins J, Kossoff G, Reeve TS: Detection and classification of liquid-filled masses in the breast by gray-scale echography. Radiology 1977;125:205

65. Kimme-Smith C, Rothschild PA, Bassett LW et al: Ultrasound artifacts affecting the diagnosis of breast masses. Ultrasound Med Biol, suppl. 1, 1988;14:203

66. Kobayashi T: Gray-scale echography for breast cancer. Radiology 1977;122:207

67. Harper AP, Kelly-Fry E, Noe JS et al: Ultrasound in the evaluation of solid breast masses. Radiology 1983;146:731

68. Fornage BD, Lorigan JB, Andry E: Fibroadenoma of the breast: sonographic appearance. Radiology 1989;172:671

69. Nishimura S, Matsusue S, Koizumi S, Kashihara S: Size of breast cancer on ultrasonography, cut-surface of resected specimen, and palpation. Ultrasound Med Biol, suppl. 1, 1988;14:139

70. Schoenberger SG, Sutherland CM, Robinson AE: Breast neoplasms: duplex sonographic imaging as an adjunct in diagnosis. Radiology 1988;168:665

71. Adler DD, Carson PL, Rubin JM, Quinn-Reid D: Doppler ultrasound color flow imaging in the study of breast cancer: preliminary findings. Ultrasound Med Biol 1990;16:553

72. Cosgrove DO, Bamber JC, Davey JB et al: Color doppler signals from breast tumors. Work in progress. Radiology 1990;176:175

73. Jackson VP: Duplex sonography of the breast. Ultrasound Med Biol, Suppl. 1, 1988;14:131

74. Scoutt L, Ramos I, Taylor KJW et al: CW doppler examination of breast masses. Radiology, suppl. 1988;169:21

75. Cole-Beuglet C, Soriano RZ, Kurtz AB, Goldberg BB: Ultrasound analysis of 104 primary breast carcinomas classified according to histopathologic type. Radiology 1983;147:191

76. Meyer JE, Amin E, Lindfors KK et al: Medullary carcinoma of the breast: mammographic and US appearance. Radiology 1989;170:79

77. Schneider JA: Invasive papillary breast carcinoma: mammographic and sonographic appearance. Radiology 1989;171:377

78. Cole-Beuglet C, Soriano R, Kurtz AB et al: Ultrasound, x-ray mammography, and histopathology of cystosarcoma phylloides. Radiology 1983;146:481

79. Jellins J, Hughes C, Ryan J et al: A comparative evaluation of a case of cystosarcoma phylloides: ultrasound, xeroradiography and thermography. Radiology 1977;124:803

80. Kobayashi T: Clinical Ultrasound of the Breast. Plenum, New York; 1978

81. Derchi LE, Rizzato G, Guiseppetti GM et al: Metastatic tumors of the breast: sonographic findings. J Ultrasound Med 1985;4:69

82. Jackson VP: Sonography of malignant breast disease. Semin US CT MR 1989;10:119

83. Grant EG, Holt RW, Chun B et al: Angiosarcoma of the breast: sonographic, xeromammographic, and pathologic appearance. AJR 1983;141:691

84. Tassin GB, Fornage BD, Sneige N: Primary multifocal angiosarcoma of the breast: sonographic evaluation with pathologic correlation. J Ultrasound Med 1990;9:481

85. Cole-Beuglet C, Soriano RZ, Kurtz AB, Goldberg BB. Fibroadenoma of the breast: sonomammography correlated with pathology in 122 patients. Radiology 1983;140:369

86. Adler DD, Jeffries DO, Helvie MA: Sonographic features of breast hamartomas. J Ultrasound Med 1990;9:85

87. Guyer PB, Dewbury KC: Sonomammography: An Atlas of Comparative Breast Ultrasound. John Wiley & Sons, New York, 1987

88. Kersschot EAJ, Hermans M, Pauwels C et al: Juvenile papillomatosis of the breast: sonographic appearance. Radiology 1988;169:631

89. Adler DD: Ultrasound of benign breast conditions. Semin US CT MR 1989;10:106

90. Muller JWTh: Diagnosis of breast cysts with mammography, ultrasound and puncture. A review. Diagn Imag Clin Med 1985;54:170

91. Fornage BD, Faroux MJ, Sumatos A: Breast masses: ultrasound guided fine-needle aspiration biopsy. Radiology 1987;162:409

92. Harper AP: Fine needle aspiration biopsy of the breast using ultrasound techniques—superficial localization and direct visualization. Ultrasound Med Biol, suppl. 1, 1988;14:5

93. Hogg JP, Harris KM, Skolnick ML: The role of ultrasound-guided needle aspiration of breast masses. Ultrasound Med Biol, suppl. 1, 1988;14:13

94. Laing FC, Feffrey RB, Minagi H: Ultrasound localization of occult breast lesions. Radiology 1984;151:795

95. Ueno E, Aryoshi Y, Imamura A et al: Ultrasonographically guided biopsy of nonpalpable lesions of the breast by the spot method. Surg Gynecol Obstet 1990;170:153

96. Kopans DB, Meyer JE: Versatile springhook-wire breast lesion localizer. AJR 1982;138:586

97. Tabar L, Pentek Z, Dean PB: The diagnostic and therapeutic value of breast cyst puncture and pneumocystography. Radiology 1981;141:659

98. Zajadela A, Ghossein NA, Pilleron JP, Ehnuyer A: The value of aspiration cytology in the diagnosis of breast cancer: experience at the Foundation Curie. Cancer 1975;35:499

3

Thyroid and Parathyroid

Gretchen A.W. Gooding

With the advent of higher frequency transducers and better resolution, ultrasound has come to the fore as an appropriate study to define the morphology of the thyroid gland and, with enlargement, parathyroid pathology in a noninvasive way, at reasonable cost, and without the use of contrast agents.

In the thyroid, ultrasound offers an extension to the physical examination as to the confirmation of mass lesions, the character of the gland, and the response to therapy. In hyperparathyroidism, the study offers confirmatory evidence that a lesion consistent with parathyroid either exists in the neck or does not, so that the clinician can adjust the further workup to meet the needs of the patient expeditiously.

THYROID

The advantages of thyroid sonography are that it is safe, simple, of low cost, accurate, and well tolerated, with no radiation hazard.

Thyroid sonography is used to define the morphology of the gland rather than the functional state as determined by scintigraphy. However, the overactivity of Graves' disease is manifested sonographically by increased vascularity on color Doppler.[1] Conversely, a small hypoechoic gland in autoimmune thyroiditis suggests hypothyroidism.[2]

Thyroid ultrasound is often utilized to determine the nature of a nodule (single or multiple, solid or cystic, complex or calcified). The size and location of the thyroid lesion are demarcated and note is made whether there are signs of local extension, adjacent adenopathy, or even invasion of the carotid artery[3] and jugular veins. Ultrasound guidance of fine needle aspiration is another use and when both solid and cystic components of a mass exist, aspiration cytology of both components can be obtained. This is a definite advantage over a blind pass. In conjunction with scintigraphy, cold, nonfunc-tioning nodules can be further characterized morphologically by sonography. Cold nodules of the thyroid have an incidence of malignancy of 10 to 25 percent.[4] Multiple nodules reduce that risk to less than 4 percent. Because the resolution is superior, sonography may be used to identify nodules of the thyroid not apparent by scintigraphy. Sonography is also appropriate for the delineation of a thyroid nodule during pregnancy when scintigraphy poses potential risk to the patient.[5] Pregnancy itself is associated with a slight increase in thyroid volume, which is noted sonographically.[6,7]

Patients appropriately followed by ultrasound are those receiving thyroxine (T4) suppression therapy (i.e., those receiving thyroid medication to inhibit the growth of the gland as a whole or who take the hormone to deter the progression of a nodule), as well as patients who have a history of cervical radiation therapy and who are at increased risk for nodules of the thyroid, both benign and malignant. Sonography is also performed to delineate the nature of a neck mass as thyroidal or extrathyroidal, to screen for occult malignancy, and for detection of recurrence in patients who have had prior surgery to treat thyroid cancer.

In children, thyroid sonography has value as a diagnostic tool in the differential diagnosis of thyroid disorders.[8] Normal thyroid gland volume as a function of height can be determined by ultrasound.[9] In adults, thyroid volume is positively related to body weight.[10]

TECHNIQUE

Before the examination, the ultrasonographer should get an appropriate history from the patient about general health, thyroid medications, imaging studies already performed, family history of hyperparathyroidism or medullary thyroid carcinoma, previous neck irradiation or neck surgery, and the reason for the referral.

Successful thyroid sonography requires meticulous technique. A high resolution linear array 7- to 10-MHz transducer that provides 4 to 5 cm of penetration can detect 1- to 2-mm focal abnormalities in the thyroid. Although sonography can be performed with 2.25- to 5-MHz transducers, the information provided is suboptimal and significant pathology can be unrecognized. A near field of view is essential. Also, a water path interface between the transducer and the skin of the neck becomes necessary if the focus of the transducer used is in the midrange rather than a short range of penetration since the tissues of the neck are shallow.

Using a contact gel, scans in sagittal, longitudinal, and transverse planes are performed throughout the entire gland. The scans should extend superiorly to the level of the submandibular glands, inferiorly to the level of the clavicles, and laterally to beyond the internal jugular vein. This allows for the detection of other abnormalities of the anterior neck, such as branchial cleft cyst, thyroglossal duct cyst, parathyroid adenoma, cervical adenopathy, or myositis (Figs. 3-1 and 3-2). Specifically, each lobe of the thyroid is examined in both the transverse and parasagittal planes and labeled as either right or left for the permanent record. The upper, mid, and lower part of each lobe is examined in the transverse plane and so labeled and the lateral, mid, and sagittal portions are examined in the parasagittal plane and so labeled. The study is photographed or put on disk for film development, or in the case of color Doppler, color printed and videotaped.

The patient lies supine with the neck hyperextended, resting on a pillow nestled under the shoulders and the lower neck, which exaggerates the extension and allows the neck to be somewhat stretched and fixed. In this position, the lower lobes of the thyroid are usually noted. If they are hidden below the sternal notch, the transducer is angled caudally posterior to the clavicles to try to visualize the inferior border. In addition, swallowing by the patient will often cause a low-lying thyroid to rise up briefly into the neck and allow visualization of the previously obscured border. The examination takes about 30 minutes.

Problems in visualization arise when the thyroid inferior poles are hidden in the upper mediastinum. In such

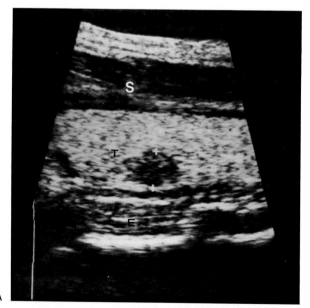

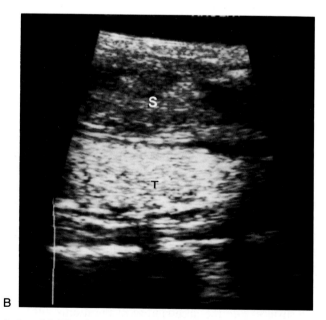

A   B

Fig. 3-1. **(A)** A 7.5-MHz longitudinal sonogram of the left thyroid *(T)* defines a hypoechoic mass (dots), which on aspiration proved to be a thyroid adenoma. The esophagus *(E)* is well seen immediately behind the thyroid gland. This mass was occult, found during the examination of the neck. (*S*, strap muscle.) **(B)** On the right in the same patient, a hugely swollen sternothyroid muscle *(S)* is seen anterior to the thyroid; the enlargement is secondary to myositis in a drug abuser.

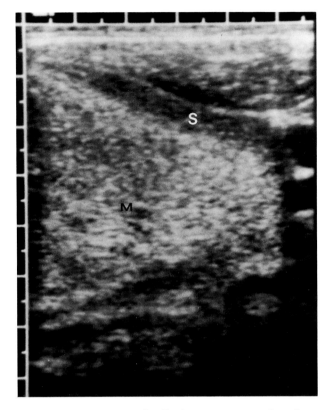

Fig. 3-2. A 5-MHz longitudinal sonogram was thought to show a large thyroid nodule but was false positive. The mass *(M)* was actually a lipoma anterior to the thyroid. (*S,* strap muscle.)

cases computed tomography (CT), magnetic resonance imaging (MRI), or scintigraphy are the only options to evaluate this portion of the gland. Patients with ankylosing spondylitis and other conditions that interfere with hyperextension of the neck may also have a limited evaluation because of a poor sonographic window.

Needle Biopsy

The needle size in fine needle aspiration of the neck varies from 20 to 25 gauge. The needle length is 1 1/2 to 1 5/8 in. Local anesthesia is not required for needle aspiration with higher gauge needles but, if desired, a fraction of a milliliter of 1 percent lidocaine can be injected with a fine needle of 25 to 28 gauge. With sonographic guidance, biopsies of lesions of a few millimeters in size and not palpable can be performed. Successful aspiration depends on the experience of the physician, the size and location of the lesion, the depth of the abnormality from the surface, and the accessibility of the lesion.[11,12] For instance, aspiration of lesions behind the carotid and jugular may be difficult because of the possibility of hitting a major vessel (the resultant blood will dilute the cytologic sample).

If an actual core of tissue is desired, a larger (usually 16 to 19) gauge needle is required. Anesthesia is recommended. Depending on the material obtained, smears and direct staining may be done or the sample may be fixed for histologic sectioning. Cutting-needle biopsies with large 12- to 16-gauge needles are not usually necessary in the neck.

Technique

After signing a consent form, the patient lies supine with the neck hyperextended, which tends to fix the thyroid in a stationary position. The skin is cleaned with alcohol or an iodine solution. Initially, the lesion to be biopsied is identified by sonography and the depth from the surface identified. This depth can be marked on the needle with a Steri-strip or a needle guide. If palpable, the lesion is fixed between two fingers. If the biopsy is to be done blindly, care should be taken to go in with the needle at the same angle to the skin as the transducer was, so as to localize the mass precisely.

If the transducer is used during the actual biopsy procedure to follow the needle into the mass, it is covered with a sterile sheath and sterile gel is applied to the prepared site for good sound transmission. Care should be taken that no air bubbles, which will degrade the image, are present. Some transducers have biopsy-guided devices that allow the needle to track along a predetermined path for appropriate visualization during the procedure. This usually requires one person wearing sterile gloves to hold the transducer in proper position, while the person with the biopsy needle directs its course. If a biopsy guide is not used and the examiner wishes to follow the needle to the lesion, the needle, as it enters the skin, is placed in a path along the shortest axis of the transducer. The patient is asked not to swallow during the procedure, since the thyroid can move significantly when that occurs. When the lesion has been reached by the needle, the transducer is removed. A syringe is attached to the needle and suction is applied while the needle is vigorously moved up and down in the mass in a rotary fashion several times. Suction is then released; while the needle is still in the soft tissues it is separated from the syringe to prevent aspirating material into it, and then removed. If blood appears in the syringe, the needle and syringe are removed at once since this dilutes the material and tends to decrease the yield. The material from the needle and syringe is dropped onto a slide or several slides. This fine needle aspiration technique provides a monolayer of smears available for direct staining. Air-dried slides are stained with Wright stain or fixed in 95 percent alcohol for a Papanicolaou preparation.[13] The aspiration site is compressed for a few minutes to avoid any hematoma. The patient is observed for about 20 minutes and then released.

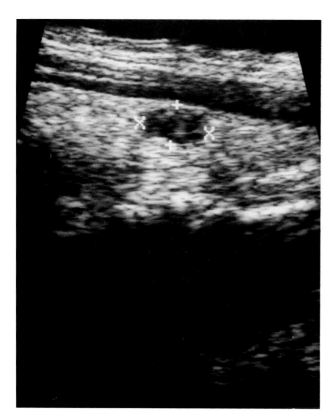

Fig. 3-3. A 10-MHz longitudinal sonogram demonstrates an anterior hypoechoic thyroid lesion (dots), which by aspiration was benign.

An aspiration syringe holder enhances the ability to develop suction rapidly and effectively. Certain needles have been developed with crosshatches to be more echo producing and therefore more visible in the soft tissues.

The requisition forms for the pathology department need to define the problem and the preliminary diagnosis.

Fine needle aspirations are well tolerated, relatively easy to perform, and quick (Fig. 3-3). Successful aspirations of the thyroid occur in 90 percent of the aspirations performed by those experienced in retrieving the sample and interpreting the cytologic material[13-16] (Fig. 3-4).

With mixed lesions of both solid and cystic components, a sample of the solid component may eliminate the possibility of a false-negative fluid aspiration[17] (Fig. 3-5). Complications are unusual, with a small hematoma being the most common. The patients are often outpatients and return home after the procedure and a short period of observation. Occasionally, the carotid artery will be inadvertently punctured. This is not a serious problem in patients with normal hemostasis, although blood in the syringe will dilute any cytologic material. If the carotid artery is punctured, the vessel is firmly compressed for about 5 minutes to prevent a hematoma and then the aspiration procedure is resumed.

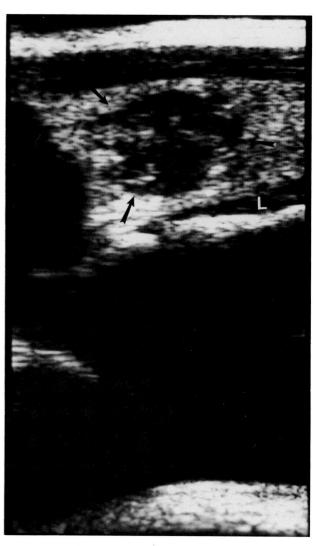

Fig. 3-4. A 10-MHz longitudinal sonogram shows an inhomogeneous thyroid lesion (arrows). The young female patient had had a cystic lesion aspirated previously at the same site and was on suppression therapy without change in a palpable nodule. At surgery, a benign follicular nodule was found. (*L*, longus coli.)

NORMAL ANATOMY

The thyroid by sonography is a homogeneous hyperechoic gland that straddles the trachea anteriorly. The bilateral lobes extend on either side and are bound laterally by the carotid arteries. The thyroid cartilage marks the superior border of the gland. The midline portion, the isthmus, is a narrow band of glandular tissue of similar echotexture to the lateral right and left lobes (Fig. 3-6). Sometimes noted is a pyramidal lobe that extends superiorly from the isthmus.

With color Doppler, both the inferior and superior thyroidal artery branches can be found as they enter the

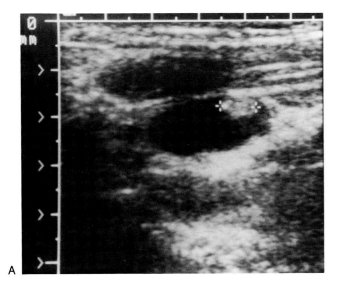

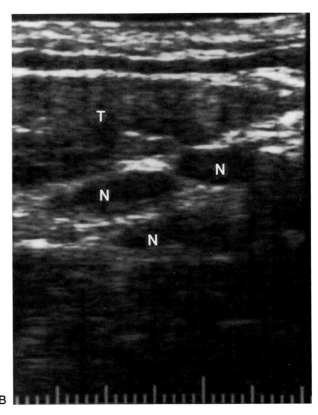

Fig. 3-5. **(A)** A longitudinal 5-MHz sonogram of the right thyroid demonstrates a cystic lesion with a solid component (dots), which, at surgery, proved to be a papillary thyroid carcinoma. Fine needle aspirate was suspicious for malignancy. **(B)** A longitudinal 10-MHz sonogram of the same patient shows ipsilateral adenopathy *(N)*. (*T,* thyroid.)

gland but in the euthyroid patient the vascularity of the glandular tissue itself is minimal.

The esophagus is a hypoechoic linear structure that is usually noted posteriorly next to the air column of the trachea on the left. On transverse image, the esophagus appears to have concentric rings. With swallowing, flashes of hyperechoic saliva are noted passing through it (Fig. 3-7). More lateral, as well as posterior and bilateral, the hypoechoic longus coli muscle is apparent, transversely as a triangular structure behind the lateral thyroid and the carotid and longitudinally as a long homogeneous column behind the lateral thyroid (Fig. 3-8). Occasionally noted is a much thinner hypoechoic linear band that runs longitudinally and is noted posteromedial to the thyroid that is thought to be the recurrent laryngeal nerve[18] (Figs. 3-9 and 3-10).

CONGENITAL ABNORMALITIES

Sonography in congenital hypothyroidism is less accurate than scintigraphy when an absent thyroid gland is the cause of the disorder, or when the thyroid tissue is in an ectopic locale (usually the lingual area at the base of

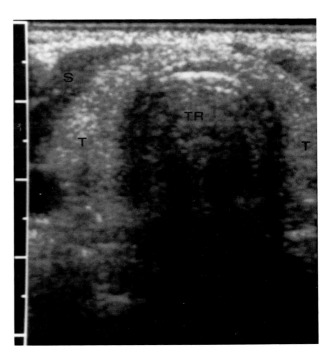

Fig. 3-6. A 7-MHz transverse sonogram of the thyroid shows a normal isthmus of the thyroid *(T)* anterior to the trachea *(TR),* which is an air column characterized by recurrent reverberation echoes. (*S,* strap muscle.)

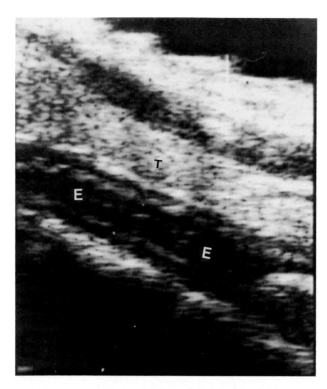

Fig. 3-7. A 10-MHz sonogram of the neck shows a normal esophagus *(E)* behind the normal thyroid gland *(T)*.

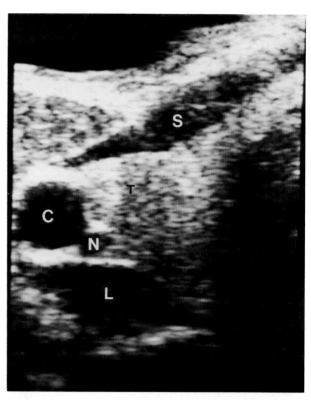

Fig. 3-9. A 10-MHz transverse sonogram of the right thyroid demonstrates normal hyperechoic tissue *(T)* including the isthmus, normal strap muscles *(S)* anteriorly, normal hypoechoic longus coli *(L)* posterior to the carotid artery *(C)*, and just medial and inferior to the carotid is a tiny hypoechoic nonvascular structure thought to represent the recurrent laryngeal nerve *(N)*.

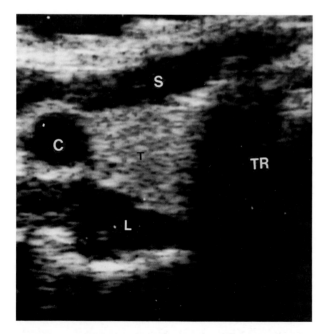

Fig. 3-8. A 10-MHz transverse sonogram of the right thyroid *(T)* shows normal gland sitting on a hypoechoic longus coli *(L)*. The carotid artery *(C)* is lateral. The strap muscles *(S)* are anterior. The shadow medially is the trachea *(TR)*.

the tongue).[19] On the other hand, congenital hypothyroidism caused by an inborn metabolic error results in a goiter, which can be well defined sonographically. Three cases of sonographically detected thyroid enlargement in utero suggest new horizons in the detection of goitrous hypothyroidism in fetuses.[20]

Thyroid hemiagenesis is unusual but can be detected by sonography and is associated with compensatory hypertrophy of the opposite side.[21]

Embryologically, the thyroid gland migrates from the foramen cecum at the base of the tongue to the lower neck. Thyroglossal duct cysts are midline structures that can originate anywhere along that migratory path (Fig. 3-11). Sonographically, the appearance is usually cystic but it may be complex if the cyst has become infected. An infection is more likely if there is a sinus tract to the foramen cecum. A sinus tract or fistula is not seen by ultrasound. Thyroid cancer can develop within the cystic wall and is usually papillary in nature.[22] Heterotopic thyroid tissue can also occur along this midline path, but is best recognized by scintigraphy.

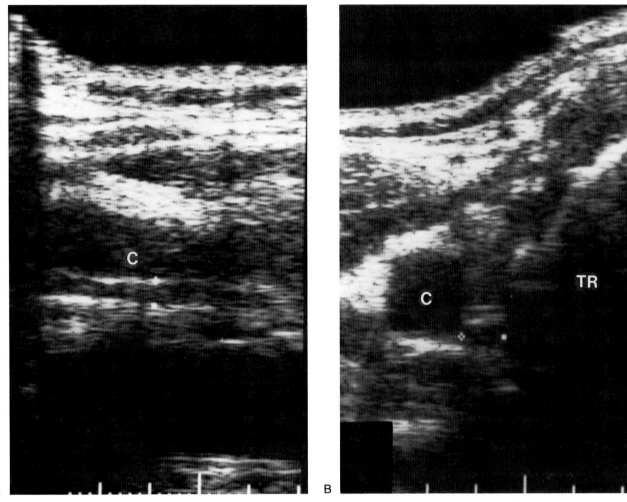

Fig. 3-10. **(A)** A 10-MHz longitudinal sonogram of the neck shows a linear structure along the carotid artery *(C)* that is typical for the recurrent laryngeal nerve (dots) which is occasionally noted by ultrasound. **(B)** On transverse sonogram, the recurrent laryngeal nerve (dots) is medial to the carotid *(C)* artery, immediately adjacent to it, and posterior. (*TR*, trachea.)

THYROIDITIS

Acute thyroiditis is infectious in nature. Clinically swollen and tender, the thyroid is enlarged and hypoechoic by sonography.

Subacute thyroiditis (granulomatous thyroiditis or de Quervain's thyroiditis) also causes tenderness and enlargement of the gland, which may be asymmetric. Two characteristic findings are a high erythrocyte sedimentation rate and a low radioactive iodine uptake. The disease is idiopathic. Sonographically, multiple hypoechoic areas are noted in the thyroid, which tend to decrease in size over time. Thyroid volume also decreases over time.[23-25] Other granulomatous infections include tuberculosis, mycosis, and syphilis.

Sonography in autoimmune thyroiditis is associated with diffuse dramatic hypoechogenicity of the gland. The thyroid volume in those patients with confirmed hypothyroidism tends to be reduced.[26] Sonographically, these volume estimations are best estimated with planimetry of cross sections through the gland.[27]

Hashimoto's thyroiditis (autoimmune thyroiditis) predominantly affects women over age 40 (Fig. 3-12). The initial presentation may be that of hyperthyroidism followed by hypothyroidism. The gland is enlarged, may be multinodular, and is characteristically hypoechoic by sonography[28] (Fig. 3-13). Hypoechogenicity suggests hypothyroidism and severe thyroidal follicular degeneration.[2] Circulating autoantibodies against thyroglobulin and other thyroid antigens develop.[29] Occasionally,

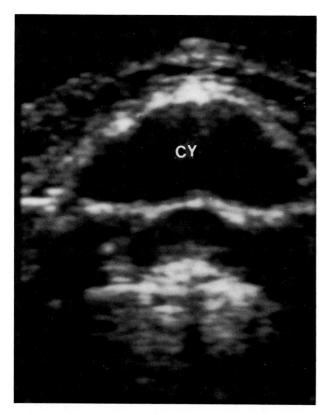

Fig. 3-11. A 10-MHz transverse sonogram of the anterior midline above the thyroid demonstrates a thyroglossal duct cyst *(CY)*.

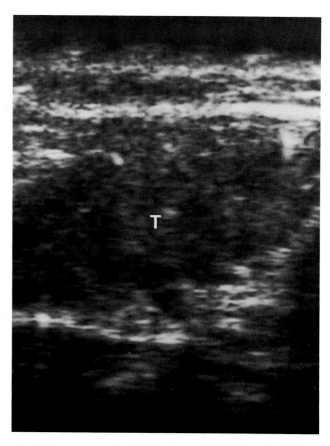

Fig. 3-12. A 10-MHz longitudinal sonogram shows typical Hashimoto's thyroiditis, a small thyroid lobe *(T)* with inhomogeneity, and marked decrease in echogenicity.

spontaneous remission of the resultant hypothyroidism occurs.[30] Patients with Hashimoto's thyroiditis are at risk to develop malignant lymphoma, leukemia, papillary carcinoma, and Hürthle cell neoplasms.[29]

Lymphocytic thyroiditis usually presents as an asymptomatic goiter with low radioactive iodine uptake. Hypoechoic areas have been reported by ultrasound.[31] This is believed to be a different manifestation of the same process as Hashimoto's thyroditis.[32]

Reidel's thyroiditis (Reidel struma) is a rare, asymmetric, focal fibrosclerosis of the thyroid.

DIFFUSE HYPERPLASIA

Hyperplasia of the thyroid is either diffuse or nodular.[33-35]

Graves' disease (thyrotoxicosis) causes diffuse hyperplasia of the thyroid. The thyroid hyperfunction is manifested by elevations of serum triiodothyronine (T_3) and T_4 and an increased uptake of radioactive iodine.

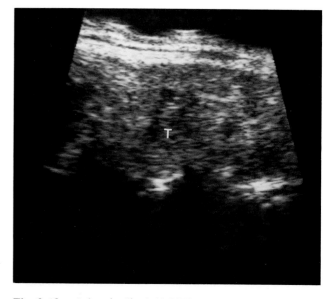

Fig. 3-13. A longitudinal 10-MHz sonogram demonstrates an enlarged inhomogeneous thyroid gland *(T)* with decreased echogenicity, Hashimoto's thyroiditis.

By sonography, the gland is usually but not always either homogeneously or heterogeneously enlarged.[36] Heterogeneous enlargement is more apt to occur with greater severity of disease and higher levels of T_3, T_4, and free T_4.[37] The typical appearance of thyrotoxicosis by color Doppler, first described by Ralls et al,[1] is that of an extremely vascular enlarged gland.

The classic signs and symptoms of nervousness, heat intolerance, weight loss, tachycardia, irritability, weakness, goiter, and exophthalmos may be associated with atrial fibrillation, pretibial myxedema, and periosteal new bone formation, the so-called thyroid acropachy. The cause of the disorder is not known.

Patients with Graves' disease develop various degrees of eye signs and symptoms, including exophthalmos, and are at risk for optic neuropathy. Thyroid hyperfunction causes enlargement of the medial rectus muscle, which can be detected and followed with orbital sonography.[38]

Amiodarone is a cardiac antiarrythmic drug but also a goitrogen; its ingestion may trigger thyrotoxicosis.[39] Paradoxically, it is also associated with iodide-induced hypothyroidism.[40]

Initial treatment of hyperthyroidism begins with antithyroid drugs such as propylthiouracil, methimazole, and carbimazole, followed by radioactive iodine or subtotal thyroidectomy.

Nodular hyperplasia, multinodular goiter, and adenomatous hyperplasia are some of the terms used to describe goiter, which is the most common thyroid abnormality.[29] Endemic goiter is associated with inadequate dietary iodine intake. The common sporadic nodular goiter or nontoxic goiter refers to thyroid enlargement in a patient without thyrotoxicosis, myxedema, inflammation, or neoplasia (Figs. 3-14 and 3-15). Usually the cause is not known. Toxic nodular goiter, a disease of the elderly, refers to an enlarged thyroid gland with areas of functional autonomy. By sonography, the goitrous gland is usually enlarged, nodular, and may be inhomogeneous with solid and cystic components (Figs. 3-16 and 3-17). As the nodules enlarge, the thyroid may expand into the upper mediastinum. In these cases, the inferior margins cannot be identified by sonography and the referring clinician should be notified that further studies (CT, scintigraphy, or MRI) will be required to define the mediastinal extent.

FOCAL HYPERPLASIA

Pathologic data suggest that by the fifth decade over half of adults have thyroid nodules.[29] Even though suppression therapy for thyroid nodules is common prac-

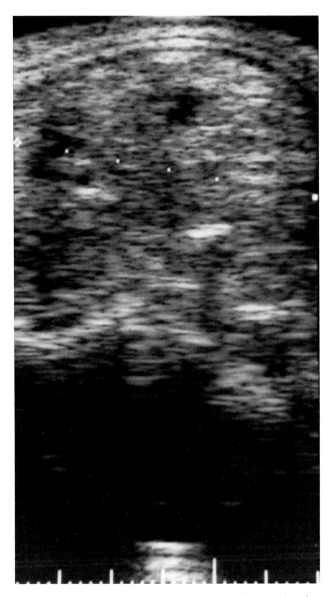

Fig. 3-14. A transverse 10-MHz sonogram shows a huge inhomogeneous thyroid, a multinodular goiter (dots).

tice, in one study, no appreciable effect was noted by sonography in those treated with T_4 over a 6-month period.[41] Focal nodular changes of the thyroid gland are particularly common in middle-aged women.[42]

The most common focal thyroid abnormality is adenomatous hyperplasia. Other common thyroid nodules are thyroid adenoma, cyst, involutional nodule, cancer, and focal thyroiditis (M. D. Okerlund, personal communication, 1986). Much less common are lymphoma, metastatic cancer, granulomas, and abscess. The malignant thyroid neoplasms are papillary carcinoma; follicular carcinoma, including clear and Hürthle cell types

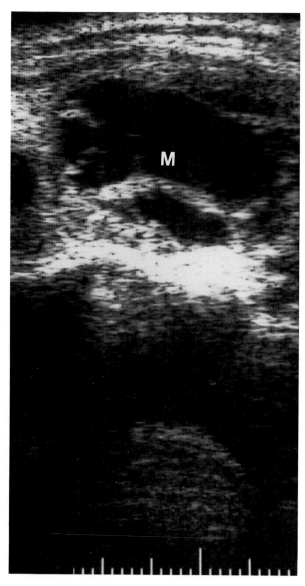

Fig. 3-15. A 10-MHz longitudinal sonogram shows a multi-septated cystic mass *(M)* of the lower thyroid, which proved to be benign colloid goiter.

(Fig. 3-18); occult sclerosing carcinoma; anaplastic carcinoma; medullary carcinoma; epidermal and mucinous carcinoma; sarcomas (rare); and metastases.[13]

Benign

Focal nodules of adenomatous hyperplasia typically have a hypoechoic rim demarcating them from the neighboring gland (Fig. 3-19). This rim appears vascular by color Doppler.[43] This halo is not pathognomonic for a benign lesion, however, since occasional malignancies present with such a halo.

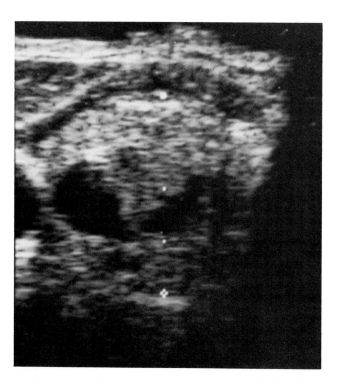

Fig. 3-16. A 10-MHz sonogram demonstrates a solid thyroid nodule with cystic components (dots).

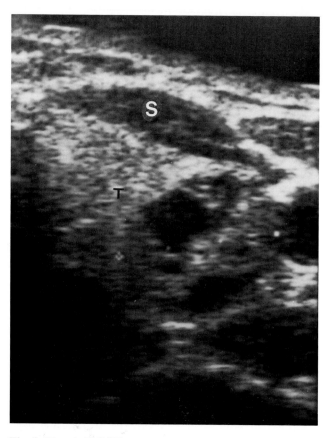

Fig. 3-17. A 10-MHz transverse sonogram shows a mass in the thyroid *(T)* that is solid with a few little cystic components, which on aspiration was benign goiter (dots). (*S*, strap muscle.)

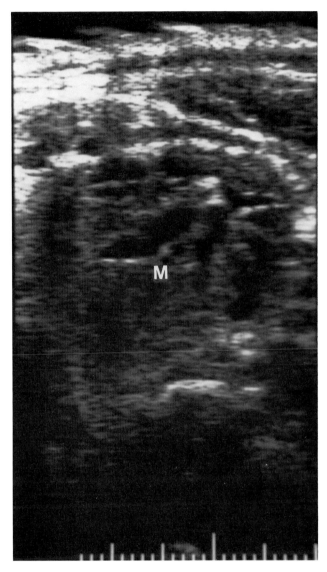

Fig. 3-18. A longitudinal 10-MHz sonogram demonstrates a large irregular mass *(M)* of the left thyroid, a Hürthle cell carcinoma.

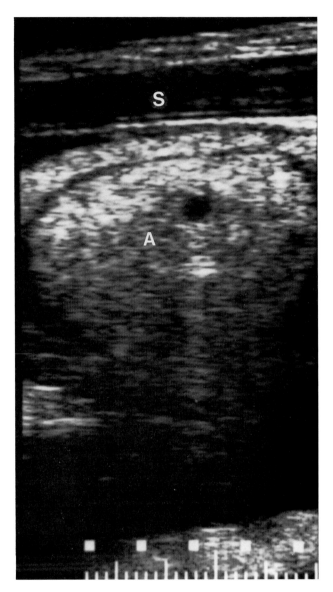

Fig. 3-19. A longitudinal 10-MHz sonogram demonstrates a solid thyroid mass with a hypoechoic rim, very typical but not pathognomonic for a thyroid adenoma *(A)*. A tiny cyst is within the tumor. (*S*, strap muscle.)

The follicular adenoma is a benign, often single, encapsulated tumor, which by scintigraphy typically is nonfunctioning, but occasionally is warm, or rarely, hot.[29] Cold, nonfunctioning nodules by scintigraphy may be identified as cysts by ultrasound in 11 percent of cases. Limited experience with color Doppler suggests that autonomous hot nodules have increased vascularity, as do those of thyroid carcinoma. This is in contrast to simple nodular goiter, in which vascularity is usually not prominent.[43]

Thyroid cysts are not usually true cysts, but are more likely degenerating adenomatous hyperplastic lesions, retention cysts, and giant thyroid follicles (Figs. 3-20 and 3-21). Aspiration yields yellow, hemorrhagic, or chocolate-colored fluid. About 40 percent of cysts will be elim-

inated by aspiration.[44,45] The fluid in a thyroid cyst has elevated thyroid hormone, even though the patient is usually euthyroid. Clear fluid aspirate suggests a parathyroid cyst. Sonographically, both parathyroid and thyroid cysts appear as anechoic structures with smooth walls and posterior echo enhancement beyond the cyst boundaries.

Malignant

Most thyroid tumors are benign. A solitary nodule may be malignant in 10 to 25 percent of cases, but the risk of malignancy decreases with the presence of multi-

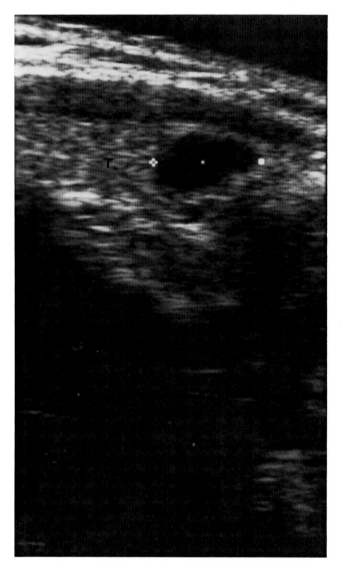

Fig. 3-20. A longitudinal 10-MHz sonogram demonstrates a simple inferior pole thyroid *(T)* cyst (dots).

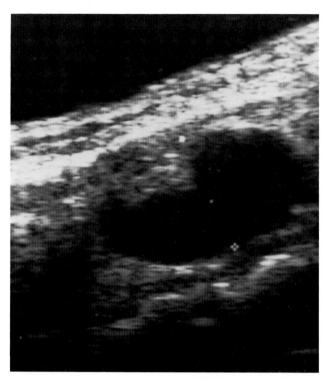

Fig. 3-21. A 10-MHz longitudinal sonogram demonstrates a cystic lesion of the thyroid gland with solid components (dots), which proved to be cystic degeneration of adenomatous hyperplasia.

ple nodules.[4] Thyroid malignancy is more common in men. A solitary thyroid nodule in the presence of cervical adenopathy on the same side suggests malignancy. Autonomous nodules functioning by scintigraphy (iodine-123 [I[123]]) tend to be benign. Simple cystic lesions by sonography are almost always benign. Hyperechoic lesions by ultrasound have a low incidence of malignancy. Thyroid cancer is commonly isoechoic or hypoechoic by ultrasound, but fine needle aspiration is the final arbiter in the diagnosis since morphologic appearance alone cannot differentiate between a benign and a malignant mass.

Papillary thyroid cancer is the most common of the thyroid malignancies (Figs. 3-5 and 3-22) and is the predominant cause of thyroid cancer in children. Women

between the ages of 25 and 35 years are more likely to be affected. About 25 percent of these patients will have metastatic cervical adenopathy, and some may present with adenopathy as the only finding clinically (Fig. 3-23). These involved nodes have a tendency to cystic degeneration[29] (Fig. 3-24). Distant metastases are not frequent, with spread to the lung being the most likely.

Follicular carcinoma of the thyroid is usually a solitary mass of the thyroid. This neoplasm is not occult and is more likely to metastasize primarily to lung or bone rather than to cervical nodes.

Hürthle cell neoplasms can be benign or malignant. Metastases have a similar pattern of spread as follicular cell carcinoma.

Undifferentiated carcinoma, a disease of the elderly, is highly aggressive locally and distantly. Although carotid invasion is rare and is associated with a poor prognosis, sonography is effective in determining whether that possibility should be considered.[2]

Medullary carcinoma (C-cell carcinoma), which accounts for 10 percent of thyroid malignancies,[46] arises from the parafollicular C cells of neural crest origin[29] and can be sporadic or familial. Of the 80 percent that are sporadic, a single nodule is the most likely presentation in a middle-aged adult. The familial type, which occurs

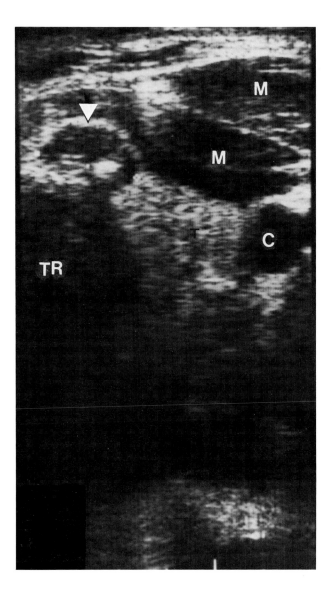

Fig. 3-22. A transverse 10-MHz sonogram of a single thyroid nodule (white arrowhead) of the isthmus with a fleck of calcification in a middle-aged man proved to be papillary thyroid carcinoma on fine needle aspiration, confirmed at surgery. (*C*, carotid artery; *M*, strap muscle and sternocleidomastoid muscle (anterior); *TR*, trachea.)

in younger patients and children who have inherited an autosomal dominant trait, can be multiple and bilateral. The precursor premalignant lesion in these families is C-cell hyperplasia and the patients are followed for elevations of calcitonin or carcinoembryonic antigen (CEA), which indicate disease.[29,47] Focal clumps of coarse calcification surrounded by amyloid are common in this tumor (83 percent) and are noted sonographically as a mass with bright interfaces generating marked acoustic shadowing. However, calcification is not a specific marker, since other thyroid lesions, both benign and malignant, calcify[46] (Fig. 3-25).

Locally invasive, this cancer spreads to cervical lymph nodes, and metastasizes distantly to the lung, liver, and bone[48] (Fig. 3-26). Nodal calcifications also may calcify (75 percent), but this development is not specific as it is also noted in granulomatous disease (Fig. 3-27). Medul-

lary thyroid carcinoma is a constituent of multiple endocrine neoplasia (MEN) types II and III (Fig. 3-28). The treatment is total thyroidectomy and cervical lymph node dissection.

An occasional unsuspected parathyroid adenoma may be noted on sonography of the thyroid in a patient with a history suspicious for MEN who is being examined for a thyroid nodule.

Patients with Hashimoto's thyroiditis have a predilection to develop primary thyroid lymphoma. This presents sonographically as focal, well-differentiated hypoechoic masses of the thyroid and may be associated with cervical adenopathy.[49,50]

Cervical radiation affects the thyroid gland, which over many years tends to develop nodules, both benign and malignant, in response[51] (Fig. 3-29). Sonography, because is is noninvasive, is useful in long range follow-

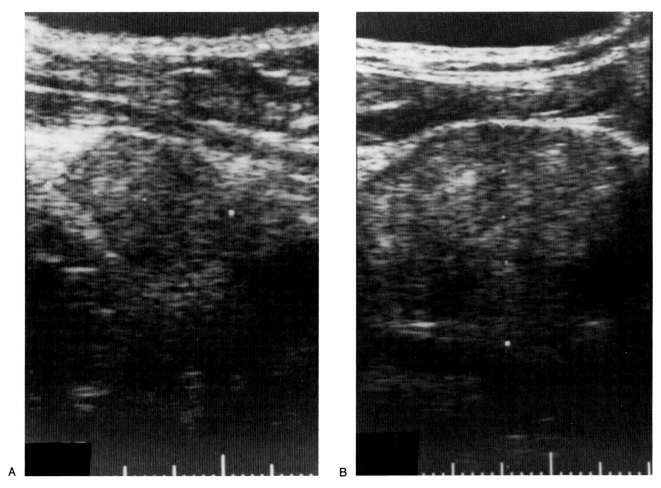

Fig. 3-23. **(A)** A 10-MHz longitudinal sonogram of a pregnant patient who had had a right thyroid lobectomy for papillary thyroid carcinoma shows a solid homogeneous mass in the left thyroid (dots). **(B)** A 10-MHz longitudinal sonogram of the same pregnant patient who had had a right thyroid lobectomy for papillary thyroid carcinoma shows a similar extrathyroidal mass in the lateral neck (dots), also papillary thyroid cancer at surgery.

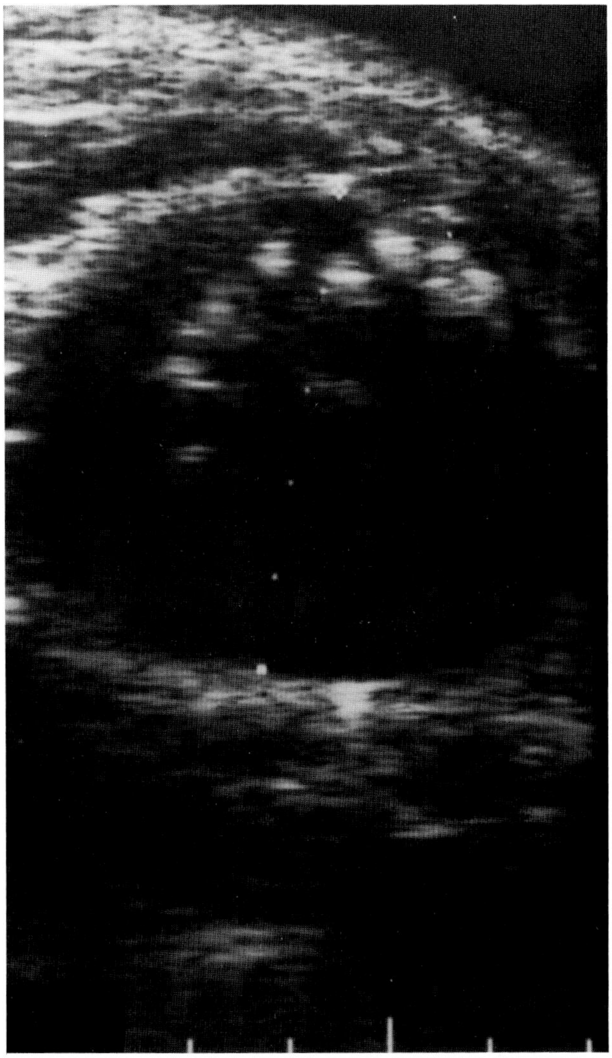

Fig. 3-24. A 10-MHz sonogram of the neck lateral to the jugular vein demonstrates a predominantly cystic metastasis (dots) from papillary cancer of the thyroid.

up of these patients and in the localization for fine needle aspiration. The prevalence of thyroid cancer is about 7 percent in patients with a history of neck irradiation[52,53] (Fig. 3-30A & B).

Treatment

The definitive treatment of thyroid cancer is surgical. Whether patients with papillary and follicular neoplasms should also be treated with postsurgical radioactive iodine therapy is controversial.

An alternative is ablation of both thyroid and parathyroid nodules with percutaneous ethanol injection. Although experience with this treatment is limited, early studies suggest its feasibility, while recognizing that injury to the recurrent laryngeal nerve, with vocal cord paralysis, is a potential risk.[54]

Postoperatively, patients who have had thyroid cancer resected can be followed with sonography to detect clinically occult thyroid bed tumor recurrence and lymph node metastases.[55] After thyroid surgery, the carotid artery is noted close to the trachea with little soft tissue intervening and no discrete mass of tissue, other than the superficial muscles, is seen. Recurrent tumor, which can occur anywhere in the neck and appears as a discrete mass sonographically, can be categorically defined with ease by fine needle aspiration with or without sonographic guidance.[56] In experienced hands, the sensitivity of sonographic detection in these cases is 96 percent and the specificity 83 percent.[55] Palpation is a poor prognosticator of recurrent cervical thyroid cancer.

Thyroid cancer does not have a unique pathognomonic appearance by sonography,[57] buy may present in a variety of ways. Simple cystic lesions are unlikely to

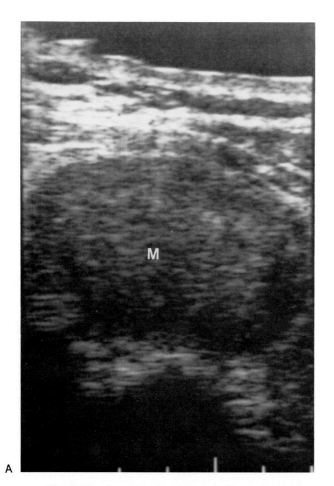

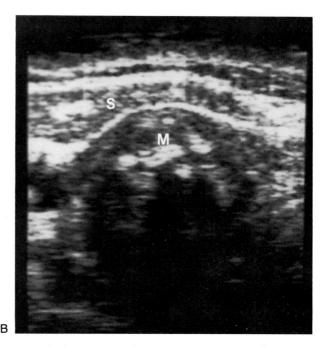

A   B

Fig. 3-25. **(A)** A longitudinal 10-MHz sonogram demonstrates on the left a sharply circumscribed solid mass of the thyroid, medullary thyroid carcinoma *(M)*. **(B)** On the right side, another focus is identified with the characteristic clumps of calcification, also medullary thyroid carcinoma, that abuts the strap muscles *(S)*.

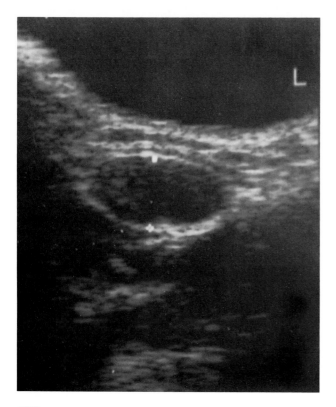

Fig. 3-26. A 10-MHz longitudinal sonogram of the upper neck defines an oval hypoechoic lymph node (dots) in a patient suspected of recurrent medullary thyroid cancer. The patient has no residual thyroid tissue.

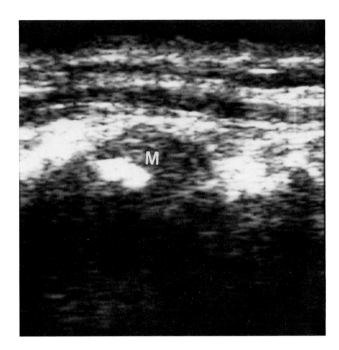

Fig. 3-27. A 10-MHz longitudinal sonogram of the neck in a patient with a total thyroidectomy for medullary thyroid carcinoma *(M)* shows a recurrent superficial metastasis with a clump of calcification within.

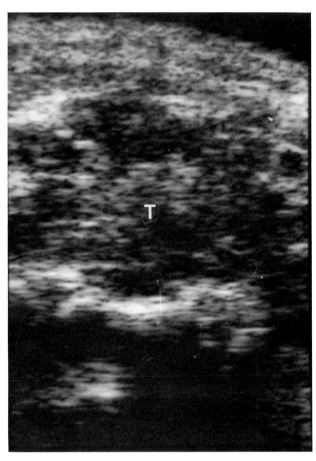

Fig. 3-29. A 10-MHz longitudinal sonogram defines an abnormal heterogeneous hypoechoic gland with irregular margination. The patient had irradiation therapy to the neck following a tonsillectomy 35 years prior and is at risk for malignant degeneration of the thyroid *(T)*.

harbor cancer. Lesions with both cystic and solid components have about an 11 percent likelihood of malignancy, usually involving papillary, follicular, and metastatic neoplasms[58] (Figs. 3-5, 3-31, and 3-32). Hyperechoic thyroid masses are usually benign (96 per-

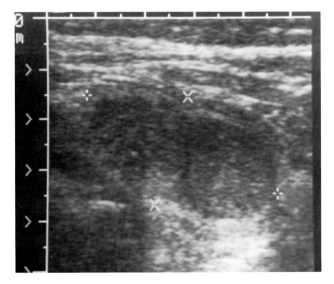

Fig. 3-28. A 5-MHz longitudinal sonogram of the left thyroid shows a solid nodular mass, a medullary thyroid carcinoma (crosshatches). This patient is the father of the patient in Fig. 3-25.

cent). Thyroid cancer tends to be hypoechoic (63 percent) or isoechoic (26 percent)[58] (Fig. 3-33). Calcifications occur in both benign and malignant disease of the thyroid, but some discrete clumps of calcification are associated with medullary thyroid carcinoma.[46] Boundaries may be discrete or irregular. Invasive cancer may extend into the adjacent soft tissues and muscle with cervical adenopathy and involvement with progressive invasion of the jugular vein or, rarely, the carotid artery[2] (Fig. 3-34). Solbiati et al[59] in a large series, have shown sonographically that microcalcifications smaller than 2 mm in diameter that have acoustic shadowing are more likely to be associated with malignant (61.8 percent) than with benign (1.6 percent) lesions. The sonographic findings were proven correct by fine needle aspiration. These calcifications correspond to those of psammoma bodies, which occur in both papillary and medullary carcinomas.

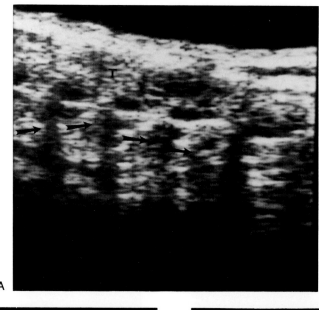

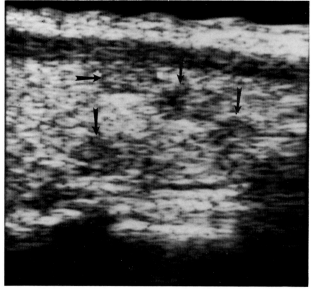

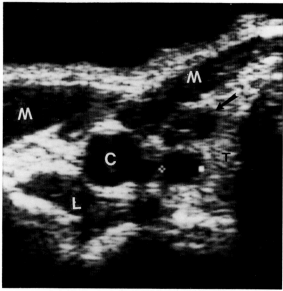

Fig. 3-30. **(A)** A 10-MHz longitudinal sonogram of the midline neck demonstrates a narrow band of normal thyroid isthmus *(T)* and recurrent acoustic shadows (arrows) from the normal tracheal rings. **(B)** A longitudinal 10-MHz sonogram of this woman's thyroid shows multiple thyroid nodules (arrows). She is 31 and had radiation treatment for acne at age 16. **(C)** A transverse sonogram of the thyroid shows both a cystic (dots) and an anterior solid lesion (arrow). (*L*, longus coli; *M*, sternocleidomastoid muscle and strap muscle; *T*, thyroid; *C*, carotid artery.)

With the development of color Doppler, the delineation of thyroid masses and their vascularity has the potential to generate additional information about these lesions.[60] Thyroid lesions 0.5 cm or less tend to be avascular, developing increased vascularity with increases in size. Cystic thyroid lesions are avascular.[61] Thyroid adenomas characteristically have a halo, which is a vascular boundary, but cancers can present similarly.[43,62]

Patients who have hyperparathyroidism often have a sonogram for localization prior to surgery. Thyroid lesions are common in this group (40 percent),[63] and malignancy occurs in 6 to 11 percent of these patients.[64] Thyroid lesions of a few millimeters or intrathyroidal parathyroid tumors noted by sonography are not always appreciated at surgery unless the surgeon actually incises the thyroid gland. Thyroid lesions are also frequently

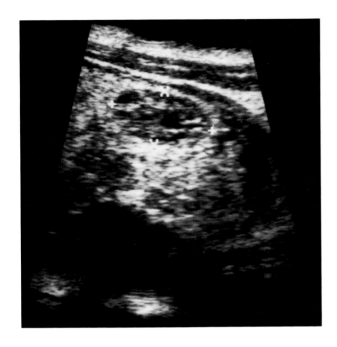

Fig. 3-31. A 10-MHz longitudinal sonogram of the thyroid shows an oval solid thyroid lesion with tiny cystic areas in a man (dots).

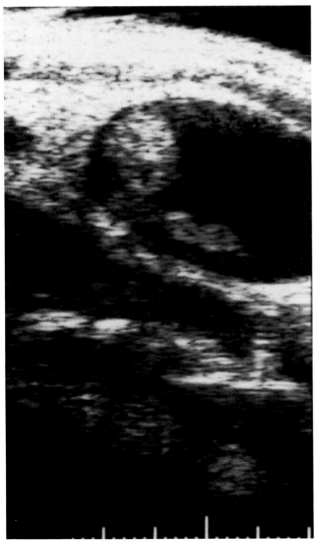

Fig. 3-32. A longitudinal sonogram demonstrates a largely cystic thyroid lesion with solid components. Overall, these types of lesions have about an 11 percent chance of malignancy (see Solbiati et al[58]).

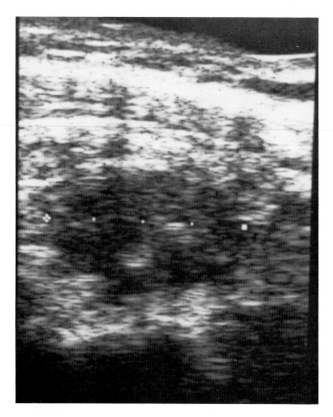

Fig. 3-33. A 10-MHz sonogram demonstrates on longitudinal plane an irregular hypoechoic mass (dots) in the left lobe of the thyroid, with a few tiny calcifications, a papillary thyroid carcinoma.

noted in passing by those who do sonography of the carotid artery.[65]

Metastases to the thyroid present as thyroid nodules, both discrete and diffuse, and develop secondary to lung cancer, malignant melanoma, renal cell carcinoma, and breast carcinoma.[66] Also, they sometimes develop in association with cervical adenopathy and jugular vein invasion. Fine needle aspiration yields material for the definitive diagnosis.[67]

COMPARISON STUDIES

Thyroid nodules are common and some clinicians aspirate palpable nodules without any localizing studies.

Scintigraphy is the study of choice for thyroid function. Poor resolution limits its ability to define morphology, whereas sonography has a distinct advantage.[68] With high resolution transducers, sonography can detect lesions of a few millimeters,[63] while scintigraphy is dependent on a size of at least 1 or 1.5 cm for reliable detection. Scintigraphy has greater detectability for peripheral lesions and those not hidden by superimposed radionuclide activity. This is analogous, in my mind, to the detection of renal cysts by intravenous

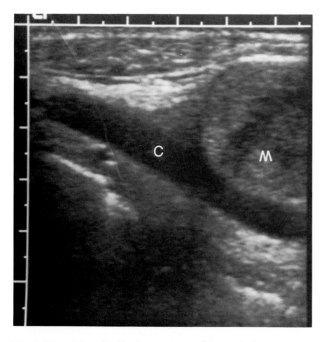

Fig. 3-34. A longitudinal sonogram of the neck demonstrates a mass *(M)*, which is a recurrent follicular cell carcinoma of the thyroid, compressing, but not actually invading, the carotid artery *(C)*.

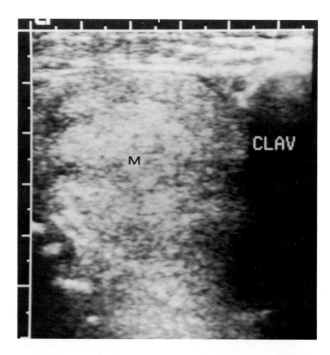

Fig. 3-35. A 5-MHz longitudinal sonogram of a large solid thyroid mass *(M)* shows that it extends below the clavicle (CLAV) and, therefore, cannot be seen in its entirety by ultrasound. CT or MRI would be indicated to see the morphology in the mediastinum.

urography, which has largely been supplanted by sonography.

Computed tomography, scintigraphy, and MRI are all effective localizers of thyroid pathology in the mediastinum.[16,64,69] Sonography is not (Fig. 3-35). CT has poor discrimination of thyroid lesions within the gland as well as motion and streak artifact from the shoulders.[69]

Limited experience suggests that MRI can be used to detect thyroid lesions but cannot distinguish thyroid from parathyroid abnormality within the gland.[70] Also, MRI has the potential to differentiate abnormal tissue due to tumor recurrence from postoperative fibrosis on the basis of differences in signal contrast.[71]

PARATHYROID

TECHNIQUE

High resolution, ideally obtained using a 10-MHz linear array transducer, is the key to successful sonographic detection of parathyroid abnormality. A good near field of view is necessary; therefore when a transducer with a longer focus is used a water path interface may be necessary. The average parathyroid tumor is about 1 cm in length and can be easily overlooked by the inexperienced (Fig. 3-36). If no lesion is seen, a lower frequency trans-

ducer (7.5 or 5 MHz) with greater penetration may allow detection of a deeper parathyroid tumor, which can be missed by the exclusive 4- to 5-cm near field of view that the 10-MHz transducer provides (Fig. 3-37).

The patient is scanned supine with the neck hyperextended, using an aqueous gel as a couplant. Transverse and longitudinal scans are taken from the upper neck at the level of the submandibular glands down to the sternal notch. The patient is asked to swallow in order to elevate by a few millimeters the soft tissues hidden behind the

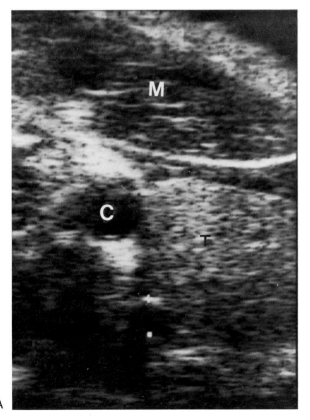

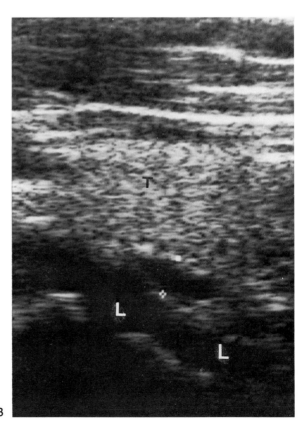

A   B

Fig. 3-36.   **(A)** A 10-MHz transverse sonogram demonstrates a small anechoic parathyroid adenoma posteriorly (dots). (*T*, thyroid; *M*, sternocleidomastoid muscle; *C*, carotid artery.) **(B)** A longitudinal 10-MHz sonogram demonstrates the parathyroid adenoma (dots) above the longus coli *(L)*. (*T*, thyroid.)

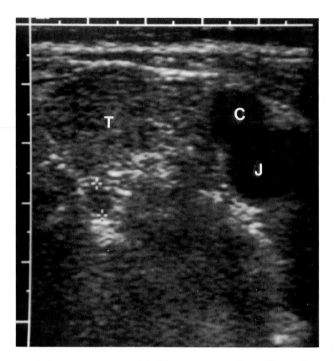

Fig. 3-37. A transverse 5-MHz sonogram of a small parathyroid adenoma (dots) illustrates the difficulties in visualization using lower frequency transducers to identify small lesions. (*T*, thyroid; *C*, carotid artery; *J*, jugular vein.)

sternum. This also helps to define the esophagus, which usually is posterior and medial, and just lateral to the midline trachea on the left. The esophagus appears as a linear structure that is hypoechoic with linear echoes within it. Occasionally, a bright focus of saliva will be seen flashing down it as the patient swallows. On transverse scan, the esophagus is oval or circular (Fig. 3-38).

The longus coli muscle lies posterior to the thyroid and the carotid artery bilaterally. As striated muscle, it appears hypoechoic with striations. Longitudinally, it runs the length of the thyroid gland, which is homogeneous and hyperechoic. On transverse scan the longus coli appears triangular. Parathyroid adenomas commonly lie along the longus coli adjacent to the thyroid, and sometimes can be confused with the longus coli, particularly when elongated.

Scans of the anterior neck are continued to the jugular veins, since about 1.6 percent of parathyroid adenomas may reside in the area of the carotid or jugular vessels. Masses lateral to the internal jugular vein are more likely to be nodes than parathyroid adenoma[72] (Fig. 3-39).

In patients who have had a thyroidectomy for thyroid cancer and have hyperparathyroidism, a small hypoechoic mass in the residual thyroid bed can be parathyroid adenoma or recurrent thyroid tumor. Aspiration biopsy serves to distinguish the two.

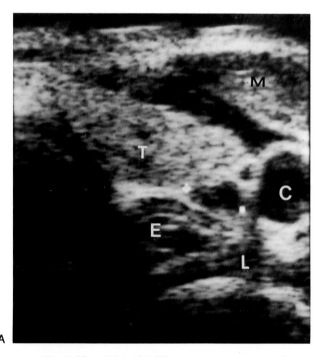

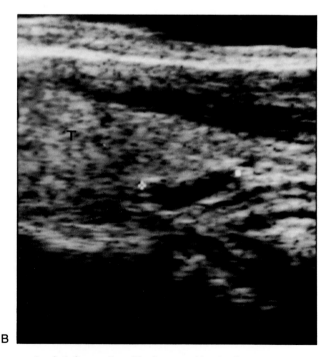

A   B

Fig. 3-38. **(A)** A 10-MHz transverse sonogram demonstrates a classic left parathyroid adenoma (dots) adjacent and lateral to the esophagus *(E)* on transverse image. (*C*, carotid artery; *M*, sternocleidomastoid muscle; *L*, longus coli.) **(B)** A 10-MHz longitudinal sonogram demonstrates a classic left parathyroid adenoma (dots) posteroinferior to the thyroid *(T)*.

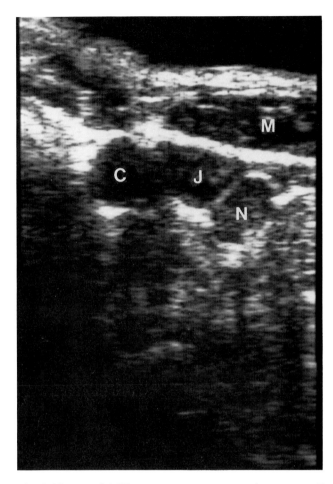

Fig. 3-39. A 10-MHz transverse sonogram shows a small solid mass *(N)* adjacent to and lateral to the jugular vein *(J)*. On dual tracer scintigraphy, this was thought to be a parathyroid adenoma. By sonography it has an appearance consistent with node because of the location, although parathyroid could not be excluded by the morphology alone. At surgery, this was a lymph node. (*N*, node; *C*, carotid artery; *M*, sternocleidomastoid muscle.)

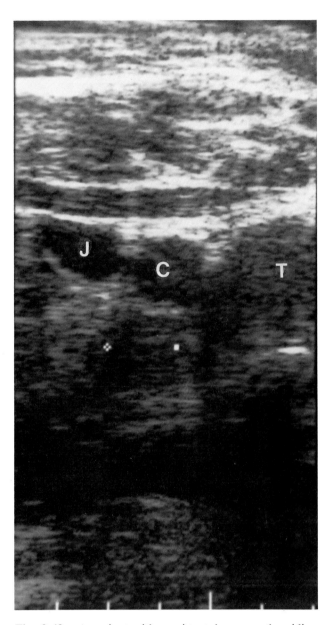

Fig. 3-40. A patient with persistent hyperparathyroidism after several parathyroidectomies has a hypoechoic lesion behind the carotid *(C)* on a transverse 10-MHz sonogram, which by aspiration under ultrasonic guidance proved to be a parathyroid adenoma. Lesions behind the great vessels are difficult to aspirate because of the risk of significant blood diluting the sample, so a path that avoids that possibility is necessary. (*J*, jugular; *T*, thyroid.)

Biopsy

Parathyroid biopsy is particularly helpful in patients who, despite prior parathyroid surgery, have not only recurrent or persistent disease but also a mass suspicious for parathyroid adenoma identified in the neck[73,74] (Fig. 3-40). If parathyroid tumor can be confirmed before surgery, the surgeon can explore that area as a first priority.[75-77]

Technique

With the neck hyperextended, the lesion is defined sonographically in two planes at right angles to one another and the distance marked from the skin surface to the midpoint of the mass. After a wheal of lidocaine 2 percent is injected in the superficial soft tissues, a short 22-gauge standard needle attached to a 10-ml syringe is directed into the lesion. With either a suction device for the syringe or hand-generated suction, the needle is pushed forward and back in the lesion several times, suction is released, the needle and syringe are removed, and the drop of cytologic material is smeared on a slide. The slides are prepared for cytologic examination as well as radioimmunoassay. In addition, parathyroid hormone (PTH) bioassay of selected material confirms the diagnosis. Because it may be difficult to differentiate cells of thyroid origin from those of parathyroid, the use of a parathyroid hormone antibody in an immunochemical system confirms the parathyroid origin of the cells in smears of fine needle aspirate.[78,94] This fine needle technique is simple to perform and without complication except for an occasional minor hematoma.

NORMAL ANATOMY

The parathyroid glands arise from endodermal derivatives, are about 4 by 3 by 1.5 mm,[79] and weigh from 117 to 131 mg.[80] The upper two glands originate from the fourth branchial cleft and descend into the neck during gestation, to rest posteriorly at about the level of the middle third of the thyroid gland. If the migration is anomalous, these upper glands may be found in other areas such as in the carotid sheath (1.6 percent)[81] or a retroesophageal locale. The lower two parathyroid glands arise from the third branchial cleft, as does the thymus, and descend into the neck in a more ventral position than the upper glands to rest in the area of the inferior thyroid, near the inferior thyroidal artery, which supplies them. Occasionally, the lower glands migrate with the thymus into the superior mediastinum, an ectopic location. Ectopic locales represent about 10 to 13 percent of the total. Intrathyroidal parathyroid adenomas occur in about 1 to 6 percent of cases.[82,83] Rare locations include the pharyngeal mucosa, the esophageal wall, and the pericardium, none of which are detected sonographically.[84,85]

The parathyroid glands are usually symmetric and intimately associated with the thyroid, and are often posterior in location. Most patients (84 percent) have four, a few (3 percent) have three parathyroid glands. In about 13 percent, five or more glands may be present.[86,87]

The four normal parathyroid glands are usually not seen by ultrasound, but occasionally a single one may be noted as a flat hypoechoic structure posterior to the thyroid and immediately adjacent to it (Fig. 3-41). Primarily oval or bean-shaped (83 percent), parathyroid glands are elongated in 11 percent. With adenomatous enlargement, elongated parathyroid glands can be confused sonographically with other linear structures such as the longus coli muscle. Bilobed or multilobed glands occur in 6 percent.[86]

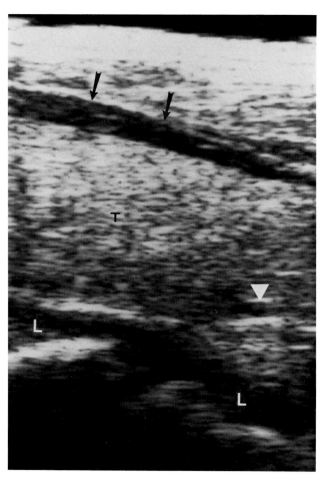

Fig. 3-41. A 10-MHz longitudinal sonogram of a normal thyroid *(T)* demonstrates the hypoechoic anterior strap muscles (arrows), the hypoechoic posterior longus coli muscle *(L),* and possibly a normal parathyroid gland (white arrowhead) inferoposterior to the thyroid.

HYPERPARATHYROIDISM

The basic histologic component of the parathyroid is the chief cell, which secretes parathyrin. With neoplastic change of the parathyroid (Fig. 3-42), patients develop hyperparathyroidism demonstrated by elevated serum calcium, elevated parathyrin levels, hypophosphatemia in 50 percent, and hypercalciuria.

Normal serum calcium ranges from 8.5 to 10.5 mg/dl. Routine screening examinations with determination of serum calcium elevations have detected increasing numbers of asymptomatic patients with primary hyperparathyroidism.

Radioimmunoassays for PTH vary in sensitivity. A reliable specific in vitro radioimmunoassay for PTH

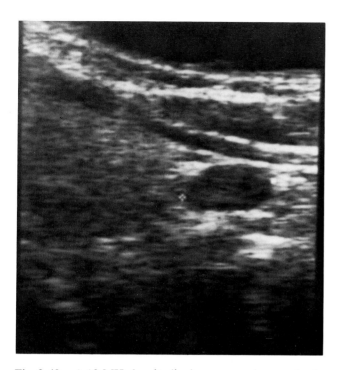

Fig. 3-42. A 10-MHz longitudinal sonogram shows a classic hypoechoic oval parathyroid adenoma inferior to the thyroid gland (dots).

confirms the diagnosis of hyperparathyroidism by detecting elevated circulating concentrations of iPTH. These concentrations are above the upper limit of the normal range in 90 percent of patients. Abbott and Arnaud[88] have shown that in the remaining 10 percent, formal discriminative analyses of serum iPTH and serum calcium distinguish 100 percent of hyperparathyroid patients from normal subjects.

C-terminal assays are superior to N-terminal assays in discriminating normal subjects from those with hyperparathyroidism. When primary hyperparathyroidism coexists with one of the nonparathyroid hypercalcemic states, C-terminal immunoreactive serum iPTH is increased, which permits a correct diagnosis. Patients with hypercalcemia due to causes other than parathyroid disease, such as malignancy, sarcoidosis, multiple myeloma, and vitamin D intoxication, have low or undetectable concentrations of parathyrin. In such cases the secretion is suppressed because of hypercalcemia.

With widespread screening of blood chemistry, patients with hyperparathyroidism may be asymptomatic at the time of diagnosis, although mild depression and lethargy are very common. Renal calculi and osseous changes of generalized osteopenia, subperiosteal resorption, and cystic lesions of bone develop over time. Skeletal lesions, the brown tumors, tend to resolve rapidly

after parathyroidectomy. Pancreatitis and peptic ulcer have also been associated with the disease.

Hyperparathyroidism may be primary, secondary, or tertiary. Most patients with overactivity of the parathyroid have primary hyperparathyroidism. Usually, this is related to a single benign parathyroid adenoma (85 percent), although in 3 percent of patients multiple adenomas may be present. A small number of patients with primary hyperparathyroidism (12 percent) will have parathyroid hyperplasia.[82] A few will present with a parathyroid cyst as the cause of their elevated parathyrin or will have a parathyroid cancer (4 percent).

Primary hyperparathyroidism occurs in about 1 in 700, with a preponderance of women (3:1),[79] and typically appears in the fourth decade. Children and the elderly may also be affected, although this is uncommon. The cause of primary hyperparathyroidism is not known.

Secondary hyperparathyroidism develops from chronic renal disease or intestinal malabsorption. Serum phosphorus rises and serum calcium falls, which precipitate chief cell hyperplasia and concomitant elevation of parathyrin in the parathyroid glands. Bone density increases and soft tissue calcifications develop. Patients typically develop enlargement of all the parathyroid glands (Fig. 3-43). Tertiary hyperparathyroidism refers to the entity of an autonomous parathyroid gland or glands that develop in the setting of secondary hyperparathyroidism.

Familial hyperparathyroidism is an autosomal dominant inherited trait associated with hyperplasia of all the parathyroid glands. Parathyroid chief cell hyperplasia is characteristic of both familial hyperparathyroidism and MEN types I and IIa. Those with MEN type IIa may have a concomitant medullary thyroid carcinoma amenable to detection by sonography. Patients with these inherited traits are at increased risk for recurrent and persistent disease following parathyroidectomy.[82]

The MEN syndromes are also inherited as autosomal dominant traits. MEN type I, or Wermer syndrome, is associated with parathyroid hyperplasia or multiple parathyroid adenomas, as well as pancreatic tumors of endocrine origin (insulinomas, gastrinomas), pituitary tumors, and a variety of miscellaneous neoplasms including carcinoid,[89] bronchial adenomas, lipomas, adrenal and ovarian tumors, melanoma, and differentiated thyroid cancer.[82]

Multiple endocrine neoplasia type II, or Sipple syndrome, has two categories: IIa includes medullary thyroid carcinoma and C-cell hyperplasia of the thyroid, parathyroid hyperplasia or adenomas, and pheochromocytoma; IIb refers to a category of medullary thyroid carcinoma, pheochromocytoma, ganglineuromatosis,

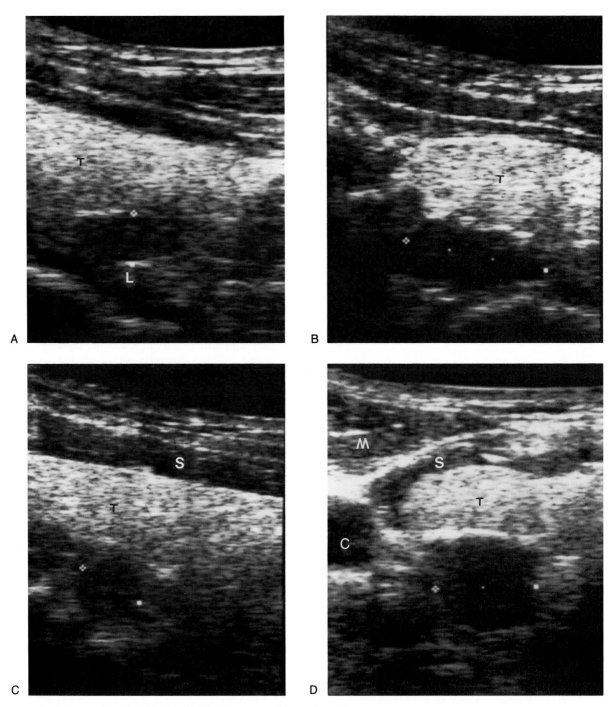

Fig. 3-43. **(A)** A 10-MHz longitudinal sonogram in a patient with secondary hyperparathyroidism and parathyroid hyperplasia (dots) shows a left lower parathyroid hyperplastic lesion. **(B)** A 10-MHz longitudinal sonogram in the same patient with secondary hyperparathyroidism and parathyroid hyperplasia (dots) shows a left upper hyperplastic parathyroid gland. **(C)** A 10-MHz longitudinal sonogram in the same patient with secondary hyperparathyroidism and parathyroid hyperplasia (dots) shows a right lower hyperplastic parathyroid gland. (*L*, longus coli; *T*, thyroid; *S*, strap muscle.) **(D)** A transverse 10-MHz sonogram in the same patient shows the right lower parathyroid hyperplastic lesion. (*M*, sternocleidomastoid muscle; *C*, carotid artery.)

mucosal neuromas, and marfanoid habitus with pectus excavatum.[82] In patients with MEN type II, close attention to both thyroid and parathyroid abnormalities is essential since ultrasound is used not only in the initial diagnosis of parathyroid hyperplasia and the detection of thyroid mass, but also in the follow-up of recurrent or persistent disease.

Parathyroid hyperplasia occurs in multiple endocrine neoplasia (MEN) types I and IIa. All the glands may enlarge, one may be predominant, or they may appear normal in size but be hyperplastic by pathologic examination.[90]

Low-dose radiation has also been implicated as a cause of hyperparathyroidism. Those who have been exposed to low-dose radiation have a higher incidence of both thyroid cancer and hyperparathyroidism.[91] Oral lithium therapy is associated with the development of hypercalcemia in 10 percent of cases and parathyroid adenoma has been found in some patients.[92]

Although parathyroid adenomas develop in both upper and lower glands, it may be that the superior glands, which tend to migrate posteriorly and inferiorly, are miscalled lower when ectopic.[82] Ectopic glands in the posterior mediastinum are likely to be superior glands, ectopic inferior glands migrate to the anterior mediastinum, usually in the thymus.

Parathyroid pathology is not usually palpable, al-though giant glands can be appreciated. However, ultrasound is not typically used as a screening test for the presence of parathyroid pathology. The patient is referred after a diagnosis of hyperparathyroidism has been reached as a result of abnormal elevated serum calcium levels and elevated serum parathyrin assays. These patients are evaluated by ultrasound primarily for localization prior to surgical removal. Sonography is not used to distinguish hypercalcemia of sarcoidosis, hyperthyroidism, multiple myeloma, milk alkali syndrome, vitamin A and D intoxication, or familial hypercalcemic hypocalciuria from parathyroid adenoma or hyperplasia. Serum biochemical studies can clarify those considerations.

Sonographic Appearance

First described sonographically by Sample et al,[93] most parathyroid adenomas are intimately associated with the thyroid gland. Of the 13 percent in ectopic locations, most are in the superior mediastinum and, although not amenable to sonographic detection, can be removed without a sternal-splitting incision.

The typical parathyroid adenoma is in the neck and by sonography is about 1 cm in length, oval, hypoechoic or anechoic without through transmission of enhanced

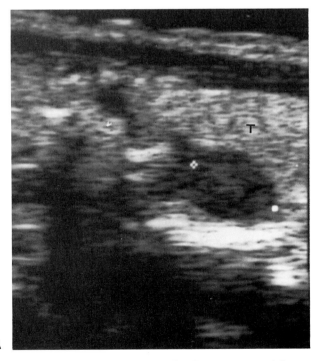
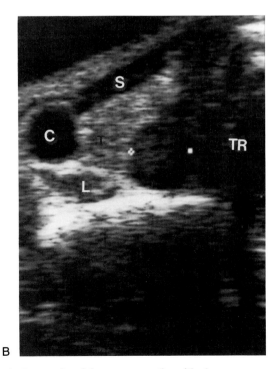

Fig. 3-44. **(A)** A 10-MHz longitudinal sonogram defines a typical posterior right upper parathyroid adenoma (dots). **(B)** A 10-MHz transverse sonogram of the same patient shows it medial to the trachea. (*L*, longus coli; *T*, thyroid; *S*, strap muscle; *TR*, trachea; *C*, carotid artery.)

echoes beyond its posterior boundaries (Figs. 3-38 and 3-44), and is oriented in a cranial-caudal direction, usually posterior to the thyroid. A position lateral to the adjacent thyroid and medial to the carotid artery is another common locale (Fig. 3-45). The discrete nature of the parathyroid adenoma is probably related to its encapsulation and the homogeneity of the sonographic appearance, to the sheets of cells (predominately chief cells) noted on pathologic examination. The parathyroid gland, classically hypoechoic and oval, is almost never more echoic than the thyroid, although with hemorrhage and fatty infiltration inhomogeneity may occur.

Although the relationship is not directly linear, larger parathyroid tumors tend to have higher calcium and parathyrin levels,[56] and are more likely to be detected. By sonography, glands as small as 3 to 4 mm are occasionally noted and the question arises as to whether these are normal parathyroid glands or hyperplastic tumors. Sonography is not as effective in delineating primary parathyroid hyperplasia. Sonographers must always be on the alert for more than one parathyroid gland, since primary hyperplasia occurs in 12 percent of cases and multiple adenomas in primary hyperparathyroidism occur in 3 percent of cases. In our experience with one patient,

to date, 10 hyperfunctioning parathyroid glands have been removed. Sonographically, primary parathyroid hyperplasia is difficult to assess correctly because although several glands are involved, one may be dominant, leading the examiner erroneously to the diagnosis of a single parathyroid adenoma. Also, primary hyperplastic glands tend to be small, often less than 200 mg, and may be undetected by ultrasound or any other imaging method. With 5-MHz transducers, these parathyroid abnormalities may not even be recognized as present. With MEN as a possibility, parathyroid hyperplasia is likely and medullary thyroid cancer should also be sought. This thyroid malignancy presents as a mass lesion within the thyroid and is sometimes with associated cervical adenopathy. Clumps of calcification are common in these particular neoplasms.

An intrathyroidal parathyroid adenoma (Figs. 3-46 and 3-47) can be detected with sonography but distinguishing it from other thyroid lesions is not always possible without confirmation by aspiration biopsy. A large thyroid gland will tend to obscure a small posteriorly located parathyroid adenoma. Multiple thyroid nodules tend to confuse the examiner in distinguishing thyroid from parathyroid when the findings are not classic.

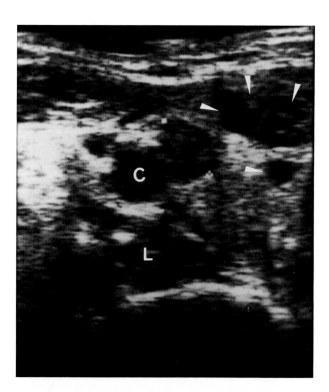

Fig. 3-45. A transverse 10-MHz sonogram of the neck defines an anterior parathyroid adenoma (dots) medial to the carotid artery *(C)* and, in addition, there are two hypoechoic thyroid lesions more medial and also anterior (arrowheads). (L, longus coli.)

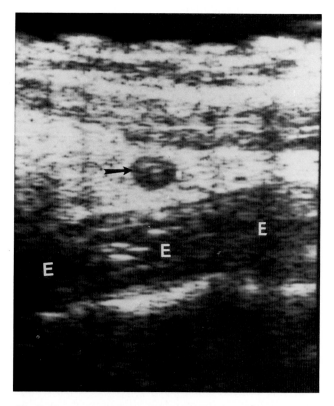

Fig. 3-46. A 10-MHz longitudinal sonogram demonstrates a typical hypoechoic 4-mm intrathyroidal parathyroid adenoma (arrow) in the left lower thyroid gland anterior to the hypoechoic esophagus *(E)*.

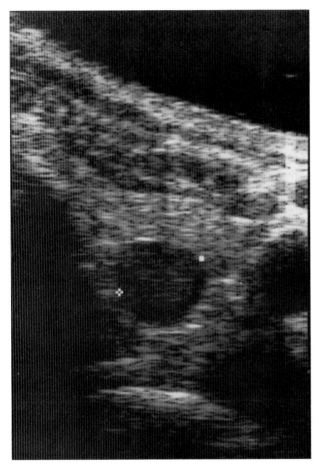

Fig. 3-47. A well-circumscribed intrathyroidal parathyroid adenoma (dots) is noted transversely on this 10-MHz sonogram, with echogenicity markedly lower than that of the normal surrounding thyroid tissue.

Small adjacent lymph nodes adjacent to the superior or inferior thyroid gland can also be difficult to differentiate from parathyroid adenoma, although false-positive designations are much less common than false-negative ones (Fig. 3-48).

The normal thyroid gland is relatively avascular, although with color Doppler the inferior and superior thyroidal arteries and veins can be identified. With color Doppler, parathyroid tumors up to 1 cm tend to be avascular, while those greater than that usually have some vascular component (Fig. 3-49 and Plates 3-1 and 3-2). The vascularity appears to be dependent on the size.[61] Focal hemorrhage in a parathyroid adenoma produces cystic areas sonographically. Calcification, so common in thyroid disease, is distinctly uncommon in parathyroid pathology. As the glands enlarge, increases in lobulation occur as well as both cystic changes and increased heterogeneity. In a series of 235 parathyroid glands, a simple parathyroid cyst was identified in 0.4 percent (Fig. 3-50), cystic changes in a solid gland in 3.8 percent, giant size of 3 cm or greater in 4.6 percent (Fig. 3-51), a multilobulated configuration in 2 percent, an inhomogeneous gland in 2 percent, and calcification in the gland in only 2.5 percent[95] (Figs. 3-52 and 3-53).

Parathyroid carcinoma may appear sonographically as a typical parathyroid adenoma (oval, hypoechoic, and well circumscribed) or may exhibit characteristics of heterogeneity and local soft tissue invasion[96,97] (Fig. 3-54). While these patients may present with mildly elevated serum calcium levels so typical of parathyroid adenoma, they are more likely to present with markedly elevated serum calcium in the range of 14 to 15 mg/ml or even in the 20 mg/ml range. With aggressive enlargement, a palpable cervical mass may develop with vocal cord paralysis secondary to local invasion. Parathyroid carcinoma and hyperplasia can coexist.[98]

Parathyroid cysts are distinctly uncommon as compared with the frequent incidence of thyroid cysts but are sonographically indistinguishable from thyroid cysts.[45,99-101] Usually the patient is normocalcemic. The cyst aspirate is clear, colorless, and contains parathyrin. Infrequently, a patient with hyperparathyroidism has a parathyroid cyst as the cause; other cases represent cystic degeneration in a parathyroid adenoma.[102]

Thyroid nodules are extremely common in patients with hyperparathyroidism (46 percent)[63] (Fig. 3-55). Of these, approximately 6 to 11 percent may be thyroid carcinoma.[103,104]

Obviously, a single parathyroid adenoma adjacent to an otherwise normal thyroid gland will be more likely to be detected accurately with sonography than several hyperplastic parathyroid adenomas in the matrix of an enlarged thyroid with multiple thyroid nodules. When several nodules are present and the question of thyroid versus parathyroid arises, only aspiration biopsy can ultimately separate categorically one from the other.

Under sonographic guidance, fine needle aspiration can confirm the diagnosis of parathyroid neoplasia by cytology, using the immunoperioxidase technique and bioassay.

Diagnostic Imaging

Hyperparathyroidism is a common disease associated with morbidity, including hypertension, renal stones, gout, peptic ulcers, pancreatitis, weakness, depression, and lethargy. Accurate and reliable, noninvasive preoperative localization studies have the potential at the time of surgery to decrease tissue dissection, allow for unilateral dissection in selected cases, shorten the surgery, and eventually may reduce the number of patients with persistent or recurrent disease. A highly sensitive noninva-

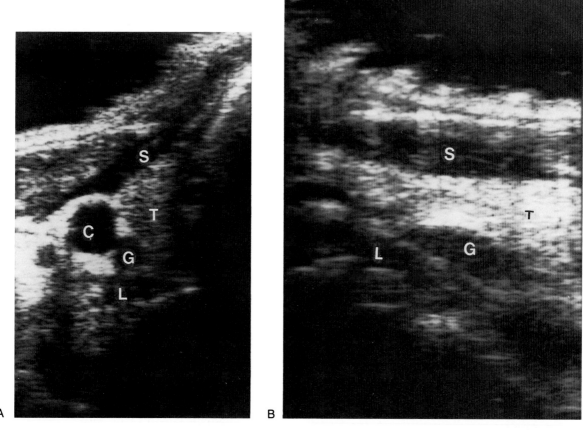

Fig. 3-48. **(A)** A transverse 10-MHz sonogram of the right thyroid gland *(T)* defines a small hypoechoic mass *(G)* medial to the carotid, which was thought to represent a possible parathyroid adenoma, but which at surgery proved to be an enlarged sympathetic ganglion. (*L*, longus coli; *C*, carotid artery; *S*, strap muscle.) **(B)** This oval hypoechoic ganglion *(G),* mimicking a parathyroid adenoma is also noted anterior to the longus coli *(L)* on longitudinal scan. (*T*, thyroid; *S*, strap muscle.)

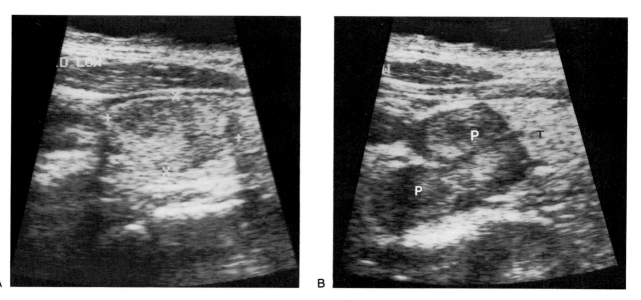

Fig. 3-49. **(A)** A 10-MHz longitudinal sonogram of the thyroid shows a well-circumscribed thyroid adenoma (crosshatches) with a faint halo. **(B)** This same patient also had a large lobulated parathyroid adenoma *(P).* Typically, as parathyroid adenomas increase in size, the echogenicity increases, as noted in this case. (*T*, thyroid.) (See also Plates 3-1 & 3-2.)

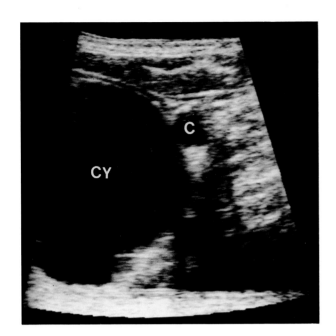

Fig. 3-50. A 10-MHz transverse sonogram demonstrates a large left parathyroid cyst *(CY)* just medial to the carotid artery *(C)*.

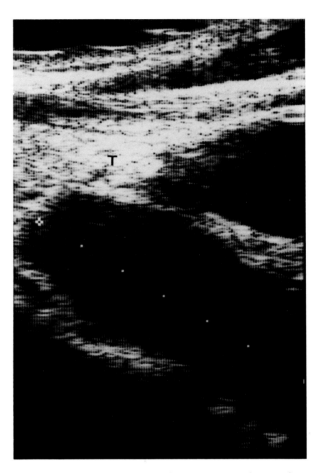

Fig. 3-51. A 10-MHz longitudinal sonogram shows a huge hypoechoic elongated parathyroid adenoma (dots). (*T*, thyroid.)

sive imaging modality can decrease patient morbidity, which eventually is reflected in decreased costs in the care of these patients.

If high resolution instrumentation and an experienced clinician are available, the first study to be considered in the evaluation of hyperparathyroidism is high resolution ultrasound. If that is positive and typical, the patient may then undergo surgery. Sensitivity of sonographic detection depends not only on the experience of the examiner and the interpreter, but also on the resolution of the transducers used, as well as the size of the parathyroid glands and the presence of concomitant thyroid disease or adenopathy. Patients with persistent and recurrent disease and those with hereditary susceptibility for parathyroid hyperplasia will offer the greatest challenge (Fig. 3-56). Sensitivity figures for the detection of parathyroid lesions by sonography range from 36 percent to 88 percent.[105-109]

In our hands, from 48 to 82 percent of all cases, depending on the patient mix, will be appropriately identified, with the lower figures for detection of primary parathyroid hyperplasia, and the higher for parathyroid adenoma[110-112] (Fig. 3-56). In another study, overall sensitivities in the detection of parathyroid disease in a prospective comparison of 100 patients were 73 percent using double tracer scintigraphy, 68 percent using CT, 55 percent using ultrasound, 57 percent using MRI, with specificities of 87 percent or higher.[105] Parathyroid tumors of less than 250 mg in this series had poor detec-

tion rates and small hyperplastic glands with multiple gland disease were not detected by any modality.[105]

A significant increase in sensitivity occurs when an additional diagnostic imaging study is added to a single one. If the initial sonographic study is equivocal or a confirmation is in order, another study is obtained (dual tracer scintigraphy with thallium 201 and technetium 99m pertechnetate, CT, or MRI.[110,113-115] The choice depends on the resources available and the expertise of the examiner. Sonography is not the tool to identify lesions in the mediastinum.

Scintigraphy has the disadvantage of only one plane of visualization, as opposed to sonography. However scintigraphy compares favorably with ultrasound, with the same limitations of poor detection rates for primary hyperplasia. The advantage of scintigraphy is that it provides a mediastinal window. Ultrasound is not effective for localization in the mediastinum or in areas where air or bone interfere with visualization (e.g., the retroesophageal locale or a location posterior to inferior clavicle).

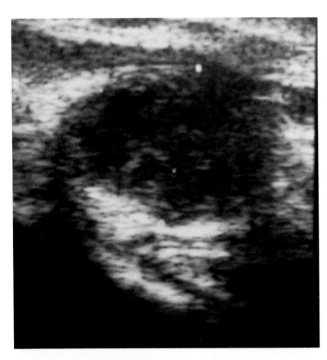

Fig. 3-52. A 10-MHz longitudinal sonogram of an inhomogeneous parathyroid adenoma (dots), which had tiny cystic areas on pathologic examination.

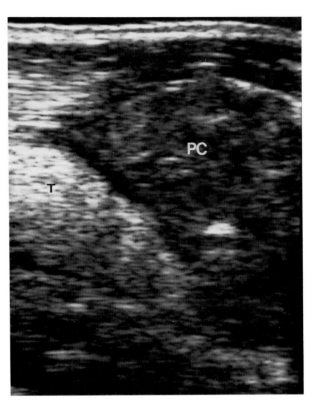

Fig. 3-54. A longitudinal 10-MHz sonogram shows inferior to normal thyroid *(T)* a hypoechoic mass extending into the anterior musculature, a parathyroid cancer *(PC)*.

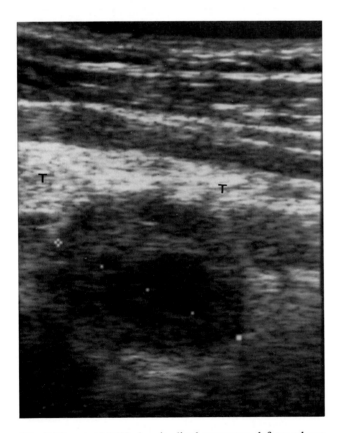

Fig. 3-53. A 10-MHz longitudinal sonogram defines a large parathyroid adenoma (dots) with a central cystic component. (*T*, thyroid.)

Double tracer scintigraphy (thallium 201 and technetium 99m pertechnetate), CT, and MRI are all appropriate for mediastinal parathyroid detection. When an additional study is added to the ultrasound examination (scintigraphy, CT, or MRI), the sensitivity of detection rises.[105,111,112,115,116] High resolution ultrasound and scintigraphy in combination allow detection of 91 percent of parathyroid adenomas.[110] High resolution ultrasound and MRI in combination have been used effectively for parathyroid detection with an 86 percent sensitivity prospectively, and a 95 percent detection rate retrospectively.[111]

Often, a definitive diagnosis can be accurately made when a combination of the above modalities are used. However, if results are still problematic, the patient may then undergo highly selective venous catheterization with sampling of the inferior thyroidal and innominate veins in hope of defining a step-up of twice normal immunoreactive parathyrin concentration, which in effect localizes the parathyroid tumor. While this is an invasive, time-consuming, and expensive procedure, it may positively localize the parathyroid mass (57 percent) whereas the other studies may not have been able to do so[115]; it also has an overall sensitivity of 70 to 80 percent for some sonographers.[115,117] For PTH assay, venous

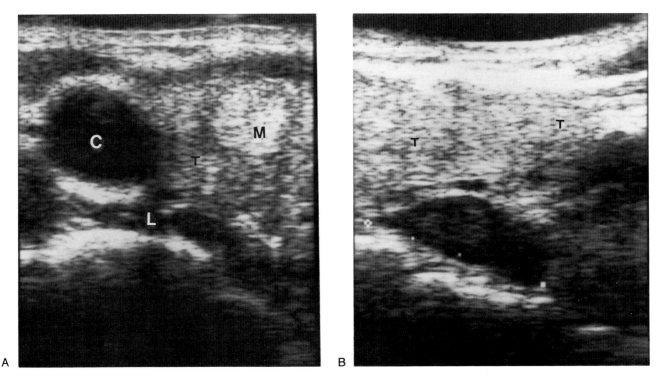

Fig. 3-55. (A) A transverse 10-MHz sonogram demonstrates a hyperechoic discrete mass *(M)* in the anterior upper right thyroid *(T)* that proved to be a thyroid adenoma in a thyroid with Hashimoto's thyroiditis, which accounts for the decreased echoes of the rest of the thyroid gland. (*C*, carotid artery; *L*, longus coli.) **(B)** A longitudinal 10-MHz sonogram in the same patient shows a right lower posterior parathyroid adenoma (dots).

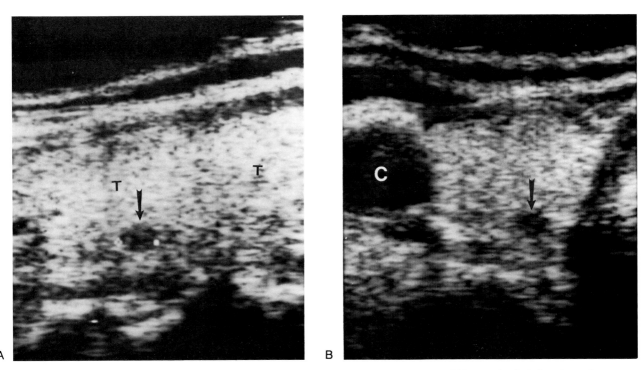

Fig. 3-56. (A) A 10-MHz longitudinal sonogram demonstrates a small parathyroid hyperplastic lesion (arrow) in a patient with multiple endocrine neoplasia. She also had a thyroid adenoma. Her daughter had a large unsuspected parathyroid adenoma and a benign thyroid lesion. Her two grandchildren had normal sonograms. (*T*, thyroid.) **(B)** A 10-MHz transverse sonogram in the same case demonstrates a small parathyroid hyperplastic lesion (arrow) in a patient with multiple endocrine neoplasia. (*C*, carotid artery.)

sampling should include specimens from both right and left inferior thyroidal veins and the major drainage from both superior and inferior parathyroid glands. If possible, other samples should include superior thyroidal, middle thyroidal, vertebral, thymic, and internal mammary veins.[118] Inferior thyroidal vein gradients are not pathognomonic for localization, for although they actually define the side, both neck and mediastinal adenomas may drain into the vessel. Venous drainage from the mediastinal parathyroid glands ascends via the thymic veins to the left innominate vein, or the vein may drain laterally into the internal mammary vein. Alternatively, the veins may drain back into the inferior thyroidal veins in the neck. A left innominate venous sampling alone in the presence of a gradient greater than two does not identify either the laterality (right versus left) or the location (neck versus mediastinum), since right and left inferior thyroidal and thymic veins will all drain into it. The more specific the sampling, the more precise the localization is likely to be.

Since parathyroid tumors tend to be highly vascular,[119] as an alternative in difficult cases, others have used angiography and intra-arterial digital subtraction angiography with fair results,[117] particularly when noninvasive tests are negative and the patient has recurrent disease. Invasive procedures such as venous sampling and angiography have an inherently higher risk of significant complications.

Intraoperative parathyroid localization is a further step in the localization process and has a sensitivity of 78 percent when performed by an experienced sonographer.[117] Because the incision is relatively limited, small high resolution transducers covered by a sterile sheath are necessary. Saline is the contact agent.

Computed tomography with contrast agents is also effective when performed by experienced sonographers, provided a positioning device is available to reduce the problems with the shoulder artifact interfering with visualization of the lower neck.[83,120] Parathyroid enhancement following contrast is variable. CT is not effective in intrathyroidal detection because the enhancement of the thyroid obscures the parathyroid lesions.[83]

With MRI, the typical parathyroid adenoma has low to medium signal intensity on short TR/TE images (T_1-weighted), and high signal intensity on long TR/TE images (T_2-weighted), but this varies from the norm when degenerative changes and hemorrhage exist within the parathyroid adenoma.[64,121]

Naturally, the imaging studies of choice will depend on what technology is available and the expertise of the technicians and radiologists who perform and evaluate the studies. Sonography is the least expensive and the fastest to perform, it does not require contrast agents, and no radiation is involved. Overall, diagnostic imaging, including sonography, has about a 76 percent sensitivity for detection of parathyroid pathology.[122]

Cost considerations limit the use of diagnostic imaging in every case, but in recurrent and persistent hyperparathyroidism, imaging studies allow a more precise approach and may prevent the necessity of exploration of the mediastinum. Before diagnostic imaging modalities were available, reoperation for parathyroid neoplasm was successful in finding the lesion in only 65 percent of cases.[123]

Treatment

Surgery is the conventional treatment for hyperparathyroidism, particularly in symptomatic patients and those with calcium serum levels over 11 mg/dl.[82] Surgeons are 95 percent accurate in removing the parathyroid adenoma on the first try. However, when the patient has recurrent or persistent hyperparathyroidism, and the next attempt is made without localizing studies, the chances of surgical intervention yielding a positive identification of the offending tumor is significantly reduced.[123] That is why localizing studies have gained such popularity. They have the potential to guide the surgeon to the correct site in the neck, or with MRI, CT, and scintigraphy to ectopic locations in the mediastinum.

Primary parathyroid hyperplasia is treated with subtotal parathyroidectomy of 3.5 glands.[124] Autotransplantation of parathyroid tissue into the forearm with removal of all parathyroid tissue from the neck is another approach. This transplant can be functionally identified with double tracer scintigraphy and is occasionally defined with sonography.

Secondary hyperparathyroidism is treated medically. Sonography has a sensitivity of about 76 percent in this category of parathyroid disease[125,126] and it can be helpful in the management of patients on chronic hemodialysis, where it is used to follow the size of the parathyroid glands.[127] The parathyroid hyperplastic glands of secondary hyperparathyroidism tend to be larger than those of primary hyperplasia and more reliably detected by diagnostic imaging. Surgery for secondary hyperparathyroidism is recommended in 5 to 10 percent of cases[128] when hypercalcemia is marked or osseous disease is debilitating. Subtotal parathyroidectomy or total parathyroidectomy with parathyroid autotransplantation into the forearm are the options.

Following parathyroid surgery, recurrent hyperparathyroidism is common in patients with familial hyperparathyroidism and in MEN type I.[82]

Following surgical removal, pathologic examination of parathyroid tissue is complicated because review of the material does not always delineate clearly normal from abnormal parathyroid, or even parathyroid adenoma from chief cell hyperplasia.[79] Therefore the final diagnosis sometimes must be made by the surgeon who relies on the appearance of the gland in relation to the adjacent tissue.

Interventional angiographic techniques have been used to embolize mediastinal parathyroid adenomas in poor-risk patients.[129,130]

Recent experience, although limited, suggests that parathyroid ablation with ethanol injection of the parathyroid tumor, applied under sonographic localization, has the potential to ameliorate the disease in some instances. As such it is a possible alternative to surgery in elderly or high-risk patients. The major risk for this approach is the possibility of both transient and permanent vocal cord paralysis by injection near or into the recurrent laryngeal nerve, which is in close proximity to the lesion.[131,132]

Summary

Parathyroid localizing tests are helpful before the initial parathyroidectomy procedure to define the appropriate side and to indicate the possibility of mediastinal disease, but they are most important in patients with persistent or recurrent disease. In these patients, scarring and fibrosis may be evident. Surgical planes are not as well defined. Successful resection is much more problematic. Diagnostic imaging adds a measure of certainty, particularly when two or more of the studies (ultrasound, CT, scintigraphy, or MRI) suggest a similar site. Successful preliminary localization of parathyroid pathology permits a shortened exploration time. Therefore, less anesthetic is required and there is potential for decreased risk to the patient.

REFERENCES

1. Ralls PW, Mayekawa DS, Lee KP et al: Color-flow Doppler sonography in Graves disease: "thyroid inferno." AJR 1988;150:781
2. Hayashi N, Tamaki N, Konishi J et al: Sonography of Hashimoto's thyroiditis. J Clin Ultrasound 1986;14:123
3. Gooding GAW, Langman AL, Dillon WP et al: Malignant carotid artery invasion: sonographic detection. Radiology 1989;171:435
4. Clark OH (ed): Thyroid nodules and thyroid cancer. p. 56. In Endocrine Surgery of the Thyroid and Parathyroid Glands. 1st Ed. CV Mosby, St. Louis, 1985
5. Vinatier D, Cosson M, Proye C et al: Thyroid cancer and pregnancy. Rev Fr Gynecol Obstet 1989;84:919
6. Brander A, Kivisaari L: Ultrasonography of the thyroid during pregnancy. J Clin Ultrasound 1989;17:403
7. Rasmussen NG, Hornnes PJ, Hegedus L: Ultrasonographically determined thyroid size in pregnancy and post partum: the goitrogenic effect of pregnancy. Am J Obstet Gynecol 1989;160:1216
8. Ivarsson SA, Ericsson UB, Fredriksson B et al: Ultrasonic imaging in the differential diagnosis of diffuse thyroid disorders in children. Am J Dis Child 1989;143:1369
9. Ueda D: Sonographic measurement of the volume of the thyroid gland in healthy children. Acta Paediatr Jpn 1989;31:352
10. Berghout Z, Wiersinga WM, Smits NJ et al: Determinants of thyroid volume as measured by ultrasonography in healthy adults in a non-iodine deficient area. Clin Endocrinol 1987;26:273
11. Reading CC, Charboneau JW, James EM et al: Sonographically guided percutaneous biopsy of small (3 cm or less) masses. AJR 1988;151:189
12. Rizzatto G, Solbiati L, Croce F et al: Aspiration biopsy of superficial lesions: ultrasonic guidance with a linear-array probe. AJR 1987;148:623
13. Abele JS, Miller TR: Fine-needle aspiration of the thyroid nodule: clinical applications. p. 293. In Clark OH (ed): Endocrine Surgery of the Thyroid and Parathyroid Glands. 1st Ed. CV Mosby, St. Louis, 1985
14. Akerman M, Tennvall J, Bjorklund A et al: Sensitivity and specificity of fine needle aspiration cytology in the diagnosis of tumor of the thyroid gland. Acta Cytol 1985;29:850
15. Ramacciotti CE, Pretorius HT, Chu EW et al: Diagnostic accuracy and use of aspiration biopsy in the rapid diagnosis and management of thyroid neoplasm. Arch Intern Med 1984;144:1699
16. Suen KCH, Quenville NF: Fine needle aspiration biopsy of the thyroid gland. J Clin Pathol 1983;36:1036
17. Muller N, Cooperberg PL, Suen KCH et al: Needle aspiration biopsy in cystic papillary carcinoma of the thyroid. AJR 1985;144:252
18. Solbiati L, Pra LD, Ierace T et al: High-resolution sonography of the recurrent laryngeal nerve: anatomic and pathologic considerations. AJR 1985;145:989
19. Muir A, Daneman D, Daneman A et al: Thyroid scanning, ultrasound, and serum thyroglobulin in determining the origin of congenital hypothyroidism. Am J Dis Child 1988;142:214
20. Leger J, Le Guern H, Plouhinec C et al: Antenatal diagnosis of goiter by ultrasonography. Presse Med 1987;16:1521
21. Vazquez-Chaves C, Acevedo-Rivera K, Sartorius C et al: Thyroid hemiagenesis. Report of 3 cases and review of the literature. Gac Med Mex 1989;125:395
22. Jaques DA, Chambers RG, Oertel JE: Thyroglossal tract carcinoma. A review of the literature and addition of eighteen cases. Am J Surg 1970;120:439
23. Birchall IW, Chow CC, Metreweli C: Ultrasound appearances of De Quervain's thyroiditis. Clin Radiol 1990;41:57
24. Tokuda Y, Kasagi K, Tida Y et al: Sonography of subacute thyroiditis: changes in the findings during the course of the disease. J Clin Ultrasound 1990;18:21

25. Benker G, Olbricht T, Windeck R et al: The sonographical and functional sequelae of De Quervain's subacute thyroiditis: long-term follow-up. Acta Endocrinol 1988;117:435

26. Nordmeyer JP, Shafeh TA, Heckmann C: Thyroid sonography in autoimmune thyroiditis. A prospective study on 123 patients. Acta Endocrinol 1990;122:391

27. Azagra JS, Frederic N, Demeester-Mirkine N et al: Value of echography for measuring the volume of the thyroid and its lesions. J Radiol 1990;71:109

28. Scheible W, Leopold GR, Woo VL et al: High-resolution real-time ultrasonography of thyroid nodules. Radiology 1979;133:413

29. Rosai J: Thyroid gland. p. 391. In Ackerman's Surgical Pathology. 7th Ed. CV Mosby, St. Louis, 1989

30. Yamamoto T, Sakamoto H: Spontaneous remission from primary hypothyroidism. Ann Intern Med 1978;88:808

31. Gutekunst R, Hafermann W, Mansky T et al: Ultrasonography related to clinical and laboratory findings in lymphocytic thyroiditis. Acta Endocrinol 1989;121:129

32. Nikolai TF, Brosseau J, Kettrick MA et al: Lymphocytic thyroiditis with spontaneously resolving hyperthyroidism (silent thyroiditis). Arch Intern Med 1980;140:478

33. Rojeski MT, Gharib H: Nodular thyroid disease. Evaluation and management. N Engl J Med 1985;313:428

34. Simeone JF, Daniels GH, Mueller PR et al: High-resolution real-time sonography of the thyroid. Radiology 1982;145:431

35. Katz JF, Kane RA, Reyes J et al: Thyroid nodules: sonographic pathologic correlation. Radiology 1984;151:741

36. Hegedus L, Hansen JE, Veiergang D et al: Thyroid size and goitre frequency in hyperthyroidism. Dan Med Bull 1987;34:121

37. Iwasawa T, Takebayashi S, Ozawa Y et al: High-resolution ultrasound of the thyroid in patients with Graves' disease. Nippon Igaku Hoshasen Gakkai Zasshi 1989;49:249

38. Given-Wilson R, Pope RM, Michell MJ et al: The use of real-time orbital ultrasound in Graves' ophthalmopathy: a comparison with computed tomography. Br J Radiol 1989;62:705

39. Smyrk TC, Goeliner JR, Brennan MD et al: Pathology of the thyroid in amiodarone-associated thyrotoxicosis. Am J Surg Pathol 1987;11:197

40. Rapoport B: Hypothyroidism. p. 144. In Clark OH (ed): Endocrine Surgery of the Thyroid and Parathyroid Glands. 1st Ed. CV Mosby, St. Louis, 1985

41. Gharib HK, James EM, Charboneau JW et al: Suppressive therapy with levothyroxine for solitary thyroid nodules. A double-blind controlled clinical study. N Engl J Med 1987;317:70

42. Brander A, Viikinkoski P, Nickels J et al: Thyroid gland: US screening in middle-aged women with no previous thyroid disease. Radiology 1989;173:507

43. Fobbe F, Finke R, Reichenstein E et al: Appearance of thyroid diseases using colour-coded duplex sonography. Eur J Radiol 1989;9:29

44. Hegedus L, Hansen JM, Karstrup S et al: Tetracycline for sclerosis of thyroid cysts. A randomized study. Arch Intern Med 1988;148:1116

45. Clark OH, Okerlund MD, Cavalieri RR et al: Diagnosis and treatment of thyroid, parathyroid, and thyroglossal duct cysts. J Clin Endocrinol Metab 1979;48:963

46. Gorman B, Charboneau JW, James EM et al: Medullary thyroid carcinoma: role of high-resolution US. Radiology 1987;162:147

47. Wells SA Jr, Baylin SB, Leight GS et al: The importance of early diagnosis in patients with hereditary medullary thyroid carcinoma. Ann Surg 1982;195:595

48. Fletcher JR: Medullary (solid) carcinoma of the thyroid gland. A review of 249 cases. Arch Surg 1970;100:257

49. Takashima S, Morimoto S, Ikezoe J et al: Primary thyroid lymphoma: comparison of CT and US assessment. Radiology 1989;171:439

50. Parulekar SG, Katzman RA: Primary malignant lymphoma of the thyroid: sonographic appearance. J Clin Ultrasound 1986;14:60

51. Stewart RR, David CL, Eftekhari F et al: Thyroid gland: US in patients with Hodgkins disease treated with radiation therapy in childhood. Radiology 1989;172:159

52. Refetoff S, Harrison J, Karanfilski BT et al: Continuing occurrence of thyroid carcinoma after irradiation to the neck in infancy and childhood. N Engl J Med 1975;292:171

53. Favus MJ, Schneider AB, Stachura ME et al: Thyroid cancer occurring as a late consequence of head-and-neck irradiation. Evaluation of 1056 patients. N Engl J Med 1976;294:1019

54. Livraghi T, Paracchi A, Ferrari C et al: Treatment of autonomous thyroid nodules with percutaneous ethanol injection: preliminary results. Work in Progress. Radiology 1990;175:827

55. Simeone JF, Daniels GH, Hall DA et al: Sonography in the follow-up of 100 patients with thyroid carcinoma. AJR 1987;148:45

56. Sutton RT, Reading CC, Charboneau JW et al: US-guided biopsy of neck masses in postoperative management of patients with thyroid cancer. Radiology 1988;168:769

57. Hayashi N, Tamaki N, Yamamoto K et al: Real-time ultrasonography of thyroid nodules. Acta Radiol 1986;27:403

58. Solbiati L, Volterrani L, Rizzato G et al: Thyroid gland with low uptake lesions: evaluation by US. Radiology 1985;155:187

59. Solbiati L, Arsizio B, Ballarati E et al: Microcalcifications: a clue in the diagnosis of thyroid malignancies. Radiology, suppl. 1990;177:140

60. Woodcock JP, Owen GM, Shedden EJ et al: Duplex scanning of the thyroid. Ultrasound Med Biol 1985;11:659

61. Gooding GAW, Clark OH: Color coded Doppler imaging in the distinction between thyroid and parathyroid lesions. Am J Surg (in press)

62. Propper RA, Skolnick ML, Weinstein BJ et al: The nonspecificity of the thyroid halo sign. J Clin Ultrasound 1980;8:129

63. Stark DD, Clark OH, Gooding GAW et al: High resolution ultrasound and computerized tomography of thyroid lesions in patients with hyperparathyroidism. Surgery 1983;94:863

64. Stark DD, Moss AA, Gamsu G et al: Nuclear magnetic resonance imaging of the neck: pathologic findings. Radiology 1984;150:455

65. Hubert JP Jr, Kiernan PD, Beahrs OH et al: Occult papillary carcinoma of the thyroid. Arch Surg 1980; 115:394

66. Shimaoka K, Sokal JE, Pickren JW: Metastatic neoplasms in the thyroid gland. Pathological and Clinical findings. Cancer 1962;15:557

67. Eftekhari F, Peuchot M: Thyroid metastases: combined role of ultrasonography and fine needle aspiration biopsy. J Clin Ultrasound 1989;17:657

68. Ikekubo K, Higa T, Hirasa M et al: Evaluation of radionuclide imaging and echography in the diagnosis of thyroid abnormalities. Clin Nucl Med 1986;11:145

69. Carroll BA: Asymptomatic thyroid nodules: incidental sonographic detection. AJR 1981;133:499

70. Gegter WB, Spritzer CE, Eisenberg B et al: Thyroid imaging with high-field strength surface-coil MR. Radiology 1987;164:483

71. Aufferman W, Clark OH, Thurnher S et al: Recurrent thyroid carcinoma: characteristics on MR images. Radiology 1988;168:753

72. Sutton RT, Reading CC, Charboneau JW et al: US-guided biopsy of neck masses in postoperative management of patients with thyroid cancer. Radiology 1988;168:769

73. Clark OH, Gooding GAW, Ljung BM: Locating a parathyroid adenoma by ultrasonography and aspiration biopsy cytology. West J Med 1981;135:154

74. Gooding GAW, Okerlund MD, Stark DD et al: Parathyroid imaging: comparison of double tracer (thallium-201 technetium-99m) scintigraphy and high resolution sonography. Radiology 1986;161:57

75. Karstrup S, Glenthoj A, Hainau B et al: Ultrasound-guided histological, fine-needle biopsy from suspect parathyroid tumours: success-rate and reliability of histological diagnosis. Br J Radiol 1989;62:981

76. Kahaly G, Krause U, Dienes HP et al: Fine-needle biopsy of parathyroid adenomas. Klin Wochenschr 1986;64:1176

77. Solbiati L, Montali G, Croce F et al: Parathyroid tumors detected by fine needle aspiration biopsy under ultrasonic guidance. Radiology 1983;148:793

78. Winkler V, Gooding GAW, Montgomery CK et al: Immunoperoxidase confirmation of parathyroid origin of ultrasound-guided fine needle aspirates of the parathyroid glands. Acta Cytol 1987;31:40

79. Rosai J: Parathyroid glands. p. 449. In Ackerman's Surgical Pathology. 7th Ed. CV Mosby, St. Louis, 1989

80. Gilmour JR, Maring WJ: The weight of the parathyroid glands. J Pathol Bacteriol 1937;44:431

81. Wang C: The anatomic basis of parathyroid surgery. Ann Surg 1975;183:271

82. Clark OH (ed): Hyperparathyroidism. p. 172. In Endocrine Surgery of the Thyroid and Parathyroid Glands. CV Mosby, St. Louis, 1985

83. Stark DD, Gooding GAW, Moss AA et al: Parathyroid imaging: comparison of high-resolution CT and high-resolution sonography. AJR 1983;141:633

84. Herrold KM, Rabson AS, Ketcham AS: Aberrant parathyroid gland in pharyngeal submucosa. Arch Pathol 1962;73:60

85. Sloane JA, Moody HC: Parathyroid adenoma in submucosa of esophagus. Arch Pathol Lab Med 1978;102:242

86. Akerstrom G, Malmaeus J, Bergstrom R: Surgical anatomy of human parathyroid glands. Surgery 1984;95:14

87. Russel CF, Grant SS, van Heerden JA: Hyperfunctioning supernumerary parathyroid glands. An occasional cause of hyperparathyroidism. Mayo Clin Proc 1982;57:122

88. Abbott SR, Arnaud CD: Calcium regulating hormones —parathyroid hormone, calcitonin, vitamin D. p. 224. In Rothfield BM (ed): Nuclear Medicine In Vitro. JB Lippincott, Philadelphia, 1983

89. Duh Q-Y, Hybarger CP, Geist R et al: Carcinoids with multiple endocrine neoplasia syndromes. Am J Surg 1987;154:142

90. Black WD III, Haff RC: The surgical pathology of parathyroid chief cell hyperplasia. Am J Clin Pathol 1970;53:565

91. Prinz RA, Paloyan E, Lawrence AM et al: Radiation-associated hyperparathyroidism: a new syndrome? Surgery 1977;82:296

92. Braunwald EE, Isselbacher KJ, Petersdorf RG et al: Diseases of the parathyroid gland and other hyper- and hypocalcemic disorders. p. 1870. In Potts JT Jr (ed): Harrison's Principles of Internal Medicine. McGraw-Hill, New York, 1988

93. Sample FW, Mitchell SP, Bledsoe RC: Parathyroid ultrasonography. Radiology 1978;127:485

94. Gooding GAW, Clark OH, Stark DD et al: Parathyroid aspiration biopsy under ultrasonic guidance in the postoperative hyperparathyroid patient. Radiology 1985;155:193

95. Randel SB, Gooding GAW, Clark OH et al: Parathyroid variants, US evaluation. Radiology 1987;165:191

96. Edmunson GR, Charboneau JW, James EM et al: Parathyroid carcinoma: high frequency sonographic features. Radiology 1986;161:65

97. Kinishita Y, Fukase M, Uchihashi M et al: Significance of preoperative use of ultrasonography in parathyroid neoplasms: comparison of sonographic textures with histologic findings. J Clin Ultrasound 1985;13:457

98. Haghighi P, Astarita RW, Wepsic T et al: Concurrent primary parathyroid hyperplasia and parathyroid carcinoma. Arch Pathol Lab Med 1983;107:349

99. Clark OH: Parathyroid cysts. Am J Surg 1978;135:395

100. Graif M, Itzchak Y, Strauss S et al: Parathyroid sonography: diagnostic accuracy related to shape, location, and texture of the gland. Br J Radiol 1987;60:439

101. Calandra DB, Shah KH, Prinz RA et al: Parathyroid cysts: a report of eleven cases including two associated with hyperparathyroid crisis. Surgery 1983;94:887

102. Rogers LA, Fetter BF, Peele WPJ: Parathyroid cyst and

cystic degeneration of parathyroid adenoma. Arch Pathol 1969;88:476

103. Prinz RA, Barbato AL, Braithwaite SS et al: Simultaneous primary hyperparathyroidism and nodular thyroid disease. Surgery 1982;92:454

104. LiVolsi VA, Feind CR: Parathyroid adenoma and nonmedullary thyroid carcinoma. Cancer 1976;38:1391

105. Krubsack AJ, Wilson SD, Lawson TL et al: Prospective comparison of radionuclide, computed tomographic, sonographic, and magnetic resonance localization of parathyroid tumors. Surgery 1989;106:639

106. Uden P, Aspelin P, Berglund J et al: Preoperative localization in unilateral parathyroid surgery. A cost benefit study on ultrasound, computed tomography, and scintigraphy. Acta Chir Scand 1990;156:29

107. Miller DL, Doppman JL, Shawker TH et al: Localization of parathyroid adenomas in patients who have undergone surgery. Part I. Noninvasive imaging methods. Radiology 1987;162:133

108. Moreau JF, Chigot JP, De Feraudy MN et al: Preoperative parathyroid ultrasonography: 45 recent verified cases. Presse Med 1987;16:804

109. Simeone JF, Mueller PR, Ferucci JT et al: High-resolution real-time sonography of the parathyroid. Radiology 1981;141:745

110. Udien P, Aspelin P, Berglund J et al: Preoperative localization in unilateral parathyroid surgery. A cost-benefit study on ultrasound, computed tomography, and scintigraphy. Acta Surg Scand 1990;156:29

111. Auffermann W, Gooding GAW, Okerlund MD et al: Diagnosis of recurrent hyper-parathyroidism: comparison of MR to other imaging techniques. AJR 1988;150:1027

112. Winzelberg GG, Hydrovitz JD, O'Hara KR et al: Parathyroid adenomas evaluated by Tl-201/Tc-99m pertechnetate subtraction scintigraphy and high-resolution ultrasonography. Radiology 1985;155:231

113. Stark DD, Gooding GAW, Clark OH: Noninvasive parathyroid imaging. Semin Ultrasound CT MR 1985;6:310

114. Clark OH, Okerlund MD, Moss AA et al: Localization studies in patients with persistent or recurrent hyperparathyroidism. Surgery 1985;98:1083

115. Levin KE, Gooding GAW, Okerlund MD et al: Localizing studies in patients with persistent or recurrent hyperparathyroidism. Surgery 1987;102:917

116. Erdman WA, Breslau NA, Weinreb JC et al: Noninvasive localization of parathyroid adenomas: a comparison of x-ray computerized tomography, ultrasound, scintigraphy, and MRI. Magn Reson Imaging 1989;7:187

117. Miller DL, Doppman JL, Krudy AG et al: Localization of parathyroid adenomas in patients who have undergone surgery. Part II. Invasive procedures. Radiology 1987;162:138

118. Shimkin PM, Powell D, Doppman JL et al: Parathyroid venous sampling. Radiology 1972;104:571

119. Doppman JL: Parathyroid localization. Arteriography and venous sampling. Radiol Clin North Am 1976;14:163

120. Stark DD, Moss AA, Gooding GAW et al: Parathyroid scanning by computed tomography. Radiology 1983;148:297

121. Aufferman W, Guis M, Tavares NJ et al: MR signal intensity of parathyroid adenomas: correlation with histopatology. AJR 1989;153:873

122. Clark OH, Stark DD, Gooding GAW et al: Localization procedures in patients requiring reoperation for hyperparathyroidism. World J Surg 1984;8:466

123. Satava RM Jr, Beahrs HO, Scholz DA: Success rate of cervical exploration for hyperparathyroidism. Arch Surg 1975;110:625

124. Wang C, Castleman B, Cope O: Surgical management of hyperparathyroidism due to primary hyperplasia. A clinical and pathologic study of 104 cases. Ann Surg 1982;195:384

125. Clark OH, Stark DD, Duh D et al: Value of high resolution real-time ultrasonography in secondary hyper-parathyroidism. Am J Surg 1985;150:9

126. Takebayashi S, Matsui K, Onohara Y et al: Sonography for early diagnosis of enlarged parathyroid glands in patients with secondary hyperparathyroidism. AJR 1987;148:911

127. Tomic C, Brzac H, Pavlovic D et al: Parathyroid sonography in secondary hyperparathyroidism:correlation with clinical findings. Nephrol Dial Transplant 1989;4:45

128. Clark OH (ed): Secondary hyperparathyroidism. p. 241. In Endocrine Surgery of the Thyroid and Parathyroid Glands. CV Mosby, St. Louis, 1985

129. Geelhoed GW, Krudy AG, Doppman JL: Long-term follow-up of patients with hyperparathyroidism treated by transcatheter staining with contrast agent. Surgery 1983;94:849

130. Doppman JL, Marx SJ, Spiegel AM et al: Treatment of hyperparathyroidism by percutaneous embolization of a mediastinal adenoma. Radiology 1975;115:37

131. Karstrup S, Holm HH, Glenthoj A et al: Nonsurgical treatment of primary hyperparathyroidism with sonographically guided percutaneous injection of ethanol: results in a selected series of patients. AJR 1990;154:1087

132. Karstrup S, Transbol IB, Holm HH et al: Ultrasound-guided chemical parathyroidectomy in patients with primary hyperparathyroidism: a prospective study. Br J Radiol 1989;62:1037

4

Carotid, Vertebral, and Jugular Evaluation

Barbara A. Carroll

Stroke is the third leading cause of death in the United States; approximately 50 percent of strokes are due to atherosclerotic disease in the extracranial carotid artery, usually within 2 cm of the carotid bifurcation.[1] For many years, diagnosis of suspected extracranial carotid arterial disease consisted of a physical examination and conventional arteriography. Currently, intra-arterial digital subtraction angiography (IADSA) has assumed this screening role. However, IADSA is expensive and invasive and therefore, over the last decade, numerous noninvasive, less expensive imaging techniques have been developed; these have had a major impact on the diagnostic approach to suspected carotid atherosclerotic disease. They can be grouped into two large categories: indirect and direct.

Indirect noninvasive tests study blood flow in the ophthalmic and the periorbital arteries as a means of indirectly evaluating significant carotid occlusive disease.[2,3] One common indirect noninvasive test is oculoplethysmography (OPG). OPG measures systolic pressure in the ophthalmic arteries and analyzes differences in pressures and pulse arrival times. Significant asymmetry of systolic pressures or a major delay in pulse arrival time indicates a flow-limiting carotid artery lesion. Bidirectional periorbital Doppler involves the use of continuous-wave (CW) Doppler technology to study flow in the supratrochlear and supraorbital vessels. The direction of flow in these vessels can indicate the presence of severe occlusive disease, as well as the formation of significant collateral-flow channels.[1] These indirect tests provide an accurate assessment of flow-limiting lesions in the internal carotid artery (ICA).[4] However, these tests cannot localize the site, extent, or number of lesions within the carotid artery, nor can they detect lower grades of stenosis or characterize plaque.[2]

Transcranial Doppler uses lower-frequency ultrasound to image vessels in the circle of Willis.[5,6] This technology provides indirect information about the presence of extracranial carotid artery stenoses and can also detect collateral pathways that have opened up along the circle of Willis. TCD may also detect intracranial carotid stenosis and allow assessment of vertebral basilar insufficiency.[7] Other applications include the detection of vasospasm following subarachnoid hemorrhage and the assessment of infants undergoing extracorporeal membrane oxygenation or with suspected brain death.[8-12]

Although these indirect tests have useful applications, they lack the sensitivity and specificity necessary for a screening test designed to detect a wide range of carotid arterial disease. Furthermore, indirect tests such as OPG or periorbital Doppler cannot distinguish between extremely high grade lesions and stenoses and may be invalidated by significant bilateral carotid occlusive disease. For these reasons, indirect tests are most effective when used in conjunction with direct noninvasive tests if the direct test is inconclusive.

Direct noninvasive tests use Doppler technology to directly image the extracranial carotid artery and evaluate blood flow within these vessels.[2] CW and pulsed

Doppler imaging techniques can be used to quantify the degree of carotid stenosis in terms of the peak frequency shift or velocity shift produced in the area of stenosis. CW Doppler uses two transducers, one that transmits the Doppler signal and one that receives it. Since the transmitted Doppler signal is continuous in CW Doppler, this technology is not limited by aliasing and thus can detect a wider range of frequencies than can pulsed Doppler. The major limitation of CW Doppler is its lack of range resolution. If more than one vessel is in the Doppler plane, it is impossible to determine with certainty the vessel from which the Doppler signal has arisen. Pulsed Doppler, however, allows one to sample discrete depths, and thus the vessel of choice can be selected for Doppler interrogation. Pulsed Doppler has better depth (range) resolution than CW Doppler.[2-13] However, a discrete pulse repetition frequency (PRF) must be used in order to receive Doppler signals from only a certain depth. Thus the highest detectable frequency cannot exceed half the PRF. If the frequencies (velocities) within a vessel exceed half the PRF, aliasing results.[13]

Duplex sonography combines high-frequency real-time imaging with physiologic blood flow information provided by Doppler. Most duplex systems combine steerable Doppler technology and the availability of "si-multaneous" Doppler and imaging studies. Two-dimensional color Doppler is the latest improvement in carotid duplex imaging.[13,14] Color Doppler allows one to view real-time flow information as well as gray-scale anatomy over a variable cross-sectional area. This allows one to quickly identify areas of abnormal color flow within vessels, thus greatly speeding the carotid examination. In addition to speeding the examination, color Doppler increases the confidence of diagnoses and allows a more uniform, reproducible carotid examination.

Although duplex examinations are performed most frequently to evaluate suspected atherosclerotic disease involving the extracranial carotid arteries, sonography can play a useful role in the evaluation of vertebral arterial disease as well as of internal jugular vein abnormalities. The focus in this chapter is on carotid atherosclerotic disease evaluation; however, other applications of duplex sonography to cervical vascular disease are discussed, including evaluation of patients during and/or after surgery; preoperative screening before major vascular surgery; monitoring of progression or regression of known atherosclerotic disease; and evaluation of nonatherosclerotic carotid diseases including fibromuscular dysplasia, malignant carotid artery invasion, and carotid body tumors.[15-19]

CAROTID ARTERY

A carotid ultrasound examination actually consists of three parts: visual inspection of the gray-scale image of the vessel, Doppler spectral analysis of flowing blood, and color Doppler analysis. Each aspect of the carotid ultrasound examination is important in the final determination of the presence and extent of disease. The image and Doppler assessments are usually in close agreement, but if there are discrepancies every attempt should be made to uncover the source of the disagreement. The more closely the Doppler and image findings agree, the higher the degree of confidence in the diagnosis. Generally speaking, gray-scale images detect and quantify low-grade stenoses better than high-grade occlusive disease, which is more accurately assessed by Doppler spectral analysis. Color Doppler facilitates both imaging and Doppler determinations of stenosis and often helps explain apparent discrepancies between image and Doppler information.[20] If the source of a discrepancy cannot be found, the final report should reflect the disagreement between the Doppler and image information because it may relate to additional cardiovascular abnormalities proximal or distal to the extracranial carotid.

TECHNIQUE

Carotid artery examinations are performed with the patient supine. For best visualization of the vessels, the neck should be slightly extended and the head turned away from the side being examined. Some carotid arteries are best approached by scanning anterior to the sternocleidomastoid muscles, whereas others are imaged more easily from an approach posterior to the sterno-cleidomastoid muscles. Some examiners prefer to sit at the patient's head to perform the examination, and others prefer to scan at the patient's side, in a manner analogous to ultrasound examinations of the abdomen or pelvis. A 5- to 10-MHz transducer is preferred for imaging; a 3- to 7.5-MHz transducer is preferred for Doppler with transducer selection governed by the pa-

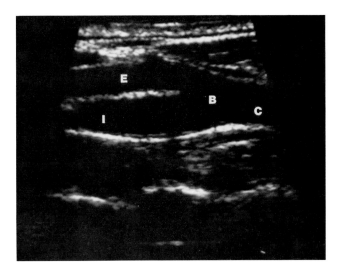

Fig. 4-1. Longitudinal sonogram of the carotid bifurcation. (*C*, common carotid artery; *B*, carotid bulb; *E*, external carotid artery; *I*, internal carotid artery.)

tient's body habitus and the technical features of the ultrasound equipment.

A complete ultrasound examination consists of gray-scale imaging and Doppler analysis of the entire extracranial carotid. It is usually easiest to begin examination in the transverse projection, obtaining scans along the entire course of the carotid artery from the supraclavicular notch all the way to the angle of the mandible. Caudal angulation of the transducer in the supraclavicular area

frequently images the right common carotid artery (CCA) origin; the left CCA origin is deeper and less frequently imaged than the right. Just before the bifurcation, the CCA widens into the carotid bulb (Fig. 4-1). Transverse views of the carotid bifurcation help establish the orientation of the ICA and external carotid artery (ECA) and allow the examiner to determine the optimal longitudinal plane in which to perform Doppler spectral analysis (Fig. 4-2). This rapid initial transverse scan can also detect atherosclerotic disease. If disease is detected, the percent diameter or area of stenosis can be calculated directly by using electronic calipers and software analytic algorithms, which are available in most duplex instruments. Color Doppler can also be used during this initial transverse scan since it can readily demonstrate flow abnormalities and give a rough estimation of the patent lumen in areas of stenosis. Atherosclerotic plaques should be carefully evaluated to determine their extent and location relative to the bifurcation, as well as to assess their surface contour and texture in both transverse and longitudinal planes.

Measurements in the longitudinal plane may overestimate the severity of a stenosis by partial voluming through an eccentric plaque (Figs. 4-3 and 4-4). Thus, most accurate measurements of diameter and area stenosis are obtained in a transverse plane perpendicular to the long axis of the carotid (Fig. 4-5). Since the percent diameter and area stenoses are not always linearly related, particularly in eccentric or irregular plaques, clinical reports should always state the type of stenosis mea-

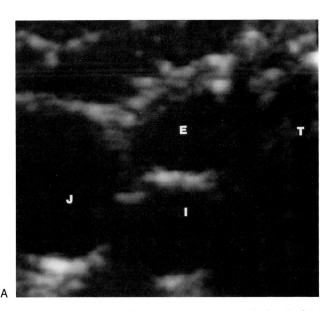

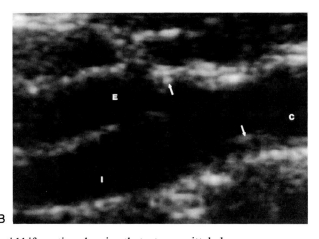

A   B

Fig. 4-2. **(A)** Transverse sonogram at the level of the carotid bifurcation showing that a true sagittal plane scan (Fig. B) should visualize both carotid branches in the same plane with the CCA. (*E*, external carotid artery; *I*, internal carotid artery; *J*, internal jugular vein; *T*, trachea.) **(B)** Subsequent sagittal scan showing both the external carotid artery *(E)* and internal carotid artery *(I)* in the same plane as the common carotid artery *(C)*. Plaque (arrows) is present in the distal common carotid and proximal external carotid arteries.

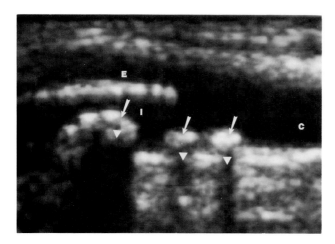

Fig. 4-3. Longitudinal scan through the carotid bifurcation demonstrating several areas of plaque with calcification (arrows) at the origin of the internal carotid artery *(I)*. Posterior acoustic shadowing (arrowheads) is seen posterior to the calcific plaque. (*C*, common carotid artery; *E*, external carotid artery.)

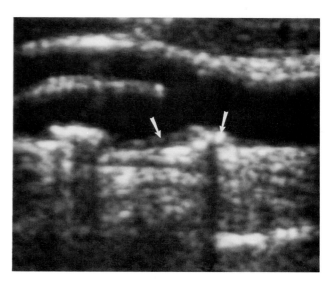

Fig. 4-4. Longitudinal scan of the same carotid bifurcation seen in Fig. 4-3 demonstrating heterogeneous plaque (arrows) at the origin of the ICA. This heterogeneous plaque, which has relatively homogeneous hypoechoic components as well as echogenic calcific components, is unlikely to contain intraplaque hemorrhage. Furthermore, this image of the carotid bifurcation demonstrates the importance of careful scanning to avoid overestimating the degree of carotid stenosis by obtaining a scan too close to the wall of a vessel with an eccentric plaque and in effect "partial voluming" the true maximum diameter of the vessel lumen.

surement that has been made. Theoretically, eccentric, asymmetric stenoses are most appropriately quantified by using area stenosis measurements. However, these measurements are often time-consuming and technically difficult, and it may be difficult to relate them to diameter stenosis measurements obtained on angiography. The cephalocaudal extent and length of plaques should be noted, as should the presence of tandem lesions.

Although high-resolution real-time imaging is probably the best method for imaging minimal, early atherosclerotic changes, some of which may go undetected at arteriography, the quality of the real-time imaging deteriorates as stenosis increases. Several factors contribute to image degradation in high-grade stenoses. Irregular plaque or plaque containing calcification may produce shadowing that obscures the vessel lumen. "Soft plaque" or thrombus with acoustic properties similar to that of the flowing blood may appear anechoic and be almost invisible. In some cases, a vessel may show little visible plaque and yet be totally occluded. In such situations, color Doppler is useful in distinguishing between hypoechoic occlusive lesions and flowing blood (Plate 4-1). Gray-scale ultrasound imaging is best suited for the evaluation of low-grade stenoses, whereas Doppler spectral analysis and color Doppler can more accurately quantify high-grade stenoses.

Following the initial transverse survey, longitudinal scans are obtained. The optimal longitudinal scan plane has already been determined by the transverse scans. Optimal longitudinal orientation can range from nearly

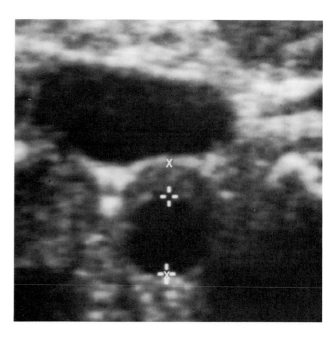

Fig. 4-5. Transverse CCA with homogeneous plaque as an example of how to measure diameter stenosis. The patent lumen measurement (calipers) is subtracted from the entire vessel lumen measurement *(x)* to yield a percent diameter stenosis, in this case 30 percent.

coronal to almost sagittal; however, in most cases the optimal scan plane will be oblique and intermediate between sagittal and coronal. Roughly 50 to 60 percent of patients have a carotid bifurcation orientation that allows both vessels to be visualized in the same plane as the distal CCA (Fig. 4-2). In the remainder, orientation of the vessels of the bifurcation allows only a single vessel to be imaged in the same plane as the CCA.[1] Images should be obtained to display the orientation of vessels at the carotid bifurcation, as well as to visualize the cephalocaudal extent of plaque.

Doppler Spectral Analysis and Color Doppler Examination

The extent of the Doppler spectral examination required depends on whether color Doppler is available. If color Doppler is not available, a rapid initial Doppler spectral analysis of the entire extracranial carotid is made with the Doppler range gate expanded to include the entire vessel lumen. The Doppler range gate is then narrowed to a smaller volume (1.5 mm³), and frequency or velocity spectral analysis is performed. Blood flow velocities are obtained and spectral analysis performed below, at, and just beyond the region of maximal visible stenoses and at 1-cm intervals distal to the visualized plaque until the vessel becomes intracranial or a signal can no longer be obtained.

Color Doppler technology greatly speeds spectral analysis. A quick transverse and longitudinal color Doppler survey pinpoints areas of high-velocity and/or disturbed flow, which are manifested as areas of less saturated, inhomogeneous color.[14,20] Once these areas of abnormal color flow are identified, one can place the pulsed Doppler sample volume in the area of color Doppler abnormality and obtain spectral traces. Using color Doppler in this fashion shortens the examination. If both gray-scale and color Doppler images of the entire carotid artery are normal, only representative spectral traces from the CCA, ICA, and ECA are necessary to complete the examination.

Angle theta, or the Doppler angle, is defined as the angle between the Doppler transducer line of sight and the direction of blood flow (Fig. 4-6). The ideal angle theta is 0 degrees (cosine angle theta = 1), which allows the greatest possible detectable frequency shift. However, this angle is difficult to achieve in carotid examination, where the vessels parallel the skin surface. Therefore, a range of Doppler angles from 30 to 60 degrees is considered acceptable for carotid spectral analysis. When angle theta exceeds 60 to 70 degrees, the accuracy of velocity and frequency determinations declines precipitously to the point where virtually no velocity change can be detected at angle theta 90 degrees. Also, as Doppler angles approach 90 degrees, a mirror image artifact begins to appear around the zero-velocity baseline (Fig. 4-7). This artifact is often angle related and, when present, should alert one to a suboptimal Doppler angle with suspect velocity readings. Positioning the Doppler angle cursor parallel to the vessel walls determines the angle theta used to convert frequency information into velocity values. The entire course of the CCA and ICA should be interrogated with a relatively consistent angle theta maintained throughout the examination when possible. Generally, only the origin of the ECA is sub-

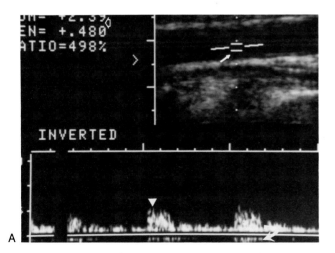
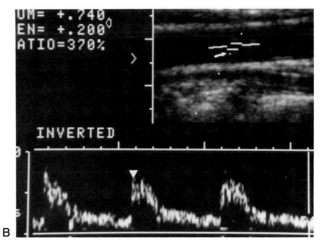

Fig. 4-6. **(A)** Suboptimal angle theta (arrow) (Doppler angle). This results in an abnormal waveform shape in the CCA (arrowhead), spuriously elevated systolic velocity (open arrow), and a hint of mirror imaging (curved arrow). **(B)** More appropriate Doppler angle (arrow) of 50 degrees. This results in a normal-appearing carotid waveform (arrowhead), normal velocities (open arrow), and no mirror image.

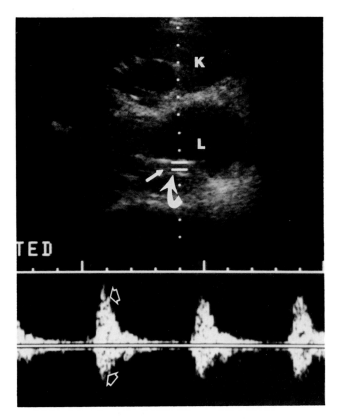

Fig. 4-7. More graphic demonstration of a mirror image artifact (open arrows) in an internal iliac artery (arrow) supplying a renal transplant. The Doppler angle (curved arrow) is almost 90 degrees. The mirror image is not exactly symmetric. This characteristic finding should suggest that the Doppler velocities are very suspect and prompt a change to a more appropriate Doppler angle. (*L*, lymphocele; *K*, renal allograft.)

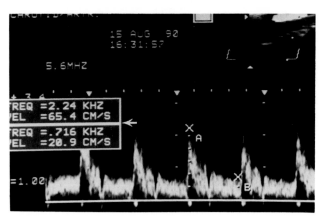

Fig. 4-8. Normal CCA waveforms demonstrating the level at which peak systolic *(A)* and end-diastolic *(B)* measurements should be made. Both frequency and velocity information are presented in this format (arrow).

jected to spectral analysis, because occlusive plaque in the ECA is less common than in the ICA and is rarely of clinical significance. Still, a significant stenosis of the ECA should be noted, particularly when it may account for a worrisome cervical bruit in the setting of a normal ICA.

Carotid Spectral Analysis

Normal Doppler Spectrum. The Doppler spectrum is a quantitative, graphic display of the velocities and directions of moving blood present in the Doppler sample volume. Although the exact source of the Doppler signal is uncertain, red blood cells or red blood cell interfaces are believed to represent the reflectors that produce the Doppler signal. Doppler assessment of carotid occlusive disease can be performed by using either frequency or velocity information (Fig. 4-8). However, velocity calculations are potentially more accurate than frequency

shift measurements because they allow angle theta between the transducer line of sight and the blood flow vector to be used to convert a frequency shift to a velocity.[21] Frequency shifts vary according to both angle theta and the incident Doppler frequency; velocity measurements take both of these factors into account. Furthermore, velocity values readily translate from transducer to transducer and machine to machine, allowing a more universal standardization of Doppler spectral analysis. The Doppler shift ΔF, measured in hertz, is given by the *Doppler equation:*

$$\Delta F = 2F_0\, V\cos\theta/C$$

where F_0 is the frequency of the transmitted ultrasound in hertz, C is the velocity of sound in blood (1,560 m/s), V is the velocity of blood flow, and $\cos\theta$ is the cosine of the angle between the blood flow vector and the direction of Doppler insonification (angle theta or Doppler angle [Fig. 4-6]). The Doppler equation clearly shows that the major Doppler shift, ΔF, and subsequent velocity determinations are extremely dependent on the Doppler angle. It is important that the Doppler angles be as small as can be consistently obtained throughout the carotid; ideally, they should never exceed 60 degrees. Doppler angles in excess of 60 degrees are associated with a markedly inaccurate representation of true blood flow velocity.

The Doppler spectral display depicts velocities on the *y* axis and time on the *x* axis. By convention, flow toward the transducer is displayed above the zero-velocity baseline, while flow away from the transducer is displayed below. If one wishes, spectra that project below the baseline (which originate in vessels in which blood is flowing away from the Doppler transducer) can be inverted and placed above the baseline for ease of spectral analysis, always remembering the true direction of blood flow within the vessel (Fig. 4-9). Note that the direction of blood flow is toward the Doppler transducer in Figure 4-9A and away from the transducer in Figure 4-9B. Doppler spectra are inverted (see notation on the image in Fig. 4-9B indicating that this has been done) to maintain a consistent orientation. The amplitude of each velocity component within the Doppler frequency spectrum determines the brightness of the traces; this is known as a gray-scale velocity plot. The normal carotid artery shows a relatively narrow frequency spectrum in systole and a somewhat wider spectrum in early and late diastole. A normal black area between the spectral trace and the zero-velocity baseline is termed the *spectral window* (Fig. 4-10). Filling in of this black spectral window with frequency spectral information is termed *spectral broadening.*

The ICA and ECA have distinctive Doppler flow velocity waveforms (Fig. 4-10). The ICA supplies the low-resistance circulation of the brain and hence has a flow waveform pattern similar to that seen in vessels that supply other "blood-hungry" organs, such as the liver, kidneys, and fetus. The characteristic feature of low-resistance arterial waveforms is a large quantity of continuous forward flow throughout diastole. The ECA, which supplies the high-resistance vascular bed of the facial muscles, has a flow velocity waveform similar to that of other peripheral arteries. Flow velocity rises sharply during systole and falls rapidly toward diastole, approaching zero or transiently reversing direction in

diastole. The CCA waveform is a composite of the ICA and ECA waveforms, but most often resembles ICA patterns more closely than ECA patterns, with persistent diastolic blood flow above the zero-velocity baseline. Roughly 80 percent of the CCA blood flow enters the ICA en route to the brain, while 20 percent enters the ECA to supply the facial musculature.

Doppler Spectral Analysis. Doppler spectral analysis is founded on the principle that blood flow velocities increase in areas of stenosis in proportion to the degree of luminal narrowing. These increased velocities are most marked immediately distal to the area of maximum stenosis, emphasizing the importance of sampling directly in the areas that are most narrowed. Normal blood flow patterns and velocities begin to reconstitute as one moves further distal from an area of stenosis unless there is a tandem lesion distal to the initial stenosis or unless the degree of stenosis is preocclusive. Systolic and diastolic velocity measurements are the main parameters used to assess stenosis by Doppler.[21-32] Peak systolic velocity was the initial parameter used to quantify high-grade stenoses. This parameter is easily measured and reproducible, and numerous studies have shown that it has a predictable relationship with the degree of luminal narrowing.[21,23,26] End-diastolic velocity measurements, peak systolic ICA/CCA ratios, and peak end-diastolic ICA/CCA ratios have been shown to be additional reliable parameters for assessing hemodynamically significant stenoses.[22,27] End-diastolic velocity ratios are particularly useful in distinguishing among degrees of

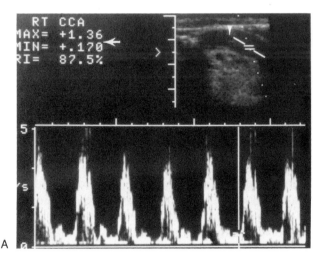
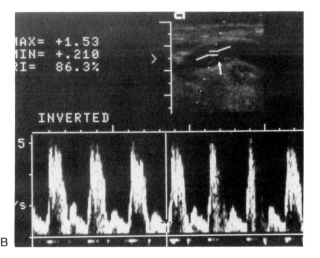

Fig. 4-9. **(A)** Right CCA demonstrating high-velocity systolic flow of 136 cm/s and end-diastolic flow of 17 cm/s (arrow). Although reverberation artifacts (arrowhead) are noted within the proximal CCA, there was no evidence of plaque in this region. **(B)** Proximal ICA in the same patient demonstrating plaque (arrow) producing less than 50 percent stenosis. However, increased systolic velocity of 153 cm/s is noted in this vessel in a fashion analogous to that seen in the more proximal CCA. The disproportionate elevation of systolic velocity without a concomitant elevation of end-diastolic velocity is due to severe chronic, uncontrolled hypertension. Color Doppler confirmed the absence of significant vascular stenosis (see Plate 4-10).

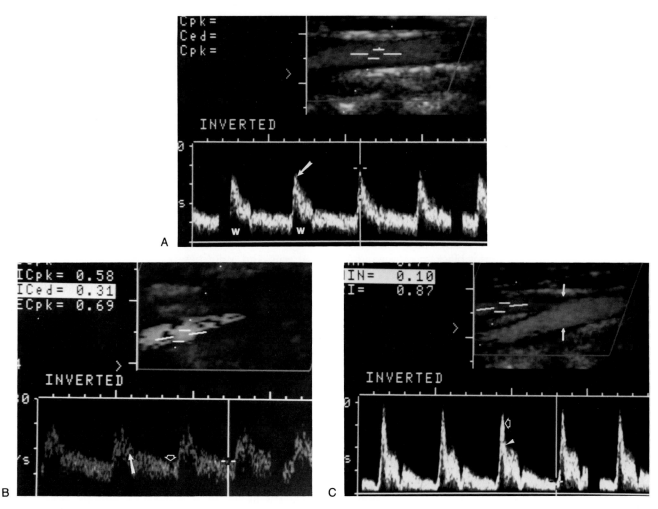

Fig. 4-10. **(A)** Longitudinal scan demonstrating normal CCA flow velocity waveforms (arrow). Note the wide spectral window *(W)* indicating a lack of significant spectral broadening. **(B)** Longitudinal image demonstrating normal ICA flow velocity waveforms (arrow). Note the large amount of end-diastolic flow (open arrow). **(C)** Longitudinal scan at the region of the carotid bifurcation (arrows) demonstrating a normal ECA waveform (open arrow). Note the relatively small amount of end-diastolic flow (caliper) and the sharp systolic downswing (arrowhead). This is consistent with a relatively high-resistance vascular bed.

high-grade carotid stenoses. In addition, a comparison of peak systolic velocities in the two carotid arteries may provide information about carotid disease proximal or distal to the readily visualized portion of the extracranial carotid. A right/left CCA peak systolic average velocity ratio less than 0.7 or greater than 1.3 correlates with a greater than 50 percent diameter stenosis in the right and left ICA, respectively.[29] Table 4-1 is a composite of numerous published Doppler criteria for assessing carotid artery stenoses.

Carotid stenoses usually begin to reduce blood flow (become hemodynamically significant) when they exceed 50 percent of the diameter of the artery (70 percent cross-sectional area reduction).[21,33,34] There is a progres-

sive decrease in blood flow until a critical level of 70 percent diameter reduction (90 percent area reduction) is reached; beyond this point there is a precipitous decrease in blood flow as the percent stenosis approaches that of complete occlusion (100 percent). Clinical studies have shown that risk of stroke due to compromised blood flow secondary to high-grade stenoses (not due to embolic phenomena) does not increase until stenoses exceed 75 to 80 percent. For this reason, it is critical to distinguish these high-grade narrowings from other "hemodynamically significant" stenoses.[33,34] However, the hemodynamic significance of a narrowing in the carotid artery of a patient who is both supine and resting is difficult to assess.

TABLE 4-1.   Doppler Spectral Analysis

Diameter Stenosis (%)	ICA/CCA Peak Systolic Velocity Ratio	ICA/CCA Peak Diastolic Velocity Ratio	Peak Systolic Velocity (cm/s)	Peak Diastolic Velocity (cm/s)
0-40	<1.5	<2.6	<110 > 25	<40
41-59	<1.8	<2.6	>120	<40
60-79	>1.8	>2.6	>130	>40
80-99	>3.7	>5.5	>250 < 25	>80-135
100 (occlusion)	Unilateral damped flow in CCA; no flow or reversed flow proximal to ICA occlusion			

Spectral Broadening.   When atherosclerotic plaques project into the arterial lumen, the normal smooth laminar flow of erythrocytes is disturbed. This results in a wider range of velocities in the flowing blood, which produces spectral broadening. Spectral broadening is manifested by filling in the normally black spectral window that exists under the narrow band of velocities in normal vessels (Fig. 4-11). Spectral broadening increases in proportion to the severity of carotid artery stenosis, and some investigators have attempted to use a measure of spectral broadening to assess the degree of stenosis.[24,35]

Some duplex instruments allow the operator to measure spectral width between a maximum and minimum velocity (bandwidth), thereby quantitating spectral broadening. No investigations have yet proven that quantitative spectral broadening measurements are more accurate than peak systolic or diastolic velocity measurements; further correlative studies are needed to document the relationship of quantitative spectral broadening to carotid stenosis. However, recognition of spectral window obliteration and color Doppler heterogeneity, provides a useful, if not quantitative, predictor of the severity of flow disturbance.

Color Doppler

Normal.   Color Doppler is a welcome addition to duplex sonography and has been quickly incorporated into the routine diagnostic work-up of suspected carotid disease.[14,20,36,37] Color Doppler displays flow information in real-time over either an entire two-dimensional real-time image or a selected smaller region. Stationary soft tissue structures that lack phase or frequency shift are assigned an amplitude value and displayed in a standard gray-scale format (Plate 4-2). In areas of the cross-sectional image where there is flowing blood that has a phase and frequency shift, a color assignment is superimposed on the gray-scale image. The color assignment depends on the direction of blood flow relative to the Doppler transducer. The color assignment is also a function of both the mean frequency shift produced by moving red blood cells within a given pixel and the Doppler angle. Thus blood flow toward the Doppler transducer will have one color, whereas flow away from the transducer will have another (Plate 4-3). If a vessel is tortuous or diving, the Doppler angle will change along the course of the vessel, resulting in changing color assignments that are relatively unrelated to a true change in red blood

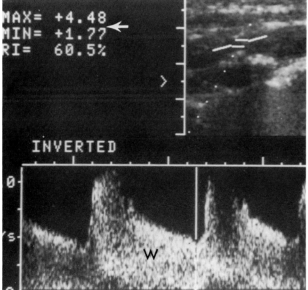

Fig. 4-11.   Duplex sonogram through a proximal ICA stenosis of greater than 80 percent demonstrating elevated systolic and end-diastolic velocities (arrow) as well as spectral broadening filling in the spectral window *(W)*.

cell velocity. Furthermore, color assignment in a tortuous vessel may reverse if the blood flow direction changes with respect to the Doppler transducer, even though the true direction of blood flow in the vessel is unchanged. When a portion of the vessel is normal to the interrogating Doppler beam, the Doppler angle is roughly 90 degrees and little or no frequency shift will be detected; hence no color Doppler will be displayed in this area of the vessel even though blood flow is present. As with pulsed Doppler, when the Doppler angle approaches 90 degrees, color Doppler velocity assignments are relatively inaccurate.

Color assignment in color Doppler is arbitrary and may be set up to represent any anatomic configuration. Color saturation is directly related to blood flow velocity. More intensely saturated shades indicate lower velocities; as velocities increase, the color shades become lighter or less saturated. Some systems feature selected frequency shifts in a contrasting color (i.e., green). Such "green tagging" can provide a real-time estimation of the blood flow velocities above or at a certain value (Plate 4-4).

Color Doppler examinations should be performed with optimal flow sensitivity and gain settings. The system should be adjusted until color fills the entire vessel lumen but does not spill over into the adjacent soft tissues. The frame rate and pulse repetition frequency (PRF) should be set to provide visualization of the flow phenomena that are expected in a given vessel.[38] Frame rates vary as a function of the width of the area selected for color Doppler display, as well as the depth of the region of interest. The larger the color Doppler image area, the slower the image frame rate will be. The deeper the back wall of the color Doppler image box, the slower the PRF will be. Color Doppler sensitivity should be appropriate for the vessel sampled. For example, if one is hoping to detect a trickle of flow in a preocclusive carotid stenosis, low flow settings with decreased sampling rates should be used. However, the color Doppler system will then alias at lower velocities owing to a decrease in the PRF.

In color Doppler, flowing blood becomes in effect a contrast agent that outlines the patent vessel lumen. Color Doppler identifies areas of disturbed flow and spectral broadening, and high-velocity color jets can be quickly identified so that the Doppler gate can be positioned in these regions for subsequent Doppler spectral analysis. These colored jets define both the presence of a high-velocity abnormality and the direction of flow in this region, which facilitates optimal spectral analysis by using color Doppler to direct Doppler angle corrections. Although no studies that validate the concept of using color Doppler to position the Doppler cursor within a stenotic jet have been performed, it is reasonable to assume that this is a useful way of optimizing spectral

analysis. Although color Doppler readily demonstrates spectral broadening as areas of heterogeneous color, the degree of color heterogeneity and the degree of pulsed Doppler spectral broadening may not always coincide (Plate 4-5 and Fig. 4-12). Since the color Doppler pixel color assignments are based on mean velocity values, spectral broadening may be masked if the means of broadened spectra are relatively homogeneous across a vessel lumen. Use of velocity variant mapping may accentuate differences in blood flow velocity spectra. Color Doppler manifestations of spectral broadening are also related to the portion of the cardiac cycle in which the color cardiac cycle in which the color image is obtained.

Color Doppler greatly speeds the examination of the carotid arteries by demonstrating the presence and direction of blood flow within the vessels, as well as identifying branches of the ECA, which facilitates differentiation of the ECA from the ICA, particularly if the ICA is occluded. Color Doppler also identifies the normal blood flow separation that occurs in the carotid bifurcation. There is a transient flow reversal opposite the origin of the ECA, which is graphically displayed by color Doppler as areas of intensely saturated reversed flow located along the outer wall of the carotid bulb. This transient flow reversal appears either at early systole or at peak systole and persists for a variable length of time into

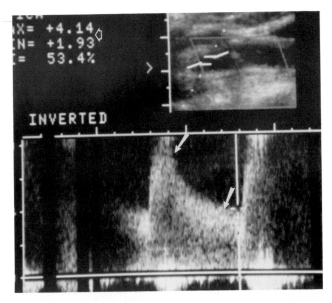

4-12. Pulsed Doppler spectral trace in the region of a high-grade stenosis in the same patient as in Plate 4-5, demonstrating marked spectral broadening (arrows) as well as elevated systolic and diastolic velocities (open arrow). The apparent mismatch in spectral broadening as seen by color (see Plate 4-5) and spectral analysis occurs because color Doppler reflects mean velocity within a pixel. If the mean velocities are all similar, despite a wide range of velocities within the pixel, the color assignments may be relatively homogeneous.

the diastolic portion of the cardiac cycle[39,40] (Plate 4-6). This normal flow reversal demonstrates a distinctly different color pattern from that of aliasing. In true flow reversal, the reversed flow and the forward flow both demonstrate intensely saturated colors. Conversely, in aliasing, the contiguous forward and reverse color flow pixel assignments demonstrate less saturated color patterns. Some investigators suggest that failure to detect this characteristic flow reversal in the carotid bifurcation is abnormal and that it may represent one of the earliest changes of atherosclerotic disease. Failure to demonstrate normal flow reversal at the carotid bifurcation should initiate a careful search for subtle abnormalities at the origin of the ICA.[40]

NORMAL ANATOMY

The right CCA arises from the innominate or brachiocephalic artery, the first major branch off of the aortic arch. The innominate artery divides into the right subclavian artery and right CCA. The left CCA, the second major branch off of the aortic arch, usually arises directly from the arch separate from the left subclavian artery, the third major branch (Fig. 4-13). The CCAs course cephalad in the neck posterolateral to the thyroid gland, posteromedial to the jugular vein, and posterior to the sternocleidomastoid muscle. The CCA widens in the region of the carotid bulb, just proximal to the carotid bifurcation. The level of the carotid bifurcation is vari-

able. The CCA bifurcates into two major branches, the ICA and the ECA. The ICA is usually the larger and more posterolateral of the two vessels. Approximately 5 percent of individuals have an anomalous orientation of the vessels above the bifurcation. The ECA, which supplies the facial musculature, has multiple branches in its extracranial portion, whereas the ICA has no branches in the neck.

Normal Vessel Walls

Longitudinal images of the normal carotid wall demonstrate two roughly parallel echogenic lines, separated by a hypoechoic to anechoic region (Fig. 4-14). The first echo, which abuts the vessel lumen, represents the lumen–intima interface. The second echo, distal to the hypoechoic zone, is caused by the media–adventitia interface.[41-43] The media is the anechoic or hypoechoic zone between these two echogenic lines. The distance between these lines represents the combined thickness of the intima and media; widening of this distance beyond 1.2 mm is considered abnormal (Fig. 4-15). Detection of this sort of widening or focal plaque, however minimal, correlates with an increased risk for subsequent cardiovascular events.[41] Thus detection of these gray-scale abnormalities should initiate a search for other risk factors, such as hypertension, increased plasma lipoprotein levels, and a family history positive for cardiovascular disease. Investigations continue into the significance of intimal-medial thickness within the carotid arteries. One recent article has even raised the concern that these findings may be artifactual.[44] However, numerous investigators have shown that subtle changes in the vessel wall can

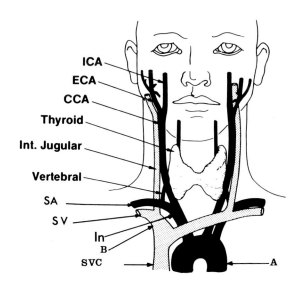

Fig. 4-13. Diagram of normal cervical arterial and venous anatomy. (*ICA,* internal carotid artery; *ECA,* external carotid artery; *CCA,* common carotid artery; *SA,* subclavian artery; *SV,* subclavian vein; *In,* innominate artery; *B,* brachiocephalic vein; *SVC,* superior vena cava; *A,* aorta; *Thyroid,* thyroid gland; *Int. jugular,* internal jugular vein; *vertebral,* vertebral artery.)

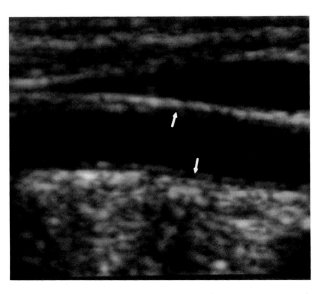

Fig. 4-14. Longitudinal images of the CCA. Note the normal intimal-medial arterial wall echocomplex (arrows).

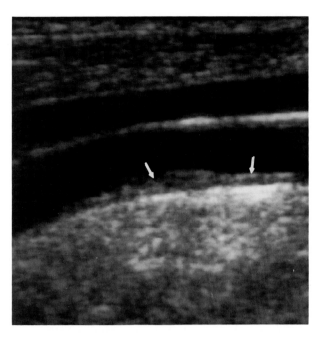

Fig. 4-15. Longitudinal scan of the distal CCA. Note the early intimal-medial thickening and plaque formation (arrows).

be imaged, and many believe that evaluation of intimal-medial thickening may be a useful tool for monitoring progression or regression of early atherosclerosis.[41,42]

ABNORMALITIES

Plaque

All carotid plaques should be evaluated to determine their extent, location, surface contour, and texture, as well as to assess the diameter stenosis that they produce. Several studies have shown that fewer than half of patients with documented transient ischemic attacks (TIAs) have hemodynamically significant carotid stenoses.[45,46] Ulcerated carotid plaques can serve as a nidus for emboli, which may cause TIAs and stroke.[47,48] From 50 to 70 percent of patients with cerebral vascular symptoms demonstrate hemorrhagic and/or ulcerated plaque. Analysis of plaque from carotid endarterectomy specimens has implicated intraplaque hemorrhage as an important factor in the development of neurologic symptoms.[41-44,48-56] However, there is controversy about the exact relationship of hemorrhagic changes to the onset of symptoms.[51,52]

High-resolution gray-scale imaging allows noninvasive plaque characterization. The most important distinction in plaque evaluation is classification of its tex-

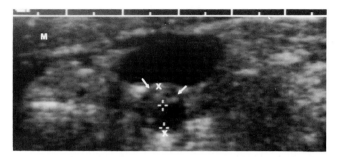

Fig. 4-16. Transverse image of the right CCA demonstrating a relatively homogeneous plaque (arrows) with echogenicity similar to that of adjacent muscles *(M)*. The plaque produces a 50 percent diameter stenosis (calipers). (calipers, patent lumen; *x*, entire lumen.)

ture as homogeneous or heterogeneous. Homogeneous plaques usually have a relatively uniform echotexture and a smooth surface.[41,55,57] This uniform acoustic texture corresponds pathologically to dense fibrous connective tissue (Fig. 4-16). Such homogeneous fibrous plaques are common in asymptomatic elderly individuals. Calcified plaques, which produce posterior acoustic shadowing, are also common in asymptomatic individuals and are generally considered stable (Fig. 4-3). Occasionally plaques that are otherwise homogeneous in echotexture contain focal echogenic regions. These echogenic regions usually correspond to areas of fatty or calcific deposition (Fig. 4-4). Such heterogeneous plaques are usually stable and not associated with neurologic symptoms.

Conversely, heterogeneous plaques, which are characteristic of intraplaque hemorrhage, have a complex internal echopattern that contains at least one focal sonolucent region (Fig. 4-17). The surface of the plaque may be smooth or irregular or may demonstrate features that suggest frank ulceration. This heterogeneous acoustic appearance corresponds to the histopathologic findings of intraplaque hemorrhage, clot, fibrosis, and irregular calcification. Hemorrhagic plaque is considered unstable and is subject to an abrupt increase in plaque size following intraplaque hemorrhage. In addition, virtually all ulcerated plaques are superimposed on a substrate of intraplaque hemorrhage. Sonography has been reported to identify the presence or absence of intraplaque hemorrhage with a sensitivity ranging from 90 to 94 percent and a specificity ranging from 75 to 88 percent. False-positive diagnoses of intraplaque hemorrhage are occasionally made if there are large deposits of lipid within the plaque.

Although most investigators believe that sonography can identify intraplaque hemorrhage, there is much disagreement about the ability of sonography to reliably

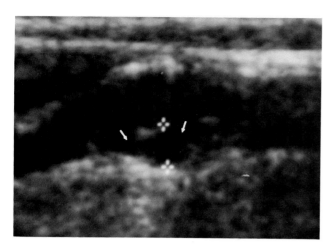

Fig. 4-17. Longitudinal scan through the origin of the left ICA demonstrating heterogeneous plaque on the posterior wall of the carotid bulb (calipers). This plaque demonstrates multiple anechoic or hypoechoic "Swiss cheese" defects (arrows). These types of heterogeneous plaque are likely to contain intraplaque hemorrhage.

and reproducibly predict plaque ulceration.[58-61] No universally accepted criteria exist for the sonographic diagnosis of ulceration. Findings that suggest ulceration include a continuous contour of a plaque surface with a focal depression, a well-defined break in the plaque surface, and an anechoic region that extends all the way to the plaque surface with no intimal echoes seen between the anechoic area and the vascular lumen. Some researchers believe that color Doppler demonstration of slow-moving eddying regions of color within an anechoic plaque suggests ulceration and that color Doppler may therefore be able to help improve sonographic detection of ulceration[62] (Plate 4-7). However, at present, it seems that neither arteriography nor real-time ultrasound is highly accurate in identifying ulcerated plaque.[63] Although the ability of sonography to diagnose ulceration is controversial, its ability to predict intraplaque hemorrhage, which has definite associated clinical implications, stresses the importance of ultrasound plaque characterization. The presence of heterogeneous irregular plaque that contains multiple "Swiss cheese" anechoic areas should always be noted in a report, because hemorrhagic plaque in a stenosis of less than 50 percent may be considered a "surgical lesion" in the appropriate clinical setting.

ICA Occlusion

Duplex ultrasound and spectral analysis have proven useful and accurate, when compared with arteriography, for the detection and quantification of carotid stenoses;

sensitivities and specificities ranging from 84 to 99 percent and overall accuracies ranging from 90 to 95 percent have been reported for the differentiation of greater or less than 50 percent stenosis.[21-32] However, although the accuracy of duplex ultrasound is high for predicting stenoses, early studies show that it is less accurate in differentiating occlusion from severe stenosis than in grading lesser degrees of stenosis. One reason for this is that as a stenosis approaches occlusion, the high-velocity blood flow is reduced to a mere trickle. Early pulsed Doppler systems were unable to detect the low-amplitude, low-flow velocities (below 2 to 4 cm/s) present in these preocclusive stenoses. It may also be difficult to locate the small string of the residual lumen, particularly if adjacent plaque or thrombus is anechoic, making it difficult to differentiate residual lumen from plaque or, if the plaque is calcified, obscuring visualization of the vessel. The recent introduction of color Doppler units and the advent of slower-flow detection capabilities in Doppler systems may facilitate more accurate diagnosis of occlusion and allow easier identification of a residual string of blood flow in the area of a preocclusive stenosis. Still, if a lesion is considered potentially operable, 100 percent accuracy is desirable for the diagnosis of a complete ICA occlusion; if a vessel is truly occluded, it is usually inoperable, but restoration of normal circulation may be possible in vessels where only a tiny string of flow remains. Angiography or IADSA is usually indicated in any person who is a candidate for surgery and who demonstrates an apparent ICA occlusion on ultrasound examination.

Carotid artery occlusion is diagnosed when no flow is detected in a vessel by pulsed Doppler or color Doppler (Plate 4-1). However, several indirect findings frequently coexist with carotid artery occlusion. An extremely high-grade ICA stenosis or occlusion usually produces asymmetric, damped blood flow (high-resistance waveforms) in the ipsilateral CCA and ICA proximal to the occlusion (Fig. 4-18). Decreased, absent, or reversed end-diastolic flow may be seen in these vessels unless there has been significant collateralization of ECA blood flow to the intracranial circulation. If such ECA collateralization has occurred, one may be faced with another pitfall in the diagnosis of a totally occluded ICA (i.e., mistaking a patent ECA or one of its branches for the ICA). When ECA collaterals open up in response to long-standing ICA disease, the ECA acquires a low-resistance flow waveform (Fig. 4-19). If only a single vessel is detected above the carotid bifurcation and it has low-resistance waveforms, one must determine whether it is the ECA or the ICA. One technique that can identify the ECA is scanning at the ECA origin while simultaneously tapping the temporal artery (Fig. 4-20). This maneuver can alter flow in the ECA, whereas the ICA

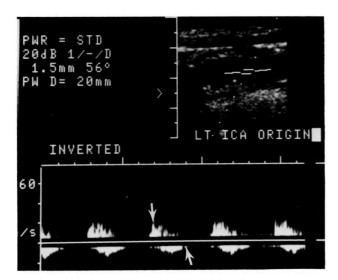

Fig. 4-18. Longitudinal duplex scan at the origin of the ICA demonstrating markedly damped abnormal flow (arrows) characteristic of that seen immediately proximal to either a complete occlusion or an extremely high-grade ("string sign") narrowing.

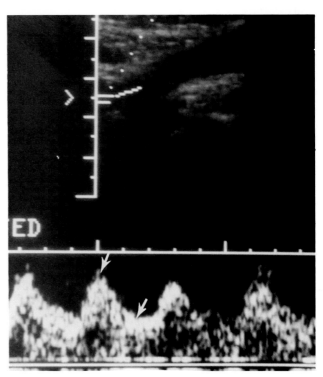

Fig. 4-19. Longitudinal duplex scan of the ECA in a patient with ICA occlusion demonstrating internalization (arrows) of the ECA waveform. The ECA now demonstrates a low-resistance pattern.

should be unaffected.[21,64,65] Branching vessels are unique to the ECA, and detection of such branches should readily differentiate this vessel from the ICA. Color Doppler may also aid in the identification of ECA branches (Plate 4-8).

Another problem in the evaluation of potential ICA occlusion is transmitted pulsations. The Doppler cursor should be located directly in the center of the ICA lumen, and the blood flow identified in this location should be carefully evaluated to assess the direction of flow as well as the shape of the flow velocity waveforms. The sample volume should be decreased to a minimum, and true center-stream sampling locations should be documented on both transverse and longitudinal images. Extraneous pulsations usually demonstrate aberrant waveforms, which are not characteristic of ICA flow and are seldom transmitted to the center of a thrombosed ICA.

Distal propagation almost always follows a proximal ICA occlusion. However, CCA occlusions are often localized. Flow may be maintained about the carotid bifurcation in both the ECA and ICA; however, this flow must be reversed in one of these two vessels. Usually, retrograde ECA flow into the carotid bulb will supply antegrade flow in the ICA (Plate 4-9). Rarely, the opposite flow pattern is encountered.[66,67]

Pitfalls in Spectral Analysis

Although velocity measurements have proven valuable in assessing the degree of vascular stenosis, there are times when absolute velocity determinations are less re-

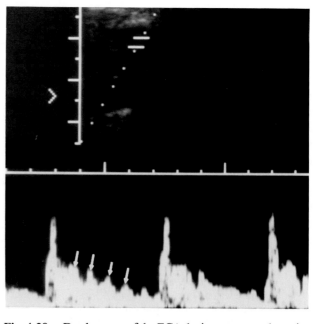

Fig. 4-20. Duplex scan of the ECA during a temporal tapping maneuver, demonstrating characteristic tapping defects in the ECA trace (arrows).

liable.[20,64,65] Cardiac arrhythmias, aortic valvular lesions, and severe cardiomyopathies can produce significant aberrations in the shape of carotid artery flow waveforms and alter systolic and diastolic velocity readings in a manner unrelated to carotid artery abnormalities. These alterations can invalidate standard Doppler spectral analysis as a means of quantifying stenoses. For example, bradycardia produces increased stroke volume, resulting in increased systolic velocities, whereas prolonged diastolic runoff produces spuriously decreased end-diastolic values. Any process that significantly alters cardiovascular physiology may affect carotid velocity measurements. Carotid artery velocity readings in a hypertensive patient may be higher than those in a normotensive individual with a comparable degree of carotid artery narrowing (Fig. 4-9 and Plate 4-10). Conversely, significantly decreased cardiac output or profound hypotension can decrease both systolic and diastolic velocities. Color Doppler can be particularly useful in overcoming the diagnostic uncertainties produced by cardiovascular abnormalities. The use of "cineloop" playback capabilities is particularly helpful. Cineloop allows the ultrasound computer to store up to 10 seconds of the previous color Doppler examination for playback at real-time rates or frame by frame. If one moves through the previous 10 seconds of the examination at a frame by frame rate, one can assess the filling of all parts of the vessel lumen, even if they are not all filled simultaneously.

High-grade stenoses or occlusions in one carotid artery can have a significant effect on velocities in a contralateral vessel. Severe unilateral ICA stenosis or occlusion can produce collateral shunting of increased blood flow through the contralateral carotid artery (Fig. 4-21 and Plate 4-11). This increased blood flow may artifactually increase velocity measurements in the contralateral vessel, particularly in areas of stenosis. Although one might expect that the velocity ratios in the carotid ar-

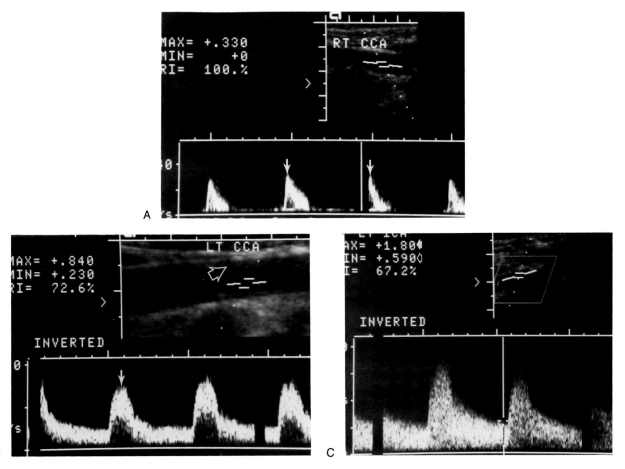

Fig. 4-21. (A) Markedly damped flow (arrows) in the right CCA in a patient with left hemispheric symptoms. There was no evidence of right ICA flow by pulsed or color Doppler (see Plate 4-11). (B) The left CCA demonstrates a normal spectral waveform (arrow). Note thickening of the intimal-medial complex (open arrow). (C) The left ICA demonstrates elevation of the peak systolic (arrow) and end-diastolic (open arrow) flow velocities, suggesting a 60 to 79 percent stenosis. Peak systolic ICA/CCA velocity ratios support this degree of stenosis, whereas the ICA/CCA end-diastolic velocity ratio suggests a lesser degree of stenosis.

teries contralateral to a high-grade narrowing would remain normal in the face of the velocity elevations, this is not always the case. Velocity ratios frequently are abnormal as a result of a disproportionate increase in velocities in areas of moderate narrowing compared with those in a completely patent vessel. A high-grade proximal CCA or innominate artery stenosis may reduce flow and produce spuriously decreased velocity measurements in stenoses distal to the point of the proximal narrowing ("tandem lesion").

The use of velocity ratios, which compare velocities in the ICA with those in the ipsilateral CCA, can help avoid some of the pitfalls involved in absolute velocity determinations.[20,21] The velocities obtained to compute ICA/CCA ratios should be obtained in the optimal location. ICA values should be obtained at or just distal to the point of maximum visible stenosis (greatest color Doppler spectral abnormality), and CCA values should be obtained proximal to the widening of the CCA in the region of the carotid bulb. Velocity ratios are particularly helpful when unusually high or low CCA flow velocities are found. Color Doppler is extremely valuable in avoiding pitfalls related to spurious pulsed Doppler spectral information (see below).

Although high-grade stenoses usually produce increased velocities in and distal to an area of narrowing, the presence of an additional high-grade narrowing, whether intracranial or extracranial, in tandem with a second high-grade stenosis may reduce expected velocity abnormalities. For this reason, it is extremely important that Doppler interrogation of vessels should be performed as far proximal and distal as possible to avoid missing a distal "tandem" lesion. Flow in and immediately distal to stenoses with greater than 95 percent narrowing is often damped with an abnormal waveform and small, if any, increase in velocity (Fig. 4-22). High-grade circumferential, long-segment vascular narrowings may also produce damped carotid artery waveforms that lack the expected high-velocity shift. Although no velocity elevations may be present in such long circumferential narrowings, spectral broadening and disturbed flow distal to these lesions is usually apparent. Color Doppler is particularly useful in detecting these fusiform narrowings in real-time (Fig. 4-18).

Aliasing, another potential source of error in pulsed Doppler ultrasound analysis, is caused by the inability to detect the true peak velocities in a vessel because of too low a Doppler sampling rate (PRF). The classic visual analogy of aliasing can be seen in Western movies, with an apparent reversal of stagecoach wheel spokes when the wagon wheel rotations exceed the film frame rate. The maximum detectable frequency shift cannot exceed half the PRF. Aliasing produces a characteristic appearance: the top of the time velocity spectrum (the highest velocities) is cut off and wraps around to emerge below

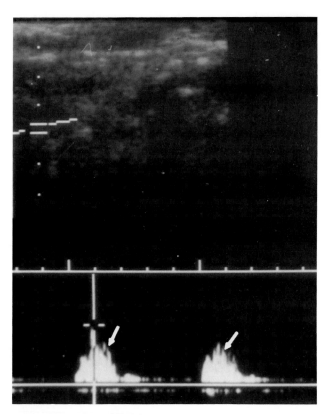

Fig. 4-22. Markedly abnormal low-velocity damped flow (arrows) in a right ICA with a long segment of greater than 95 percent stenosis.

the baseline (Fig. 4-23). It is easy to recognize that the negative-velocity spectrum does not represent true negative flow because the peaks of the negative flow point toward the zero baseline rather than away from it as should be the case with true negative-velocity spectra. CW ultrasound probes can be used in conjunction with duplex pulsed sonography to demonstrate the true peak velocity shift since CW Doppler does not have the PRF limitation inherent in pulsed Doppler. Aliasing can also be decreased or eliminated by increasing angle theta (the angle of Doppler insonation), thereby decreasing the detected Doppler shift, or by decreasing the insonating sound beam frequency. Increasing the PRF will increase the detectable frequency shift; however, the PRF increase is limited by the depth of the vessel as well as the center frequency of the transducer.[13] Aliasing can also be eliminated by shifting the zero baseline and reassigning a larger range of velocities to forward flow. It is valid to add velocities above and below the baseline in aliasing to obtain an accurate velocity, provided, however, that multiple wraparounds do not occur. Aliasing also occurs in color Doppler images and may be particularly useful in accenting the severity of flow disturbances.[14,62]

Although spectral broadening is a common feature of

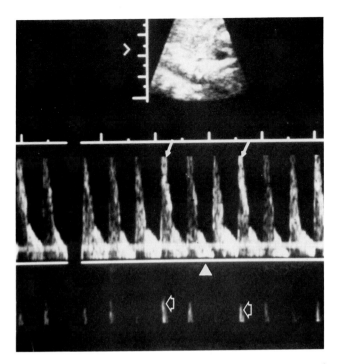

Fig. 4-23. Spectral waveforms demonstrating an example of aliasing. Note that the tops of the systolic peaks (arrows) are chopped off and appear as a wraparound flow velocity signal (open arrows) that points toward the zero-velocity baseline (arrowhead).

carotid stenosis, "pseudo spectral broadening" can be produced by numerous technical factors, including Doppler gain settings that are too high. When this happens, spurious background noise will be superimposed on the Doppler spectral waveform. Whenever spectral broadening is suspected, the gain should be optimized to eliminate background noise and to see whether the spectral window clears. Spectral broadening may also occur secondary to vessel wall motion when the Doppler sample volume is too large or positioned too close to a vessel wall. Decreasing the sample volume size and placing the sample volume midstream should eliminate this potential pitfall.

Flow separation, resulting in altered blood flow, is normal in branching vessels or at sites where there is an abrupt change in vessel diameter. For example, it is normal to see flow separation in the carotid bulb as the CCA branches into the ECA and ICA[39,40] (Plate 4-6). Spectral broadening may be detected in a normal carotid bulb in a localized area of dilatation prior to the carotid bifurcation. It is due to normal flow separation, not to abnormalities. Flow separation, with subsequent spectral broadening and increased velocity, may also occur in tortuous carotid vessels in the absence of atherosclerotic disease. Disturbed blood flow patterns in the ECA can also be seen in nonatheromatous abnormalities, includ-

ing carotid artery aneurysms, arterial dissections, and fibromuscular dysplasia.[15,68]

Spectral broadening has a tendency to increase in direct proportion to the velocity of blood flow. For example, it is seen in normal ECAs, in vertebral arteries, and in vessels carrying increased collateral circulation owing to occlusion of another major carotid branch. Increased velocities may also account for the disturbed flow sometimes observed in the carotid arteries of healthy athletes with normal cardiac outputs or in patients with pathologically increased cardiac output states. Such spectral broadening is frequently seen in areas of arteriovenous (AV) fistulas or AV malformations. Postoperative spectral broadening often persists for months following carotid endarterectomy in the absence of significant residual or recurrent disease[20,69,70] (Plate 4-12). Postoperative spectral broadening is particularly striking in cases of vein patch graft carotid surgery. This may be due to differences in wall compliance between the artery and vein patch, as well as to the relatively pronounced change in the diameter of the vessel in the area of the patch graft. In addition to marked spectral broadening, spectral analysis may demonstrate discordantly high or low velocities in the area of the vein patch graft. These discordant velocity readings obtained in the region of the patch graft can occur even though color Doppler shows a widely patent graft. However, color Doppler also shows the markedly disturbed patterns of flow within the area of the vein patch. The abnormal spectral velocity traces are high probably due to inappropriate assumptions regarding the true Doppler angle of the abnormal flow swirling within the patch graft. Incorrect assumptions about Doppler angles can result in inappropriate increases or decreases in subsequent velocity determinations. Fortunately, CCA flow proximal to these grafts and ICA flow distal to the grafts demonstrate relatively normal flow velocity waveforms and velocities.

Correlation of image and Doppler information with the Doppler spectrum usually defines the cause of spectral broadening. One should remember that spectral broadening is a nonspecific finding, which does not necessarily imply vascular pathology. Familiarity with normal Doppler flow patterns and the use of appropriate Doppler techniques will eliminate many potential diagnostic pitfalls.

Benefits of Color Doppler

Color Doppler clearly delineates the patent vessel lumen and may allow one to visualize subtle vessel wall irregularities and hypoechoic plaque better than with gray-scale imaging and Doppler alone (Plate 4-1). Plaque ulcerations within hypoechoic plaque that are not readily appreciated on conventional gray-scale imaging may be better demonstrated by color Doppler, which shows relatively low-velocity eddying flow within the plaque ulcerations (Plate 4-7). Doppler spectral analysis is speeded by using color Doppler, which readily identifies flow abnormalities for subsequent pulsed Doppler spectral analysis. Heterogeneous color changes within a vessel, as well as apparent visible luminal narrowing demonstrated on color Doppler, suggest a major stenosis (Plate 4-13). A severe stenosis may produce a bruit or a thrill; the perivascular tissue vibrations can actually be visualized by color Doppler as artifactual transient red and blue speckles in the tissue adjacent to the stenosis.[71] Although changes in the color pattern are useful for identifying flow abnormalities for subsequent pulsed Doppler analysis, one must be cautious not to equate color saturation with velocity as determined by pulsed Doppler spectral analysis.[38] The color assignment within a vessel is corrected for only one angle along the course of a vessel. Therefore, it may change independently of velocities within a vessel if the Doppler angle in a vessel changes relative to the Doppler transducer. For example, desaturated color or "green-tagged" flow in a vessel may represent abnormally elevated velocities; however, it may also represent a region of flow that is at a more acute Doppler angle relative to the transducer than are other parts of the vessel (Plate 4-14). Furthermore, color systems generally compute the mean velocity to assign colors to each pixel in the image. However, the maximum velocity is required for spectral analysis that is used to assess the degree of stenosis. Thus, Doppler spectral sampling remains necessary for precise quantitation of hemodynamically significant stenoses.

There are several areas in which color Doppler may help avoid potential pitfalls in the duplex ultrasound examination. When there are alterations in cardiovascular physiology, tandem lesions within vessels, or obstructive lesions in ipsilateral or contralateral vessels,[72] or when vessels are extremely tortuous, color Doppler may be particularly useful in directing spectral analysis or clarifying the source of a discrepancy between image and Doppler data. Furthermore, color Doppler appears to have particular value in detecting small channels of flow in areas of a high-grade carotid stenosis[73,74] (Plate 4-15). These small strings of flow can be easily missed by duplex scanning if the sample volume is not placed precisely in the area of the channel. This could result in a misdiagnosis of complete occlusion when actually a surgically correctable high-grade stenosis is present. In high-grade stenoses (≥ 90 percent), with markedly decreased peak ICA velocities, standard color Doppler sensitivity settings may fail to demonstrate residual flow. "Slow-flow" sensitivity settings should always be used to discriminate between critical stenoses and occlu-

sions.[71,73] Carotid artery occlusion is diagnosed when no color flow is identified within the carotid even with "slow-flow" settings. Early diastolic flow reversal at the orifice of an occluded ICA can further support the diagnosis of complete occlusion. However, such flow reversal is occasionally seen in extremely high-grade stenoses, and normal flow reversal may also exist at the carotid bifurcation. The presence of a high-grade stenosis or occlusion can also be inferred from color Doppler flow patterns within the ipsilateral CCA, which show color flow in systole but a marked, asymmetric decrease or absence of color flow in diastole.[75] This is the color Doppler analogy of the damped waveform seen in pulsed Doppler spectral analysis proximal to a high-grade occlusive lesion.

Preliminary studies comparing color Doppler with conventional duplex ultrasound and angiography show that they have similar accuracy, sensitivity, and specificity.[73-76] Although color Doppler may facilitate differentiation of high-grade stenosis from occlusions better than pulsed Doppler spectral analysis does, 100 percent accuracy in the color Doppler distinction between these two conditions has not been documented. Still, color Doppler improves confidence in diagnosis by clarifying confusing situations that may arise from apparent conflicts between Doppler and image information. It greatly speeds the carotid Doppler examination

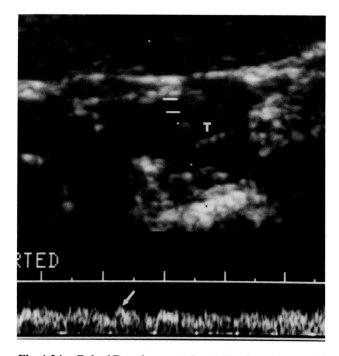

Fig. 4-24. Pulsed Doppler spectral analysis of another carotid body tumor *(T),* demonstrating a characteristic high-velocity AV shunt-type waveform (arrow), consistent with the very vascular nature of this tumor. (See also Plate 4-18.)

and improves the reproducibility of Doppler spectral analyses.[77]

Nonatherosclerotic Carotid Pathology

Atherosclerotic carotid disease is far more common than nonatherosclerotic carotid pathology. However, Doppler, and particularly color Doppler, may be useful in the evaluation of nonatherosclerotic carotid diseases. Fibromuscular dysplasia (FMD) results from hypertrophy of muscular and fibrous arterial walls, separated by abnormal zones of fragmentation. This noninflammatory process involves the ICA more often than other segments of the vessel. Although a characteristic "string-of-beads" appearance has been described for FMD on angiography, ultrasound descriptions of the appearance of this lesion are limited[68] (Plate 4-16). FMD may result in carotid dissections, and in such cases an intimal flap may be seen waving in the vessel lumen on real-time sonography. Autoimmune processes, such as

Takayasu's arteritis or temporal arteritis, or radiation damage may produce diffuse concentric thickening of vessel walls. The arteritides most frequently involve the CCA.[78] Cervical trauma can produce carotid dissections or aneurysms. Experience of using color Doppler and pulsed Doppler to investigate these abnormalities is limited, but it appears that color Doppler may be particularly useful in detecting channels of flow within a carotid dissection[15] (Plate 4-17).

Carotid body tumors, one of a group of paragangliomas that involve the head and neck, are characteristically benign, well-encapsulated masses located at the carotid bifurcation. These very vascular tumors often produce a bruit and may demonstrate peritumoral AV shunt-type Doppler flow patterns (Plate 4-18 and Fig. 4-24). They may be bilateral, and some produce catecholamines, resulting in precipitous changes in blood pressure postoperatively. Extravascular masses, including tumors, hematomas, and abscesses, may compress or displace the carotid; these can be readily distinguished from primary vascular masses, such as aneurysms, by real-time ultrasound and color Doppler.

VERTEBRAL ARTERY

The vertebral arteries provide the main blood supply to the posterior brain circulation. They also provide a source of collateral circulation to other portions of the brain via the circle of Willis when significant carotid occlusive disease is present. Although evaluation of the extracranial vertebral artery seems a natural extension of the carotid duplex examination, these arteries have not been studied as intensively as the carotids. This may in part be because vertebral arteries demonstrate many anatomic variations. In addition, they are relatively small vessels with a deep course and visualization is limited by overlying transverse processes and the base of the skull. Symptoms of vertebrobasilar insufficiency tend to be vague and poorly defined compared with symptoms referable to carotid pathology; therefore it is difficult to correlate suspected vertebral abnormalities with patient symptoms. Finally, there has been limited interest in surgical correction of vertebral lesions.[79] Despite these drawbacks, duplex ultrasound and color Doppler have established a clear-cut role in screening for subclavian steal syndrome.[75,80,81] The clinical utility of vertebral sonography for detecting vertebral artery stenoses and occlusions is less well established, since only anecdotal reports of visualization of vertebral artery aneurysms and dissections detected by sonography have been published.

TECHNIQUE

Vertebral arteries can be visualized, and Doppler flow can be detected in some portion of over 95 percent of cases.[80,81,84] Color Doppler facilitates rapid detection of vertebral arteries and can help establish the direction of blood flow within these vessels. The vertebral artery duplex examination is performed as follows. First the CCA is located in the longitudinal plane. Then direction of flow in the CCA and jugular vein is determined. A gradual angulation of the transducer laterally will demonstrate the vertebral artery and usually the vertebral vein coursing between the transverse processes of C6 to C2 (Plate 4-19). These transverse processes, which are identified by their periodic posterior acoustic shadows, prevent a complete analysis of the vertebral arteries. Angling the transducer inferiorly at the level of the clavicles allows one to visualize the vertebral artery origin 80 percent of the time on the right side and roughly 50 to 60 percent of the time on the left. This discrepancy is probably because the left vertebral artery origin is deeper, and in 6 to 8 percent of patients it arises directly from the aortic arch.

The presence and direction of blood flow within the vertebral artery should be determined. Transverse scanning with color Doppler may allow the examiner to visualize the carotid artery, jugular vein, and vertebral artery at the same time. The presence and direction of flow within the vertebral artery should be documented, as should any visible plaque disease. Care should be taken not to mistake flow in a pulsatile vertebral vein for that in the adjacent vertebral artery. If an intermittent or partial subclavian steal syndrome is suspected, procedures may be performed to provoke a complete subclavian steal.

NORMAL ANATOMY

The vertebral artery is usually the first branch off of the subclavian artery. However, variation in the vertebral artery origin is common. The left vertebral artery arises directly from the aortic arch proximal to the left subclavian artery in 6 to 8 percent of individuals. The proximal vertebral artery courses superomedially, passing anterior to the transverse process of C7 and entering

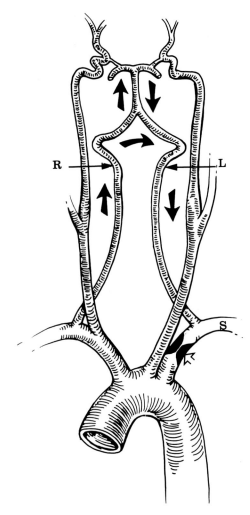

Fig. 4-26. Diagram of the mechanisms involved in the subclavian steal syndrome. The arrows demonstrate the aberrant flow pathways that result from a high-grade proximal left subclavian artery (*S*) stenosis (open arrow). (*R*, right vertebral artery; *L*, left vertebral artery.)

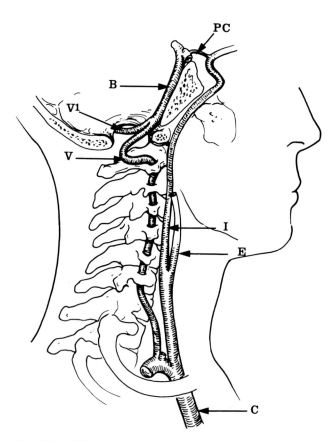

Fig. 4-25. Diagram of normal vertebral and carotid circulation with intracranial communications. (*C*, common carotid artery; *I*, internal carotid artery; *E*, external carotid artery; *V*, vertebral artery; *V1*, contralateral vertebral artery; *B*, basilar artery; *PC*, posterior communicating artery.)

the transverse foramen at the C6 level in 90 percent of individuals. However, vertebral arteries may enter the transverse foramina anywhere from the C7 to C4 level. The size of the vertebral arteries is variable. The left is larger than the right in 42 percent of individuals, the two arteries are equal in size in 26 percent, and the right is larger than the left in 32 percent. Occasionally, a vertebral artery is congenitally absent or hypoplastic. Vertebral arteries unite within the posterior fossa to form the basilar artery and supply most of the posterior brain circulation. In addition, these arteries may provide collateral circulation via the circle of Willis to the anterior brain in cases of carotid occlusive disease (Fig. 4-25).

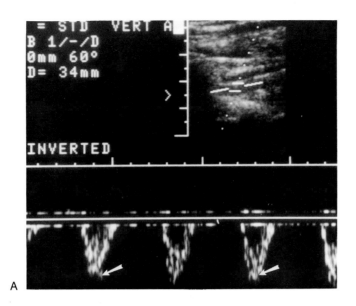

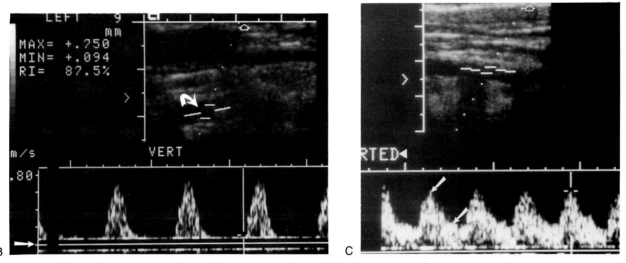

Fig. 4-27. **(A)** Duplex scan of the left vertebral artery in a patient with subclavian steal syndrome, demonstrating a high-resistance reversed arterial flow pattern (arrows). This pattern is consistent with subclavian steal syndrome. **(B)** Duplex scan in the same left vertebral artery, demonstrating the importance of paying attention to the appropriate direction of blood flow in vessels. In this scan the flow in the vertebral artery is above the zero-velocity baseline (arrow) (toward the Doppler transducer). However, in this particular scan, flow in the vertebral artery (curved arrow) should be directed away from the Doppler transducer (open arrow). Flow would be directed below the zero-velocity baseline if this vertebral artery were normal. When Doppler flow in a vessel is directed away from the Doppler transducer, the only way that flow velocity waveforms can be depicted above the zero-velocity baseline is by inverting the Doppler waveforms, as has been done in Fig. A. **(C)** Flow velocity waveforms in the right vertebral artery in this patient with a left subclavian steal, demonstrating increased cephalic flow (arrows). Note that flow in the vertebral artery is again directed away from the Doppler transducer (open arrow). However, flow velocity waveforms are depicted above the baseline, because the signal has been inverted (arrowhead). Flow in this vertebral artery is in the correct direction. *(Figure continues.)*

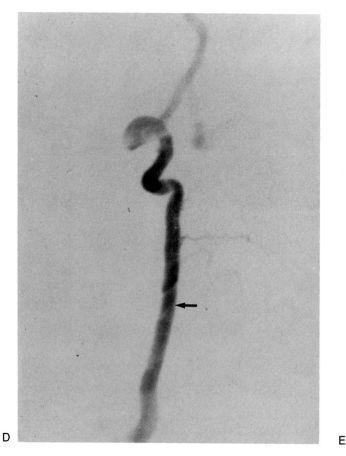

D

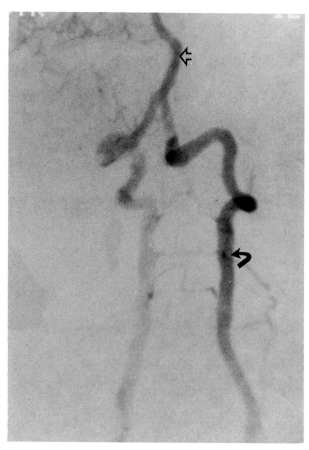

E

Fig. 4-27 *(Continued).* **(D & E)** Angiographic findings of subclavian steal syndrome. There is initial filling of the right vertebral artery (arrow, Fig. D). The subsequent steal into the left subclavian artery (curved arrow) via the basilar artery (open arrow) is seen in Fig. E.

ABNORMALITIES

Subclavian Steal Syndrome

Subclavian steal syndrome results when the proximal subclavian artery is stenotic or occluded. The ischemic arm "steals" blood flow from the basilar circulation via retrograde vertebral artery flow, producing symptoms of vertebral basilar insufficiency (Fig. 4-26). These symptoms are usually most pronounced during arm exercise, although occasionally positioning of the head exacerbates symptoms. Subclavian steal is readily identified by detecting reversed vertebral artery flow on Doppler spectral tracings or color Doppler images (Fig. 4-27). Not all subclavian steals are complete, however. Occult or incomplete subclavian steals may not demonstrate reversed vertebral artery flow unless provocative maneuvers are performed. Five minutes of ipsilateral arm exercise or of sphygmomanometer inflation to just above systolic pressures to produce postocclusive hyperemia

can convert these occult subclavian steals to complete steals. Thus these maneuvers should be a routine part of the evaluation of a suspected subclavian steal unless a frank subclavian steal is demonstrated at the beginning of the examination. A partial subclavian steal phenomenon may also be demonstrated by Doppler. This consists of retrograde flow in systole and antegrade flow in diastole[82] (Fig. 4-28). Such partial steals may also be converted to complete steals by provocative maneuvers if desired.

Pulsed Doppler analysis demonstrates retrograde, high-resistance vertebral artery blood flow. Color Doppler may show two similarly color-coded vessels running between the transverse processes of the cervical spine, representing reversed flow in the vertebral artery and normal flow in the adjacent vertebral vein. If only a single vessel is seen coursing between the transverse processes and it demonstrates retrograde color Doppler flow and coding, it is essential to perform pulsed Doppler spectral analysis to avoid mistaking the flow reversal of a

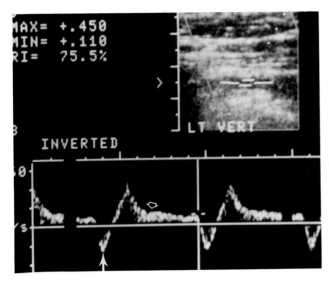

Fig. 4-28. Duplex scan in a left vertebral artery demonstrating characteristic flow velocity waveforms in a patient with a partial or incomplete subclavian steal syndrome. Note the transient reversal of flow (arrow) in early systole with subsequent antegrade flow through the remainder of the cardiac cycle (open arrow).

subclavian steal for normal pulsatile vertebral venous flow (Fig. 4-29). It has been suggested that visualizing only a vertebral vein is suggestive of occlusion or congenital absence of the vertebral artery.[75] Demonstration of clear-cut flow reversal in any portion of the vertebral artery is sufficient to make the diagnosis of subclavian steal syndrome.

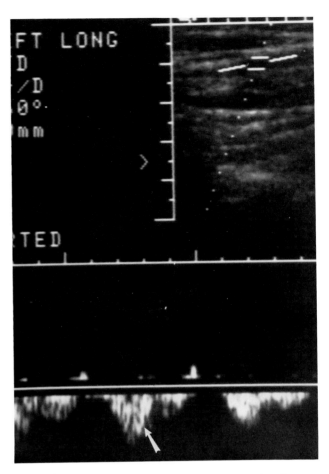

Fig. 4-29. Longitudinal duplex scan demonstrating the normal, pulsatile appearance of vertebral veins (arrow).

Stenosis and Occlusion

Diagnosis of vertebral artery stenosis is more difficult than diagnosis of subclavian steal. Most vertebral artery stenoses occur at the origin of the vessel, which is located deep in the upper thorax and can be visualized in only 60 to 70 percent of patients. Furthermore, the deep location of the vertebral artery origin may make optimal adjustments of the Doppler angle and velocity measurements difficult. A large part of the vertebral artery cannot be visualized because of overlying transverse processes and the skull. Although transcranial Doppler may provide information about the intracranial blood flow within the vertebral arteries, no universally accepted reproducible criteria for evaluating vertebral artery stenoses exist. Since blood flow within the vertebral arteries typically demonstrates spectral broadening, that criteria cannot be used as a reliable indicator of stenosis. The wide range of variability in vertebral artery diameters makes absolute velocity measurements less reliable as criteria for stenosis. Although velocities exceeding 100 cm/s often indicate stenosis, they have been demonstrated in angiographically normal vessels.[83,84] Some investigators suggest that a focal increase in velocity of at least 50 percent and/or visible stenosis on gray-scale or color Doppler may indicate significant vertebral stenoses. The variability of resistivity indices (RIs) in normal and abnormal vertebral arteries precludes the use of this parameter as an indicator of vertebral stenosis.[84]

Vertebral artery occlusion is also difficult to diagnose. Hypoplastic or congenitally absent vertebral arteries cannot be distinguished from occluded vessels. Furthermore, differentiation of a high-grade stenosis from an occlusion in the vertebral artery is even more difficult than in the ICA. Nevertheless, if one is capable of detecting vertebral venous flow and no arterial flow is detected adjacent to venous flow, an obstructed, extremely narrowed, or congenitally absent vertebral artery is likely.

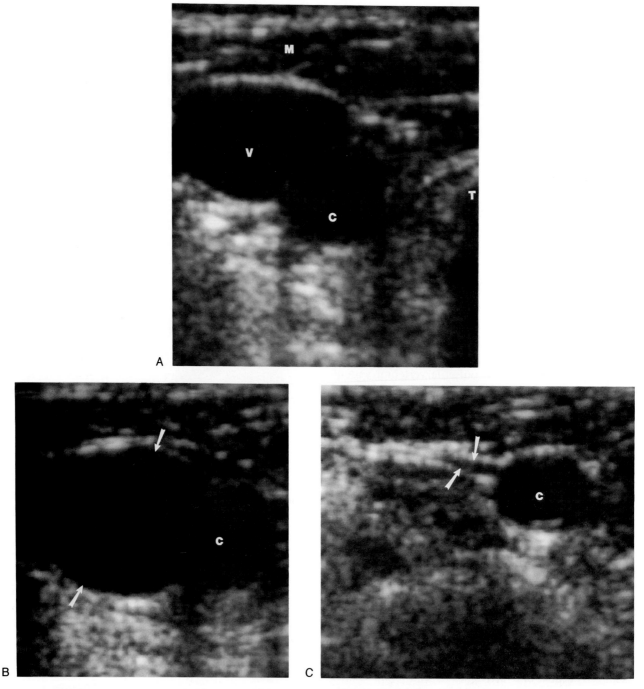

Fig. 4-30. **(A)** Transverse scan demonstrating a normal, prominent right internal jugular vein *(V)*. (*C*, common carotid artery; *M*, sternocleidomastoid muscle; *T*, trachea.) **(B)** Transverse image of the same internal jugular vein during a Valsalva maneuver demonstrating a marked increase in diameter (arrows). (*C*, common carotid artery.) **(C)** Transducer compression of the same internal jugular vein, producing complete coaptation of the walls of the vein (arrows). (*C*, common carotid artery.)

INTERNAL JUGULAR VEIN

The internal jugular vein is responsible for the return of the majority of venous blood from the brain. Duplex sonography and color Doppler of the internal jugular vein are most commonly performed to evaluate suspected jugular vein thrombosis.[85-88] Sonography is also useful in the evaluation of jugular venous ectasia[89-91] and for directing catheterization of the internal jugular vein, particularly in situations in which the vascular anatomy is distorted.[92-94] Sonography is also used to assess subclavian vein patency and to guide subclavian venopuncture.[94]

TECHNIQUE

The jugular vein is scanned with the patient's neck extended and the head turned away from the side being examined. Longitudinal and transverse scans should be obtained with minimal transducer pressure on the neck to avoid compressing and collapsing the vein. An attempt should be made to visualize the lower segment of the internal jugular vein and the medial segment of the subclavian vein as they join to form the brachiocephalic vein in the supraclavicular fossa. Real-time sonography should demonstrate venous pulsations relative to right-heart contractions, as well as changes in venous diameter in response to respiration. With inspiration, decreased intrathoracic pressure causes flow toward the heart and the jugular veins decrease in diameter. During expiration and with Valsalva maneuvers, increased intrathoracic pressure decreases blood return and causes venous enlargement and a marked decrease in venous flow. If venous thrombosis is suspected, moderate transducer pressure should be applied to the jugular vein; the walls of a patent jugular vein should coapt completely with such maneuvers (Fig. 4-30). Furthermore, sniffing techniques that reduce intrathoracic pressure produce transient venous collapse on real-time sonography. Doppler and color Doppler provide additional insight into venous patency (Fig. 4-31). Furthermore, color Doppler may outline the extent of nonocclusive thrombus within jugular or subclavian veins. Visualization of moving valves within the distal internal jugular or subclavian vein may further assist in the determination of venous patency (Fig. 4-32).

ANATOMY

The internal jugular vein drains the majority of blood from the brain, face, and neck. It courses inferiorly in the neck, lying anterolateral to the ICA and CCA. In the retroclavicular region, it unites with the subclavian vein

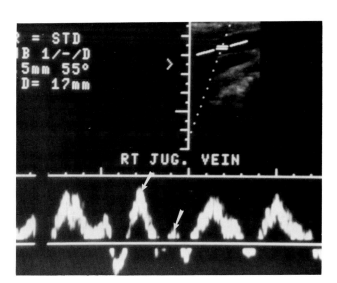

Fig. 4-31. Normal right internal jugular vein demonstrating a pulsatile waveform reflecting right-heart contractions (arrows).

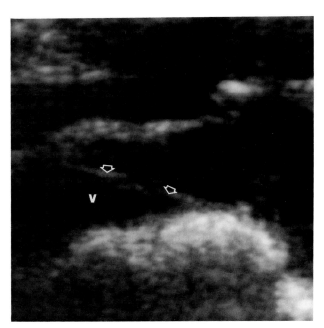

Fig. 4-32. Transverse scan through the right subclavian vein (*V*) demonstrating paired venous valves (open arrows), which move with venous pulsations.

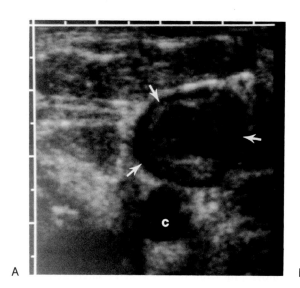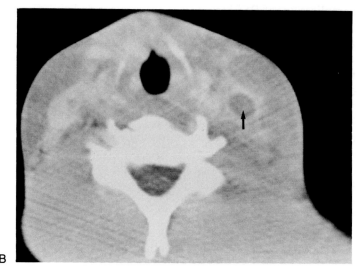

Fig. 4-33. (A) Transverse sonogram in a patient with swelling and pain in the left neck associated with intravenous drug abuse, demonstrating a distended, noncompressible, thrombus-filled left internal jugular vein (arrows). (*C*, common carotid artery.) **(B)** CT scan demonstrating the large, low-density filling defect in the left internal jugular vein (arrow).

to form the brachiocephalic vein (Fig. 4-13). The right internal jugular vein usually crosses over the subclavian artery as it is joining the subclavian vein, whereas the left internal jugular vein usually overlaps the proximal CCA before it unites with the left subclavian vein. Both internal jugular veins contain a pair of valves located about 2.5 cm above their junction with the subclavian veins. The right internal jugular vein is usually larger than the left.

ABNORMALITY

Jugular Vein Thrombosis

Jugular vein thrombosis (JVT) presents clinically with a tender, erythematous, ill-defined mass or swelling. The clinical presentation can be very confusing, and the source of the abnormalities may not be immediately apparent.[85] Internal JVT can be asymptomatic because of the relatively deep position of the vein and the presence of abundant cervical collaterals. Before the advent of duplex sonography, JVT was diagnosed by venography. This is an invasive procedure and thus was performed only when there was a high index of clinical suspicion. Now that noninvasive imaging techniques, including ultrasound, computed tomography (CT), and magnetic resonance imaging (MRI), are available, JVT is being diagnosed more frequently. The most common cause of internal JVT is central venous catheteriza-

tion.[85,88] JVT may also be caused by intravenous drug abuse, hypercoagulable states, mediastinal tumors, prior head and neck surgery and/or radiation, and the presence of local infectious or inflammatory processes or adenopathy. Occasionally, JVT is idiopathic. Potential

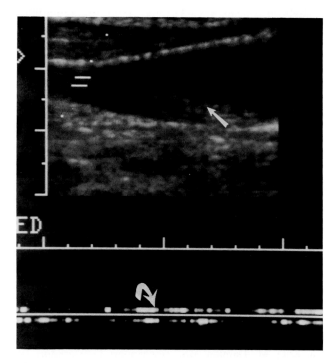

Fig. 4-34. Duplex scan in the same patient as shown in Plate 4-20, with internal jugular vein thrombus (arrow), demonstrating the absence of pulsed Doppler flow (curved arrow).

complications of JVT include clot propagation and pulmonary embolism, as well as suppurative thrombophlebitis and abscess formation.[95]

Sonographic features of JVT include an enlarged, noncompressible jugular vein that may contain visible echogenic thrombus (Fig. 4-33). Acute thrombus may be anechoic and indistinguishable from flowing blood; however, the jugular vein should still be dilated and lack compressibility on real-time examination. Furthermore, absent flow on Doppler or color Doppler examination quickly distinguishes between anechoic thrombus and flowing blood, as well as demonstrating the extent of nonocclusive venous thrombus (Fig. 4-34 and Plate 4-20). Thrombosed jugular veins also lose their response to respiratory maneuvers and lack normal cardiothoracic variability and pulsation. Venous collaterals, particularly prominent in chronic internal JVT, are readily identified by color Doppler. Chronic JVT may organize, resulting in an echogenic venous lumen that may be difficult to distinguish from surrounding echogenic perivascular fatty tissue.[88] Although chronic venous thrombi are frequently echogenic, clot echogenicity is not a reliable means of distinguishing acute from chronic venous thrombosis.

Sonography is a quick, noninvasive, and accurate method of diagnosing JVT. However, it has limited access and cannot image all portions of the jugular vein and subclavian vein, particularly those located behind the clavicle or mandible. Still, since demonstration of the full extent of thrombus is usually not critical in planning treatment, sonography offers a valuable screen for detecting pathology in this area. Color Doppler is particularly useful in the evaluation of subclavian vein thrombosis, where compression techniques cannot be readily applied, to assess the presence of venous thrombosis. Serial sonographic examinations can be safely and inexpensively performed to evaluate response to anticoagulant therapy.[96,97]

CONCLUSION

Color Doppler and duplex sonography provide accurate, noninvasive vascular imaging and have had a major impact on the diagnostic approach to vascular diseases. They provide an ideal screening test for suspected extracranial artery disease. Subclavian steal syndrome and venous thrombosis are also diagnosed quickly and noninvasively. Because sonography is noninvasive and relatively inexpensive, it can be used repeatedly to follow up the response to therapy for arterial or venous diseases. Improved Doppler technology and a broader understanding of blood flow patterns in normal and diseased vessels should yield even greater advances in vascular imaging diagnosis.

REFERENCES

1. Carroll BA: "Duplex" Doppler carotid sonography. p. 762. In Fleischer AC, James AE (eds): Diagnostic Sonography: Principles and Clinical Applications. WB Saunders, Philadelphia, 1989

2. Strandness DE Jr: Noninvasive evaluation of arteriosclerosis—comparison of methods. Arteriosclerosis 1983;3:103

3. O'Leary DH, Persson AV, Clouse ME: Noninvasive testing for carotid artery stenosis. 1. Prospective analysis of three methods. AJR 1981;137:1189

4. Sumner DS, Russell JB, Ramsey DE et al: Noninvasive diagnosis of extracranial carotid arterial disease—a prospective evaluation of pulsed-Doppler imaging and oculoplethysmography. Arch Surg 1979;114:1222

5. de Bray JM, Joseph PA, Jeanvoine H et al: Transcranial Doppler evaluation of middle cerebral artery stenosis. J Ultrasound Med 1988;7:611

6. Kaps M, Damian MS, Teschendorf U, Dorndorf W: Transcranial Doppler ultrasound findings in middle cerebral artery occlusion. Stroke 1990;21:532

7. Niederkorn K, Myers LG, Nunn CL et al: Three-dimensional transcranial Doppler blood flow mapping in patients with cerebrovascular disorders. Stroke 1988; 19:1335

8. Aaslid R, Huber P, Nornes H: Evaluation of cerebrovascular spasm with transcranial Doppler ultrasound. J Neurosurg 1984;60:37

9. Grant EG, White EM, Schellinger D et al: Cranial duplex sonography of the infant. Radiology 1987;163:177

10. Mitchell DG, Merton D, Desai H et al: Neonatal brain: color Doppler imaging. Part II. Altered flow patterns from extracorporeal membrane oxygenation. Radiology 1988;167:307

11. Matsumoto JS, Babcock DS, Brody AS et al: Right common carotid artery ligation for extracorporeal membrane oxygenation: cerebral blood flow velocity measurement with Doppler duplex US. Radiology 1990; 175:757

12. Glasier CM, Seibert JJ, Chadduck WM et al: Brain death in infants: evaluation with Doppler US. Radiology 1989;172:377

13. Carroll BA, von Ramm CT: Fundamentals of current Doppler technology. Ultrasound 1988;6:275

14. Merritt CRB: Doppler color flow imaging. J Clin Ultrasound 1987;15:591

15. Bluth EI, Shyn PB, Sullivan MA, Merritt CRB: Doppler color flow imaging of carotid artery dissection. J Ultrasound Med 1989;8:149

16. Steinke W, Hennerici M, Anlick A: Doppler color flow imaging of carotid body tumors. Stroke 1989;20:1574

17. Gooding GAW, Langman AW, Dillon WP, Kaplan MJ: Malignant carotid artery invasion: sonographic detection. Radiology 1989;171:435

18. Russell D, Bakke SJ, Wiberg J et al: Patency and flow velocity profiles in the internal carotid artery assessed by digital subtraction angiography and Doppler studies three months following endarterectomy. J Nerol Neurosurg Psychiatry 1986;49:183

19. Glover JL, Bendick PJ, Dilley RS et al: Restenosis following carotid endarterectomy—evaluation by duplex ultrasonography. Arch Surg 1985;120:678

20. Carroll BA: Carotid sonography: pitfalls and color flow. Appl Radiol 1988;Oct:15

21. Zwiebel WJ: Spectrum analysis in carotid sonography. Ultrasound Med Biol 1987;13:623

22. Bluth EI, Wetzner SM, Stavros AT et al: Carotid duplex sonography: a multicenter recommendation for standardized imaging and Doppler criteria. RadioGraphics 1988;8:487

23. Robinson ML, Sacks D, Perlmutter GS, Marinelli : Diagnostic criteria for carotid duplex sonography. AJR 1988;15:1045

24. Garth KE, Carroll BA, Sommer FG, Oppenheimer DA: Duplex ultrasound scanning of the carotid arteries with velocity spectrum analysis. Radiology 1983;147:823

25. Jackson VP, Kuehn DS, Bendick PJ et al: Duplex carotid sonography: correlation with digital subtraction angiography and conventional angiography. J Ultrasound Med 1985;4:239

26. Blackshear WM, Phillips DJ, Chikos PM et al: Carotid artery velocity patterns in normal and stenotic vessels. Stroke 1980;11:67

27. Friedman SG, Hainline B, Feinberg AW et al: Use of diastolic velocity ratios to predict significant carotid artery stenosis. Stroke 1988;19:910

28. Dreisbach JN, Seibert CE, Smazal SF et al: Duplex sonography in the evaluation of carotid artery disease. AJNR 1983;4:678

29. Vaisman U, Wojciechowski M: Carotid artery disease: new criteria for evaluation by sonographic duplex scanning. Radiology 1986;158:253

30. Kotval PS: Doppler waveform parvus and tardus—a sign of proximal flow obstruction. J Ultrasound Med 1989;8:435

31. Withers CE, Gosink BB, Keightley AM et al: Duplex carotid sonography—peak systolic velocity in quantifying internal carotid artery stenosis. J Ultrasound Med 1990;9:345

32. Taylor DC, Strandness DE: Carotid artery duplex scanning. J Clin Ultrasound 1987;15:635

33. Eklof BO, Schwartz SI: Effects of critical stenosis of the carotid artery and compromised cephalic blood flow. Arch Surg 1969;99:695

34. Moneta GL, Taylor DC, Ziesler E et al: Asymptomatic high-grade internal carotid artery stenosis: is stratification according to risk factors or duplex spectral analysis possible? J Vasc Surg 1989;10:475

35. Kassam M, Kohnston KW, Cobbold RSC: Quantitative estimation of spectral broadening for the diagnosis of carotid arterial disease: method and in vitro results. Ultrasound Med Biol 1985;11:425

36. Sumner DS: Use of color-flow imaging technique in carotid artery disease. Surg Clin North Am 1990;70:201

37. Grant EG, Tessler FN, Perrella RR: Clinical Doppler imaging. AJR 1989;152:707

38. Mitchell DG: Color Doppler imaging: principles, limitations and artifacts. Radiology 1990;177:1

39. Phillips DJ, Greene FM, Langlois Y et al: Flow velocity patterns in the carotid bifurcation of young, presumed normal subjects. Ultrasound Med Biol 1983;9:39

40. Middleton WD, Foley WD, Lawson TL: Flow reversal in the normal carotid bifurcation: color Doppler flow imaging analysis. Radiology 1988;167:207

41. O'Leary DH, Polak JF: High-resolution carotid sonography: past, present, and future. AJR 1989;153:699

42. Poli A, Tremoli E, Colombo A et al: Ultrasonographic measurement of the common carotid artery wall thickness in hypercholesterolemic patients. A new model for the quantitation and follow-up of preclinical atherosclerosis in living human subjects. Atherosclerosis 1988;70:253

43. Pignoli PP, Tremoli ET, Poli A et al: Intimal plus medial thickness of the arterial wall: a direct measurement with ultrasound imaging. Circulation 1986;74:1399

44. Nolsoe CP, Engel U, Karstrup S et al: The aortic wall: an in vitro study of the double-line pattern in high-resolution US. Radiology 1990;175:387

45. Carroll BA: Duplex sonography in patients with hemispheric symptoms. J Ultrasound Med 1989;8:535

46. Brown PB, Zwiebel WJ, Call GK: Degree of cervical carotid artery stenosis and hemispheric stroke: duplex US findings. Radiology 1989;170:541

47. Dixon S, Pais SO, Raviola C et al: Natural history of nonstenotic asymptomatic ulcerative lesions of the carotid artery, a further analysis. Arch Surg 1982;17:1493

48. Langsfield M, Gray-Weale AC, Lusky RJ: The role of plaque morphology and diameter reduction in the development of new symptoms in asymptomatic carotid arteries. J Vasc Surg 1989;9:548

49. Leaky AL, McCollum PT, Feeley TM et al: Duplex ultrasonography and selection of patients for carotid endarterectomy: plaque morphology or luminal narrowing. J Vasc Surg 1988;8:558

50. Harward TRS, Kroener JM, Wickbom IG, Bernstein EF: Natural history of asymptomatic ulcerative plaques of the carotid bifurcation. Am J Surg 1983;146:208

51. Bassiouny HS, Davis H, Massawa N et al: Critical carotid stenoses: morphologic and clinical similarity between symptomatic and asymptomatic plaques. J Vasc Surg 1989;9:202

52. Lennehan L, Kupsky WJ, Mohr JP et al: Lack of association between carotid plaque hematoma and ischemic cerebral symptoms. Stroke 1987;18:879

53. Lusby RJ, Ferrell LD, Ehrenfeld WK et al: Carotid plaque

hemorrhage — its role in production of cerebral ischemia. Arch Surg 1982;117:1479

54. Reilly LM, Lusby RJ, Hughes L et al: Carotid plaque histology using real-time ultrasonography — clinical and therapeutic implications. Am J Surg 1983;146:188

55. Bluth EI, Kay D, Merritt CRB et al: Sonographic characterization of carotid plaque: detection of hemorrhage. AJR 1986;146:1061

56. Imparto A, Riles T, Mintzer R, Baumann F: The importance of hemorrhage in the relationship between gross morphologic characteristics and cerebral symptoms in 376 carotid artery plaques. Am Surg 1983;197:195

57. O'Donnell TF, Erdoes L, Mackey WC et al: Correlation of B-mode ultrasound imaging and arteriography with pathologic findings at carotid endarterectomy. Arch Surg 1985;120:443

58. O'Leary DH, Holen J, Ricotta JJ et al: Carotid bifurcation disease: prediction of ulceration with B-mode US. Radiology 1987;162:523

59. Bluth EI, McVay LV, Merritt CRB, Sullivan MA: The identification of ulcerative plaque with high resolution duplex carotid scanning. J Ultrasound Med 1988;7:73

60. Comerota AJ, Katz ML, White JV, Grosh JD: The preoperative diagnosis of the ulcerated carotid atheroma. J Vasc Surg 1990;11:505

61. Eikelboom BC, Riles TR, Mintzer R et al: Inaccuracy of angiography in the diagnosis of carotid ulceration. Stroke 1983;14:882

62. Middleton WD, Foley WD, Lawson TL: Color-flow Doppler imaging of carotid artery abnormalities. AJR 1988;150:419

63. Edwards JH, Kricheff II, Riles T, Imparto A: Angiographically undetected ulceration of the carotid bifurcation as a cause of embolic stroke. Radiology 1979;132:369

64. Zwiebel WJ, Crummy AB: Sources of error in Doppler diagnosis of carotid occlusive disease. AJR 1981;137:1

65. Jacobs NM, Grant EG, Schellinger D et al: Duplex carotid sonography: criteria for stenosis, accuracy, and pitfalls. Radiology 1985;154:385

66. Bebry AJ, Hines GL: Total occlusion of the common carotid artery with a patent internal carotid artery: report of a case. J Vasc Surg 1989;10:469

67. Blackshear WM, Phillips DJ, Bodily KC, Strandness DE: Ultrasonic demonstration of external and internal carotid patency with common carotid occlusion: a preliminary report. Stroke 1980;11:249

68. Kliewer MA, Carroll BA: Carotid web. RadioGraphics 1991;11:504

69. Healy DA, Zierler RE, Nicholls SC et al: Long-term follow-up and clinical outcome of carotid restenosis. J Vasc Surg 1989;10:662

70. Zbornikova V, Elfstrom J, Lassvik C et al: Restenosis and occlusion after carotid surgery assessed by duplex scanning and digital subtraction angiography. Stroke 1986;17:1137

71. Middleton WD, Erickson S, Melson GL: Perivascular color artifact: pathologic significance and appearance on color Doppler US images. Radiology 1989;171:647

72. Hayes AC, Johnston W, Baker WH et al: The effect of

contralateral disease on carotid Doppler frequency. Surgery 1988;103:19

73. Steinke W, Kloetzsch C, Hennerici M: Carotid artery disease assessed by color Doppler flow imaging: correlation with standard Doppler sonography and angiography. AJNR 1990;11:259

74. Erickson SJ, Mewissen MW, Foley WD et al: Stenosis of the internal carotid artery: assessment using color Doppler imaging compared with angiography. AJR 1989;152:1299

75. Erickson SJ, Middleton WD, Mewissen MW et al: Color Doppler evaluation of arterial stenoses and occlusions involving the neck and thoracic inlet. RadioGraphics 1989;9:389

76. Hallam MJ, Reid JM, Cooperberg PL: Color-flow Doppler and conventional duplex scanning of the carotid bifurcation: prospective, double-blind, correlative study. AJR 1989;152:1101

77. Polak JF, Dobkin GR, O'Leary RH et al: Internal carotid artery stenosis: accuracy and reproducibility of color-Doppler-assisted duplex imaging. Radiology 1989;173:793

78. Bond JR, Charboneau JW, Stanson AW: Takayasu's arteritis: carotid duplex sonographic appearance, including color Doppler imaging. J Ultrasound Med 1990;9:625

79. Grant EG, Wong W, Tessler F, Perrella R: Cerebrovascular ultrasound imaging. Radiol Clin North Am 1988;26:1111

80. Davis PC, Nilsen B, Braun IF, Hoffman JC: A prospective comparison of duplex sonography vs angiography of the vertebral arteries. AJNR 1986;7:1059

81. Bluth EI, Merritt CRB, Sullivan MA et al: Usefulness of duplex ultrasound in evaluating vertebral arteries. J Ultrasound Med 1989;8:229

82. Kotval PS, Babu SC, Shah PM: Doppler diagnosis of partial vertebral/subclavian steals convertible to full steals with physiologic maneuvers. J Ultrasound Med 1990;9:207

83. Bendick PJ, Jackson VP: Evaluation of the vertebral arteries with duplex sonography. J Vasc Surg 1986;3:523

84. Carroll BA, Holder CA: Vertebral artery duplex sonography, abstracted. J Ultrasound Med 1990;9:S27

85. Williams CE, Lamb GHR, Roberts D, Davies J: Venous thrombosis in the neck: the role of real time ultrasound. Eur J Radiol 1989;9:32

86. Gaitini D, Kaftori JK, Perry M, Engel A: High-resolution real-time ultrasonography: diagnosis and follow-up of jugular and subclavian vein thrombosis. J Ultrasound Med 1988;7:621

87. Balk RL, Smith DF: Thrombosis of upper extremity thoracic inlet veins: diagnosis with duplex Doppler sonography. AJR 1987;149:677

88. Weissleder R, Elizondo G, Start DD: Sonographic diagnosis of subclavian and internal jugular vein thrombosis. J Ultrasound Med 1987;6:577

89. Gribbin C, Raghavendra BN, Ginsburg HB: Ultrasound diagnosis of jugular venous ectasia. NY State J Med 1989;9:532

90. Hughes PL, Qureshi SA, Galloway RW: Jugular venous aneurysm in children. Br J Radiol 1988;61:1082

91. Jasinski RW, Rubin JM: CT and ultrasonographic findings in jugular vein ectasis. J Ultrasound Med 1984;3:417

92. Lee W, Leduc L, Cotton DB: Ultrasonographic guidance for central venous access during pregnancy. Am J Obstet Gynecol 1989;161:1012

93. Bond DM, Nolan R: Real-time ultrasound imaging aids jugular venipuncture. Anesth Analg 1989;68:700

94. Machi J, Takeda J, Kakegawa T: Safe jugular and subclavian venipuncture under ultrasonographic guidance. Am J Surg 1987;153:321

95. Albertyn LE, Alcock MK: Diagnosis of internal jugular vein thrombosis. Radiology 1987;162:505

96. Grassi CJ, Polak JF: Axillary and subclavian venous thrombosis: follow-up evaluation with color Doppler flow US and venography. Radiology 1990;175:651

97. Knudson GJ, Wiedmeyer DA, Erickson SJ et al: Color Doppler sonographic imaging in the assessment of upper-extremity deep venous thrombosis. AJR 1990;154:399

5

Liver

Edward G. Grant

The liver is the largest abdominal organ and the largest structure in the reticuloendothelial system. Despite this, clinical evaluation is difficult because the superior aspect of the liver lies beneath the diaphragm and the remainder of the organ is surrounded by the ribs. Even the seemingly simple assessment of liver size is problematic. Detection of the edge of the liver beneath the costal margin does not always indicate hepatomegaly, because the position of the liver is variable and it may be displaced inferiorly by a low or depressed diaphragm. The detection of large hepatic masses by physical examination is also impossible in most cases. Furthermore, the symptoms of liver disease are often nonspecific (anorexia, dyspepsia, malaise, or abdominal discomfort) and clinical signs of liver disease such as jaundice and hepatomegaly may not occur until liver failure is advanced. Biochemical tests can be used to quantitate impaired liver function but are of limited use in narrowing the differential diagnosis in diffuse liver disease. As a result, ultrasound and other imaging techniques are essential in the evaluation of both focal and diffuse liver disease.

TECHNIQUE

No preparation is necessary for an ultrasound examination directed specifically at the liver. The surface of the liver lies directly beneath the skin in most cases, and when the inter- or subcostal approach is used, the parenchyma literally serves as its own sonic window. In most cases, examination of the liver is not limited by bowel gas because the colon and small intestines are usually infe-

rior to the liver. In patients with cirrhosis, however, there is an increased frequency of colonic interposition,[1] which may render the examination more challenging in this population. If, as is usually the case, the gallbladder and pancreas are to be evaluated in addition to the liver, it is preferable to have the patient fast overnight. The fasting technique allows for greater dilatation of the gallbladder and is likely to decrease the amount of bowel gas. In the evaluation of the pancreas, food and other nonliquid material in the stomach markedly diminish the ability to image the gland.

The key to the sonographic examination of the liver is adherence to strict protocol. The *Standards and Guidelines for the Performance of the Abdominal and Retroperitoneal Examinations* published by the American Institute of Ultrasound in Medicine (AIUM) provides an excellent framework for a basic examination.[2] One must examine all portions of the liver parenchyma carefully and identify specific anatomic landmarks, including the various segments and fissures, the portal and hepatic venous structures and their branches, and the common bile duct. The technical considerations for real-time examination of the liver are similar to those for the general abdominal scan. The highest-frequency transducer possible should be used to afford the best resolution. If adequate penetration to the posterior liver cannot be obtained with a high-frequency transducer, a lower-frequency transducer should be used as well. In most adults, the liver can be examined with a 3- to 5-MHz transducer. In children and thin adults, a 5-MHz transducer should be sufficient for the entire examination. Use of a 5-MHz transducer should probably be considered a routine part of the examination even if the liver cannot be penetrated in its entirety, because subtle masses may be missed by a 3-MHz transducer. In obese patients or those with fatty infiltration of the liver, a lower-frequency transducer (usually 2.25 MHz) may be necessary and, depending on the manufacturer, may yield a relatively satisfactory scan. The time-gain-compensation (TGC) settings and the overall output (system gain) should be adjusted to yield a uniform representation of the hepatic parenchyma from the anterior to the posterior liver. TGC and system gain are adjustable on all machines; less universal methods of optimizing hepatic images exist and often vary from one manufacturer or machine to the next. A thorough familiarity with the characteristics of individual machines is therefore essential. Because the sonographic diagnosis of hepatic parenchymal disease is often dependent on relatively subjective criteria, a definite attempt should be made to standardize all images as much as possible.

The scan itself is generally performed in deep inspiration to bring as much of the liver below the costal margin or sternum as possible; the right lobe is often best imaged from an intercostal approach. A sector format transducer is essential for scanning between the ribs and provides a wide field of view yet requires a small sonic window. At times, one may need to scan with the patient in the left lateral decubitus position or even sitting up. One should never be limited by convention if better images can be obtained by changing the patient's position. The liver should always be evaluated in both longitudinal and transverse planes. Representative images should be obtained at regular intervals, and important anatomic landmarks should be included in the hard copy as well. If color Doppler is a part of the examination, images of specific vessels (these will vary depending on the history) should be made to document the presence or absence of pathology. In many cases the color images should be supplemented with spectral tracings to define flow patterns.

NORMAL ANATOMY

The liver is composed of three cell types: biliary epithelial cells, Kupffer cells, and hepatocytes. In each liver lobule, hepatocytes radiate out to the periphery around a central vein and synthesize, metabolize, and excrete a variety of compounds. The outer margins of the lobule are incompletely demarcated by portal triads, which are surrounded by connective tissue septa and contain branches of the hepatic artery, hepatic vein, and bile duct. The vascular sinusoids are lined with endothelial cells and Kupffer cells. The Kupffer cells (which are part

of the reticuloendothelial system) phagocytize bacteria and foreign material. The normal adult liver weighs 1,400 to 1,600 g; the right lobe is approximately six times larger than the left.[3] The right lobe is usually 15 to 17 cm in length, with its upper border generally at the level of the nipples and its lower border at the level of the costal cartilage of the eighth to ninth ribs. The hepatic flexure of the colon lies in immediate proximity to the free margin of the right lobe. The position of the left lobe is more variable, with its inferior margin lying in close proximity to the body and antrum of the stomach. The left lobe frequently lies immediately adjacent to the body of the pancreas.

Lobes

The liver is divided into lobes by anatomic landmarks, which are clearly visible by ultrasound (Fig. 5-1). Lobar division has clinical relevance in planning surgical resection of primary hepatic neoplasms, solitary metastatic lesions, and nonmalignant hepatic processes as well. By identifying specific anatomic features, it is possible to define the segmental anatomy of the liver.

The right lobe is the portion of the liver located to the right of a line intersecting the gallbladder fossa inferiorly, the middle hepatic vein superiorly, and the sulcus for the inferior vena cava (IVC) posteriorly[4] (Fig. 5-2). The right lobe is further subdivided into anterior and posterior segments by the right hepatic vein (RHV).[5] Riedel's lobe, more common in women, is a tonguelike projection of the right lobe that may extend to the iliac crest. This normal variant is composed of both anterior and posterior segments of the right lobe (Fig. 5-3). The left lobe of the liver is normally smaller than the right but varies considerably in size.[6] The medial segment of the left lobe (quadrate lobe) lies between the fissure for the ligamentum teres and the gallbladder fossa, anterior to the porta hepatis.[4,5] The lateral segment of the left lobe lies to the left to the fissure of the ligamentum teres inferiorly and the left hepatic vein (LHV) superiorly (Fig. 5-4).

In rare instances, there is a congenital absence of either the right or left lobe of the liver. Agenesis of the right lobe should be considered only after lobar atrophy secondary to cirrhosis or hilar cholangiocarcinoma has been excluded. The hallmark of this unusual anomaly is the absence of the RHV.[7] Unfortunately, the RHV may be difficult to identify in patients with severe atrophy by real-time sonography alone; color Doppler should be considered in such cases. On the other hand, failure to identify liver tissue to the left of the gallbladder fossa and the falciform ligament should raise the suspicion of congenital absence of the left lobe.[8]

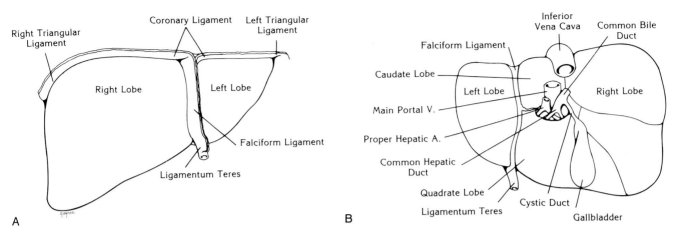

Fig. 5-1. Lobar anatomy. **(A)** Anterior and **(B)** posterior views. Using the traditional anatomic system for lobar division, the left lobe is considered that portion of the liver to the left of the falciform ligament with the remainder of the liver subdivided into the right, caudate, and quadrate lobes. Using the functional system for lobar division based on vessels, the "traditional" left lobe represents the lateral segment of the left lobe with the quadrate lobe representing the medial segment of the left lobe. With this system, the right and left lobes are divided with the plane of separation from the inferior vena cava to the gallbladder fossa.

The caudate lobe is located posterior to the porta hepatis between the fissure for the ligamentum venosum and the IVC[4,9,10] (Fig. 5-5). The left margin of the caudate lobe forms the hepatic boundary of the superior recess of the lesser sac. The right margin of the caudate extends in a tonguelike projection called the caudate or papillary process and lies between the IVC, the main portal vein (MPV), and the medial portion of the right hepatic lobe.[5,6,9-12] The papillary process may extend for some distance inferiorly and appears to be separate from the rest of the caudate lobe in transverse sections in 15.5

percent of scans according to the study of Donoso et al.[12] In some cases, a prominent caudate appendage mimics a mass on the anterior aspect of the pancreatic head (Fig. 5-6). Awareness of this normal variant and careful scanning of the longitudinal plane should allow this potential pitfall to be avoided. The caudate may also appear more hypoechoic than the adjacent liver because it lies immediately posterior to the fissure of the ligamentum venosum and the fat and fibrous tissue in the fissure attenuate the sound beam. This normal, relatively hypoechoic appearance should not be mistaken for a mass.[10]

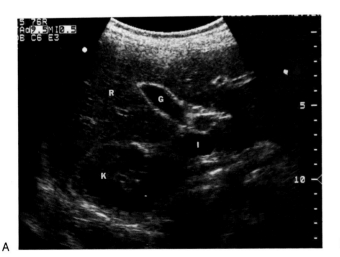

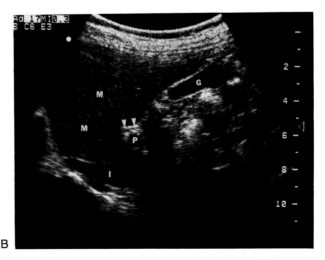

Fig. 5-2. Right lobe. **(A)** Transverse section showing the right lobe of the liver *(R)* anterior to the right kidney *(K)* and lateral to the gallbladder *(G)* and inferior vena cava *(I)*. **(B)** Longitudinal section demonstrating landmarks dividing the right and left lobes, including the middle hepatic vein *(M)*, inferior vena cava *(I)*, and gallbladder *(G)*. (*P*, portal vein; arrowheads, common hepatic duct.)

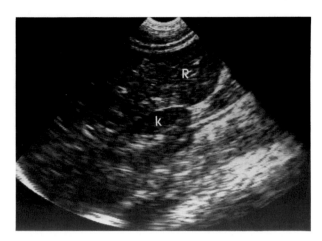

Fig. 5-3. Riedel's lobe. Longitudinal real-time scan. Note the inferior aspect of the liver extends inferior to the kidney *(k).* This represents Riedel's lobe *(R).*

Ligaments and Fissures

The ligaments and fissures of the liver are brightly echogenic because of the collagen and fat in and around them. The falciform ligament extends from the umbilicus to the diaphragm in an oblique parasagittal plane; contained between its layers are the ligamentum teres and the umbilical vein remnant. In the anterior-posterior axis the falciform ligament extends from the right rectus muscle to the bare area of the liver, where its reflections separate to contribute to the hepatic coronary ligaments.[13] The falciform ligament and the ligamentum teres divide the lateral and medial segments of the left lobe.[4,5] On a transverse ultrasound section, the ligamentum teres hepatis is seen as a round hyperechoic area immediately to the right of the midline[13,14] (Fig. 5-4A). The ligament is linear in longitudinal sections and extends from the anteroinferior surface of the liver to the left portal vein. When scanning is performed in a transverse orientation, the falciform ligament occasionally mimics a mass. In such cases one should turn the transducer longitudinally and watch the "mass" elongate.[15] The falciform ligament may be affected by several disease processes, although this is unusual. Most are benign; lipoma, cyst, paraganglioma, and leiomyosarcoma have been reported.[16,17]

The major fissure of the liver divides the left and right lobes and is seen on longitudinal scans as a linear echogenic structure that extends from the gallbladder to the porta hepatis (Fig. 5-7). Identification of the major fissure may be of value in the identification of a contracted gallbladder when it is otherwise impossible to find.[18] A third commonly identified hepatic fissure is that of the ligamentum venosum. This fissure contains the hepatogastric ligament and is located between the caudate lobe and the lateral segment of the left lobe[4,9,14] (Fig. 5-5). Other, less constant fissures have been found in the liver. These accessory fissures are usually located near the dome of the liver and are thought to represent invaginations of the diaphragm. Accessory fissures are identified with various degrees of frequency and are reported to be present on as many as 25 percent of computed tomography (CT) scans.[19] These structures have no clinical significance and should not be confused with echogenic masses when sectioned transversely.

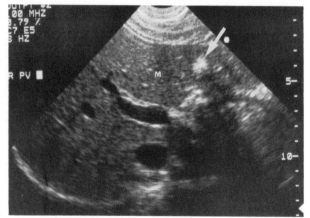

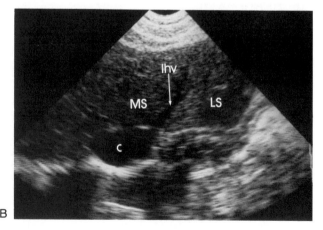

Fig. 5-4. Left lobe. **(A)** Medial segment of the left lobe *(M)* lies between the ligamentum teres (arrow) and porta hepatis. **(B)** Lateral segment *(LS)* lies to the left of the left hepatic vein *(lhv),* which runs in left segmental fissure. *(MS,* medial segment of left lobe; *c,* inferior vena cava.)

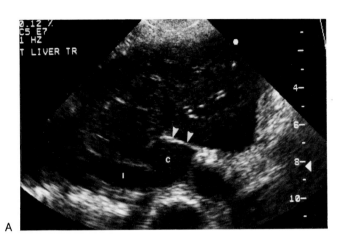
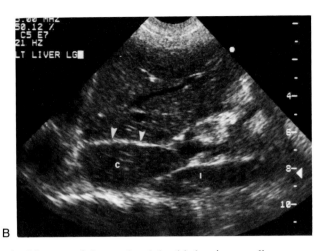

Fig. 5-5. Caudate lobe. **(A)** Transverse and **(B)** longitudinal images of the caudate lobe *(c)* showing a well-defined anterior border provided by the specular reflections of the ligamentum venosum (arrowheads). (*I*, IVC.)

Vascular Anatomy

The liver receives its nutrients via the hepatic artery and the portal vein; blood exits the liver via the hepatic veins. The portal vein blood is 80 percent saturated with oxygen and supplies 50 to 60 percent of the oxygen requirement of the hepatocytes.[3] Overall, the portal vein supplies 70 to 75 percent of the total volume of incoming blood to the liver.[20] With this dual blood supply, infarcts are rare. The hepatic artery of the normal native liver, in fact, can be completely thrombosed with little or no sequelae. The portal and hepatic veins, on the other hand, are essential to hepatic vascular integrity and may be involved in several significant disease processes. In

addition, these veins are used as a "road map" in localizing pathologic abnormalities in patients being considered for hepatic resection and serve as landmarks for orientation in follow-up studies. It is therefore important to be able to properly identify these vessels and their branches and differentiate between the two. A number of well-known methods exist to do this.

Portal veins lie adjacent to the hepatic artery and bile duct in the portal triad. Because the portal triad is encased in a collagenous sheath, its margins tend to be echodense. Echogenic walls may be used to differentiate portal veins from hepatic veins, which have minimal collagen in their walls and, as such, have imperceptible margins.[4,21] Another way of differentiating between he-

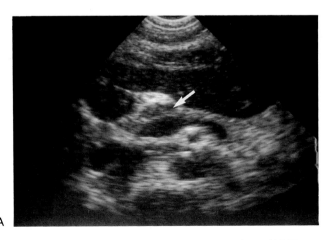
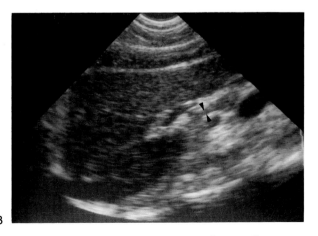

Fig. 5-6. Prominent caudate appendage. **(A)** Transverse section at the level of the pancreas showing a well-defined, hypoechoic structure (arrow) anterior to the body of the gland. **(B)** Longitudinal section identifying the structure as the caudate appendage. Note the narrow connection to the inferior caudate lobe (arrowheads).

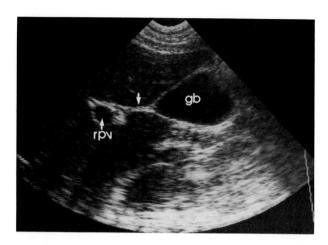

Fig. 5-7. Major fissure. The fissure appears as a linear echogenicity (arrow) extending from the gallbladder *(gb)* to the right portal vein *(rpv)*. It divides the right and left lobes of the liver.

patic veins and portal veins is to use real-time ultrasound to simply trace the vessel back to its origin at either the MPV or IVC. Within the liver itself, the portal and hepatic veins also have different branching patterns. The apex of the angle of portal vein bifurcations is horizontal and points toward the porta hepatis. The apex of hepatic vein bifurcations, on the other hand, is vertical and points toward the IVC.[4,21] The caliber of the hepatic veins also increases as they course toward the diaphragm and IVC, whereas the caliber of the portal veins increases toward the porta hepatis (Fig. 5-8).

If a question exists about the nature of any vascular structure in the liver, color and spectral Doppler should provide the definitive answer rapidly. The anatomic appearance of these vessels on color Doppler should be sufficient to make their differentiation quite clear. In addition, their flow runs in opposite directions. Portal vein flow comes into the liver and toward the transducer

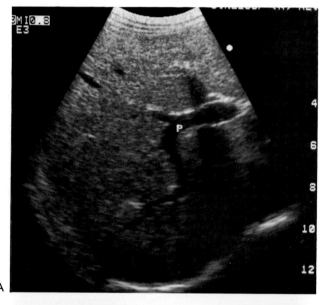

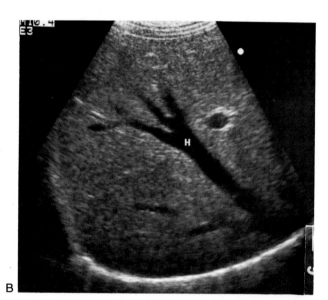

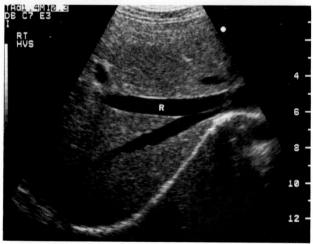

Fig. 5-8. Hepatic venous anatomy. **(A)** Transverse image through the right lobe of the liver demonstrating a normal right portal vein *(P)*. Note the brightly echogenic walls; the apex of bifurcation points toward the porta hepatis. Portal veins tend to be oriented horizontally. **(B)** Hepatic veins *(H)* are without brightly echogenic walls, and bifurcations point toward the diaphragm and inferior vena cava. Branches of the middle and left hepatic veins have a vertical orientation. **(C)** The right hepatic vein *(R)* tends to have a horizontal orientation. Large, central hepatic vein walls may be somewhat echogenic when they lie perpendicular to the incident sound beam.

during scanning through the anterior or lateral abdomen; hepatic venous flow is always away from the transducer. When using a red toward/blue away color scheme, portal venous flow should be displayed in red and hepatic veins in blue. This is, of course, an oversimplification because all color assignment is completely angle dependent. For example, while flow in the MPV is invariably toward the transducer (when scanning from an anterior approach) and displayed in red, portal branches going away from the transducer may be displayed in blue. A blue color assignment is typical of the posterior branch of the right portal vein (RPV); its color and orientation can cause it to be mistaken for the middle hepatic vein (MHV) or RHV (Plate 5-1). Although color Doppler is of considerable use in liver examinations, its technical complexities are considerable and are beyond the scope of this chapter. Several texts and articles are available on this subject.[22-24]

Spectral analysis is also an excellent method for differentiating among the hepatic vessels.[23] The portal vein is part of an isolated vascular unit and, as such, has monophasic, low-velocity flow. The hepatic veins are systemic veins and are in open communication with the right heart. The hepatic veins therefore exhibit choppy, triphasic flow patterns, which are easily distinguished from those of the portal vein. Both portal and hepatic vein signals should also be easily distinguished from those arising in the hepatic artery, which displays typical low-resistance arterial patterns (Fig. 5-9).

The MPV emerges to the right of the midline at the junction of the superior mesenteric and splenic veins; an ampullary dilatation is commonly seen at this juncture (Fig. 5-10). The MPV courses cephalad and slightly to the right, lying anterior to the IVC. Its normal diameter is 11.2 mm.[25] Once beyond the porta hepatis, the MPV divides into a smaller left portal vein (LPV), which courses in an anterior and cranial direction and the larger RPV, which runs in a posterior and caudal direction (Fig. 5-11). Elongation of the MPV at the origin of the LPV defines the precise location of the porta hepatis. The LPV then branches into medial and lateral divisions

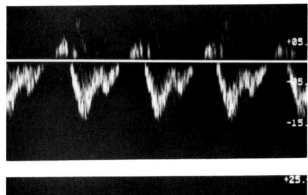

A

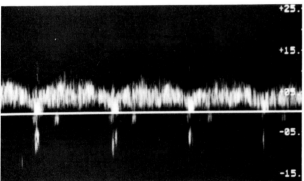

B

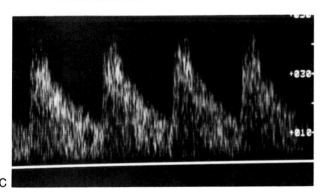

C

Fig. 5-9. Spectral analysis. **(A)** Hepatic vein shows a "choppy" triphasic signal with two forward phases of flow (below baseline) corresponding to two phases of right atrial filling. Note the periodic flow reversal with right atrial contraction. **(B)** Portal vein flow is relatively monophasic. Changes secondary to cardiac activity or respiratory motion are minimal. **(C)** Hepatic artery exhibits typical low-resistance flow observed in arteries supplying parenchymal organs. (From Grant et al,[23] with permission.)

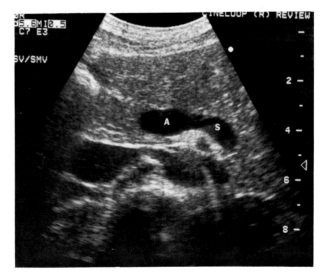

Fig. 5-10. Splenic vein. The normal splenic vein *(S)* is oriented transversely and joined by the superior mesenteric vein to form the portal vein. The region of their junction is identified by a mild ampullary dilatation *(A)*.

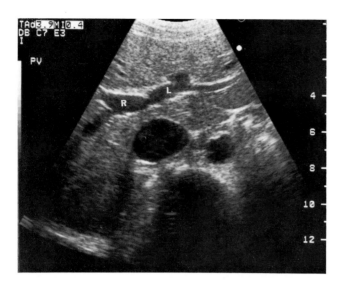

Fig. 5-11. Intrahepatic portal vein anatomy. Beyond the porta hepatis, the main portal vein divides into the smaller left portal vein *(L)*, which has an anterior and cranial orientation, and the larger right portal vein *(R)*, which runs in a posterior and caudal direction.

and the RPV into anterior and posterior divisions. At this point they become intrasegmental in their course.[6] The LPV, which arises to the right of midline, proceeds cranially along the anterior surface of the caudate and then arches back anteriorly and to the left. It gives branches to the caudate lobe and divides into medial and lateral branches. The umbilical vein is also a branch of the LPV. At times, the size of the LPV and the angle at which it travels from the MPV vary.[26] The LPV and its surrounding connective tissue may also mimic the posterior margin of the lateral segment of the left lobe on the transverse scan.[27] In addition, similar to what is seen in the caudate lobe, the attenuation of the sound beam by the fibrous tissue around the LPV may cause the posterior portion of the left lobe to appear somewhat hypoechoic when compared with the anterior segment. The RPV travels posteriorly and has a long, horizontal course. Its anatomy is relatively constant.[26]

The hepatic veins branch directly off the superior aspect of the IVC just below the diaphragm. The hepatic veins are best visualized on a high transverse section through the liver with mild cranial angulation. The RHV is located in the right intersegmental fissure coursing between the anterior and posterior branches of the RPV.[14,22] The RHV divides the superior aspect of the anterior and posterior segments of the right hepatic lobe.[14] The MHV is located in the main lobar fissure separating the right and left lobes.[14] Located in the left intersegmental fissure, the LHV divides the cephalic aspects of the medial and lateral segments of the left

lobe.[5,6,28] Real-time scans often adequately image all three hepatic veins on a single transverse subxiphoid section. This, however, is not the case with Doppler imaging, in which optimum signal reception is from a parallel vantage point. The RHV lies at 90 degrees to the ultrasound beam during scanning from a subxiphoid position, and little or no signal may be received. To optimize the Doppler angle for this vessel, one should scan from a right lateral intercostal position[23] (Fig. 5-12 and Plate 5-2).

The courses of the three main hepatic veins are relatively constant. In one series of 269 patients, however, 10 percent demonstrated an inferior or accessory RHV. The identification of this vessel may be significant in patients who are being considered for hepatectomy or have Budd-Chiari syndrome. The preoperative visualization of a hypertrophied inferior RHV would facilitate preservation of both the vein and the right posteroinferior area of the liver during a resection. In patients with Budd-Chiari syndrome, the main draining vein of the right lobe of the liver may be the accessory RHV.[29] To identify the inferior RHV, it is necessary only to see the vessel posterior to the RPV and trace it back medially to the IVC (Fig. 5-12). It should not be confused with the posterior RPV branch, which courses more caudally than the main RHV. Again, if a question exists, spectral Doppler should facilitate differentiation.

Although the hepatic artery is not commonly involved in specific disease processes, sonography of the hepatic artery is of interest as this vessel may be confused with dilated or even normal bile ducts[30] and its identification is essential in patients with transplanted livers.[31] The common hepatic artery emerges from the celiac axis,

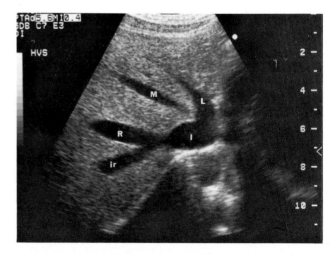

Fig. 5-12. Normal hepatic veins. Real-time image showing right *(R)*, middle *(M)*, and left *(L)* hepatic veins entering the inferior vena cava *(I)*. Note the inferior right hepatic vein *(ir)*. Color Doppler imaging requires a slightly different technique to optimally visualize all three vessels. (See also Plate 5-2.)

crosses to the right along the superoanterior border of the pancreas at the porta hepatis, and lies adjacent to the portal vein and common bile duct. The gastroduodenal artery, a branch of the common hepatic artery, curves caudally and runs along the right anterolateral surface of the head of the pancreas. This vessel serves as an important landmark and separates the head of the gland from the posteromedial duodenum[32,33] (Fig. 5-13 and Plate 5-3). The proper hepatic artery is the continuation of the common hepatic artery distal to the origin of the gastroduodenal artery. The vessel turns anterior and cephalad and runs along the free edge of the lesser omentum (hepatoduodenal ligament) toward the porta hepatis. In the region of the porta, the proper hepatic artery divides into the right, middle, and left hepatic arteries (Fig. 5-14). The right hepatic artery runs in the right intersegmental fissure, where it is posterior to the bile duct and between the duct and portal vein.

The hepatic artery is the most variable of all abdominal arteries, with as many as 12.5 percent of patients showing some form of departure from the expected course.[34] The most common variant, known as a replaced hepatic artery, may be diagnosed by identifying two main hepatic arteries. One vessel, usually the smaller, follows the expected course along the superior edge of the pancreas, while the second arises from the superior mesenteric artery and loops behind the portal vein. The two arteries then join as they course toward the porta hepatis (Fig. 5-15). Two-thirds of the patients also have a right hepatic artery that crosses behind the common bile duct or right hepatic duct, whereas the left hepatic artery crosses anterior to the left hepatic duct.[32]

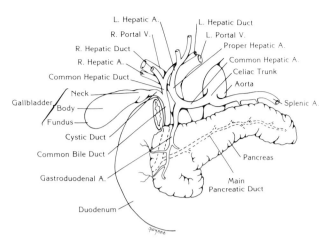

Fig. 5-14. Hepatic duct, hepatic artery, and portal vein. Note the relationships of the hepatic ducts, hepatic arteries, and portal veins. On the right, the right hepatic artery is between the right portal vein and right hepatic duct, with the duct anterior. On the left, the left hepatic artery is anterior to the left hepatic duct and left portal vein. (Modified from Sauerbrei,[248] with permission.)

In most patients, the right hepatic artery is anterior to the RPV.

The common bile duct is said to lie anterolateral to the portal vein and the hepatic artery anteromedial.[35] On the basis of this anatomic tenet, the common hepatic duct at the level of the RPV can be routinely visualized by scanning obliquely through the ribs. Such an image is an essential part of every hepatobiliary sonogram and is the primary method of identifying dilatation of the biliary tree (Fig. 5-16). Although this technique is adequate in most patients, it is well known that the hepatic artery often follows a meandering course and may even become ectatic in older or cirrhotic patients, leading to difficulty in differentiating between the two. Luckily, both spectral and color Doppler can be applied to this situation and can easily determine whether flow is present (hepatic artery) or not (duct)[36,37] (Fig. 5-17). This ability to differentiate between duct and vessel may also be of assistance in imaging the liver itself, because dilated hepatic arteries may be seen in both normal individuals and patients with cirrhosis[38] and may be indistinguishable from dilated ducts. Again, color or spectral Doppler can make this distinction quite easily (Fig. 5-18 and Plate 5-4).

Although hepatic vascularity is usually discussed in terms of its three main vessel systems (hepatic artery, portal vein, and hepatic veins), the caudate lobe has a unique circulation and deserves separate attention. Both left and right portal triads give off portal venous and hepatic arterial branches to the caudate lobe. The cau-

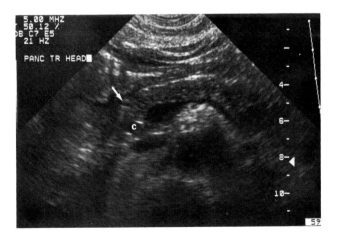

Fig. 5-13. Hepatic artery. At the anterolateral border of the pancreas, the hepatic artery turns cephalad and parallels the portal vein. An inferior branch, the gastroduodenal artery (arrow), courses along the anterolateral border of the pancreatic head. Note the normal common bile duct *(c)* on the posterolateral border of the pancreatic head. (See also Plate 5-3.)

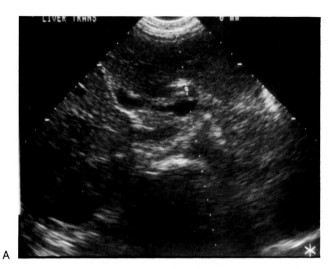
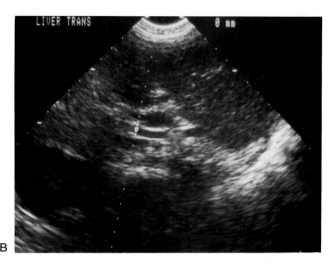

Fig. 5-15. Replaced hepatic artery. **(A)** In this common normal variant, one branch of hepatic artery arises in normal position from celiac trunk (caliper). **(B)** The second branch originates from superior mesenteric artery and courses behind portal vein as shown (caliper).

date is also drained by a series of short venous channels that extend directly from its posterior aspect into the IVC. This unusual blood supply is postulated to have several important clinical implications. The short intra-hepatic course of the caudate lobe afferent vessels favors less attenuation of the caudate lobe vasculature by adjacent hepatic fibrosis. A discrepancy between perfusion of the caudate lobe and perfusion of the right hepatic lobe may be responsible for the caudate lobe enlargement and right hepatic lobe shrinkage seen in cirrhotic patients. Caudate enlargement with compression of the underlying IVC is also implicated in the development of various cirrhotic complications including IVC hypertension, ascites, portacaval shunt failure, and, possibly, hepatorenal syndrome.[3,9] In addition, its independent venous drainage renders the caudate less susceptible to hepatic

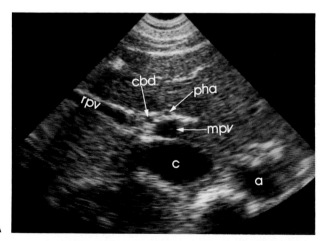
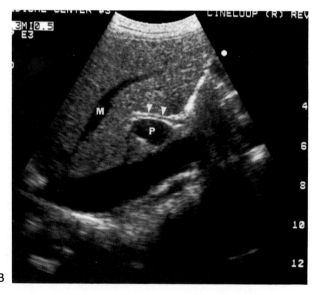

Fig. 5-16. Porta hepatis. **(A)** Transverse image through the region of the porta hepatis demonstrating the normal anatomic relationship of the main portal vein *(mpv),* proper hepatic artery *(pha),* and common hepatic duct *(cbd). (a,* aorta; *c,* inferior vena cava; *rpv,* right portal vein.) **(B)** Typically, the hepatic artery lies medial to the portal vein *(P)* while the duct (arrowheads) lies laterally, allowing the latter to be imaged via a longitudinal intercostal approach. *(M,* middle hepatic vein.)

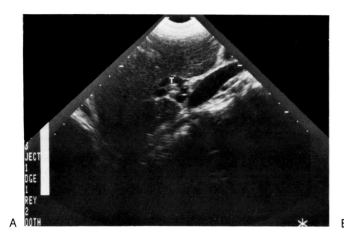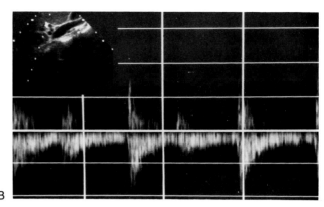

Fig. 5-17. Ectatic hepatic artery. **(A)** Tubular structure *(T)* anterior to the portal vein in the porta hepatis could represent either an ectatic hepatic artery or a mildly dilated common bile duct. **(B)** Spectral Doppler applied to the structure clearly defines its vascular nature.

vein thrombosis. The caudate lobe may be the only area of the liver to be spared in Budd-Chiari syndrome and may account for the association of caudate lobe enlargement with hepatic vein thrombosis. When scanning patients suspected of having Budd-Chiari syndrome, one should not mistake a large, patent caudate vein for the MHV[39] (Plate 5-5).

Echopattern

The appearance of the hepatic parenchyma is so typical in normal patients that it is often used as the standard for setting up overall scan parameters for the entire ab-

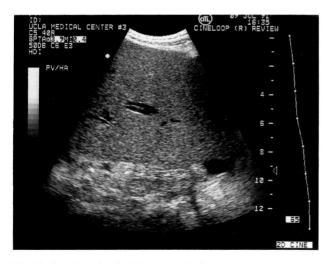

Fig. 5-18. Pseudo double-channel sign. Hepatic arteries of patients with cirrhosis may enlarge and mimic the "double-duct" sign of biliary dilatation. (See also Plate 5-4.)

domen.[2] The parenchyma of the liver is moderately echogenic and has a relatively fine echotexture, which (assuming proper adjustment of TGC) should be homogeneous throughout. The liver is isoechoic (or almost so) with the spleen, more echogenic than the renal parenchyma, and less echogenic than the pancreas.[4] Interspersed within the parenchyma are well-defined, fluid-filled vessels (see Fig. 5-26A below).

Size

Numerous techniques exist for determining the size of the liver. Most rely on a simple longitudinal measurement; others advocate measuring the liver in two planes.[40] On a longitudinal scan obtained at the midhepatic line, the liver is measured from its superior (dome of the diaphragm) to inferior margin. The liver is usually measured transversely from the midspine to the corresponding lateral surface. According to an early article by Gosink and Leymaster,[41] which has seemingly stood the test of time, the longitudinal measurement alone is 87 percent accurate in determining the presence or absence of hepatomegaly. If the liver is 13 cm or less in the midhepatic line, it is normal in 93 percent of cases. If the liver is 15.5 cm or greater, it is enlarged in 75 percent of cases.

More recent work by Niederau et al[42] has considered several parameters in the sonographic evaluation of hepatomegaly. This work confirmed the superiority of the longitudinal measurement at the midclavicular line and was in reasonably close agreement with the work of Gosink and Leymaster[41] described above. Their investigations[40,42] also suggested that an anteroposterior (AP) measurement of the right lobe may be of value in pa-

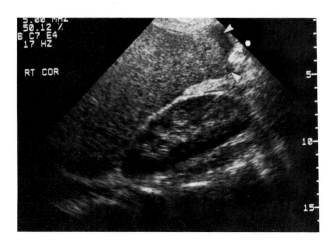

Fig. 5-19. Hepatomegaly. The liver measured approximately 15.6 cm. Other findings suggesting hepatomegaly include extension of the liver to or beyond the lower pole of the right kidney and a rounded edge (arrowheads).

tients who are either obese or quite thin. In the former, the liver tends to be larger in the AP dimension, whereas in the latter, the liver tends to be long and narrow. When obtaining liver measurements, most sonographers are aware that the entire right lobe may be impossible to image in a single longitudinal section. In such cases, an approximation or the use of contiguous dual images may be the only option.

Two additional signs of hepatomegaly exist and, although they are subjective, may be of value in selected cases. Extension of the right lobe below the level of the inferior pole of the kidney may indicate enlargement and may be useful in examinations of short or pediatric patients. Unfortunately, the variable relationship of the right kidney, liver, and diaphragm makes universal application of this sign impossible. Hepatomagaly should also be considered when the inferior border of the liver takes on a rounded appearance (Fig. 5-19). This sign is caused by swelling of the hepatic parenchyma against the relatively nondistensible capsule; it can be of value and is often overlooked.

DIFFUSE PARENCHYMAL DISEASE

Hepatocellular disease can be defined as a pathologic process that affects the hepatocytes and interferes with liver function. "Liver function tests" themselves are estimates of deranged hepatic activity, and when the results are abnormal, they are usually indicative of specific abnormalities. With cell necrosis, the hepatic enzyme levels are elevated. With cholestasis or inhibition of bile secretion, alkaline phosphatase and direct bilirubin

levels increase. When there are defects in protein synthesis, there may be elevated serum bilirubin levels and decreased serum albumin and clotting factor levels.

Major categories of diffuse parenchymal disease include fatty infiltration and acute and chronic hepatitis. Cirrhosis, on the other hand, although usually classified among diffuse parenchymal disease, is actually the result or end point of other pathologic processes and is usually not the primary liver disease. Imaging of many forms of diffuse disease is often complicated by the presence of various degrees of cirrhosis or hepatic fibrosis along with the primary pathologic process. Although one might be tempted to classify all patients with a diffuse alteration of the liver architecture as having "hepatocullular disease" or "parenchymal disease," specific patterns have been described and should be familiar to the medical imager.

Fatty Infiltration

Fatty infiltration implies increased lipid accumulation in the hepatocytes and is the result of significant injury to the liver or a systemic disorder leading to impaired or excessive metabolism of fat.[3] Fatty infiltration can be seen in patients with diabetes mellitus, ethanol abuse, obesity, tuberculosis, ulcerative colitis, kwashiorkor, excessive overeating, starvation, corticosteroid therapy, hyperlipidemia, parenteral nutrition, Reye syndrome, severe hepatitis, glycogen storage disease, cystic fibrosis, or jejunoileal bypass for obesity.[43] Although fatty infiltration is a benign process in many instances and may be completely and rapidly reversible, it is particularly significant in chronic alcoholism.[3] If an echodense liver is demonstrated in a child who is not malnourished or receiving parenteral hyperalimentation or treatment with chemotherapy, metabolic disease should be suspected.[44]

Most patients with histologically moderate or severe fatty infiltration have abnormally echogenic livers on ultrasound[45,46] (Fig. 5-20). According to the study of Behan and Kazam,[46] the high-level echoes are due to an increase in the collagen content of the liver rather than to the fat. The study of Taylor et al,[47] however, attributed increases in hepatic parenchymal echogenicity to lipid accumulation, implying that increased hepatic echogenicity should be specific for fatty infiltration. The ability to actually identify subtle increases in echogenicity, however, seems to be variable. Foster et al[45] were able to detect only 60 percent of patients with fatty infiltration of the liver. The sensitivity of detection by recognition of a bright liver echopattern was related to the degree of infiltration and increased to 90 percent in moderate and severe cases; the false-positive rate was very low.[45] The study of Scatrige et al[43] correlated the ability of ultra-

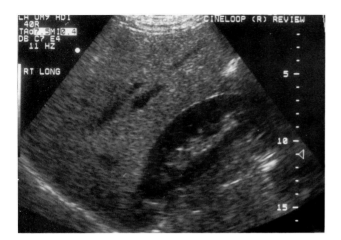

Fig. 5-20. Fatty infiltration. The liver is increased in overall echogenicity, and normal vascular markings are absent. Note the blackened, featureless appearance of renal parenchyma.

sound and CT to detect fatty infiltration of the liver. The overall accuracy of ultrasound was 85 percent with a 100 percent sensitivity and a 56 percent specificity. Three grades were defined for fatty infiltration: grade 1 (mild), slight diffuse increase in the fine echoes in the hepatic parenchyma with normal visualization of the diaphragm and intrahepatic vessel borders; grade 2 (moderate), moderate diffuse increase in the fine echoes with slightly impaired visualization of the intrahepatic vessels and diaphragm; and grade 3 (severe), marked increase in fine echoes with poor or no visualization of the intrahepatic vessel borders, diaphragm, and posterior portion of the

right lobe of the liver. A coarser, more scattered increase in echogenicity and an altered shape of the cirrhotic liver was sufficiently characteristic to permit differentiation from fatty infiltration, but there was some overlap.

Fatty infiltration of the liver is not uniform in all patients. Nonuniform distribution of fat has been reported with alcohol abuse, administration of exogenous steroids, and malnutrition accompanying cancer, among other causes.[48,49] Sometimes there is a patchy distribution of the fat throughout the liver. Cases of nonuniform distribution predominantly involve the right lobe and may cause a problem in diagnosis. The reason for the nonuniformity is not known. Most cases of focal fatty infiltration, however, have a characteristic appearance. Bandlike areas of increased echogenicity with relatively linear or angular edges are typical[50] (Fig. 5-21). As opposed to true neoplastic masses, fatty infiltration also tends to produce little or no displacement of the regional hepatic vessels. Rounded, masslike areas of focal fatty infiltration, however, are problematic and may require CT correlation for confident differentiation from neoplastic lesions (Fig. 5-22).

Focal sparing is also characteristic of fatty infiltration.[51,52] Although, again, the etiology is not entirely clear, the predilection for specific areas of the liver has led some to postulate a vascular cause.[53] Focal sparing should be suspected in patients who have masslike hypoechoic areas in typical locations in a liver that is otherwise increased in echogenicity. The appearance of a focally spared area should be sufficiently characteristic that neoplasm is not considered. The most common area to be affected is the hepatic parenchyma anterior to the

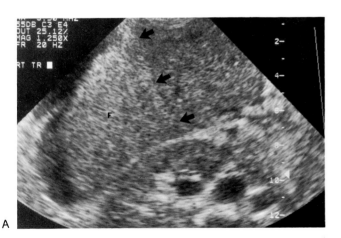

A

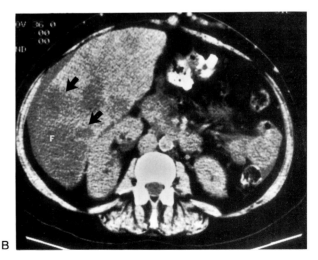

B

Fig. 5-21. Focal fatty infiltration. (A) The common geographic pattern of focal fatty infiltration *(F)* is typified by a peripheral area of increased echogenicity having a relatively linear demarcation (arrows) from the normal liver. (B) CT scan confirming the sonographic findings. Note the low-density region of fatty infiltration (*F*, arrows) in area corresponding to the ultrasound abnormality.

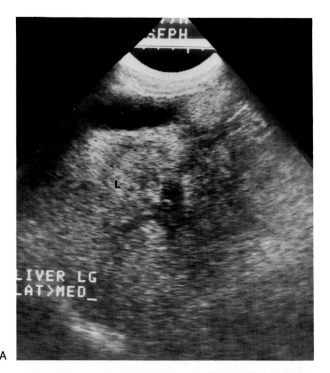

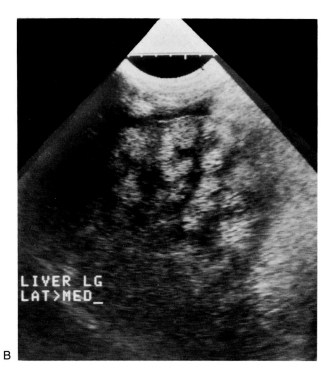

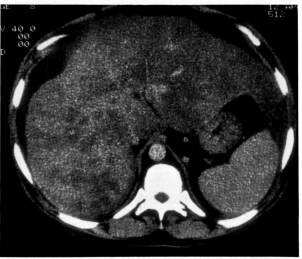

Fig. 5-22. Focal fatty infiltration. This patient with long history of alcohol abuse presented with hepatomegaly. **(A)** Left lobe of the liver *(L)* is homogeneously echogenic in a pattern typical of fatty metamorphosis. **(B)** The right lobe contains numerous rounded echogenic masses thought to represent focal fatty change. **(C)** CT scan confirming the sonographic findings. Note the diffuse fatty metamorphosis in the left lobe and rounded focal lesions in the right lobe. The patient had a repeat scan after 1 month of abstinence, and the liver appearance had improved markedly.

gallbladder or the portal vein (Fig. 5-23). The posterior portion of the left lobe of the liver is also commonly affected; the sonographic appearance may be quite striking (Fig. 5-24). In addition, focal fatty infiltration may be identified adjacent to the falciform ligament and, again, has a characteristic appearance.[54]

Hepatitis

Hepatitis is broadly defined as inflammation of the liver. In cases of viral hepatitis, the offending organism is generally hepatitis A, B, or C virus. The incubation pe-

riod for hepatitis A virus is 2 to 6 weeks; the period for hepatitis B virus is 2 to 6 months. Hepatitis A virus is transmitted from person to person via the fecal-oral route, whereas the source of hepatitis B virus is a chronic carrier or, rarely, a patient with acute hepatitis B. Hepatitis B virus may be transmitted vertically via parenteral inoculation. The extent of the liver injury in acute hepatitis may range from mild and subclinical disease to massive necrosis and liver failure. There is diffuse hepatocellular disarray and necrosis without portal or periportal abnormality. The severity and extent of the necrosis appear to vary with the level of immune response evoked by the infected hepatocytes. The pathologic

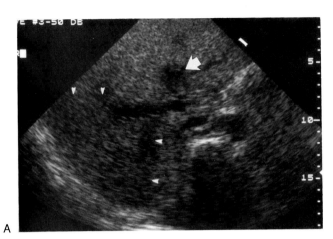
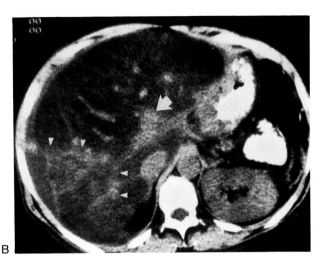

A   B

Fig. 5-23. Focal sparing. **(A)** This patient with diffuse fatty infiltration has two regions of relative sparing within the liver. The more prominent (arrow) is in a typical location anterior to the portal vein. Note the somewhat more subtle difference in echogenicity in the posterior right lobe (arrowheads). **(B)** CT scan is confirming focal sparing anterior to the portal vein (arrow) and in the posterior right lobe (arrowheads).

changes seen include (1) liver cell injury, swelling of the hepatocytes, and hepatocyte degeneration which may lead to cell necrosis; (2) reticuloendothelial and lymphocytic response with Kupffer cells enlarging; and (3) regeneration. With chronic hepatitis, there is portal inflammatory infiltration without extension across the portal limiting plate and preservation of the lobular architecture. In chronic active hepatitis, there is more extensive change than in chronic persistent hepatitis, with inflammation extending across the limiting plate, spreading out in a perilobular fashion, and causing piecemeal necrosis,[55] which is frequently accompanied

by fibrosis. The outcome of hepatitis A is typically complete recovery following 4 to 6 weeks of illness. Hepatitis B tends to be more prolonged. If the hepatitis becomes fulminant, massive necrosis may ensue, with the entire liver shrinking. Although chronic persistent hepatitis is a benign, self-limiting process, chronic active hepatitis usually progresses to cirrhosis and liver failure.[3]

Specific sonographic patterns associated with hepatitis have been described. With acute hepatitis, the predominant findings are accentuated brightness and more extensive demonstration of the portal vein radicle walls, accompanied by overall decreased echogenicity of the

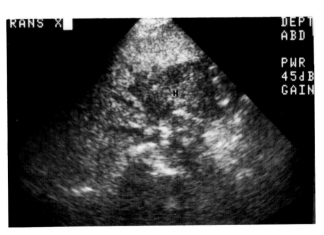
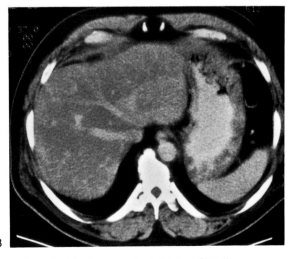

A   B

Fig. 5-24. Focal sparing. **(A)** A well-defined hypoechoic region is identified in the posterior left lobe of the liver *(H)*. Note the linear demarcation from fatty infiltrated liver anteriorly. **(B)** CT scan confirming focal sparing.

liver parenchyma (Fig. 5-25). With chronic hepatitis, the liver exhibits a coarse echopattern. The patterns of acute and chronic hepatitis appear to be specific, with a confidence level of 95 percent in a retrospective study. The probability in detecting acute and chronic hepatitis patterns is thus reported to be 93 percent.[55]

Cirrhosis

Cirrhosis is a diffuse process characterized by fibrosis and conversion of normal liver architecture into structurally abnormal nodules. The essential feature is concurrent parenchymal necrosis, regeneration, and diffuse fibrosis resulting in disorganization of lobular architecture. The process is chronic and progressive, and liver cell failure and portal hypertension result. In the United States, cirrhosis is the third most common cause of death in 25- to 65-year-old persons and the fifth most common cause of death overall. Thirty to sixty percent of cirrhosis is secondary to alcohol abuse (Laennec, portal, and nutritional cirrhosis); 2 to 5 percent represents pigment cirrhosis (cirrhosis associated with hemochromatosis and Wilson's disease); 10 to 30 percent, postnecrotic cirrhosis; and 10 to 20 percent, biliary cirrhosis.[3] In children, the causes of cirrhosis include infection (neonatal and viral hepatitis, ascending cholangitis), metabolic abnormalities, obstructive biliary disease, vascular disease, drugs, and toxins.[56]

Numerous investigators have evaluated the sonographic patterns associated with cirrhosis. Ultrasound is certainly helpful in evaluating liver size, increased echogenicity, ascites, and obstruction of the biliary tract. The specific diagnosis of cirrhosis, however, remains elusive and, for the most part, still requires biopsy. In addition, sonography is unable to give any quantitative estimate of the severity of the histologic change.[57] Sonographic findings, however, can be suggestive and should be familiar because ultrasound is often the first examination performed when right upper quadrant disease is suspected. The classic finding in cirrhosis is "coarsening" of the hepatic echopattern. The normal liver parenchyma is quite homogeneous and should retain consistent midlevel echoes. With cirrhosis, the fibrosis and nodularity lead to a diffuse alteration in the echopattern, ranging from an almost imperceptible coarsening of the echogenicity to gross nodularity (Fig. 5-26).

Considering the subjective and nonspecific (many entities, including diffuse metastatic disease, can lead to similar findings) nature of "coarsened" echogenicity, investigators have studied changes in hepatic morphology in an attempt to diagnose cirrhosis objectively. The demonstration of surface nodularity by using high-resolution linear array transducers is reported to be 88 percent sensitive in identifying patients with cirrhosis[58] (Fig. 5-27). More widely applied in the diagnosis of cirrhosis, however, is the comparison of the size of the right lobe with that of the caudate lobe. It is well known that as cirrhosis becomes manifest, the right lobe shrinks in comparison with the caudate. By using a ratio of caudate to right lobe width (C/RL ratio), cirrhotic livers can be distinguished from noncirrhotic livers with an acceptable degree of success. The C/RL ratio is determined by dividing the transverse dimension of the caudate lobe (from the lateral margin of the MPV to the outside of the caudate) by that of the right lobe (lateral margin to

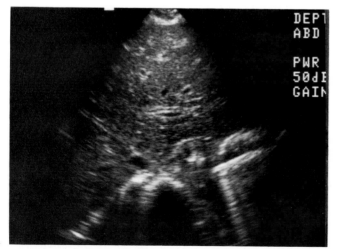
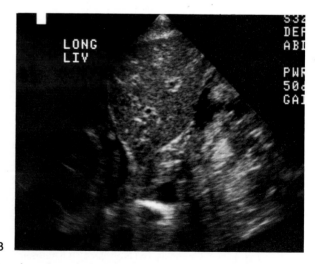

A   B

Fig. 5-25. Hepatitis. **(A)** Transverse and **(B)** longitudinal sections through the left lobe of the liver demonstrating accentuation of portal vein walls. The patient had markedly abnormal enzyme levels and proved to have acute viral hepatitis.

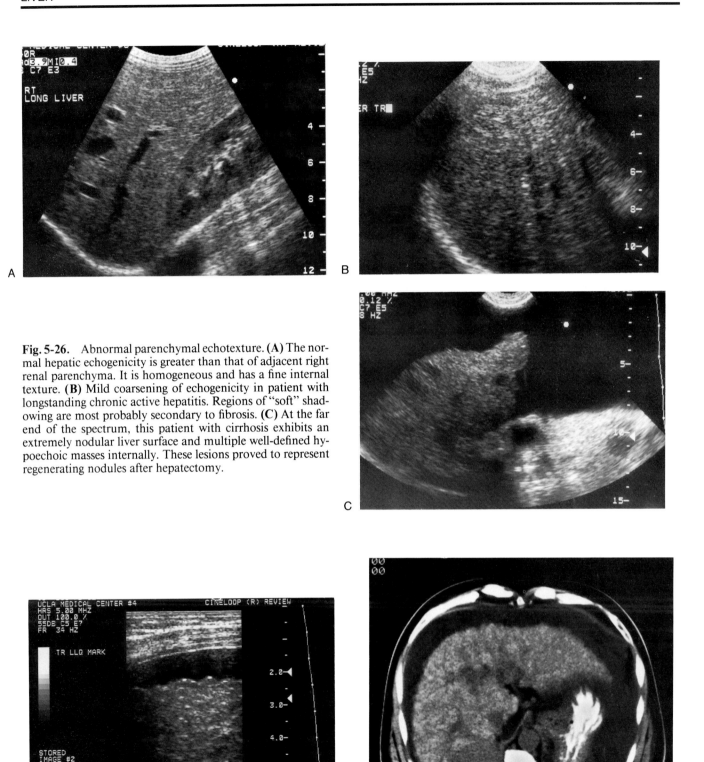

Fig. 5-26. Abnormal parenchymal echotexture. **(A)** The normal hepatic echogenicity is greater than that of adjacent right renal parenchyma. It is homogeneous and has a fine internal texture. **(B)** Mild coarsening of echogenicity in patient with longstanding chronic active hepatitis. Regions of "soft" shadowing are most probably secondary to fibrosis. **(C)** At the far end of the spectrum, this patient with cirrhosis exhibits an extremely nodular liver surface and multiple well-defined hypoechoic masses internally. These lesions proved to represent regenerating nodules after hepatectomy.

Fig. 5-27. Cirrhosis. **(A)** Nodularity is a hallmark of cirrhosis and is best demonstrated by evaluating the surface of the liver by using a high-resolution transducer with optimum focus in the near field. **(B)** CT scan confirming the nodularity of the liver surface. Note the low-density mass in the posterior right lobe *(M)*. A biopsy demonstrated hepatocellular carcinoma.

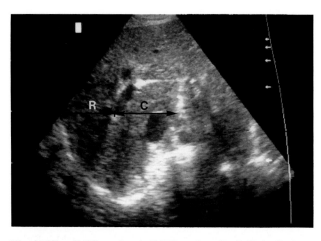

Fig. 5-28. C/RL ratio. A C/RL ratio of >0.65 is likely to indicate cirrhosis. The C/RL ratio is calculated by comparing the transverse dimension of the caudate lobe *(C)* with that of the right lobe at the level of the portal vein *(R)*.

the lateral edge of the MPV) (Fig. 5-28). According to the study of Harbin et al[59] if the C/RL ratio is greater than 0.65, cirrhosis can be diagnosed with 96 percent confidence. If the ratio is greater than 0.73, cirrhosis can be diagnosed with 99 percent confidence, and if it is less than 0.6, cirrhosis is unlikely. When using the C/RL ratio of greater than 0.65 as positive for cirrhosis, the diagnosis from this ratio alone has a sensitivity of 84 percent, a specificity of 100 percent, and an accuracy of 93 percent.[59] A ratio of 0.6 to 0.65 is borderline. Giorgio et al,[60] using the same criteria, corroborated the high sensitivity of Harbin et al,[59] but found lower specificity (43 percent).

Glycogen Storage Disease

Glycogen storage disease, or glycogenosis, is an autosomal recessive genetic disorder of carbohydrate metabolism characterized by a derangement of synthesis or degradation of glycogen and its subsequent utilization.[56,61,62] There are six categories of glycogen storage disease, divided on the basis of clinical symptoms and specific enzymatic defects. Type I glycogen storage disease (von Gierke's disease) is the most prevalent kind[56] and is characterized by impairment of the activity of the enzyme glucose-6-phosphatase, preventing glycogenolysis and release of glucose. Excess glycogen accumulates in the hepatocytes and, together with fatty metamorphosis, accounts for the hepatomegaly.[56,61] Sonographically, the livers of patients with glycogen storage disease are enlarged and brightly echogenic.[61] This disease is associated with hepatic adenomas, focal nodular hyperplasia, and hepatomegaly.[56] There is an overall 8 percent incidence of adenomas in these patients, which rises to 40 percent in patients with type I disease[62] (Fig. 5-29).

Congenital Generalized Lipodystrophy

Congenital generalized lipodystrophy is a rare hereditary disease characterized by muscular hypertrophy and lack of adipose tissue throughout the body. The characteristics of this disease include increased basal metabolic rate, hypertriglyceridemia, hepatomegaly with impaired liver function, and insulin-resistant diabetes without ketosis. Enlargement of the liver is particularly marked

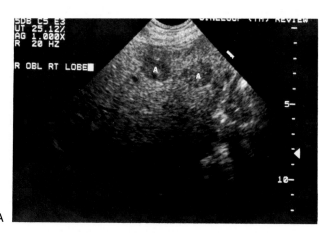

A

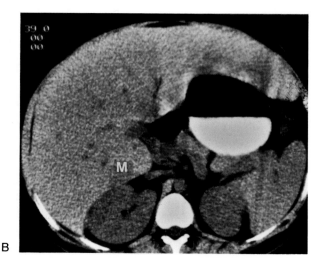

B

Fig. 5-29. Glycogen storage disease. **(A)** This patient with glycogen storage disease exhibits markedly increased echogenicity throughout the liver. Two hypoechoic adenomas *(A)* are present anteriorly. **(B)** CT scan confirming marked hepatomegaly and multiple small masses *(M)*. Considerably more masses were identified by ultrasound than by CT.

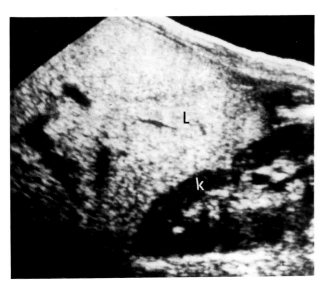

Fig. 5-30. Congenital generalized lipodystrophy. Longitudinal static scan. An echodense pattern compatible with fatty infiltration of the liver is noted. The liver *(L)* is much greater in density than the renal *(k)* cortex. (From Smevik et al,[63] with permission.)

during the first year of life. Investigators have described a hyperechoic pattern on ultrasound[63] (Fig. 5-30).

Schistosomiasis

Schistosomiasis, or bilharziasis, is an endemic disease in some parts of the world. *Schistosoma haematobium* involves primarily the lower urinary tract, and *S. mansoni* and *S. japonicum* involve mainly the colonic mucosa. The immature worm, or cercaria, lives in fresh water, and infection occurs when it punctures the skin of the human host and migrates via the lymphatics or venous system to the general circulation. In the liver, it matures into the adult form and lives in pairs. The female worm, once fertilized, migrates in a retrograde fashion into the terminal venous radicles of the bladder, ureters, and colon. The ova deposited by the female worm penetrate the mucosa and infect the urine and feces. The discharge of infected excreta into the water allows the cycle to continue.[64]

Ova may also travel back via the portal venous system to the liver, where they penetrate the walls of the smaller vessels and lodge in the periportal connective tissue. This causes an intense fibrotic response, resulting in obstruction of the portal venous system and in portal hypertension. This process evolves slowly over a period of years. The liver may be normal in size or small with foci of increased echoes secondary to diffuse fibrosis.[64] Dense echogenic bands are seen when scanning along the long

axis of the intrahepatic portal vein radicles as well as along the central and peripheral bifurcation points of the portal vein[65] (Fig. 5-31).

VASCULAR ABNORMALITIES

Portal Hypertension

Portal hypertension is due to cirrhosis in more than 90 percent of cases.[3] The disease can also be caused by obstruction of the portal vein, hepatic veins, and/or IVC or even prolonged congestive heart failure. There are two types of portal hypertension: presinusoidal and intrahepatic. The presinusoidal type includes sinusoidal obstruction by Kupffer and other cells and is generally associated with relatively normal hepatocellular function. It can be divided into extrahepatic presinusoidal and intrahepatic presinusoidal. Extrahepatic presinusoidal hypertension is caused by obstruction of the portal vein and is more common in children than adults. The causes of the portal vein obstruction include neonatal sepsis, pylephlebitis, tumor, and hypercoagulable states. One-third of children with extrahepatic obstruction have a history of omphalitis, sepsis, dehydration, and umbilical vein catheters. In the remainder, it is idiopathic. The intrahepatic presinusoidal category of portal hypertension is due to lesions of the portal zone, including schistosomiasis, primary biliary cirrhosis, congenital hepatic fibrosis, sarcoidosis, and reticuloendothelial disease within the sinusoids of liver.[3,28]

The intrahepatic forms of portal hypertension are associated with hepatocellular disease (most notably cirrhosis), and often patients suffer both gastrointestinal hemorrhage and liver failure. In cirrhosis, obstruction to portal venous blood flow occurs at all levels in the liver, resulting in a decreased intrahepatic portal vascular bed, compressed venous radicles and sinusoids as a result of regenerating nodules, and obstruction to hepatic venous outflow from the portal zones to the sinusoids. Portal hypertension leads to ascites (46 percent), splenomegaly, gastrointestinal bleeding as a consequence of abnormal venous collaterals (23 percent), signs and symptoms of hepatic failure (19 percent), and jaundice (9 percent). Of patients with advanced cirrhosis, 67 percent have varices and 25 percent have hematemesis.[3]

Portal hypertension develops when hepatopetal flow within the portal system is impeded. Simply stated, portal flow cannot get through the liver to the systemic veins and must be diverted around it via collateral pathways. The collaterals that develop represent closed or partially closed embryonic channels that reopen, connecting portal and systemic venous systems. The most common

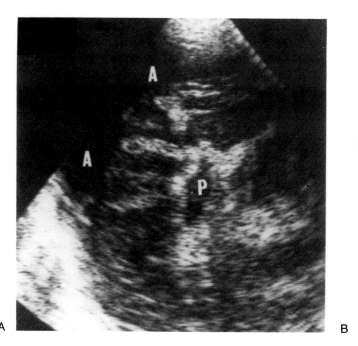
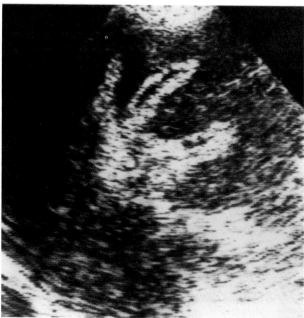

Fig. 5-31. Schistosomiasis. **(A & B)** Dense echogenic bands are identified when scanning along the axis of the intrahepatic portal vein radicals and bifurcation points. (*A*, ascites; *P*, porta hepatis.) (From Fataar et al,[65] with permission.)

pathway is the coronary-esophageal route, found in 80 to 90 percent of patients with portal hypertension.[66,67] The coronary vein runs between the two layers of the lesser omentum and cephalad toward the esophageal hiatus. At angiography, it is normally 1.3 to 3.8 mm in diameter; if it is greater than 5 mm, it is abnormal.[28,67] Other, less commonly encountered, portosystemic collateral pathways include a recanalized umbilical or paraumbilical vein[68] and splenorenal, gastrorenal, retroperitoneal, hemorrhoidal, and intestinal collaterals[69] (Fig. 5-32). Dilated coronary veins are typically imaged as venous structures arising from the MPV in the area of the splenic/superior mesenteric venous confluence (Plate 5-6) or about the stomach. The recanalized umbilical vein runs in the falciform ligament from the LPV to the epigastric veins in the anterior abdominal wall at the umbilicus (Plate 5-7). The veins in the abdominal wall are responsible for the "caput medusae" found on clinical examination. Splenorenal collaterals extend from splenic hilar or capsular veins via the pancreatic and the retroperitoneal veins into the left renal vein[69] (Plate 5-8). The pancreaticoduodenal veins drain the retroperitoneal structures such as the duodenum, pancreas, ascending and descending colon, and spleen. These veins are seen in the region of the descending duodenum and the head of the pancreas and often coexist with gastroesophageal varices.[67] The retroperitoneal-paravertebral veins lie below the level of the duodenum and may be either to

the left or right of the midline (see Plate 5-13). Gastrorenal collaterals connect the short gastric vein or coronary vein via gastric varices to the left adrenal vein, which empties into the left renal vein. Not infrequently, collat-

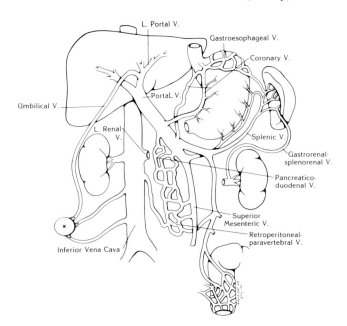

Fig. 5-32. Diagram of the common portosystemic collateral venous pathways in portal hypertension. (Modified from Subramanyam et al,[67] as modified from Orloff[250] with permission.)

erals from more than one of the last four groups coexist. The hemorrhoidal collaterals extend from the inferior mesenteric vein via the hemorrhoidal plexus into the systemic veins. The intestinal collaterals arise from the superior mesenteric vein and divert blood to the IVC.[69]

Absolute documentation of portal hypertension requires invasive procedures such as arteriography or direct portovenography. Such procedures, however, can result in significant morbidity in patients with coagulopathies and other medical problems.[69] A noninvasive alternative such as ultrasound would therefore be most attractive. Most studies thus far have used real-time ultrasound,[25,66-72] and many investigators initially considered portal vein dilatation to be a predictor of portal hypertension. The normal portal vein has been found to measure 1.1 to 1.3 cm[25,70] and can be identified in as many as 97 percent of examinations by the real-time technique.[25] Unfortunately, portal vein diameter alone has not proven a sufficiently accurate predictor of portal hypertension. Bolondi et al[70] found only a 41.8 percent sensitivity when portal vein size was considered alone. The normal portal vein varies markedly in size and may actually be small in individuals with severe portal hypertension if enough blood is diverted away by collaterals. Another method of diagnosing portal hypertension was based on an evaluation of the caliber variation of the splenic and superior mesenteric veins during respiration. With this technique, the sensitivity of ultrasound in the diagnosis of portal hypertension was purported to be 79.7 percent with a specificity of 100 percent.[70] Although this method of diagnosing portal hypertension is attractive from a physiologic standpoint (and quite accurate in the hands of the authors), it is not commonly used (Fig. 5-33). Duplex sonography has also been considered in the diagnosis of portal hypertension,[73] and a slowing of portal vein velocity seemed a logical predictor of the disease. Unfortunately, normal portal vein flow velocity is quite variable and is affected by many factors unassociated with portal hypertension. Further detracting from the possible use of duplex sonography is that shunting through a patent umbilical vein may allow portal vein blood flow velocity to become normal or even high.

Practically speaking, it is the identification of reversal of portal vein flow (Fig. 5-34 and Plate 5-9) or of collaterals that allows the sonographic diagnosis of portal hypertension. Therefore, a thorough search through the entire upper abdomen should be undertaken with particular attention to the expected areas of collateralization. Although no comparative series has yet appeared in the literature, color Doppler should be used when possible because it will facilitate the identification of vessels that might otherwise be hidden by bowel gas or mesentery.[39] The coronary veins are best seen on a longitudinal scan just medial to the point where the splenic vein joins the superior mesenteric vein. When the coronary veins are acting as collaterals, their internal diameter should be greater than 4 to 5 mm.[28] When the umbilical vein serves as a collateral, the classic "bull's-eye" pattern is seen in the area of the ligamentum teres as a result of echodense fat surrounding the dilated, fluid-filled vessel; this sign is seen in 11 percent of patients with cirrhosis.[28,74] To be significant, a patent umbilical vein must be at least 3 mm in diameter, because a small, hypoechoic center may occasionally be seen in the ligament of normal patients.[74-76] Color or spectral Doppler simplifies this task, and we no longer diagnose recanalization of the umbilical vein unless Doppler confirms flow in the presumed lumen. Esophageal varices are seen on a transverse scan with the transducer angled cranially through the left lobe of the liver. However, these important collaterals may be better identified by endoscopic ultrasound.[77] Gastrorenal, splenorenal, and dilated short gastric veins are best seen on a longitudinal scan through the spleen with the patient in the right lateral decubitus position.[28]

Ultrasound can also be used to evaluate surgically created portosystemic shunts; duplex sonography or color Doppler is essential for an adequate examination.[78] There are three main types of shunts; the scan technique will vary with each. Portacaval shunts join the end or side of the MPV to the adjacent IVC (Fig. 5-35 and Plate 5-10). Such shunts are historically the most common type constructed and are the easiest to see by ultrasound because the liver usually acts as a sonic window. As surgical techniques have improved and the potential for liver transplantation dictates that the portal vein be left intact, selective shunts (mesocaval and distal splenorenal) are becoming more commonplace. Mesocaval shunts allow decompression of the portal system via an interposition graft connecting the mid/distal superior vena cava to the IVC. These shunts may be difficult to identify by ultrasound because they lie in the central or right lower abdomen and may be shrouded by bowel gas and mesentery. We generally recommend scanning with real-time ultrasound until the serrated walls of the synthetic graft are identified. The presence or absence of flow can then be assessed using Doppler (Fig. 5-36 and Plate 5-11). Alternatively, using color Doppler, one may follow the distal IVC proximally and identify its junction with the graft by demonstrating flow from a perpendicular direction (shown by the opposite color). With continued pressure on the transducer, the bowel gas may be parted sufficiently to afford better visualization of the shunt and its characteristic walls.

With distal splenorenal (Warren) shunts, the splenic vein is severed and its tail anastomosed to the left renal vein. These shunts are popular because they divert only splenic flow and (theoretically) allow enough oxygen-

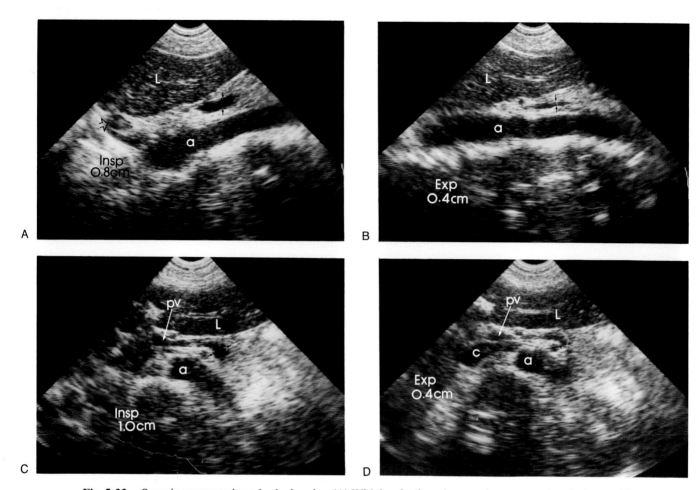

Fig. 5-33. Superior mesenteric and splenic veins. **(A)** With inspiration, the superior mesenteric vein (arrows) is measured on this longitudinal scan. (*a*, aorta; *L*, liver; open arrow, diaphragm level.) **(B)** With expiration, the superior mesenteric vein (arrows) is seen to decrease in size. (*a*, aorta; *L*, liver.) **(C)** With inspiration, the splenic vein (arrows) is measured on this transverse scan (*pv*, portal vein; *L*, liver, *a*, aorta). **(D)** With expiration, the splenic vein (arrows) is seen to decrease in size. (*pv*, portal vein; *L*, liver; *a*, aorta; *c*, inferior vena cava). In portal hypertension, there is lack of caliber variation in the superior mesenteric and splenic veins between expiration and inspiration.

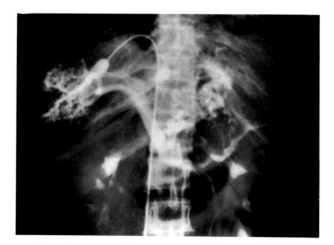

Fig. 5-34. Reversed portal vein flow. The portal vein *(P)* could not be visualized by usual arterial injection. Reversal of flow was confirmed by using wedged hepatic venography. (See also Plate 5-9.)

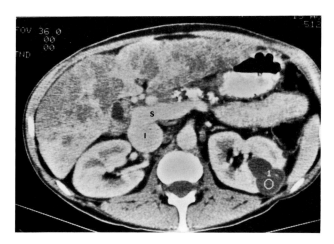

Fig. 5-35. Portacaval shunt. CT scan illustrating the shunt anatomy well. The splenic/portal vein *(S)* is anastomosed to the anterior inferior vena cava *(I)*. Multiple regions of fatty infiltration are seen throughout the liver in this patient with a history of alcohol abuse. (See also Plate 5-10).

rich blood to reach the liver from the gut to discourage encephalopathy. Warren shunts can be challenging to assess by ultrasound, and our recent study has shown that color is essential in their evaluation.[78] Spectral Doppler is simply not adequate, because the splenic limb and anastomosis are often hidden by bowel gas.[79] Although the basic scanning approach is via a coronal or oblique left intercostal window, reception of Doppler signals is often maximized by scanning first from an anterior approach via the spleen to identify the splenic

limb and then laterally to define the renal vein (Fig. 5-37 and Plate 5-12). In practice, various scanning maneuvers may be necessary to depict the anastomosis, and even then it may not be seen in every patient. Properly directed flow in well-defined splenic and renal limbs and an absence of significant left upper collaterals should imply that the shunt is patent (Fig. 5-38 and Plate 5-13).

Portal Vein Thrombosis

Portal vein thrombosis is often a relatively silent process; the liver is neither enlarged nor tender and jaundice is frequently absent as well. Ascites may be the major complaint. In adults, portal vein thrombosis is most often related to neoplastic processes (hepatocellular, pancreatic, or gastric carcinoma, or lymphoma), inflammation secondary to intra-abdominal or pelvic infection (appendicitis, diverticulitis, inflammatory bowel disease, omphalitis, and sepsis), cirrhosis, trauma, and blood dyscrasias (polycythemia rubra vera, thrombocytosis). In a significant number of cases it is also idiopathic.

The older literature teaches that the inability to identify the portal vein on a real-time examination is strong

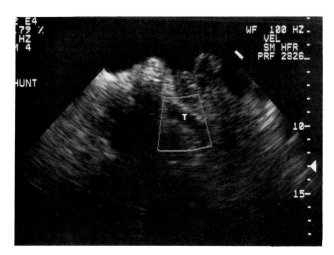

Fig. 5-36. Mesocaval shunt. This patient with a thrombosed mesocaval shunt *(T)* has no flow in the graft. Mesocaval shunts may be difficult to evaluate because the graft is frequently surrounded by bowel gas. In cases in which the shunt cannot be identified, reversed flow in the superior mesenteric vein may be used to imply patency. (See also Plate 5-11.)

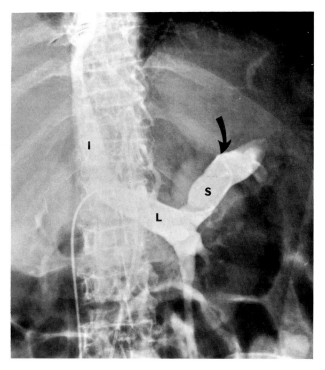

Fig. 5-37. Splenorenal shunt. Angiogram illustrating the anatomy of a normal splenorenal shunt. The procedure was performed via an inferior vena caval approach; the tip of the catheter (curved arrow) is in the splenic limb *(S)*. (*L*, left renal vein; *I*, inferior vena cava.) (See also Plate 5-12.)

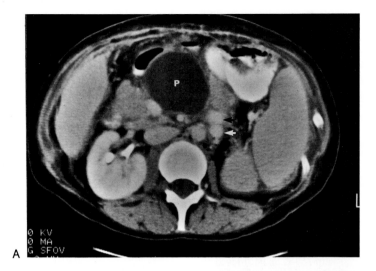

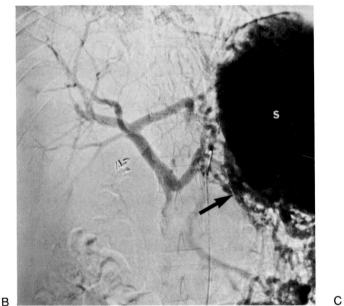

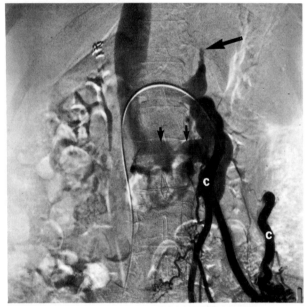

Fig. 5-38. Abnormal splenorenal shunts. **(A)** CT scan confirming the pseudocyst *(P)* in Plate 5-13. Note the collateral vessels in the left retroperitoneum (arrows). **(B)** Late phase of selective splenic arteriogram showing an enlarged spleen *(S)* drained by numerous collaterals. The splenic vein terminates abruptly at the region of the thrombosis (arrow). **(C)** Injection through the left renal vein showing shunt occlusion from the opposite vantage point (arrow). Opacified vessels are large retroperitoneal collaterals *(C)*. Note the second, retroaortic renal vein (arrows). (See also Plate 5-13.)

inferential evidence of portal vein occlusion, because the vessel is seen in a high percentage of cases.[66,80] Optimally, however, color Doppler should be used for this purpose; our recent study has demonstrated excellent results when color was compared with angiography and surgery.[81] We found that a normal study virtually excluded the possibility of thrombosis; in positive cases flow was absent or the vein was expanded by hypoechoic clot (Fig. 5-39 and Plate 5-14). Patients with severe portal hyper-

tension, however, may have sufficiently reduced flow velocity that Doppler signals are not returned even though the vein is patent (Fig. 5-40 and Plate 5-15). Such patients are unusual in the general population and should undergo further studies by MRI or angiography before it is assumed that the vein is thrombosed. It should also be noted that the "gold standard" of angiography is not always accurate; the isolated portal system is often difficult to opacify, and false-positive studies may possible because focal areas of thrombosis away from the MPV occur occasionally (Plate 5-16).

In some cases of idiopathic portal vein thrombosis, complete resolution will occur and the patient may return to normal. If portal vein occlusion occurs in infancy or the neonatal period, extensive collateral development may occur in the porta hepatis. This collection of vessels is termed cavernomatous transformation of the portal vein, and the sonographic findings are characteristic.[82-84] The normal single portal vein is not seen; pathologically, it is found to be replaced by a fibrotic band. Visualization of multiple serpiginous channels in the porta should be diagnostic, and their vascular nature can be confirmed by spectral or color Doppler[84] (Fig. 5-41 and Plate 5-17).

Portal Vein Aneurysm/Congenital Vascular Lesions

The portal venous system develops from the vitelline and umbilical veins that drain the primitive intestine. Several congenital abnormalities involving the portal vein may occur, including duplication, anomalous pulmonary venous drainage, atresia, an abnormal ventral

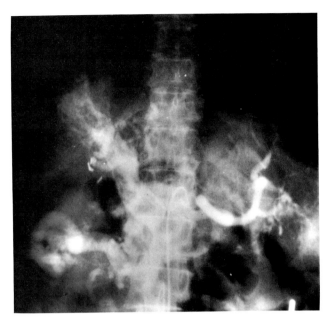

Fig. 5-39. Portal vein thrombosis. Late phase of superior mesenteric arteriogram confirming the sonographic findings in Plate 5-14.

occur. Although color Doppler is not specific in all cases, the high negative predictive value (0.98) in our series implies that it is an excellent screening procedure for portal vein thrombosis.[81] When examining such patients, as much of the portal system should be scanned as

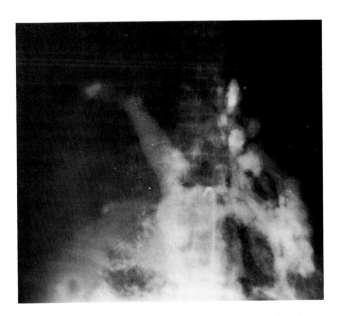

Fig. 5-40. Late phase of a mesenteric angiogram showing a patent portal vein. Note the presence of an extensive collateral bed, which facilitated reduction of portal vein flow. (See also Plate 5-15.)

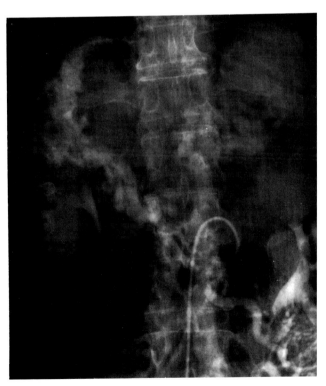

Fig. 5-41. Cavernous transformation of the portal vein. Mesenteric arteriogram confirming the presence of cavernous transformation in Plate 5-17. Note the prominent varices extending to the left upper quadrant. (See also Plate 5-17.)

position,[85] and various types of fistulae. Portal vein aneurysms occur either proximally at the junction of the superior mesenteric vein and splenic vein or distally in the portal vein radicles.[85] The ampullary dilatation at the junction of the superior mesenteric vein and the splenic vein, however, may be considerable and should not be considered abnormal. Portal vein aneurysms may be congenital or acquired secondary to portal hypertension (Plate 5-18).

Portal Vein Gas

In infants, portal vein gas is typically associated with necrotizing enterocolitis. If not diagnosed and treated early, necrotizing enterocolitis leads to sepsis, bowel per-

foration, and eventually death. These patients have abdominal distension, feeding intolerance, and bloody diarrhea. Radiographic findings include dilated bowel loops, pneumatosis intestinalis, a foamy bowel gas pattern, pneumoperitoneum, and portal vein and hepatic parenchymal gas. In adults, portal vein air has typically been considered a bad prognostic sign and strongly associated with bowel infarction. Recently, however, several groups have reported portal vein gas in patients after liver transplantation. In this population, the finding seems to be of little prognostic significance.[86]

The most characteristic ultrasound pattern of portal vein gas is that of highly echogenic particles (probable microbubbles) flowing within the portal vein[86,87] (Fig. 5-42). These moving reflectors are far more echogenic

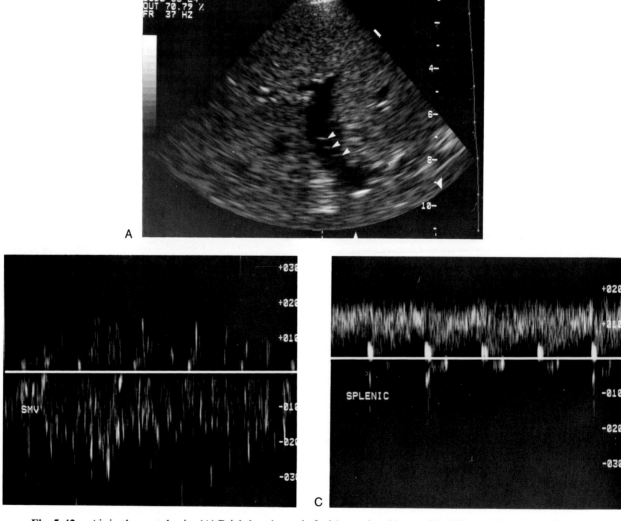

Fig. 5-42.   Air in the portal vein. **(A)** Brightly echogenic foci (arrowheads) were identified coursing through the portal vein 7 weeks after liver transplantation. **(B)** Spectral Doppler from the portal vein and superior mesenteric vein *(SMV)* showing unusual "pinging" sound; note the spikelike spectral tracing. Findings are typical of air in the portal vein. **(C)** Doppler evaluation of the splenic vein was normal, implying that the air originated in the gut.

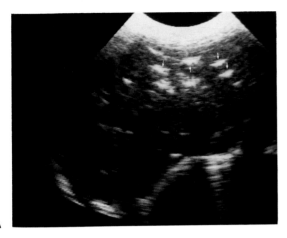
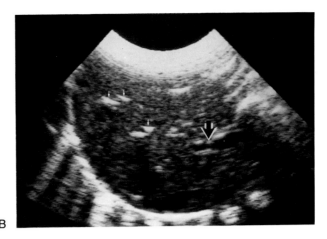

A   B

Fig. 5-43.   Portal vein gas. Necrotizing enterocolitis. **(A)** Transverse and **(B)** longitudinal scans of an infant with necrotizing enterocolitis. Numerous echogenic patches (arrows) in the hepatic parenchyma tend to occupy the nondependent parts of the liver. In Fig. B, there is a microbubble within the portal vein (large arrow). (From Merritt et al,[87] with permission.)

than those normally seen in slow-moving venous blood and should not cause confusion. If any question exists, spectral analysis can be used to confirm that air is present by demonstrating a characteristic "pinging" sound.[86] Gas in the portal vein may be intermittent and is not associated with acoustic shadowing. Once in the liver, portal air causes poorly defined, highly echogenic patches within the hepatic parenchyma, which are most apparent in the nondependent part of the liver and fade with time[87] (Fig. 5-43). These findings are frequently observed before the characteristics of the disease process are noted on the radiograph and permit earlier aggressive therapy with the potential of reducing mortality and complications.

Hepatic Fistulae

Hepatic artery-to-portal vein fistulae are uncommon lesions that may be congenital or secondary to rupture of a preexisting hepatic artery aneurysm into the portal vein, trauma, biopsy, cirrhosis, or hepatic neoplasm eroding into the artery and portal vein. Most clinically significant cases arise from rupture of an aneurysm; 75 percent of the aneurysms are extrahepatic, and 63 percent involve the common hepatic artery. Portal hypertension tends to be severe because of the large quantity of high-pressure blood being delivered into the portal system.[88] Sonographically, large hepatic artery-to-portal vein fistulae should be striking. When they are small, the Doppler features may be subtle and limited to the identification of a localized high-speed jet or bruit with marked turbulence (Plate 5-19 and Fig. 5-44). Secondary fea-

tures include reversal of portal vein flow, large varices, and an arterialized flow pattern by spectral analysis.

Hepatic vein-to-portal vein fistulae are also unusual and, again, may be congenital or acquired. They are most often asymptomatic but may cause hepatic encephalopathy. Sonographically, cystlike, anechoic structures that demonstrate flow on Doppler examination are identified within the liver (Fig. 5-45 and Plate 5-20).

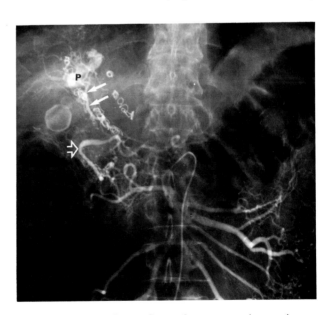

Fig. 5-44.   Late phase of superior mesenteric arteriogram confirming the sonographic findings of Plate 5-19. The abnormal artery in the sonogram corresponded to the feeder (arrows) arising from the pancreaticoduodenal artery (open arrow). Note the retrograde filling of the portal vein *(P)*. (See also Plate 5-19.)

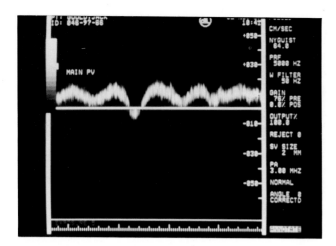

Fig. 5-45. Hepatic vein-to-portal vein fistula. Spectral analysis of the portal vein revealing marked pulsatility. A pulsatile portal vein is to be expected secondary to portosystemic communication. (See also Plate 5-20.)

These "varices" should be easily followed to their connection with the hepatic and portal veins.[89] Hepatic vein-to-portal vein fistulae are an unusual cause of pulsatile flow in the portal vein.[90] More common causes of portal pulsatility tend to be cardiac (Fig. 5-46). Recent reports implicate both elevated right heart pressure[90] and tricuspid regurgitation.[91]

Budd-Chiari Syndrome

Budd-Chiari syndrome involves obstruction to hepatic venous outflow; the offending lesion may be anywhere from the level of the hepatic venules (hepatic veno-occlusive disease) to the IVC. The liver becomes enlarged and tender; intractable ascites is typical. In one-third of cases, the etiology of Budd-Chiari syndrome is never determined. Thrombosis of the hepatic veins, however, is associated with hypercoagulable states (especially polycythemia vera), paroxysmal nocturnal hemoglobinuria, collagen vascular diseases, oral contraceptives, hepatic tumors (in particular hepatocellular carcinoma), renal and adrenal carcinoma, radiation, and congenital hepatic webs.[92-96] Pathologically, centrilobular congestion and necrosis are seen early and central fibrosis and periportal regenerating nodules occur later. Three major forms of Budd-Chiari syndrome have been described: (1) occlusion of the IVC, with or without secondary occlusion of the hepatic vein; (2) occlusion of the major hepatic veins, with or without occlusion of the IVC; and (3) veno-occlusive disease of the liver, a progressive thrombotic occlusion of small centrilobar veins that is typically associated with drugs or radiation. Hepatic veno-occlusive disease has become more common recently and is a recognized possible complication of the conditioning regimen for bone marrow transplants.[95]

With acute thrombosis, absence of hepatic venous flow may be the only color Doppler abnormality present. The entire liver should be carefully evaluated in every case, since thrombosis may not affect all three major veins. The caudate lobe has a separate venous drainage from the rest of the liver, and a single large vessel draining this area may be identified. The caudate vein should not be mistaken for a patent MHV (Plate 5-5).

Following the acute thrombotic episode, collateral veins open in and about the liver. Intrahepatic collaterals are essentially diagnostic of hepatic venous occlusion, and their demonstration by color Doppler should pro-

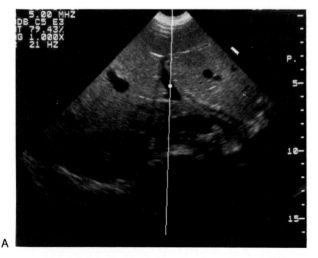

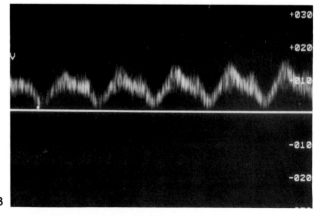

A   B

Fig. 5-46. Pulsatile portal vein. This patient with right heart failure and abnormal liver function tests was evaluated to exclude intrinsic hepatic abnormality. **(A)** The real-time evaluation was normal. **(B)** Spectral analysis showing pulsatile portal vein flow. Such portal venous patterns are often associated with right heart abnormalities; passive congestion may be the etiology of abnormal liver function tests.

vide a definitive diagnosis. The most striking manifestation of this is the abrupt central termination of peripheral veins and reversal of their flow into adjacent branches, resulting in the striking bicolored appearance unique to this disease[97] (Plate 5-21). The identification of small, often serpiginous central collaterals that do not appear to lead directly to the IVC should also strongly suggest Budd-Chiari syndrome (Fig. 5-47 and Plate 5-22); this picture is the sonographic correlate of the classic "spider web appearance" well known to angiographers.[96]

In addition to a thorough evaluation of the hepatic veins and any attendant abnormal intrahepatic circulatory patterns, the portal vein and IVC should be examined. The careful evaluation of these vessels should be emphasized because either or both may be compromised as part of Budd-Chiari syndrome and knowledge of their status is essential in planning therapy. Portal vein thrombosis has been reported to occur in as many as 20 percent of patients with Budd-Chiari syndrome,[93] and this vessel may serve as an essential conduit to decompress hepatic vascular congestion if it is patent.[98,99] If it is thrombosed, surgical decompression is not possible and the only options are medical therapy (which may control the ascites but not the progressive liver damage) or liver transplantation.

Evaluation of the IVC is also necessary because com-

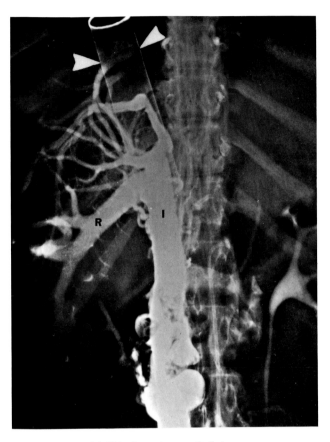

Fig. 5-48. Budd-Chiari syndrome. Inferior vena cavagram confirming the findings in Plates 5-22 and 5-23. Note the complete occlusion of the proximal inferior vena cava *(I)*, numerous intrahepatic collaterals, and a large patent right hepatic vein *(R)*. The large cylindrical structure is a mesoatrial shunt (arrowheads).

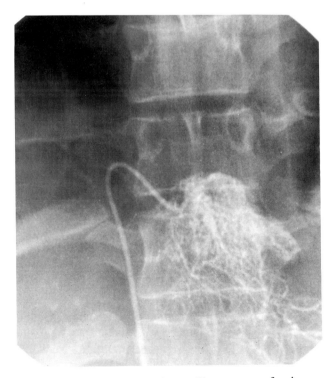

Fig. 5-47. Budd-Chiari syndrome. Venogram confirming sonographic findings in Plate 5-22 and demonstrating the "spider web" sign. (See also Plates 5-22 and 5-23.)

promise of this vessel may be the etiology of the syndrome itself. The underlying IVC abnormality may be a congenital web; compression or invasion by tumor thrombus, either bland or neoplastic; or compression by an enlarged caudate lobe (Fig. 5-48 and Plate 5-23). Another reason for assessment of the IVC is that the surgical procedure of choice will be altered if a significant gradient exists between the right heart and the IVC. Patients with a widely patent IVC may undergo a simple portocaval shunt. Those having a significant gradient will require a mesoatrial shunt, which is far more difficult to construct and has a higher incidence of complications. Portocaval and mesoatrial shunts (Fig. 5-49 and Plate 5-24) are easily evaluated by duplex sonography or color Doppler imaging, and sonography should be considered the primary examination when thrombosis is suspected.[78,97]

Obstruction of the hepatic veins may also occur at the microscopic level, but symptoms are similar to those caused by macroscopic thrombosis. Hepatic veno-occlusive disease was rarely reported until recently. The

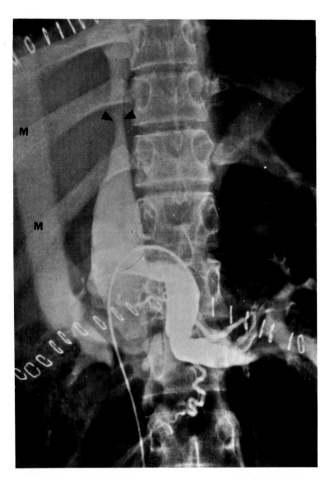

Fig. 5-49. Mesoatrial shunt. Contrast study showing the mesoatrial shunt *(M)* to good advantage. The inferior vena cava is compressed (arrowheads) by an enlarged caudate lobe. (See also Plate 5-24.)

incidence, however, has increased since the advent of bone marrow transplantation. In these patients, the chemotherapeutic conditioning regimens cause a chemical inflammation leading to blockage of hepatic venous outflow at the venule level. Unfortunately, hepatic veno-occlusive disease is difficult to diagnose since the larger, visible vessels remain patent and flow moves in and out of the vessels in relation to right atrial and systemic venous pulsations. Brown et al,[100] however, have reported certain associated abnormalities in this group of patients, which may be useful in diagnosis. Blockage of the hepatic veins will decrease or even reverse portal venous flow. In such cases, decreased portal vein velocity may be diagnostic but the variation requires a baseline sonogram for comparison. Hepatic veno-occlusive disease, however, may be definitively diagnosed in patients with bone marrow transplantation if reversal of portal vein flow is identified without a well-established diagnosis of cirrhosis and portal hypertension (Plate 5-25).

Hereditary Hemorrhagic Telangiectasia

Hereditary hemorrhagic telangiectasia (Osler-Weber-Rendu disease) is an autosomal dominant disorder that may involve every organ. Liver abnormalities include angiodysplasia, fibrosis, cirrhosis, portosystemic encephalopathy, and hepatocellular carcinoma. Classically, there is a familial incidence with multiple telangiectasias and recurrent episodes of bleeding. The most serious sequelae are cardiovascular complications and gastrointestinal bleeding. On ultrasound, an abnormally dilated common hepatic artery with multiple arteriovenous malformations and an abnormal echogenicity of the liver are noted[101] (Fig. 5-50). Large feeding arteries, prominent pulsations, ectatic vascular structures, and large draining veins may be seen.

FOCAL ABNORMALITIES

Nonparasitic Cysts

Liver cysts may be congenital, traumatic, parasitic, or inflammatory in origin. In most cases, however, no etiology is evident. Congenital cysts arise from developmental defects in the formation of bile ducts.[3,102] Cysts vary in diameter (average size, 3 cm), tend to be superficial, and are lined with cuboidal epithelium. The right lobe is affected twice as often as the left. The incidence of hepatic cysts is said to be 17 in 10,000 at abdominal exploration[101,103] and 1 in 600 at laparotomy.[103] Most cysts, however, are not identified by these procedures. Sonographically, hepatic cysts are quite common in the older population, although the exact incidence has never been determined.[104] Hepatic cysts are typically asymptomatic; they usually do not cause hepatomegaly and are rarely palpable.[3] Cysts may cause epigastric pain or mass effect, suggesting a more serious condition such as an infected cyst, abscess, or neoplasm. Fifty-five percent of symptomatic patients present with an abdominal mass, 40 percent with hepatomegaly, 33 percent with abdominal pain, and 9 percent with jaundice.[105] There is a slight female predominance (4:1),[103] and the clinical presentation is typically in the fifth to seventh decades. From 25 to 50 percent of patients with autosomal dominant polycystic kidney disease have one or more cysts in the liver. On the other hand, 60 percent of patients with polycystic liver have renal cysts.[106]

Sonographically, a cyst should be anechoic, exhibit posterior acoustic enhancement, and have thin, well-defined walls (Fig. 5-51). Many cysts contain several fine internal septae; these are not of clinical concern unless a history of a cystic cancer (e.g., ovarian carcinoma) is present (Fig. 5-52). The accuracy of ultrasound in diag-

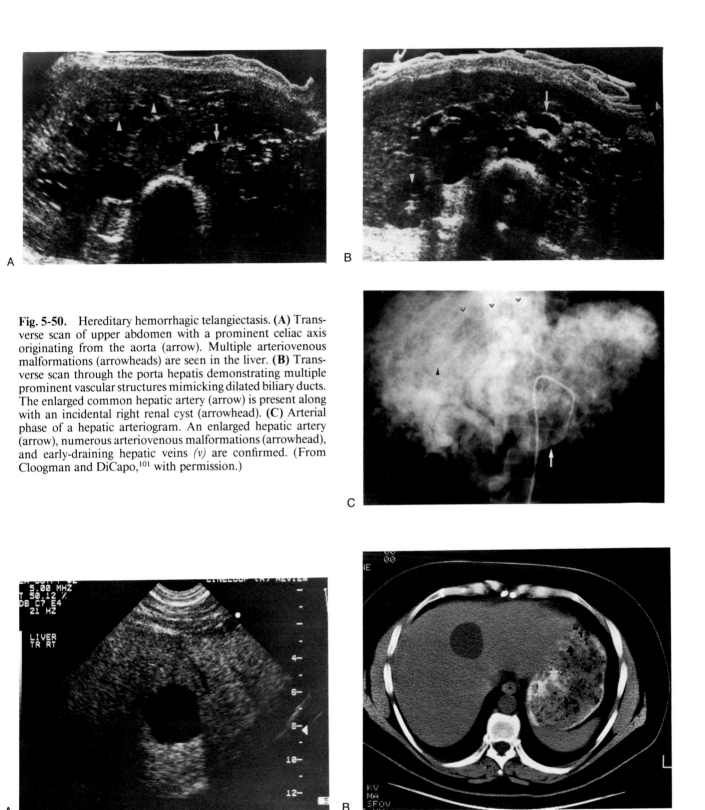

Fig. 5-50. Hereditary hemorrhagic telangiectasis. **(A)** Transverse scan of upper abdomen with a prominent celiac axis originating from the aorta (arrow). Multiple arteriovenous malformations (arrowheads) are seen in the liver. **(B)** Transverse scan through the porta hepatis demonstrating multiple prominent vascular structures mimicking dilated biliary ducts. The enlarged common hepatic artery (arrow) is present along with an incidental right renal cyst (arrowhead). **(C)** Arterial phase of a hepatic arteriogram. An enlarged hepatic artery (arrow), numerous arteriovenous malformations (arrowhead), and early-draining hepatic veins *(v)* are confirmed. (From Cloogman and DiCapo,[101] with permission.)

Fig. 5-51. Liver cyst. **(A)** Simple cysts of the liver are common in older people. The lesion is anechoic internally, has smooth walls, and exhibits good through transmission posteriorly. **(B)** CT scan confirming a simple liver cyst.

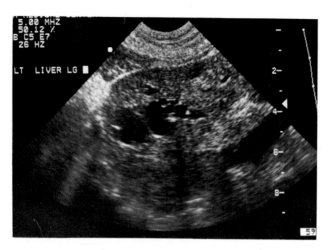

Fig. 5-52. Multiple cysts. Multiple or clustered cysts may be encountered and need not be associated with polycystic kidney disease or cancer. Note the wall irregularity and internal septations.

nosing hepatic cysts is said to be 95 to 100 percent,[102] although small, peripheral lesions are easily overlooked unless a specific search for their presence is undertaken. In this regard, the study of Brick et al[107] showed ultrasound to be an excellent method of determining whether small indeterminate lesions found on CT are simple cysts or solid metastases. The differential diagnosis for cystic liver lesions includes simple cyst, necrotic metastasis, echinococcal cyst, hematoma, hepatic cystadenocarcinoma, and abscess. The appearance of most benign, simple cysts, however, is usually sufficiently characteristic to avoid further studies. If the diagnosis of a cyst is in

doubt, an ultrasound-guided percutaneous cyst aspiration may be performed.[103] Although percutaneous aspiration is effective as a primary diagnostic maneuver, it lacks permanent therapeutic benefit.[108] In one series of 13 patients who underwent cyst aspiration, all cysts recurred within 2 years.[108] Definitive therapy requires surgical or chemical ablation of the cyst lining,[109] sclerosis,[110] or internal drainage by marsupialization.[108]

Inflammatory Processes

Echinococcal Disease

Echinococcal cysts (hydatid disease) are common in regions of the world where the parasite *Echinococcus* is endemic. The highest incidence is in countries where dogs are used to herd sheep and cattle.[111] Increased travel and immigration, however, has resulted in dissemination, and *Echinococcus* (as well as most other "tropical" diseases) may now be encountered almost anywhere in the world. The eggs of the worm (*Echinococcus granulosis* and *E. multilocularis*) are excreted in the feces of infected dogs; cattle, sheep, hogs, and humans serve as the intermediate host.[64] The eggs hatch in the lumen of the proximal small intestine, and embryos penetrate the mucosa, eventually entering the blood vessels and hence traveling throughout the body. Larvae lodge in capillaries and incite an inflammatory reaction composed principally of mononuclear leukocytes and eosinophils. Many such larvae are destroyed, but others encyst. The cyst is initially microscopic but may enlarge, taking 5 years or more to reach massive size.[3] Most cysts grow at a

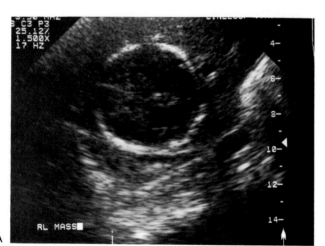

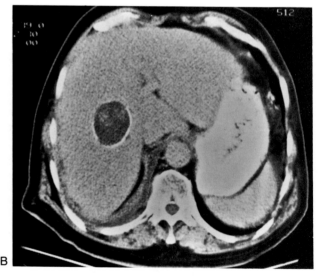

A   B

Fig. 5-53. Echinococcal cyst. **(A)** The lesion is well-defined and round and has curvilinear calcifications in the wall. **(B)** CT scan confirming sonographic findings.

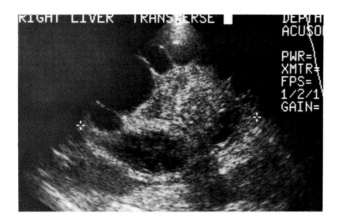

Fig. 5-54. Echinococcal cyst. Classic thick-walled echinococcal cyst demonstrating multiple rounded internal compartments representing "daughter" cysts.

rate of 0.25 to 1.00 cm/yr and remain asymptomatic for 5 to 10 years. Enclosing the fluid within the cyst is an inner, nucleated, germinative layer, which gives rise to the brood capsules, and an outer opaque nonnucleated layer.[111] The outer layer is quite distinctive, with innumerable delicate laminations like fine tissue paper. Outside the opaque layer is an inflammatory reaction, which produces a layer of fibroblasts, giant cells, and mononuclear and eosinophilic infiltration.[3] When cysts have been present for about 6 months, daughter cysts develop within them, arising from the germinal epithelium. Impingement on blood vessels can lead to vascular thrombosis and infarction. The cyst may rupture and fluid may escape, evoking a massive anaphylactic reaction.[111,112] In humans, more than 50 percent of cysts are in the liver.[3]

Other sites, in decreasing order, include the lungs, bones, brain, and pancreas.[113]

Numerous articles have described the sonographic findings of echinococcal cysts.[111-121] The patterns identified include (1) discrete simple cysts (with or without calcification) (Fig. 5-53); (2) multiple cysts or cysts within cysts (typical of so-called daughter cysts) (Fig. 5-54); (3) honeycomb cysts (fluid collection with septa) (Fig. 5-55); and (4) solid-appearing masses (Fig. 5-56). An oval or spherical shape and smooth walls are common.[114] Esfahani et al[115] have described several other signs thought to be fairly specific, including the "double-line" sign (the identification of pericyst and laminated membrane) and arc-shaped curvilinear calcifications (Fig. 5-57). The number and size of the cysts vary considerably. Identification of daughter cysts is not indispensable to the diagnosis but is highly suggestive of this disease.[116] If there are no daughter cells, the cyst may be inactive, with disintegration of the daughter cysts. A shell-like calcification in the thick wall around a cyst is also typical of true hydatid disease. In some instances, the liver may contain multiple parent cysts situated in both lobes, producing hepatomegaly.[64] To make the diagnosis of echinococcal disease in such a case, cysts with thick walls occupying different parts of the liver must be seen. The presence of tissue between the cysts indicates that each cyst is a separate parent cyst and are not daughter cysts (Fig. 5-55). Calcification may occur in the wall many years after the initial infection. Complete cyst wall calcification usually indicates an inactive lesion, but other viable noncalcified cysts may be present.[64] An ultrasonic "water lily" sign has been described and results from the detachment and collapse of the germinal layer or laminated membrane. This sign is

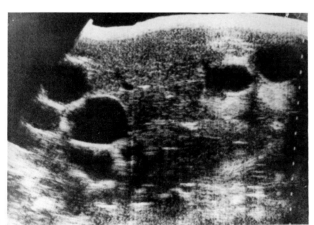
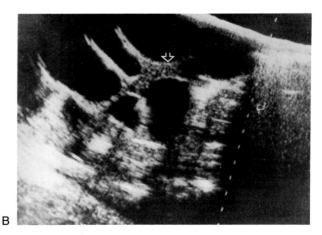

A   B

Fig. 5-55. Echinococcal cyst—multiple parents. **(A)** Multiple well-defined separate fluid-filled cysts of various sizes are present within the liver. **(B)** Some cysts are compressed by others and lose their rounded appearance. There is liver tissue between the cysts (arrow), indicating that they are multiple parent cysts and not daughter cysts. (From Itzchuk et al,[249] with permission.)

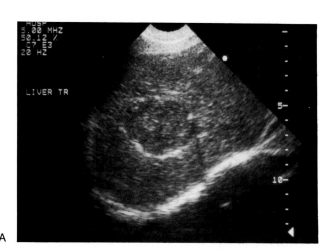

A

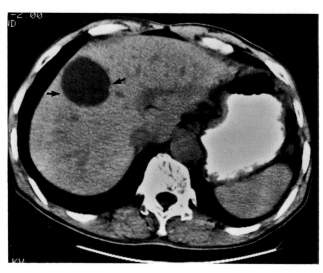

B

Fig. 5-56. Echinococcal disease. **(A)** Transverse image through the dome of the liver showing a well-defined solid mass with echogenic borders. Several areas of discrete shadowing imply calcifications. **(B)** CT scan showing similar features. Note the calcific nodules in the periphery (arrows).

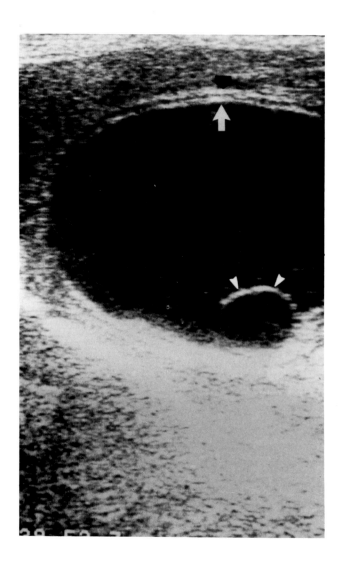

Fig. 5-57. Echinococcal cyst. "Double-line" sign (arrows) is a specific sign of echinococcal disease and is secondary to the presence of inner laminated membrane. Note the rounded daughter cyst posteriorly (arrowheads). (From Esfahani et al,[115] with permission.)

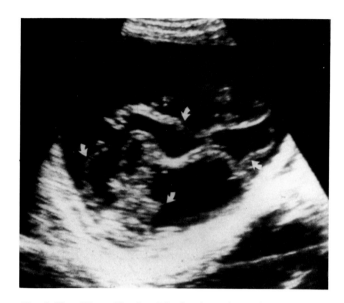

Fig. 5-58. Water lily sign. The laminated membrane (curved arrows) has fallen away from the outer pericyst and lies in the dependent portion of the cyst. The double-line sign is no longer seen. Such undulating membranes have been described as the water lily sign and are pathognomic of echinococcal cysts. (From Esfahani et al,[115] with permission.)

analogous to that on chest radiographs. The collapsed germinal layer is seen as an undulating linear collection of echoes either floating in the cyst fluid or lying in the most dependent portion of the cyst[117] (Fig. 5-58).

Although cystic lesions are typical of hydatid disease of the liver, several authors have described solid-appearing lesions as well[118,119] (Fig. 5-56). Garcia et al,[119] in fact, found that 17 percent of their patients with hydatid cysts had solid lesions. It is postulated that in cases in which the cysts appear solid, the germinative membranes of the cysts are very active, giving rise to many daughter cysts; pieces of the membrane may even detach, fall into such a cyst, and continue to proliferate. The presence of daughter cells within hydatid cysts depends on many factors, such as resistance of the organs where cysts grow and natural or acquired mechanisms of immunity of the host.[118] *E. alveolaris,* which produces a different disease from the more common *E. multilocularis,* typically produces multinodular solid lesions in the liver and should be considered in the differential of solid masses in endemic areas[120] (Fig. 5-59 and Plate 5-26).

When hydatid cysts become secondarily infected or are treated medically, a different pattern may be seen on ultrasound. In either case the number of internal echoes may increase, giving rise to the appearance of a solid mass (Fig. 5-60). The laminated membrane or the mem-

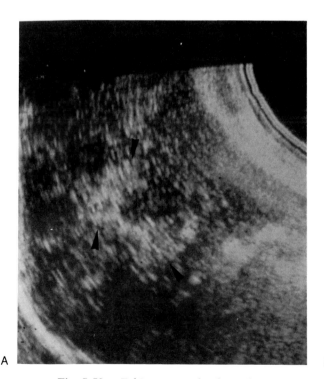

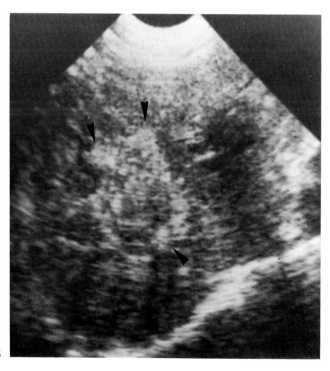

A　　　　　　　　　　　　　　　　　　　　B

Fig. 5-59. *Echinococcus alveolaris* disease. **(A & B)** Solid mass in the right lobe of the liver consisting of a conglomerate of multiple small echogenic nodules (arrowheads) is typical. (See Plate 5-26). (From Didier et al,[120] with permission.)

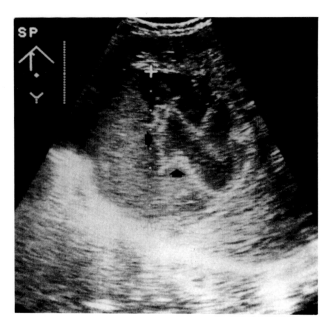

Fig. 5-60. Superinfected cyst. Such cysts tend to contain inhomogeneous echogenic material. The laminated membrane (arrows) is frequently detached. (From Esfahani et al,[115] with permission.)

brane of the daughter cysts may disintegrate and take on a bizarre appearance.[64,121] Large cysts may be surgically removed in some cases; omentoplasty is usually used in conjunction with removal of the cyst.[122] In this procedure the cavity of the lesion is "unroofed" and a piece of omentum with its blood supply preserved is mobilized, spread into the cavity, and fixed to the walls. The use of omental patching of the space has decreased bile leaks and infection of the operative space and has shortened

the hospital stay. Sonographically, a well-circumscribed, sharply angulated echogenic focus is seen within the liver. The large size, sharply angulated margins, and internal echopattern of the lesion should help to distinguish it from most naturally occurring abnormalities of the liver[116,122] (Fig. 5-61). When omentoplasty is not used, a large cystic cavity may be seen in the area of the previously resected echinococcal cyst (Fig. 5-62). When discussing treatment of echinococcal cysts, it is worth noting a recent article by Khuroo et al[123] in which 21 echinococcal cysts in 12 patients were drained percutaneously. Medical dogma has taught us to avoid puncture of such lesions lest anaphylactic reaction occur. Their experience with percutaneous drainage has been excellent, with no evidence of allergic reaction in any patient. Should further studies corroborate these results, percutaneous drainage of echinococcal cysts may become the preferred treatment.

Pyogenic Abscess

Bacteria gain access to the liver from the biliary tree, portal vein, hepatic artery, contiguous infection, and trauma.[102,124] Most infections, however, arise from the biliary tree and obstruction, hepatic cyst, and biliary tumor are all predisposing conditions.[124,125] Frequently, the source of infection is never found. The most common agents are *Escherichia coli* and anaerobic bacteria such as *Clostridium* or *Bacteroides,* suggesting some form of association with the bowel.[3]

Clinically, the presentation of hepatic abscess is varied, with fever, pain, pleuritis, nausea, vomiting, and diarrhea the most common symptoms. Leukocytosis, elevated liver function tests, and anemia are also usually

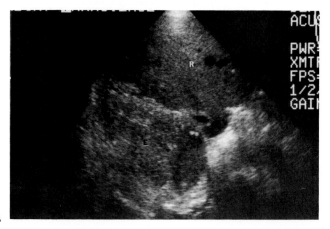

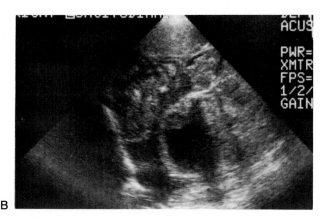

A   B

Fig. 5-61. Omentoplasty. This patient had undergone cystectomy with omental packing of the space. **(A)** Right transverse image showing well-demarcated echogenic structure *(E)* posterior to the right lobe of the liver *(R).* **(B)** Longitudinal view taken further to the left showing a more undulating internal pattern of hyper- and hypoechogenicity. This finding is the result of alternating fatty and fibrous layers of omentum.

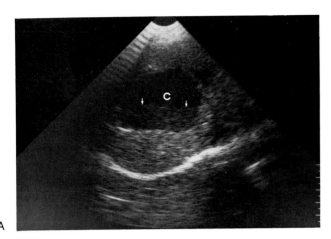
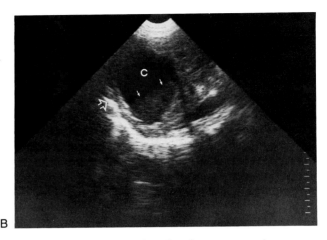

A   B

Fig. 5-62. Postoperative hydatid cyst. **(A)** Transverse and **(B)** longitudinal scans of the liver in a postoperative patient for hydatid cyst removal. A cystic (lucent) mass *(c)* is seen in the area of the previously resected cyst. It has a fluid-fluid level (arrows) within it. This was monitored by ultrasound and serologic titers. By 1 year, it had disappeared. (open arrow, diaphragm.)

present. Rapid diagnosis and therapy are vital since up to 100 percent mortality has been described with untreated liver abscess.[124,125] Liver abscesses vary considerably in size; 80 percent are located in the right lobe, and they may be single or multiple (10 percent). In rare instances, an abscess occurs in the falciform ligament because its layers represent a potential space providing communication with the gallbladder.[126] Sonographically, abscesses are usually round or ovoid with irregular thick walls (90 percent) and poor outer definition. Internally, these lesions are typically hypoechoic (Fig. 5-63) and may demonstrate fluid-debris levels[124,125] (Figs. 5-64 and

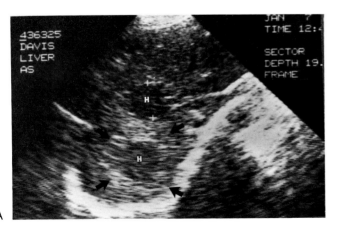
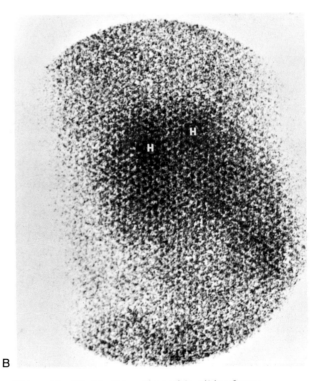

A   B

Fig. 5-63. Pyogenic abscesses. **(A)** Two hypoechoic masses *(H)* are identified in this patient with spiking fevers. Note the relatively echogenic area (arrows) around the posterior lesion, probably representing parenchymal inflammation. **(B)** Right lateral image of gallium 67 (^{67}Ga) scintigram demonstrating uptake in two discrete areas *(H)*. Findings are suggestive of abscess. Percutaneous puncture of the more anterior lesion yielded *E. coli.*

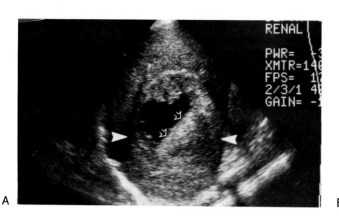
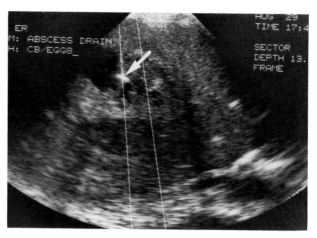

Fig. 5-64. Pyogenic abscess. **(A)** The patient was a 31-year-old Cambodian man with acute-onset right upper quadrant pain and fevers. Sonogram through right lobe of liver showing a large mass with thick walls (arrowheads). Note the fluid-debris level posteriorly (open arrows). **(B)** Sonographically guided percutaneous puncture (arrow, needle tip) yielded gross pus. The lesion was successfully treated by percutaneous catheter drainage.

5-65). Abscesses with brightly echogenic foci may contain air or microbubbles[127,128] (Fig. 5-66); acoustic shadowing is a reliable indicator of a gas-containing abscess. Real-time ultrasound can be used to guide puncture of an abscess for diagnosis and/or catheter drainage.[125,129]

Amebic Abscess

Although primarily an infection of the colon, amebiasis can spread to the liver, lungs, and brain. Amebic abscesses are a common complication and one of the most widespread diseases in the world. The parasites

(Entamoeba histolytica) reach the liver through the portal vein. They may burrow through the subdiaphragmatic space to enter the thorax. Amebiasis is contracted by ingesting the cysts in contaminated food or water. The wall of the cyst dissolves in the alkaline content of the small bowel, and the trophozoite emerges to colonize and ulcerate the colon. The cecum and ascending colon are the most common areas affected. Most patients are asymptomatic, and the organism remains confined to the gastrointestinal tract. Patients may have clinical symptoms of abdominal pain, diarrhea, and melena.[3] In some cases amebas invade the colonic mucosa and are

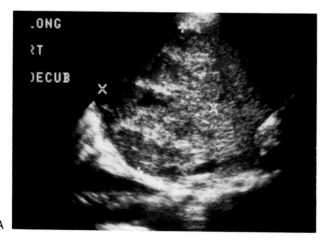
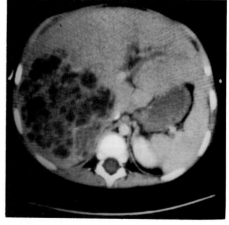

Fig. 5-65. Pyogenic abscess. **(A)** Section through the right lobe of the liver in a child with pain, fevers, and chills showing a large, solid-appearing mass (calipers). **(B)** CT scan showing a multiseptate lesion. A biopsy specimen of the suspected neoplasm yielded purulent material. Pathologic evaluation of the lesion after surgical removal showed no evidence of malignancy. (Case contributed by Inez Boechat, M.D., UCLA Medical Center.)

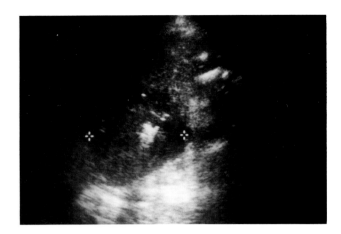

Fig. 5-66. Pyogenic abscess. Patient with advanced cervical carcinoma and multiple hepatic metastases. Note the hyperechoic region in the center of the mass. Fluoroscopic examination at the time of percutaneous drainage revealed clustered air bubbles in the corresponding area. Drainage was successful and provided palliative relief of infectious symptoms.

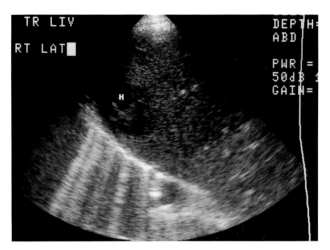

Fig. 5-67. Amebic abscess. This Hispanic male with hepatomegaly and right upper quadrant pain is demonstrated to have a hypoechoic mass *(H)* beneath the dome of the liver. Note the poorly defined region of relative increased echogenicity about the hypoechoic lesion. The patient responded well to medical therapy; serial sonograms showed complete resolution of the lesion.

carried to the liver via the portal venous system. The liver can be affected without overt colonic involvement.[64] Deposition in the capillaries of the portal vein presumably accounts for the peripheral predilection of the abscesses. When the infection has been established, there is liquefaction necrosis of the hepatocytes with little leukocytic or fibrotic response, which, when coupled with hemorrhage into partially digested debris, results in the diagnostic chocolate-colored "anchovy paste" material within.[64,130] Complications of amebic abscess include rupture into pleuropulmonary structures (15.8 percent) or into the peritoneal cavity (6 percent).[124]

Numerous descriptions of the ultrasound features of amebic abscesses of the liver may be found in the literature.[64,118,126,127,130–137] Forty percent of patients exhibit findings suggestive of the diagnosis including lack of significant wall echoes; a round or oval configuration; echogenicity less than normal liver parenchyma, with fine, homogeneous, low-level echoes at high gain; location contiguous with liver capsule; and distal sonic enhancement[64,132] (Fig. 5-67). Fifty percent of the above 40 percent were found to exhibit all but one or two characteristics.[132] Unfortunately, although the imaging features may be suggestive, Ralls et al[133] found that pyogenic abscesses could not be distinguished from amebic abscesses in a significant number of cases. When a question exists, however, an ultrasound-guided aspiration should be considered.[134] One series reported 7 of 74 amebic abscesses that appeared partly or predominantly hyperechoic.[135] On follow-up examination after a course of therapy, the appearance of four of six changed to a more typical hypoechoic form, probably secondary to

tissue liquefaction. After successful therapy, complete resolution of the ultrasound abnormality may be expected in a period of 6 weeks to 23 months (median, 7 months)[132,136]; occasionally, a cystic residuum remains[132,136,137] (Fig. 5-68). With therapy, ultrasound findings vary; the cyst may enlarge, shrink, or remain unchanged.[64] It is important that a transient persistent abnormality seen after successful treatment not prompt reinstitution of therapy or further diagnostic testing.[136]

Aspiration of amebic abscesses is rarely indicated, as the diagnosis can be confirmed by hemagglutination titers and response to specific therapy. Percutaneous aspiration, however, is safe and may be considered when the diagnosis is uncertain, superimposed pyogenic infection is suspected, response to drug therapy is inadequate, or impending rupture is considered likely.[133] Untreated, the mortality of amebic abscess is almost 100 percent; even treated, the mortality is 10 percent. Early and accurate diagnosis followed by adequate therapy is essential.[64]

Candidiasis

Noncutaneous candidiasis is uncommon and occurs almost invariably in immunologically compromised hosts. The disease should therefore be considered in patients undergoing chemotherapy or organ transplantation or in those with chronic granulomatous disease or human immunodeficiency virus (HIV) infection. Once in the bloodstream, the *Candida* infection may occur in

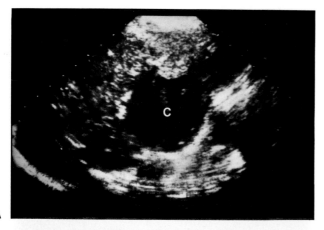

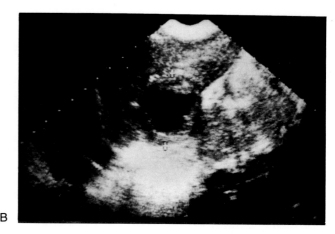

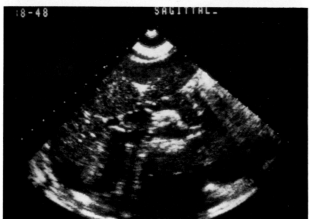

Fig. 5-68. Amebic abscess. **(A)** Large, multiseptate fluid collection *(C)* is demonstrated on the inferior edge of the left lobe of the liver. An amebic abscess was suspected clinically, and the patient was treated medically. **(B)** Follow-up scan after 2 weeks demonstrating a decrease in the size of the lesion and development of a thick wall. **(C)** A scan at 3 months was normal. (Case contributed by Inez Boechat, M.D., UCLA Medical Center.)

any organ, with the kidneys, heart, and brain the most commonly affected.[138] The presenting symptoms are nonspecific, with fever and pain referable to the area of involvement.[139] On ultrasound, a hypoechoic area with a central focus of increased echogenicity (bull's-eye or target) has been described as characteristic[138,140] (Fig. 5-69). Such target lesions are not entirely specific, however, and may also appear with lymphoma and several other opportunistic infections. Pastakia et al[141] have described four patterns in hepatic candidiasis including "wheel within wheel," bull's-eye, and two different hypoechoic patterns. A diagnosis of candidiasis is quickly made by percutaneous fine-needle aspiration although the small size of the lesions may render the procedure rather difficult.

Chronic Granulomatous Disease

Chronic granulomatous disease is an X-linked recessive trait related to a congenital defect in the leukocyte, which renders it unable to inactivate catalase-positive, previously phagocytized bacteria.[142] Clinically, when a child presents with recurrent infection of the lungs,

paranasal sinuses, bone, lymph nodes, or liver, the diagnosis should be suggested. The catalase-positive bacterium involved is usually *Staphylococcus aureus* or *Escherichia coli,* but may also be *Serratia marcescens;* the fungus *Aspergillus* is another possible cause. On ultrasound, hypoechoic, poorly marginated areas are seen with posterior enhancement[142] (Fig. 5-70). These lesions may be single or multiple. They are usually less well defined than true abscesses. Early recognition of the disease is important, because antibiotics are especially effective at this stage. An aspiration biopsy may be needed for a definitive diagnosis. Ultrasound may be used to monitor lesions after treatment.

Miscellaneous Infectious Processes

The ultrasound features of several other infectious processes affecting the liver have been described. In patients with acquired immunodeficiency syndrome (AIDS), numerous liver abnormalities may be found. Many such patients will present with generalized increased echogenicity (presumed fatty metamorphosis)

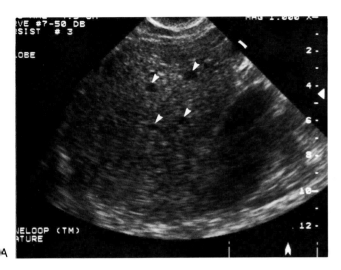

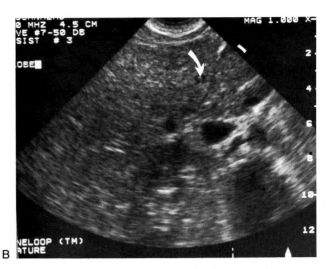

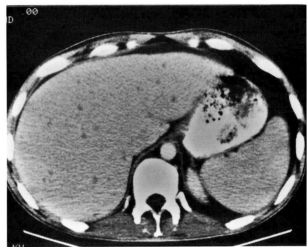

Fig. 5-69. Candidiasis. This patient was immunosuppressed from chemotherapy for chronic myelogenous leukemia. **(A)** Multiple small hypoechoic lesions were found in the liver (arrowheads). **(B)** Several lesions contained an umbilicated hyperechoic central focus (curved arrow). **(C)** CT scan confirming multiple small low-density lesions. A biopsy specimen yielded *Candida*.

and hepatomegaly. However, *Pneumocystis carinii* has recently been described as producing numerous small, hyperechoic foci in the liver that are thought to be secondary to an inflammatory reaction surrounding the organism (see Fig. 16-27). These lesions may become more prevalent with increasing use of aerosol pentamidine as a prophylactic treatment for pulmonary disease; the systemic infection may remain untreated.[143] Cytomegalovirus has also been implicated as a cause of focal echogenic lesions in this population,[144] but is considerably less common than biliary tract involvement.[145] Among granulomatous diseases, leprosy can produce poorly defined echogenic foci in the liver[146] and tuberculosis may cause hypoechoic masses with or without calcifications.[147] *Actinomyces,* a gram-positive bacterium may also affect the liver and cause abscess formation. A unique feature, similar to what is found in thoracic involvement, is extension to the abdominal wall.[148]

Neoplasms of Infancy and Childhood

Hepatoblastoma

Hepatoblastoma is a rare malignant tumor that is seen in infancy and childhood. The patient presents with abdominal enlargement with hepatomegaly. Coarse calcifications may be seen on radiographs,[149] and the α-fetoprotein (AFP) level is increased. There are two types of hepatoblastoma: (1) epithelial sheets of cells resembling fetal liver cells or undifferentiated "embryonal" cells and (2) mixed epithelial, mesenchymal connective tissue and other elements, particularly osteoid tissue. On ultrasound, these lesions are echogenic with hypoechoic or anechoic areas of necrosis or hemorrhage. By imaging alone, however, the lesion cannot be definitively differentiated from other infantile liver tumors[149] (Fig. 5-71). Bates et al[150] have recently described specific spectral

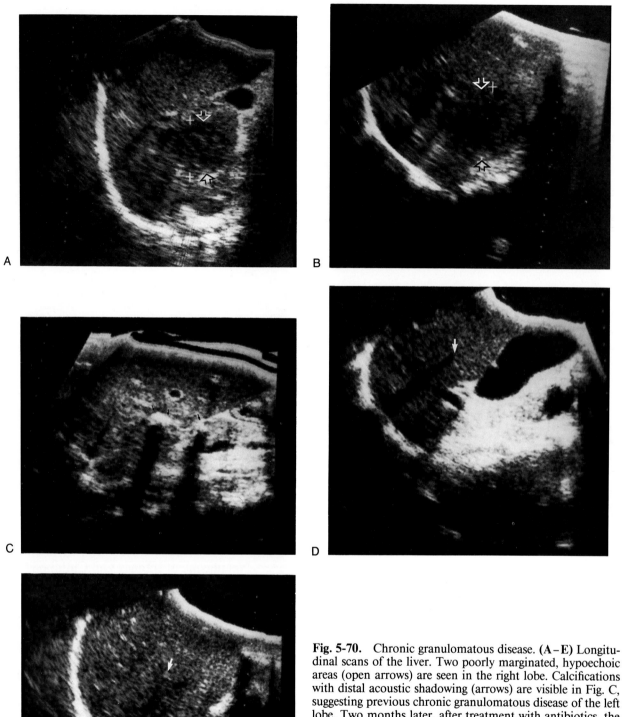

Fig. 5-70. Chronic granulomatous disease. (A–E) Longitudinal scans of the liver. Two poorly marginated, hypoechoic areas (open arrows) are seen in the right lobe. Calcifications with distal acoustic shadowing (arrows) are visible in Fig. C, suggesting previous chronic granulomatous disease of the left lobe. Two months later, after treatment with antibiotics, the hypoechoic areas have subsided (Figs. D & E). Scars are still visible (arrows) with a single calcification, which remained unchanged 2 years later. (From Garel et al,[142] with permission.)

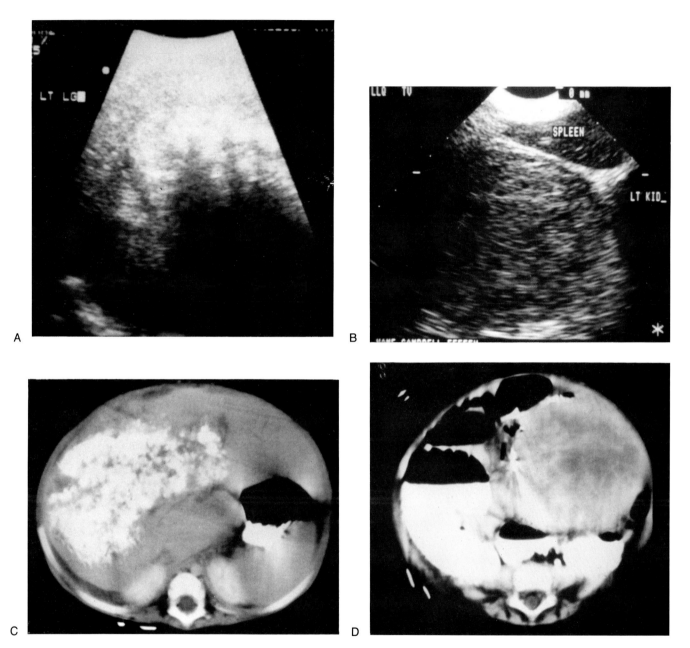

Fig. 5-71. Hepatoblastoma. Child with a large abdominal mass. (**A**) Longitudinal section through the left lobe of the liver showing numerous calcific foci. (**B**) Section through the left midabdomen demonstrating a homogeneously echogenic mass. (**C**) CT scan confirming extensive calcifications in the upper portion of the mass. (**D**) CT section through the midabdomen showing a large, round mass on the left. Hepatoblastoma was found at surgery. (Case contributed by Theodore Hall, M.D., UCLA Medical Center.)

Doppler signals (> 4 kHz) in this lesion, but this finding must be corroborated by other groups before dispensing with biopsy.

Mesenchymal Hamartoma

Mesenchymal hamartomas are rare, occur in children less than 2 years of age, and may enlarge to produce an abdominal mass. These unusual lesions are composed of well-differentiated ductal structures surrounded by loose mesenchymal connective tissue and are thought to be developmental rather than neoplastic.[151,152] On ultrasound, a mass that is either well-defined and predominantly anechoic with peripheral trabeculation, or reticular and lacelike throughout is seen[151-153] (Fig. 5-72).

Infantile Hemangioendothelioma

Infantile hemangioendothelioma is the most common symptomatic vascular liver tumor of infancy.[154] Eighty-five percent occur before 6 months of age, with a female preponderance of 2:1.[154,155] A normal AFP level effectively excludes hepatoblastoma from the differential diagnosis. Hemangioendothelioma usually grows rapidly after presentation and then gradually regresses.[155] Spontaneous regression of infantile hemangioendotheliomatosis of the liver has been reported as well.[156] The child typically presents with an abdominal mass and high cardiac output failure secondary to arteriovenous shunting throughout the tumor.[150,157] Congestive heart failure associated with this mass is not as common as once thought.[155] Complications of this lesion include thrombocytopenia, angiopathic anemia, gastrointesti-

nal bleeding, and intra-abdominal rupture with hemorrhage.[150,156]

Pathologically, the mass is round and tends to be well demarcated. In large lesions central areas of infarction, hemorrhage, fibrosis, and foci of dysmorphic calcification may be seen.[155] Two types have been described. The first contains variable-sized vascular spaces lined with relatively immature, plump endothelial cells with supporting fibrous stroma and some foci of less well-differentiated myxomatous tissue. Between the vascular spaces are scattered bile ducts, which may contain hematopoietic cells. The second type consists of more immature, bigger pleomorphic cells that reflect the more aggressive end of the spectrum and may mimic hemangioendothelial sarcoma (generally seen in older adults) with poorly formed vascular spaces and branching structures.[155,156]

Plain film shows hepatomegaly and, rarely, calcifications, which may be numerous and spongelike or in the form of spicules radiating from a central core.[156] On ultrasound, the lesion has been described as hyperechoic, hypoechoic, and diffuse[155,157] (Fig. 5-73 and Plate 5-27). Multiple lucent lesions varying from 1 to 3 cm with scattered low-level echoes and hyperechoic margins may also be seen. Large draining veins and a dilated proximal abdominal aorta may be seen secondary to arteriovenous shunting.[153]

Metastatic Disease

In children, the most common neoplasms to metastasize to the liver include neuroblastoma, Wilms' tumor, and leukemia.[157,158] Neuroblastoma, which is a malig-

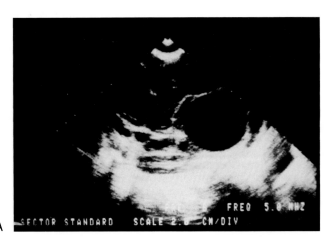
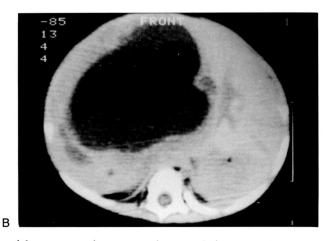

Fig. 5-72. Mesenchymal hamartoma. Child with a large right upper quadrant mass who was relatively asymptomatic. **(A)** Longitudinal section through the right upper quadrant showing a multiseptate, cystic mass replacing almost all the right lobe of the liver. **(B)** CT scan confirming the presence of a large cystic mass. Septa are seen to better advantage on ultrasound. (Case contributed by Theodore Hall, M.D., UCLA Medical Center.)

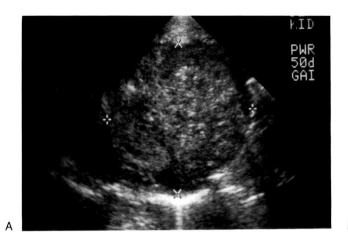

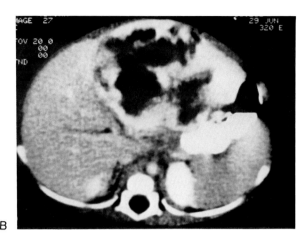

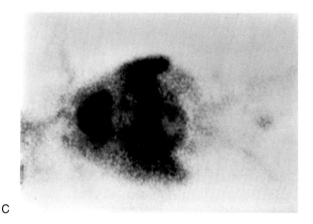

Fig. 5-73. Infantile hemangioendothelioma. (A) Ultrasound through the left lobe of the liver in a 7-week-old infant with a clinical impression of hepatomegaly, showing a well-defined, large, solid mass. The internal echopattern was relatively inhomogeneous. (B) Contrast-enhanced CT scan showing peripheral enhancement but no other specific features. (C) Nuclear medicine scan showing patchy uptake of tracer. (See also Plate 5-27).

nant neoplasm of sympathetic nerve cell origin, produces a densely reflective pattern of liver involvement that may be indistinguishable from hepatoma, hepatoblastoma, and Wilms' tumor (Fig. 5-74). With neuroblastoma the liver is commonly involved, by contrast to Wilms' tumor, in which the lungs are the most frequent site of involvement. Metastatic Wilms' tumor produces a densely reflective pattern with hypoechoic areas resulting from necrosis.[151,158] Metastatic adenocarcinoma is unusual in a child.

Benign Neoplasms of Adulthood

Cavernous Hemangioma

Cavernous hemangioma is the most common benign tumor of the liver; the incidence is as high as 7.3 percent in one autopsy series.[159] Hemangiomas are composed of a large network of vascular endothelium-lined spaces filled with blood. They are more frequent in women and increase with age. Hemangiomas may enlarge slowly and undergo degeneration, fibrosis, and calcification,[160,161]

although the study of Gibney et al[162] demonstrated that only 18 percent showed significant change in sonographic appearance when monitored over time. When they are larger than 4 cm they are classified as giant hemangiomas.[163]

Most hemangiomas are in the posterior right lobe of the liver[164,165]; 73 percent are in the right lobe, with 27 percent in the left lobe.[166] These lesions tend to be subcapsular (70 percent), 32 percent are smaller than 2 cm, and 35 percent are multiple.[167] Hemangiomas have been described as round (75.5 percent), oval (13.5 percent), or lobulated (11 percent). The contours were well defined in 92 percent.[166] Most authors describe a homogeneous echodense (70 to 94 percent) pattern that is sharply marginated.[154,159,163,165] The high level of echogenicity in hemangiomas is postulated to be due to the multiple interfaces between the walls of the cavernous sinuses and blood within them.[164] One series described a 76.5 percent incidence of posterior acoustic enhancement in hemangiomas, with all lesions greater than 25 mm in diameter demonstrating increased through transmission[166] (Fig. 5-75). The zone of distal enhancement results from less attenuation of sound in a largely fluid-

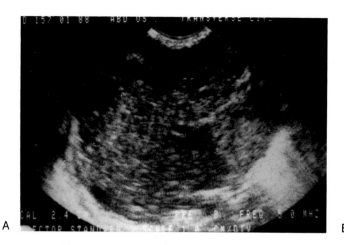

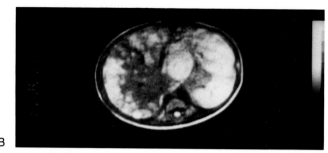

Fig. 5-74. Metastatic disease. **(A)** The liver of this child with hepatomegaly had a coarsened echopattern on ultrasound examination. Biopsy showed diffusely infiltrating metastatic neuroblastoma. **(B)** MR scan taken several months later showing numerous small metastatic foci throughout the liver.

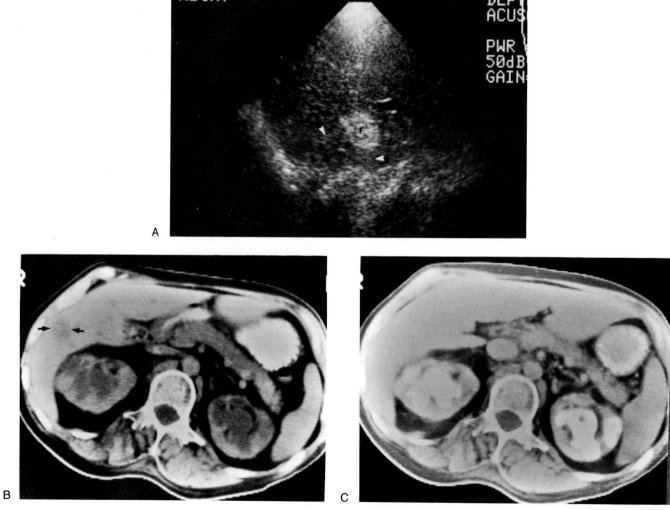

Fig. 5-75. Hemangioma. **(A)** Sonogram performed to evaluate the gallbladder showing a small, brightly echogenic focus in the periphery of the right lobe of the liver (*F*). Note the posterior acoustic enhancement (arrowheads). CT with and without contrast confirmed lesion as hemangioma. **(B)** Note the relatively low density of the lesion on a precontrast scan (arrows) and **(C)** "filling in" on a postcontrast study.

filled mass than in the liver. As the hemangioma undergoes degeneration and fibrous replacement, the echopattern may become more heterogeneous.[164] Some lesions may be calcified, complex, or anechoic.[161,168] Spectral Doppler has also been investigated as a potential method of diagnosing hemangiomas and differentiating them from neoplastic lesions.[169] Unfortunately, both hemangiomas (flow too slow to produce Doppler signals) and metastasis may be "avascular" to the Doppler examination, rendering it of little value in narrowing the differential diagnosis in suspected hepatic hemangiomas.

The sonographic features of hemangiomas are not specific (Figs. 5-76 and 5-77). A solitary echogenic mass in the liver has a differential diagnosis including not only hemangioma but also hepatocellular carcinoma, solitary metastasis, and liver cell adenoma. Therefore, a definitive diagnosis cannot be made with ultrasound alone, and a correlative imaging modality should be considered. Currently a scintigraphic evaluation involving tagged red blood cells is recommended for evaluating lesions greater than 2.5 cm while MRI can be considered for smaller masses. According to Nelson et al,[163] a classic or near-classic appearance on any two imaging modali-

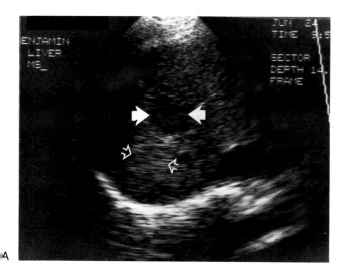

A

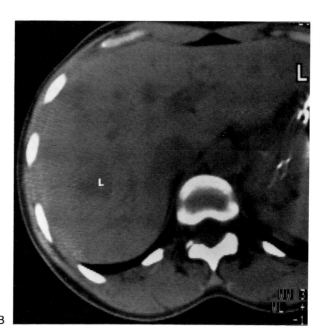

B

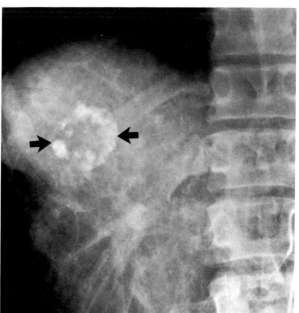

C

Fig. 5-76. Hemangioma. **(A)** Patient undergoing obstetric sonogram in whom the obstetrician noted hypoechoic mass (arrows) in the right lobe of the liver. Note the posterior acoustic enhancement (open arrows). **(B)** CT scan demonstrating a low-density lesion *(L),* but a bolus injection failed to confirm hemangioma. **(C)** Late phase of a hepatic arteriogram showing pooling of contrast (arrows) in a pattern diagnostic of hemangioma.

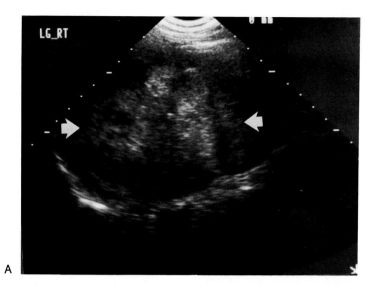

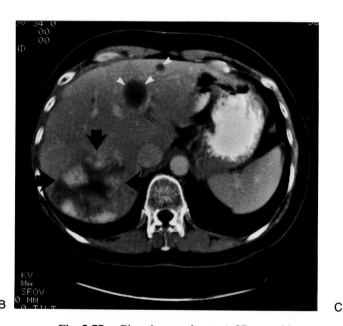

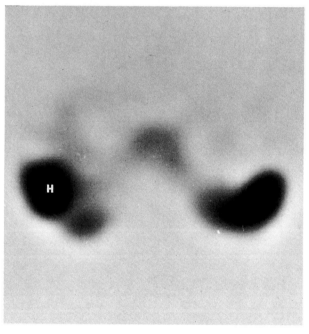

Fig. 5-77. Giant hemangioma. A 37-year-old woman with vague right upper quadrant pain. **(A)** Ultrasound demonstrating a large, lobulated, relatively echogenic mass in the posterior right lobe of the liver (arrows). **(B)** CT scan with contrast confirmed the lesion (arrows), but findings were not specific for hemangioma. Note the presence of two other lesions (arrowheads), confirmed as cysts on ultrasound. **(C)** Nuclear medicine tagged red blood cell scan using SPECT imaging diagnosed hemangioma *(H)*.

ties (ultrasound, CT, MRI, or single photon emission CT [SPECT] scan) should be considered diagnostic and the work-up ended. However, for patients with small lesions who have no history of cancer, hepatic dysfunction, or predisposing factors with a classic appearance for hepatocellular carcinoma, an argument can be made for just monitoring the lesion by ultrasound alone to ensure sta-

bility.[170] In cases in which imaging findings are inconclusive (MRI findings in hemangiomas are not entirely specific and lesions less than 2.5 cm may not be seen on the scintigram), biopsy might also be considered in patients with a history of cancer. Although a definitive diagnosis of hemangioma may be difficult to obtain with biopsy, neoplastic lesions should be identified with an acceptable degree of accuracy. Fine-needle biopsy is safe in evaluating hemangiomas, and the vascular nature of these lesions should not discourage the procedure if it may be of clinical value.[170]

Focal Nodular Hyperplasia

Focal nodular hyperplasia (FNH) is an unusual benign tumor that is often discovered serendipitously by imaging procedures. This lesion is most common in women younger than 40 years of age and has an increased incidence with the use of oral contraceptives. FNH is usually asymptomatic and is most frequently located near the free edge of the liver in a subcapsular location. Typically, the mass is located in the right lobe or in the lateral segment of the left lobe; 13 percent are multiple. FNHs are usually solitary, well-circumscribed, nonencapsulated tumors. The tumor itself is composed of normal hepatocytes, Kupffer cells, bile duct elements, and fibrous connective tissue.[171,172] Pathologically, multiple nodules are separated by bands of fibrous tissue often radiating from a large central scar. Others describe a well-circumscribed nodular, almost cirrhotic mass. The characteristic depressed central or eccentric stellate scar is composed of dense fibrous connective tissue, proliferating bile ducts, and thin-walled blood vessels.[172,173] Malignant transformation is not reported, and intraperitoneal bleeding is rare.[171,172] The rarity of complications has led to conservative management. Biopsy or nuclear medicine scan should be diagnostic and may be the only procedure required.[174]

On ultrasound, FNH is most often homogeneous and slightly less echogenic than the rest of the liver[171] (Fig. 5-78). These masses are very similar to the normal liver pathologically, and therefore many are almost isoechoic to it and are evidenced only by mass effect on the surrounding parenchyma or vessels.[172-175] A dense nonshadowing linear or stellate group of echoes in a solitary hepatic mass has been described as diagnostic but is quite unusual. A 100 percent sensitivity for ultrasound in detecting FNH has been reported, whereas CT has a 78 percent sensitivity, angiography an 82 percent sensitivity, and nuclear medicine a 55 to 70 percent sensitivity. Normal colloid uptake by a focal hepatic mass is virtually diagnostic of this entity.[172-174]

A separate entity, nodular regenerative hyperplasia, should not be confused with FNH. Unlike FNH, nodular regenerative hyperplasia is composed of normal hepatocytes forming hyperplastic nodules. This lesion is said to be present in as many as 0.6 percent of autopsy specimens and is probably underdiagnosed because it is not well known and biopsy results can easily be misinterpreted. Nodular regenerative hyperplasia may bleed and is often associated with portal hypertension; underlying conditions include myelo/lymphoproliferative disease and various immune diseases. Imaging findings are not specific; ultrasound most often reveals a hypo- or isoechoic nodule with an anechoic center.[176]

Liver Cell Adenoma

Liver cell adenoma is composed of normal or slightly atypical hepatocytes frequently containing areas of bile stasis and focal hemorrhage or necrosis, but not contain-

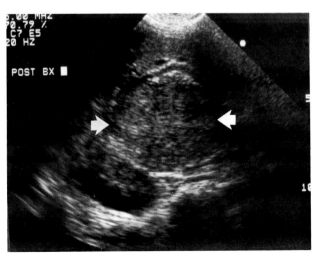
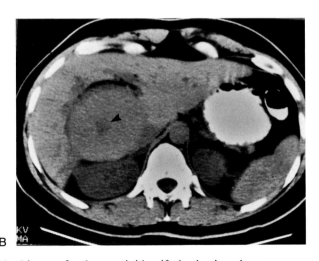

Fig. 5-78.   Focal nodular hyperplasia. **(A)** This patient with a history of melanoma is identified as having a large hypoechoic mass in the right lobe of the liver (arrows). **(B)** CT scan confirming the presence of a solitary lesion; note the central stellate area (arrowhead) of low density typical of focal nodular hyperplasia. The scintigram was not specific; ultrasound-guided biopsy revealed focal nodular hyperplasia.

ing bile ducts or Kupffer cells.[177] These lesions usually present as a solitary, marginated, encapsulated mass; are more common in women; and have been linked to oral contraceptives. They are not usually symptomatic but may present with a palpable mass or severe right upper quadrant pain as a result of rupture with hemoperitoneum or bleeding into the tumor.[102] The ultrasound pattern is variable; if bleeding has occurred, the mass may be hypoechoic (if old) or echogenic[102,137,150,165,166,174-177] (Fig. 5-79). Adenomas and FNH may appear similar on ultrasound.[177] In glycogen storage disease, there is an 8 percent incidence of adenomas (Fig. 5-29), with a frequency of 40 percent in type I disease.[62]

Lipomas/Fatty Tumors of the Liver

Lipomas are rare, benign primary tumors of the liver that are derived from mesenchymal elements. They are nonencapsulated and are in continuity with the normal liver parenchyma. They are invariably hyperechoic[178]

(Fig. 5-80), and a "shadow conus" is seen as a result of the diminished penetration of the sound beam to the posterior liver. Because sound travels through fat at a different speed from that through the normal liver parenchyma, the diaphragm may appear artifactually misplaced behind the tumor as well.[179] All fatty hepatic masses, however, are not lipomas. Angiomyolipomas (Fig. 5-81) typically have fatty elements and have been reported to occur in the liver, but almost invariably as part of tuberous sclerosis.[180] Hepatoma, like normal liver, may also undergo fatty degeneration[181] and should be considered in patients having a fatty hepatic tumor but no history of tuberous sclerosis (Fig. 5-82).

Malignant Tumors of Adulthood

Hepatocellular Carcinoma

Hepatocellular carcinoma (HCC) appears to be related to cirrhosis, chronic hepatitis B virus infection, and

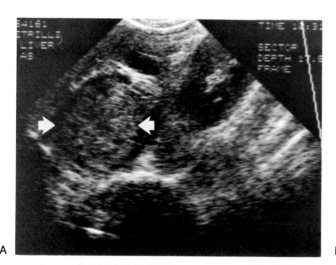

A

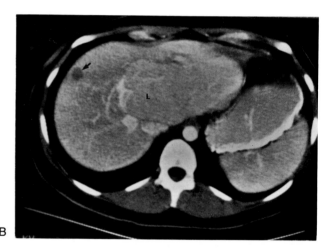

B

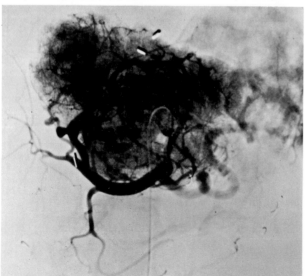

C

Fig. 5-79. Hepatic adenoma. This 27-year-old woman with a history of ovarian carcinoma was found to have multiple liver masses. **(A)** Oblique, longitudinal section through the left lobe of the liver showing a poorly defined, relatively hyperechoic mass posteriorly (arrows). **(B)** CT scan with contrast confirming a large enhancing lesion in the left lobe of the liver *(L)*. Note the smaller hypodense mass (arrow) in the anterior right lobe. **(C)** Selective hepatic arteriogram confirming the hypervascular nature of the mass. At laparotomy, the larger left lobe mass proved to represent hepatic adenoma. The small right lobe lesion was hemangioma.

hepatocarcinogens in food. Eighty percent of HCCs occur in livers with preexisting cirrhosis, most frequently in those with postnecrotic or macronodular cirrhosis (13 to 24 percent) and less commonly in those with alcoholic cirrhosis (3.2 percent). The overall incidence of HCC with cirrhosis in the United States is 5 percent, although the tumor is far more common in Asia. Morphologically, there are three patterns of HCC: a solitary tumor, multiple nodules throughout the liver, and diffuse infiltration. All of these may cause hepatic enlargement, and in several series, 90 percent of patients with HCC had clinical hepatomegaly.[182] HCC tends to invade the hepatic veins (13 percent of cases), the biliary tree, and the portal veins. Thrombosis or tumor invasion of the portal system is seen in 30 to 68 percent of HCCs and is so characteristic that a presumptive diagnosis of HCC can be considered in any patient with a solitary hepatic mass causing portal vein invasion. HCC has a distinct tend-

ency to destroy the portal venous radicle walls and invade the vessel lumen. The tumor then grows within the vessel, deriving its blood supply from the capillary bed, surrounding vein, and/or adjacent bile duct. Vascular invasion can be an early event and does not indicate inoperability.[183]

Clinically, patients present with a palpable mass in the liver, rapid liver enlargement, or an unexplained mild fever. One should suspect HCC when the condition of a patient with cirrhosis suddenly worsens or there is a progressive enlargement of the liver with bloody ascites. Liver function tests often disclose surprisingly little abnormality; the underlying cirrhosis itself usually explains any abnormality found. Measurement of the AFP level may be helpful in determining the diagnosis; 70 percent of patients with HCC have elevated levels. AFP is synthesized by HCC, but elevation of the AFP level can be seen in severe liver necrosis as well. Most investi-

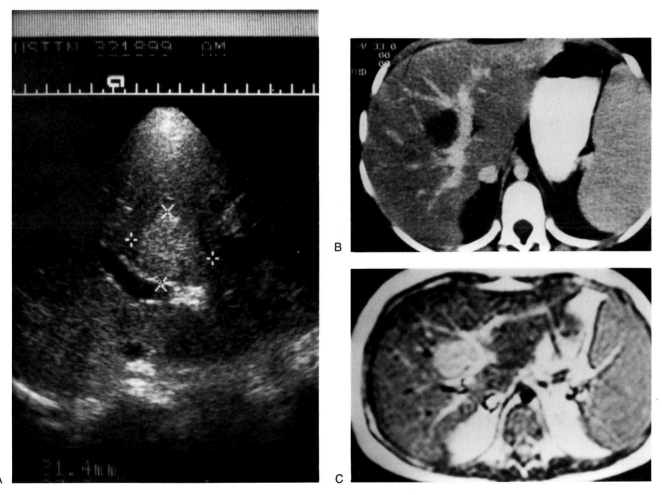

Fig. 5-80. Hepatic lipoma. **(A)** Oblique section through the right lobe of the liver in a child being evaluated for renal reflux showing a brightly echogenic mass (calipers) anterior to the portal vein. **(B)** CT scan showing fat density lesion. **(C)** MR scan is also consistent with lipoma. (Case contributed by Inez Boechat, M.D., UCLA Medical Center.)

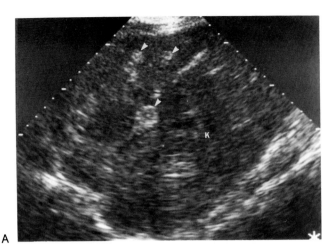
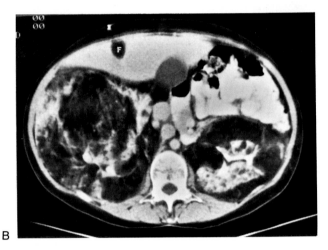

Fig. 5-81. Hepatic angiomyolipoma. **(A)** Patient with tuberous sclerosis and multiple echogenic lesions (arrowheads) in the liver. Note the massive enlargement of the right kidney *(K)*. **(B)** CT scan confirming several fatty lesions *(F)* in the liver. The renal architecture is markedly distorted by angiomyolipomas bilaterally.

gators currently recommend screening patients with chronic active hepatitis for HCC by yearly AFP measurement and ultrasound examination.[184,185]

Numerous ultrasound patterns have been found in patients with HCC: discrete hypoechoic, discrete echogenic, mixed, isoechoic, and diffusely infiltrative (Figs. 5-83 and 5-84). Several studies suggest a close relationship between the echopattern, size, and histologic findings.[186-188] The hypoechoic tumors were without necrosis and were hypoechoic presumably because of a lack of any structure within the tumor to serve as a reflective source. The hyperechoic lesion was the site of nonliquefactive necrosis. The anechoic lesion was the

site of extensive liquefactive necrosis. Fatty metamorphosis, as well as severe sinusoidal dilatation, was visualized as hyperechoic.[181,188] The ultrasound appearance also may be associated with the age of the tumor. The study of Sheu et al[188] demonstrated that HCCs tend to evolve from small hypo- or isoechoic masses to large hyperechoic, inhomogeneous lesions with time.

A 90 percent sensitivity for ultrasound in detecting HCC, with a specificity of 93 percent, has been reported.[189] Ultrasound was found to be the most sensitive method for the detection of small tumors and is currently the most commonly used screening technique. In one series of 36 tumors smaller than 3 cm, real-time

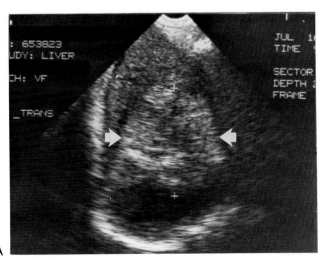
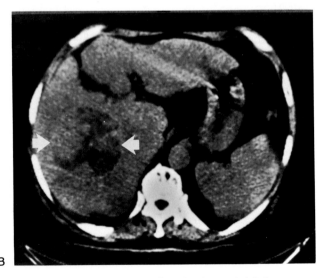

Fig. 5-82. Hepatocellular carcinoma. **(A)** This 67-year-old man with hepatomegaly was found to have a brightly echogenic mass in the right lobe of the liver (arrows). **(B)** CT scan confirming fatty elements (arrows). Biopsy revealed hepatocellular carcinoma.

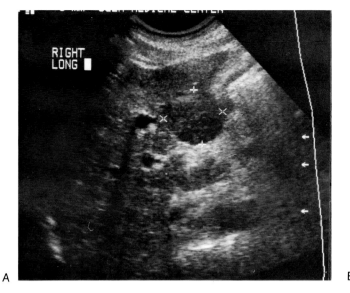

A

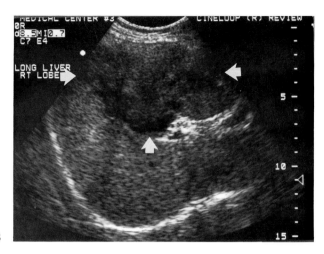

B

Fig. 5-83. Hepatocellular carcinoma. **(A)** Yearly screening ultrasound in this patient with a history of hepatitis B and cirrhosis revealed a well-defined isoechoic mass (calipers) in the periphery of the liver. **(B)** Longitudinal section in a different patient showing a large bilobed mass (arrows) with considerable internal inhomogeneity. Both were cases of hepatocellular carcinoma.

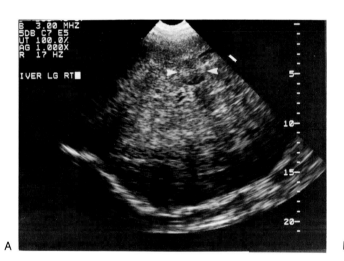

A

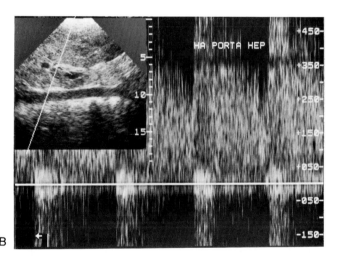

B

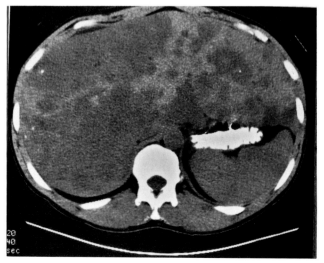

C

Fig. 5-84. Hepatocellular carcinoma. **(A)** Ultrasound in a patient with hepatomegaly confirming that the liver was markedly enlarged. Several small discrete masses were present (arrowheads); the overall echogenicity was quite coarsened. **(B)** Spectral tracing from the main hepatic artery was remarkable for high-velocity, turbulent flow. **(C)** CT scan showing innumerable low-density lesions throughout both lobes of the liver. Biopsy demonstrated hepatocellular carcinoma. Spectral tracings were postulated to be secondary to either arterial compression from tumor or the hypervascular nature of hepatocellular carcinoma.

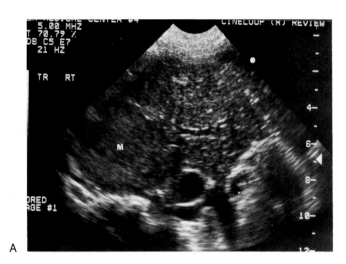
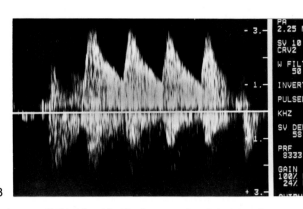

Fig. 5-85. Hepatocellular carcinoma. **(A)** A large hypoechoic mass *(M)* is identified in the posterior right lobe of liver (see Fig. 5-82B for the CT scan of this lesion) in a patient with long-standing, severe cirrhosis. **(B)** Color and spectral analysis showing hypervascular tumor. Maximum Doppler shifts, however, did not exceed 3 kHz.

scans revealed 93.9 percent of the small tumors, CT revealed 84.3 percent (those missed were 2 cm or less), angiography revealed 75.7 percent, and nuclear medicine revealed 12.1 percent.[190] According to Gandolfi et al,[191] ultrasound is also superior to laparoscopy. Although several studies advocate using two imaging modalities (ultrasound and CT or ultrasound and nuclear medicine SPECT scan),[192] the minimal increase in sensi-

tivity is probably not cost-effective, and most investigators would recommend the use of ultrasound and AFP levels.

Color and spectral Doppler have also been used in the evaluation of HCC. Taylor et al[169] found that Doppler shifts of greater than 5 MHz were specific for this lesion, and Tanaka et al[193] used color and described a "basket" pattern in 75 percent and internal vascularity in 65 per-

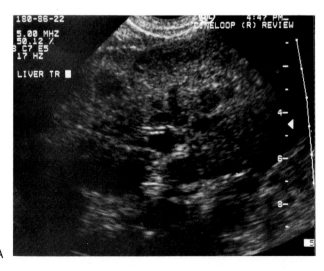
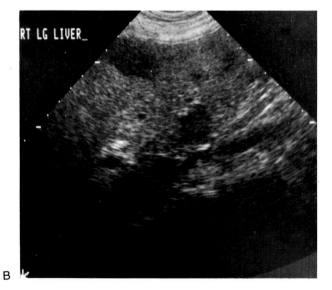

Fig. 5-86. Hypoechoic metastases. **(A)** This 54-year-old man with primary lung carcinoma is noted to have numerous small hypoechoic masses throughout the liver. **(B)** This 69-year-old woman with a history of colon carcinoma is found to have several discrete hypoechoic masses in the liver. Ultrasonically guided biopsy confirmed metastatic disease in both cases.

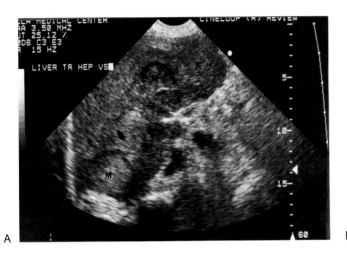
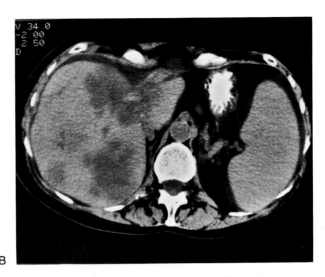

Fig. 5-87. Echogenic metastases. **(A)** Transverse section through the right lobe of the liver in a patient with metastatic carcinoid. Multiple hyperechoic masses *(M)* were identified in both lobes of the liver. **(B)** CT scan confirming multiple low-density lesions.

cent. The combination of the two was considered specific for HCC. Unfortunately, neither of these techniques has gained widespread acceptance. In our experience, the finding of Doppler shifts greater than 5 kHz is extremely unusual (Fig. 5-85), and the study of Ralls[194] found that the color Doppler patterns described by Tanaka et al[193] were not sufficiently specific to be of value. One specific type of HCC, fibrolamellar HCC, deserves mention because it is pathologically and prognostically distinct, having a better prognosis than other

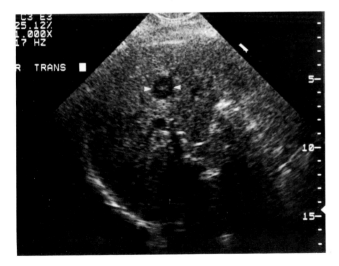

Fig. 5-88. Target pattern. Patient with metastatic melanoma and multiple masses in the liver. Note the target lesion with a relatively hypoechoic periphery and an echogenic focus centrally (arrowheads).

varieties. These lesions tend to have a central scar (80 percent) and calcification.[195]

Metastases

Metastases are the most common neoplasm to involve the liver. The usual primary sites are the gastrointestinal tract (particularly colon), breast, and lung. The tumor is disseminated to the liver via the portal vein, lymphatics, and hepatic artery and, less frequently, by direct extension (e.g., from the gallbladder or stomach). Widespread metastatic disease usually causes liver enlargement. Multiple nodules throughout both lobes are typical, but solitary lesions may occur as well.

Four major ultrasound patterns have been described with metastasis: (1) discrete hypoechoic (Fig. 5-86), (2) discrete echogenic (Fig. 5-87), (3) target (Fig. 5-88), and (4) diffusely inhomogeneous (Fig. 5-89).[179-181] The ultrasound appearance is not specific in defining the organ of origin.[196-198] Besides identifying the lesions, ultrasound can be used to monitor the lesions when assessing chemotherapeutic response. A change in echopattern does not seem to be clinically significant; assessment is based on change in the number or size of lesions.[199] Metastases are also occasionally cystic or calcified. When they are cystic, the primary cancer itself is usually cystic, such as ovarian carcinoma, or the tumor has undergone extensive necrosis or hemorrhage (Fig. 5-90). With calcified metastases, the primary may vary and often has more to do with tumor degeneration than cell type. Calcification of metastases is always associated

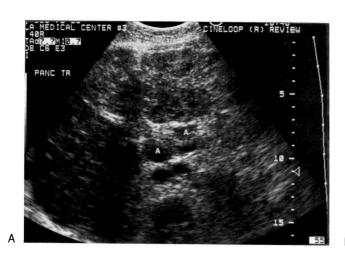

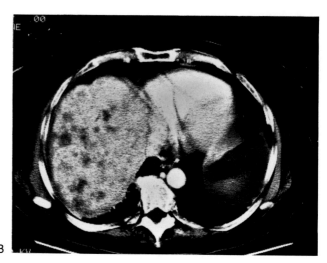

Fig. 5-89. Diffuse metastatic disease. This patient with a history of cirrhosis and shrunken liver presented with new onset of right upper quadrant pain and hepatomegaly. **(A)** Sonogram showing diffuse alteration of hepatic echogenicity. The presence of several hypoechoic regions suggested discrete masses. The possibility of metastatic disease was further suggested by identification of adenopathy *(A)*. **(B)** CT scan confirming the presence of multiple hypoechoic masses. Biopsy revealed diffuse adenocarcinoma of unknown primary.

with a polymetastatic hepatic condition but does not affect the prognosis. One ultrasound series revealed 13 cases of calcified metastases; the calcification had been identified on radiographs in only 9 cases.[200] As expected, metastatic calcifications appear as brightly echogenic foci with acoustic shadowing (Fig. 5-91). Cancer of the colon is the cell type most frequently associated with calcification. Less frequently associated are endocrine

tumors of the pancreas, leiomyosarcoma, malignant melanoma, cystadenocarcinoma of the ovary, adenocarcinoma of the stomach, lymphoma, osteosarcoma, pleural mesothelioma, neuroblastoma, and breast cancer.[200-202]

Although CT or MRI is preferred over ultrasound as the primary screening procedure in patients with possible metastatic disease, interest in intraoperative ultra-

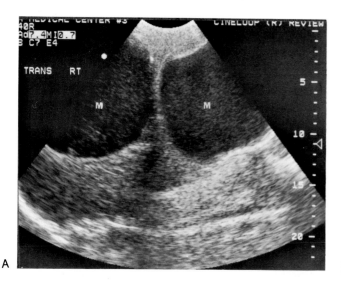

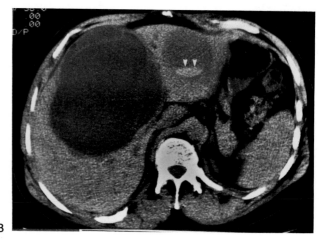

Fig. 5-90. Cystic metastasis. This patient with mixed teratocarcinoma and embryonal carcinoma of testes presented with massive hepatomegaly. **(A)** Sonogram showing several large cystic masses in the liver *(M)*. Moving low-level hypoechoic material internally suggested blood. **(B)** CT scan confirming the presence of masses. Note the posterior layering of high-density hemoglobin (arrowheads).

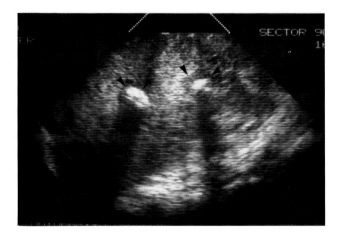

Fig. 5-91. Calcified metastases. Patient with history of breast carcinoma and stable hepatic metastatic disease who is receiving chemotherapy. Note the internal calcifications. Solid tissue can still be identified about the periphery of the masses (arrowheads).

sound has increased in recent years. Some surgeons now consider patients with primary HCC or three or fewer metastatic lesions from selected primaries (usually colon cancer) candidates for resection, and precise characterization of the number, size, and location of these lesions is essential.[203,204] Intraoperative ultrasound has shown considerable promise in this area and should probably be used routinely in patients undergoing hepatic resection. According to the study of Seltzer and Holman,[204] intraoperative ultrasound identified 25 percent more lesions than did any other technique. This impression now seems well established and has been corroborated by several other groups.[205,206]

The ultrasound patterns in hepatic lymphoma have also been studied; almost all these lesions are hypoechoic (Fig. 5-92). Hypoechoic and diffuse patterns have been found in both Hodgkin's and non-Hodgkin's lymphoma, whereas target and echogenic patterns have been found only in non-Hodgkin's lymphoma.[207,208] Intrahe-

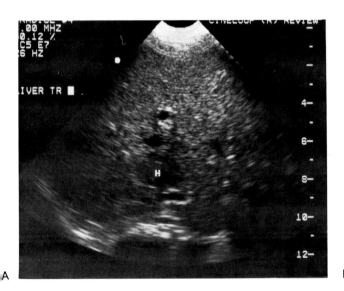

A

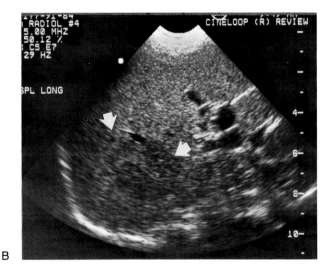

B

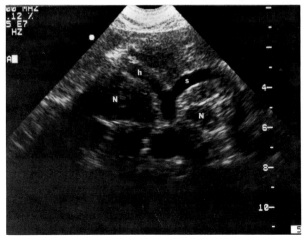

C

Fig. 5-92. Lymphoma. Patient with advanced Hodgkin's lymphoma and hepatosplenomegaly. **(A)** Sonogram showing multiple hypoechoic masses in the liver *(H)*. **(B)** A large mass is also identified in the spleen (arrows), and **(C)** extensive adenopathy is identified in the region of the celiac axis. (*N*, lymph nodes; *h*, hepatic artery; *s*, splenic artery.)

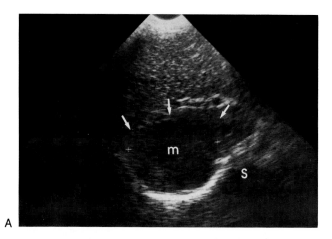
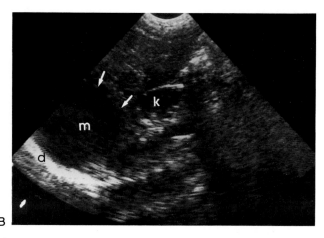

Fig. 5-93. Burkitt's lymphoma. Hypoechoic pattern. **(A)** Transverse and **(B)** longitudinal scans demonstrating a well-defined hypoechoic mass (*m*, arrows) in the posterior right lobe. (*S*, spine; *d*, diaphragm, *k*, right kidney.)

patic hypoechoic lesions have also been described with Burkitt's lymphoma[209] (Fig. 5-93). There is, however, no correlation between the type of lymphoma and the ultrasound appearance. In autopsy series, the liver is often found to be invaded by lymphoma. Sonographically, however, lymphomatous involvement of the liver is unusual and is identified in less than 5 percent of patients.[210]

In leukemia, multiple discrete hepatic masses known as chloromas are identified occasionally. These lesions have been described as hypoechoic with no acoustic enhancement[211] (Fig. 5-94). Many may exhibit a bull's-eye appearance with a dense center resulting from necrosis

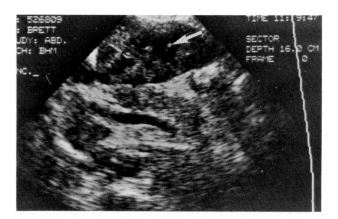

Fig. 5-94. Leukemic infiltration. Leukemic infiltration of the liver may be diffuse and result in simple hepatomegaly or form discrete masses known as chloromas. This patient with chronic lymphocytic leukemia presented with hepatomegaly. Numerous hypoechoic masses were found in the liver. Several were umbilicated (arrow), raising question of candidiasis. Biopsy revealed leukemic infiltration.

and, as such, may be indistinguishable from candidiasis. Gross liver involvement with leukemia is uncommon; microscopic infiltration is more common, and the only ultrasound abnormality may be hepatomegaly.[211]

Miscellaneous Masses

The sonographic features of several additional rare hepatic tumorous conditions have been reported and are worth including for the sake of completeness; some occur de novo and others are part of an overall systemic condition. Among the former, epithelioid hemangioendothelioma,[212] undifferentiated (embryonal) sarcoma[213] (Fig. 5-95), and bile duct hamartomas[214] (Fig. 5-96) have been described, but, again, radiographic features are not specific. Extramedullary hematopoiesis,[215,216] peliosis hepatis,[217] and focal masses secondary to erythromycin-induced hepatitis[218] have been reported. Extramedullary hematopoiesis should be considered in patients with a suggestive history (severe anemia, myelofibrosis, polycythemia vera, hepatosplenomegaly, etc) and single or multiple inhomogeneous liver masses (Fig. 5-97). Peliosis hepatitis is most often associated with wasting diseases such as tuberculosis or cancer and with androgenic steroid administration; it is characterized by blood-filled cystic spaces within the liver ranging from 1 to 5 mm in diameter. Hepatomegaly is often present. The ultrasound pattern is not specific, but has been described as patchy with echopoor and echogenic areas (Fig. 5-98).[217] Erythromycin-induced hepatitis, on the other hand, may produce multiple, poorly demarcated hyperechoic lesions that are indistinguishable from other truly neoplastic processes. Although this condition is unusual (incidence, 1 in 1,000 to 1 in 150,000), it should be consid-

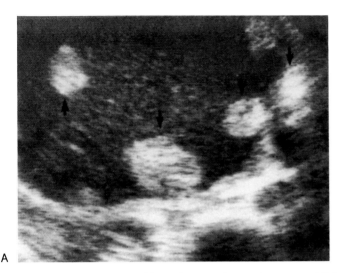

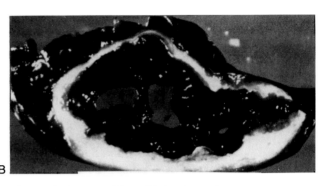

A   B

Fig. 5-95. Undifferentiated embryonal sarcoma. **(A)** Large, hypoechoic mass with multiple echogenic nodules peripherally (arrows). **(B)** Pathologic specimen showing a predominantly cystic lesion with a thick wall. Echogenic masses correspond to solid, hemorrhagic masses (arrows). (From Ros et al,[213] with permission.)

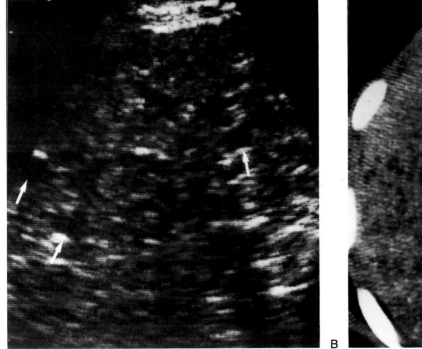

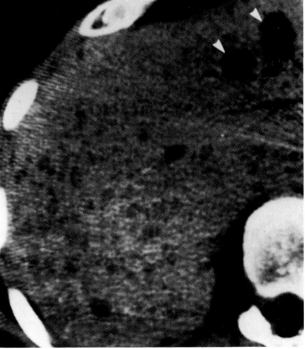

A   B

Fig. 5-96. Bile duct hamartomas. **(A)** Sonogram showing multiple, small hypoechoic lesions in the liver (arrows). **(B)** Confirmatory CT scan demonstrating numerous small, low-density masses. Larger lesions (arrowheads) are simple cysts. Biopsy revealed bile duct hamartomas. (From Eisenberg et al,[214] with permission.)

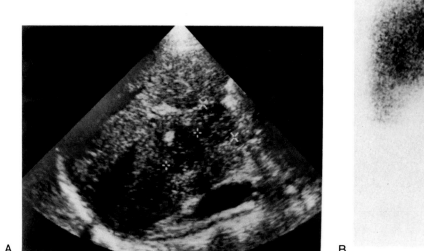

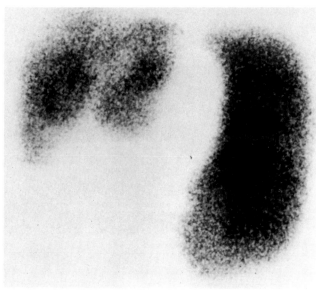

A

B

Fig. 5-97. Extramedullary hematopoiesis. Patient with a long history of polycythemia rubra vera. **(A)** Sonogram demonstrating two hypoechoic lesions (calipers) in the right lobe of the liver. **(B)** Nuclear medicine scan with bone marrow agent confirming extramedullary hematopoiesis; the lesions took up colloid. (From Abbitt and Teates,[216] with permission.)

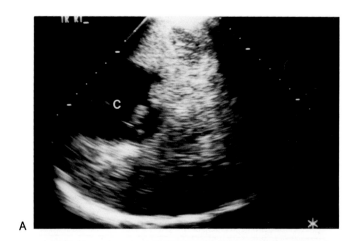

A

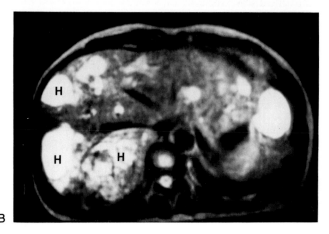

B

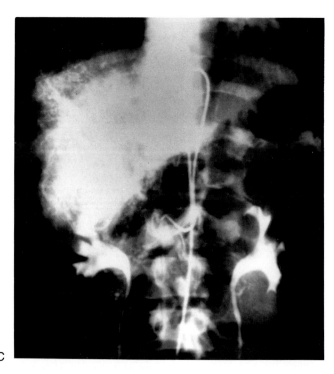

C

Fig. 5-98. Peliosis hepatis. Patient with no pertinent history of systemic disease. A question of anabolic steroid ingestion was raised. **(A)** Sonogram showing multiple cystic spaces *(C)* in the liver, with irregular walls. **(B)** MRI demonstrating high-intensity lesions *(H)* as shown. **(C)** Angiogram showing numerous ectatic vascular spaces, and confirming the presence of peliosis hepatis.

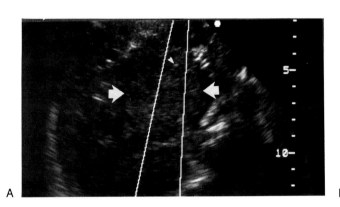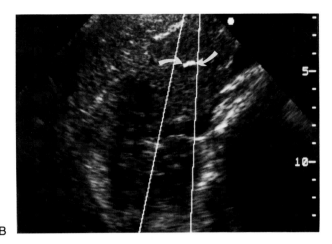

A   B

Fig. 5-99. Electronic enhancement of a needle tip. **(A)** Patient with a right hepatic mass (arrows) is undergoing ultrasound-guided biopsy. The needle tip (arrowhead) is poorly visible. **(B)** Electronic enhancement of the needle tip (curved arrows) clearly shows a large, brightly visible focus corresponding to the location of needle within mass.

ered in patients who are taking this drug. The masses will spontaneously regress after erythromycin is withdrawn.[218]

Biopsy/Aspiration

Ultrasound is excellent for biopsy localization of lesions larger than 2 cm; CT may be more desirable for smaller lesions or those for which the approach is not clearly defined with ultrasound. A series of 23 tumors biopsied has been reported in which there were no false-positive findings and only one complication when a pneumothorax was found. The risk of serious complication increases with the caliber of the cannula. The yield of a single pass was 75 percent, with greater than 90 percent accuracy in diagnosing malignancy or benignancy.[219] Some investigators report an 83 percent yield in obtaining enough cytologic material to correctly make a diagnosis without significant complication.[220] Others report an accuracy in cytohistologic evaluation of 91.6 percent with a sensitivity of 92.2 percent, a specificity of 88.9 percent, and a high positive predictive value.[221] When comparing liver biopsy using 18- and 22-gauge needles, the overall accuracy of the 18-gauge needle was 98 percent whereas the accuracy of the 22-gauge needle was 84 percent.[222] In that particular series, there were no complications with either needle. The major advantage of the 18-gauge needle was a more consistent retrieval of adequate cellular material. The decision to use histologic versus fine-needle aspiration technique will depend on the expertise of the pathologist, whether a specific diagnosis of cell type is required, and the disease in question

(lymphoma may be impossible to diagnose by the aspiration technique). As experience has grown, there has been a tendency toward the use of larger-bore needles. In addition, newer "spring-loaded" biopsy guns, both reusable and disposable, are particularly well suited for use with ultrasound guidance and yield a clean core of material suitable for histologic evaluation in almost every case.[223] A promising new adjunct to sonographic guidance is electronic enhancement of the needle tip.[224] This adaptation allows the needle tip to flash as it passes through the ultrasound beam. This facilitates the ability to monitor the needle position, and may considerably increase the desirability of ultrasound as a guidance technique in the future (Fig. 5-99).

Percutaneous aspiration with ultrasound guidance is a safe, useful, highly accurate method. Compared with CT, real-time ultrasound usually is more practical, requires no ionizing radiation, and is widely applicable. Real-time ultrasound also allows real-time visualization of the procedure. Ultrasound guidance should be considered first in the biopsy of hepatic masses because of its simplicity, safety, and accuracy.[225,226] Besides assisting in the biopsy of tumors, ultrasound can guide successful aspiration and localization for catheter drainage of abscesses.

Hematomas

The etiology of a liver hematoma (Fig. 5-100) may be trauma or rupture of a pseudoaneurysm or neoplasm such as an adenoma, metastatic choriocarcinoma, or cavernous hemangioma.[227] Subscapsular hematomas

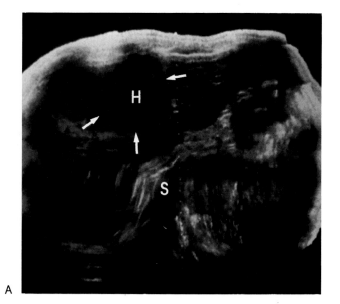

A

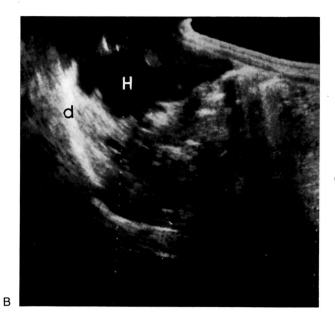

B

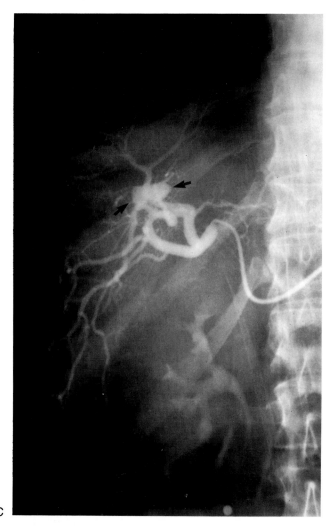

C

Fig. 5-100. Intrahepatic hematoma. (A) Transverse static scan at 18 cm above the iliac crest. An anechoic area (*H*, arrows) is seen within the anterior aspect of the liver. (*S*, spine.) (B) Longitudinal static scan at 5 cm to the right of the midline. The anechoic area *(H)* is seen with some acoustic enhancement. (*d*, diaphragm.) (C) Angiogram demonstrating a false aneurysm (arrows) of the distal hepatic artery. This had bled into the liver.

are also known to occur in association with eclampsia in what is termed HELLP syndrome[228] (Fig. 5-101). There are three categories of liver trauma: (1) rupture of the liver and its capsule, (2) separation of the capsule by a subcapsular hematoma, and (3) central rupture of the liver. In the past, aggressive treatment was advocated. However, newer imaging modalities have allowed a more conservative approach. If the patient's clinical status is stable, the liver may be evaluated by CT initially and monitored serially with ultrasound.[229]

Generally, hepatic hematomas have been described as hypoechoic with poorly defined margins. With an acute bleed, the pattern tends to be echogenic as a result of deposition of fibrin and erythrocytes[230] (Fig. 5-102). If the hematoma is subcapsular, the fluid borders the liver; if it ruptures, it is difficult to identify or may appear similar to ascites. When monitoring hematomas on a serial basis, there may be a significant increase in the cystic component before reduction in size and complete resolution occur.[229,230]

Several other non-neoplastic abnormalities may also cause focal lesions in the liver. Echodensities with strong

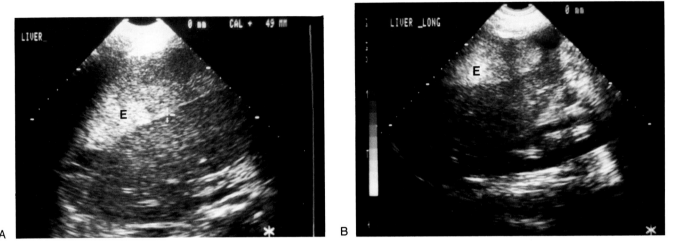

Fig. 5-101. HELLP syndrome. **(A)** Transverse and **(B)** longitudinal images through the right upper quadrant of this patient with severe eclampsia. Note the well-defined region of increased echogenicity *(E)* anteriorly, representing a large subcapsular hematoma. A small amount of free intraperitoneal blood is present (arrow).

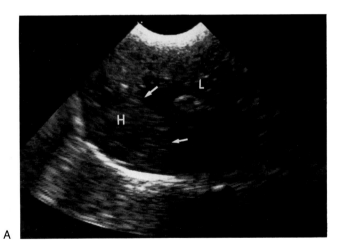

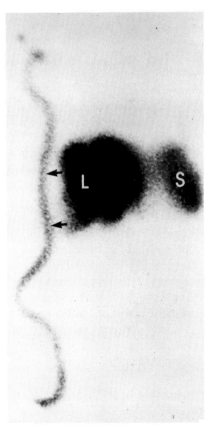

Fig. 5-102. Subcapsular hepatic hematoma. "Fresh." Neonate with a traumatic delivery and decreased hematocrit. **(A)** Transverse view of the liver demonstrating the subtle difference between the liver *(L)* parenchyma and the "fresh" subcapsular hematoma *(H,* arrows). **(B)** Anterior view of a sulfur colloid liver-spleen scan verifying the separation between the liver *(L)* and the skin (arrows). *(S,* spleen.)

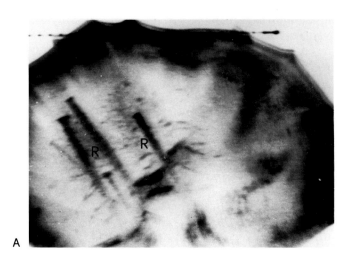

A

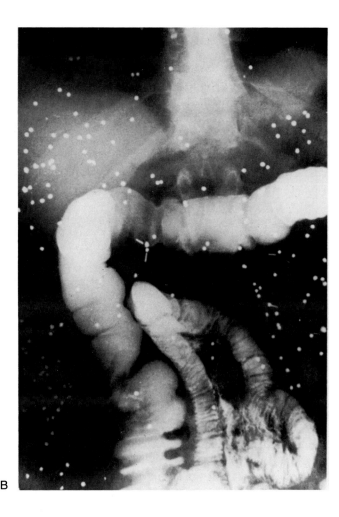

B

Fig. 5-103. Metallic foreign body. **(A)** Transverse scan of the upper portion of the abdomen demonstrating numerous intrahepatic echodensities with posterior reverberations *(R)*. **(B)** Selected film from a barium enema examination showing several lead shot pellets. (From Wendell and Athey,[231] with permission.)

posterior reverberation echoes can be seen with metallic foreign bodies in the liver[231] (Fig. 5-103). Calcified granulomas seen with trauma, tuberculosis, syphilis, and parasitic and bacterial diseases can produce echogenic foci within the liver[232] (Fig. 5-104). With biliary tract air, linear echodensities may be scattered throughout the liver[127] (Fig. 5-105) and may or may not produce a shadow or reverberation artifact. Air in the biliary system is most commonly an incidental finding and is secondary to a surgically created biliary tract anastomosis or sphincterotomy. Other significant causes include passage of a stone through the duct, a spontaneous fistula, or choledochoenteric communication. Portal venous gas is also seen as linear echogenicities within the hepatic parenchyma but is said to lie in a more peripheral location than biliary air[127] (Fig. 5-43).

Ultrasound in Liver Transplantation

Sonography plays a major role in the pre- and postoperative evaluation of hepatic transplantation. As orthotopic liver transplantation (OLT) becomes more widely accepted, the necessity to perform sonography in this population has become commonplace and no is longer limited to the university setting. With today's improved technique, the expected survival rate at 1 year is 70 to 83 percent.[233] Improvements in survival rate can be attributed to several factors, including the ability to more optimally preserve the liver prior to transplantation, the availability of more effective immunosuppressive agents, improved surgical technique and anesthesia, and better postoperative care.

Preoperatively, duplex sonography and color Doppler are the pivotal screening examinations and are performed on all potential recipients. The main function of these examinations is the evaluation of the portal vein. A preoperative knowledge of size or patency is essential because a small or thrombosed vessel will render the surgery more difficult or exclude the patient as an operative candidate altogether.[233-235] As a screening procedure, a normal sonogram of the portal vein should be sufficient to exclude a significant abnormality.[81] Any patient in whom the sonogram is not entirely normal with respect to portal anatomy, however, should un-

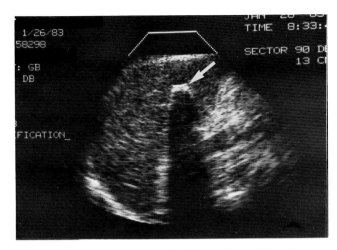

Fig. 5-104. Intrahepatic calcification. Patient with no known history of hepatic granulomatous disease. A history of liver biopsy raises the possibility that calcification (arrow) represents a calcified hematoma.

dergo MRI or angiography to further define vascular anatomy. In addition to the portal vein, the hepatic artery, hepatic veins, and IVC should be assessed. A careful evaluation of the hepatic parenchyma must be undertaken to identify hepatic masses, because the incidence of hepatoma is increased in this usually cirrhotic population. Finally, biliary dilatation and the presence or absence of portosystemic collaterals should be noted as well.

In the pediatric age group, biliary atresia is the most common indication for hepatic transplantation, and associated anomalies (polysplenia, hepatic vascular ab-

normalities, abnormalities of the IVC and kidneys) should be sought.[236,237] The study of Bisset et al[236] has found MRI to be more efficacious in this group because of the frequency of coexisting abnormalities that may be difficult to visualize by ultrasound. In the general population, however, ultrasound remains the initial imaging technique. In addition to evaluating the liver and upper abdominal vasculature, an assessment of splenic size and of both kidneys is an essential part of all pretransplant evaluations.

Postoperatively, hepatic artery thrombosis is the most serious complication of the early post-transplant period. Hepatic artery thrombosis occurs most frequently in the first weeks following transplantation. The incidence of thrombosis is described as 3 to 12 percent in adults and 11 to 42 percent in children[233] and is increased in pediatric patients with small arteries or in adults with a history of primary biliary cirrhosis in whom the recipient hepatic artery may be brittle.[238] Complex surgical procedures increase the risk of thrombosis and complicate the sonographic evaluation; therefore, knowledge of any unusual vascular anatomy is essential. Hepatic artery reconstruction is variable, and the anastomotic site will depend on numerous factors. An end-to-end anastomosis is preferred, but unusual surgical reconstructions, including hepatic artery-aortic anastomoses, dual arterial blood supplies, and even synthetic vascular grafts, may be necessary.[233,238]

Duplex and color Doppler evaluation of the hepatic artery is usually initially undertaken in the region of the porta hepatis. In this location the hepatic artery is normally large and is easily visualized by color Doppler; the vessel also maintains a relatively constant relationship

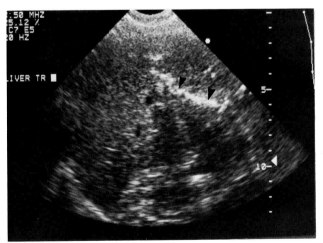

A

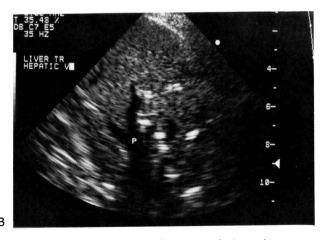

B

Fig. 5-105. Pneumobilia. Patient with history of biliary bypass. **(A)** Brightly echogenic, linear area of echogenicity (arrowheads) is identified in the location of the common bile duct. Note the poorly defined posterior shadowing. **(B)** Scanning in the periphery of the liver demonstrating numerous linear echogenic areas adjacent to the portal veins *(P)*. Findings are typical of pneumobilia.

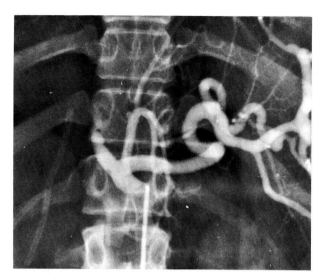

Fig. 5-106. Hepatic artery thrombosis. Selective celiac arteriogram confirming hepatic artery thrombosis in the patient in Plate 5-28.

with the portal vein, assuming that an unusual arterial reconstruction has not been necessary. A well-defined, low-resistance arterial signal in the region of the porta hepatis is considered indicative of vascular patency. Thrombosis of the hepatic artery, as implied by absent hepatic arterial signal, is a poor prognostic sign and almost invariably dictates retransplantation (Fig. 5-106 and Plate 5-28). Unlike in the normal liver, potential collateral pathways are absent and do not develop for a considerable period, if ever. Compromise of the hepatic arterial circulation is typically associated with parenchymal infarction or ischemic damage to the biliary tree.

The former leads to focal hypoechoic lesions, whereas the latter causes segmental intrahepatic strictures. According to the study of Worzney et al,[239] the incidence of hepatic artery thrombosis was 86 percent in patients with such lesions.

At some institutions, routine Doppler evaluation of the hepatic artery is performed on specific postoperative days. As our own experience has increased, however, the rate of vascular complication has fallen to the point that in adults without complex anastomoses we no longer perform routine ultrasound examinations or we reserve the examination for patients with evidence of hepatic dysfunction, abscess, infarction, delayed biliary leak, or massive hepatic necrosis. Patients with focal abnormalities or intrahepatic biliary dilatation, in fact, are so strongly suspected to have hepatic artery compromise that arteriography should be considered even if the sonogram reveals intrahepatic arterial signals.[239] The Doppler study should be quite accurate in most cases; however, the study of Flint et al[240] demonstrated 92 percent accuracy in identifying hepatic artery thrombosis.

The ability to form collateral vessels is limited after transplantation but may occur in children; only rarely will collaterals form in adults. Flint et al,[240] however, concluded that flow in these patients was sufficiently reduced that Doppler signals should remain undetectable. Our experience has been the opposite,[241] and we have clearly identified hepatic arterial signals within the livers of such patients (Fig. 5-107 and Plate 5-29). Although arterial collateralization brings flow to the liver, it is insufficient and ischemia remains. These children, therefore, are typically troubled by recurrent bouts of sepsis and persistent intrahepatic biliary dilatation. Both our experience[241] and that of Hoffer et al[242] indicate that

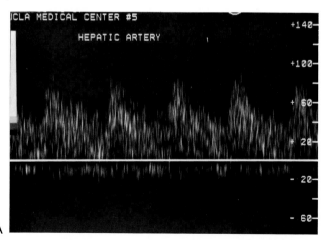

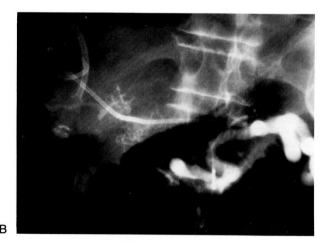

Fig. 5-107. Hepatic artery thrombosis. **(A)** Doppler evaluation of the patient in Plate 5-29 showing weak arterial signals within the liver. Note the extremely high diastolic flow. **(B)** Arteriogram demonstrating that the hepatic artery was occluded. Collaterals had formed and were responsible for Doppler signals.

such children may survive for long periods without re-transplantation despite the ischemic damage. Our study indicates that pediatric patients with evidence of hepatic artery ischemia should be considered for arteriography even if arterial signals are found. A review of the spectral tracings from these children shows that in general, the resistive index of the hepatic artery is low as a collateral bed is being sampled. Because of the potential for hepatic artery thrombosis with subsequent collateral formation in children, we do scan our pediatric transplant patients on a regular basis. Generally, the child is examined at 24 and 48 hours post-transplant and weekly thereafter. In this way the acute thrombotic episode will be manifest by virtue of absent Doppler signals even if symptoms are absent.

Another potential problem affecting the hepatic artery is the development of anastomotic stenoses. Although relatively uncommon, this complication is yet another cause of ischemia and can produce findings similar to those of chronic or acute thrombosis. On this basis, pa-tients with parenchymal abnormalities or bile duct strictures should be thoroughly evaluated by color Doppler (monitoring the entire hepatic artery may be difficult with duplex sonography alone) to identify any potential area of hepatic artery stenosis. Turbulent high-velocity flow has been described as typical of focal hepatic artery stenosis.[243] Unfortunately, abnormal hepatic arteries without stenosis may produce similar signals in our experience (Fig. 5-108 and Plate 5-30). Although ultrasound may not be specific, arteriography is indicated in either situation, so an unnecessary invasive procedure is not performed. Early identification of hepatic artery stenosis is essential if complete thrombosis and extensive parenchymal damage are to be avoided. Once identified, hepatic artery stenosis can be treated successfully by angioplasty, thereby avoiding a surgical procedure.

Several authors have also studied hepatic arterial waveforms in an effort to diagnose transplant rejection. Certainly it is common to find instances in which little or no diastolic flow is present in this normally low-

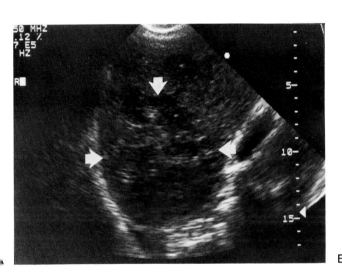

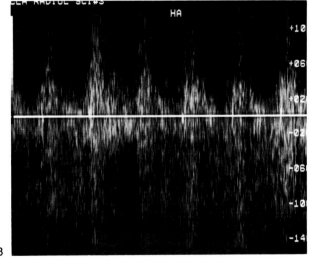

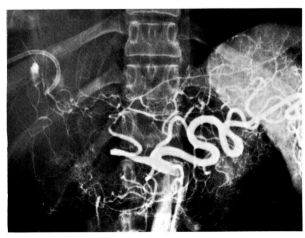

Fig. 5-108. Abnormal hepatic artery. **(A)** This patient with fever and chills is noted to have a large hypoechoic lesion occupying much of the posterior right lobe (arrows). **(B)** Signals in the hepatic artery were extremely abnormal, raising suspicion of stenosis. Note the marked spectral broadening and loss of the normal waveform. **(C)** Hepatic arteriogram confirming abnormal hepatic artery. Stenosis was not present. Such findings may be secondary to severe rejection and simply a poor prognosis. (See also Plate 5-30.)

resistance artery (Fig. 5-109 and Plate 5-31). The studies of Longley et al[244] and Marder et al,[245] however, have shown no correlation between absent diastolic flow and rejection. The reasons for the wide variations in the hepatic arterial flow patterns remain unclear; however, both studies concluded that decreased diastolic flow has no apparent clinical significance.

Portal vein thrombosis may also occur following transplantation, and its sonographic features are similar to those in the native liver (Fig. 5-39 and Plate 5-14). In our experience, this entity is most unusual, although Dalen et al[246] report a 7.1 percent frequency. Like hepatic arterial thrombosis, thrombosis of the portal vein is a devastating vascular complication, also usually requiring retransplantation. The large, normal portal vein should be easily visualized in all transplants. A narrow waist with perivascular echogenic foci secondary to surgical clips is frequently noted at the region of the anastomosis, and a region of moderate postanastomotic dilatation may be present as well. Unusual spectral patterns with an almost gurgling sound are common and are most probably secondary to turbulence originating in the region of the anastomosis (Fig. 5-110 and Plate 5-32). Anastomotic narrowing is occasionally severe enough to cause high-velocity flow, implying that significant stenosis exists (Plate 5-33). The clinical implications of such stenoses, however, remain uncertain, but these patients do not appear to progress to frank thrombosis.

Air in the portal vein is also common after transplantation. Although the exact etiology is uncertain in this population, it should not be considered a grave prognostic sign as it would in nontransplant patients (Plate

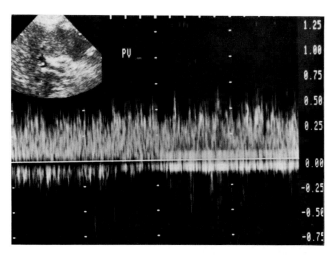

Fig. 5-110. Portal vein. Spectral Doppler tracings showing a spiked appearance, which has a characteristic "gurgling" sound probably secondary to turbulence created by the anastomotic narrowing. (See also Plate 5-32.)

5-18). Moving, brightly echogenic foci within the portal vein and a bubbly sound on spectral Doppler are typical of air in the portal vein.[86]

Although hepatic artery and portal vein thromboses are the most clinically significant vascular abnormalities following transplantation, compromise of the IVC is common as well.[246] Moderate compromise of the proximal IVC in the region of the surgical anastomosis has been sufficiently common in our population that it is typically not considered clinically significant (Fig. 5-111

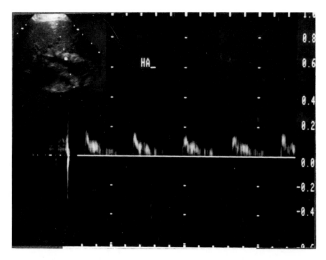

Fig. 5-109. Hepatic artery spectral patterns. Patient in Plate 5-31 scanned portably 24 hours after transplant fails to show diastolic flow in the hepatic artery. The significance of loss of diastolic flow is uncertain but does not correlate with rejection.

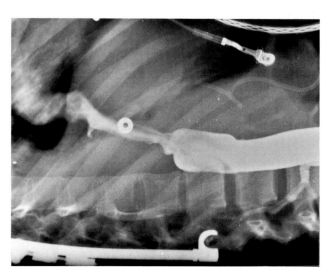

Fig. 5-111. Thrombosis of the inferior vena cava. Inferior vena cavagram confirming the sonographic findings in Plate 5-34. Although such patients were initially a cause of concern, experience has shown that most do well.

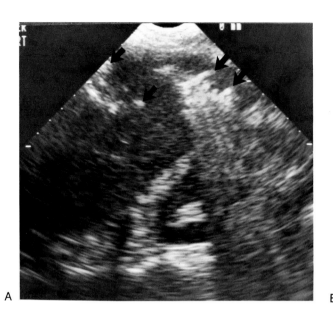
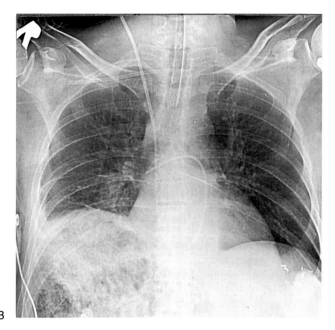

Fig. 5-112. Massive hepatic necrosis. Patient with sepsis following transplantation. Color Doppler imaging failed to reveal flow in either the portal vein or hepatic artery. (A) Real-time evaluation of the liver identified numerous regions of bright echogenicity with posterior shadowing (arrows), suggesting air within the parenchyma. (B) Portable chest film confirming the sonographic findings of massive hepatic necrosis.

and Plate 5-34). Even complete thrombosis can be monitored, and most patients seem to do relatively well. Although compromise or thrombosis of the IVC is common post-transplantation, hepatic vein thrombosis is quite unusual. Three patent hepatic veins, however, should be visible in all transplant recipients, although color may be required to define the flow because minor degrees of swelling can compress the vessels and render them invisible on real-time examination. Rarely, one or more (usually the middle and left) veins are compro-

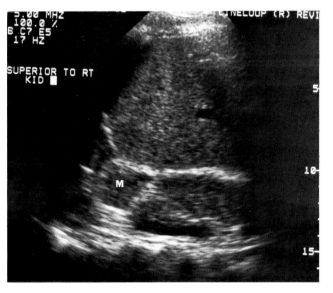
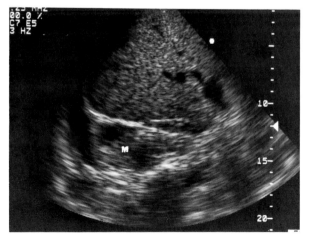

Fig. 5-113. Adrenal hemorrhage. (A) A solid, triangular mass (M) is identified above the right kidney in a patient who is status-post transplant. Adrenal hemorrhage was suspected. (B) Follow-up sonogram after 2 weeks showing mild enlargement of the lesion (M) but a considerable decrease in echogenicity as the hematoma liquefies.

mised at their junction with the IVC (Plate 5-35). Such focal narrowing of the hepatic veins is probably mechanical and most likely to be encountered in patients in whom a large liver was placed into a relatively small cavity.

Several miscellaneous abnormalities also affect the liver and deserve inclusion in this discussion. Among the most deadly is massive hepatic necrosis. This abnormality is typically associated with thrombosis of either the hepatic artery or the portal vein or both. Massive hepatic necrosis is essentially gangrene of the liver, and air in the hepatic parenchyma should be diagnostic (Fig. 5-112). The condition is often fatal, although retransplantation may be considered if it is discovered early. Right adrenal hemorrhage has also been reported in association with hepatic transplantation. Etiologically, right adrenal hemorrhage is thought to be secondary to the ligation and division of the right adrenal vein during hepatectomy. Typically, an echogenic mass is identified in the expected position of the right adrenal gland (Fig. 5-113). CT should not be necessary, because follow-up ultrasound should be confirmatory when the hematoma liquefies over time. Adrenal hemorrhage is of no clinical significance and should not be mistaken for an adrenal neoplasm.[247]

REFERENCES

1. Gore RM, Ghahremani GG, Joseph AE et al: Radiology 1989;171:739
2. Standards and Guidelines for Performance of the Abdominal and Retroperitoneal Examination. American Institute of Ultrasound in Medicine, 1990
3. O'Brien MJ, Gottlieb LS: The liver and biliary tract. p. 1009. In Robbins SL, Cotran RS (eds): Pathologic Basis of Disease. WB Saunders, Philadelphia, 1979
4. Kane RA: Sonographic anatomy of the liver. Semin Ultrasound CT MR 1981;2:190
5. Sexton CC, Zeman RK: Correlation of computed tomography, sonography and gross anatomy of liver. AJR 1983;141:711
6. Marks WM, Filly RA, Callen PW: Ultrasonic anatomy of the liver: a review with new applications. J Clin Ultrasound 1979;7:137
7. Radin DR, Colletti PM, Ralls PW et al: Agenesis of right lobe of the liver. Radiology 1987;164:639
8. Belton RL, VanZandt TF: Congenital absence of the left lobe of the liver: a radiologic diagnosis. Radiology 1983;147:184
9. Brown BM, Filly RA, Callen PW: Ultrasonographic anatomy of the caudate lobe. J Ultrasound Med 1982;1:189
10. Mitchell SE, Gross BH, Spitz HB: The hypoechoic caudate lobe: an ultrasonic pseudolesion. Radiology 1982;144:569
11. Dodds WJ, Erickson SJ, Taylor AJ et al: Caudate lobe of the liver: anatomy, embryology, and pathology. AJR 1990;154:87
12. Donoso L, Martinez-Noguera A, Zidan A et al: Papillary process of the caudate lobe of the liver: sonographic appearance. Radiology 1989;173:631
13. Hillman BJ, D'Orsi CJ, Smith EH et al: Ultrasonic appearance of the falciform ligament. AJR 1979;132:205
14. Parulekar SG: Ligaments and fissures of the liver: sonographic anatomy. Radiology 1977;130:409
15. Sones PJ, Torres WE: Normal ultrasonic appearance of the ligamentum teres and falciform ligament. J Clin Ultrasound 1978;6:392
16. Enterline DS, Rauch RE, Silverman PM et al: Cyst of the falciform ligament of the liver. AJR 1984;142:327
17. Delbridge L, Connolly J: Paraganglioma of the falciform ligament: a case report. Aust NZ J Surg 1982;52:315
18. Fried AM, Kreel L, Cosgrove DO: The hepatic interlobar fissure: combined in vitro and in vivo study. AJR 1984;143:561
19. Auh YH, Rubenstein WA, Zirinsky K et al: Accessory fissures of the liver: CT and sonographic appearance. AJR 1984;143:565
20. Schenk WG, McDonald JC, McDonald K et al: Direct measurement of hepatic blood flow in surgical patients. Ann Surg 1962;156:463
21. Chafetz N, Filly RA: Portal and hepatic veins: accuracy of margin echoes for distinguishing intrahepatic vessels. Radiology 1979;130:725
22. Foley WD (ed): Color Doppler Flow Imaging. Andover Medical Publishers, Boston, 1991
23. Grant EG, Tessler FN, Perrella RR: Clinical Doppler imaging. AJR 1989;152:707
24. Ralls RW: Color Doppler sonography of the hepatic artery and portal venous system. AJR 1988;155:517
25. Weinreb J, Kumari S, Phillips G et al: Portal vein measurements by real-time sonography. AJR 1982;139:497
26. Filly RA, Laing FC: Anatomic variation of portal venous anatomy in the porta hepatis: ultrasonographic evaluation. J Clin Ultrasound 1978;6:83
27. Callen PW, Filly RA, DeMartini WJ: The left portal vein: a possible source of confusion on ultrasonograms. Radiology 1979;130:205
28. Hill MC, Sanders RC: Sonography of the upper abdominal venous system. p. 289. In Sanders RC, Hill MC (eds): Ultrasound Annual 1983. Raven Press, New York, 1983
29. Makunchi M, Hasegawa H, Yamazaki S et al: The inferior right hepatic vein: ultrasonic demonstration. Radiology 1983;148:213
30. Bressler EL, Rubin JM, McCracken S: Sonographic parallel channel sign: a reappraisal. Radiology 1987;164:343
31. Davis PL, Van Thiel DH, Zajko AB et al: Imaging in hepatic transplantation. Semin Liver Dis 1989;9:90
32. Willi UV, Teele RL: Hepatic arteries and the parallel-channel sign. J Clin Ultrasound 1979;7:125
33. Ralls PW, Quinn MF, Rogers W et al: Sonographic anatomy of hepatic artery. AJR 1981;136:1059
34. Michels NA: In: Blood Supply and Anatomy of the Upper Abdominal Organs. JB Lippincott, Philadelphia, 1955

35. Behan M, Kazam E: Sonography of the common bile duct: value of the right anterior oblique view. AJR 1978;130:701

36. Berland LL, Lawson TL, Foley WD: Porta hepatis: sonographic discrimination of bile ducts from arteries with pulsed Doppler with new anatomic criteria. AJR 1982;138:833

37. Berland LL, Lawson TL, Foley WD: Portal hepatis: sonographic discrimination of bile ducts from arteries with pulsed Doppler with new anatomic criteria. AJR 1982;138:833

38. Wing VW, Laing FC, Jeffrey RB et al: Sonographic differentiation of enlarged hepatic arteries from dilated intrahepatic bile ducts. AJR 1985;145:57

39. Grant EG: Parenchymal disease of the liver. In Rifkin MD, Charboneau JW, Laing FC (eds): Ultrasound 1991 Syllabus: Special Course. RSNA Publications, Oak Brook, IL, 1991

40. Niederau C, Sonnenberg A: Liver size evaluated by ultrasound: ROC curves for hepatitis and alcoholism. Radiology 1984;153:503

41. Gosink BB, Leymaster CE: Ultrasonic determination of hepatomegaly. J Clin Ultrasound 1981;9:37

42. Niederau C, Sonnenberg A, Muller JE et al: Sonographic measurements of the normal liver, spleen, pancreas and portal vein. Radiology 1983;149:537

43. Scatarige JC, Scott WW, Donovan PJ et al: Fatty infiltration of the liver: ultrasonographic and computed tomographic correlation. J Ultrasound Med 1984;3:9

44. Henschke CI, Goldman H, Teele RL: The hyperechogenic liver in children: cause and sonographic appearance. AJR 1982;138:841

45. Foster KJ, Dewbury KC, Griffin AH et al: The accuracy of ultrasound in the detection of fatty infiltration of the liver. Br J Radiol 1980;53:440

46. Behan M, Kazam E: The echographic characteristics of fatty tissues and tumors. Radiology 1978;129:143

47. Taylor KJW, Riely CA, Hammers L et al: Quantitative US attenuation in normal liver and in patients with diffuse liver disease: importance of fat. Radiology 1986;160:65

48. Scott WW, Sanders RC, Siegelman SS: Irregular fatty infiltration of the liver: diagnostic dilemmas. AJR 1980;135:67

49. Wilson SR, Rosen IE, Chin-Sang HB et al: Fatty infiltration of the liver: an imaging challenge. J Can Assoc Radiol 1982;33:227

50. Quinn SF, Gosink BB: Characteristic sonographic signs of hepatic fatty infiltration. AJR 1985;145:753

51. White M, Simeone J, Mueller P et al: Focal periportal sparing in hepatic fatty infiltration: a cause for hepatic pseudomass on US. Radiology 1987;162:57

52. Sauerbrei EE, Lopez M: Pseudotumor of the quadrate lobe in hepatic sonography: a sign of generalized fatty infiltration. AJR 1986;147:923

53. Arai K, Matsui O, Takashima T et al: Focal spared areas in fatty liver caused by regional decreased portal flow. AJR 1988;151:300

54. Yoshikawa J, Matsui O, Takashima T et al: Focal fatty change of the liver adjacent to the falciform ligament: CT and sonographic findings in five surgically confirmed cases. AJR 1987;149:491

55. Kurtz AB, Rubin CS, Cooper HS et al: Ultrasound findings in hepatitis. Radiology 1980;136:717

56. Gates GF: The liver, gallbladder and biliary tree. p. 56. In Haller JO, Shkolnik A (eds): Clinics in Diagnostic Ultrasound: Diagnostic Ultrasound in Pediatrics. Vol. 8. Churchill Livingstone, New York, 1981

57. Taylor KJW, Gorelick FS, Rosenfield AT et al: Ultrasonography of alcoholic liver disease with histological correlation. Radiology 1981;141:157

58. DiLeio A, Cestari C, Lomazzi A et al: Diagnosis with sonographic study of the liver surface. Radiology 1989;172:389

59. Harbin WP, Robert NJ, Ferrucci JT: Diagnosis of cirrhosis based on regional changes in hepatic morphology. Radiology 1980;135:273

60. Giorgio A, Pietro A, Lettieri G et al: Cirrhosis: value of caudate to right lobe ration in diagnosis with US. Radiology 1986;161:443

61. Grossman H, Ram PC, Coleman RA et al: Hepatic ultrasonography in type I glycogen storage disease (von Gierke disease). Radiology 1981;141:753

62. Brunelle F, Tammam S, Odievre M et al: Liver adenomas in glycogen storage disease of children: ultrasound and angiographic study. Pediatr Radiol 1984;14:94

63. Smevik B, Swensen T, Kolbenstvedt A et al: Computed tomography and ultrasonography of the abdomen in congenital generalized lipodystrophy. Radiology 1982;142:687

64. Itzchuk Y, Rubinstein Z, Shilo R: Ultrasound in tropical diseases. p. 69. In Sanders RC, Hill MC (eds): Ultrasound Annual 1983. Raven Press, New York, 1983

65. Fataar S, Bassiony H, Satyanath S et al: Characteristic sonographic features of schistosomal periportal fibrosis. AJR 1984;143:69

66. Kane RA, Katz SG: The spectrum of sonographic findings in portal hypertension: a subject review and new observations. Radiology 1982;142:453

67. Subramanyam BR, Balthazar EJ, Madamba MR et al: Sonography of portosystemic venous collaterals in portal hypertension. Radiology 1983;146:161

68. Lafortune M, Constantin A, Breton G et al: The recanalized umbilical vein in portal hypertension: a myth. AJR 1985;144:549

69. Juttner H-V, Jeeney JM, Ralls PW et al: Ultrasound demonstration of portosystemic collaterals in cirrhosis and portal hypertension. Radiology 1982;142:459

70. Bolondi L, Gandolfi L, Arienti V et al: Ultrasonography in the diagnosis of portal hypertension: diminished response of portal vessels to respiration. Radiology 1982;142:167

71. Dach JL, Hill MC, Pelaez JC et al: Sonography of hypertensive portal venous system: correlation with arterial portography. AJR 1981;137:511

72. Dokmeci AK, Kimura K, Matsutani S et al: Collateral veins in portal hypertension: demonstration by sonography. AJR 1981;137:1173

73. Patriquin H, Lafortune M, Burns P et al: The duplex Doppler examination of children and adults with

portal hypertension: technique and anatomy. AJR 1987;
149:71

74. Schabel SI, Rittenberg GM, Javid LH et al: The "bull's-eye" falciform ligament: a sonographic finding of portal hypertension. Radiology 1980;136:157

75. Glazer GM, Laing FC, Brown TW et al: Sonographic demonstration of portal hypertension: the patent umbilical vein. Radiology 1980;136:161

76. Saddekni S, Hutchinson DE, Cooperberg PL: The sonographically patent umbilical vein in portal hypertension. Radiology 1982;145:441

77. Caletti G, Brocchi E, Baraldini M et al: Assessment of portal hypertension by endoscopie ultrasonography. Gastrointest Endosc 1990;36:S21

78. Grant EG, Tessler FN, Gomes AS et al: Color Doppler imaging of portosystemic shunts. AJR 1990;154:393

79. Foley WD, Gleysteen JJ, Lawson TL et al: Dynamic computed tomography and pulsed Doppler ultrasonography in the evaluation of splenorenal shunt patency. J Comput Assist Tomogr 1983;7:106

80. Miller EI, Thomas RH: Portal vein invasion demonstrated by ultrasound. J Clin Ultrasound 1979;7:57

81. Tessler FT, Gehring BJ, Gomes A et al: Diagnosis of portal vein thrombosis: value of color Doppler imaging. AJR 1991;157:293

82. Grand MP, Remy J: Ultrasound diagnosis of extrahepatic portal vein obstruction in childhood. Pediatr Radiol 1979;8:155

83. Marx M, Scheible W: Cavernous transformation of the portal vein. J Ultrasound Med 1982;1:167

84. Weltin G, Taylor KJW, Carter AR et al: Duplex Doppler: identification of cavernous transformation of the portal vein. AJR 1985;144:999

85. Vine HS, Sequeira JC, Widrich WC et al: Portal vein aneurysm. AJR 1979;132:557

86. Chezmar JL, Nelson RC, Bernardino ME: Portal venous gas after hepatic transplantation: sonographic detection and clinical significance. AJR 1989;153:1203

87. Merritt CRB, Goldsmith JP, Sharp MJ: Sonographic detection of portal venous gas in infants with necrotizing enterocolitis. AJR 1984;143:1059

88. Ramchandani P, Goldenberg NJ, Soulen RL et al: Isobutyl 2-cyanoacrylate embolization of a hepatoportal fistula. AJR 1983;140:137

89. Bezzi M, Mitchell DG, Needleman L et al: Iatrogenic aneurysmal portal-hepatic venous fistula. Diagnosis by color Doppler imaging. J Ultrasound Med 1988;7:457

90. Duerinckx A, Grant E, Perrella R et al: The pulsatile portal vein: correlation of duplex Doppler with right atrial pressures. Radiology 1990;176:655

91. Abu-Yousef MM, Milam SG, Farner RM: Pulsatile portal vein flow: a sign of tricuspid regurgitation on duplex Doppler sonography. AJR 1990;155:785

92. Clain D, Freston J, Kreel L et al: Clinical diagnosis of the Budd-Chiari syndrome. Am J Med 1967;43:544

93. Parker RGF: Occlusion of the hepatic veins in man. Medicine 1959;38:369

94. Hirooka M: Embryonic abnormality as the pathogenesis of membranous obliteration of the inferior vena cava in the hepatic portion. Acta Hepat Jpn 1969;10:566

95. Tisnado J, Cho S-R, Carithers RL et al: The Budd-Chiari syndrome: angiographic-pathologic correlation. RadioGraphics 1983;3:155

96. Brink AJ, Botha D: Budd-Chiari syndrome: diagnosis by hepatic venography. Br J Radiol 1955;28:330

97. Grant EG, Perrella RR, Tessler FN et al: Budd-Chiari syndrome: the results of duplex and color Doppler imaging. AJR 1989;152:377

98. Longer B, Stone RM, Colapinto RF et al: Clinical spectrum of the Budd-Chiari syndrome and its surgical management. Am J Surg 1975;129:137

99. Cameron JL, Kadir S, Pierce WS: Mesoatrial shunt: a prosthesis modification. Surgery 1984;96:114

100. Brown BP, Abu-Yousef MM, Farner R et al: Doppler sonography: a non-invasive method for evaluation of hepatic venocclusive disease. AJR 1990;154:721

101. Cloogman HM, DiCapo RD: Hereditary hemorrhagic telangiectasia: sonographic findings in the liver. Radiology 1984;150:521

102. Sandler MA, Marks DS, Hricak H et al: Benign focal diseases of the liver. Semin Ultrasound CT MR 1981;2:202

103. Taylor KJW, Viscomi GN: Ultrasound diagnosis of cystic disease of the liver. J Clin Gastroenterol 1980;2:197

104. Weaver RM, Goldstein HM, Green B et al: Gray scale ultrasonographic evaluation of hepatic cystic disease. AJR 1978;130:849

105. Roemer CE, Ferrucci JT, Mueller PR et al: Hepatic cysts: diagnosis and therapy by sonographic needle aspiration. AJR 1981;136:1065

106. Spiegel RM, King DL, Green WM: Ultrasonography of primary cysts of liver. AJR 1978;131:235

107. Brick SH, Hill MC, Lande IM: The mistaken or indeterminate CT diagnosis of hepatic metastases: the value of sonography. AJR 1987;148:723

108. Saini S, Mueller PR, Ferrucci JT et al: Percutaneous aspiration of hepatic cysts does not provide definitive therapy. AJR 1983;141:559

109. Bean WJ, Rodan BA: Hepatic cysts: treatment with alcohol. AJR 1985;144:237

110. Shiina S, Tagawa K, Unuma T et al: Percutaneous ethanol injection therapy for neoplasms located on the surface of the liver. AJR 1990;155:507

111. Fulton AJ, Picker RH, Cooper RA: Ultrasonic appearance of hydatid cysts of the liver. Australas Radiol 1982;26:64

112. Lewall DB, McCorkell SJ: Rupture of echinococcal cysts: diagnosis, classification, and clinical implications. AJR 1986;146:391

113. Andrew WK, Thomas RG: Hydatid cyst of the pancreatic tail: ultrasonic features including application of the Escudero-Nemenow sign. S Afr Med J 1981;59:235

114. Beggs I: The radiology of hydatid disease. AJR 1985;145:639

115. Esfahani F, Rooholamini SA, Vessal K: Ultrasonography of hepatic hydatid cysts: new diagnostic signs. J Ultrasound Med 1988;7:443

116. Itzchyk Y, Rubinstein Z, Heyman Z et al: Role of ultrasound in the diagnosis of abdominal hydatid disease. J Clin Ultrasound 1980;8:341

117. Niron EA, Ozer H: Ultrasound appearances of liver hydatid disease. Br J Radiol 1981;54:335

118. Barriga P, Cruz F, Lepe V et al: An ultrasonographically solid tumor-like appearance of echinococcal cysts in the liver. J Ultrasound Med 1983;2:123

119. Garcia FJ, Marti-Bonmati L, Menor F et al: Echogenic forms of hydatid cysts: sonographic diagnosis. J Clin Ultrasound 1988;16:305

120. Didier D, Weiler S, Rohmer P et al: Hepatic alveolar echinococcosis: correlative US and CT study. Radiology 1985;154:179

121. Bezzi M, Teggi A, DeRosa F et al: Abdominal hydatid disease: US findings during medical treatment. Radiology 1987;162:91

122. Papanicolaou N, Mueller PR, Simeone JF et al: The sonographic appearance of omentoplasty in the surgical treatment of large cystic lesions of the liver. J Ultrasound Med 1984;3:181

123. Khuroo MS, Zargar SA, Mahajan R: Echinococcus granulosus cysts in the liver: management with percutaneous drainage. Radiology 1991;180:141

124. Kuligowska E, Noble J: Sonography of hepatic abscesses. Semin Ultrasound CT MR 1983;4:102

125. Kuligowska E, Conners SK, Shapiro JH: Liver abscess: sonography in diagnosis and treatment. AJR 1982;138:253

126. Sones PJ, Thomas BM, Masand PP: Falciform ligament abscess: appearance on computed tomography and sonography. AJR 1981;137:161

127. Gosink BB: Intrahepatic gas: differential diagnosis. AJR 1981;137:763

128. Powers TA, Jones TB, Karl JH: Echogenic hepatic abscess without radiographic evidence of gas. AJR 1981;137:159

129. Johnson RD, Mueller PR, Ferrucci JT Jr et al: Percutaneous drainage of pyogenic liver abscesses. AJR 1985;144:463

130. Ralls PW, Colletti PM, Quinn MF et al: Sonographic findings in hepatic amebic abscess. Radiology 1982;145:123

131. Abul-Khair MH, Kenawi MM, Korasky EE et al: Ultrasonography and amoebic liver abscesses. Ann Surg 1981;193:221

132. Ralls PW, Mikity VG, Colletti P et al: Sonography in the diagnosis and management of hepatic abscesses in children. Pediatr Radiol 1982;12:239

133. Ralls PW, Barnes PF, Radin DR et al: Sonographic features of amebic and pyogenic liver abscesses: a blinded comparison. AJR 1987;149:499

134. vanSonnenberg E, Mueller PR, Schiffman HR et al: Intrahepatic amebic abscesses: indications for and results of percutaneous catheter drainage. Radiology 1985;156:631

135. Dalrymple RB, Fataar S, Goodman A et al: Hyperechoic amoebic liver abscesses: an unusual ultrasonic appearance. Clin Radiol 1982;33:541

136. Ralls PW, Quinn MF, Bowswell WD Jr et al: Patterns of resolution in successfully treated hepatic amebic abscess: sonographic evaluation. Radiology 1983;149:541

137. Gooding GAW: Amebic abscess: sonographic follow-up of persistent hepatic defects in two patients one year after successful treatment for amebiasis of the liver. J Clin Ultrasound 1981;9:451

138. Ho B, Cooperberg PL, Li DKB et al: Ultrasonography and computed tomography of hepatic candidiasis in immunosuppressed patients. J Ultrasound Med 1982;1:157

139. Miller JH, Greenfield LD, Wald BR: Candidiasis of the liver and spleen in childhood. Radiology 1982;142:375

140. Callen PW, Filly RA, Marcus FS: Ultrasonography and computed tomography in the evaluation of hepatic microabscesses in the immunosuppressed patient. Radiology 1980;136:433

141. Pastakia B, Shawker TH, Thaler M et al: Hepatosplenic candidiasis: wheels within wheels. Radiology 1988;166:417

142. Garel LA, Pariente DM, Nezelop C et al: Liver involvement in chronic granulomatous disease: the role of ultrasound in diagnosis and treatment. Radiology 1984;153:117

143. Spouge AR, Wilson SR, Gopinath N et al: Extrapulmonary *Pneumocystis carinii* in a patient with AIDS: sonographic findings. AJR 1990;155:76

144. Vieco PT, Rochon L, Lisbona A: Multifocal cytomegalovirus-associated hepatic lesions simulating metastases in AIDS. Radiology 1990;176:123

145. Dolmatch BL, Laing FC, Federle MP et al: AIDS-related cholangitis: radiographic findings in nine patients. Radiology 1987;163:313

146. Doehring E, Reider F, Eittrich M et al: Ultrasonographic findings in the livers of patients with lepromatous leprosy. J Clin Ultrasound 1986;14:179

147. Brauner M, Buffard MD, Jeantils V et al: Sonography and computed tomography of macroscopic tuberculosis of the liver. J Clin Ultrasound 1989;17:563

148. Sheth S, Fishman EK, Sanders R: Actinomycosis involving the liver: computed tomography/ultrasound correlation. J Ultrasound Med 1987;6:329

149. Dachman AH, Pakter RL, Ros PR et al: Hepatoblastoma: radiologic-pathologic correlation in 50 cases. Radiology 1987;164:15

150. Bates SM, Keller MS, Ramos IM et al: Hepatoblastoma: detection of tumor vascularity with duplex Doppler US. Radiology 1990;176:505

151. Gates GF: Liver and spleen. p. 16. In: Atlas of Abdominal Ultrasonography in Children. Churchill Livingstone, New York, 1978

152. Ros PR, Goodman ZD, Ishak KG et al: Mesenchymal hamartoma of the liver: radiologic-pathologic correlation. Radiology 1986;158:619

153. Stanley P, Hall TR, Woolley MM et al: Mesenchymal hamartomas of the liver in childhood: sonographic and CT findings. AJR 1986;147:1035

154. Abramson SJ, Lack EE, Teele RL: Benign vascular tumors of the liver in infants: sonographic appearance. AJR 1982;138:629

155. Dachman AH, Lichtenstein JE, Friedman AC et al: Infantile hemangioendothelioma of the liver: a radiologic-pathologic-clinical correlation. AJR 1983;140:1091

156. Pardes JG, Bryan PJ, Gauderer MWL: Spontaneous regression of infantile hemangioendotheliomatosis of the liver: demonstration by ultrasound. J Ultrasound Med 1982;1:349

157. Kassner EG, Friedman AP: Liver masses. p. 80. In Haller JO, Shkolnik A (eds): Clinics in Diagnostic Ultrasound: Diagnostic Ultrasound in Pediatrics. Vol. 8. Churchill Livingstone, New York, 1981

158. Filiatrault D, Garel L, Tournade MF et al: Echographic aspects of hepatic metastases of nephroblastomas. Pediatr Radiol 1982;12:72

159. Onodera H, Ohta K, Oikawa M et al: Correlation of the real-time ultrasonographic appearance of hepatic hemangiomas with angiography. J Clin Ultrasound 1983;11:421

160. McArdle CR: Ultrasonic appearances of a hepatic hemangioma. J Clin Ultrasound 1978;6:124

161. Mirk P, Rubaltelli L, Bazzocchi M et al: Ultrasonographic patterns in hepatic hemangiomas. J Clin Ultrasound 1982;10:373

162. Gibney RG, Hendin AP, Cooperberg PL: Sonographically detected hepatic hemangiomas: absence of change over time. AJR 1987;149:953

163. Nelson RC, Chezmar JL: Diagnostic approach to hepatic hemangiomas. Radiology 1990;176:11

164. Bree RL, Schuab RE, Neiman HL: Solitary echogenic spot in the liver: is it diagnostic of a hemangioma? AJR 1983;140:41

165. Bruneton JN, Drouillard J, Fenart D et al: Ultrasonography of hepatic cavernous haemangiomas. Br J Radiol 1983;56:791

166. Taboury J, Porcel A, Tubiana J-M et al: Cavernous hemangiomas of the liver studied by ultrasound: enhancement posterior to a hyperechoic mass as a sign of hypervascularity. Radiology 1983;149:781

167. Marchal G, Baert AL, Fevery J et al: Ultrasonography of liver haemangioma. Fortschr Rontgenstr 1983;138:201

168. Wiener SN, Parulekar SG: Scintigraphy and ultrasonography of hepatic hemangioma. Radiology 1979;132:149

169. Taylor KJW, Ramos I, Morse SS et al: Focal liver masses: differential diagnosis with pulsed Doppler US. Radiology 1987;164:643

170. Cronan JJ, Esparza AR, Dorfman GS et al: Cavernous hemangioma of the liver: role of percutaneous biopsy. Radiology 1988;166:135

171. Atkinson GO, Kodroff M, Sones PJ et al: Focal nodular hyperplasia of the liver in children: a report of three new cases. Radiology 1980;137:171

172. Rogers JV, Mack LA, Freeny PC et al: Hepatic focal nodular hyperplasia: angiography, CT, sonography, and scintigraphy. AJR 1981;137:983

173. Scatarige JC, Fishman EK, Sanders RC: The sonographic "scar sign" in focal nodular hyperplasia of the liver. J Ultrasound Med 1982;1:275

174. Welch TJ, Sheedy PF II, Johnson CM et al: Focal nodular hyperplasia and hepatic adenoma: comparison of angiography, CT, US and scintigraphy. Radiology 1985;156:593

175. Majaewski A, Gratz KF, Brolsch C et al: Sonographic pattern of focal nodular hyperplasia of the liver. Eur J Radiol 1984;4:52

176. Dachman AH, Ros PR, Goodman ZD et al: Nodular regenerative hyperplasia of the liver: clinical and radiologic observations. AJR 1987;148:717

177. Sandler MA, Petrocelli RD, Marks DS et al: Ultrasonic features and radionuclide correlation in liver cell adenoma and focal nodular hyperplasia. Radiology 1980;135:393

178. Marti-Gonmati L, Menor F, Vizcaino I et al: Lipoma of the liver: US, CT, and MRI appearance. Gastrointest Radiol 1989;14:155

179. Roberts JL, Fishman EK, Hartman DS et al: Lipomatous tumors of the liver: evaluation with CT and US. Radiology 1986;158:613

180. Robinson JD, Grant EG, Haller JO et al: Hepatic angiomyolipomas in tuberous sclerosis. Report of two cases. J Ultrasound Med 1989;8:575

181. Yoshikawa J, Matsui O, Takashima T et al: Fatty metamorphosis in hepatocellular carcinoma: radiologic features in 10 cases. AJR 1988;15:717

182. Kamin PD, Bernardino ME, Green B: Ultrasound manifestations of hepatocellular carcinoma. Radiology 1979;131:459

183. Jackson VP, Martin-Simmerman P, Becker GJ et al: Real-time ultrasonographic demonstration of vascular invasion by hepatocellular carcinoma. J Ultrasound Med 1983;2:277

184. Takashima T, Matsui O, Suzuki M et al: Diagnosis and screening of small hepatocellular carcinomas. Radiology 1982;145:635

185. Takayasu K, Moriyama N, Muramatsu Y et al: The diagnosis of small hepatocellular carcinomas: efficacy of various imaging procedures in 100 patients. AJR 1990;155:49

186. Tanaka S, Kitamura T, Imaoka S et al: Hepatocellular carcinoma: sonographic and histologic correlation. AJR 1983;140:701

187. Choi BI, Kim C-W, Han MC et al: Sonographic characteristics of small hepatocellular carcinoma. Gastrointest Radiol 1989;14:255

188. Sheu J-C, Chen D-S, Sung J-L et al: Hepatocellular carcinoma: US evolution in the early stage. Radiology 1985;155:463

189. Cottone M, Marceno MP, Maringhini A et al: Ultrasound in the diagnosis of hepatocellular carcinoma associated with cirrhosis. Radiology 1983;147:517

190. Sheu J-C, Sung J-L, Chen D-S et al: Ultrasonography of small hepatic tumors using high resolution linear-array real-time instruments. Radiology 1984;150:797

191. Gandolfi L, Muratori R, Solmi L et al: Laparoscopy compared with ultrasonography in the diagnosis of hepatocellular carcinoma. Gastrointest Endosc 1989;35:508

192. Kudo M, Hirasa M, Takakuwa H et al: Small hepatocellular carcinomas in chronic liver disease: detection with SPECT. Radiology 1986;159:697

193. Tanaka S, Kitamura T, Fujita M et al: Color Doppler flow imaging of liver tumors. AJR 1990;154:509

194. Ralls PW: Focal hepatic and pancreatic disease. p. 293. In

Rifkin MD, Charboneau JW, Laing FC (eds): Ultrasound 1991 Syllabus: Special Course. RSNA Publications, Oak Brook, IL, 1991

195. Brandt DJ, Johnson CD, Stephens DH et al: Imaging of fibrolamellar hepatocellular carcinoma. AJR 1988; 151:295

196. Green B, Bree RL, Goldstein HM, Stanley C: Gray scale ultrasound evaluation of hepatic neoplasms: patterns and correlations. Radiology 1977;124:203

197. Scheible W, Gosink BB, Leopold GR: Gray scale echographic patterns of hepatic metastatic disease. AJR 1977;129:983

198. Hillman BJ, Smith EH, Gammelgaard J et al: Ultrasonographic-pathologic correlation of malignant hepatic masses. Gastrointest Radiol 1979;4:361

199. Bernardino ME, Green B: Ultrasonographic evaluation of chemotherapeutic response in hepatic metastases. Radiology 1979;133:437

200. Bruneton JN, Ladree D, Caramella E et al: Ultrasonographic study of calcified hepatic metastases: a report of 13 cases. Gastrointest Radiol 1982;7:61

201. Viscomi GN, Gonzalez R, Taylor KJW: Histopathological correlation of ultrasound appearances of liver metastases. J Clin Gastroenterol 1981;3:395

202. Katrugadda CS, Goldstein HM, Green B: Gray scale ultrasonography of calcified liver metastases. AJR 1977;129:591

203. Ferrucci JT: Liver tumor imaging: current concepts. AJR 1990;155:473

204. Seltzer SE, Holman BL: Imaging hepatic metastases from colorectal carcinoma: identification of candidates for partial hepatectomy. AJR 1989;152:917

205. Hayashi N, Yamamoto K, Tamaki N et al: Metastatic nodules of hepatocellular carcinoma: detection with angiography, CT, and US. Radiology 1987;165:61

206. Machi J, Isomoto H, Yamashita Y et al: Intraoperative ultrasonography in screening for liver metastases from colorectal cancer: comparative accuracy with traditional procedures. Surgery 1987;101:678

207. Wernecke K, Peters PE, Kruger K-G: Ultrasonographic patterns of focal hepatic and splenic lesions in Hodgkin's and non-Hodgkin's lymphoma. Br J Radiol 1987;60:655

208. Ginaldi S, Bernardino ME, Jing BS et al: Ultrasonographic patterns of hepatic lymphoma. Radiology 1980;136:427

209. Siegal MJ, Melson GL: Sonographic demonstration of hepatic Burkitt's lymphoma. Pediatr Radiol 1981;11:166

210. Carroll BA, Ta HN: The ultrasonic appearance of extranodal abdominal lymphoma. Radiology 1980; 136:419

211. Lepke R, Pagani JJ: Sonography of hepatic chloromas. AJR 1982;138:1176

212. Furui S, Itai Y, Ohtomo K et al: Hepatic epithelioid hemangioendothelioma: report of five cases. Radiology 1989;171:63

213. Ros PR, Olmsted WW, Dachman AH et al: Undifferentiated (embryonal) sarcoma of the liver: radiologic-pathologic correlation. Radiology 1986;161:141

214. Eisenberg D, Hurwitz L, Yu AC: CT and sonography of multiple bile-duct hamartomas simulating malignant liver disease (case report). AJR 1986;147:279

215. Wiener MD, Halvorsen RA Jr, Vollmer RT et al: Focal intrahepatic extramedullary hematopoiesis mimicking neoplasm. AJR 1987;149:1171

216. Abbitt PL, Teates CD: The sonographic appearance of extramedullary hematopoiesis in the liver. J Clin Ultrasound 1989;17:280

217. Lloyd RL, Lyons EA, Levi CS et al: The sonographic appearance of peliosis hepatis. J Ultrasound Med 1982;1:293

218. Rigauts HD, Selleslag DL, Van Eyken PL et al: Erythromycin-induced hepatitis: simulator of malignancy. Radiology 1988;169:661

219. Nosher JL, Plafker J: Fine-needle aspiration of the liver with ultrasound guidance. Radiology 1980;136:177

220. Zornoza J, Wallace S, Ordonez N et al: Fine-needle aspiration biopsy of the liver. AJR 1980;134:331

221. Schwerk WB, Schmitz-Moorman P: Ultrasonically guided fine-needle biopsies in neoplastic liver disease: cytohistologic diagnoses and echopattern of lesions. Cancer 1981;48:1469

222. Pagani JJ: Biopsy of focal hepatic lesions: comparison of 18 and 22 gauge needles. Radiology 1983;147:673

223. Parker SH, Hopper KD, Yakes WF et al: Image-directed percutaneous biopsies with a biopsy gun. Radiology 1989;171:663

224. Perrella R, Kimme-Smith C, Tessler FN et al: A new electronically enhanced biopsy system: value for improving needle tip visibility during interventional procedures. AJR 1992;158:195

225. Charboneau JW, Reading CC, Welch TJ: CT and sonographically guided needle biopsy: current techniques and new innovations. AJR 1990;154:1

226. Matalon TAS, Silver B: US guidance of interventional procedures. Radiology 1990;174:43

227. Green B, Goldstein HM: Hepatic ultrasonography. p. 62. In Sarti DA, Sample WF (eds): Diagnostic Ultrasound Text and Cases. GK Hall, Boston, 1980

228. Rachner T, Grant EG: Unknown case 3: subcapsular liver hematoma. J Ultrasound Med 1988;7:649

229. Lam AH, Shulman L: Ultrasonography in the management of liver trauma in children. J Ultrasound Med 1984;3:199

230. Van Sonnenberg E, Simeone JF, Meuller PR et al: Sonographic appearance of hematomas in the liver, spleen and kidneys: a clinical, pathologic and animal study. Radiology 1983;147:507

231. Wendell BA, Athey PA: Ultrasonic appearance of metallic foreign bodies in parenchymal organs. J Clin Ultrasound 1981;9:133

232. Weeks LE, McCune BR, Martin JF, O'Brein TF: Differential diagnosis of intrahepatic shadowing on ultrasound examination. J Clin Ultrasound 1978;6:399

233. Morton MJ, James EM, Wiesner RH, Krom RAF: Applications of duplex ultrasonography in the liver transplant patient. Mayo Clin Proc 1990;65:360

234. Taylor KJW, Morse SS, Weltin GG et al: Liver transplant

recipients: portable duplex US with correlative angiography. Radiology 1986;159:357

235. Longley DG, Skolnick ML, Zajko AB, Bron KM: Duplex Doppler sonography in the evaluation of adult patients before and after liver transplantation. AJR 1988;151:687

236. Bisset GS III, Strife JL, Balistreri WF: Evaluation of children for liver transplantation: value of MR imaging and sonography. AJR 1990;155:351

237. Ledesma-Medina J, Dominguez R, Bowen AD et al: Pediatric liver transplantation. Part I. Standardization of preoperative diagnostic imaging. Radiology 1985;157:335

238. Davis PL, Van Thiel DH, Zajko AB et al: Imaging in hepatic transplantation. Semin Liver Dis 1989;9:90

239. Worzney P, Zajko AB, Bron KM et al: Vascular complications after liver transplantation: a 5-year experience. AJR 1986;147:657

240. Flint EW, Sumkin JH, Zajko AB, Bowen AD: Duplex sonography of hepatic artery thrombosis after liver transplantation. AJR 1988;151:481

241. Hall TR, McDiarmid SU, Grant EG et al: False-negative duplex Doppler studies in children with hepatic artery thrombosis after liver transplantation. AJR 1990;154:573

242. Hoffer FA, Teele RL, Lillehei CW, Vacanti JP: Infected bilomas and hepatic artery thrombosis in infant recipients of liver transplants. Interventional radiology and medical therapy as an alternative to retransplantation. Radiology 1988;169:435

243. Cantarero JM, LLorente JG, San Millian JM et al: Duplex Doppler in the diagnosis of hepatic artery stenosis after liver transplantation. J Ultrasound Med 1990;9:S1

244. Longley DG, Skolnick ML, Sheahan DG: Acute allograft rejection in liver transplant recipients: lack of correlation with loss of hepatic artery diastolic flow. Radiology 1988;169:417

245. Marder DM, DeMarino GB, Sumkin JH, Sheahan DG: Liver transplant rejection: value of the resistive index in Doppler US of hepatic arteries. Radiology 1989;173:127

246. Dalen K, Day DL, Ascher NL et al: Imaging of vascular complications after hepatic transplantation. AJR 1988;150:1285

247. Bowen A, Keslar PJ, Newman B, Hashida Y: Adrenal hemorrhage after liver transplantation. Radiology 1990;176:85

248. Sauerbrei E: Ultrasound of the common bile duct. p. 1. In Sanders RC, Hill MC (eds): Ultrasound Annual 1983. Raven Press, New York, 1983

249. Itzchuk Y, Rubinstein Z, Shilo R: Ultrasound in tropical diseases. p. 69. In Sarder RC, Hill MC (eds): Ultrasound Annual 1983. Raven Press, New York, 1983

250. Orloff MJ: The liver. p. 1009. In Davis C (ed): Textbook of Surgery. 10th Ed. WB Saunders, Philadelphia

6

Biliary System

Carol A. Mittelstaedt

The biliary system became one of the primary areas for evaluation by ultrasound in the 1980s. With the use of the newer high-resolution sector real-time ultrasound systems, the gallbladder and extrahepatic ducts can be identified in most patients despite their body habitus or clinical condition. Unlike radiographic evaluation, ultrasound may be performed rapidly, repeatedly (if necessary), without radiation or contrast administration, and at the bedside in critically ill patients. As a result, ultrasound has become the primary tool in evaluation of the gallbladder and the jaundiced patient. It is also an accurate and reliable technique for evaluating the common bile duct and intrahepatic ducts and is effective for evaluating neighboring structures (e.g., the liver and pancreas).

TECHNIQUE

Preparation

For an optimal examination of the gallbladder, the patient should fast for at least 6 hours prior to the ultrasound study. It is desirable to perform the gallbladder ultrasound after an overnight fast whenever possible. This fasting allows for maximum distension of the gallbladder, which promotes better visualization not only of the gallbladder but also of intraluminal and/or wall abnormalities. A satisfactory gallbladder examination can usually still be performed in an emergency or a critically ill patient, as many of these patients have eaten little to nothing anyway.

It is also helpful for the patient to have been fasting when the extrahepatic ducts are studied. Because one study is rarely performed without the other, this fasting is needed mainly for gallbladder distension.

Scan Technique

Evaluation of the biliary system by real-time ultrasound can average 10 to 15 minutes in trained hands. The gallbladder can be quickly identified and meticulously scanned in various scan planes and body positions. In addition, with sector real-time systems, one can quickly identify the extrahepatic ducts because the real-time system has the advantage of easy maneuverability of the scanhead.

Gallbladder and Ducts

Examination of the gallbladder begins with the patient supine. In the sagittal plane, the gallbladder is located by identifying the major fissure of the liver (Fig. 6-1). Once located, the gallbladder is scanned very slowly from its medial to lateral borders, with at least three freeze-frame images taken. It is then scanned transversely from its inferior to superior extent (Fig. 6-1). The transducer frequently used for the examination depends on the patient's body habitus. The highest-frequency transducer possible should be used, as this affords better resolution. The depth of the gallbladder should be matched to the focal zone of the transducer.

249

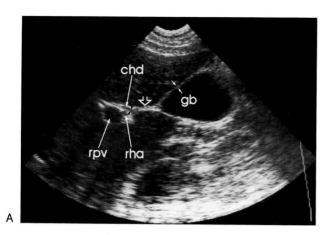
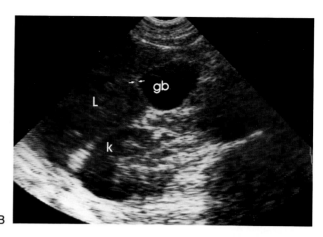

Fig. 6-1.   Normal gallbladder. **(A)** Sagittal supine real-time scan. The gallbladder *(gb)* is seen as an oval anechoic structure with a thin wall (small arrows). It is located by identifying the major fissure (open arrow) of the liver. The internal diameter (arrowheads) of the common hepatic duct *(chd)* is measured anterior to the right portal vein *(rpv)*. *(rha,* right hepatic artery). **(B)** Transverse supine scan. The gallbladder *(gb)* is seen as a thin-walled (arrows) anechoic structure in the area of the major fissure. The gallbladder wall is most easily measured next to the liver *(L)*. *(k,* right kidney.)

During examination of the gallbladder, the extrahepatic ducts are always evaluated. With the patient in the same supine position as above, several sagittal scans of the common hepatic duct are obtained following sagittal scans of the gallbladder. The common hepatic duct can be seen as a small anechoic tubular structure anterior to the right portal vein on this projection (Fig. 6-1). Although it is impossible to tell exactly where the common hepatic duct ends and the common bile duct begins (the cystic duct is not generally identified), there is a general rule that the common hepatic duct is the portion of the common duct located above the level of the gallbladder on sagittal scans and the common bile duct is the portion located inferiorly.

When examining in the transverse plane, the common bile duct can be quickly identified by finding the long axes of the main and right portal veins. The duct can be seen anterior to the portal vein (Fig. 6-2). This plane parallels the costal margin in most patients. As such, the transducer is placed in an oblique position. In a straight transverse plane, the bile duct can be seen anterior and lateral to the portal vein, with the common hepatic artery anterior and medial to the portal vein (Fig. 6-2C & D). The bile duct and hepatic artery should not be confused. If there is a question, the common hepatic artery can be followed back to its origin in the celiac artery by using the real-time system.

Once supine views are obtained, the patient is positioned in the left lateral decubitus position, which often affords improved clarity and visualization of abnormalities.[1] No gallbladder examination should be done in only one position unless the patient is clinically not able to be

moved. Sagittal and transverse views of the gallbladder are also obtained with the patient in the decubitus position. If stones were suspected in the supine views, evaluation for movement of the stones is necessary (Fig. 6-3). As with examination of the gallbladder, views of the extrahepatic ducts are again obtained in this position by the technique described above. Sometimes the ducts are poorly imaged in the supine position and can be seen only in the decubitus position. Some investigators report an accuracy of 96 percent in identifying the common bile duct in the decubitus view.[2]

If the gallbladder is quite high or there is still a question after the decubitus examination, the gallbladder may be examined with the patient upright (Fig. 6-3C). Once again, the sagittal and transverse views are obtained. This change in position may demonstrate a shifting position of stones, which confirms their presence.[3] It may also allow a different view of the extrahepatic ducts.

Examining the patient in the prone position can be helpful in the diagnosis of stones, sludge, or polyps in the gallbladder.[4] These abnormalities are best (or exclusively) demonstrated in the prone position in some cases[4] (Fig. 6-4). Examination in the prone position is particularly helpful to avoid reverberation artifacts from the abdominal wall or bowel.[4] When performing the examination with the patient in this position, the examiner scans in the lateral intercostal space at the right midaxillary line. Sometimes the transducer must be moved more anteriorly or posteriorly until the gallbladder is demonstrated, using the liver as an acoustic window.[4] To obtain the long axis of the gallbladder, it may be necessary to scan in oblique planes.[4]

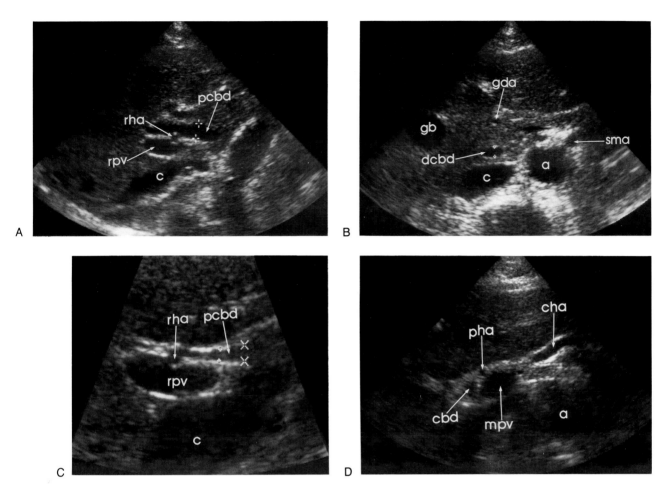

Fig. 6-2. Common bile duct. Case 1. **(A)** The normal proximal common bile duct (*pcbd*, 6 mm) is seen anterior to the right hepatic artery *(rha)* and right portal vein *(rpv)* on a long-axis view. (*c*, inferior vena cava.) **(B)** On transverse view, the distal common bile duct (*dcbd*, 4.1 mm) is seen within the pancreatic head. (*gb*, gallbladder; *gda*, gastroduodenal artery; *sma*, superior mesenteric artery; *a*, aorta; *c*, inferior vena cava.) **(C)** Case 2. Transverse cone-down view showing the normal proximal duct (*pcbd*, calipers, 2–4 mm) anterior to the right hepatic artery *(rha)* and right portal vein *(rpv)*. (*c*, inferior vena cava.) **(D)** Case 3. Transverse oblique scan showing the common hepatic artery *(cha)* extending from the area of the celiac artery and running toward the main portal vein *(mpv)*. The common bile duct *(cbd)* is seen anterolateral to the main portal vein, with the proper hepatic artery *(pha)* more anteromedial. (*a*, aorta.)

Cystic Duct

If the examiner is specifically interested in evaluating the cystic duct, the patient may be placed in Trendelenburg's position (with the head lower than the feet). Since most ultrasound tables do not tilt, this position may be achieved by placing a pillow and/or rolled sheets under the patient's hips. Then the gallbladder and cystic duct may be scanned in the sagittal and transverse planes. In addition, it may be helpful to scan the cystic duct with the patient in the left and/or right lateral decubitus position (with the patient still in Trendelenburg's position). These positions appear to improve visualization of the long axis of the cystic duct for maximum visualization

(Fig. 6-5). Still, in many patients, a complete evaluation of the cystic duct cannot be obtained.

With careful examination, the normal cystic duct may be demonstrated in 51 percent of patients with a normal common bile duct and a normal gallbladder.[5] It is seen much more often when the common bile duct is dilated.[5] To visualize the distal cystic duct, the examiner scans sagittally with the patient supine and in the right lateral decubitus position[5] (Fig. 6-6). The distal cystic duct is located posterior to the common bile duct in 95 percent of patients and anterior to the common bile duct in 5 percent.[5]

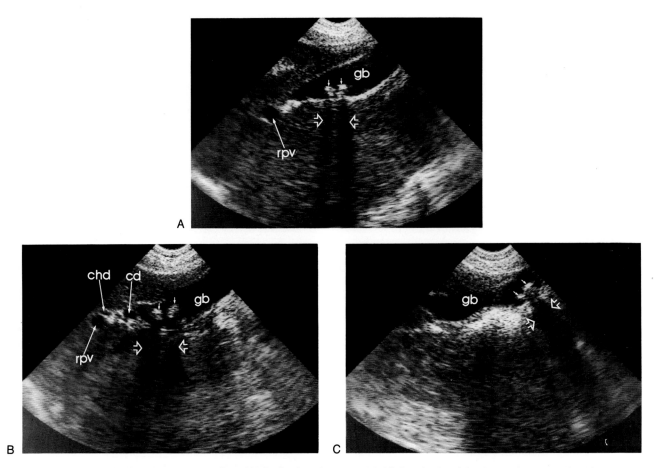

Fig. 6-3. Gallbladder, stone motion. **(A)** Sagittal supine scan. Multiple echodensities (arrows) are seen layering within the posterior gallbladder *(gb)*. There is shadowing (open arrows) posterior to the stones. *(rpv,* right portal vein.) **(B)** Left lateral decubitus sagittal scan. The stones (arrows) have moved to the dependent portion of the gallbladder *(gb)* toward the gallbladder neck. The stones are associated with shadowing (open arrows). *(chd,* common hepatic duct; *cd,* cystic duct; *rpv,* right portal vein.) **(C)** Upright sagittal scan. The stones (arrows) are seen layering out in the dependent portion (fundus) of the gallbladder *(gb)* in this position. (open arrows, shadowing.)

Gallbladder Dynamics

Gallbladder contractility has been investigated.[6] For evaluation of gallbladder contraction, the subject undergoes an overnight fast of 8 to 12 hours, with the gallbladder volume measured before and 45 to 60 minutes after (residual gallbladder volume) a standard fatty meal consisting of 60 ml of Neo-Cholex. The volume measurements are made by using the following formula: volume = 0.52 (width × height × length).[6] By using the equation, 100 percent × (fasting gallbladder volume − residual gallbladder volume)/(fasting gallbladder volume), the percent gallbladder contraction is calculated.[6]

The gallbladder volume may be calculated by using the sum-of-cylinders method, but this technique is mod-

erately cumbersome and time-consuming.[7] Instead, a simple ellipsoid method may be applied to the gallbladder images; this yields a reasonable volume approximation.[7] This volume is nearly identical to that obtained by the sum-of-cylinders method.[7] The ellipsoid method uses the following formula: $V = \pi/6(L \times W \times H)$, where L is the length, W is the width, and H is the height or depth.[7] This method may be readily used for clinical or investigational assessment of the gallbladder volume.[7]

The degree of gallbladder contraction has been shown to vary widely in a given person, and a single recording may be misleading.[6] A wide range of normal values have been demonstrated, with the fasting gallbladder volume ranging from 1.9 to 45.5 ml, the residual gallbladder volume from 0.1 to 21.0 ml, and the percent gallbladder

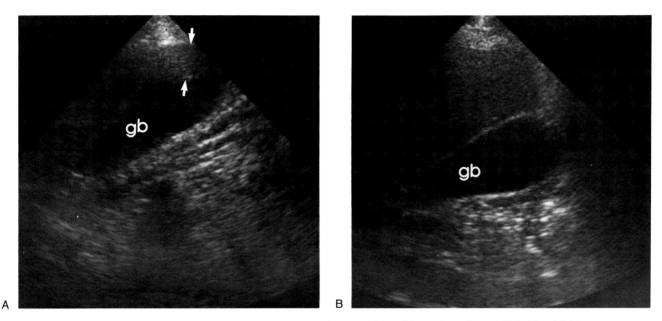

Fig. 6-4. Gallbladder, prone view. **(A)** Sagittal supine scan in a thin patient. The gallbladder *(gb)* is very superficial, and there is reverberation artifact (arrows) within the fundus anteriorly. **(B)** Sagittal prone scan of the same gallbladder *(gb).* The anterior gallbladder wall is much better defined without any artifact.

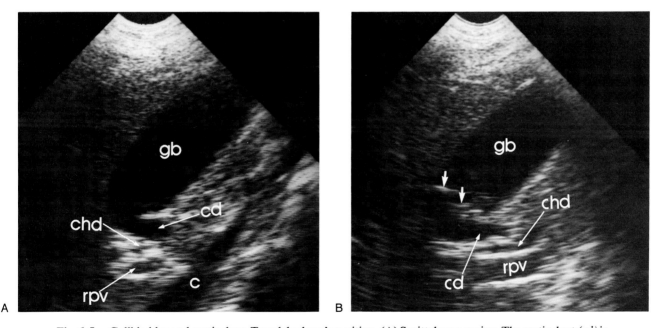

Fig. 6-5. Gallbladder and cystic duct, Trendelenburg's position. **(A)** Sagittal scan supine. The cystic duct *(cd)* is clearly identified medial to the gallbladder *(gb).* (*chd,* common hepatic duct; *rpv,* right portal vein; *c,* inferior vena cava.) **(B)** Sagittal scan slightly right lateral decubitus. The cystic duct *(cd)* is seen anterior to the common hepatic duct *(chd)* and right portal vein *(rpv).* There were stones in the gallbladder *(gb);* the interface with the lateral edge of the stones (arrows) is noted.

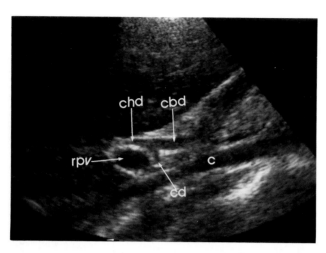

Fig. 6-6. Normal cystic duct. Sagittal left lateral decubitus view demonstrating the normal distal cystic duct *(cd)* posterior to the common bile duct *(cbd)*. *(chd,* common hepatic duct; *rpv,* right portal vein; *c,* inferior vena cava.)

contraction from −10 to 99 percent.[6] The percent of gallbladder contraction varies from 60 to 87 percent in 60 percent of subjects.[6] The percent gallbladder contraction values then vary by more than 20 percent; in 20 percent of the subjects, it varies by more than 40 percent.[6] Use of a contraction value of 20 percent as a cutoff level to indicate cystic duct patency remains justifiable as a means of assessing eligibility for either oral dissolution therapy or biliary lithotripsy.[6]

It may be desirable to measure the contraction of the gallbladder in response to cholecystokinin (CCK) when cystic duct obstruction is suspected.[8] Although the demonstration of significant contraction after CCK administration is strong evidence of cystic duct patency, the converse does not always hold true. Failure of contraction is not specific.[8,9]

The effects of fatty meals and CCK have been assessed.[10] Although the peak levels of CCK (a potent stimulant of gallbladder contraction) are significantly higher after administration of CCK than after the ingestion of a fatty meal, this does not significantly affect the emptying rate or maximal contraction.[10] As such, the administration of intravenous CCK does not offer any advantage over the ingestion of fatty meals in radiographic studies of the gallbladder involving induced contraction.[10]

Other investigations have also studied the pharmacologic effects on gallbladder contraction. With ceruletide administration, a significant contraction occurs earlier than after a fatty meal (40 versus 25 minutes) and leads to a much more marked reduction in area (69 versus 53 percent).[11] However, the end of the contraction does not differ (50 versus 45 minutes).[11]

Ductal Evaluation with Cholelithiasis/Choledocholithiasis

If stones are identified in the gallbladder, careful evaluation of the extrahepatic ducts, as well as of the pancreas, must be performed. The bile duct is scrutinized for stones with the patient in the supine and left and right lateral decubitus positions (Figs. 6-1 and 6-2 to 6-4). Some investigators recommend the 45 or 90 degree right anterior oblique position to better demonstrate the duct.[12] Visualization of the distal common duct is improved by placing the patient in the upright or semiupright position[13] (Fig. 6-7). At times, the patient may be given 32 oz (four glasses) of water to drink to better evaluate the distal common duct (the retroduodenal and intrapancreatic parts). The scans may then be performed transversely in the upright and/or right lateral decubitus position (Fig. 6-8). (The right lateral decubitus position allows the air in the stomach to float to the fundus, and the second portion of the duodenum tends to fill with fluid, nicely outlining the head of the pancreas.)

Visualization of choledocholithiasis may be improved by using certain alterations in the technique: filling the duodenum and gastric antrum with drinking water (right lateral decubitus position), scanning 45 to 60 minutes after a fatty meal, and changing the patient's position during scanning.[14] Additionally, the patient may be placed in the knee-chest position or Trendelenburg's position.[14] In this position, it may be possible to move stones from the distal to the dependent proximal position of the common duct, where they are more easily detected.[14]

Ultrasound may successfully identify choledocholithiasis with a sensitivity of 75 percent.[14] False-negative results may be produced by (1) obscuration of the distal duct by overlying bowel gas, (2) missing a small stone in a nondilated bile duct, or (3) misdiagnosing soft pigment or an impacted stone with an atypical hypoechoic image in the distal duct as a tumor.[14] The specificity is 83 percent, with false-positive results produced by various hyperechoic lesions in the neck of the gallbladder, cystic duct, and periampullary region.[14] The overall diagnostic accuracy of gallstones in the extrahepatic bile duct by ultrasound is 80 percent.[14]

Since stones in the gallbladder and/or duct may be associated with pancreatitis, the pancreas should be evaluated for its parenchymal echopattern, mass effect, and ductal size and configuration. With careful scanning, the main pancreatic duct can be identified in the body of the pancreas on a transverse scan (Fig. 6-9). The parenchymal pattern of the pancreas should be similar to or denser than that of the liver. If the pancreas is lucent or a mass effect is identified, pancreatitis should be considered.

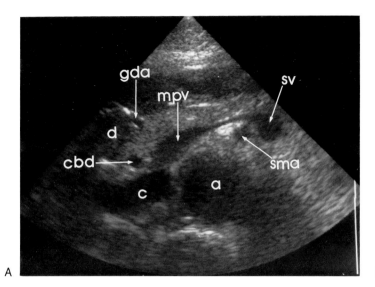

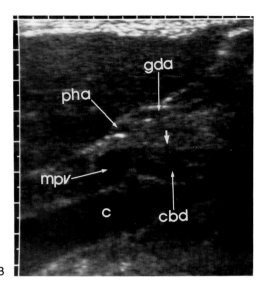

A

B

Fig. 6-7. Distal common bile duct. Upright. **(A)** Transverse scan. The distal common bile duct *(cbd)* can be seen within the inferolateral portion of the pancreatic head. The fluid within the duodenum *(d)* improves the visualization of the lateral border of the pancreatic head. (*gda,* gastroduodenal artery; *mpv,* main portal vein; *sv,* splenic vein; *sma,* superior mesenteric artery; *a,* aorta; *c,* inferior vena cava.) **(B)** Sagittal scan, magnified. The distal common bile duct *(cbd)* is noted to be running posterior to the pancreatic head with the gastroduodenal artery *(gda)* running anteriorly. The proper hepatic artery *(pha)* is at the superior margin of the pancreas with the main portal vein *(mpv).* The pancreatic duct (arrow) can be seen in the center of the pancreatic head. (*c,* inferior vena cava.)

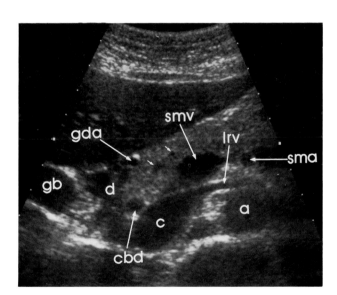

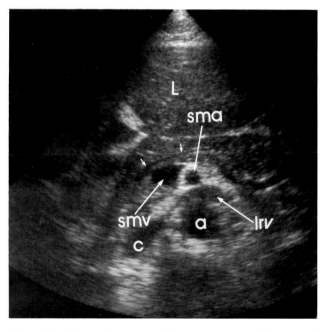

Fig. 6-8. Distal common bile duct, water technique. Right lateral decubitus view. The pancreatic head is seen outlined by the fluid-filled duodenum *(d)* with the inferior vena cava *(c)* posterior and the superior mesenteric vein *(smv)* medial. (*sma,* superior mesenteric artery; *a,* aorta; *gb,* gallbladder; small arrows, pancreatic duct; *gda,* gastroduodenal artery; *lrv,* left renal vein; *cbd,* common bile duct.)

Fig. 6-9. Normal pancreas. Transverse scan. The normal pancreas is seen, with the pancreatic duct (arrows) seen as a tubular lucency within the body (and head) of the pancreas. The pancreas is isoechoic to the liver *(L).* (*c,* inferior vena cava; *a,* aorta; *sma,* superior mesenteric artery; *smv,* superior mesenteric vein; *lrv,* left renal vein.)

Ductal Evaluation with Dilated Ducts

If no gallstones are identified but dilated intra- or extrahepatic ducts are seen, a careful search for the etiology should be undertaken. One should identify the level of obstruction (e.g., distal common bile duct or common hepatic duct, intrahepatic dilatation without common bile duct dilatation) and then search for the etiology. The pancreas should always be evaluated for mass effect. Unfortunately, not all pancreases can be visualized, because of overlying bowel gas and/or body habitus. (Evaluation of the pancreas is thoroughly discussed in Ch. 7.) The examination is not complete until an evaluation for lymphadenopathy in the porta hepatis and metastatic liver disease has been undertaken.

Biliary Dynamics

Dynamic changes have been demonstrated with biliary dilatation. The common hepatic duct can be evaluated before and after fat ingestion.[15] In normal patients, the common hepatic duct remains the same or decreases in caliber after a fatty meal. A response is abnormal if a normal-sized duct increases in size or a slightly dilated duct remains the same size or increases in size. Evaluation before and after a fatty meal may aid in evaluation of a common hepatic duct that is equivocally or mildly dilated and can indicate the need for further invasive studies. After the fat enters the duodenum, CCK is released by the intestinal mucosa. The release of bile into the duodenum is mediated by CCK. It produces gall-bladder contraction, relaxation of the sphincter of Oddi, and increased bile flow from the liver.[15]

A number of investigators have studied the effect of a fatty meal on biliary dynamics.[16-18] The common duct diameter has been studied after a fatty meal of Lipomul (1.5 ml/lb).[16] The rationale for this study is as follows: (1) ingested fat causes the release of endogenous CCK into the bloodstream; (2) circulating CCK causes gallbladder contraction, increases hepatic bile flow, and relaxes the sphincter of Oddi; and (3) the net effect of these actions is enhanced bile flow through the common duct without any increase in its intraluminal pressure or caliber.[16] The fatty meal acts as a stress test when there is partial common duct obstruction. This is because the pressure of the increased bile flow enlarges the bile duct proximal to the area of obstruction, which unmasks the partial common duct obstruction.[16] It is proposed that in the presence of partial common duct obstruction, fat-induced increases in bile flow related to increased circulating levels of CCK are associated with an increase in diameter of the common bile duct.[16]

The study is performed as follows: (1) the patient is given a standardized fatty meal after control measurements of common duct diameter; (2) repeat measurements of the duct are made after 45 minutes; (3) if the duct has increased or decreased by more than 1 mm, the test is complete and is interpreted as positive or negative; and (4) if the 45-minute measurement differs from the premeal value by 1 mm or more, the measurement is repeated at 60 minutes and the test is then considered complete[16] (Fig. 6.10). A true change in common duct diameter occurs only if the size change is 2 mm or

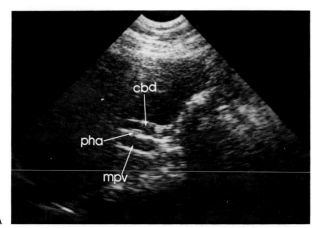 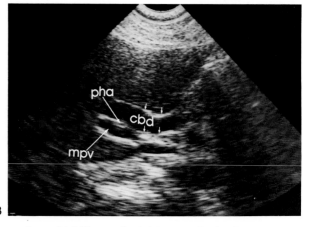

A   B

Fig. 6-10. Dilated common bile duct. Postcholecystectomy patient with biliary colic. **(A)** Long-axis view in the left lateral decubitus position. The proximal common bile duct *(cbd)* seen anterior to the main portal vein *(mpv)* measures 6 mm. (*pha,* proper hepatic artery.) **(B)** Long-axis left lateral decubitus scan (same location and magnification as in Fig. A). Ten minutes after a fatty meal, the duct *(cbd)* is rescanned; it has dilated to 10 mm. This represents an abnormal response. The convex ventral configuration (arrows) is more pronounced on this view. At ERCP, the patient was found to have ampullary stenosis. (*mpv,* main portal vein; *pha,* proper hepatic artery.)

more.[16] The ductal diameter must be monitored for at least 45 to 60 minutes.[16]

This test can also be used on postoperative cholecystectomy patients. In these patients, the diameter of the common hepatic duct is 5 mm or less; the response to a fatty meal is helpful in evaluating those whose common hepatic duct is 5 mm or greater.[15] With the gallbladder removed, the response of the normal duct should remain the same. Even if the common duct is mildly dilated (6 to 10 mm) before a fatty meal, a decrease of 5 mm or less seems to indicate normal bile duct dynamics and excludes the possibility of obstruction.[15] If the duct is of normal caliber or slightly dilated before fat ingestion and increases in caliber after fat ingestion, this is a strong indicator of bile duct abnormality[15] (Fig. 6-10).

Although fatty-meal stimulation significantly improves the diagnostic accuracy of ductal evaluation, there are problems.[17] The problem is in the situation when the duct does not change in size after fatty-meal stimulation. Investigations have shown that 84 percent of those with no change have no obstruction.[17] As such, a dilated common bile duct that does not change in size after a fatty meal is not a specific indicator of obstruction.[17] Perhaps in these patients, the increased bile flow produced by the stimulation by the fatty meal is balanced by sphincter relaxation.[17] The most probable explanation for these findings is the loss of elasticity of the duct wall owing to chronic dilatation, inflammation, or aging.[17]

In cases of suspected partial common duct obstruction, the specificity of the fatty meal is found to be 100 percent with a sensitivity of 74 percent.[16] Others have reported a sensitivity of 84 percent, an accuracy of a positive test of 84 percent and an accuracy of a negative test of 93 percent.[18] A positive finding always indicates partial common duct obstruction.[16] This test has been believed to have a greater sensitivity for accurately identifying patients with sphincter of Oddi dysfunction than patients with common bile duct stones.[16] The former patients appear to have an abnormality that is either persistent (stenosis, types of dyskinesia); or provoked by the challenge of a fatty meal (certain types of dyskinesia).[16] A fatty-meal sonogram is thought to be a useful screening test for evaluating patients for suspected partial common duct obstruction.[16]

Other

If the patient is referred to ultrasound for right upper quadrant pain and the biliary examination is negative, careful examination of other structures (e.g., right kidney, diaphragm, liver, and vessels) should be performed. Liver or kidney abnormalities may then be identified.

Utility of Oral Cholecystogram

What is the future of oral cholecystography (OCG)? Has gallbladder sonography completely replaced this procedure as the technique of choice for all gallbladder examinations? OCG is not as sensitive as ultrasound in the detection of small stones and cannot be performed as expeditiously as radionuclide examinations in the prompt diagnosis of cystic duct obstruction, nor is it as accurate as computed tomography (CT) in the determination of gallstone composition and detection of calcifications.[19] However, OCG does provide sufficient information regarding cystic duct patency and gallbladder function and is accurate in determining the number and size of stones.[19]

The approval by the Food and Drug Administration in 1988 of ursodeoxycholic acid for clinical use for oral dissolution of cholesterol gallstones ensures the continued use of OCG.[19] Although not commonly used in the past, its prognostic information regarding the integrity of the gallbladder wall (i.e., function) may be valid in this era of emphasis on conservative management of gallstones.[19] To perform and interpret an OCG, the radiologist must have a basic knowledge of pharmacology of biliary contrast agents, proper patient preparation, the use of meticulous radiographic techniques, and an understanding of interpretive principles enabling the understanding of the role of OCG in current clinical imaging and management alternatives of nonemergent gallstone disease.[19]

NORMAL ANATOMY

Gallbladder

The gallbladder is a conical musculomembranous sac lying in a fossa under the liver.[20] Its segments include (1) the fundus—a hemispheric blind end, (2) the body—the portion between the fundus and neck, and (3) the neck—a narrow tubelike structure that tapers to the cystic duct[20] (Fig. 6-11). The fundus is usually close to the hepatic flexure of the colon and duodenum.[21] The neck of the gallbladder is oriented posteromedially toward the porta hepatis, with the fundus situated lateral, caudal, and anterior to the neck.[21] The size and shape of the gallbladder are variable. When relaxed, the gallbladder is 7 to 10 cm in length and 2 to 3 cm in width.[20] It has a capacity of 30 to 50 ml.[20] The Rokitansky-Aschoff sinuses of the gallbladder are small outpouchings of the mucosa of the gallbladder that extend into the underlying connective tissue and sometimes into the muscular layer.[20] They communicate directly with the lumen of the gallbladder.[20]

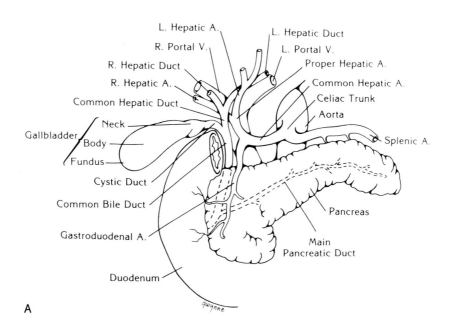

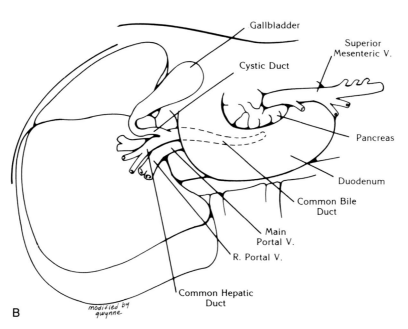

Fig. 6-11. Gallbladder and bile ducts. The relationship of the hepatic vessels, ducts, and pancreas is shown in **(A)** a frontal and **(B)** a lateral projection. (Fig. A modified from Sauerbrei,[32] and Fig. B modified from Mueller et al.,[393] with permission.)

Bile secreted by the liver contains water, cholesterol, bile salts, bile acids, bilirubin, lecithin in micellar complexes, inorganic ions, and mucoproteins secreted by epithelium. Bile salts (sodium salts of taurocholic and glycocholic acids) aid in maintaining cholesterol in solution. The gallbladder concentrates bile by selective absorption of water, inorganic ions, and small amounts of bile salts. Contraction and partial emptying of the gallbladder occur when foods, especially fatty ones, or other stimulants enter the duodenum. The gallbladder activity is mediated through CCK, a hormone that is released from the duodenum into the blood.[20]

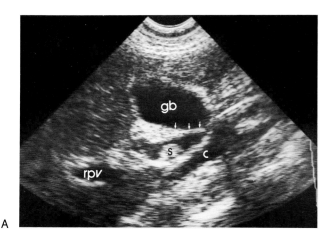 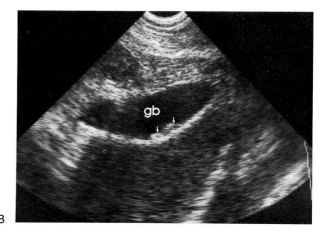

Fig. 6-12. Gallbladder, folded neck. **(A)** Sagittal left lateral decubitus scan. There is a stone *(S)* in the neck of the gallbladder *(gb)*. The gallbladder is folded (arrows) on itself in the region of the neck. (*rpv,* right portal vein; *c,* inferior vena cava.) **(B)** Transverse long-axis view of the gallbladder *(gb)* in the right lateral decubitus position. In this view, the gallbladder is unfolded and the stones (arrows) are clearly seen within the gallbladder.

Ultrasound Appearance

On ultrasound, the gallbladder is seen as an anechoic fluid-filled ellipsoid structure adjacent to and indenting the inferomedial aspect of the right lobe of the liver (Fig. 6-1). It is situated along the junction of the medial segment of the left lobe and the right lobe.[22] A linear echodensity connecting the gallbladder to the right or main portal vein is seen on ultrasound in 68 percent of cases[23] (Fig. 6-1A). This linear echodensity is the main lobar fissure of the liver and appears to be a reliable anatomic indicator of gallbladder location.[23] The gallbladder lies in the posterior and caudal aspect of this fissure, with the right portal vein under the medial segment of the left hepatic lobe before it bifurcates and enters the parenchyma of the right lobe.[23] The neck of the gallbladder usually is in contact with the main segment of the right portal vein or the main portal vein near the origin of the left portal vein.[23] A redundant or folded neck of the gallbladder should not be confused with a dilated common bile duct[24] (Fig. 6-12). Ninety-eight percent of gallbladders can be visualized by ultrasound.[25]

In its distended state, the gallbladder has a smooth wall that is usually not measurable. The anterior wall is normally seen as a thin, strongly reflective structure, whereas the posterior wall may be difficult to evaluate because of transmission of sound and its contact with the bowel[26] (Fig. 6-1A). The wall is never more than 3-mm thick, even in children.[27] The gallbladder wall measurement is most accurate if it is obtained along the portion of the wall that is perpendicular to the sound beam[28] (Fig. 6-1). In addition, it is best to measure the anterior wall adjacent to the liver.

The gallbladder may vary in size and shape. It is usu-

ally 8 cm in length and less than 3.5 cm in diameter in adults and children.[21,27] In neonates, the mean gallbladder width/length ratio is 0.37.[29] It may be dilated in diabetics, bedridden patients with protracted illness or pancreatitis, and patients taking anticholinergics.[21]

Contracted Gallbladder

A well-contracted gallbladder has a striking appearance on ultrasound.[26] It changes from a single to a double concentric structure with three components: (1) a strongly reflective outer contour, (2) a poorly reflective inner contour, and (3) an anechoic area between the two contours[26] (Fig. 6-13). After a fatty meal, 69 percent of

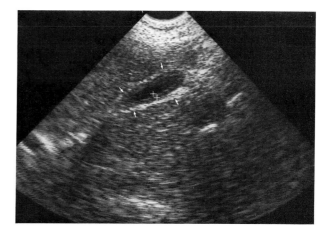

Fig. 6-13. Contracted gallbladder. Sagittal scan. The contracted gallbladder is seen as a double concentric structure with a strongly reflective outer contour (arrows), a poorly reflective inner contour, and an anechoic area between the two.

gallbladders completely contract, while 31 percent incompletely contract.[26]

Cystic Duct

The junction of the cystic duct and common bile duct is usually visualized immediately below the porta hepatis, but it may be at a considerably lower (distal) level[5] (Fig. 6-6). In most patients (95 percent), the distal cystic duct is posterior to the common bile duct.[5] It has an average diameter of 1.8 mm with average length of 1 to 2 cm demonstrated.[5]

Normal Variants

A variety of folds and kinks are noted in the body of 14.5 percent of gallbladders[30] (Figs. 6-12, 6-14, and 6-15); the most common is at the incisura between the body and infundibulum analogous to the junctional fold[30] (Fig. 6-14). Care should be taken not to mistake septations or a phrygian cap for stones.[31] The phrygian cap is a fold toward the fundus of the gallbladder in the distal segment[22] (Fig. 6-15). It may be caused by angulation, kinking, or circumferential constriction of the body of the gallbladder, producing an apparently expanded bulbous end to the fundus.[20]

Bile Ducts

The extrahepatic biliary system (gallbladder and extrahepatic ducts) maintains direct connection between the liver and the gastrointestinal tract and serves as an essential link in the enterohepatic circulation.[20] The

ducts passively transfer bile from the liver to the duodenum, directly or via the gallbladder.[20] The extrahepatic duct system has two functions: the storage and concentration of bile and the delivery of bile to the duodenum.[20] Bile flows if the intraductal pressure is lower than the hepatic secretory pressure. Pressure differences are affected by (1) activity of the sphincter at the distal end of the common bile duct, (2) gallbladder filling and resorption of bile in the gallbladder, and (3) bile flow from the liver.[32] Contractility at the distal sphincter is probably the most important dynamic factor in affecting intraductal pressure. Normally, there is a regular cycle of contractions and relaxations causing flow of bile into the duodenum. The common bile duct has no motor role in bile flow.

The right and left hepatic ducts emerge from the liver parenchyma in the porta hepatis and unite to form the common hepatic duct, which passes caudal and medial (Fig. 6-11). It is joined by the cystic duct to form the common bile duct, which descends along the free border of the lesser omentum for a variable distance, crossing behind the first portion of the duodenum and entering the parenchyma of the head of the pancreas. It then turns somewhat toward the right and enters the second portion of the duodenum, where it ends at the ampulla of Vater (Fig. 6-11). In its supraduodenal segment, the common bile duct is situated lateral to the hepatic artery and anterior to the portal vein (Fig. 6-2). As it descends behind the duodenal bulb and enters the pancreas, the duct becomes more posterior, lying close to the anterior margin of the inferior vena cava (Figs. 6-7 and 6-8). Within the liver parenchyma, the bile ducts follow the same course as the portal venous and hepatic arterial branches. All are encased in a common collagenous sheath, forming

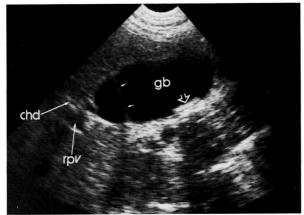

A

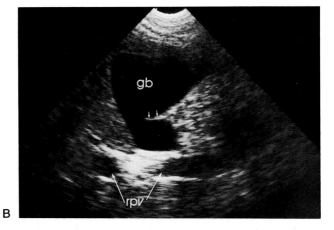

B

Fig. 6-14. Gallbladder, junctional fold. **(A)** Sagittal scan. A fold (arrows) or kink is seen at the incisura between the body and infundibulum of the gallbladder *(gb)*. On this view, it appears more like a septum. *(rpv,* right portal vein; *chd,* common hepatic duct; open arrow, stones.) **(B)** Transverse oblique scan. The fold (arrows) in the gallbladder *(gb)* is more clearly defined in this view. *(rpv,* right portal vein.)

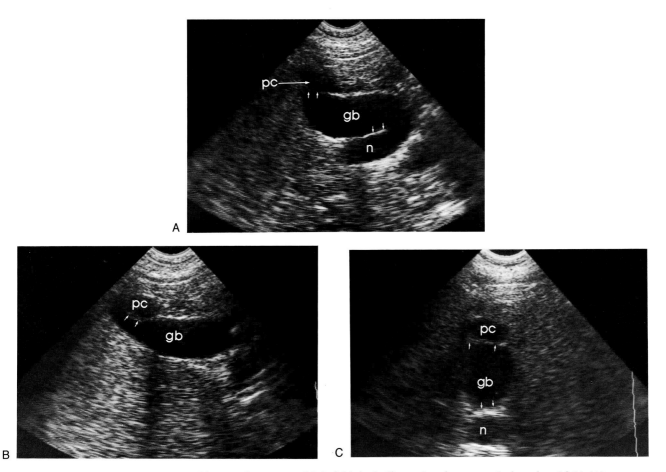

Fig. 6-15. Phrygian cap. In this case, there are multiple folds including a phrygian cap and a junctional fold. **(A)** Left lateral decubitus sagittal scan. Folds (arrows) are demonstrated in the fundus and neck *(n)* ends of the gallbladder *(gb)*. A phrygian cap *(pc)* is a fold in the distal segment toward the fundus. **(B)** Oblique longitudinal view performed to open the folds demonstrate the phrygian cap *(pc)* *(gb,* gallbladder; arrows, folds.) **(C)** Upright sagittal view. With the folds (arrows), there is the appearance of three cystic structures. The more anterior one is the phrygian cap *(pc)*, and the more posterior one is the neck *(n)*, the middle section being the body of the gallbladder *(gb)*.

the so-called portal triad. The common bile duct is tethered superiorly to the liver, where the left and right hepatic ducts converge, and inferiorly, where it enters the posterior portion of the head of the pancreas. The rest of the common bile duct is relatively unfixed as it passes along the lateral edge of the hepatoduodenal ligament, with the main portal vein and proper hepatic artery superior to the pancreas.[32] The main right and left bile ducts nearly always lie anterior to the corresponding portal vein trunk. The hepatic artery may lie anterior to the portal vein, although the left hepatic artery is often posterior to the left portal vein. In the periphery of the liver, the orientation of ducts and vessels is variable.[21]

On a section at the level of the hepatoduodenal ligament (just below the porta hepatis and just above the head of the pancreas), the portal vein lies immediately anterior to the inferior vena cava and the common bile duct is situated anterolateral to the portal vein (Fig. 6-2). Slightly more inferior, the common bile duct is more posterior as it courses through the head of the pancreas. This distal duct is best seen on a transverse scan inferior to the level of the superior mesenteric vein in the region of the uncinate process[13] (Figs. 6-7 and 6-8). An anterior-to-posterior course of the common bile duct is seen on a sagittal scan, which allows differentiation of the common bile duct from the superior mesenteric vein (Fig. 6-7B). The superior mesenteric vein is slightly to the left and pursues a relatively horizontal course. The cystic duct itself is seldom visualized because of its small size.

Contours

The common bile duct may take on various contours. The normal duct courses dorsally as it goes inferiorly, making a sharp dorsal bend as it passes over the portal vein (Figs. 6-2 and 6-7B). Most dilated common bile ducts display a convex ventral configuration that allows easy differentiation from the portal vein (Fig. 6-16). The common bile duct courses caudally, medially, and dorsally in the hepatoduodenal ligament, ventral and lateral to the portal vein. At the termination of the hepatoduodenal ligament, the duct runs dorsally and continues through the dorsal part of the pancreatic head until it empties into the duodenum. As described above, the proximal end of the common bile duct is tethered by its intrahepatic tributary ducts as it merges from the porta and the distal end is fixed by surrounding pancreatic tissue. In patients with a dilated duct, the ventral convex configuration of the prepancreatic segment (hepatoduodenal ligament) occurs in most cases (Fig. 6-16). Since the duct is tethered both inferiorly and superiorly and is constrained dorsally by the portal vein, the dilated duct bows ventrally. Therefore, when a ventrally convex large tubular structure is noted in the hepatoduodenal ligament region, it may be confidently identified as a dilated duct, even when other anatomic landmarks are not imaged.[33]

In reviewing intraoperative cholangiograms, investigators have found that the transverse segment of the common bile duct is longer than 35 mm in 18 percent of dilated extrahepatic ducts and 6 percent of normal-caliber ducts. When dilated, the transverse segment may be confused with the portal and splenic veins on ultrasound. The course of the extrahepatic duct is dependent largely on the positions of the porta hepatis and the head of the pancreas and on the site of insertion of the duct into the duodenum. In 6 percent of normal patients, the extrahepatic duct has a long transverse segment that may reach or extend beyond the midline.[34]

Size

Many studies have been performed with high-resolution real-time equipment to evaluate the normal size of the extrahepatic ducts. In 98 percent of normal individuals, the common hepatic duct measures 4 mm or less as it passes anterior to the right portal vein[35] (Fig. 6-1A). This and all measurements reflect the internal dimension of the duct or the lucency and not an external measurement, which could be affected by technique. The upper limits of normal size for the common bile and hepatic ducts are thus 4 to 8 mm. In children, the lumen of the common hepatic duct increases with age but never exceeds 4 mm.[27] In neonates, the common bile duct is less than or equal to 1 mm.[29] A measurement of 6 to 8 mm in adults is equivocal.

Some investigators believe that if the common hepatic duct is greater than 4 mm, biliary obstruction is probably present; therefore, a measurement of 5 mm is considered borderline and a measurement of 6 mm is consistent with obstruction.[36] With these measurements, a sensitivity of 99 percent and a specificity of 87 percent are achieved.[36] The range of size considered normal is greater if the patient has had prior biliary surgery; the upper limit is then 10 mm.

There is a discrepancy between the radiographic and sonographic bile duct measurements.[37] The ultrasound measurement is smaller than the radiographic one (11 mm) as a result of several factors: (1) radiographic magnification, (2) ultrasound underestimation due to wall reverberation causing underestimation of lumen size, (3) possible choleretic effect of radiographic contrast material, and (4) the use of different techniques to measure different regions of the duct.[37] The choleretic effect of contrast material has been shown to significantly increase ductal size in a small percentage of cases. The radiographic magnification factor is usually 1.3. The ultrasound diameter is generally 1.5 to 2.0 mm smaller than the true size. The most important cause of the discrepancy between the ultrasound and radiographic values is the measurement of different regions of the duct by different techniques. Some investigators recommend always measuring the common hepatic duct anterior to the right portal vein.[37] Although the ultrasound measurements are generally assumed to be accu-

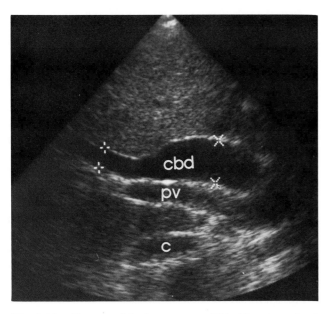

Fig. 6-16. Common bile duct contour. This dilated proximal common bile duct (*cbd,* 18 mm) is projecting ventrally as it courses inferiorly. (*pv,* portal vein; *c,* inferior vena cava.)

rate, reverberation and other artifacts can cause a slight increase or decrease in size. The artifactual thickening of the duct wall encroaches on the lumen of the fluid-filled duct, which makes the duct smaller.[37]

Distensibility

Some authors have studied the distensibility of the common bile duct.[38] Initially, the grossly dilated common hepatic duct returns to normal size within minutes. This rapid size change probably occurs only in patients without a normally functioning gallbladder. The wall of the duct is composed largely of fibroelastic tissue, and the stretch potential of the elastic fibers permits duct dilatation; the elastic recoil of the fibers is responsible for the return of the duct to normal size after relief of the obstruction.[38] In humans, the size of the common bile duct is largely determined by intraductal pressure. With an increase in intraductal pressure, the common bile duct progressively dilates to a limit governed by the elastic properties of the ductal wall.[39] Some obstructive lesions affect the elastic tone of the duct, creating irreversible damage and effectively converting the duct to a passive or "floppy tube." On ultrasound, this duct may appear normal. On direct cholangiogram, the duct quickly dilates to an abnormal size. It is postulated that in these cases the elastic network is damaged or distorted and an actual "floppy duct" phenomenon develops. The discrepancies between individual static measurements of duct caliber underscore the need for assessment by other techniques.[38]

Relationship of Ducts to Vessels

At times it may be difficult to differentiate bile ducts from vessels. Some investigators have offered suggestions in making this distinction. The "parallel-channel" sign is used to describe the image of a dilated duct. It refers to the simultaneous visualization on a transverse or sagittal scan of the right portal vein and the right hepatic duct and/or the left portal vein and the left hepatic duct. The common hepatic artery normally emerges from the celiac axis and crosses to the right to run adjacent to the portal vein and common bile duct at the porta hepatis (Figs. 6-2 and 6-11A). There it branches into the right and left hepatic arteries. In two-thirds of patients, the right hepatic artery crosses behind the common bile duct or right hepatic duct, whereas the left hepatic artery crosses anterior to the left hepatic duct (Fig. 6-11A). In most patients, on cross-section the right hepatic artery is anterior to the right portal vein (Fig. 6-1A). When the common hepatic artery arises from the superior mesenteric artery, it runs between the portal vein and common bile duct to join the superior mesenteric artery.[40] Duplex scanning of the porta hepatis may be performed to help in the identification of the common bile duct and common hepatic artery (Fig. 6-17). In 59 percent of patients, the hepatic artery is as large as or larger than the duct. Ultrasound signs that help differentiate the two structures include (1) intrinsic pulsations of the arteries; (2) indentation or displacement of structures by arteries; (3) change in the caliber of the duct during real-time ultrasound; and (4) the orientation, contour, caliber, and curvature of the tubular structures in the porta hepatis.[41]

The anatomic relationship of bile ducts to portal veins has been reassessed.[42] It has been found that the relationship of the bile ducts to the portal veins is variable. For example, it was found that within the lateral segment of the left lobe, the bile ducts were anterior to the portal vein in 41 percent of cases, posterior in 41 percent, and tortuous in 18 percent.[42] In the medial segment of the left lobe, the bile ducts were anterior in 23 percent of cases, posterior in 23 percent, tortuous in 18 percent, and not seen in 36 percent.[42] In the right lobe, the bile ducts were anterior in 53 percent of cases, posterior in 29 percent, tortuous in 6 percent, and not seen in 12 percent.[42] Within the porta hepatis, the bile ducts were anterior in 59 percent of cases, posterior in 6 percent, tortuous in 29 percent, and not seen in 6 percent.[42] Histologic examinations confirmed all these findings. In conclusion, it was found that the bile duct is more anterior in only 50 percent of cases, with the portal vein anterior in 30 percent and the two structures interlaced in 20 percent[42] (Figs. 6-18 and 6-19). As such, these findings contradict the commonly held view that the intrahepatic ducts are anterior to the portal vein and may be clinically significant for techniques such as bile duct drainage.[42]

Although tubular structures proximal to the right and left hepatic ducts are generally considered to be abnormally dilated ducts, this may no longer be true.[43] With newer, electronically focused transducers, it is now possible to reveal peripheral tubular structures paralleling portal venous branches[43] (Figs. 6-18 and 6-19). The following ducts have been visualized normally: right hepatic (100 percent), right anterior (100 percent), right posterior (88 percent), left hepatic (98 percent), left medial (62 percent), left lateral (96 percent), left lateral superior (54 percent), and left lateral inferior (54 percent).[43] Ducts proximal to the right and left hepatic ducts are 2 mm or less in diameter, and those proximal to the common hepatic ducts average 20 percent of the diameters of their accompanying portal veins.[43] No ducts proximal to the common hepatic ducts are more than 40 percent of the diameter of their respective portal vein branches, except for 4 percent of the left lateral inferior ducts.[43] As such, the visualization of parallel channels

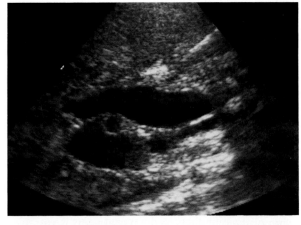

A

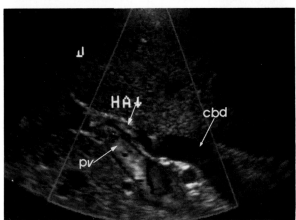

C

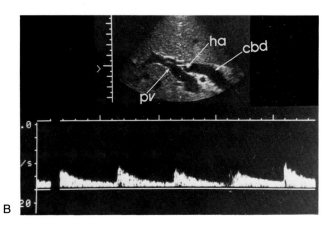

B

Fig. 6-17. Doppler of duct versus vessel. **(A)** Sagittal view of the porta hepatis showing three lucent structures, with the more anterior one measuring 14 mm. To further assess these structures, Doppler evaluation was performed. **(B)** The middle tubular structure is noted to have an arterial waveform consistent with the hepatic artery *(ha)*. (*pv*, portal vein; *cbd*, common bile duct.) **(C)** With color Doppler, flow (white) is demonstrated within the posterior tubular structure (*pv*, right portal vein) and within the hepatic artery *(HA)*. No flow is demonstrated within the more anterior structure. This represented a dilated proximal common bile duct *(cbd)*.

proximal to the right and left hepatic ducts is by itself no longer evidence for biliary dilatation.[43]

Doppler may be used to help distinguish bile ducts from vascular structures (Fig. 6-17). Sample-volume Doppler is technically difficult and tedious in evaluating suspected intrahepatic tubular abnormalities.[44] However, Duplex ultrasound may be used to distinguish prominent intrahepatic arterial branches from mild intrahepatic ductal dilatation.[45] With color Doppler, flow information is passively displayed, which facilitates the differentiation of ducts from vessels[44] (Fig. 6-18). Although there are inherent limitations of the color Doppler system, definite information may be obtained.[44]

Differentiation of the umbilical portion of the left portal vein and intrahepatic bile ducts may also be difficult. The left branch of the portal vein courses horizontally as a transverse portion and then veers anteriorly at an acute angle to form the umbilical portion. This can be demonstrated in normal and 95 percent of jaundiced patients (Fig. 6-19). The left hepatic duct does not curve anteriorly at an acute angle, but branches off to the lateral

segment, running superior to the umbilical portion. This anatomic relationship and characteristic form of the umbilical portion is useful in differentiating the portal vein from the bile duct[46] (Figs. 6-18 and 6-19).

GALLBLADDER ABNORMALITIES

Normally, the gallbladder is an elongated, smoothly marginated, anechoic structure in the right upper quadrant. Its anterior wall is a single thin, strongly reflective structure. Its posterior wall is difficult to evaluate because of sound transmission and because it is in contact with the bowel. After a fatty meal, 69 percent of gallbladders demonstrates complete contraction, with 31 percent demonstrating incomplete contraction. The most striking finding of a well-contracted gallbladder is its appearance, which changes from a single to a double concentric structure with three components: (1) a strongly reflective outer contour, (2) a poorly reflective inner contour, and (3) an anechoic area between the two[26] (Fig. 6-13).

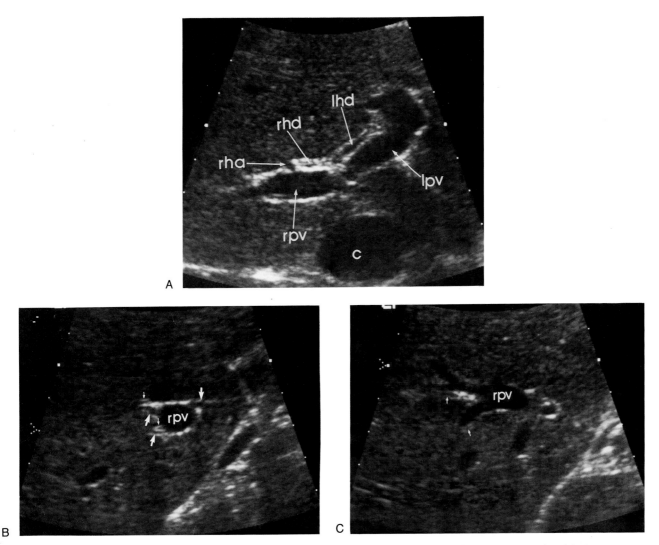

Fig. 6-18. Relationship of normal ducts to vessels, right. **(A)** Cone-down view of the porta hepatis with the normal right hepatic duct *(rhd)* seen anterior to the right portal vein *(rpv)*. The normal left hepatic duct *(lhd)* is also seen anterior to the left portal vein *(lpv)*. (*c*, inferior vena cava; *rha,* right hepatic artery.) **(B)** Magnified sagittal view of a right portal vein branch *(rpv)* (posterior) demonstrating the relationship to the segmental hepatic ducts (small arrows) and hepatic arterial branches (large arrows). **(C)** Long-axis view of an anterior right portal vein branch *(rpv)* demonstrating right anterior segmental ducts posteriorly (arrows).

The gallbladder, as a fluid-filled structure, is an ideal sonographic subject. Ultrasound evaluation of the gallbladder has become more sophisticated with the advances in technology and an increased understanding of sonographic appearances of various gallbladder disease processes. In evaluating the gallbladder for abnormalities, one must search for more than just gallstones; the gallbladder should be evaluated for size, wall thickness, intraluminal echopattern, and pericholecystic area. In addition, one must recognize the limitations of the nonspecific ultrasound findings; often ultrasound may be used as an adjunct with other imaging modalities, specifically hepatobiliary nuclear medicine.[47]

Anomalies

Developmental anomalies of the gallbladder take many forms and are of varied clinical significance. There may be agenesis, hypoplasia, hyperplasia, total reduplication to form a double gallbladder, or subtotal division of the fundus and body to create a bilobed structure.[20]

The extrahepatic biliary tract probably has more structural anomalies that result during embryologic development than does any other area of the body.[48] The embryo develops an entodermal diverticulum from the primitive gastrointestinal tract at the junction of the distal foregut and midgut in the fifth week of intrauterine

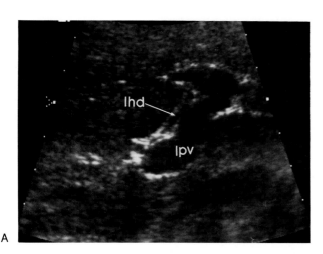
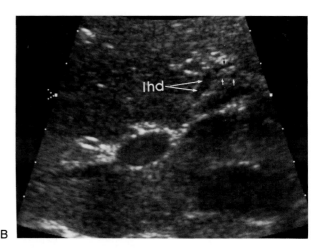

A   B

Fig. 6-19. Relationship of normal ducts to vessels, left. **(A)** Cone-down magnified view of the porta hepatis angling more toward the long axis of the left portal vein *(lpv)* than in Fig. 6-18A. The left hepatic duct *(lhd)* is seen anterior to the ascending left portal vein. **(B)** By angling the transducer slightly more to the left and cephalad, the left lateral segmental duct *(lhd)* can be seen to be branching into lateral superior (black arrow) and inferior (white arrows) subsegmental ducts.

life.[48] The primordium for the liver, extrahepatic biliary ducts, gallbladder, and ventral pancreatic bud is the diverticulum.[48] The diverticulum sacculates into a cranial and caudal bud, with the caudal sacculation responsible for the formation of the gallbladder and cystic duct. Congenital gallbladder agenesis is due to either failure of the caudal portion of the original hepatic sacculation to develop or lack of proper vacuolization of the gallbladder primordium.[48] With improper migration of the original gallbladder diverticulum, the gallbladder may be located in the abdominal wall, falciform ligament, or liver or on the left side or retroperitoneally.

Agenesis

Gallbladder agenesis may occur alone or in association with various other developmental anomalies.[48] This is a rare congenital anomaly with a reported incidence of 0.01 to 0.04 percent.[48,49] At least half of the reports are from necropsy studies.[48] This condition is usually asymptomatic until later in life when it is present as an isolated defect.[48] Approximately 23 percent of patients will develop symptoms suggestive of biliary tract disease during their lifetime.

The diagnosis of gallbladder agenesis is difficult since the gallbladder would be nonvisualized on ultrasound or other imaging modalities. This diagnosis must be considered in patients with atypical symptoms of biliary tract disease and a nonvisualized gallbladder by ultrasound or OCG.[48]

Ectopic Gallbladder

An aberrant gallbladder might have originated from abnormal migration of the gallbladder bud.[50] The cephalic bud becomes the liver and the hepatic biliary tree, while the caudal branch becomes the gallbladder and cystic duct.[50] Both branches undergo a cephalic migration and remain bound with the primitive intestine by a solid cord.[50] The most common location for an aberrant gallbladder is under the left hepatic lobe.[50] The second most common location is within the liver.[50] As such, it is important that a very thorough examination of the right upper quadrant be performed to search for the gallbladder. Its diagnosis may be inferred if the cystic intrahepatic area is pear-shaped and contracts after a fatty meal.

Bicameral Gallbladder

A bicameral gallbladder is one in which the organ's lumen is partitioned, often nearly completely, into two chambers (fundal and ductal) that are usually of approximately equal size.[51] The prevalence of this anomaly has been reported to be 4 to 7.5 percent.[51] Some classify these divided gallbladders as congenital folds, kinks due to posture, and adenomyomatous strictures.[51] This gallbladder configuration results in stagnant bile in the fundal chamber with complications of calculi and cholecystitis.[51] With an OCG, the contrast material concentrates in the ductal chamber, with the fundal chamber overlooked. Ultrasound has the advantage of visualizing both portions of the bicameral gallbladder as well as the septation between two chambers[51] (Fig. 6-20).

Double Gallbladder

Double gallbladder is a rare anomaly, occurring with an incidence of 1 in 3,000 to 4,000 with a 2:1 female/male ratio.[52-54] Only 15 percent of 150 cases of double gallbladder proven at surgery had been demonstrated radiologically.[52] It is surprising that there have been only two previous sonographic descriptions, given the frequency with which ultrasound is used to evaluate gallbladder disease.[53] OCG has a low diagnostic rate as a result of both nonvisualization of the diseased gallbladder and the difficulty in distinguishing true duplication from various anatomic anomalies, either congenital or acquired.[52]

The classification of a double gallbladder includes (1) bilobed incomplete gallbladder division with one cystic duct; (2) complete gallbladder duplication with separate cystic ducts entering the common hepatic duct; and (3) complete gallbladder duplication with a common cystic duct entering the common hepatic duct.[53] Differentiation of the different types is not possible with ultrasound.[53]

With a double gallbladder, two parallel pear-shaped cystic structures are seen in the gallbladder fossa[28] (Figs. 6-21 and 6-22). When ultrasound detects two gallbladders in the gallbladder fossa, the following diagnoses should be entertained: folded gallbladder, phrygian cap, focal adenomyomatosis, pericholecystic fluid, gallbladder diverticulum, choledochal cyst, or Ladd's bands dividing the gallbladder.[52,53] A positive diagnosis of a dou-

ble gallbladder can definitely be made if two cystic ducts are identified.[52,53] Inference of true duplication can be made if ultrasound establishes the confinement of stones to only one of the two visualized lumina[52] (Fig. 6-21). Alternatively, the presence of stones in both cystic structures does not exclude gallbladder duplication.[52] A more specific sign may be the isolated contraction of the nondiseased lobe with absent contraction of a diseased lobe[53] (Fig. 6-22).

Multiseptate Gallbladder

One of the rarest congenital malformations of the gallbladder is the multiseptate gallbladder.[55] There are only 11 cases reported in the literature.[56] All reported cases have been in females aged 15.5 to 45 years, with the presenting symptoms being pain, sometimes colicky in nature, in the right upper quadrant or in the epigastrium.[56] It is thought to be a congenital malformation, although the embryogenetic mechanism is not clear.[55] The anomaly may be due to incomplete vacuolization of the developing gallbladder bud or to persistent "wrinkling" of the gallbladder wall.[55] At pathologic examination, such a gallbladder is found to be crisscrossed by septa, creating a honeycomb pattern with intercommunicating lobules.[56]

On ultrasound, the multiseptate gallbladder is seen to contain multiple fine septations projecting into the lumen and arising perpendicularly from the wall of the gallbladder[55] (Fig. 6-23). The essential diagnostic features are multiple fine, nonshadowing septations that bridge the gallbladder lumen.[55,56] The differential diagnosis of such an abnormality would include desqua-

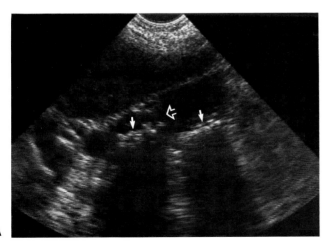
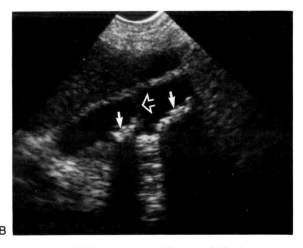

Fig. 6-20. Bicameral gallbladder. **(A)** Sagittal supine view. Echogenic material (stones, arrows) is seen within the fundal and ductal compartments of this divided gallbladder. (open arrow, septum.) **(B)** Sagittal left lateral decubitus view demonstrating a septum (open arrow) between the two compartments. (arrows, stones.)

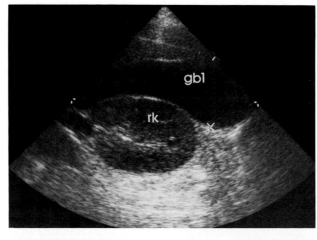

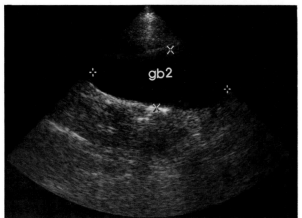

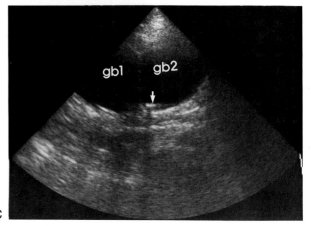

Fig. 6-21.   Double gallbladder, adult. **(A & B)** Sagittal scans of two gallbladders with Fig. A more lateral *(gb1)* and Fig. B more medial *(gb2)*. *(rk,* right kidney.) **(C)** Transverse view showing stones (arrow) within the more medial gallbladder *(gb2)*. These stones did not move to the lateral compartment *(gb1)* with a change in patient position.

mated gallbladder mucosa and the hyperplastic chole-cystoses.[55]

Gallstones

There is a 10 to 20 percent incidence of gallstones in adults. The occurrence increases progressively and reaches a peak in the sixth and seventh decades. It is more common in females than males, with a 4 : 1 ratio. It has been said that the perfect candidate for gallstones is "fat, fertile, female, and forty." There is a predisposition for the formation of pigment stones in biliary infection, alcoholic cirrhosis, and anemias characterized by abnormal hemolysis and increased production of bilirubin pigment.[20]

The pathogenesis for gallstones is varied depending on the type. There is an increased risk of cholesterol stones in patients with ileal disease or ileal resection, females

receiving estrogens, intestinal bypass for morbid obesity, and type IV hyperlipidemia, as well as obesity, pregnancy, diabetes, and clofibrate therapy. The three most important factors affecting gallstone formation are abnormal bile composition, stasis, and infection. The abnormalities of composition of the bile appear to be the most important.[20]

Gallstone formation occurs in three stages: (1) formation of saturated bile, (2) nucleation (initiation of stone formation), and (3) growth of the gallstone to a detectable size. Inflammation can be caused by chemical irritation secondary to alteration in bile caused by invasion of bacteria. Stasis may result from obstruction to outflow, which predisposes to infection.[20]

Gallstone composition is variable. They may be composed of cholesterol, calcium bilirubinate (pigment stones), and/or calcium carbonate. Most are either bilirubin or cholesterol; pure calcium carbonate stones are very rare. Cholesterol stones are usually mixtures of cho-

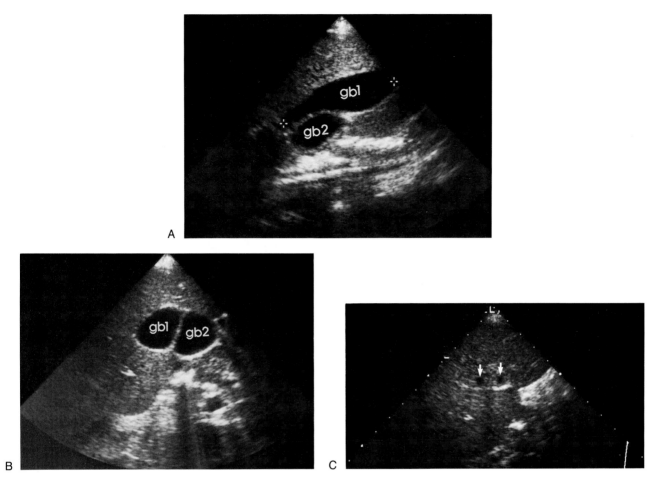

Fig. 6-22. Double gallbladder, child. On **(A)** sagittal and **(B)** transverse views, two gallbladders *(gb1, gb2)* are seen. **(C)** After a fatty meal, the two gallbladders (arrows) are seen to contract on a transverse view similar to Fig. B.

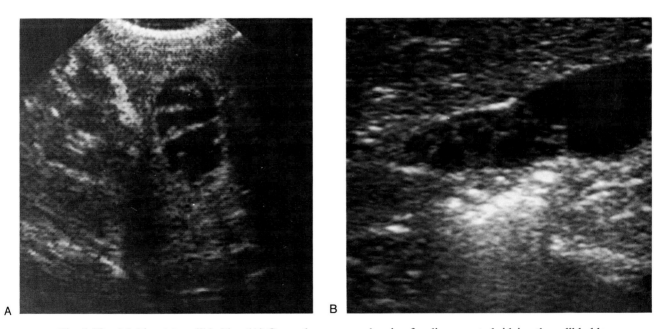

Fig. 6-23. Multiseptate gallbladder. **(A)** Coronal sonogram showing fine linear septa bridging the gallbladder lumen. **(B)** Sagittal sonographic appearance of "honeycomb" septation pattern most prominent in body and neck of gallbladder. (From Lev-Toaff et al,[55] with permission.)

lesterol with pigment and carbonate.[20] Pure cholesterol stones represent 10 percent of all stones. Calcium bilirubinate stones (pigment stones) are less common than pure cholesterol in the Western countries but are more common in the Asiatic ones. Ninety percent of all gallstones are mixed or combined. Mixed stones are those having various proportions of the three stone-forming constituents. Combined stones have a central core or external layer that is pure, with the remainder being mixed.[20]

The clinical implications of gallstones are varied. In 80 percent of cases, the gallbladder stones evoke no clinical manifestations. The most serious consequence of calculous disease is obstruction of the cystic duct or common bile duct. With complete blockage of the cystic duct, hydrops of the gallbladder results. In calculous obstruction, the gallbladder is often not distended and may be small (fibrotic gallbladder); in neoplastic obstruction of the common bile duct, an association with chronic cholecystitis is less likely and so continual formation of bile results in a distended gallbladder (Courvoisier's law). Calculous obstruction of the cystic or common bile duct predisposes to bacterial infection, which may lead to cholangitis and ascending cholangitis. Presumably, stasis, distension of the biliary system, impaired lymphatic drainage and vascular supply, and chemical irritation are operative factors. Rarely, in patients with gallstones and acute inflammatory disease, a stone erodes through the gallbladder wall and adherent intestinal loop to create a cholecystointestinal fistula. Most stones pass unnoticed through the gastrointestinal tract. Large ones, however, may impact at the ileocecal valve, resulting in gallstone ileus. There is a high incidence (65 to 95 percent) of stones associated with a cancerous gallbladder.[20]

Ultrasound Properties

Several ultrasound studies have been performed to evaluate the sonographic characteristics of gallstones. Stones have been shown to be echodense with a posterior acoustic shadow[57-60] (Fig. 6-24). It has been shown that all stones larger than 3 mm demonstrate a shadow.[61,62] This acoustic shadow does not relate to the calcium content, shape, surface characteristics, or specific gravity of the stone.[61,62] It is due to the high reflectivity of the near surface of the gallstone and absorption by the stone of the remainder of the sound that is reflected.[22] Further, it has been shown that stones containing more than 88 percent cholesterol float and produce a shadow.[62] If, however, nonshadowing echogenic foci smaller than 5 mm are seen in the gallbladder, 81 percent of these will represent stones[63] (Fig. 6-25). In addition, any echogenic structure within the gallbladder lumen that causes a posterior shadow and moves with gravity will be a gallstone in all cases.[63,64]

Shadow. The ability to demonstrate the acoustic shadow is highly dependent on the relationship between the stone and the acoustic beam.[22,58,65-68] If the transducer is situated such that the peripheral edge of the acoustic beam encounters the stone, no shadow is demonstrated. If sound waves at or near the center or focal zone of the beam strike the same stone and the stone is large in comparison with the beam width or wavelength used, an acoustic shadow will be easily perceived.[65,67]

By using in vivo and in vitro techniques, stones with higher attenuation have been shown to demonstrate the most shadowing.[69] Attenuation is correlated with physical structure; more highly attenuating stones tend to

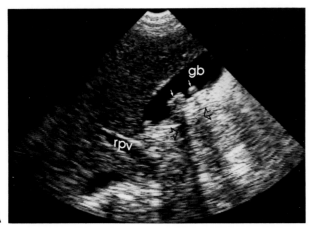
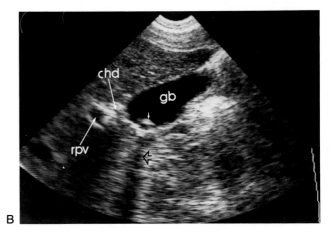

Fig. 6-24. Gallstones, typical. **(A & B)** Sagittal left lateral decubitus scans in two patients. Echodense stones (arrows) are seen in the dependent portion of the gallbladder *(gb)* with associated posterior acoustic shadowing (open arrows). (*rpv,* right portal vein; *chd,* common hepatic duct.)

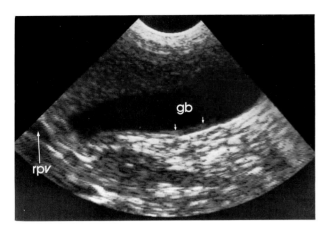

Fig. 6-25.   Gallstones, nonshadowing. Sagittal left lateral decubitus scan. Multiple small echodensities (arrows) are seen within the dependent portion of the gallbladder *(gb)*. There is no associated shadow. At surgery, small stones (2 to 4 mm) were found. *(rpv,* right portal vein.) (From Durrell et al,[47] with permission.)

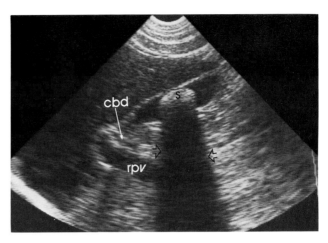

Fig. 6-26.   Gallstone, "clean shadow." Slightly oblique sagittal left lateral decubitus scan. The shadow associated with this gallstone *(S)* has distinct margins (open arrows) and lacks reverberation echoes. *(rpv,* right portal vein; *cbd,* common bile duct.)

have the largest percentage of crystalline material, a larger average crystal size, and more rigid structure. Use of a higher-frequency transducer is recommended if no shadow is demonstrated. A shadow occurs when the attenuation of the stone is greater than that of an equivalent amount of tissue. The difference increases with frequency, and so a greater shadow is seen with a higher frequency.[69] The high attenuation of the gallstone results in the formation of a shadow on ultrasound. The shadow is best seen when the stone lies within the focal zone of the transducer and is large in comparison with the beam width or wavelength used.[67]

The characteristics of the acoustic shadow associated with gallstones have been investigated.[70] The shadow is described as a "clean shadow" if there are distinct margins and a lack of reverberation echoes (Fig. 6-26). Because calcification in stones reflects a much larger percent of the incident sound beam, reverberation echoes are seen within this shadow. The heavier the calcification, the stronger the reverberations are within this shadow (Fig. 6-27). The lack of reverberation echoes does not exclude calcification because its production is dependent on the size and shape of the stone and its orientation with respect to the sound beam. The in vitro ultrasound compositional analysis of stones for detection of calcification might influence the therapeutic decision regarding selection of patients for chemodeoxycholic acid therapy for stone dissolution.[70]

Two shadowing patterns have been described: "clean" and "dirty."[71] The shadowing produced by sound-absorbing materials (e.g., stones) is called "clean," whereas that produced by sound-reflecting materials (e.g., abdominal gas) is called "dirty," but these properties are not always consistent.[71] It has been found that the rougher and/or smaller the radius of the curvature of the surface insonified by the sound beam, the cleaner the shadow, independent of the composition of the underlying reflecting medium.[71] As such, these shadowing patterns appear to be related primarily to the properties of the surface of the shadowing object and provide little information about its structure.[71]

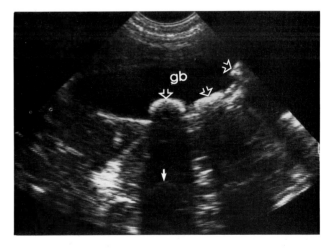

Fig. 6-27.   Gallstone, reverberations in shadow. Sagittal scan. With the central gallstone (left open arrow), there are reverberations (arrow) within the acoustic shadow. The heavier the calcification, the stronger the reverberations are within the shadow. There are many other stones (open arrows) that are not in the center of the sound beam. (*gb,* gallbladder.)

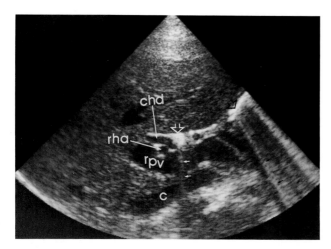

Fig. 6-28. Ring-down and comet-tail artifacts. In this post-cholecystectomy patient, an echogenic area caused by a metallic clip (white open arrow) is seen in the region of the gallbladder bed. Posterior to the echogenic area is seen a series of parallel bands (small white arrows) radiating from the metallic clip. This comet-tail artifact appears similar to the ring-down artifact (small black arrows) posterior to the gas (open black arrow) in the bowel inferior to the liver. (*rpv,* right portal vein; *rha,* right hepatic artery; *chd,* common hepatic duct; *c,* inferior vena cava.)

It may be difficult to differentiate the acoustic shadow due to calculi from that due to gas collections. In vitro, the acoustic shadows distal to calculi contain significantly fewer echoes and are more sharply defined than those distal to gas collection (Figs. 6-24, 6-26, and 6-27).

Artifactual reverberation echoes within the acoustic shadows distal to gas collection result from virtually total sound reflection at tissue-air interfaces, whereas shadows distal to calculi are primarily due to sound absorption[72] (Fig. 6-28).

Artifacts and Reverberations. A number of acoustic artifacts and reverberation shadows in the gallbladder sonogram have been evaluated.[73] Artifacts and reverberation shadows are formed when a significant difference exists between the acoustic impedance of two media.[73] These acoustic artifacts occurring in the gallbladder usually originate in the anterior wall, projecting their shadows over a favorable acoustic medium such as the bile, inferior vena cava, or ascites.[73] They may be divided into two major groups according to their anatomic location: artifacts originating from the gallbladder wall and artifacts originating in the gallbladder lumen.

The V-shaped artifact is the most commonly observed wall artifact, appearing in 80 percent of those with artifacts.[73] A cholesterol stone impacted in a gallbladder wall diverticulum may produce a V-shaped artifact, consisting of a hyperechoic focus, usually located at the gallbladder wall, and a short hyperechoic tail[73] (Fig. 6-29). It has been shown that the V-shaped artifact originates from a small intramural cholesterol stone.[74] All the gallbladders examined microscopically have shown thickened walls, and most have had stones impacted within the wall and accompanying chronic gallbladder inflammation.[74] This V-shaped artifact must be distinguished from the larger comet-tail and ring-down arti-

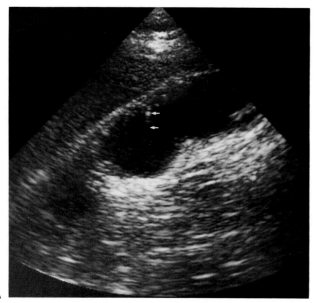

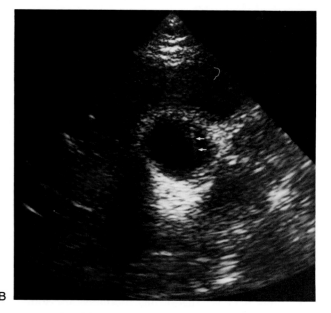

Fig. 6-29. V-shaped artifact. **(A)** Sagittal and **(B)** transverse scans of a gallbladder with a thickened wall. There is a V-shaped artifact (short echogenic tail, arrows) posterior to an echogenic focus in the gallbladder wall. This was secondary to a cholesterol stone adherent to the gallbladder wall.

facts, which arise from metal or gas.[74] The ring-down artifact appears as a long, solid hyperechoic streak or as a series of parallel bands radiating away from gas collections[74] (Fig. 6-28). The comet-tail artifact may appear identical to the ring-down artifact, even though its origin is a metallic object rather than air[74] (Fig. 6-28).

These acoustic artifacts and reverberation shadows observed during gallbladder sonography may be variable and related to multiple conditions.[73] There may be associated pathologic gallbladder findings in 80 percent of patients showing acoustic artifacts.[73] The following occur with artifacts originating from the gallbladder wall: emphysematous cholecystitis, intramural cholesterol stones, intramural diverticula and microabscesses, adenomyomatosis, and surgical metallic clips.[73] When the artifacts occur within the lumen, the following should be considered: emphysematous cholecystitis (microbubbles), biliary-enteric anastomosis or fistula, and floating cholesterol calculi[73] (Fig. 6-30).

Stone Characteristics. Several criteria must be met to diagnose gallstones clinically on an ultrasound scan. The gallbladder must be well visualized in at least two body positions and two scan planes. Intraluminal gallbladder densities that move with a change in body position should be seen. These densities must shadow and/or move rapidly with changes in body position.[47,75,76] (Figs. 6-24 to 6-27).

The type and composition of the stone and its relationship to buoyancy have been evaluated.[77] At times, these intraluminal densities may be seen to float (Fig. 6-31). Floating gallstones (on OCG) are cholesterol stones, with a significantly lower calcium salt content than that of nonfloating cholesterol stones.[77] If a patient has had a recent OCG, the contrast material raises the specific gravity of the bile and causes this phenomenon. The stones seek a level where their specific gravity equals that of the mixture of bile and contrast agent.[78,79] These floating gallstones may be difficult to see, since they will be quite superficial. Some investigators suggest that use of an OCG contrast agent in conjunction with ultrasound in cases when the ultrasound scans are equivocal; this combination facilitates the demonstration of small cholesterol stones by inducing the phenomenon of layering.[79] The identification of floating gallstones is a favorable indicator for dissolution therapy.[79] This might explain why such stones are relatively more susceptible to medical dissolution.[77]

Floating stones may also be seen with gas-containing stones[80] (Fig. 6-32). When stones are especially reflective, such as those that contain gas or are composed primarily of cholesterol crystals, posterior reverberations and/or comet-tail artifacts have been described.[81] Fissuring takes place preferentially in rapidly formed stones and can proceed eventually to complete rupture of a stone into smaller fragments. Gas may be generated by low pressure in the stone as a result of fissuring, out of the small amount of fluid that is present in the stone. At ultrasound, the gas produces floating stones in a nonopacified gallbladder[80] (Fig. 6-32). Since there is no

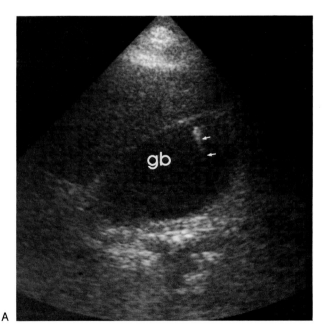

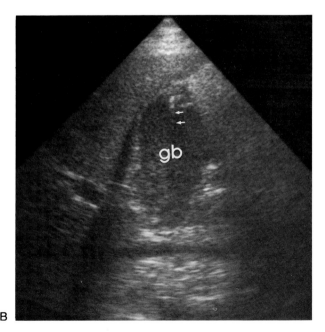

A   B

Fig. 6-30. V-shaped artifact. **(A)** Sagittal view of a gallbladder *(gb)* that had a normal wall thickness. There are several intraluminal echogenic foci within the fundus anteriorly with associated ring-down artifacts (arrows). The bile in the gallbladder is echogenic. **(B)** With a change in patient position, the bright echogenic focus within the gallbladder moved. This artifact was secondary to be cholesterol stones.

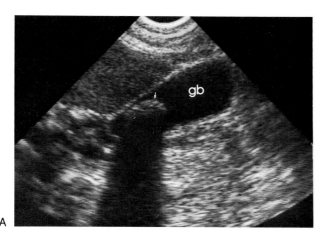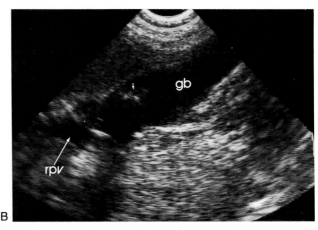

A   B

Fig. 6-31. Floating gallstone. **(A & B)** Left lateral decubitus sagittal scans. An echodense gallstone (arrow) is noted to be floating. This patient had taken an oral cholecystographic agent. The contrast material is thought to raise the specific gravity of the bile, causing the stone to float. The associated acoustic shadowing is "clean" in Fig. A but not well seen in Fig. B; in Fig. B the sound beam is visualizing only the edge of the stone. (*rpv*, right portal vein; *gb*, gallbladder.)

known significance to intracalculus gas per se, the clinical importance of the double-echo sign is uncertain.[81] This double-echo sign is composed of two parallel echoes, with one from within the stone.[81]

There has been a report of food particles in the gallbladder mimicking cholelithiasis in a patient with a cholecystojejunostomy.[82]

Evaluation of the morbidly obese for gallstones can be very difficult. However, it has been found that ultrasound is equal or superior to OCG for this diagnosis.[83]

Cholelithiasis in Children

Children. When children develop cholelithiasis, there is usually a predisposing disease or underlying circumstance. Possible predisposing diseases are hemolytic anemia, thalassemia, cystic fibrosis, metabolic disease, liver disease, neonatal septicemia, Crohn's disease, and cardiac disease. Hemolysis of transfused blood in aplastic anemia is another cause of gallstone formation.[84] Possible underlying circumstances are prior orthopaedic surgery, chemotherapy, postpartum state, and prior bowel resection or malabsorption.[75,85,86]

Two mechanisms are involved in cholelithiasis in children: interruption of the enterohepatic circulation of bile salts and bile stasis.[75] Bile is a supersaturated solution of bilirubin and cholesterol held in balance by the presence of bile salts and phospholipids. Factors such as increased secretion of cholesterol and bilirubin, decreased secretion of bile salts and phospholipids, and damage to biliary mucosa by inflammation, stasis, or abnormal pH level can alter this balance and initiate the formation of calculi. Developing gallstones require a pe-

riod in which incipient microliths increase in size without being discharged from the biliary tree, implying impairment of gallbladder contractility.[86] In one series, cholesterol stones were found most commonly and pigmented stones were less common.[86]

In sickle cell anemia, a 27 to 30 percent incidence of gallstones has been reported.[87,88] More recent investigators have reported cholelithiasis in 4.2 percent of those with sickle cell anemia.[89] This is in contrast to the range of 0.1 to 0.28 percent in children at postmortem examination.[90] The incidence of gallstones appears to increase significantly with age. In addition, these patients with gallstones appear to have a significantly higher mean bilirubin level.[88] In one series, it was found that one-third of the patients with sickle cell anemia had stones, with one-fifth demonstrating sludge.[91] The most common abnormality is gallbladder wall thickening (8.1 percent) and is found as early as 4 years of age.[89] Patients with thalassemia major also have an increased incidence of gallstones. One series reported an incidence of 23 percent in these patients.[90]

A study was done to evaluate the apparent increase in the incidence of gallstones in children. In 55 percent of these cases, there was an underlying predisposing disease or circumstance. The rest did not have predisposing factors. It is believed that if a child is at high risk for gallstones, ultrasound is mandatory to prevent complications of unrecognized gallstones.[75]

Neonates and Infants. Although cholelithiasis is rare in the newborn, it has been associated with a number of conditions. These include hemolytic anemia, congenital anomalies of the biliary tract, administration of paren-

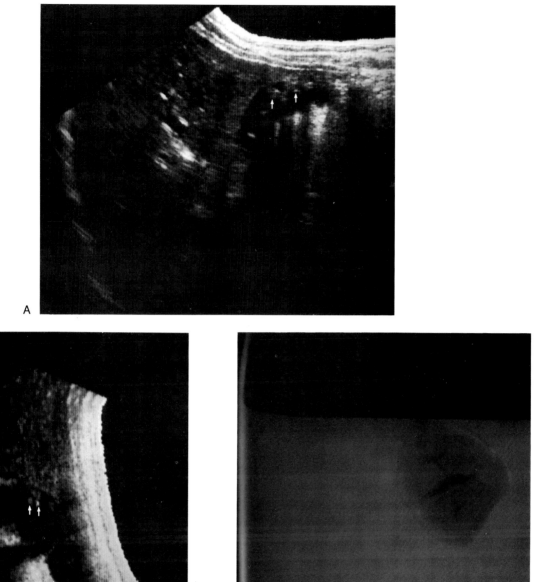

Fig. 6-32. Fissured gallstones. **(A)** Longitudinal supine scan showing multiple floating stones (arrows). **(B)** Longitudinal upright scan showing multiple floating and sedimentary stones (arrows). **(C)** Radiograph with horizontal beam of the gallstones in a container filled with saline (specific gravity, 1.006). One stone is floating under the surface, and one is lying on the bottom. (From Strijk et al,[80] with permission.)

teral nutrition, furosemide therapy, phototherapy, dehydration, infection, ileal resection, cystic fibrosis, family history of biliary disease, multiple problems associated with prematurity, and short-gut syndrome.[75,92-95] Other predisposing factors include metabolic disease, infection, prior urologic procedures, hyperparathyroidism, oxalosis, vitamin D intoxication, and various congenital anomalies in two-thirds of affected infants.[96] Furosemide has also been implicated in nephrolithiasis.[96] In infancy, cholelithiasis is usually associated with chronic hemolytic states such as sickle cell disease, Rh incompatibility, and congenital spherocytosis.[96] Cystic fibrosis, biliary tract malformations, obesity, and Wilson's disease may also predispose an infant to gallstone formation.[96]

Neonates undergoing total parenteral nutrition (TPN) have been evaluated for gallbladder diseases.[97] In these cases, it is theorized that the patients are deprived of the normal stimulatory effect of enteral nutrition and that this leads to stasis within the biliary system.[92] In addition, the hepatocellular enzyme system is immature, with disturbance in the transport of conjugated bilirubin, which impairs bile secretion. This occurrence seems to be related to three main factors: prematurity with immaturity of the enterohepatic circulation of bile acids, duration of TPN, and lack of enteral nutrition.[97] After a mean period of 10 days of TPN, gallbladder sludge is seen in 44 percent of patients.[97] The length of time on parenteral hyperalimentation, aberrant eating patterns, and prior ileal resection are predisposing elements.[96] In one series, 40 percent of infants receiving total parenteral nutrition for longer than 8 months developed cholelithiasis.[96] An evolution of sludge to "sludge balls" has been found in 12 percent.[97] Five percent developed uncomplicated gallstones, and a spontaneous resolution occurred in one of them 6 months after the examination.[97] In neonates receiving TPN, ultrasound might be helpful in monitoring the abnormal gallbladder content and rapid introduction of parenteral feeding is advisable upon its identification.[97] As such, this finding indicates conservative management.[97]

Patients who have respiratory distress syndrome complicated by bronchopulmonary dysplasia are often treated with assisted ventilation, TPN, and furosemide. Furosemide enhances the excretion of calcium into the urine. It is not known whether it has similar actions on bile.[92]

When stasis occurs in the gallbladder secondary to obstruction or failure of the gallbladder to contract, the microliths increase in size.[95] It takes time for gallstones to develop. The observation of cholelithiasis and its subsequent spontaneous disappearance in infants with multiple reasons for jaundice suggests that cholelithiasis in such infants may resolve with remission of cholestatic

liver disease, and an initial conservative approach is therefore recommended.[94] The defects demonstrated may have been caused by tumefactive sludge with acoustic shadowing.[94]

Contracted or Nonvisualized Gallbladder

There are numerous causes of nonvisualization of a gallbladder on ultrasound; these include (1) gallbladder disease obliterating the lumen; (2) nonfasting patient; (3) obstruction of the biliary tree proximal to the cystic duct; and (4) congenital absence of the gallbladder. The nonvisualization may also be due to a small gallbladder, a technical error, or floating stones containing gas.[98] Fissuring takes place preferentially in rapidly formed stones and can proceed eventually to complete rupture of the stone into smaller fragments that can pass. The gas in the stones causes them to float. The gas is generated by low pressure in the stone as a result of fissuring, out of the small amount of fluid that is present in the stone.[80]

In some instances, gallstones may prevent ultrasound visualization of the gallbladder. In 15 to 25 percent of patients with stones, there is gallbladder nonvisualization.[99] If many strong echoes that cast a large shadow are seen in the gallbladder area, the probability of gallbladder stones is high (Fig. 6-33). This may represent a gallbladder that is contracted or simply packed with stones; the anterior layer of stones casts a shadow that prevents the visualization of the gallbladder.[100] A specific image may also be observed — that of two parallel arcuate echogenic lines separated by a thin anechoic space with distal acoustic shadowing[99,101] (Fig. 6-34). The proximal arc represents the near wall of the gallbladder, the anechoic space is bile, and the distal arc is secondary to gallstones. This "double-arc" sign or "WES triad" (W, the wall; E, the stone; and S, the shadow) can increase the confidence of the examiner in differentiating the gallbladder from a bowel loop.[101] Care must be taken in such cases to examine the gallbladder in various body positions, particularly the left lateral decubitus position. An echogenic focus and an associated shadow that persist in the same location provide more evidence suggestive of gallstones.[102] In addition, the patient may be examined on a subsequent day. If the findings persist, a diagnosis of cholelithiasis may be made.

When there is nonvisualization of the gallbladder by ultrasound in a fasting patient, there is usually calculous gallbladder disease.[103] A number of other less common conditions can prevent gallbladder visualization or recognition.[103] This occurs when the morphology of the gallbladder is so altered that the gallbladder is difficult to identify; these conditions include (1) congenital anomalies; (2) gallbladder contraction not due to stones; (3) conditions that cause shadowing or reverberation from

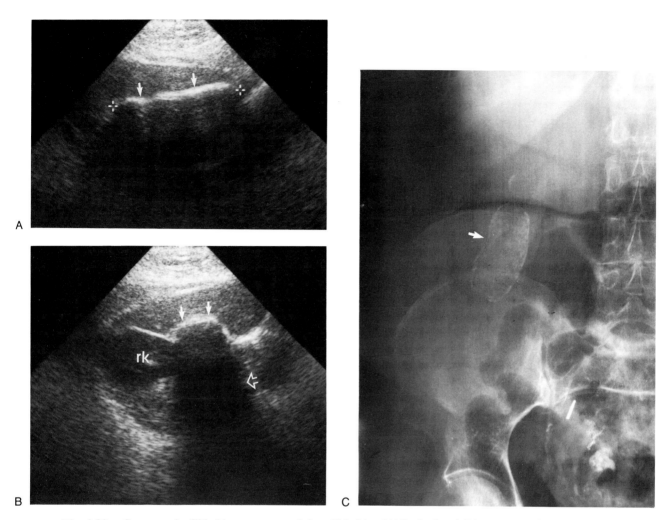

Fig. 6-33. Contracted gallbladder versus porcelain gallbladder. **(A)** Sagittal and **(B)** transverse views of the right upper quadrant demonstrating a strongly echogenic structure (arrows) in the gallbladder fossa. No gallbladder lumen is seen. There is posterior acoustic shadowing (open arrow). This appearance could be seen with a contracted gallbladder full of stones or a porcelain gallbladder with a densely calcified anterior wall producing the shadow. (*rk*, right kidney.) **(C)** Plain film. A porcelain gallbladder (arrow) is seen.

the near wall of the gallbladder; and (4) the solid gallbladder pattern.[103]

A contracted gallbladder can be an associated finding with hepatic dysfunction.[104] Despite adequate fasting, these patients may have contracted gallbladders.[104] Normal gallbladders may be visualized on ultrasound after the acute phase of hepatitis.[104] Acute hepatic dysfunction may decrease the flow of bile into the gallbladder, resulting in a gallbladder that is transiently contracted or is not visualized on ultrasound.[104]

Gallbladder Volume

Most patients with gallstones exhibit a higher resting gallbladder volume, less fractional emptying after a fatty meal, and a higher postmeal residual volume.[105] These findings may result from an abnormally high resting gallbladder volume.[105] In some patients decreased gallbladder contractility may contribute to gallstone development or proliferation.[105]

Acute viral hepatitis may result in altered gallbladder motor activity. Two patterns are recognized. The first involves normal wall thickness usually associated with greater volume, and diminished response to a stimulating meal; this pattern occurs in 58.4 percent.[106] This group would be characterized by a functionally hypotonic, hypokinetic gallbladder.[106] The second pattern involves a greater wall width and lower volume, indicating a hypertonic gallbladder.[106] These gallbladder abnormalities tend to disappear.[106] Therefore the examiner must be aware of the possibility of finding an abnormal ultrasound appearance of the gallbladder in the early

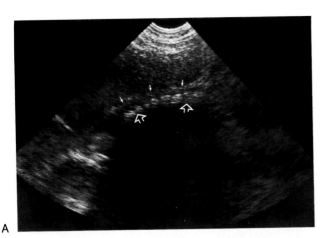 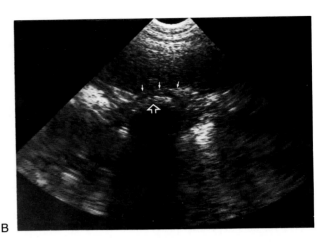

Fig. 6-34. Double-arc sign or WES triad. **(A)** Sagittal and **(B)** transverse scans. The echogenic anterior line (small arrows) represents the anterior wall of the gallbladder, with the second echogenic arc (open arrows) representing stones. A distal shadow is seen. (Fig. A from Durrell et al,[47] with permission.)

phase of acute viral hepatitis and of its transient and benign nature.[106]

Porcelain Gallbladder

The incidence of calcification in the gallbladder wall is 0.6 to 0.8 percent of cholecystectomy specimens.[107] It is associated with stones in 95 percent of cases and is more common in females, with a 5:1 female/male ratio. The pathogenesis is controversial. Some investigators speculate that obstruction of the cystic duct leads to mucosal precipitation of calcium carbonate salts, which in turn causes bile to stagnate in the gallbladder. Others believe that the calcium is a dystrophic process that results from chronic low-grade infection and/or compromised circulation due to the impacted cystic duct stone. The infection and/or compromised circulation result in hemorrhage, scarring, and hyalinization of the wall, which in turn provide the matrix for deposition of lime salts. The third theory is that chronic irritation of the wall by a stone or other foreign body produces the calcification.[107]

Histologically, there are two types of calcification.[107] In one type, there is a continuous broad band of calcification within the muscularis, which is seen on radiographs as a large plaquelike area. The second type includes numerous calcified microliths scattered diffusely throughout the mucosa and submucosa, localized within the glandular spaces and in the Rokitansky-Aschoff sinuses. On radiographs, this type appears as granular and plaquelike calcifications. Between 11 and 33 percent of carcinomas of the gallbladder are associated with calcification in the wall.

The ultrasound findings of porcelain gallbladder have been divided into three patterns: (1) type I, manifested by a hyperechoic semilunar structure with posterior acoustic shadowing; (2) type II, biconvex curvilinear echogenic structure with acoustic shadowing and gallstones; and (3) type III, irregular clumps of echoes with posterior acoustic shadowing[107,108] (Figs. 6-34 to 6-36). The gallbladder wall is diffusely replaced by dense fibrosis or hyalinization in type I disease.[108] Type I porcelain gallbladder does not appear to be associated with cancer of the gallbladder, probably because the mucosal epithelium is almost completely sloughed off and replaced by dense connective tissue with calcification.[108] Type II porcelain gallbladder is frequently associated with gallbladder cancer.[108] This may be because there is more mucosal epithelium left in types II and III disease.[108]

Gallbladder Neck/Cystic Duct Stone

Ultrasound is uniformly successful in the diagnosis of impacted stones within the gallbladder neck.[82] A typical appearance is seen: curved, highly reflective intraluminal echoes with a prominent acoustic shadow[109] (Figs. 6-37 and 6-38). To document that the stone is indeed impacted, the patient is rescanned in the upright position and then in the supine and/or decubitus position. If the stone is impacted, there will be no apparent change in its position (Fig. 6-37).

In contrast to scanning for gallbladder neck stones, ultrasound may be unsuccessful in the diagnosis of impacted stones in the cystic duct.[109] The normal cystic duct is not usually seen at ultrasound. Even when enlarged and containing an impacted stone, the cystic duct may not contain enough bile surrounding the stone to create the acoustic contrast necessary for definitive visualization.[109] A number of nonbiliary structures can

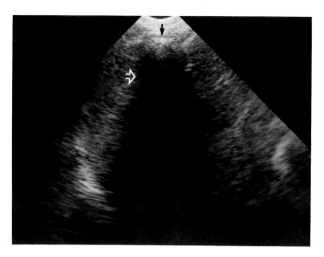
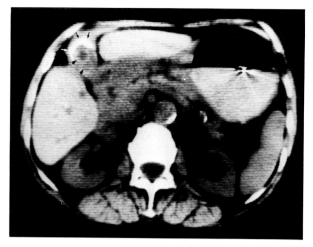

A

B

Fig. 6-35. Porcelain gallbladder. **(A)** Sagittal real-time scan. A dense line (black arrow) is seen in the gallbladder fossa with acoustic shadowing (open arrow). This finding persisted in various body positions. **(B)** CT scan. The calcification (small arrows) within the gallbladder wall is seen, as well as stones (arrowheads).

mimic a cystic duct stone: echogenic fat in the porta hepatis, duodenal gas, refractive shadow from Heister's valves, and calcification in masses in the porta hepatis.[109] If a cystic duct stone is suspected, hepatobiliary nuclear medicine is recommended.

Ultrasound may demonstrate a dilated obstructed cystic duct or "triple-channel" sign—the common hepatic duct, cystic duct, and portal vein[110] (Fig. 6-39). The diagnosis can be suggested when two tubular, parallel structures are visualized separate from the portal vein in a patient with obstructive jaundice; visualization of an echogenic stone serves as confirmation.[111] However, the typical appearance may be absent, as a result of stone penetration outside the gallbladder or biliary tract.[111]

Mirizzi Syndrome

Mirizzi syndrome is an uncommon, surgically correctable cause of extrahepatic obstruction.[112-114] The features of this syndrome include (1) the cystic duct running parallel to the common hepatic duct; (2) the presence of an impacted stone in the cystic duct, cystic duct remnant, or gallbladder neck; (3) partial mechanical obstruction of the common hepatic duct by compression or by resulting inflammatory reaction around the impacted stone; and (4) the sequelae of jaundice, recurrent cholangitis, formation of biliobiliary fistulas, or cholangitic cirrhosis.[110,112-114] The typical signs include dilatation of the common hepatic duct above the

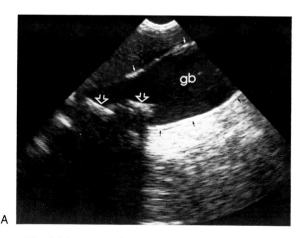
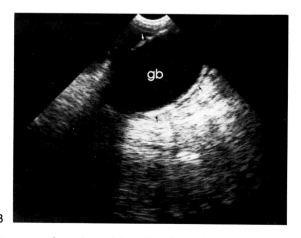

A

B

Fig. 6-36. Porcelain gallbladder. **(A & B)** Sagittal real-time scans of a patient with a palpable pelvic mass. The gallbladder *(gb)* wall (small arrows) appears denser than usual. There are gallstones (open arrows, Fig. A) associated. The palpated mass was the gallbladder. (Fig. A from Durrell et al,[47] with permission.)

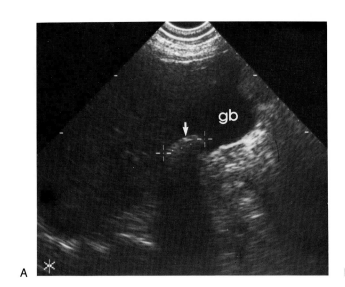
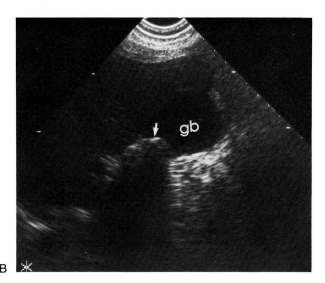

Fig. 6-37.   Impacted stone, gallbladder neck. **(A)** Supine sagittal scan. A gallstone (arrow) is seen in the area of the gallbladder *(gb)* neck. **(B)** Left lateral decubitus sagittal scan. The stone (arrow) has not moved, which is consistent with an impacted stone. (*gb*, gallbladder.)

level of the gallstone impacted in the cystic duct, with a normal duct width below the stone.[113] In most cases, there is an anomalous insertion of the cystic duct or gallbladder neck allowing a parallel arrangement of the cystic duct adjacent to the common hepatic duct.[112,114] When ultrasound demonstrates two parallel tubular structures in the position of the common bile duct, the diagnosis should be suggested[114] (Figs. 6-40 and 6-41).

The differential diagnosis based on visualization of a smooth, generally curved segmental stenosis of the common hepatic duct would include metastatic adenopathy

in the porta, gallbladder carcinoma, focal sclerosing cholangitis, primary liver tumor, or tumor of the duct. In the proper situation, the ultrasound appearance of dilated intrahepatic ducts, normal-caliber common bile duct, and stone in the neck of the gallbladder or cystic duct should suggest the diagnosis[112-114] (Figs. 6-40 and 6-41). It is important to exclude the presence of a mass in the porta hepatis or secondary signs of cancer as possibilities. Direct cholangiography is often necessary because cholecystobiliary fistula secondary to stone penetration into the common bile duct can be demonstrated only by

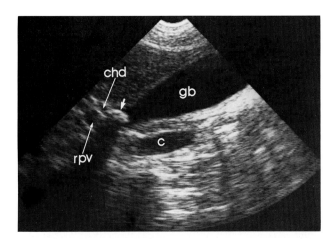

Fig. 6-38.   Impacted stone, gallbladder neck. Sagittal supine scan. A stone (arrow) is seen in the area of the gallbladder *(gb)* neck. It does not move with a change in position. (*c*, inferior vena cava; *rpv*, right portal vein; *chd*, common hepatic duct.)

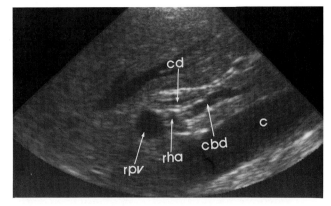

Fig. 6-39.   "Triple-channel" sign. This patient had acute cholecystitis with stones and pericholecystic fluid. On a magnified view through the region of the distal cystic duct *(cd)*, an anterior duct with thickened walls is seen. The normal-sized common duct *(cbd)* is seen posteriorly. (*rpv*, right portal vein; *c*, inferior vena cava; *rha*, right hepatic artery.)

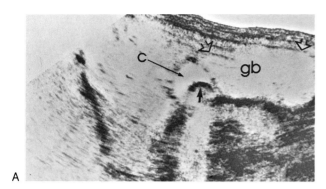

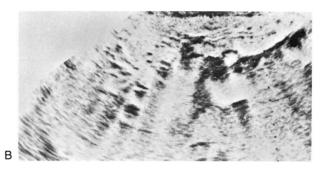

Fig. 6-40. Mirizzi syndrome. (**A**) Sagittal scan. A distended gallbladder (*gb*, open arrows) is seen, as well as a large stone (arrow) within the dilated cystic duct *(c)*. (**B**) Transverse scan of the liver demonstrating intrahepatic biliary dilatation. The common bile duct was of normal caliber. (From Jackson and Lappas,[112] with permission.)

cholangiography.[113] The main features of Mirizzi syndrome at direct cholangiography include partial common hepatic duct obstruction due either to external compression at the level of the cystic duct or to the partly or completely eroded calculus.[113] The findings may mimic cholangiocarcinoma.

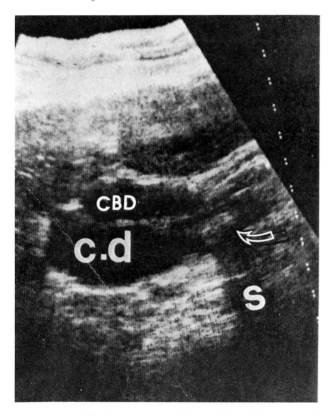

Fig. 6-41. Mirizzi syndrome. Right anterior oblique. Transverse section demonstrating a dilated cystic duct *(c.d)* and a dilated common bile duct *(CBD)* separated by a septum. A cystic duct stone (curved arrow) with distal acoustic shadow *(S)* is also demonstrated. (From Joseph et al,[110] with permission.)

Cholecystosonography Accuracy

The accuracy of ultrasound in diagnosing cholelithiasis has been compared with that of other gallbladder imaging techniques. The accuracies of the various ultrasound criteria for gallstones have been reported to be (1) shadowing moving intraluminal densities, 100 percent; (2) nonvisualization of the gallbladder lumen, 96 percent; and (3) nonshadowing opacities within the gallbladder, 61 percent.[64,115-118] An accuracy of 98.6 percent for diagnosing cholelithiasis by ultrasound has been reported when using the following criteria: (1) the gallbladder is well visualized in at least two projections; (2) intraluminal gallbladder densities are well defined; and (3) densities shadow and/or move rapidly with change in patient position.[76] Early studies with static and real-time ultrasound reported accuracies of 89 to 93 percent.[119-123] Later studies have demonstrated an overall accuracy of 96 to 98.9 percent, with a sensitivity of 98 percent, a specificity of 93.5 to 97.7 percent, a false-negative rate of 2.2 to 4 percent, and a false-positive rate of 2.8 percent.[115,118,124] The accuracy of the oral cholecystogram has been reported to be 93 to 93.2 percent.[118,125]

There is therefore much evidence suggesting that ultrasound is the modality of choice for an accurate evaluation of many pathologic states of the gallbladder, since it is an ideal organ for ultrasound evaluation. Although OCG is one of the most trusted radiographic procedures, various protocols proposed for film and pill taking probably reflect dissatisfaction with the procedure. Ultrasound allows a rapid examination to obtain a definitive diagnosis. Also, many ultrasound studies have shown stones that were not demonstrated by OCG.[126] In addition, ultrasound is more sensitive than CT for detecting the presence of gallstones because of the partial-volume averaging errors that occur with CT.[127] Because of its high accuracy, minimal preparation, speed of diagnosis, and cost-effectiveness, real-time ultrasound is recommended for screening patients with suspected gallbladder disease.[76,115]

The number and size of gallstones have a direct impact on the eligibility and expected success of extracorporeal shock wave lithotripsy and oral bile acid therapy, so a correct diagnosis is important. Stones of a uniform size are correctly detected in 92 percent of patients.[128] Stones of two different sizes are identified in only 30 percent, with the smaller stones missed in 79 percent.[128] When preoperative sonograms are analyzed, the size and number of stones are determined correctly in only 21 percent of cases. The accuracy is only 34 percent among gallbladders with single stone families; stone size and number are underestimated as often as they are overestimated.[128] Larger stones (> 2.0 cm) are underestimated in size in 88 percent of missed cases.[128] Sonography can be used to detect gallstones with 28 percent greater sensitivity than is possible with OCG, but it is less accurate for counting stones when more than three to five stones are present in a gallbladder.[128] With multiple gallstones, direct correlation with OCG findings is necessary to determine best the number and size of gallstones.[128]

For selection of patients for treatment by lithotripsy and for the evaluation of therapeutic results, accurate knowledge of the number and size of gallstones is required.[129] The sonographic stone counts and measurements were accurate in all 16 patients who had fewer than six stones in one study.[129] Ultrasound can be used to count and measure gallstones accurately when fewer than six stones are present, can reliably determine when six or more stones are present, and, in many cases, can determine the size of the largest fragments remaining after lithotripsy.[129]

With regard to the gallbladder neck/cystic duct area, ultrasound has been reported to have a sensitivity of 30 percent, a specificity of 100 percent, and an accuracy of 74 percent.[109] It is generally not a good method for diagnosis of cystic duct obstruction.

Sludge

Echogenic bile or sludge is identified in many cases. The source of the echoes in the biliary sludge particles is predominantly pigment granules with lesser amounts of cholesterol crystals.[130] The sludge consists mainly of calcium bilirubinate.[130] Echogenic bile is most often found in patients with extrahepatic biliary obstruction and acute and chronic cholecystitis and in patients undergoing a fast or hyperalimentation.[130,131] The common factor in all instances is stasis of bile in the gallbladder.

Sludge is probably formed from inspissated bile, multiple tiny nonshadowing calculi, pigment granules or cholesterol crystals, hemobilia, and purulent bile or pus.[132] As a rule, it is not accompanied by an acoustic shadow. Changes in the position of the patient result in different images, which are dependent on gravity.[132]

Sludge is visualized as nonshadowing low-amplitude echoes that layer in the dependent part of the gallblad-

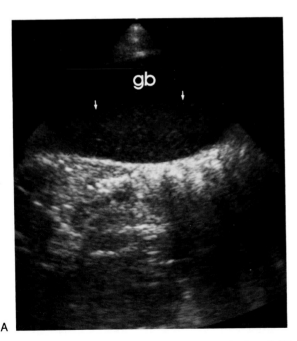
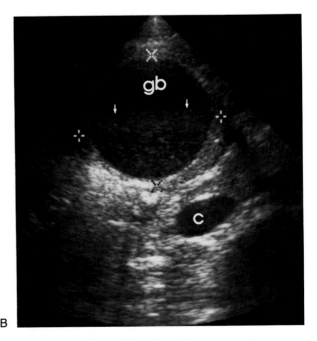

A   B

Fig. 6-42. Gallbladder sludge. **(A)** Sagittal and **(B)** transverse views of the gallbladder *(gb)* demonstrating a fluid-fluid level (arrows) with the denser component (sludge) posteriorly. *(c,* inferior vena cava.)

der.[133] Because of its high specific gravity, sludge forms a fluid-fluid level that moves slowly with changes in patient position[130] (Fig. 6-42). The nondependence of the straight horizontal line on receiver gain and the lack of change in height of debris between transverse and sagittal scans are important clues that help differentiate true sludge from debris due to slice thickness artifact.[131]

Pseudosludge

"Pseudosludge" is indistinguishable on ultrasound from true sludge and is seen as low-amplitude echoes in the posterior portion of the gallbladder.[134] Its appearance is created by a beam-averaging effect or "partial-volume phenomenon" at the diverging portion of the ultrasound beam. The overall appearance is due to an averaging of echoes from the liver adjacent to the gallbladder, containing normally anechoic bile. It must be differentiated from sedimented calcium bilirubinate granules and cholesterol crystals. On the decubitus view, the location of the sludge changes to the dependent portion of the gallbladder. The interface of the sludge and the bile is oblique to the beam, while the interface of the pseudosludge and the bile remains perpendicular to the beam.[134]

Cholesterol

One group of investigators has evaluated the sonography of cholesterol in the biliary system.[135] Cholesterol causes highly reflective echoes and may cause shadowing, but its ability to cause reverberatory artifactual echoes have only recently been reported.[135] These findings favor the diagnosis of cholesterol stones and cholesterol polyps.[135]

Hematobilia

Many entities may simulate sludge. Hematobilia (bleeding into the biliary tree) is associated with a variety of disorders including rupture of a hepatic artery aneurysm, blunt abdominal trauma, and, rarely, percutaneous liver biopsy.[136] Although hematobilia has a variety of causes, it is due to trauma more than 50 percent of the time.[137] The iatrogenic causes of traumatic hematobilia have increased as a result of increasing utilization of percutaneous transhepatic cholangiography and biliary drainage procedures.[137] When there is disease or trauma resulting in an abnormal communication between blood vessels and bile ducts, hematobilia occurs.[138] The diagnosis remains difficult, with the patient presenting with gastrointestinal bleeding, right upper quadrant pain, and jaundice.[137] Early diagnosis of hematobilia may be lifesaving, because bleeding may be intermittent and massive hemorrhage may not occur until weeks following biopsy.

On ultrasound several findings are demonstrated, ranging from scattered intraluminal echoes to an even distribution of an ovoid hypoechoic mass with smooth borders that moves freely within the gallbladder.[137] Blood seen with hematobilia may cause echogenic bile[139] (Fig. 6-43). Clot may be seen within the gallbladder. A characteristic sonographic picture of a well-

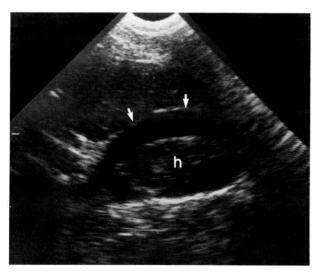

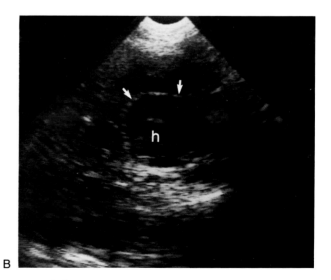

Fig. 6-43. Hematobilia. **(A)** Longitudinal and **(B)** transverse real-time scans demonstrating a smooth, ovoid, relatively hypoechoic mass within the gallbladder lumen, representing a hematoma *(h)*. The gallbladder wall (arrows) is of normal caliber, and the remaining portion of the gallbladder lumen is echofree. (From Grant and Smirniotopoulos,[136] with permission.)

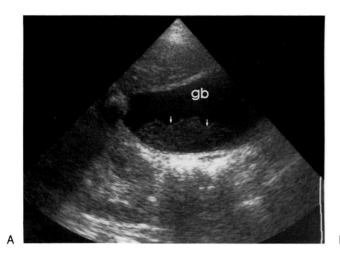

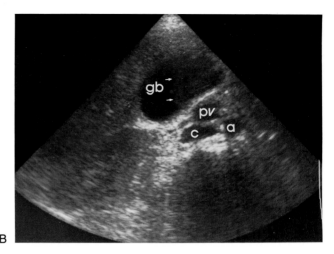

A   B

Fig. 6-44. Gallbladder mass, sludge. **(A)** Sagittal supine and **(B)** transverse left lateral decubitus scans. A mass effect (arrows) is seen within the posterior gallbladder *(gb)* in Fig. A. In Fig. B a fluid-fluid level (arrows) is demonstrated, making a mass less likely. (*a*, aorta; *c*, inferior vena cava; *pv*, portal vein.)

defined, movable, nonshadowing mass within the gallbladder may be seen with an intraluminal gallbladder hematoma.[138] Coagulated blood usually diminishes in size because of the fibrinolytic quality of bile, but does not dissolve entirely.[138] Other findings may include clot within the gallbladder and the extrahepatic ducts, liver hematoma, and aneurysm in the hepatic artery.[137]

As with any echogenic foci in the gallbladder lumen, the differential diagnosis includes stone, tumor, polyp, and sludge. Parasitic infestation, blood clot, and aggregate material containing pus or sludge may be seen.[140] These may produce mobile intraluminal gallbladder masses.

Tumor Simulation

At times biliary sludge may simulate tumor. Sludge forms layers within the gallbladder as a result of thick or inspissated bile, multiple tiny nonshadowing calculi, pigment granules, cholesterol crystal formation, hemobilia, or purulent bile. A mass effect due to temporary clumping of highly viscous material resulting from bile stasis may be seen[131,141] (Fig. 6-44). Tumefactive biliary sludge has a characteristic appearance, dispersing into small particles when the gallbladder is tapped and then reforming into a mass when the gallbladder is left at rest.[132] Upon reexamination, the "mass" is seen to disappear, further confirming the "pseudotumor" nature.[131]

At times, a gallbladder full of sludge simulates a solid mass.[142] This has been described in a Courvoisier gallbladder with a long duration of obstruction. "Tumefactive biliary sludge" and "sludge balls" are echogenic masses that more closely resemble masses or stones than sludge[143] (Figs. 6-45 and 6-46). These nonshadowing sludge balls eventually attenuate enough sound to cause a distal shadow and prove to be calculi.

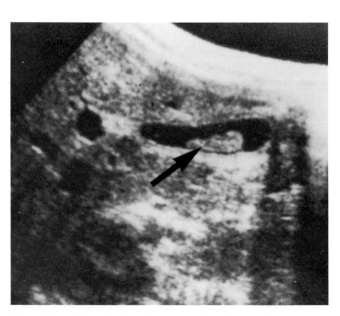

Fig. 6-45. Tumefactive sludge. Longitudinal supine scan. A polypoid mass (arrow) is seen within the lumen of the gallbladder. A repeat examination 1 day later demonstrated that the mass was no longer present. (From Fakhry,[131] with permission.)

Milk of Calcium Bile

The sonographic appearance of milk of calcium bile has been described by several authors.[144-146] Pathologically the gallbladder appears chronically inflamed, is functionless, and contains thickened bile with a high calcium content (usually as calcium carbonate). The calcium carbonate can be deposited on already existing stones, which are commonly associated with this condition, or can settle out as a semifluid or a puttylike mass.[145] There is cystic duct obstruction in most cases. Clinically, this entity is indistinguishable from chronic cholecystitis.

Milk of calcium opacity results from aggregation of small crystals of lime.[146] The crystals form in association with partial or complete obstruction of the cystic duct.[146] Stratification of bile creates a layering effect on ultrasound, with two zones separated by a fluid-fluid level. The less-dependent fraction has a lower specific gravity and appears lucent, simulating normal bile (Figs. 6-47 and 6-48). On ultrasound, an echogenic shadowing flat fluid-fluid level, a convex meniscus, or an unusually shaped area in the gallbladder is consistent with limy bile.[146] The dependent layer is dense, contains dissolved calcium, and absorbs and reflects the sound, causing a shadow. On ultrasound, the findings are similar to those of the floating gallstone.[144,145]

Clinical Implications

The clinical implications of sludge are difficult to assess. When the gallbladder bile contains cholesterol crystals or calcium bilirubinate granules in moderate to large amounts, there is a strong correlation with the presence of gallstones or other abnormalities such as cholesterolosis.[130] It can, however, be seen in normal individuals.[130] Sludge is an indicator of abnormal biliary dynamics and a possible precursor of cholecystitis.[134] One cannot distinguish thick bile from multiple nonshadowing calculi, pus, cholesterol crystals, and possibly abnormal mucus in the gallbladder.[133]

Cholecystitis

Cholecystitis represents inflammation of the gallbladder, which may be acute or chronic. The acute stage is subdivided on the basis of the severity of the inflamma-

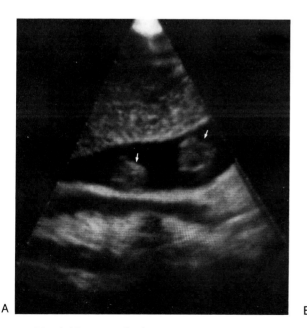
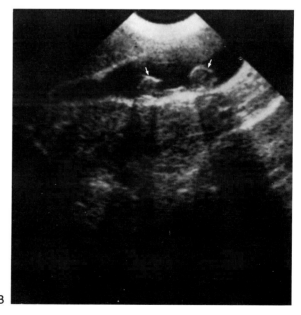

A

B

Fig. 6-46. Tumefactive sludge. **(A)** Longitudinal real-time scan with two nonshadowing "sludge balls" (arrows). **(B)** Longitudinal real-time scan 2 years after Fig. A showing clear-cut shadowing deep to the masses (arrows). At surgery, these were found to be gallstones, largely aggregations of calcium bilirubinate crystals with a much smaller component of cholesterol crystals. The sludge ball matrix was approximately 5 percent calcium. (From Britten et al,[143] with permission.)

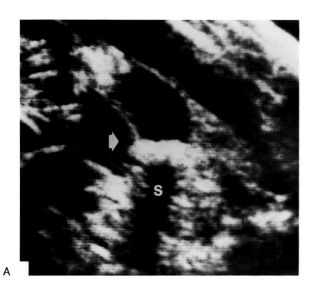

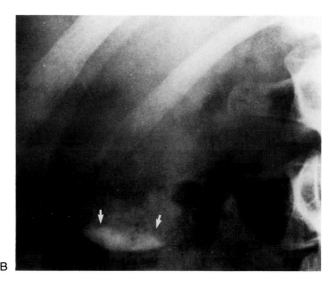

Fig. 6-47. Milk of calcium bile. **(A)** Transverse scan in the left lateral decubitus position. High-amplitude reflections (arrow) are demonstrated within the dependent portion of the gallbladder. Prominent posterior acoustic shadowing *(S)* is noted. **(B)** Upright radiograph of the right upper quadrant demonstrating the characteristic appearance of milk of calcium layering (arrows) within the dependent portion of the gallbladder. (From Chun et al,[145] with permission.)

tory response into acute supportive and gangrenous cholecystitis. There is a 70 percent incidence of cholecystitis in adults, but it does not occur in significant numbers until the mid-30s and reaches a peak in the fifth and sixth decades. There is a female/male ratio of 3:1, with the typical clinical pattern being "female, fat, forty, and fertile."[20]

Several factors affect the pathogenesis of cholecystitis. These include chemical irritation by concentrated bile, bacterial infection, and pancreatic reflux.[20,147] Stones obstructing the cystic duct are implicated in 80 to 95 percent of cases of acute cholecystitis.[20,147] Venous or lymphatic stasis may play a contributory role in the chemical irritation; an impacted stone or extrinsic pressure may interfere with the blood supply to the gallbladder and predispose patients to an acute inflammatory reaction. Such patients are likely to develop secondary bacterial infection. As such, there is a strong association (75 percent of cases of acute cholecystitis) with bacterial infection.[147] Most commonly, the offending microorganisms are staphylococci, enterococci, and gram-negative rods. Evidence of bacterial infection as the initiating etiologic factor is seen in a minority (5 to 10 percent) of patients, and there is usually concomitant septicemia or severe infection elsewhere in the body.[20] Pancreatic reflux also creates an inflammatory response. The evolution of chronic cholecystitis is very obscure, but only rarely is it preceded by a well-defined bout of acute cholecystitis.[20]

Several distinct changes are seen pathologically in cholecystitis. In acute cholecystitis, the gallbladder is enlarged and tense with serosal hemorrhages and a serosal covering layered with fibrin, and at times there is a definite suppurative coagulated exudate.[20] There is increased vascular permeability with edema, extravasation of blood in the wall, and initially monocytic and later polymorphonuclear infiltration.[147] With acute inflammation, there is edema, leukocytic infiltration, vascular congestion, frank abscess formation, or gangrenous necrosis when vascular stasis complicates the edematous inflammatory response. In more severe cases, the mucous membrane is completely destroyed.[147] The pathologic changes depend on the severity of involvement and the duration of the process. The lumen may be filled with cloudy or turbid bile containing large amounts of fibrin and pus. If there is deposition of calcium within the gallbladder wall, a calcified gallbladder or porcelain gallbladder results.

With empyema of the gallbladder, there is pure pus in the lumen and gallstones are present in up to 80 percent of cases. The gallbladder wall is up to 10 times its normal thickness and has a rubbery consistency with edema fluid, exudate, and hemorrhage.

In gangrenous cholecystitis, the mucosa of the gallbladder is patchily or totally hyperemic with a necrotic surface, small ulcerations, or desquamation.[20,147] These ulcerations may penetrate the wall to give rise to a pericholecystic abscess or generalized peritonitis.

In chronic cholecystitis, the gallbladder is contracted, normal, or enlarged. The size depends on the balance

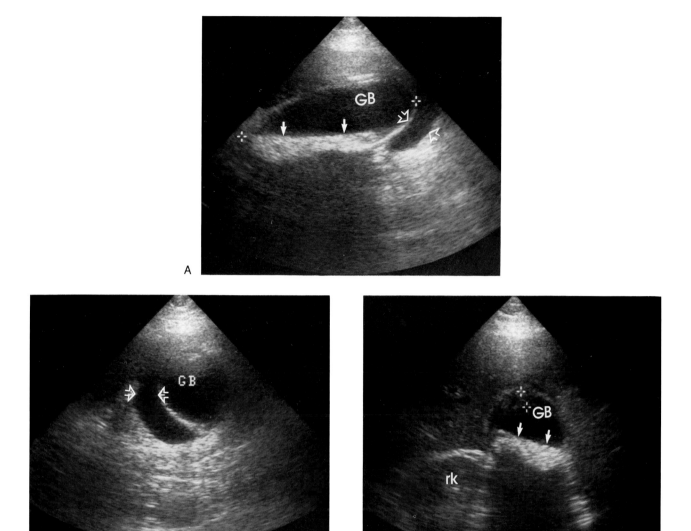

Fig. 6-48. Milk of calcium bile, cholecystitis, and pericholecystic fluid. **(A)** Sagittal and **(B & C)** transverse views of the gallbladder *(GB)* showing a very echogenic posterior fluid level (arrows) with acoustic shadowing. There is gallbladder wall thickening (calipers, Fig. C) and pericholecystic fluid (open arrows). (*rk*, right kidney.)

between the development of fibrosis in the wall and the element of obstruction in the genesis of inflammation. Ninety percent of these patients have associated gallstones. The wall is variably thickened but is rarely more than five times its normal size. In extreme cases, the wall is permeated by fibrosis seen with a considerable obliteration of the smooth musculature. Rokitansky-Aschoff sinuses are seen in 90 percent of chronically inflamed gallbladders. This is presumably because inflammatory damage to the wall predisposes to herniation of the lining epithelium.[20]

The clinical course associated with cholecystitis can be variable. Acute right upper quadrant pain may be referred to the shoulder when inflammatory exudate tracks up beneath the diaphragm, causing irritation of the phrenic nerve. Fever, nausea, vomiting, leukocytosis, and a rigid abdominal wall may be seen. Jaundice is found in 25 percent of cases. Complications of an acute attack include pericholecystic abscess due to permeative infection or perforation of the gallbladder, generalized peritonitis, ascending cholangitis, liver abscess, subdiaphragmatic abscess, and septicemia. Chronic cholecystitis is a vague insidious disorder with intolerance to fatty food, belching, postcibal epigastric distress, nausea, and vomiting. Complications of chronic cholecystitis and gallstones are a development of carcinoma of the gallbladder and passage of gallstones into the common bile duct.[20]

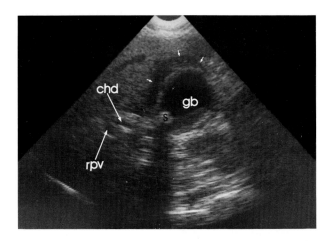

Fig. 6-49. Acute cholecystitis. Sagittal scan in a patient with pain over the gallbladder *(gb)* when scanning. Gallstones *(S)* are present in a gallbladder that has a thickened wall (arrows), an oval shape, and a transverse diameter of 5 cm. (*rpv,* right portal vein; *chd,* common hepatic duct.) (From Durrell et al,[47] with permission.)

Ultrasound Signs

To make an accurate diagnosis of cholecystitis by using ultrasound, it is necessary to adhere to specific criteria (Fig. 6-49). The major criteria are visualization or nonvisualization of a fluid-filled gallbladder in the right upper quadrant and presence or absence of stones. The minor criteria are (1) a gallbladder wall thickness, measured at a point perpendicular to the beam, of greater than 4 mm; (2) a round or oval gallbladder; and (3) a greatest transverse diameter of the gallbladder of greater than 5 cm (Fig. 6-50). The most common minor

criterion for acute cholecystitis is increased wall thickness.[148,149] In one study of patients with acute cholecystitis, 70 percent met all of the following ultrasound criteria: (1) gallbladder wall thickening of 5 mm or greater, (2) gallbladder wall anechoicity, (3) gallbladder distension as determined by external anteroposterior width of 5 cm or greater, and (4) cholelithiasis.[150] Gallbladder distension (4 cm) is seen in 87 percent of patients with cholecystitis.[150]

Right Upper Quadrant Pain

Several groups have investigated the role of ultrasound in evaluating acute right upper quadrant pain.[148,151,152] The diagnosis of acute cholecystitis is based on the highly significant observations of focal gallbladder tenderness and calculi; sludge and wall thickness are statistically significant, but to a lesser degree.[152] In one study, maximum tenderness was found over the gallbladder in 85 percent of patients with acute cholecystitis.[148] The accuracy of the sonographic Murphy sign is 87.2 percent with a sensitivity of 63 percent, a specificity of 93.6 percent, a predictive value for a positive test of 72.5 percent, and a predictive value for a negative test of 90.5 percent.[153]

In patients with normal-appearing, nontender gallbladders, ultrasound may be able to localize the site of the disease or may direct the patient's workup. When screening patients with right upper quadrant pain, ultrasound is able to detect nonbiliary abnormalities in 21 percent of patients.[151] The limiting feature of ultrasound is that it requires substantial technical expertise to obtain satisfactory images. With the introduction of high-

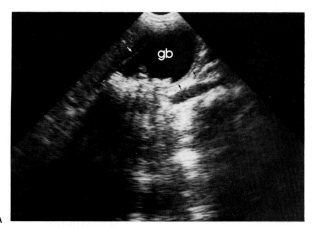

A

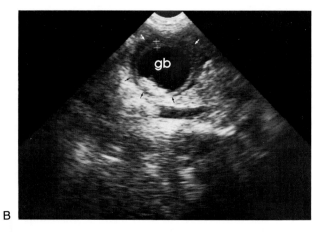

B

Fig. 6-50. Gallbladder wall thickening. **(A)** Sagittal and **(B)** transverse scans of the gallbladder *(gb)* demonstrating wall thickening (arrows) as well as cholelithiasis. It is easier to define the gallbladder wall laterally, medially, and superiorly.

resolution real-time equipment, it is possible to perform accurate examinations with considerably less operator dependence. Because of its multiorgan imaging capability and its ability to localize areas of maximum tenderness, ultrasound is the imaging technique of choice in evaluation of patients with right upper quadrant pain.[152] The diagnosis of acute cholecystitis is confirmed if calculi are visualized in a tender gallbladder. The diagnosis is further supported if the gallbladder contains sludge and has a thickened wall. If the gallbladder is nontender and stones are present, a diagnosis of chronic cholecystitis is made. If the gallbladder is normal and not tender, gallbladder disease is unlikely and clinical attention should be directed away from the gallbladder and biliary system.[152]

Gallbladder Contraction

At times, it may be desirable to measure the contraction of the gallbladder in response to CCK when cystic duct obstruction is suspected.[8] Although the demonstration of significant contraction after CCK is strong evidence of cystic duct patency, the converse does not always hold true. Failure of contraction is not specific.[8,9]

Gallbladder Wall Thickening

One of the sonographic findings in cholecystitis is an increase in the thickness of the gallbladder wall[28,154,155]

(Figs. 6-49 to 6-52). A wall thickness of greater than 3.5 mm is said to be highly accurate in predicting disease.[148,156-159] If the wall is less than 3 mm thick, cholecystitis cannot be excluded.[157] However, no patients with acute cholecystitis have had a gallbladder wall less than 5 mm thick.[150] The average gallbladder wall thickness has been reported to be less than or equal to 2 mm in 97 percent of asymptomatic patients without gallstones[160,161] (Fig. 6-1). It was noted to be 3 mm or greater in 45 percent of patients with stones in that same series.[161] Although increased wall thickness is a hallmark of chronic cholecystitis, only 55 percent of these patients were found to exhibit this at surgery in one series.[161] The mean gallbladder wall thickness is 9 mm in patients with acute cholecystitis and 5 mm in patients with chronic cholecystitis.[162]

It should be noted that wall thickness varies with transducer placement and angulation.[28,163] It is necessary to locate the true central long axis of the gallbladder for an accurate wall measurement. The wall measurement is most accurate if the region of the gallbladder wall perpendicular to the sound beam is measured[28] (Fig. 6-1). Measuring the anterior wall adjacent to the liver is most accurate, correlating within 1 mm to that found at surgery in 90 percent of cases.[28] Real-time ultrasound is the most accurate method of measuring the gallbladder wall thickness.[163] Minor angulation or decentering of the sound beam with respect to the true central long axis of the gallbladder can cause pseudothickening of the gallbladder wall.[163]

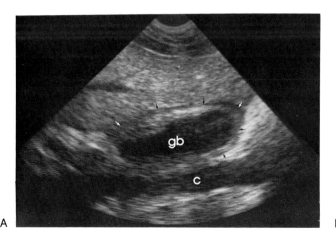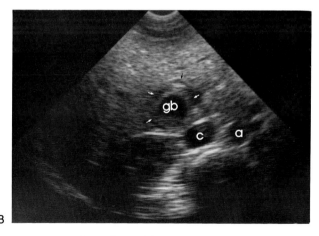

A   B

Fig. 6-51. Gallbladder "halo." **(A)** Sagittal and **(B)** transverse scans of a patient with acute cholecystitis. A thickened gallbladder *(gb)* wall (arrows) is seen. There is an inner hyperreflective layer representing the lamina propria and muscularis, with the outer poorly defined hypoechoic layer representing edema and cellular infiltration in the subserosa and adjacent liver. (*c*, inferior vena cava; *a*, aorta.) (From Durrell et al,[47] with permission.)

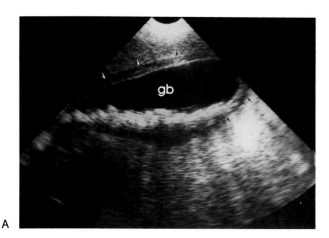
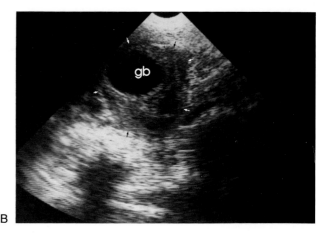

Fig. 6-52. Gallbladder wall thickening. **(A)** Sagittal and **(B)** transverse left lateral decubitus scans of the gall-bladder *(gb)* demonstrating echodense gallstones in Fig. A with wall thickening (arrows). The gallbladder wall is thickest in the fundic area as seen in Fig. B. At surgery, there were changes of both acute and chronic cholecystitis with a hematoma in the wall of the fundus.

Halo. More specific than just gallbladder wall thickening in cholecystitis is a "halo" around the gallbladder[148] (Figs. 6-49 to 6-52). In acute cholecystitis, there is diffuse hyperreflective wall thickening, hazy wall delineation, and gallbladder distension. Additionally, there is a hyporeflective or lucent layer, which is continuous or interrupted within the hyperreflective, thickened gall-bladder wall. On follow-up, this lucency represents subserosal edema and necrosis. The inner, hyperreflective contour coincides with the lamina propria and muscularis, with the thickness of irregularity of the outer contour probably related to the degree of edema and cellular infiltration in the subserosa and adjacent liver parenchyma.[164] This halo has been demonstrated in 26 percent of patients with acute cholecystitis.[148]

Striated Wall Thickening. An additional pattern has been described for gallbladder wall thickening: striated intramural lucencies.[162] This "striated" wall thickening consists of several alternating, irregular, discontinuous lucent and echogenic bands[162] (Figs. 6-53 and 6-54). It is seen in 62 percent of patients with acute cholecystitis and is not encountered in any patients who do not have acute cholecystitis.[162] The halo sign or "three-layer" thickening consists of a single circumferential lucent zone between two relatively uniform echogenic layers and is seen in only 8 percent of patients with acute cholecystitis and in 29 percent of patients with other diagnoses.[162]

As such, the various patterns described are (1) type 1, manifested by "striated" lucencies (i.e., irregular alternating, discontinuous bands of echogenicity and lucency); and (2) type 2, three-layer lucencies (i.e., a circumferential nearly continuous lucent zone interposed

between two echogenic bands).[162] When the type 2 pattern is visualized, especially in the absence of other abnormalities, noninflammatory thickening is more likely.[162]

Specificities of more than 90 percent for the diagnosis of acute cholecystitis can be achieved in the presence of echogenic foci within the gallbladder wall, wall irregularities, intraluminal membranes, and wall asymmetry.[162]

More recently, a second group of investigators have evaluated the striated wall thickening.[165] They found that this pattern is no more specific for cholecystitis than is the observation of gallbladder thickening by itself and may occur in a variety of diseases.[165] In the clinical setting of acute cholecystitis, the striations suggest gangrenous changes in the gallbladder.[165] The extent of the striations is not useful in predicting the cause of the wall thickening.[165] It cannot be explained why edema alone causes striated thickening without evidence of primary gallbladder disease, whereas in acute cholecystitis the appearance correlates with gangrene.[165] In gangrenous cholecystitis, coagulation necrosis involves all layers of the gallbladder wall, while in uncomplicated acute cholecystitis, inflammation is limited primarily to the submucosal layer of the wall.[165] It is the full-thickness involvement of the wall that produces the striations observed at ultrasound.[165]

Other Causes. Although increased gallbladder wall thickness has been associated with cholecystitis, it is also associated with other abnormalities.[157,160,166] A thickened wall may be seen with hepatitis, ascites, alcoholic liver disease, hypoproteinemia, hypoalbuminemia,

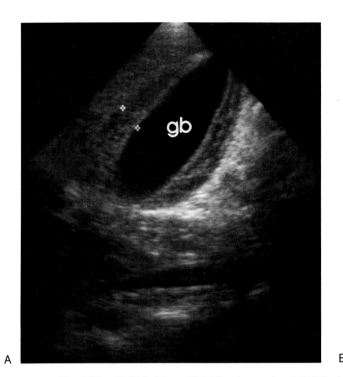

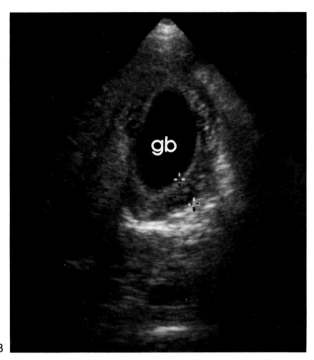

A

B

Fig. 6-53. Gallbladder wall thickening, striated. **(A)** Sagittal and **(B)** transverse views demonstrating gallbladder *(gb)* wall thickening (8 to 10 mm) in this patient with a positive Murphy sign. The wall is hypoechoic with internal densities.

heart failure, systemic venous hypertension, renal disease, multiple myeloma, and physiologic thickening resulting from partial wall contraction.[156,160,167] The mean gallbladder wall thickness is significantly increased in patients with liver cirrhosis, viral hepatitis, chronic congestive heart failure, hypoalbuminemia, and chronic renal failure.[166] An increased gallbladder wall thickness has also been seen in patients with adenomyomatosis, gallbladder tumor, pericholecystic abscess, and, possibly, varices resulting from portal hypertension.[157] A variety of nonbiliary disorders are associated with significant thickening of gallbladder walls, and this finding is not caused by incomplete gallbladder contraction.[166]

In hepatitis, excretion of the virus into the biliary system may produce a mild pericholecystic inflammation.[156,167] There is a strong correlation between gallbladder wall thickening and hypoalbuminemia.[163] In one series, all patients with ascites demonstrated gallbladder wall thickening[168] (Fig. 6-54). With ascites formation, the plasma colloid oncotic pressure and portal venous pressure seem to influence the wall thickness.[169] Hypoproteinemia states probably produce this condition by a decreased intravascular osmotic effect, just as in the bowel wall.

The gallbladder thickening in patients with ascites has been attributed to the associated hypoalbuminemia and not to the presence of ascites.[170] It has been postulated that the cause of thickening of the gallbladder wall in patients with hypoalbuminemia was edema of the wall as a result of reduced plasma oncotic pressure and increased portal pressure.[170] In one series, patients with hypoalbuminemia were studied and all were found to have a gallbladder wall of normal thickness (less than 3 mm).[170] There appeared to be no correlation between gallbladder wall thickness and the serum levels of albumin in this study.[170] As such, hypoalbuminemia may not be the cause of thickening, even when peritoneal fluid is present.[170]

Different patterns of gallbladder wall thickening have been described in malignant versus cirrhotic ascites.[171] The three patterns described were (1) single-layered nonthickened wall; (2) single-layered thickened wall; and (3) double-layered thickened wall[171] (Figs. 6-55 and 6-56). In patients with malignant ascites, the single-layered nonthickened wall pattern was more commonly observed, with the single-layered, thickened wall pattern also seen.[171] In patients with cirrhotic ascites, two patterns were found: (1) single-layered thickened wall, and (2) double-layered thickened wall[171] (Fig. 6-55). Use of single-layered nonthickened wall as a criterion for prediction of malignant ascites has a sensitivity of 80.6 percent and a specificity of 98.3 percent.[171]

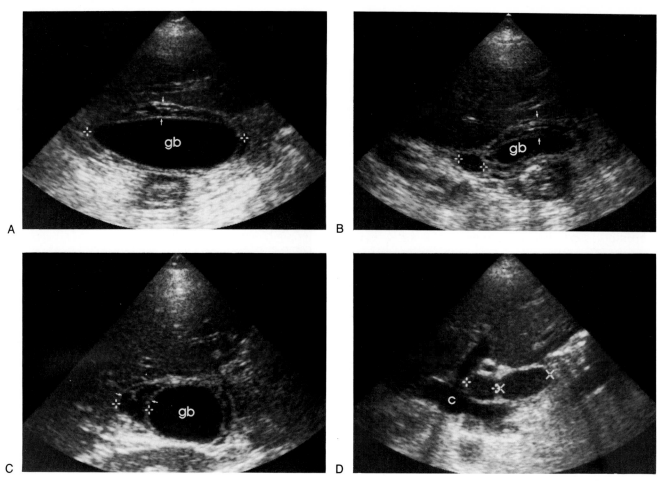

Fig. 6-54. Gallbladder wall thickening, striated. This patient with acute nonlymphocytic leukemia presented with acute right upper quadrant pain. On **(A & B)** sagittal and **(C)** transverse scans of the gallbladder *(gb),* there is striated wall thickening (14 mm, arrows). The wall is hypoechoic with internal densities. This patient had nodes (calipers) in the porta hepatis on **(D)** sagittal view and at the gallbladder neck in Fig. C. The ultrasound findings were consistent with acute cholecystitis. The patient had positive antibodies to CMV. A percutaneous cholecystostomy tube was placed, resulting in the drainage of pus. The patient died and was found at autopsy to have marked edema of the gallbladder wall with nodes (infiltrated with the patient's leukemic process) at the gallbladder neck. These were compressing the lumen, resulting in cystic duct obstruction. (*c,* inferior vena cava.)

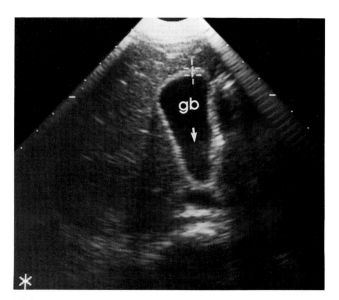

Fig. 6-55. Gallbladder wall thickening, nonmalignant ascites. Transverse scan demonstrating a gallbladder *(gb)* with a single-layered, echogenic, thickened wall (calipers, 5 mm). Ascites was demonstrated on other views. There is sludge (arrow) within the dependent portion of the gallbladder.

Varices have been reported as another cause of gallbladder wall thickening.[172] There are multiple potential collateral channels in the portal system, including small veins around the gallbladder and along the hepatoduodenal ligament.[172,173] These varices are a moderately unusual manifestation of portal hypertension, occurring in 12 percent of cases.[174] They represent a portosystemic shunt linking the cystic vein branch of the portal system to systemic anterior abdominal wall collaterals.[174] Additionally, they may act as a bypass around a focally thrombosed extrahepatic segment of the portal vein.[174] There may be retrograde flow from the cystic vein to the gallbladder varices, which may give rise to flow across the gallbladder bed directly into the hepatic parenchyma and ultimately into the right portal vein.[174] Lastly, these gallbladder varices may be due to simple back-pressure within the portal venous system.[174]

The individual dilated vessels with venous flow can be demonstrated by using high-frequency real-time ultrasound and pulsed Doppler[172,173] (Fig. 6-57). By using duplex ultrasound or color Doppler, anechoic areas within the gallbladder wall detected by ultrasound can be distinguished from intramural edema.[174] The presence of portal vein thrombosis may be implied by the visualization of gallbladder wall varices.[174] The varices may mimic a variety of diseases. Doppler appears to be the most sensitive and specific method for the detection of these varices and should be used in patients with known or suspected portal hypertension who are undergoing examinations of the liver and biliary tree.[174] The surgeons should be made aware of this finding since these varices can be a source of major blood loss.[174]

Still other causes of gallbladder wall thickening have been reported. With congestive heart failure, there is increased systemic and portal venous engorgement, which may produce edema of the wall. A thickened gallbladder wall may also be secondary to focal obstruction of the gallbladder lymphatic drainage by malignant lymphoma in portal lymph nodes.[175] Obstruction of the lymphatic drainage of an organ results in increased interstitial fluid and thickening of the tissues. This ultrasound appearance is similar to that of hemorrhagic cholecystitis, a severe inflammatory process involving the gallbladder wall, and pericholecystic fluid collections including bilomas, pancreatic pseudocyst, and abscess.[175]

Gallbladder abnormalities have been found in association with primary sclerosing cholangitis. Primary sclerosing cholangitis is a chronic cholestatic syndrome of undetermined cause and is characterized by diffuse fibrosing inflammation of the intrahepatic and extrahepatic bile ducts, resulting in bile duct obliteration, biliary cirrhosis, and hepatic failure.[176] The following gallbladder abnormalities have been found: (1) symmetric thickening of the gallbladder wall; (2) focal asymmetric thickening of the gallbladder wall; and (3) diffuse, pronounced, asymmetric thickening of the gallbladder wall.[176] Eight-nine percent of the gallbladders examined pathologically were abnormal.[176]

Specific Types of Cholecystitis

Acalculous Cholecystitis

Acalculous cholecystitis represents acute or chronic gallbladder inflammation in the absence of biliary stones. The incidence of acute cholecystitis in patients with acalculous gallbladders varies between 3.3 and 10

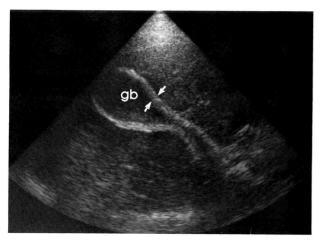
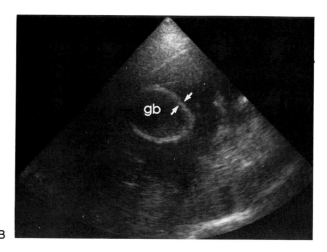

A
B

Fig. 6-56. Gallbladder wall thickening, malignant ascites. **(A)** Sagittal and **(B)** transverse views of the gallbladder *(gb)* showing a single-layered, echogenic, thickened gallbladder wall (5 mm, arrows). The ascitic fluid was positive for adenocarcinoma secondary to metastatic disease from pancreatic carcinoma.

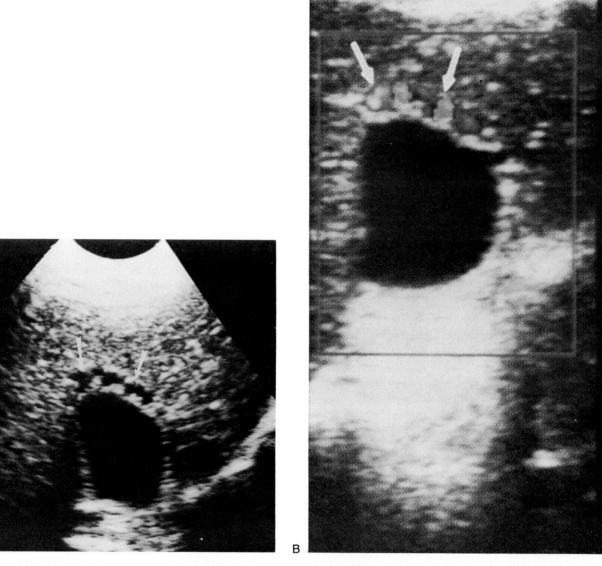

Fig. 6-57. Gallbladder varices. Images of a 12-year-old boy with chronic active hepatitis and hemobilia. **(A)** Transverse ultrasound scan through the gallbladder showing serpentine anechoic areas within the gallbladder wall (arrows). **(B)** Color Doppler image corresponding to Fig. A demonstrating flow (white on this noncolor image) within the gallbladder varices (arrows). (From West MS et al,[174] with permission.)

percent at cholecystectomy.[177] The incidence of acute acalculous cholecystitis in patients with acute cholecystitis is 5 to 10 percent.[178] It is seen in 5 to 15 percent of cases of cholecystitis and 47 percent of cases of postoperative cholecystitis.[179] Between 9 and 41 percent of cases of acalculous cholecystitis occur after an operation or severe trauma in adults.[177] In 87 percent of patients with post-traumatic and postoperative cholecystitis, acal-

culous gallbladder is found at surgery.[177] It may be associated with previous unrelated surgery, trauma, hyperalimentation, burns, cardiac arrest, diabetes, or pancreatitis. This type of cholecystitis can be associated with numerous entities and seems to be more frequent in men than in women.[177] Its pathogenesis is not completely understood. Fifty-two percent of untreated cases progress to gangrene and gallbladder rupture.

As a potentially fatal complication of prolonged critical illness, acute acalculous cholecystitis is uncommon and most probably results from a gradual increase in bile viscosity owing to prolonged stasis that leads to a functional obstruction of the cystic duct.[180] Numerous pathophysiologic mechanisms have been postulated to be the basis for acalculous cholecystitis.[179] It may be caused by substances directly toxic to the gallbladder wall such as pancreatic enzymes and hyperconcentrated bile. Pancreatitis and/or surgery for biliary tract revision may predispose patients to the reflux of pancreatic juices into the gallbladder. When organisms in the gallbladder invade the mucosa and gallbladder wall, inflammation results. Infarction of the gallbladder wall or mucosa may be due to decreased perfusion pressure or gallbladder vessel damage.[179]

The ultrasound findings with acalculous cholecystitis include (1) enlarged gallbladder, (2) diffuse or focal wall thickening, (3) focal hypoechoic regions in the wall, (4) pericholecystic fluid, (5) diffuse homogeneous echogenicity within the gallbladder lumen, and (6) a positive Murphy sign[179] (Figs. 6-51 and 6-54). With these ultrasound criteria, the sensitivity is 63 to 67 percent.[179] After a patient fasts for at least 5 hours, a positive ultrasound diagnosis may be made if at least one of the following signs is seen: (1) gallbladder wall thickening of greater than 6 mm, diffuse or focal; (2) an enlarged gallbladder with a positive Murphy sign; and (3) diffuse, homogeneous nonshadowing median level echogenicity within the gallbladder lumen, suggestive of pus in combination with a Murphy sign[179] (Fig. 6-58).

More recently a group of investigators have evaluated acalculous cholecystitis by ultrasound.[180] Their major criteria include (1) a wall thickness of 4 mm or greater when the gallbladder is distended to at least 5 cm in the longitudinal dimension and there is no evidence of ascites or hypoalbuminemia (serum protein < 3.2 mg/d); (2) the presence of pericholecystic fluid or subserosal edema, calculi, intramural gas, and/or a sloughed mucosal membrane; and/or (3) a complete lack of response to CCK.[180] The minor criteria include (1) presence of echogenic bile (sludge); (2) distension greater than 8 cm in the longitudinal dimension or 5 cm in the transverse dimension; and/or (3) a partial response (< 50 percent decrease in longitudinal and transverse dimensions) after CCK injection.[180] The study is considered positive if it includes either a minimum of two major criteria or one major and two minor criteria.[180]

The most consistent finding associated with postoperative acalculous cholecystitis in thickening of the gallbladder wall.[177] The diagnosis is more easily established if a sonolucent layer within the gallbladder wall is present.[177]

Cholecystokinin sonography has been postulated to be helpful in the diagnosis of acute acalculous cholecystitis in hospitalized patients.[181] In a study evaluating this, there was considerable variability in the gallbladder response to administration of sincalide in fasting hospitalized patients. Lack of contraction of the gallbladder after injection of CCK should not be considered a major criterion in the diagnosis of acute acalculous cholecystitis.[181]

Acalculous cholecystitis is difficult to diagnose by clinical means or contrast radiography. The sensitivity of ultrasound in detecting it is 67 percent and that of nuclear medicine is 68 percent, which is not as high as in calculous cholecystitis.[179] The overall sensitivity and specificity of hepatobiliary scintigraphy in the diagnosis of acute cholecystitis are 95 to 100 percent and 81 to 100 percent, respectively, with the sensitivity and specificity

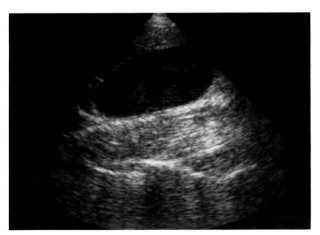
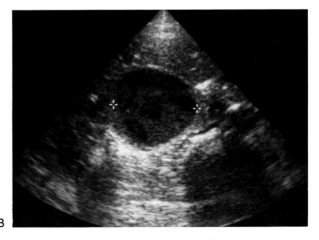

A   B

Fig. 6-58. Acalculous gangrenous cholecystitis. **(A)** Sagittal and **(B)** transverse scans in a patient with a positive Murphy sign and a palpable mass. The gallbladder (calipers) is enlarged, tense, and filled with diffuse internal echoes that do not layer. There was no wall thickening.

of ultrasound reported as 67 to 93 percent and 82 to 100 percent, respectively.[180] This series reported a sensitivity of 92 percent and a specificity of 96 percent in establishing the diagnosis of acute acalculous cholecystitis with ultrasound.[180] Ultrasound has a sensitivity equivalent to and specificity superior to cholescintigraphy. When other intra-abdominal diseases are anticipated, CT is accurate in evaluating the gallbladder for suspected acute cholecystitis.[180] Percutaneous aspiration of bile may be a valuable method of confirming the diagnosis of acute cholecystitis, but a sterile specimen without leukocytes cannot reliably exclude the diagnosis.[180]

The diagnosis of chronic acalculous gallbladder disease remains difficult. Biliary scintigraphy is the most sensitive technique (sensitivity, 89 percent) in patients with histologic changes of chronic cholecystitis.[182] OCG and ultrasound have sensitivities of 66 and 61 percent, respectively.[182] The accuracy of ultrasound, OCG, and biliary scintigraphy is 82, 86, and 38 percent, respectively, for identifying symptomatic patients who may have long-term symptomatic relief after cholecystectomy.[182] More than one study must be performed to make the correct diagnosis and to predict good results from cholecystectomy for chronic acalculous cholecystitis.[182]

Gangrenous Cholecystitis

Gangrenous cholecystitis occurs in 2 to 38 percent of patients with acute cholecystitis, and perforation occurs in 10 percent.[183] The prevalence of gangrenous cholecystitis is 1.2 percent with right upper quadrant pain.[184] Gallbladder distension and mural inflammation occur in acute nongangrenous cholecystitis, and they stimulate visceral afferent nerves in the muscular and serosal layers of the gallbladder via the autonomic nervous system.[184] Pathologically, gangrenous cholecystitis is defined as transmural hemorrhagic or liquefactive necrosis in most of the gallbladder wall.[184] It differs from acute cholecystitis by the presence of intramural hemorrhage, necrosis, and microabscesses.[183] The gallbladder wall is thickened and edematous with focal areas of exudate, hemorrhage, and even abscess.[185] Therefore there is maximal pain when the distended inflamed gallbladder is compressed. Transmural necrosis produces inflammation of the adjacent parietal peritoneum, stimulating intercostal branches of the spinal nerves and producing generalized right upper quadrant pain in the T5 to T11 dermatomes once these nerves die as they do in gangrenous cholecystitis.[184] Stones or fine gravel are seen in 80 to 95 percent of cases.[185]

There are no distinctive signs, symptoms, or laboratory findings to distinguish gangrenous cholecystitis

from uncomplicated acute cholecystitis.[186] Patients with gangrenous cholecystitis present with right upper quadrant pain, tenderness, fever, leukocytosis, and often a palpable gallbladder.[185] If surgical intervention does not take place in the early stages of gallbladder inflammation, vascular compromise will invariably lead to gangrenous changes, since the cystic artery is an end artery.[186]

Gangrenous cholecystitis and empyema of the gallbladder have been described with ultrasound.[185,187] The typical pattern is that of diffuse, medium to coarse intraluminal echoes within the gallbladder, which do not show layering or acoustic shadowing[148,183,185,187] (Fig. 6-58). Other findings include thickening of the gallbladder wall and localized peritoneal fluid collections. The echogenic debris described probably represent purulent and fibrinous debris within the gallbladder, perhaps contributed from the focal exudative and ulcerative changes in the gallbladder wall. The lack of layering effect is attributed to the markedly increased viscosity of the bile.[185] In one series, 42 percent of patients with gangrenous cholecystitis had no specific features different from those of acute cholecystitis.[183]

Atypical findings have been seen with gangrenous cholecystitis. In one study, 58 percent of patients had atypical findings, including intraluminal membranes and/or marked irregularities of the gallbladder wall. This finding is unusual in acute cholecystitis and should prompt close clinical observation for possible gangrenous cholecystitis[183] (Fig. 6-59). These linear, nonshadowing densities producing gallbladder septation seen within the gallbladder lumen represent desquamated necrotic mucosa, reflecting separation of the inflamed necrotic mucosa, which is rare in cholecystitis.[147] The sonographic findings of intraluminal membranes and irregular masslike protrusions projecting into the gall-

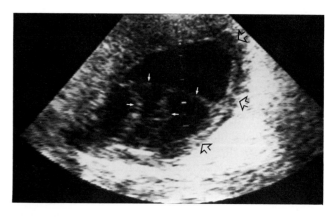

Fig. 6-59. Gangrenous cholecystitis. Membranes. A distended gallbladder with a thickened wall (open arrows) is seen sagittally with intraluminal linear densities (arrows).

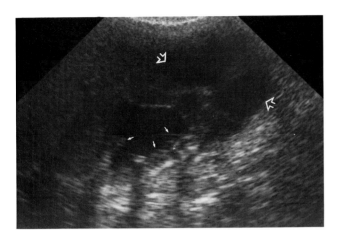

Fig. 6-60. Gangrenous cholecystitis. Heterogeneous gallbladder wall thickening. Sonogram showing a thickened gallbladder wall with irregular, masslike protrusions projecting into the gallbladder lumen (small arrows). Adjacent to the gallbladder is a large, complex pericholecystic fluid collection (type II) (open arrows). (From Teefey et al,[186] with permission.)

bladder lumen should suggest the diagnosis of gangrenous cholecystitis[186] (Fig. 6-60).

Striated thickening of the gallbladder wall frequently occurs in gangrenous cholecystitis and is the most common finding (40 percent)[186] (similar to Figs. 6-53 and 6-54). The pattern of striated thickening of the gallbladder wall, which is not associated with pericholecystic fluid, may be indicative of early gangrenous changes prior to perforation and abscess formation.[186] In the clinical setting of acute cholecystitis, mural striations are suspicious as indicators of gangrenous changes.[186]

Several patterns have been described with associated pericholecystic fluid collections: (1) type I, crescent-shaped lucent fluid collections closely adjoining the gallbladder wall with a short-axis measurement of 1 cm or less; (2) type II, larger (> 1 cm) and either anechoic or complex (thick walls, internal debris, or septations) collections; and (3) type III, complex fluid collections totally encompassing the gallbladder and resulting in an inability to delineate the gallbladder as a separate structure[186] (Fig. 6-48). Type I fluid collections are not typically associated with gallbladder wall perforation, whereas all but one of the type II or III collections in one series were the direct result of full-thickness gallbladder wall ischemia with subsequent perforation.[186]

One group of investigators have found that absence of the Murphy sign increases the possibility of gangrenous cholecystitis in patients with abdominal pain and sonographic findings of cholecystitis.[184] Only 33 percent of these patients exhibited a positive Murphy sign.[184]

Emphysematous Cholecystitis

Acute emphysematous cholecystitis is a complication or uncommon variant of acute cholecystitis and is associated with a significant increase in morbidity and mortality. With this entity, ischemia is followed by invasion of the gallbladder wall by gas-forming microorganisms. Cholelithiasis is not a major pathologic factor, and 38 percent of patients are diabetic.[188,189] This type of cholecystitis differs from the usual type of acute cholecystitis because (1) there is a definite male predilection and (2) the incidence of acalculous cholecystitis is three times as common in the emphysematous form as in acute cholecystitis.[190] Gangrene is common, and the incidence of perforation is five times greater than with acute cholecystitis.[28,189] In this form of cholecystitis, gas typically accumulates within the gallbladder wall or lumen but is occasionally found in the bile ducts or pericholecystic area.[191]

The following signs have been identified with acute emphysematous cholecystitis: (1) intraluminal gas, (a dense band of hyperreflective echoes with distal reverberations when the gallbladder is full of gas and a band of reverberations in the gas-filled portion of the gallbladder with the usual signs of cholecystitis in the bile-filled portion when the gallbladder is partially full of gas); and (2) intramural gas, (an area of high reflectivity in the gallbladder wall with reverberations that may change position with change in position of patient and a bright hyperreflective ring emanating from the whole circumference of the gallbladder)[190,191] (Fig. 6-61). The gas and its echoes may shift in response to gravity as the patient changes position.[191]

At times high-density echoes are seen within the gallbladder fossa with posterior shadowing in cases of emphysematous cholecystitis[188,189] (Fig. 6-61). Gas in the gallbladder wall may cause it to be hyperechoic with or without acoustic shadowing, depending on the amount of the gas. In most patients there are large amounts of gas in the lumen of the gallbladder. The key on ultrasound is to see reverberations within the acoustic shadow, which are produced by gas in the gallbladder (Fig. 6-61). Since reverberations are rarely seen within the shadows produced by gallstones, a "reverberation shadow" arising from the gallbladder (in the absence of biliary-enteric anastomosis or fistula) should be confirmed by abdominal radiography.[188]

Gallbladder Perforation

Perforation of the gallbladder occurs in 8 to 12 percent of patients with acute cholecystitis and typically occurs 3 to 7 days after the onset of symptoms.[192,193] The time

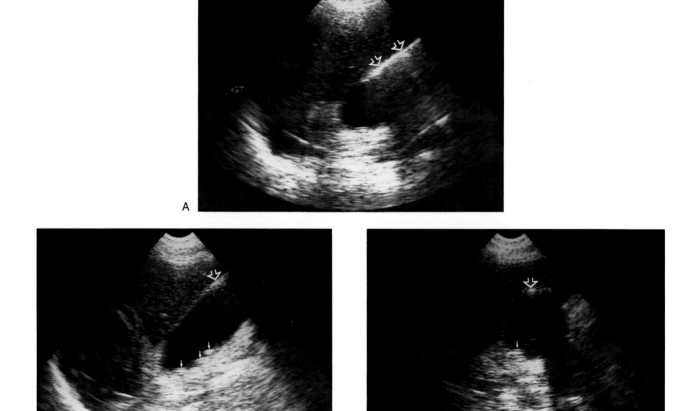

Fig. 6-61. Emphysematous cholecystitis. **(A & B)** Sagittal and **(C)** transverse real-time scans. Gallstones (small arrows) are seen in Figs. B & C, as well as a hyperreflective layer (air, open arrows) in the superficial portion of the gallbladder. (Figs. A & C from Durrell et al,[47] with permission.)

interval between the onset of symptoms and gangrene/ perforation may be as short as 24 hours or as long as 24 days.[150,194] The associated mortality has been reported to be 19 to 24 percent.[193] As a serious complication of acute cholecystitis, pericholecystic abscess has a prevalence varying from 2.1 to 19.5 percent.[195]

Predisposing factors include not only cholelithiasis but also infection, cancer, trauma, drugs (corticosteroids), and impaired vascular supply.[196] Perforation occurs as a result of calculi obstructing the cystic duct, producing mucosal injury, edema, congestion, and eventual circulatory compromise of the gallbladder wall, which leads to gangrene and perforation.[193] Detection of this complication of acute cholecystitis by clinical means is difficult since the symptoms are similar to those of uncomplicated acute cholecystitis, with a mortality with perforation of 20 percent.[195]

An accepted mechanism for perforation includes (1) impaction of a calculus in the cystic duct; (2) gallbladder distension due to secretion into its lumen by the mucous glands located in the walls of the gallbladder; (3) vascular impairment of the gallbladder due to distension of the viscus; and (4) ischemia, necrosis, and perforation of the gallbladder wall.[196] The risk of gallbladder perforation decreases the earlier cholecystectomy is performed after the onset of acute cholecystitis. The various types of perforation are (1) acute free perforation causing bile peritonitis; (2) subacute (most common) walled-off perforation causing a pericholecystic abscess; and (3) chronic perforation resulting in internal biliary fistula (cholecystoenteric or cholecystocutaneous).[193,196,197]

Perforation occurs most commonly in the gallbladder fundus because of its poor vascular supply (or in the area of gangrene) and may lead to peritonitis, pericholecystic

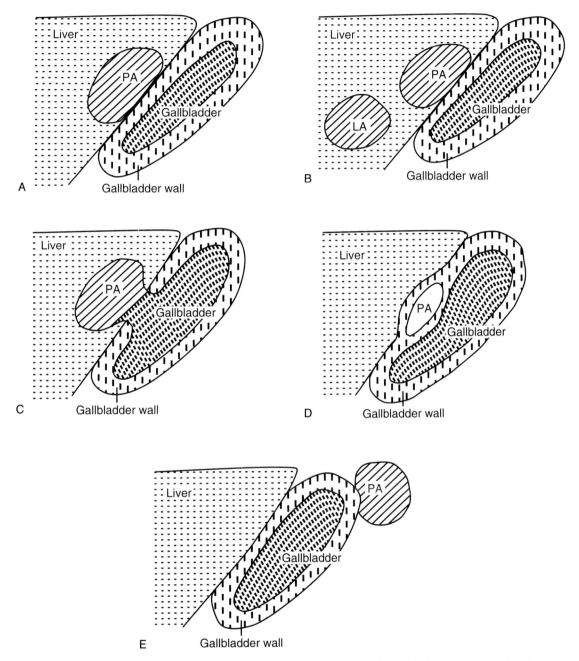

Fig. 6-62. Ultrasound classification of pericholecystic abscess *(PA)*. **(A)** Gallbladder bed group, localized abscess. **(B)** Gallbladder bed group, complicated abscess. **(C)** Gallbladder bed group, communicating abscess. **(D)** Intramural group. **(E)** Intraperitoneal group. (*LA*, liver abscess.) (From Takada et al,[195] with permission.)

abscess, or fistulous communication with adjacent viscera.[198] Peritonitis is caused by free perforation whereas fistulous communication of the gallbladder with an adjacent organ may present as chronic biliary disease or acute gallstone ileus.[198] The extraluminal fluid collection is located contiguous to a thick-walled gallbladder in the fundic region and is usually constant in location.[192] Pericholecystic fluid collections can also occur when there is inflammation in adjacent organs in such diseases as peptic ulcer disease, pancreatitis, ascites, and peritonitis.[196,199] Pericholecystic abscess usually is associated with acute inflammatory signs and symptoms.

Distension of the gallbladder and edema of its walls may be the earliest signs of impending gallbladder perforation detectable on ultrasound (Figs. 6-49 and 6-52). The gallbladder is considered dilated on ultrasound if it is greater than 3.5 to 4 cm in its anterior-posterior width. Once perforation occurs, pericholecystic collections that are easily detectable on ultrasound will develop.

The ultrasound findings in perforation of the gallbladder range from a well-defined band of low-level echoes around the gallbladder (well-encapsulated abscess) to multiple poorly defined hypoechoic masses surrounding an irregular indistinct gallbladder (extensive abscess)[196,197,200] (Figs. 6-62 to 6-66). The ultrasound findings depend on the presence or absence of inflammation or gangrene of the gallbladder wall, the size and location of the perforation, and the extent and location of the bile leakage.[193] Their internal characteristics are dependent on the duration of the pericholecystic process.[196] The residual gallbladder lumen or calculi can be identified within or peripheral to the pericholecystic process. As such, findings of perforation include (1) anechoic to complex mass; (2) gallstones; (3) coarse, nonshadowing, echogenic debris; (4) wall thickening; (5) gallbladder

distension; and (6) bile duct dilatation[198] (Figs. 6-63 to 6-66). A complex cystic mass in the gallbladder fossa with intrahepatic extension should suggest the diagnosis of perforated gallbladder with pericholecystic abscess.[198]

Pericholecystic fluid collections that develop are easily detected in sonograms but are nonspecific.[194] With careful manipulation of the transducer, the site of perforation may be demonstrated[194] (Fig. 6-65). This finding (called the "hole sign") resembles a defect in a perforated balloon and is more specific for perforation.[194]

Three different groups have been defined for pericholecystic abscess: a gallbladder group, an intramural group, and an intraperitoneal group[195] (Fig. 6-62). A pericholecystic abscess in the gallbladder bed is seen as a low-echo area in which minute echogenic patterns are observed to move with change in patient position[195] (Fig. 6-63). In the intramural group, the abscess is seen as a small, low-echo area in the thickened gallbladder wall with longitudinal scanning of the right upper part of the abdomen and with right-sided intercostal scanning[195] (Figs. 6-64 and 6-65). The intraperitoneal group is seen as minute echogenic patterns in the peritoneal cavity adjoining the gallbladder[195] (Fig. 6-66).

In one series, all patients with localized abscess in the gallbladder fossa region were adequately treated by administration of antibiotics.[195] When there was a complicated abscess with a liver abscess or with a communicating abscess with the gallbladder, the patient did not respond to antibiotic therapy because of the marked spread of the inflammation.[195] Percutaneous aspiration or drainage of the abscess was necessary.[195] In patients with an intramural abscess, close observation is necessary because perforation may occur during the therapeutic course.[195]

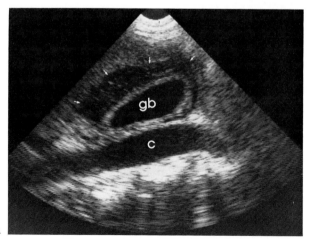

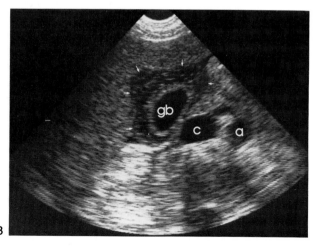

A   B

Fig. 6-63. Gallbladder perforation. **(A)** Sagittal and **(B)** transverse real-time scans. A well-defined hypoechoic layer (arrows) is seen encircling the gallbladder *(gb)* wall. This is consistent with pericholecystic fluid. (*c*, inferior vena cava; *a*, aorta.) (From Durrell et al,[47] with permission.)

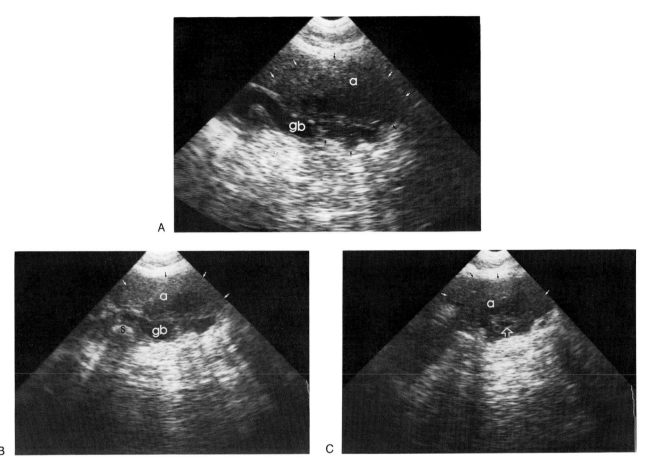

Fig. 6-64. Gallbladder perforation. **(A & B)** Sagittal and **(C)** transverse left lateral decubitus scans. An echodense stone *(s)* is seen within the neck of the gallbladder *(gb)* in Fig. B with a poorly defined mass effect (*a*, arrows) mainly in the anterior fundic region. The mass has a mixed echopattern. This proved to be a pericholecystic abscess. (open arrow, gallbladder lumen.)

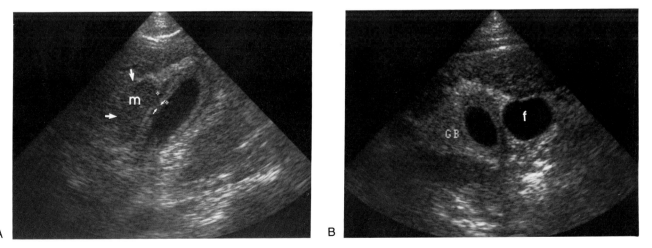

Fig. 6-65. Gallbladder perforation. **(A)** Sagittal view showing a mass (*m*, large arrows) within the gallbladder wall similar to Fig. 6-62D as well as gallbladder thickening. There is a defect (small arrows) within the gallbladder wall. **(B)** Transverse view showing pericholecystic fluid *(f)* medial to the gallbladder similar to Fig. 62E. The gallbladder *(GB)* wall is again thickened.

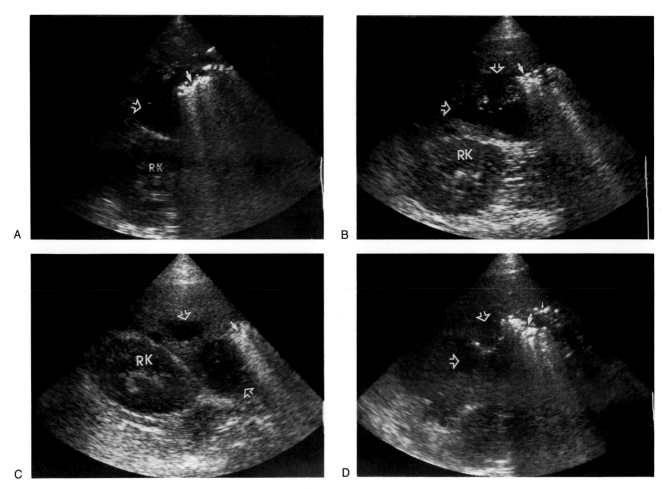

Fig. 6-66. Gallbladder perforation. This patient had presented to the emergency department 1 week prior to the ultrasound examination with right upper quadrant pain. The patient's pain had stopped the day before the ultrasound examination. **(A–C)** Transverse scans through the gallbladder fossa and porta hepatis demonstrating a poorly defined lucent area (open arrows, fluid) with air (solid arrow) medially. The gallbladder was not visualized. (*RK*, right kidney.) **(D)** After oral water, peristalsis (small arrow) could be seen medial to the air collection (large arrow) on a transverse right lateral decubitus view but it did not communicate with the large air collection. In Fig. C the fluid collection seen appears to be intrahepatic. (open arrows, fluid.) *(Figure continues.)*

Xanthogranulomatous Cholecystitis

The etiology of xanthogranulomatous cholecystitis must be similar to that of xanthogranulomatous pyelonephritis, which is a chronic infection in which the formation of calculi play a role. This disease has a prevalence of 0.7 to 10.6 percent in cholecystectomy specimens.[201] There is chronic infection and calculi associated with stasis of bile, probably causing the degeneration and necrosis of the wall and the formation of microabscesses.[201] As a rare inflammatory disease of the gallbladder, xanthogranulomatous cholecystitis is characterized histologically by the infiltration of round cells, lipid-laden histiocytes, and multinucleated giant cells and the proliferation of fibroblasts in the muscle layer.[201]

The pathologic pattern is that of lipid-containing histiocytes infiltrating the outer layer of the muscularis of the gallbladder wall.

On ultrasound, one sees a complex right upper quadrant mass containing poorly marginated, intense reflections[202] (Fig. 6-67). In these patients, a calculus or calculi are seen with moderate thickening of the gallbladder wall.[201] The appearance may be similar to that of gallbladder carcinoma.[201]

Hemorrhagic Cholecystitis

Hemorrhagic cholecystitis is a rare complication of biliary tract disease and is usually associated with cholelithiasis. It is a known complication of acute cholecysti-

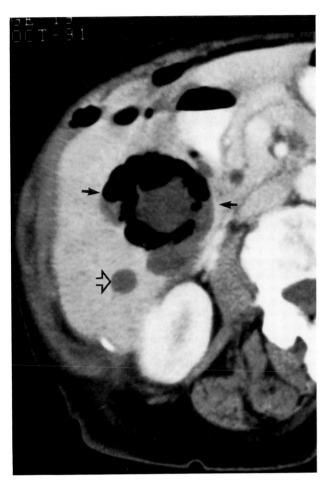

Fig. 6-66 *(Continued).* **(E)** On enhanced CT scan, a fluid collection (arrows) containing air is seen within the gallbladder fossa consistent with perforation as well as free air. There is a low-density area (open arrow) within the liver posterior to the mass.

tis.[203] Other causes include anticoagulation, biliary neoplasms, and trauma, including liver biopsy and vascular disease. Clinically, these patients may present with abdominal pain, leukocystosis, and fever.[203] There is a 13 to 25 percent incidence of occult blood in the stool in such patients.[203]

Pathologic designation of acute cholecystitis, hemorrhagic cholecystitis, and/or gangrenous cholecystitis relies on the identification of inflammation, mucosal hemorrhage, intraluminal hemorrhage, and/or gangrene.[203] These findings represent overlapping stages in a continuum of complications of acute cholecystitis leading potentially to perforation.[203] This is an earlier, less severe complication of acute cholecystitis than gangrenous cholecystitis.[203]

Patients with hemorrhagic cholecystitis may exhibit one of the following patterns: (1) focal gallbladder wall irregularity; (2) intraluminal membranes; or (3) coarse, nonshadowing, nonmobile intraluminal echoes.[203] On ultrasound, the gallbladder bile is dense, similar to what is seen with pus or thick sludge (Figs. 6-68 and 6-69). Blood clots appear as clumps of echogenic material.[204]

Cholecystitis in Children

The ultrasound signs of cholecystitis in children are the same as those in adults. These include gallbladder wall thickening, biliary sludge, gallbladder stones, Murphy sign, increased gallbladder size, and nonvisualization of the gallbladder.[27] Acalculous cholecystitis is more common in children than in adults, so one must carefully examine the gallbladder wall; 50 percent of childhood cases are not associated with stones.[27,205] In adolescents, there is a higher association with stones. In

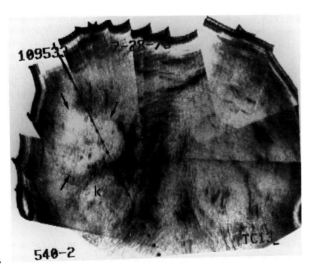

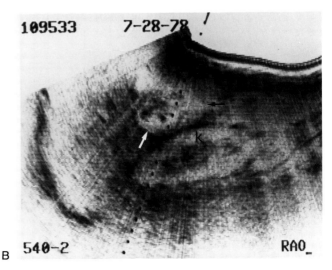

Fig. 6-67. Xanthogranulomatous cholecystitis. **(A)** Transverse and **(B)** right anterior oblique views of the abdomen 16 cm above the iliac crest. A complex mass (arrows) with internal reflections is seen just superior to the right kidney *(k)*. (From Bluth et al,[202] with permission.)

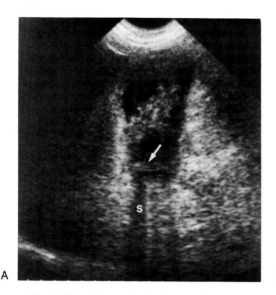 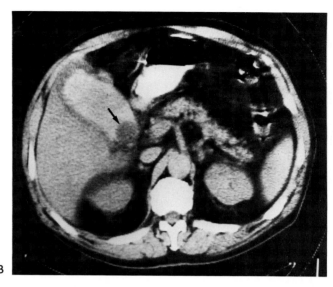

Fig. 6-68. Hemorrhagic cholecystitis. **(A)** Real-time long-axis view of the gallbladder. A thick-walled fundus is seen with an echo (arrow) and acoustic shadow *(s)* of a calculus, along with clumps of echogenic material within the gallbladder. **(B)** CT scan. A thick-walled fundus is seen with a negative filling defect (arrow) of the calculus, with increased density of blood in bile (80 CT units). (From Jenkins et al,[204] with permission.)

addition, 25 to 45 percent of children present with jaundice and only 6 percent with common bile duct stones.[205] Many cases are associated with congenital malformations of the biliary tract.[206]

Correlative Imaging and Ultrasound Accuracy in Cholecystitis

The diagnostic modality that is the method of choice for evaluation of cholecystitis is a much more controversial topic than that of cholelithiasis. Some investigators favor ultrasound because of its capabilities to view the entire right upper quadrant and to assess for pinpoint gallbladder tenderness.[154] Others favor hepatobiliary nuclear medicine because it is a better test for evaluating gallbladder function.[207,208] Most institutions do not use intravenous cholangiography because of the morbidity and mortality associated with it.[209]

Many data support the use of ultrasound as the initial imaging procedure for patients with suspected acute cholecystitis, but a comparison between ultrasound and nuclear medicine studies should be made. Rapid assessment of patients with suspected acute cholecystitis poses a difficult and important problem. Hepatobiliary nuclear medicine is useful in cases without stones, which exhibit minor criteria for gallbladder abnormality. The major diagnostic feature is the presence (cystic duct patency) or absence (cystic duct obstruction) of gallbladder visualization.[210] Although visualization of the gallblad-

der by hepatobiliary nuclear medicine usually precludes the possibility of acute cholecystitis, nonvisualization does not, and delayed views would have to be obtained. One study reported the visualization by nuclear medicine of a gallbladder in a patient with acute cholecystitis and a patent cystic duct.[211] Another reported visualization of an obstructed gallbladder via an accessory hepatic duct.[212] The visualization by nuclear medicine of two gallbladders involved with acute cholecystitis has been described.[213]

How do the accuracies of ultrasound and nuclear medicine compare with regard to acute cholecystitis? Numerous studies have reported the following statistics for nuclear medicine: accuracy of 84.7 to 88 percent, specificity of 90.2 to 100 percent, sensitivity of 95 to 98.3 percent, and false-negative rate of 5 percent.[149,214–216] The comparative values for ultrasound are accuracy of 88.1 percent, specificity of 60.2 to 100 percent, and sensitivity of 76 to 97 percent.[149,210–217] The ultrasound criterion of gallbladder roundness or a diameter of greater than 5 cm was less sensitive and less specific. When differentiating normality from all types of gallbladder disease, nuclear medicine had a sensitivity of 80 percent with a specificity of 100 percent[149]; ultrasound had a sensitivity of 100 percent with a specificity of 96 percent, with the major and minor criteria for gallbladder disease.[109] The most common minor criterion seen in acute cholecystitis is increased wall thickness.[149] Some investigators believe that the choice of the examination — nuclear medicine or ultrasound — should depend on (1)

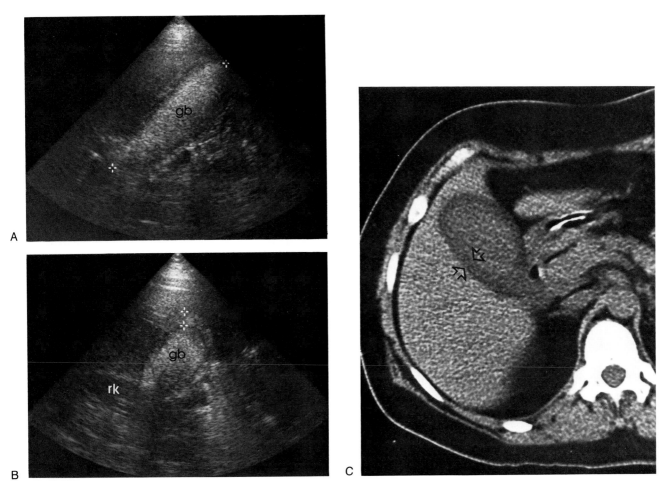

Fig. 6-69. Hemorrhagic cholecystitis. **(A)** Sagittal and **(B)** transverse views demonstrating a gallbladder *(gb)* distended with very echogenic material. The gallbladder wall (calipers, Fig. B) is thickened. (*rk,* right kidney.) **(C)** Unenhanced CT scan. The gallbladder wall thickening (open arrows) is seen as a low-density "halo." The material within the gallbladder is noted to be dense.

the quality of the available equipment, (2) the capability of the technologist to perform the examination, (3) the relative experience of the physician, and (4) the willingness of the surgeon to accept a positive result as an indication to perform emergency surgery.[214]

The reliability of the elicitation of pinpoint right upper quadrant pain in making the diagnosis of cholecystitis has also been studied. Investigators have examined the role of ultrasound in evaluating acute right upper quadrant pain in patients with a clinical suspicion of acute cholecystitis. The diagnosis of acute cholecystitis is based on the highly significant observations of focal gallbladder tenderness and calculi. Sludge and wall thickness are statistically significant, but to a lesser degree. Cholelithiasis allows differentiation of patients with chronic cholecystitis from patients with normal gallbladders; the latter patients do not have significant focal gallbladder tender-

ness, sludge, or a thickened gallbladder wall. Ultrasound has a sensitivity of 94 percent, a specificity of 85 percent, and an overall accuracy of 88 percent in diagnosing acute cholecystitis.[152] Maximum tenderness is demonstrated over the gallbladder in 85 to 87.2 percent of cases of acute cholecystitis.[148,153] The sensitivity of focal tenderness is 63 to 94 percent with a specificity of 93.6 percent, a predictive value for a positive sign of 72.5 percent, and a predictive value for a negative sign of 90.5 percent.[152,153] Focal tenderness distinguishes acute from chronic cholecystitis. With chronic cholecystitis, the sensitivity is 71 percent with a specificity of 97 percent and an overall accuracy of 88 percent.[152] Of the patients with symptoms of acute cholecystitis in this study, only 34.6 percent truly had the disease.[152] In addition, when the gallbladder wall is thicker than 3.5 mm in the absence of ascites in patients suspected of having acute acalculous cholecystitis, ultrasound can make a diagnosis with a specificity of 98 percent.[179]

More recently, the ultrasound findings in patients with suspected acute cholecystitis have been analyzed. The positive predictive values for stones combined with either a positive sonographic Murphy sign or gallbladder wall thickening are 92.2 and 95.2 percent, excellent for acute cholecystitis.[218] The positive predictive value of these signs for patients requiring cholecystectomy is 99 percent. Negative predictive values for combined use of primary and secondary signs to exclude acute cholecystitis are 95 percent for no stones and a negative sonographic Murphy sign.[219] The use of ultrasound alone can be definitive in nearly 80 percent of patients with suspected acute cholecystitis.[219] This means that cholescintigraphy could be reserved for patients who have (1) stones, a negative Murphy sign, and a normal gallbladder wall or contracted gallbladder; (2) no stones and a positive Murphy sign; (3) no stones, a negative Murphy sign, and a thickened gallbladder wall; and (4) stones, an unrecorded or unobtainable Murphy sign, and a normal wall or contracted gallbladder; or (5) equivocal finding with regard to stones.[219]

Although the accuracy of ultrasound is not as high as that of nuclear medicine, several factors support the proposition that ultrasound be performed as the initial examination in patients with acute right upper quadrant pain. They include the following: (1) two of three patients do not have acute cholecystitis; (2) ultrasound is an extremely accurate method in determining whether the gallbladder is abnormal, either acutely or chronically (sensitivity, 94 percent; specificity, 97 percent; accuracy, 96 percent); and (3) in patients with normal-appearing nontender gallbladders, ultrasound may be able to localize the site of the abnormality or may direct the work-up such that an extrabiliary site of disease will be evaluated more directly.[152] If the sonogram is normal and the pain is localized to the gallbladder fossa, a nuclear medicine scan may be performed to exclude the possibility of a stone impacted in the duct. Because of the multiorgan imaging capabilities of ultrasound and its ability to localize areas of maximum tenderness, it is considered the imaging technique of choice in evaluation of patients with right upper quadrant pain. The diagnosis of acute cholecystitis can be confirmed if calculi are visualized in a tender gallbladder; the diagnosis is further supported if the gallbladder contains sludge and has a thickened wall. If the gallbladder is not tender and stones are present, the diagnosis of chronic cholecystitis is made. If the gallbladder is not tender and appears normal, gallbladder disease is unlikely and clinical attention should be directed away from the gallbladder and biliary system. In conclusion, because acute cholecystitis is found in only a few patients with acute right upper quadrant pain, and

because ultrasound is a rapid, accurate, and noninvasive test, it should be the initial modality used to evaluate these patients.[152,219]

Oral cholecystography and gallbladder ultrasound have been compared.[220] In a double-blind study, neither ultrasound nor OCG had a diagnostic advantage in screening patients for gallbladder disease.[220] With the large numbers of false-negative examinations found on both ultrasound and OCG, the alternative study should be performed if the first examination is negative.[220]

In the prediction of acute cholecystitis, bile culture is not helpful since results are not available for a minimum for 24 to 48 hours after aspiration.[221] Gram-stained smears and bile cultures have low sensitivity, and consequently a negative test does not allow the diagnosis of acute cholecystitis to be excluded.[221]

Gallbladder Distension

Bile flow is controlled by the sphincter of Oddi. Under basal conditions and during interdigestive periods, the sphincter of Oddi is closed and bile is diverted into the gallbladder. Neural and hormonal stimuli triggered by eating cause gallbladder emptying by simultaneously stimulating gallbladder contraction and relaxation of the sphincter of Oddi. During fasting, the lack of neural and hormonal stimuli on the biliary system results in the accumulation of large amounts of bile in the gallbladder.[222] Bile viscosity and bile salt concentration are increased by water resorption and mucin secretion in the gallbladder.[223] The inspissated bile may not pass readily through the biliary tract and can cause either functional obstruction or dilatation secondary to stasis.[223]

Occasionally in an adult or a child, a distended gallbladder may cause the patient to present with a palpable mass.[85-87] This is seen while fasting and receiving parenteral hyperalimentation.[222,223] Ultrasound can quickly distinguish the gallbladder origin from other masses (Fig. 6-70).

Hydrops

In hydrops of the gallbladder, there is distension of the gallbladder, which is invariably due to total obstruction of the cystic duct. The trapped bile is resorbed, and the gallbladder is filled with a clear mucinous secretion derived from the gallbladder wall. The gallbladder is tense and enlarged, and the wall is thin (Fig. 6-70). This condition is usually asymptomatic, but some patients have epigastric pain, discomfort, nausea, and vomiting.[20]

There have been reports of children presenting with an abdominal mass that turns out to be the gallbladder. Hydrops is a rare cause of right upper quadrant pain in

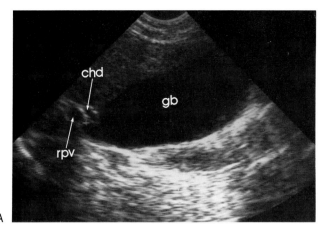 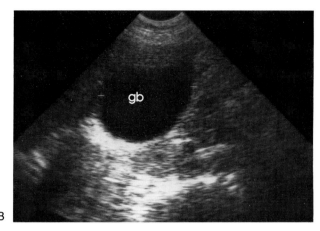

Fig. 6-70. Gallbladder hydrops. Palpable mass in the right upper quadrant. **(A)** Sagittal and **(B)** transverse scans showing a tremendously dilated gallbladder *(gb)* with a thin wall. (*rpv,* right portal vein; *chd,* common hepatic duct.)

children. It is not a form of cholecystitis, because the gallbladder is not acutely inflamed. Acute distension occurs secondary to preceding illness and a focus of infection elsewhere in the body.[204] Ultrasound can certainly identify the mass as the gallbladder in these cases.[222]

In neonates, hydrops may be associated with numerous conditions including salmonellosis, pseudomonas infection and group B streptococcal sepsis, prolonged biliary obstruction, shock, congestive heart failure, and hyperalimentation.[29] The gallbladder is also enlarged in neonates with extrahepatic biliary atresia, choledochal cyst, or inspissated bile syndrome. Fasting patients receiving total parenteral hyperalimentation develop biliary stasis, and they, too, develop gallbladder distension.[223] In a series of three premature neonates, the gallbladder distension was believed to be due to lack of enteric feeding, because it disappeared with feeding. The normal contraction of the gallbladder and simultaneous relaxation of the sphincter of Oddi are stimulated by the enteric hormone CCK with little influence from the autonomic nervous system.[224] If a follow-up ultrasound is done after initiation of oral feedings, the gallbladder size is seen to diminish.

Mucocutaneous Lymph Node Syndrome

Mucocutaneous lymph node syndrome (MLNS) is an acute febrile illness associated with cervical lymphadenopathy and involvement of the oral cavity, lips, and skin. The etiology of MLNS is unknown. Its features include (1) persistent high fever (for more than 1 week); (2) bilateral conjunctival infection; (3) abnormal mucous membranes, including erythema of the oral

cavity and dry fissured lips; (4) changes on the extremities, including indurative edema, erythema of the palms and soles, and desquamation; (5) erythematous rash; and (6) cervical lymphadenopathy.[225] Most patients are younger than 5 years of age, and more than 50 percent are younger than 2 years of age.

One of the complications of MLNS is acute hydrops of the gallbladder; this can be a major component of abdominal crisis.[225,226] The pathophysiology of hydrops in MLNS is uncertain. No organism is identified. Patients with MLNS are known to have adenopathy and vasculitis in other areas of the body, which could be the cause of the obstruction.[227] If a patient with MLNS presents with pain, distension, and/or palpable right upper quadrant mass, hydrops of the gallbladder, which can be identified on ultrasound, should be considered[225,227] (similar to the case in Fig. 6-70). The condition is usually self-limiting and transient; patients respond to conservative medical management.[225] Ultrasound is useful in evaluating complications of acute hydrops of the gallbladder, such as perforation, in which a fluid collection is demonstrated surrounding the distended gallbladder.[227]

Benign Neoplasms

Papilloma and Adenoma

Papillomas and adenomas of the gallbladder are infrequent benign epithelial tumors. They represent localized overgrowths of the lining epithelium. Papillomas grow as a pedunculated complex branching structure and adenomas as a flat sessile thickening. Papillomas may occur singly or multiply as small branching, pedunculated masses less than 1 cm in diameter that project into

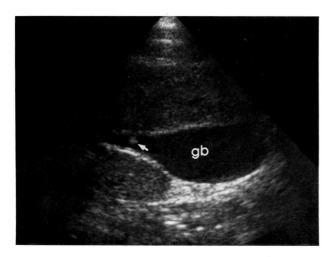

Fig. 6-71. Polyp. On sagittal view, a small (4-mm) structure (arrow) containing echoes similar to liver density is seen attached to the anterior gallbladder *(gb)* wall. Its relationship to the gallbladder wall did not change with change in patient position.

the lumen of the gallbladder. They are connected to the wall by a slender stalk. Adenomas are broad-based hemispheric elevations that are less than 1 cm in diameter and firmly attached to the underlying wall.[20] Adenomas represent the most frequent (28 percent) of benign gallbladder neoplasms with nearly half (43 percent of these) having a papillary configuration.[228]

In about 5 percent of cases in the routine population, polyps of the gallbladder are demonstrated on ultrasound.[229] The cholesterol polyp is the most common nonneoplastic type, accounting for about 33 percent of gallbladder polypoid lesions.[229] Less common is the inflammatory polyp, which has been estimated to account for about 1.1 percent.[229] These polyps may be single or,

more rarely, multiple and most often of 3 to 6 mm in diameter with a broad-based attachment to the gallbladder wall[229] (Fig. 6-71). Most inflammatory polyps are found in patients with gallstones and chronic cholecystitis, and small calculi may be missed in patients with echogenic bile.[229] A hypoechoic polypoid lesion consistent with an inflammatory polyp should raise a suspicion of chronic cholecystitis and the possible presence of gallstones.[229]

Cholesterolosis

Cholesterolosis results from the accumulation of triglycerides and esterified sterols in macrophages in the lamina propria of the gallbladder wall.[230] It represents a local disturbance in cholesterol metabolism and is not associated with any derangement in blood levels of cholesterol. Histologically, there are enlargement and distension of the mucosal folds into club shapes with aggregation of round to polyhedral histiocytes within these clubbed ends.[20] The polypoid type of cholesterolosis is associated with cholesterol polyps that are attached to the mucosa by a fragile pedicle composed of an epithelium covering a core of lipid-filled macrophages.[231] The polyps may break off (they contain no glandular elements) and form a nidus for stones. On ultrasound, one looks for nonshadowing single or multiple fixed echodense masses that project into the lumen of the gallbladder[230,231] (Fig. 6-72). Some investigators describe shadowing associated with cholesterol polyps.[232]

Adenomyomatosis

Adenomyomatosis of the gallbladder represents proliferation of the surface epithelium of the gallbladder with glandlike formation and outpouchings of mu-

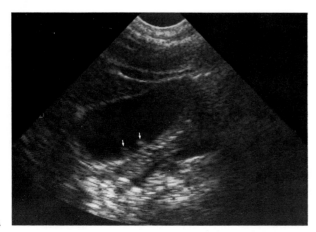

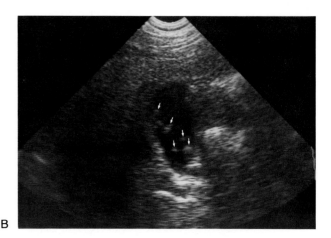

A   B

Fig. 6-72. Gallbladder cholesterolosis. **(A)** Sagittal and **(B)** transverse scans of the gallbladder. Multiple polypoid masses (arrows) are seen, and they remain attached to the wall with the change in body position.

cosa into or through a thickened muscular layer (Rokitansky-Aschoff sinuses).[231,233] Adenomyomatous hyperplasia belongs to a group of diseases known as hyperplastic cholecystoses. There are various forms of adenomyomatosis: (1) diffuse, in which the entire gallbladder is involved; (2) segmental, in which the proximal, middle, or distal third of the gallbladder is involved in a circular fashion; and (3) localized, in which the adenomyomatosis confined almost exclusively to the fundus (this occurs in most cases). This abnormality is associated with hyperplasia of the tissues of the gallbladder wall, which includes thickening of the muscular layer and proliferation of the mucosal epithelium with formation of intramural diverticula.[234] The ability to diagnose adenomyomatosis by ultrasound is dependent on the degree and nature of the gallbladder wall thickening and on identification of the intramural diverticula.[231,235]

Microscopic findings include epithelial proliferation, forming mucosal invaginations that extend into the hypertrophied muscularis layer.[234] Because of constriction in the thickened muscularis, the channels leading into the diverticula may appear sealed and these diverticula may contain stones.[234]

Adenomyomatosis of the gallbladder should be suspected when ultrasound shows diffuse or segmental thickening of the gallbladder wall and intramural diverticula are seen as anechoic or echogenic foci with or without associated acoustic shadowing or reverberation artifacts[231,235,236] (Figs. 6-73 to 6-75). The ultrasound appearance of the intramural diverticula varies depending on the size and content and whether papillary projections are present. When the intramural diverticula contain bile, they appear as anechoic spaces. Diverticula that are small or contain biliary sludge, stones, or papillary

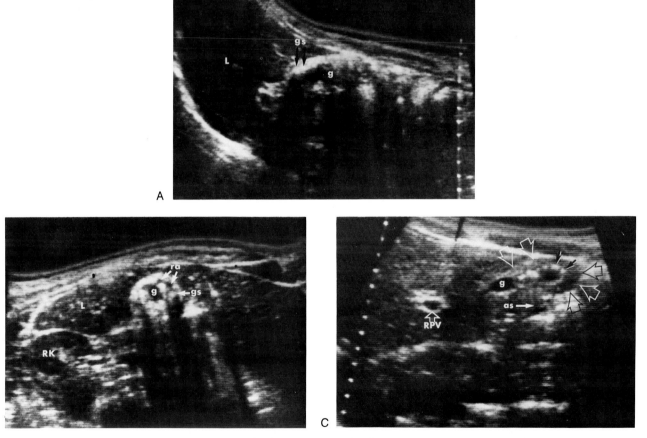

Fig. 6-73. Gallbladder adenomyomatosis. Case 1. **(A)** Longitudinal and **(B)** transverse scans of the gallbladder *(g),* with intramurally located gallstones *(gs)* and Rokitansky-Aschoff sinuses *(ra).* Mucosal hypertrophy and intramural diverticula were found on a gross specimen. *(L,* liver; *RK,* right kidney.) Case 2. **(C)** Longitudinal scan of the gallbladder *(g)* with wall thickening (open arrows) confined to the body and fundus of the gallbladder. Note the echogenic dots (closed arrows) paralleling the luminal surface in the fundus. On a gross specimen, there was marked thickening of the gallbladder wall with intramural diverticula. *(as,* acoustic shadow from gallstone; *RPV,* right portal vein.) (From Raghavendra et al,[235] with permission.)

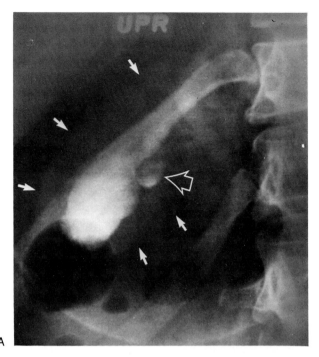

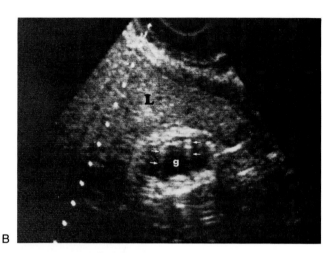

A

B

Fig. 6-74. Gallbladder adenomyomatosis. Case 1. **(A)** OCG showing markedly thickened gallbladder wall (arrows) and contrast-filled intramural diverticulum (open arrow). **(B)** Longitudinal scan of the gallbladder *(g)* showing reverberation artifacts (arrows) emanating from the thickened gallbladder wall. *(L, liver.)* Mucosal hypertrophy and intramural diverticula, were found. Frondlike projections within the diverticulum might have been responsible for the reverberation artifact. *(Figure continues.)*

projections appear as echogenic foci at various intervals within the gallbladder wall with or without acoustic shadowing or reverberation artifacts.[231,235] Diffuse adenomyomatosis has been described as a hyperechoic mass arising from the fundus of the gallbladder with a diffusely thickened wall (Fig. 6-73). The mass in such a case represents the effect of circumferential thickening of the wall.[233]

Various patterns with adenomyomatosis of the gallbladder have been described: (1) thickening of the gallbladder wall; (2) round anechoic areas in the thickened portion of the gallbladder wall, which represent the diverticular outpouchings; and (3) echogenic areas within the gallbladder wall, which could represent stone formation within the diverticula.[234] Adenomyomatosis should be suspected when examination of the gallbladder reveals multiple septations or projections.[234]

Malignant Neoplasms

Primary Neoplasm

Carcinoma of the gallbladder is the fifth most frequent gastrointestinal cancer and represents 1 to 3 percent of all cancers.[228,230-233,235-244] It is more frequent than the

aggregate of all other types of cancer and a much more common lesion than benign adenomas and papillomas. It is the most frequent cancer of the biliary system. It is more common in the sixth and seventh decades, in whites, and in women (4:1).[240-242] Gallbladder stones are present in 65 to 95 percent of cases, which strongly suggests that they play an etiologic role for inflammation.[28,240-244] In 70 to 80 percent of cases, the neoplasm is adenocarcinoma (most are well differentiated), with 15 percent of these being fungating papillary carcinoma and 65 percent being infiltrating parietal carcinoma.[245] In up to 25 percent of cases, there is calcification in the gallbladder wall.[244] The most common site is in the fundus and neck.

There are several principal forms of gallbladder carcinoma, including localized infiltrating or fungating tumors.[245] The infiltrating type is more common and is usually a poorly defined area of diffuse thickening and induration in the gallbladder wall. The fungating type grows into the lumen as an irregular cauliflower-shaped mass invading the wall. Most invade the liver centrifugally, and many have extended to the cystic duct and adjacent bile ducts. There is direct liver invasion in 69 percent of cases.[246]

Four macroscopic types of gallbladder carcinoma

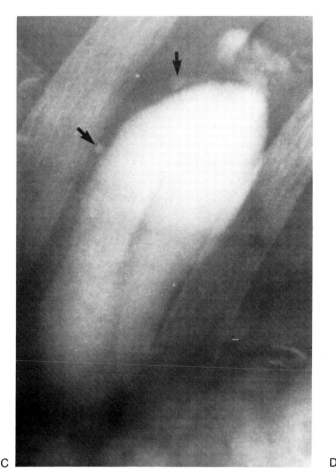

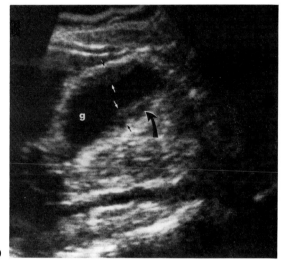

C

D

Fig. 6-74 *(Continued).* Case 2. **(C)** OCG showing at least two contrast-filled intramural diverticula (arrows). **(D)** Longitudinal scan of the gallbladder *(g)* showing segmented wall thickening (straight arrows). A rounded anechoic area representing an intramural diverticulum is seen within the thickened portion of the wall (curved arrow). (From Raghavendra et al,[235] with permission.)

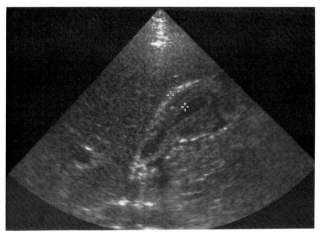

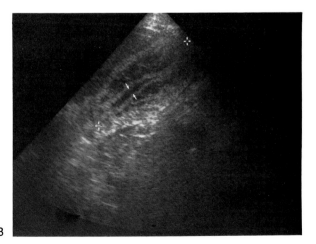

A

B

Fig. 6-75. Gallbladder adenomyomatosis. Case 1. **(A)** Sagittal scan demonstrating marked wall thickening (calipers) in the fundal region. Case 2. **(B)** Sagittal view demonstrating marked diffuse gallbladder wall thickening. The gallbladder lumen (arrows) is very narrow. (Fig. A from Mittlestaedt,[394] with permission.)

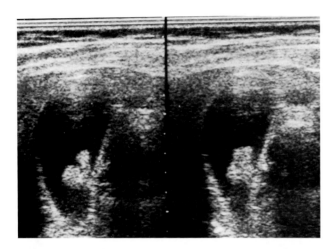

Fig. 6-76. Gallbladder carcinoma, early. Fungating mass (carcinoma in adenoma). Parasagittal right anterior oblique sonogram showing round, lobulated, and strongly hyperechoic masses in the body of the gallbladder. (From Tsuchiya,[247] with permission.)

have been described: pedunculated, sessile, superficial raised, and flat.[247] The pedunculated type is seen as a clearly protruding nonpapillary lesion with a stalk.[247] With the sessile type, a protruding papillary lesion without a stalk but with a constricted or broad base is seen.[247] With the superficial raised form, a smoothly elevated lesion rising 1.5 to 3 mm from the surrounding mucosa is seen.[247] The flat type is almost the same level as normal.[247]

The clinical course is extremely insidious, and frequently the patient is asymptomatic over long periods.

The symptoms include loss of appetite, nausea and vomiting, intolerance of fatty foods, and belching, all of which suggest some form of gallbladder involvement. Jaundice is usually not seen until there is infiltration of the major biliary ducts and extension into the liver bed. In half the cases there is a mass, and in half there is right upper quadrant pain. The diagnosis of gallbladder carcinoma is difficult. An early diagnosis is rare, because clinical signs appear late and are due to extension to contiguous structures. The average duration of life after diagnosis is 1 to 1.5 years, and rarely does survival reach 5 years.[20] The 5-year survival rate has been reported to be 4 to 12 percent.[244]

The findings of gallbladder carcinoma on ultrasound represent a spectrum that is dependent on the size of the tumor, its morphologic character, and the extent of secondary spread.[240] The early findings include (1) a localized area of thickening of the gallbladder wall; (2) a polypoid lesion with irregular borders; and/or (3) loss of the usual smooth outline of the gallbladder with replacement by an undulated configuration[240] (Figs. 6-76 to 6-79). Only 30 percent of early carcinomas are diagnosed by ultrasound.[247] It seems practical to consider that polypoid lesions greater than 1.0 cm in diameter or rapidly growing lesions should be strongly suspected of being cancers even though several cases of early cancer in this series involved lesions smaller than 1.0 cm in diameter.[247] Careful attention must be paid to mild mucosal change, because more than 50 percent of early cancers do not show apparently protruding lesions.[247]

With localized lesions, a thickened hypoechoic gallbladder wall may be seen with a gradual or abrupt junc-

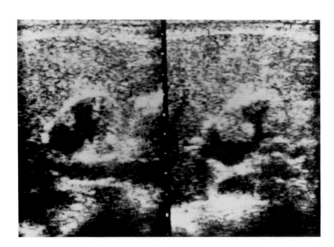

Fig. 6-77. Gallbladder carcinoma, early. Lumen-filling mass. Parasagittal right anterior oblique sonogram showing isoechoic echoes into the gallbladder lumen. (From Tsuchiya,[247] with permission.)

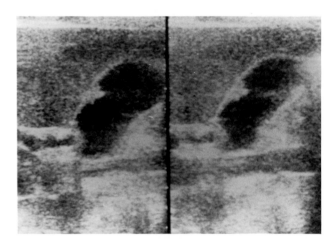

Fig. 6-78. Gallbladder carcinoma, early. Smooth raised mass. Parasagittal anterior oblique sonogram showing hyperechoic tumors in the body of the gallbladder. The height of the lesion was 6 mm as seen by ultrasound. (From Tsuchiya,[247] with permission.)

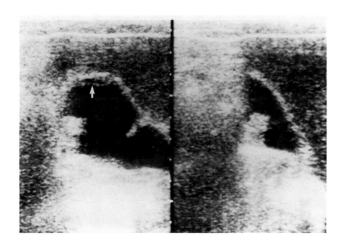

Fig. 6-79. Gallbladder carcinoma, early. Mucosal thickening. Parasagittal right anterior oblique sonogram showing mucosal thickening (arrow) in the fundus of the gallbladder. (From Tsuchiya,[247] with permission.)

tion with normal wall tissue and, later, a bilobed appearance to the gallbladder lumen[245] (Figs. 6-80 to 6-82). Localized tumors are usually located in the infundibular or fundal region and rarely involve the body of the gallbladder.[245] When such tumors are localized in the neck of the gallbladder, they are often associated with hydrops and porta hepatis invasion (Fig. 6-82).

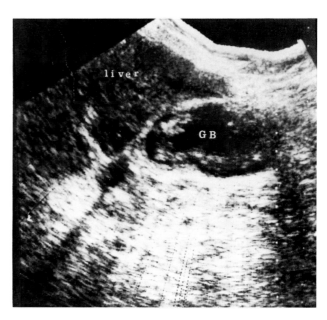

Fig. 6-81. Gallbladder carcinoma. Carcinoma infiltrating the gallbladder wall. Longitudinal left lateral decubitus scan showing a fluid-filled gallbladder *(GB)* with an asymmetrically thickened, irregular wall. (From Weiner et al,[244] with permission.)

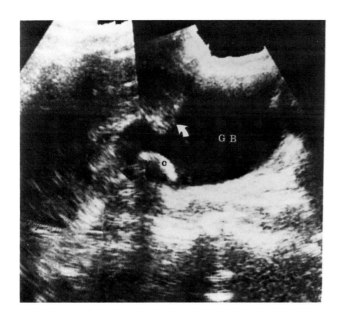

Fig. 6-80. Gallbladder carcinoma. Tumor protruding into the gallbladder lumen. Longitudinal scan showing a well-defined mass (arrow) protruding into fluid-filled gallbladder *(GB)*. Calculi *(c)* with acoustic shadowing are also noted. (From Weiner et al,[244] with permission.)

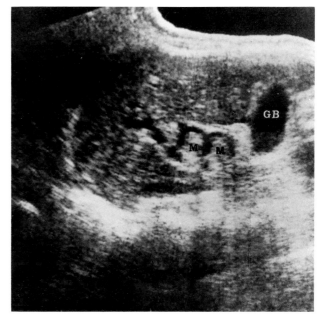

Fig. 6-82. Gallbladder carcinoma. Intraductal extension of gallbladder tumor. Longitudinal scan showing a lobulated mass *(M)* in the common bile duct. The gallbladder *(GB)* contains sludge. (From Weiner et al,[244] with permission.)

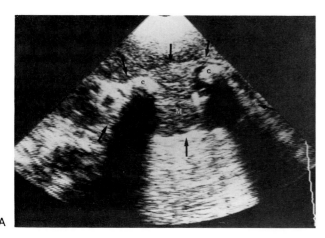 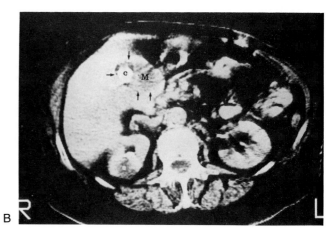

Fig. 6-83. Gallbladder carcinoma. Carcinoma replacing the gallbladder. **(A)** Longitudinal scan of the right upper quadrant and **(B)** CT scan showing a large soft-tissue mass *(M)* in the gallbladder (arrows) and calculi *(c)* with acoustic shadowing. (From Weiner et al,[244] with permission.)

Other ultrasound patterns described with gallbladder carcinoma include (1) a solid mass (with diffuse weak or strong echoes) filling the gallbladder (the most common type, occurring in 42 percent of cases); (2) an infiltrating mass with the gallbladder wall markedly thickened as a result of infiltration by carcinoma (15 percent); (3) a fungating mass on the wall, producing an intraluminal mass with an irregular contour (23 percent); and (4) a fungating or polypoid mass with a markedly thickened posterior wall[240,241,243,244,248,249] (Figs. 6-80 to 6-84). The following sonographic patterns have also been described: (1) a fungating mass type with lesions protruding into the gallbladder lumen with various echo levels and shapes;

(2) a lumen-filling mass type with a homogeneous and isoechoic image with multiple fungating masses occupying the whole lumen of the gallbladder; (3) a smooth raised mass type with slightly elevated lesions with broad bases; and (4) localized mucosal thickening with a preserved three-layer structure.[247] Another series identified a variety of patterns associated with gallbladder carcinoma: (1) gallbladder lumen identified along with a mass lesion (72.5 percent) (mass almost filling lumen, polypoidal mass projecting into the lumen, and infiltrating mass); and (2) a large mass totally replacing the gallbladder (27.5 percent).[250] The most commonly observed pattern was a mass replacing the gallbladder (39 per-

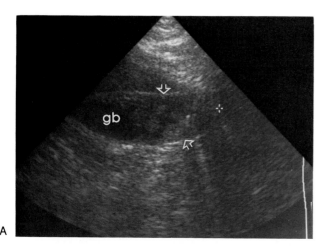 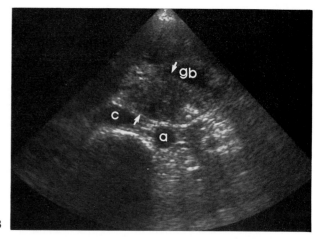

Fig. 6-84. Gallbladder carcinoma. Case 1. **(A)** Sagittal view of a gallbladder *(gb)* that was shown to contain gallstones on another view. A poorly defined echogenic mass (arrows) was seen within the gallbladder fundus. It has a similar density to sludge but did not change with a change in patient position. Case 2. **(B)** Sagittal left lateral decubitus view demonstrating a gallbladder wall mass (arrows). This patient had gallstones demonstrated on other views. (*a*, aorta; *c*, inferior vena cava; *gb*, gallbladder lumen.)

cent), followed by wall thickening and polypoid or fungating tumor.[251,252]

The gallbladder wall may be poorly distinguished from the liver. In some instances, the gallbladder wall may be hyperechoic with irregular limits and a large base of implantation. With diffuse tumor, the wall may be totally infiltrated and will appear hypoechoic and thickened (Fig. 6-81) or it may be collapsed.[245] With advanced neoplasm, a complex echogenic mass may be present, obliterating the gallbladder lumen[253] (Fig. 6-83). The presence of a stone encased within a gallbladder mass (constrained-stone sign) is almost pathognomonic for carcinoma[28] (Fig. 6-83). Other lesions such as cholesterol polyp, mucosal hyperplasia, inflammatory polyp, granulomas, and blood clot may simulate gallbladder carcinoma.[241]

Color Doppler may be helpful in making the diagnosis of gallbladder carcinoma. It may allow a confident diagnosis of gallbladder carcinoma by demonstrating flow, which eliminates the alternative diagnosis of a sludge-filled gallbladder.[254]

Various patterns of spread of gallbladder carcinoma have been described. Frequently, there is extension into the adjacent tissues as a result of the relatively thin wall.[255] When the lesions extend into the liver, the masses may lie in contact with the gallbladder or numerous tumor masses may be seen within the liver from hematogenous spread.[245] Approximately 50 to 70 percent of cases demonstrate evidence of liver extension at surgery.[255] Duodenal and colonic involvement are found in 12 and 9 percent of cases, respectively, along with gastric involvement, which can lead to cholecystoenteric fistulas.[255] Biliary obstruction can result, with contiguous growth alongside or within the cystic duct.[255]

In 84 percent of cases diagnosed preoperatively, gallbladder carcinomas are advanced.[251] With advanced gallbladder carcinoma, ultrasound allows a correct preoperative diagnosis in 70 to 82 percent of cases.[247] The most frequently observed condition that may be confused with an intraluminal gallbladder mass is sludge.[251]

Carcinoma of the gallbladder has been reported in patients who have undergone gallbladder-preserving treatments for cholelithiasis.[256] The risk of carcinoma has been reported to be 1 percent in patients undergoing cholecystectomy, and the risk of carcinoma developing in patients with asymptomatic cholelithiasis is estimated to be less than 1 percent.[256] As such, patients undergoing these procedures must have a very thorough imaging assessment both before and after treatment to ensure that a gallbladder carcinoma is not overlooked.[256]

There are a number of pitfalls and difficulties in the diagnosis of primary carcinoma of the gallbladder. The following were reported as false-negative diagnoses: 62.1 percent were diagnosed as gallbladder stones only, 20.7 percent were diagnosed as either acute or chronic cholecystitis, 6.9 percent were diagnosed as bile sludge, 6.9 percent were diagnosed as polyps, and 3.4 percent were diagnosed as liver tumors.[257] The following were reported as false-positive diagnoses: 31.8 percent were erroneously diagnosed as a mass projecting from the gallbladder wall but were pathologically proven to be polyps or bile sludge, and 36.4 percent were incorrectly diagnosed as a result of irregular thickening of the gallbladder wall but histology revealed them to be acute or chronic cholecystitis.[257]

One group of investigators has reported on the ultrasound-guided fine-needle aspiration biopsy of gallbladder masses.[258] The masses in this series were 4.8 cm in diameter.[258] With this technique, gallbladder cancer was confirmed in 88.5 of cases.[258] All of the benign lesions were properly classified.[258] One of the major drawbacks to the procedure is the occurrence of false-negative results. In four cases pain was experienced as a minor complication, with one patient developing bile peritonitis following a single-needle pass by the transperitoneal approach.[258] This group concluded that ultrasound-guided fine-needle aspiration biopsy of gallbladder masses is a safe, reliable, and accurate technique for the diagnosis of cancer.[258]

Awareness of the subtle ultrasound findings in this condition will permit its early detection. A diagnosis of gallbladder carcinoma can be made by ultrasound in 84.6 percent of patients.[241] A clear-cut solid tumor of the gallbladder, which infiltrates the liver, is highly suggestive of carcinoma.[246]

Metastatic Disease

Metastatic tumor to the gallbladder should be suspected in the presence of focal gallbladder wall thickening in association with nonshadowing intraluminal soft tissue masses. Unlike in primary carcinoma of the gallbladder, cholelithiasis is usually absent. The tumors that metastasize to the gallbladder from the stomach, pancreas, and bile duct reach the gallbladder by direct invasion, whereas metastatic disease from organs such as the lungs, kidneys, and esophagus and malignant melanoma reach the gallbladder via a blood-borne embolic phenomenon.[259,260] Several patterns have been described: (1) focal thickening of the gallbladder wall as a result of localized metastatic deposit; (2) intraluminal mass without shadowing, and with a sonographically normal gallbladder wall; (3) a combination of these two with a polypoid or irregular intraluminal mass based on an area of focal thickening of the gallbladder wall; and (4) indistinct walls that contain low-level, irregular echoes with decreased through transmission (Figs. 6-85 and 6-86).

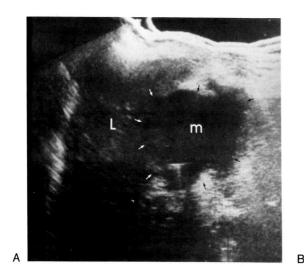
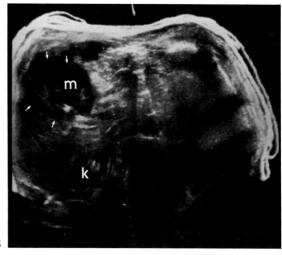

Fig. 6-85. Metastatic gallbladder disease. Squamous cell carcinoma metastatic to the gallbladder. **(A)** Longitudinal and **(B)** transverse scans demonstrating a poorly defined hypoechoic mass (*m*, arrows) in the gallbladder fossa. (*k*, right kidney; *L*, liver.)

Miscellaneous Conditions

Acquired Immunodeficiency Syndrome

Patients with AIDS are at risk for a variety of opportunistic infections and neoplasms involving the liver and biliary tract. *Crytosporidium* has been found in 6 percent of all patients with AIDS and in 21 percent of those who have diarrhea.[261] It is a protozoan parasite that infects epithelial cells of the gastrointestinal tract in a wide variety of vertebrates.[261] These patients all have the common clinical presentation of right upper quadrant pain, nausea, vomiting, fever, and biochemical evidence of anicteric cholestasis.[261]

The biliary tract abnormalities described in patients with AIDS include gallbladder wall thickening in 55 percent of these patients, dilated gallbladder in 18 percent, biliary sludge in 23 percent, and gallstones in 5 percent.[262] Two of the possible etiologies for biliary tract abnormalities include cytomegalovirus (CMV) and cryptosporidial infection.[262] Forty-two percent of those with thick gallbladder wall and 60 percent of those with dilated ducts have a diagnosis of extrabiliary CMV infection, compared with a 10 percent rate of extrabiliary CMV infection in patients with sonographically normal biliary tracts.[262] In 23 percent of patients, extrahepatic ductal dilatation is seen with both papillary stenosis and a syndrome resembling idiopathic sclerosing cholangi-

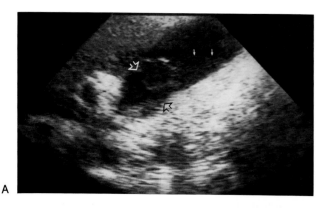
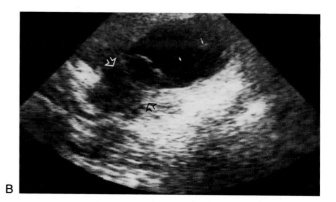

Fig. 6-86. Metastatic gallbladder disease. **(A)** Supine long-axis view of the gallbladder. Apparent debris (small arrows) are lying dependent in the gallbladder. A mass within the gallbladder is suspected (open arrows) because of the abnormal configuration of the gallbladder neck. **(B)** Upright long-axis view. A lobulated mass (open arrows) remains in the neck of the gallbladder, and debris (small arrows) layer out dependently. At surgery, there was metastatic melanoma with acute or chronic cholecystitis. (From Bundy and Ritchie,[260] with permission.)

tis.[262] Extrahepatic ductal abnormalities include uniform dilatation of the common hepatic and common bile ducts to the level of the ampulla without irregularity, beading, or strictures.[262]

Other investigators have also identified the findings of gallbladder wall thickening (which may be marked) and bile duct dilatation associated with AIDS[263] (Fig. 6-87). The gallbladder wall thickness varies from 4 to 15 mm.[263] Regional lymph obstruction by nodes is proposed as a cause of the gallbladder wall thickening.[261] None of the patients had gallstones.[261] In these patients, ultrasound shows dilatation of the biliary ducts, some with wall thickening, thickening of the gallbladder wall, and pericholecystic fluid.[261]

There appears to be an association between CMV and/or *Cryptosporidium* infection and acalculous inflammation of the biliary tract.[264] Findings similar to sclerosing cholangitis were noted with strictures, focal dilatation, and thickened duct walls.[264] The dilatation of the common bile duct varies from 12 to 15 mm.[263] Appearing unique to AIDS-related cholangitis is the combination of papillary stenosis and intrahepatic ductal strictures.[264] The pathogenesis of the bile duct dilation is most probably related to opportunistic infection and inflammation caused most frequently by *Cryptosporidium*.[263] CMV and/or *Cryptosporidium* infection is the proposed pathophysiologic mechanism.[264]

Hepatic parenchymal abnormalities include a hyperechoic parenchyma echopattern in 45.5 percent, hepatomegaly in 41 percent, and focal masses in 9 percent.[262] In livers of AIDS patients, granulomas are a very common pathologic finding, being seen in 16 to 100 percent of biopsy or autopsy specimens. Suspected or proven etiologic agents include *Mycobacterium avium-intracellulare* (MAI), *Myocbacterium tuberculosis* (MTb), cryptococcosis, histoplasmosis, toxoplasmosis, CMV infection, and drug toxicity.[262]

Gallbladder Disease in Pregnancy

Pregnancy is thought to be one possible cause of gallbladder disease.[265,266] It may be related to an alteration in the composition of the bile with a decrease in the concentration of bile salts and an increase in the cholesterol level. The gallbladder volume increases during gestation, probably as a predominant effect of progesterone or a consequence of a combined progesterone-estrogen influence, or the hormones may act directly on the gallbladder musculature. In one series of pregnant patients, 4.2 percent had abnormalities.[265] In another, 11.3 percent of obstetric patients had gallstones.[266]

Torsion

Torsion of the gallbladder is a very rare disease, with an estimated incidence of about 1 in 365,520 patient admissions.[267] It is more common in females than males (3 : 1) and occurs mostly in the sixth to eighth decades.[267] In only 20 to 33 percent are gallstones present.[267]

As a rule, the gallbladder is normally situated in the gallbladder fossa of the liver and is closely attached to the latter over the bare area of the liver, so it does not have sufficient mobility to twist.[267] About 4 percent of the population have free-lying gallbladders, usually with an asthenic habitus.[267]

Two types of floating gallbladders have been described: (1) a gallbladder with a mesentery that extends throughout the entire length or only part of the gallbladder; and (2) a gallbladder with a pedicle.[267] Because of peristaltic movement of an adjacent bowel loop or the stomach, torsion may occur.[267] More likely to be afflicted are elderly women who have lost weight, because the decreased intraperitoneal pressure renders the gallbladder mobile.[267]

The following have been defined as features of torsion of the gallbladder: (1) sign of a floating gallbladder (i.e., almost the entire gallbladder is located below the liver and is not in contact with the liver); (2) sign of a stretched and/or twisted pedicle (i.e., a conical structure that is composed of multiple linear echoes converging toward the tip of the "cone" [the conical structure represents combined cystic duct, cystic artery, and vein as well as mesentery]); and (3) signs of an inflamed and/or gangrenous gallbladder that are not specific for torsion of the gallbladder.[267] The wall of the gallbladder may be diffusely thickened and hypoechoic, although the thickening may not be uniform.[267]

Postcholecystectomy Patients

Postoperative complications are infrequent. They include wound, common duct injury, retained cystic duct, drainage tube problems, retained stones, hepatic artery injury, and fluid collections. These fluid collections represent the most frequent complications (5 to 6 percent of cases)[268] (Fig. 6-88). The fluid may be blood, bile, lymph, or peritoneal fluid. Most collections are in the area of the falciform ligament in either the right subhepatic or right subphrenic space. These areas are vulnerable to infection because the medium provided by pooling blood, lymph, bile, and a denuded liver bed is right for bacterial growth.[268]

The finding of recurrent or persistent symptoms following cholecystectomy is called *postcholecystectomy syndrome*. There is no well-defined clinical syndrome, and severe symptoms may result from a variety of different etiologic factors.[269] There are frequent anomalies associated with the cystic duct, including a low parallel position of the cystic duct and an absent or very short cystic duct, with the most common arrangement being an angular joining of the cystic and common duct.[269]

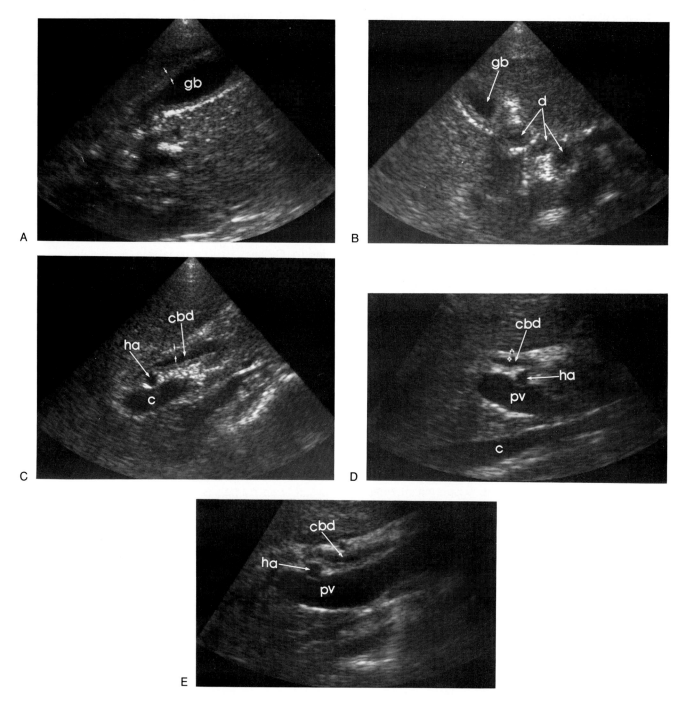

Fig. 6-87. Acquired immunodeficiency syndrome. Case 1. AIDS patient with MAI infection and abnormal liver function tests. **(A)** Sagittal view of the gallbladder *(gb)* with wall thickening (arrows). **(B)** Transverse view of porta hepatis showing the gallbladder *(gb)* wall thickening as well as ductal *(d)* wall thickening. **(C)** Long-axis view of the common duct *(cbd)* showing wall thickening (3.5 mm, arrows) with a lumen of 5 mm. *(ha,* hepatic artery; *c,* inferior vena cava.) Case 2. AIDS patient with CMV infection and elevated liver function tests. This patient had dilated intrahepatic ducts demonstrated on other views. **(D & E)** Sagittal views of the common bile duct *(cbd)* showing wall thickening (calipers on Fig. D, arrow). *(pv,* portal vein; *ha,* hepatic artery; *c,* inferior vena cava.)

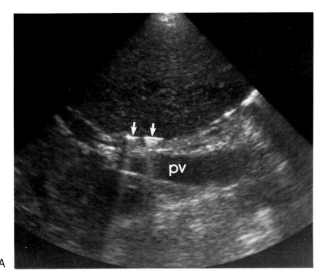 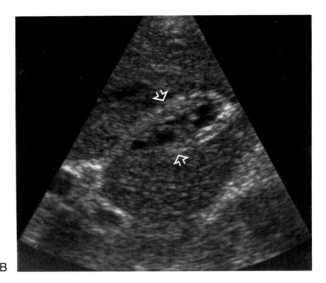

A
B

Fig. 6-88. Postlaparoscopic cholecystectomy, fluid collection. **(A)** On long-axis of the portal vein *(pv),* metallic clips (arrows) are seen as echogenic areas in the region of the gallbladder neck with associated comet-tail artifacts. **(B)** In the gallbladder bed on sagittal view, there is a structure (arrows) that appears similar to the gallbladder. This lucent fluid represented a postoperative hematoma. By ultrasound alone, infection could not be ruled out.

These anomalies result in various lengths of the cystic duct being left at surgery. There can be symptoms at any time from few months to many years following surgery.[269]

There is a higher incidence of postcholecystectomy symptoms in the setting of cystic duct remnant with stones than when the remnant is without stones.[269] With ultrasound, a 3 cm-diameter spherical cystic structure at the porta hepatis containing a highly echogenic structure 1.0 cm in diameter with a persistent shadowing is seen.[269]

One should be cautious in making a diagnosis of retained duct calculi in a postcholecystectomy patient.[270] A strong echo with distal acoustic shadowing may be seen in patients without stones (Fig. 6-89). This is assumed to be caused by a postoperative scar in the gallbladder bed.[270] If an echodense structure with an associated shadow is seen in the area of the gallbladder fossa and is surrounded by a lucency, a diagnosis of cystic duct remnant stone should be entertained (Fig. 6-90).

Percutaneous Cholecystostomy

Percutaneous ultrasound-guided puncture of the gallbladder is a new method for antegrade study of the gallbladder and common bile duct. The following represent the indications for the procedure: (1) evaluation of the common bile duct for calculi and/or obstruction; (2) aspiration of bile for Gram stain, crystal analysis, and cytologic examination; (3) evaluation of the gallbladder

lumen for intraluminal mass; and (4) identification of the anatomic site of occult abscess.[271] This technique can be successfully used to treat severely ill patients, who are at considerable surgical risk. It may be indicated as a preoperative measure in patients with known cholelithiasis or acute cholecystitis in whom prolonged anesthesia or surgery may be hazardous[271-273] (Fig. 6-91). (For further discussion, see Ch. 19.)

This percutaneous approach can be used for biliary drainage when a transhepatic approach is not possible.[274] Once the gallbladder is localized by ultrasound, a 22-gauge sheathed needle is placed into the gallbladder (by using an anterior abdominal wall approach, right axillary line) and dilute (25 to 30 percent) diatrizoate meglumine (Hypaque) can be injected into the gallbladder. Needling the gallbladder without catheterization will frequently lead to bile peritonitis.[275] Therefore it is important to introduce a pigtail catheter, which keeps the gallbladder collapsed, preventing the catheter from being pulled out.[275] Although complications with this procedure are few, they include peritonitis, fatal septic shock, and severe vasovagal reaction.[273]

BILIARY ABNORMALITIES

Anomalies

As with the gallbladder, congenital anomalies are associated with the ducts. The bile ducts may have a variety of anomalous connections. There may be agenesis of

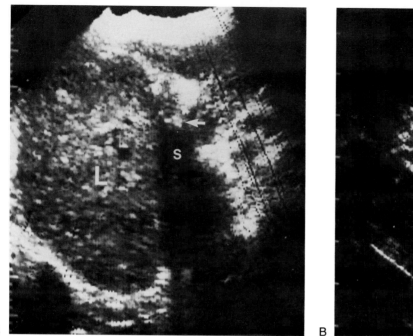
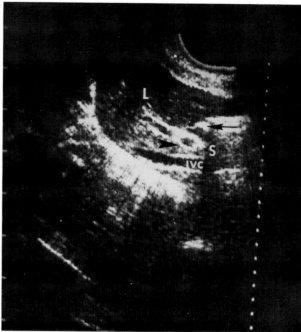

Fig. 6-89. Postcholecystectomy shadow. Pseudocalculus pattern. Longitudinal scans after cholecystectomy without (Fig. A) and with (Fig. B) surgical clips in the right upper abdomen. **(A)** Oblique scan parallel to costal margin. **(B)** Slight oblique right parasagittal scan. (arrow, strong echoes; arrowhead, portal vein; *S*, acoustic shadow; *L*, liver; *ivc,* inferior vena cava.) (From Raptopoulos,[270] with permission.)

all or a portion of the hepatic or common bile duct. Agenesis, or severe stenosis, is usually discovered shortly after birth and is incompatible with life.[20]

Congenital anomalies of the biliary system are frequent.[110] It is imperative that the modern sonographer be familiar with these anatomic variations to improve diagnostic accuracy. Low insertion of the cystic duct relative to the common hepatic duct with or without a distal common septum seems to be the most frequent.[110] Other anomalies include absence of the cystic duct, absence of the accessory bile duct, low junction of the hepatic ducts, long parallel cystic duct, diverticulum of the gallbladder, and congenital absence of the common bile duct.[110] Several variations have been found: (1) the cystic running parallel to the common hepatic duct bound in fibrous union; and (2) the cystic duct embedded in the medial wall of the common hepatic duct with a thin septum separating the two lumina.[110]

Biliary Atresia

The differentiation of biliary atresia from neonatal hepatitis is critical and is a difficult problem even with ultrasound and nuclear medicine. Whereas the bile ducts are patent in neonatal hepatitis, in biliary atresia

some or all parts of the biliary tract (usually extrahepatic ducts or intrahepatic ducts near the porta hepatis) are obliterated.[276] Differentiation between biliary atresia and neonatal hepatitis is critical because neonatal hepatitis is treated medically, whereas biliary atresia requires early surgical intervention to achieve adequate, sustained bile drainage and to avoid biliary cirrhosis.[276] Biliary atresia exists when the ducts from the hilum of the liver to the duodenum (including the gallbladder) are shown at surgery to be obliterated.[277] If a normal gallbladder (> 1.5 cm) is seen on ultrasound, the diagnosis of neonatal hepatitis is supported[277,278] (Fig. 6-92). However, gallbladders are present in 20 percent of patients with extrahepatic biliary atresia.[279] The liver may be echogenic or normal.[278]

Radionuclide scintigraphy and ultrasound play complementary roles in the attempt to differentiate biliary atresia from neonatal hepatitis.[276] If there is nonvisualization of the gallbladder or the gallbladder is small (1.5 cm) on ultrasound without evidence of excretion of the radionuclide into the gastrointestinal tract and an indeterminate hepatic biopsy, surgical exploration is indicated.[277] Ultrasound alone does not appear to be sufficient to establish the diagnosis; its principal role is to exclude other possible causes of obstructive jaundice such as choledochal cyst, biloma, or mass at the porta

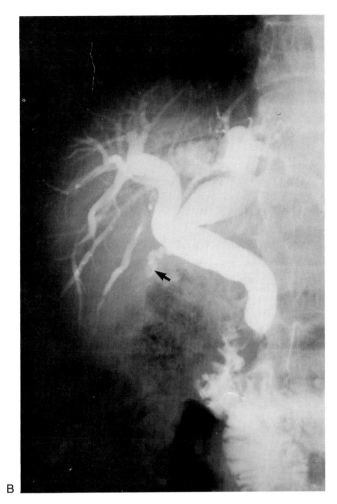

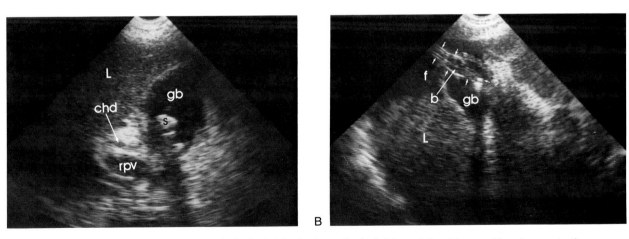

Fig. 6-90. Postcholecystectomy shadow. Retained stone. **(A)** Longitudinal scan of the gallbladder fossa. An echodense structure (arrow) with associated shadowing is seen. **(B)** Percutaneous transhepatic cholangiogram. A stone (arrow) is seen within the cystic duct remnant.

Fig. 6-91. Cholecystostomy. Cholelithiasis. **(A)** Sagittal scan in the left lateral decubitus position demonstrating echodense stones *(s)* within the gallbladder *(gb)* with shadowing. The patient was acutely ill, with a positive Murphy sign. Since the patient was not an operative candidate, a cholecystostomy tube was placed. (*L*, liver; *chd*, common hepatic duct; *rpv*, right portal vein.) **(B)** Transverse scan of the gallbladder *(gb)* with a cathether (arrows) inserted. The catheter balloon *(b)* is seen within the lumen of the gallbladder. The tip is the bright echo. Peritoneal fluid *(f)* has developed. (*L*, liver.)

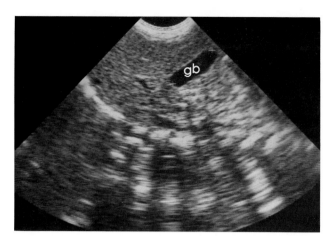

Fig. 6-92. Neonatal hepatitis. Sagittal scan in a fasting newborn. A gallbladder *(gb)* is seen, which is 2.1 cm in length.

hepatis.[276] It is most helpful to combine ultrasound and hepatobiliary nuclear medicine in these cases. Nuclear medicine has a sensitivity of 97 to 100 percent in the evaluation of neonatal jaundice with a specificity of 83 to 87 percent depending on phenobarbital stimulation.[278,279] If there is passage of the radionuclide from the liver to the gastrointestinal tract, patency of the biliary tree is noted.

One study has shown the following with regard to biliary atresia: (1) an inability of ultrasound to document the existence of a gallbladder strongly suggests the diagnosis of biliary atresia (feeding should distinguish a normal gallbladder from the atrophic gallbladder of biliary atresia when it shows a small cystic echo on the inferior hepatic surface); and (2) the presence of a cystic mass in the porta hepatis area suggests the so-called correctable biliary atresia.[280]

To differentiate biliary atresia from neonatal hepatitis, serial scans have been performed in patients before, during, and after feeding.[281] In 97 percent of normal individuals and all patients with neonatal hepatitis, the gallbladder was identified and a change in size following oral feeding was observed.[281] A small gallbladder whose size was not affected by oral feeding was observed in 67 percent of patients with biliary atresia.[281] In the remainder of the biliary atresia patients, the gallbladder was not visualized before, during or after feeding.[281] Therefore, it is believed that serial ultrasound examinations with oral feeding aids in the differential diagnosis of biliary atresia and neonatal hepatitis.[281]

In biliary atresia, there may be the absence of a visible gallbladder in the fasting state on two consecutive examinations or the presence of a small cystic structure that does not change in size with feedings, associated with an absent common bile duct or a common hepatic duct.[282] No patients with a normal visible gallbladder that contracted following oral feedings or with a normal-caliber bile duct has been found to have biliary atresia.[282]

Caroli's Disease

The pathognomonic finding of Caroli's disease is nonobstructive bile duct dilatation.[283] This abnormality is considered to be a developmental abnormality that is probably a combination of overgrowth of biliary epithelium and of its supporting portal connective tissue.[284] During the early developmental stage in normal embryology, there is a single-layered ductal plate surrounding the portal vein, followed by double-layered ductal plates and slitlike primitive bile duct lumen.[283] The final stage is produced with extensive resorption of the primitive bile duct, consisting of a network of fine bile ducts surrounding the portal vein.[283] There is insufficient resorption of the ductal plates in ductal plate malformation, which can lead to large dilated segments of primitive bile duct surrounding the central portal vein.[283] Elongation, tortuosity, and irregular dilatation of the bile ducts, with bulbar protrusion and bridge formation of the ductal walls, result from disproportionate speed and extent of growth of these two tissue components in the fetus and possibly after birth.[284] An alternative concept is that of ductal plate malformation, with arrest in the normal organogenesis of the intrahepatic biliary tree.[284] Characteristically, there is a segmental, saccular, or beaded appearance to the intrahepatic ducts, which contain bile and communicate with the biliary tree.

Communicating cavernous ectasia of the biliary tree (Caroli's disease) usually accompanies either choledochal cyst or congenital hepatic fibrosis.[285] The ectasia can range from that seen in choledochal cysts to the microscopic terminal ductal ectasia and proliferation seen in congenital hepatic fibrosis.[285] This entity is characterized by (1) segmental saccular dilatation of the intrahepatic ducts; (2) marked predisposition for biliary calculous disease, cholangitis, and liver abscesses; (3) absence of portal hypertension and cirrhosis; and (4) association with renal tubular ectasia or other forms of cystic disease of the kidney.[286] Congenital hepatic fibrosis and cystic disease of the kidney are associated with this abnormality.[283]

This condition leads to bile stasis and predisposes to bacterial growth and, by compression of parenchymal cells, impairment of liver function. It is probably a mendelian recessive trait. Also associated are infantile polycystic kidney disease, medullary sponge kidney and nephrolithiasis.[285] There has been a report of this abnormality diagnosed antenatally.[285]

Patients present with crampy pain secondary to stone formation, which in turn is believed to be secondary to bile stasis within the cyst and to cholangitis. Pain, fever, and intermittent jaundice are the most common symptoms and usually develop during childhood or young adulthood.[287]

Ultrasound permits an early diagnosis and can be used for follow-up examinations.[286] Multiple cystic structures within the liver that communicate with the biliary tree are seen (Figs. 6-93 and 6-94). With the typical pattern, there are sonolucent spaces converging toward the porta hepatis within the liver.[283] Other findings include bile duct dilatations, intraluminal bulbar protrusions, bridge formation across dilated lumina, and portal radicles partially or completely surrounded by dilated bile ducts.[284] Stones, which appear as echogenic structures, may be seen with the ducts.

Choledochal Cyst

A choledochal cyst is an uncommon abnormality with greater incidence in females and orientals.[288] It occurs four times more often in females than males.[289] The favored etiology is that of an anomalous insertion of the common bile duct into the pancreatic duct, permitting reflux of pancreatic juice into the bile duct and hence leading to cholangitis and dilatation.[288,290,291] The theory of primary weakness in the wall with a distal obstructing lesion is now less favored.[290] Choledochal cysts in neonates are congenital whereas those in older children may be acquired in association with an anomalous pancreaticobiliary union.[292] Choledochal cysts in neonates may be associated with atresia of the distal common bile duct, whereas older children may present with intermittent jaundice with nonobstructive choledochal cysts.[292]

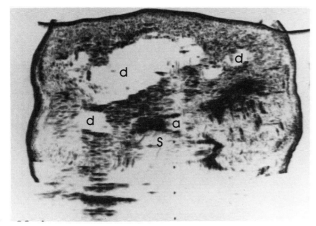

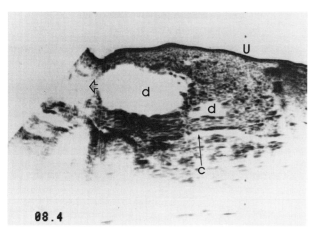

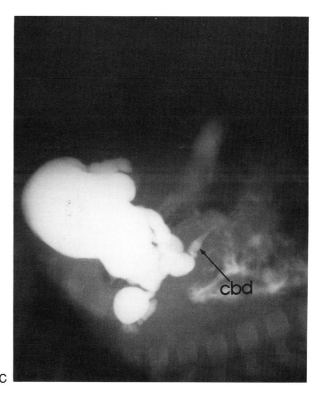

Fig. 6-93. Caroli's disease. **(A)** Transverse scan 3 cm below the xyphoid. Dilated ducts *(d)* are seen as anechoic spaces within the liver. (*a*, aorta; *S*, spine.) **(B)** Longitudinal scan 1 cm to the right of the midline. (*c*, inferior vena cava; *U*, level of the umbilicus; open arrow, level of the diaphragm; *d*, ducts.) **(C)** Transhepatic cholangiogram, lateral view. The intrahepatic ducts are dilated, but the common bile duct *(cbd)* is not dilated. (From Mittelstaedt et al,[286] with permission.)

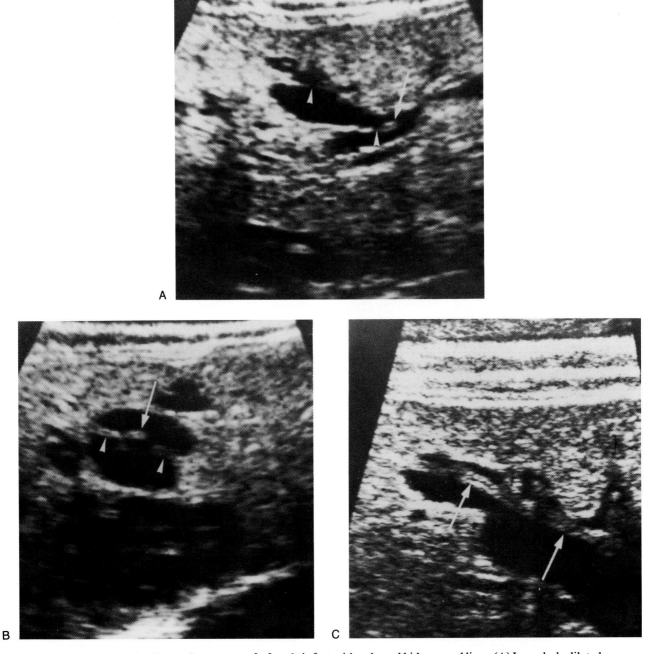

Fig. 6-94. Caroli's disease. Sonograms of a female infant with enlarged kidneys and liver. **(A)** Irregularly dilated bile ducts in the anterior portion of the liver and complete and incomplete bridging of the ductal walls (arrowheads). A small portal branch is seen at the end of an incomplete bridge (arrow). **(B)** Transverse sonogram of a large dilated bile duct demonstrating complete bridging of the ductal walls (arrowheads) and a small portal branch in the center of the bile duct (arrow). **(C)** Sagittal sonogram of a large dilated bile duct showing branching of both bile duct and intraluminal portal veins (arrows). (From Marchal et al,[284] with permission.)

Patients present in the first decade of life with pain, intermittent jaundice, and a palpable mass (in 20 to 25 percent).[290-295] Jaundice occurs in 70 percent of patients.[288] The incidence of carcinoma in a choledochal cyst is 20 times greater than that of bile duct carcinoma in the general population.[296]

There are four basic types of choledochal cysts: (1) cystic dilatation of the common bile duct (most common); (2) diverticulum of the common bile duct; (3) choledochocele; and (4) multiple intrahepatic and extrahepatic cysts.[288,290,291,294] In 50 percent of cases, there are associated dilated ducts.[297] The common hepatic duct is usually normal, with variable portions of the extrahepatic ductal system involved.[293] The preoperative diagnosis is important, because the surgical morbidity and mortality are significantly diminished in patients in whom the diagnosis is made correctly prior to surgery.[295] Prompt surgery is indicated to arrest possible complications of portal hypertension, cirrhosis, cholangitis, perforation, sepsis, and stone formation.[295]

On ultrasound, one finds a large cystic mass in the porta hepatis separate from the gallbladder, with a dilated common hepatic duct or common bile duct entering directly into the cyst[288] (Figs. 6-95 and 6-96). Calculi may be seen within the cyst.[289] These lesions have even been observed antenatally.[290] The differential diagnosis includes hepatic cyst, pancreatic pseudocyst, enteric duplication, hepatic artery aneurysm, and spontaneous perforation of the extrahepatic ducts.[288] An accurate ultrasound diagnosis may lead to early corrective surgery, which may prevent irreversible biliary cirrhosis.[291]

One group of investigators reported cases of choledochal cyst and biliary atresia.[292] All patients presented with jaundice and acholic stools. With ultrasound, a cystic structure separate from the gallbladder and representing the cyst was found.[292] With hepatobiliary scintigraphy, atresia of the distal common bile duct was diagnosed preoperatively.[292] By combining ultrasound and hepatobiliary scintigraphy, this subset of patients with persistent neonatal jaundice may be correctly identified and valuable information provided for prompt surgical management.[292]

Biliary Dilatation

Common bile duct measurement is a sensitive indicator of biliary obstruction, and its demonstration by noninvasive or invasive means is mandatory even when intrahepatic ducts appear normal.[298] The physical law of Laplace applies to the biliary system, accounting for the preferential dilatation of the extrahepatic ducts.[298] For a given pressure, the bursting force in a cylinder is directly proportional to the diameter of the cylinder. The gallbladder may also act as a reservoir and prevent dilatation of the biliary system and elevation of the bilirubin level early in the course of obstruction. The total transmural pressure applied to the intrahepatic bile ducts by adjacent hepatic parenchyma or fibrosis (as in cirrhosis) may account for the lack of ease with which they dilate. Extrahepatic duct measurement is a more sensitive measurement of biliary obstruction than is intrahepatic duct dilatation, particularly if the duration of the jaundice is less than 4 weeks.[298]

Experimental studies have been performed to evaluate biliary tract obstruction. Within 24 hours after occlusion of the distal common bile duct, there is dilatation of the common bile duct and gallbladder before elevation of the bilirubin level. After a brief interval of several hours following acute biliary obstruction, the ultrasound appearance of the ducts may be normal when nuclear medicine studies document total obstruction.[299] The ducts expand centrifugally from the obstructive point, with dilatation of the intrahepatic ducts occurring days after the onset of the obstruction. After release of the obstruction, the biliary ducts contract centripetally, with the common bile duct requiring 30 to 50 days to return to normal.[300] Others describe decompression within 43 hours after relief of acute obstruction.[301]

Some investigators have shown that a dilated common hepatic duct may return to its normal size within minutes.[39] It is postulated that the rapid size change probably occurs only in patients without a normally functioning gallbladder. The wall of the duct is composed largely of fibroelastic tissue, with the stretch potential of the elastic fibers permitting duct dilatation and their elastic recoil being responsible for return of the duct to normal size after relief of obstruction. In humans, the size of the common bile duct is determined largely by intraductal pressure. With an increase in intraductal pressure, the common bile duct progressively dilates to a limit governed by the elastic properties of the duct wall.[39] Ductal dilatation may be followed by inflammation and fibrosis and may preclude further dilatation or reduction in ductal size.[302]

Ultrasound Signs

Several ultrasound signs have been described for dilatation of the biliary system. These include (1) peripheral lucencies within the liver, which demonstrate acoustic enhancement; (2) tubular lucencies within the liver, which have an antler or stellate branching pattern; (3) lucencies within the left lobe of the liver; (4) dilated common bile duct identified as a tubular lucency anterior to the portal vein on a long-axis view of the portal vein; (5) dilated common hepatic duct identified as a

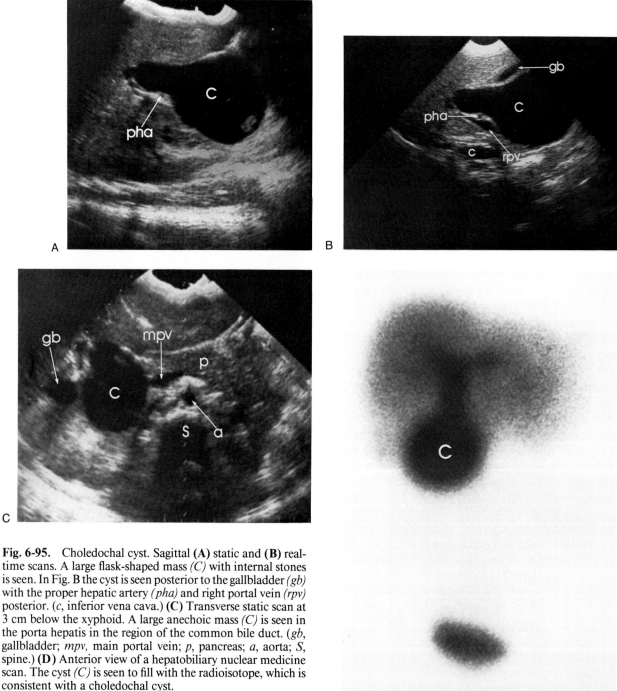

Fig. 6-95. Choledochal cyst. Sagittal (**A**) static and (**B**) real-time scans. A large flask-shaped mass *(C)* with internal stones is seen. In Fig. B the cyst is seen posterior to the gallbladder *(gb)* with the proper hepatic artery *(pha)* and right portal vein *(rpv)* posterior. (*c,* inferior vena cava.) (**C**) Transverse static scan at 3 cm below the xyphoid. A large anechoic mass *(C)* is seen in the porta hepatis in the region of the common bile duct. (*gb,* gallbladder; *mpv,* main portal vein; *p,* pancreas; *a,* aorta; *S,* spine.) (**D**) Anterior view of a hepatobiliary nuclear medicine scan. The cyst *(C)* is seen to fill with the radioisotope, which is consistent with a choledochal cyst.

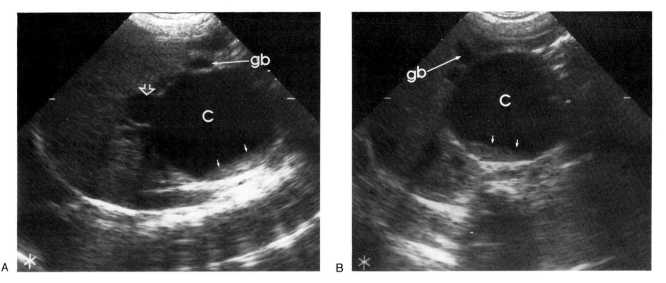

Fig. 6-96. Choledochal cyst. **(A)** Sagittal and **(B)** transverse views demonstrating a cystic structure *(C)* in the region of the common bile duct. The structure contained sludge, which layered (arrows). This structure appeared to communicate with a tubular structure (open arrow) believed to represent a duct. The gallbladder *(gb)* is seen anteriorly.

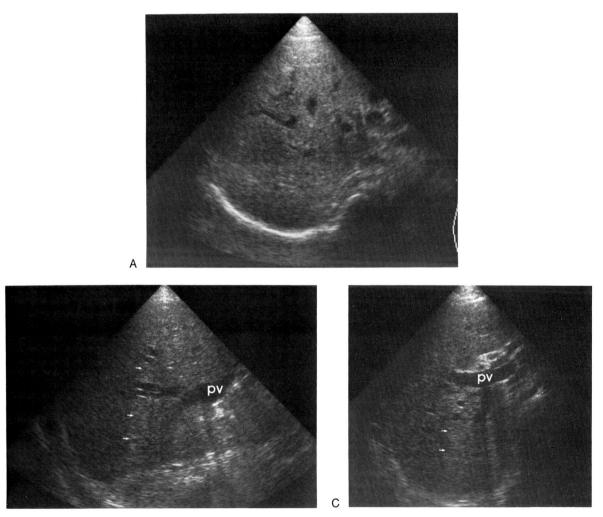

Fig. 6-97. Dilated intrahepatic ducts. Right lobe. **(A–C)** Transverse views of the right lobe of the liver demonstrating multiple lucent areas. These are associated with acoustic enhancement (arrows) characteristic of ducts. *(pv,* portal vein.)

tubular lucency anterior to the right portal vein; and (6) more than two tubular lucencies seen on a sagittal scan in the porta hepatis region[303] (Figs. 6-97 to 6-101).

Although lucencies are often seen within the right lobe of the liver on a sagittal scan, these are usually vessels and there is no acoustic enhancement. Bile, being less dense than blood, exhibits increased through transmission (Figs. 6-97 and 6-98). This sign of intrahepatic duct dilatation may be subtle. Routinely, few intrahepatic vessels are seen on a sagittal scan through the left lobe of the liver. If lucencies are seen, one should suspect dilated intrahepatic ducts (Fig. 6-98).

Abnormal common hepatic ducts have an internal dimension of more than 4 mm[36] (Fig. 6-99). A measurement of 5 mm would be borderline, with a dimension of 6 mm required to diagnose dilatation of the common hepatic duct.[36] Abnormal common bile ducts have an internal dimension of greater than 6 mm, with a dimen-

sion of 7 mm being definitely abnormal (Figs. 6-100 and 6-101).

Another finding with dilatation is the "parallel-channel" sign. This refers to the simultaneous imaging of the dilated right or left hepatic duct and adjacent contiguous main portal vein branch (Fig. 6-98). It is highly reliable in minimal duct dilatation.[304] The "shotgun" sign is similar to the parallel-channel sign. It describes the presence of two parallel ducts as pathologic.[305] As dilatation of the biliary tree progresses, the portal system becomes flattened, thus reversing the initial proportion between the diameter of the biliary junction and that of the biliary tree. With appropriate positioning, the junction of the right and left ducts can be demonstrated.[305]

Ultrasound has proved to be a more sensitive indicator of obstructive jaundice than the serum bilirubin level or biochemical profile.[306-308] Since peripheral biliary dilatation may be diagnosed as early as 4 hours after

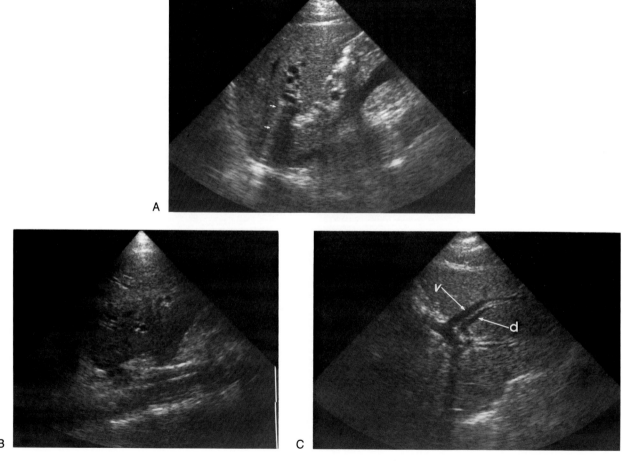

Fig. 6-98.   Dilated intrahepatic ducts. Left lobe. (A & B) Sagittal scans showing lucencies within the left lobe. There is subtle acoustic enhancement (arrows) beyond some of the ducts. (C) Transverse scan showing the relationship of the duct (d) to the vessel (v).

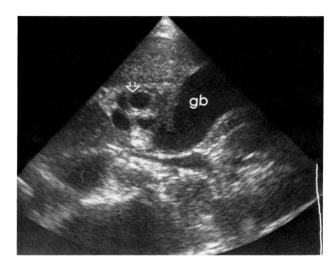

Fig. 6-99. "Too-many-tubes" sign. Sagittal view of the porta hepatis. There are too many cystic structures (arrow) visualized superior to the gallbladder *(gb)*. Some must represent dilated ducts.

biliary obstruction and before elevation of the serum bilirubin level, it has been suggested that obstruction may be diagnosed by ultrasound before the onset of icterus.[309] However, obstruction has been demonstrated in the absence of biliary dilatation.[310]

Ultrasound Accuracy

The method of choice for evaluation of biliary tract dilatation is ultrasound.[311] Ultrasound is the preferred initial screening procedure for biliary tract dilatation in jaundiced patients in whom obstruction must be differentiated from hepatocellular disease; this is because of the accuracy and sensitivity of ultrasound, although CT more precisely displays the level and cause of obstruction.[311,312] When evaluating the accuracy of ultrasound in identifying dilatation of the common hepatic duct, the sensitivity is reported to be 99 percent, with a specificity of 87 percent if the common hepatic duct is greater than 4 mm in diameter.[36] Ultrasound studies describe an ac-

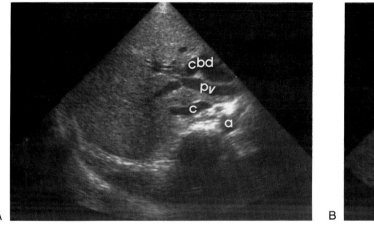

A

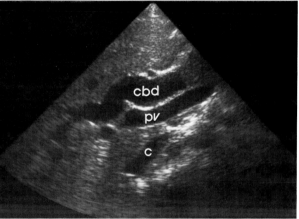

B

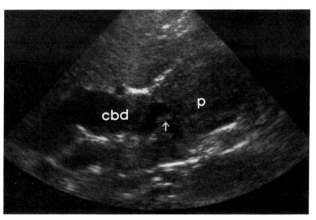

C

Fig. 6-100. Dilated common bile duct. **(A–C)** Long-axis views of the common bile duct *(cbd)* demonstrating narrowing of the distal end (arrow, Fig. C). This patient was found to have a stenosis at the distal end of the duct. *(pv,* portal vein; *p,* pancreatic head; *c,* inferior vena cava; *a,* aorta.)

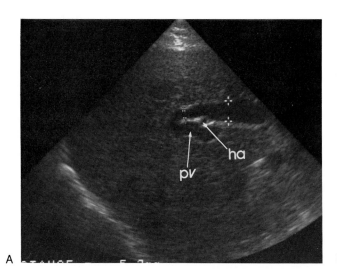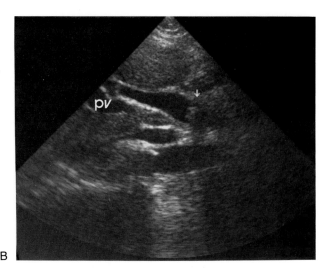

Fig. 6-101. Dilated common hepatic and bile duct. **(A)** Sagittal scan. The dilated common hepatic duct (small calipers) is seen anterior to the right portal vein *(pv)* in this postcholecystectomy patient. The proximal common bile duct (large calipers) measures 11 mm. (*ha*, right hepatic artery.) **(B)** View of the more distal common bile duct demonstrating a stone (arrow). (*pv*, portal vein.)

curacy of 86 to 97 percent for ultrasound in differentiating obstructive from nonobstructive jaundice, with a predictive value of 97 percent in obstruction and 84 percent in nonobstruction.[313–317] The level of obstruction is demonstrated in 95 percent of cases and the cause of obstruction in 68 percent.[314] When comparing ultrasound and CT, ultrasound has been reported to identify the precise level of obstruction in 60 percent and CT in 88 percent.[318] The cause of obstruction can be accurately predicted by ultrasound in 38 percent and by CT in 70 percent.[318] Although ultrasound can be used as a screen for obstructive jaundice, it is not as helpful in identifying the level of the obstruction and the cause; CT is more accurate in this respect.[318] If the ultrasound scan is normal, no further studies are needed. If there is evidence of obstruction, CT and/or percutaneous transhepatic cholangiography is performed. Markedly obese patients and patients with a biliary-enteric anastomosis are better suited to CT.[318]

Other investigators have compared ultrasound and nuclear medicine in the evaluation of biliary tract obstruction.[319] They found nuclear medicine to have a sensitivity of 18 percent with a specificity of 100 percent for large duct obstruction, whereas ultrasound had a sensitivity of 82 percent and a specificity of 86 percent, with a predictive value for a negative interpretation of 97 percent.[319]

Nonobstructive Causes

There are a number of nonobstructive causes of bile ductal dilatation. Previous inflammation and obstruction, as well as aging, may affect the elastic recoil of the duct wall, resulting in dilatation without obstruction.[320] Other causes include parenteral hyperalimentation and prolonged fasting (which result in failure of relaxation of the sphincter of Oddi from lack of stimulus to release endogenous CCK), morphine and other narcotics (which result in decreased intestinal activity and a direct effect on sphincter of Oddi, increasing its contractility and preventing its relaxation), vagus nerve stimulation (which increases upper intestinal motility and relaxes the sphincter of Oddi), and pregnant women and those taking oral contraceptives (the duct returns to normal postpartum or after administration of estrogens).[320]

Postoperatively, a statistically significant increase in the mean diameter of the hepatic duct is seen.[320] The mean diameter of the duct almost doubles, from 3.3 to 5.9 mm, in one series.[320] This is in association with a variety of conditions of intestinal hypomotility, including paralytic ileus resulting from miscellaneous abdominal and thoracic inflammatory processes or trauma.[320] Some of these patients may not respond to a fatty-meal stimulus.[320] It is postulated that this phenomenon may be due to the persistent contraction of the sphincter of Oddi that occurs when intestinal hypomotility eliminates the stimuli for CCK release.[320]

Nonobstructive biliary dilatation may be found in response to factors that inhibit the relaxation or prolong the contraction of the sphincter of Oddi.[320] Most of these factors are associated with decreased or absent intestinal motility.[320] This observation should be kept in mind to avoid misdiagnosing biliary obstruction under these conditions.[320] In the early postoperative period, biliary dilatation should be viewed as a physiologic response to the surgical trauma.[320]

Level and Cause

Each time biliary dilatation is found, the examiner should try to define the level and cause. The level of dilatation is defined as pancreatic, suprapancreatic, or at the level of the porta hepatis, with the causes including pancreatitis, choledocholithiasis, neoplasm, and stricture.[321] The most common level for obstruction is the pancreatic level (90.9 percent; most commonly caused by choledocholithiasis), followed by the suprapancreatic level (5.5 percent; most commonly caused by cancer) and then the level of the porta hepatis (most commonly caused by cancer).[321]

The technique for the examination should include examination of the distal duct initially on transverse scans obtained with the patient in a semiupright right posterior oblique position and examination of the proximal duct on a sagittal scan obtained with the patient in the supine left posterior oblique position.[321] The technique for evaluation of the common bile duct includes examining the distal common bile duct initially by obtaining transverse scans through the pancreatic head and uncinate process.[321] The scans are repeated with the patient in a semiupright position and in a right posterior oblique position. The patient is given water to drink and is placed in the right lateral decubitus position if overlying bowel gas is a problem.[321]

Accuracy. By using this technique, the level of dilatation is 91.8 percent, with the correct cause suggested in 70.9 percent.[321] With this technique, the distal obstructing lesions (which are the most common) can be optimally examined because the approach markedly improves ultrasound visualization.[321]

How does ultrasound fare in a prospective evaluation of the site and cause of obstructive jaundice? In one series, the site of obstruction could be identified in 27 percent, with 73 percent indeterminate because of the inability to visualize the complete biliary tract.[322] The cause of obstruction was determined in 23 percent, with 76 percent indeterminate.[322] The determination of the anatomic site of obstruction and its cause is critical in the management of jaundiced patients. Although ultrasound is an excellent screen for distinguishing dilated from nondilated ducts, direct cholangiography or possibly CT is necessary if stringent criteria are applied to determine the site and cause of biliary obstruction.[322]

Other investigators have evaluated the level, cause, and tumor resectability associated with bile duct obstruction.[323] In 95 percent of cases, ultrasound was able to correctly identify the level of obstruction (CT, 90 percent), and in 88 percent it correctly diagnosed the cause (CT, 63 percent).[323] Ultrasound was correct in predicting tumor resectability in 71 percent of cases, with 58 percent for direct cholangiography, 42 percent for CT and

25 percent for angiography.[323] As such, ultrasound appears to be the most useful modality in the evaluation of bile duct obstruction.[323]

Biliary Dilatation in Children

Neonates. Jaundice in neonates may develop for various reasons.[293] These include overproduction of bilirubin as a result of fetomaternal blood incompatibility, hemoglobinopathies, enzymatic and structural red blood cell defects, and polycythemia. It can also occur with hemorrhage anywhere in the body. It is seen with Hirschsprung's disease, intestinal atresia or stenoses, and meconium ileus or meconium plug syndrome. With mixed hyperbilirubinemia, there may be metabolic abnormalities, storage disease, α_1-antitrypsin deficiency, prenatal infection (toxoplasmosis, cytomegalovirus infection, herpes, syphilis), and neonatal sepsis. The leading diagnoses to be considered when all of the above have been excluded are neonatal hepatitis and biliary atresia. These entities are difficult to differentiate by ultrasound and are further discussed earlier in this chapter. In biliary atresia, the atretic segment may involve any or all parts of the biliary tree. The uninvolved part may be normal in caliber, but there may be normal-sized extrahepatic ducts with atresia.[293]

Older Children. In older children, the etiologies to be considered include choledochal cyst, Caroli's disease, cholelithiasis, cholecystitis, and hepatic and obstructive extrahepatic masses. Not only does ultrasound permit rapid detection of bile duct dilatation, but also it can permit localization for percutaneous cholangiography, which aids in the choice of surgical procedure by locating the site of obstruction.[324] Cholelithiasis, cholecystitis, choledochal cyst, and Caroli's disease have already been discussed. The major hepatic masses in infants and children are not associated with jaundice, but present with a palpable mass and are discussed in Chapter 5. Abdominal lymphoma or metastatic nodes can obstruct the biliary tree. Hepatic hemangiomas may also present with jaundice. These hemangiomas are capillary hemangiomas or hemangioendotheliomas. The jaundice is due to a low-grade hemolysis. As discussed in Chapter 5, these masses are seen on ultrasound with multiple lucent and hypoechoic areas within the liver parenchyma. Most of these patients present by 6 months of age.[293]

Postoperative Cholecystectomy Patients

There have been many reports indicating that there is dilatation of the extrahepatic ductal system following cholecystectomy. However, one study found no evidence of common bile duct dilatation in 95 percent of patients; all of their postoperative cholecystectomy patients had common bile ducts that measured 6 mm or less.[325] In most instances (84 percent), the common hepatic duct measured 4 mm or less.[326,327] If the common hepatic duct measures 6 mm or more and the common bile duct measures 8 mm or more, further studies are indicated.[326] These may include ultrasound evaluation of the biliary system before and after a fatty meal, as discussed earlier (Fig. 6-10), or a hepatobiliary nuclear medicine study.

Investigators have evaluated the effect of cholecystectomy on the common bile duct diameter.[328] The largest diameter of the common bile duct in this series postcholecystectomy was 1 cm.[328] Increases or decreases of the diameter may occur after surgery in patients with calculous gallbladder disease, with the postoperative evolution governed by the exact nature of the underlying biliary disease at the time of the index operation.[328]

Finally, the method of choice in examining postoperative cholecystectomy patients must be discussed. In these patients, endoscopic retrograde cholangiopancreatography (ERCP) is recommended as the initial diagnostic modality.[329] Ultrasound demonstrates a specificity of 87 percent in these cases; the value of a positive diagnosis is 60 percent and that of a negative diagnosis is 64 percent.[329] When comparing ultrasound and ERCP, ultrasound is 88 percent sensitive with a specificity of 93 percent.[329] The sensitivity of the sonographic measurement of the common hepatic duct as an indicator of biliary obstruction is 88 percent with a specificity of 57 percent.[326] ERCP is therefore recommended for evaluation of the postoperative gallbladder patient, even though the complication rate of the procedure is 3 percent, the mortality is 0.2 percent, and the failure rate is 12 percent.[329]

Other Causes

Mirizzi Syndrome. Mirizzi syndrome is an uncommon, surgically correctable cause of extrahepatic obstruction that was discussed earlier in this chapter.[112-114] In the proper situation, the ultrasound appearance of dilated intrahepatic ducts, normal-caliber common bile ducts, and stones in the neck of the gallbladder or cystic duct should suggest the diagnosis[112-114] (Figs. 6-40 and 6-41).

Pregnancy. The size of the bile duct during pregnancy has been evaluated.[330] The following has been concluded: (1) the greatest normal size of the common hepatic duct is 5 mm; (2) there is no correlation between the size of the common hepatic duct and the stage of pregnancy; and (3) gallstones were incidentally noted in 3.9 percent of cases.[330] During the second and third trimesters of pregnancy, pregnancy hormones, notably progesterone, are believed to cause incomplete emptying of the gallbladder.[330]

Aortic Aneurysm. Unusual causes of biliary dilatation have been reported. These include obstruction due to compression by an aortic aneurysm.[331]

Choledocholithiasis

Although ultrasound is the method of choice for diagnosing cholelithiasis and for evaluating intra- and extrahepatic biliary ductal dilatation in jaundiced patients, its role in the diagnosis of choledocholithiasis is uncertain. Ductal stones are identified by the presence of echogenic material within the duct (Figs. 6-102 to 6-106). The absence of surrounding bile makes the diagnosis difficult. Also, a high percentage of common bile duct stones do not cause shadows (probably because of their size).[332]

The echogenic nature of the calculus in the ampulla is difficult to distinguish from the pancreas and mucus in the duodenum.[109] Although the proximal common bile duct can usually be reliably identified in its long axis, the distal duct is difficult to see because of bowel gas. The administration of small amounts of water containing microbubbles, while simultaneously scanning the ampulla and pancreatic head, frequently defines the duodenum more clearly and allows better delineation of the medial aspect of the pancreas. The distal duct is best visualized in the transverse plane with the patient in the upright and/or right lateral decubitus position.[13] Occasionally, by placing the patient in Trendelenburg's position, the stone may be seen migrating cephalad into the more visible part of the duct.[109] The stones in the proximal common bile duct are best demonstrated by sagittal sections with the patient in the right anterior oblique position.[333] This evaluation is best performed by high-resolution real-time sector ultrasound. It is especially helpful to reevaluate a dilated common duct on a subsequent day if no stones are seen.[333]

The reasons for difficulties with this diagnosis of choledocholithiasis rest on these factors: (1) deeper position of the common bile duct as compared with the gallbladder; (2) difficulty in continuously observing a stone secondary to interference from changing pockets of gas within the overlying bowel; (3) reflection and refraction of the beam by the curved wall of the duct; (4) the position of the common bile duct such that it may lie out of the optimal focal zone of the transducer; and (5) the presence of a very small amount of fluid surrounding the stone, especially in the minimally dilated or normal-sized duct.[333]

Structures that create confusion include (1) air or residue in the adjacent bowel, mimicking a stone; (2) the

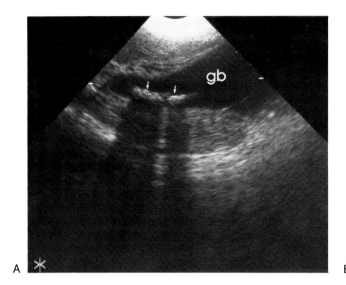

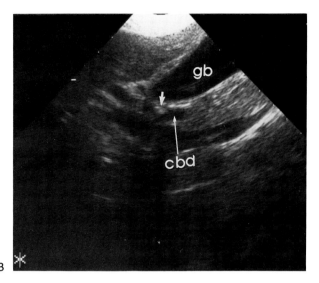

Fig. 6-102. Cholelithiasis and choledocholithiasis. **(A)** Sagittal view of the gallbladder *(gb)* demonstrating stones (arrows). **(B)** Another sagittal view demonstrating dilatation of the proximal common bile duct *(cbd)*. There is a stone (arrow) within the duct. *(gb*, gallbladder.)

right hepatic artery crossing the common bile duct and indenting it; (3) postoperative cholecystectomy clips; (4) impression on the common bile duct by the cystic duct; (5) air in the biliary tree; (6) a mucous plug; and (7) calcification in the head of the pancreas[333] (Figs. 6-28 and 6-88). As such, one should be familiar with the artifacts created by such things as clips, catheters, and air, which can lead to a false-positive diagnosis.[334] Knowl-

edge of previous surgery and the availability of a plain radiograph are also important in such cases. A positive diagnosis of choledocholithiasis can be made only if ultrasound demonstrates hyperechoic structures within the common bile duct with an associated shadow; it is especially helpful to the diagnosis if the echodense structures are seen to change position within the common bile duct as the patient changes position.[333]

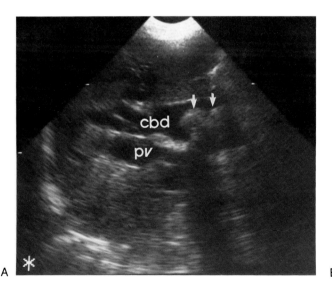

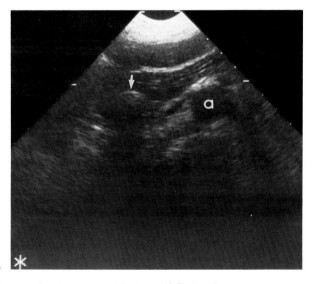

Fig. 6-103. Choledocholithiasis. **(A)** Long-axis view of the proximal common bile duct *(cbd)* showing a massively dilated common bile duct (2 to 3 cm) containing very large stones (arrows). *(pv*, portal vein.) **(B)** Transverse view of the pancreatic head showing an echogenic structure (arrow) in the region of the distal duct. This represented a large obstructing calculus. *(a*, aorta.)

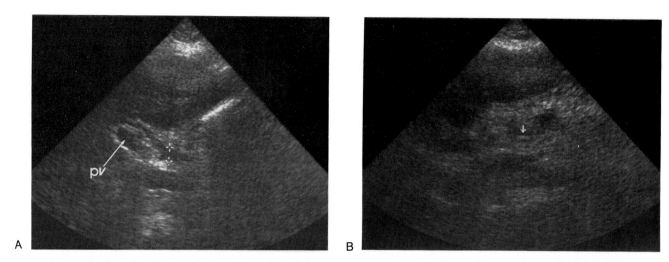

Fig. 6-104. Choledocholithiasis. This patient had cholelithiasis and was not "sonogenic." It was still possible to delineate a dilated (9-mm) proximal common bile duct (calipers) on sagittal view. (*pv*, portal vein.) **(B)** Barely visible was a stone (arrow) within the area of the distal common bile duct on transverse views through the region of the pancreatic head.

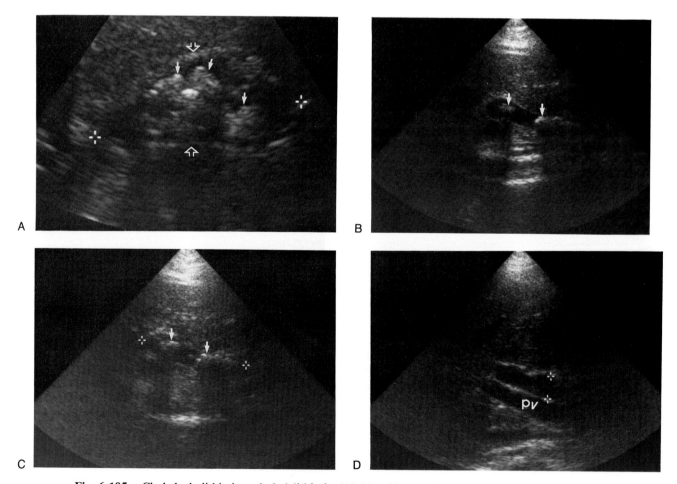

Fig. 6-105. Choledocholithiasis and cholelithiasis. **(A)** Magnified sagittal view showing multiple gallstones (arrows) within the gallbladder (open arrows). **(B & C)** Long-axis views of the proximal common bile duct showing stones (arrows). **(D)** The more distal common bile duct is seen to be dilated (calipers, 11 mm). (*pv*, portal vein.)

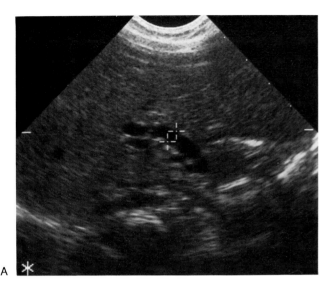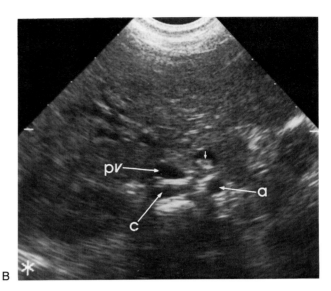

Fig. 6-106. Choledocholithiasis. Infant with short-bowel syndrome and abnormal liver function tests. **(A)** Transverse view showing a dilated proximal common bile duct (calipers, 4 mm). **(B)** Transverse view of distal common bile duct showing a stone (arrow). (*a*, aorta; *c*, inferior vena cava; *pv*, portal vein.)

At times it is difficult to distinguish gas from clips in normal postcholecystectomy sonograms. As a rule, the surgical clip artifacts emanate from short echogenic foci and are persistent, whereas gas foci are either long or short with evanescent artifacts.[335] Ninety-six percent of patients with clips and 6 percent of patients without clips demonstrate multiple reverberations artifacts.[335]

Accuracy

Several studies have demonstrated an improved accuracy in the diagnosis of choledocholithiasis by the new high-resolution real-time systems.[13,109] In one study, the earlier results demonstrated a sensitivity of 29 percent, a specificity of 91 percent, and an accuracy of 55 percent.[109] In the last part of the study using high-resolution real-time ultrasound, the sensitivity increased to 55 percent, the specificity increased to 90 percent, and the accuracy increased to 71 percent.[109] The improved results were thought to be secondary to (1) the high-resolution real-time ultrasound with flexibility and ability to display rapidly many planes of sections and (2) improved skills in imaging the common bile duct.[109] By adding an evaluation of the distal common bile duct in another study, the overall sensitivity of ultrasound for the diagnosis of choledocholithiasis was 75 percent.[13] Eighty-nine percent of proximal and 70 percent of distal common bile duct calculi were identified.[13]

CT and ultrasound have been compared for their ability to diagnose choledocholithiasis.[336] Ultrasound demonstrated a sensitivity of 18 percent with an accuracy of 19 percent.[336] CT had a sensitivity of 87 percent with an accuracy of 84 percent.[336] CT is thought to be effective in visualizing common bile duct stones and is superior to ultrasound in diagnosing the cause of obstruction. Although ultrasound is an excellent initial procedure to detect biliary dilatation, CT is effective in the definition of the level and cause of obstruction. Ultrasound is limited in its ability to image a calculus in the distal common bile duct. Percutaneous cholangiography is reserved for cases in which (1) further confirmation is required preoperatively, (2) the cause is not determined by CT, (3) ducts are not dilated on ultrasound or CT but there is clinical suspicion of obstruction, (4) percutaneous biliary decompression is indicated, and (5) ERCP sphincterotomy is the treatment of choice.[336]

One group of investigators has reevaluated the ultrasound diagnosis of choledocholithiasis.[337] This group demonstrated a 55 percent sensitivity for the detection of stones, representing more than a threefold increase over that in the previous series.[337] In 67 percent, dilated extrahepatic ducts were seen, with 77 percent having an intraluminal stone.[337] The marked improvement in detection rate probably is due to the improvements in imaging technology as well as the increased diagnostic efforts.[337]

Cholangitis and Other Infections

Oriental Cholangitis

With the recent influx of immigrants from Southeast Asia into the United States, there is an increased likelihood of encountering oriental cholangiohepatitis or pyogenic cholangitis in this country.[338] Endemic in Southeast Asia, oriental cholangiohepatis is characterized by recurrent attacks of cholangitis with abdominal pain, fever, and jaundice.[338-343] The largest number of cases occur in persons 20 to 40 years of age, with men and women affected almost equally.[338,342,344]

A number of changes are seen pathologically with this disease process. Along the periportal spaces and hepatic parenchyma there are proliferation of bile ducts and infiltration of inflammatory cells.[338] This process is characterized histologically by peribiliary fibrosis and grossly by bile duct stricture with marked ductal dilatation, duc-

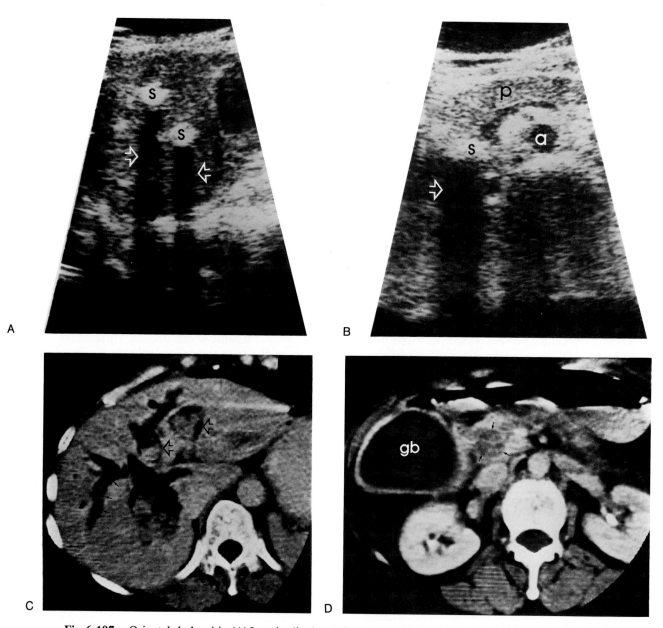

Fig. 6-107. Oriental cholangitis. **(A)** Longitudinal real-time scan with multiple highly reflective echoes *(S)* with acoustic shadowing (arrows) representing intrahepatic calculi. **(B)** Transverse scan demonstrating similar marked echoes *(S)* with posterior shadowing (arrow) in the distal common duct within the head of the pancreas *(p)*. (*a*, aorta.) **(C)** CT scan showing massive dilatation of the intrahepatic ducts with some discrete calculi (open arrows) and other intraductal debris, which form a cast of the dependent ducts (small arrows). **(D)** CT scan caudal to Fig. C, showing a dilated common bile duct (arrows) within the pancreatic head. The duct is filled with a calculus that has higher attenuation than the bile in the gallbladder *(gb)*. At surgery, numerous pigmented stones were present in the intra- and extrahepatic ducts, along with biliary mud and pus. (From Federle et al,[344] with permission.)

tal stones, local hepatic necrosis, and hepatic abscess. Fibrous tissue proliferates in the portal tracts, and the intrahepatic ducts show dilatation and stricture and may contain pigmented stones, pigmented mud, and debris and may shed epithelial cells, exudates, and frank pus.[338] The ductal stones originate in the bile ducts and are composed mostly of bile pigment with variable calcification. Stones are present in 75 to 80 percent of cases. There may be localized intrahepatic segmental ductal stenosis, especially in the lateral segment of the left lobe

or the posterior segment of the right lobe.[338] In 85 to 100 percent of cases, there is dilatation of the extrahepatic ducts and large intrahepatic ducts such as the right and left hepatic ducts.[338] There is a close relationship between recurrent pyogenic cholangitis and cholangiocarcinoma, with a prevalence ranging from 2.4 to 5 percent.[338,341]

Many possible etiologies have been cited; a combination of causes is probable.[344] These may include (1) congenital or acquired stricture; (2) coliform bacterial infec-

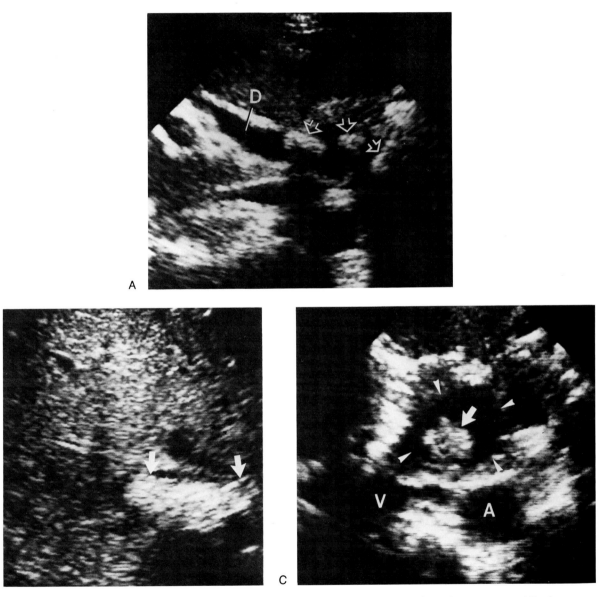

Fig. 6-108. Oriental cholangiohepatitis. **(A)** Sagittal sonogram showing dilatation of the common bile duct containing three shadowing stones (arrows). The wall of the common bile duct *(D)* is thick. **(B)** Transverse sonogram of liver showing a shadowing echogenic cast filling the posterior segmental bile duct of the right hepatic lobe (arrows). **(C)** Transverse sonogram of the common bile duct showing a round, nonshadowing stone (arrow). Proximal and distal portions of the bile duct are dilated diffusely (arrowheads). (*A*, abdominal aorta; *V*, inferior vena cava.) (From Lim,[338] with permission.)

tion of bile; and (3) parasitic infestation (commonly found), particularly by *Clonorchis sinensis.*[338,343,344] Although the cause of the disease is not known, there has been an association with clonorchiasis, ascariasis, and nutritional deficiency.[338] There may be induced ductal injury and strictures, leading to stone formation.[335] With stagnation, bacterial infection results in pyogenic cholangitis. *C. sinensis* flukes are killed when pyogenic infection occurs in the bile ducts.[335] With bile stasis and the presence of dead flukes and ova or their debris, a nucleus can be formed for gallstones or bile duct stones; this can instigate all the consequent pathologic processes, resulting in a cycle of repeated bouts of cholangitis and stone formation. If untreated, cholangitis leads to intrahepatic bile stasis and ultimately to death from liver failure. Although many of the acute attacks respond to antibiotic treatment, many require decompression of the biliary tree after control of the acute attack, especially when there are stones in or stricture of the bile ducts. The treatment is surgical decompression of the biliary tree with a permanent drainage procedure.[343]

The findings on ultrasound and CT include (1) intra- or extrahepatic duct stones, (2) dilatation of the extrahepatic duct with relatively mild or no dilatation of the intrahepatic ducts, (3) localized dilatation of the lobar or segmental bile ducts, (4) increased periportal echogenicity, (5) segmental hepatic atrophy, and (6) gallstones.[338,339] There may be diffuse, uniform dilatation of the small intrahepatic bile ducts with no focal obstructing lesion, and there can be thickening of the bile ducts.[341] The ducts may be massively dilated, frequently as large as 3 to 4 cm in diameter (Figs. 6-107 to 6-109). The common bile duct is the most frequently involved structure, followed by the left and right hepatic ducts. The gallbladder is large and palpable in 30 percent of cases. The differential diagnosis on ultrasound should include biliary obstruction and Caroli's disease.[342]

Striking dilatation of the extrahepatic ducts is seen, with the ducts packed with huge pigmented stones. Ultrasound may fail to demonstrate the ductal calculi and extrahepatic dilatation because of the soft-mud consistency of the stones.[344] In 81.1 percent of cases there are bilirubinate stones.[342] In 60 percent there are ductal stones, with cholelithiasis seen in 15 to 20 percent.[344] Floating or dependent discrete nonshadowing echogenic foci in the gallbladder lumen are produced by adult worms.[339]

Bile duct dilatation can be demonstrated by ultrasound in all patients, with the extrahepatic bile ducts being dilated in 85 to 100 percent of cases and the larger intrahepatic ducts being dilated in 66 to 79 percent.[338] In 85 to 90 percent a stone or stones are detected, and these may be intra- and/or extrahepatic. These stones may be more echogenic than liver parenchyma or isoechoic.[338] As such, the detectability of the stones depends on their size, echogenicity, shadowing characteristics, and location.[338] Isoechoic bile duct stones filling the biliary tree as a cast can be missed, as can biliary mud.[338]

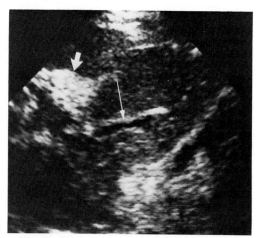
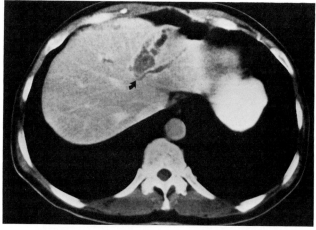

A   B

Fig. 6-109. Oriental cholangiohepatitis. Multiple intrahepatic stones in the lateral segment of the left lobe and extrahepatic stone. **(A)** Transverse sonogram of epigastrium showing echogenic foci (short arrow). Note the moderate dilatation of the subsegmental bile duct with a thick wall (long arrow). **(B)** CT scan of liver showing localized severe dilatation of lateral segmental bile duct of the left hepatic lobe as a result of a localized stricture (arrow). Multiple tiny high-density areas within the dilated duct represent small stones that might have been overlooked on the basis of CT alone. The wall of the dilated bile ducts is enhanced. (From Lim,[338] with permission.)

Acute Obstructive Suppurative Cholangitis

As a severe form of cholangitis secondary to bacterial contamination in the biliary system, acute obstructive suppurative cholangitis (AOSC) develops in the presence of bile stasis, and its clinical features are almost the same regardless of the cause, whether it is benign stenosis such as stones or inflammatory strictures, or neoplastic changes.[345] These patients present with jaundice, pain, and spiky fever of a septic nature.[345] One of the most important conditions closely associated with AOSC is choledocholithiasis, especially in the lower bile duct.[345]

Two new observations have been made with AOSC: (1) although almost no change in bile duct diameter was documented, biliary sludge appeared in the common bile duct just before the onset of AOSC; and (2) dense internal echoes were seen in the portal venous system during the most severe clinical stage.[345] Biliary drainage is recommended as soon as possible for any type of bile duct dilatation, even without jaundice. The sudden appearance of massive biliary sludge within the common bile duct requires immediate biliary drainage to prevent suppurative changes[345] (Fig. 6-110).

Sclerosing Cholangitis

The etiology of sclerosing cholangitis is unknown, but it may be secondary to either bacterial or metabolic alteration of bile acids. It is seen in fewer than 1 percent of patients with ulcerative colitis. It is also associated with Riedel struma, Crohn's disease, retroperitoneal fibrosis, and, possibly, mediastinal fibrosis.[346] It is more common in young men and is associated with findings of jaundice, pruritus, fever, pain, weight loss, and hepatomegaly.

Histologically, sclerosing cholangitis demonstrates nonspecific inflammation characterized by lymphocytic and plasma cells, bile duct proliferation, periportal fibrosis, cholestasis, and copper accumulation in the hepatic tissue.[346] Secondary cholangitis can be caused by tumors, previous surgery or trauma, and passage of large gallstones with resultant strictures.[346] On ultrasound, one sees evidence of biliary obstruction associated with marked concentric thickening of the intra- and extrahepatic biliary tree[346] (Fig. 6-111).

Hydatid Disease

Hydatid cysts may rupture into the biliary tree, with hydatid debris and daughter cysts entering the ducts and giving rise to jaundice and biliary colic.[347,348] Rupture into the biliary tract is the most common complication of hepatic echinococcal cysts, occurring in 5 to 10 percent of cases and causing biliary colic and jaundice.[349] In this disease, the cyst may suppurate and/or rupture into the biliary tree.[350] The site and incidence of intrabiliary rupture are the right hepatic duct in 55 percent of cases, left hepatic duct in 29 percent, bifurcation in 9 percent,

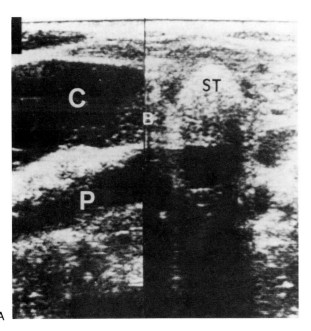

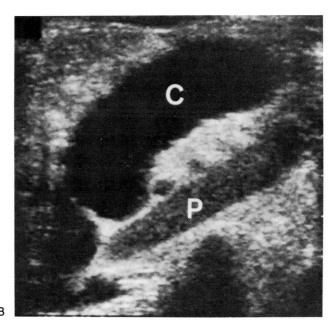

A   B

Fig. 6-110. Acute obstructive suppurative cholangitis. **(A)** Oblique section of the right upper abdomen. Biliary sludge *(B)* is seen in the common bile duct *(C)*. *(ST,* stone; *P,* portal vein.) **(B)** Oblique section of the right upper abdomen. Note the multiple internal echoes in the main porta vein *(P)*. *(C,* common bile duct.) (From Ishida et al,[345] with permission.)

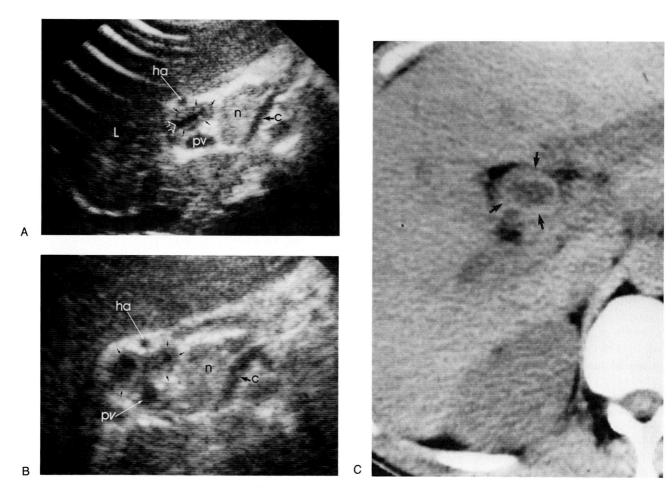

Fig. 6-111. Sclerosing cholangitis. **(A)** Longitudinal left decubitus scan through the porta hepatis. There is concentric thickening of the walls of the common hepatic and common bile duct to 1.5 cm (arrows). The lumen of the common duct (open arrow) is less than 5 mm in diameter. (*L*, liver; *pv*, portal vein; *n*, portal adenopathy; *c*, inferior vena cava; *ha*, hepatic artery.) **(B)** Oblique scan through the porta hepatis. There is concentric thickening of the walls of the right and left hepatic ducts (arrows). (*ha*, hepatic artery; *pv*, portal vein; *n*, node; *c*, inferior vena cava.) **(C)** CT scan at the level of the porta hepatis. There is concentric thickening of the dilated common bile duct (arrows). (From Carroll and Oppenheimer,[346] with permission.)

gallbladder in 6 percent, and common bile duct in 1 percent.[348] The latter is an uncommon complication showing the signs of obstructive jaundice indistinguishable from calculous disease.[350] The jaundice is caused by the accumulation of hydatid sand in the extrahepatic ducts.[348]

Direct ultrasound demonstration of hydatid material in the extrahepatic bile ducts has only very rarely been described.[349] The diagnosis should be suggested on ultrasound if a complex mass is noted to be communicating with the biliary ducts[347] (Figs. 6-112 and 6-113). The lesion may be cystic with or without septation, or it may exhibit a heterogeneous hypo- or hyperechoic pattern.[348] On ultrasound, the scoleces can be seen as filling defects

simulating stones. These echogenic intrabiliary scoleces produce echofree shadows and can be mistaken for stones.[350] Multiple small cysts and a more amorphous reflective material in the common bile duct may be demonstrated.[349] These cysts are freely movable within the dilated bile ducts, with respiration compatible with the evacuation of daughter cysts via the biliary tract.[349]

Biliary Ascariasis

In 1967, there was a report that estimated that the ascaris roundworm *(Ascaris lumbricoides)* infests one-fourth of the world's population as a result of heavy endemicity in the Far East, former USSR, Latin Amer-

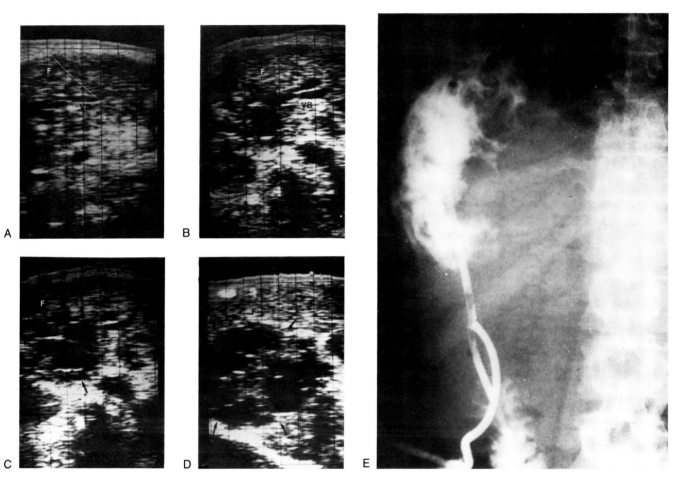

Fig. 6-112. Hydatid disease. **(A)** Transverse scan. An enlarged liver *(F)* is seen with diffuse high-level structural echoes; the biliary ducts *(VB)* are dilated. **(B)** Transverse scan. The right biliary ducts *(VB)* communicate with a rounded irregular complex mass (arrow). *(F,* liver.) **(C & D)** Oblique subcostal scans. A mass is seen with many rounded cystic spaces divided by thick septa of solid tissue. The mass measured 18 × 12 cm and was oval with polycyclic margins (arrows) clearly separated from surrounding liver. *(F,* liver.) **(E)** T-tube cholangiogram. The mass is clearly demonstrated communicating with the biliary ducts. Within the tube, hydatid debris and/or small daughter cysts can be seen. (From Biggi et al,[347] with permission.)

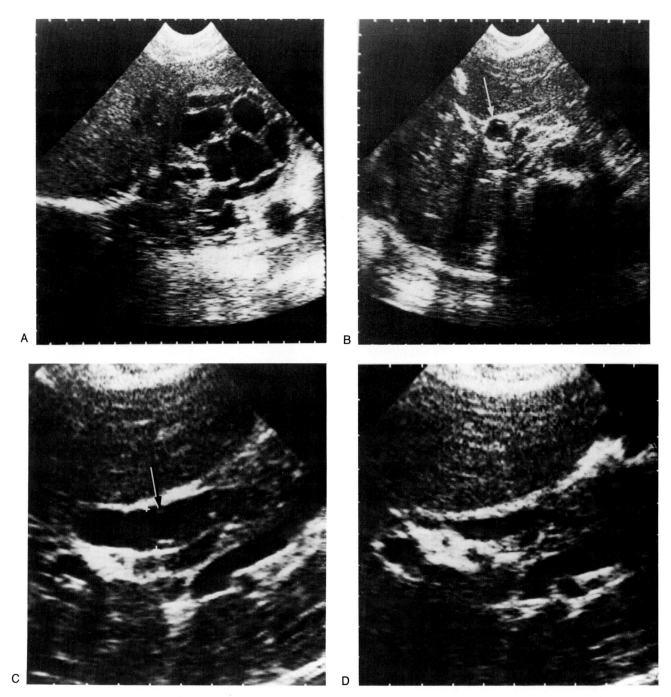

Fig. 6-113.   Biliary echinococcosis. **(A)** Transverse sonogram of the liver showing large thick-walled multilobulated hydatid cyst in the lateral segment of the left liver lobe. **(B)** Transverse sonogram at the level of the common bile duct (arrow) showing enlargement of the common bile duct in which a small cystic structure can be recognized. **(C)** Sagittal view of the common bile duct showing marked enlargement of the bile duct containing in its distal segment poorly reflective material and some small cystic structures (arrow). In real-time the contents of the bile duct were freely moving with respiration. **(D)** Follow-up ultrasound the next day. The bile duct has returned to its normal size. (From Gelin et al,[349] with permission.)

ica, and Africa. It has a lower endemicity in many other areas including the southeastern United States and Europe. The adult worm is 15 to 49 cm long and 3 to 6 mm thick and lives mainly in the jejunum. The most common clinical presentation, apart from passage per rectum or vomiting worms, is small bowel obstruction by a bolus of worms.[237] In a small number of patients, one or more ascarids migrate through the biliary tract and reach the ducts and gallbladder, causing cholecystitis, cholangitis, biliary obstruction, and hepatic ab-

scess.[237,238] The clinical manifestations are seen mainly in children.[238]

On ultrasound, these worms are seen as (1) echogenic, nonshadowing images in the main bile duct and/or gallbladder; (2) single strips (on occasion with its digestive tract seen as an anechoic "inner tube"); (3) multiple strips, giving a spaghettilike appearance; (4) coils; or (5) more amorphous fragments[237,239] (Fig. 6-114). On real-time ultrasound, one may even see a moving image of a worm in the duct.[238]

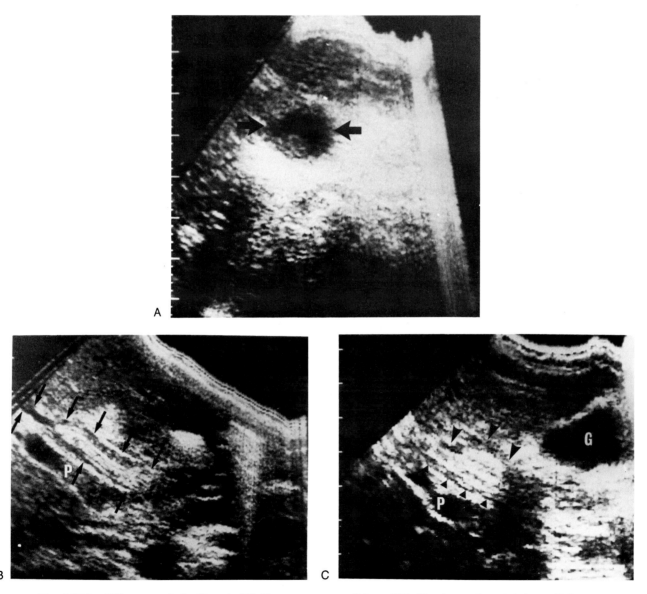

Fig. 6-114. Biliary ascariasis. Case 1. **(A)** Transverse scan of the gallbladder (arrows) containing coiled-up worms. Case 2. **(B)** Spaghetti appearance of the main bile duct worms. The main bile duct (arrows) expands to contain numerous longitudinal interfaces. (*P*, portal vein.) Case 3. **(C)** Spaghetti appearance of main bile duct worms. The lumen of the main bile duct is entirely replaced by the longitudinally disposed bundle of echogenic interfaces. (large arrowheads, anterior margin; small arrowheads, posterior margins; *P*, portal vein; *G*, gallbladder.) *(Figure continues.)*

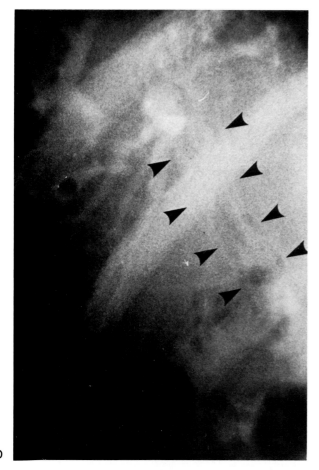

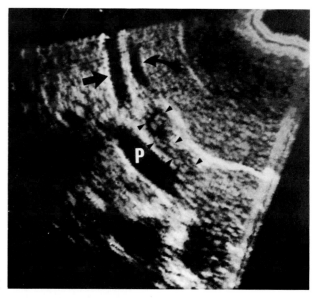

Fig. 6-114 *(Continued).* **(D)** Intravenous cholangiogram. The distended main bile duct (arrowheads) contains worms throughout its length. The intrahepatic bile ducts are also dilated. **(E)** Improved appearance 9 days later. The lumen of the main bile duct is now seen (arrowheads), but still contains echogenic fragments of worms. (curved arrow, left hepatic bile duct; straight arrow, left portal vein.) (From Schulman et al,[237] with permission.)

Biliary Neoplasm

Adenocarcinoma and Squamous Cell Carcinoma

The predisposing influences of inflammation and cholelithiasis are less established for carcinoma of the bile ducts than for carcinoma of the gallbladder.[20] Stones are found in one-third of cases. With chronic ulcerative colitis, there is also an increased incidence of this type of carcinoma. These tumors occur in the same age range as carcinoma of the gallbladder, with a greater frequency in males than females. As a primary cancer of the biliary ductal epithelium, cholangiocarcinoma is relatively rare, accounting for 0.5 to 1 percent of all cancers.[351] It is highly lethal, with an overall 1 percent 5-year survival rate and a 20 percent 5-year survival rate in patients who undergo curative resection.[351] Most are adenocarcinomas, with some squamous cell carcinomas.

There are three types: nodular, infiltrating, and papillary.[352] Most are annular infiltrating scirrhous carcinomas, which are slow-growing and usually extend along the length of the ducts, resulting in longer lesions.[353] In a few cases the tumor is papillary or polypoid.[353] The relatively inaccessible location of this carcinoma and frequent local invasion of the liver, portal vein, and hepatic artery make en bloc resection difficult.[352]

The sites of location of the tumor, in descending order of frequency, include the common bile duct (especially lower end); junction of the cystic duct, hepatic duct, and common bile duct; hepatic ducts; cystic duct; and duodenal portion of the common bile duct.[20] Cholangiocarcinoma is present in the liver in 13 percent of patients, in the common hepatic duct and bifurcation in 37 percent, in the junction of the cystic duct and common bile duct in 15 percent, in the cystic duct in 6 percent, and in the common bile duct in 33 percent.[353] These lesions are

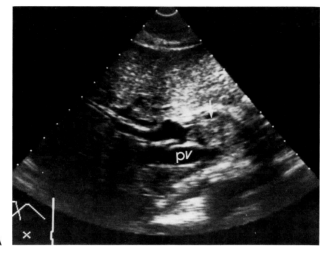

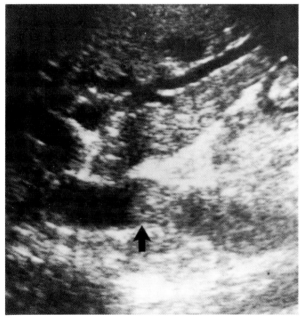

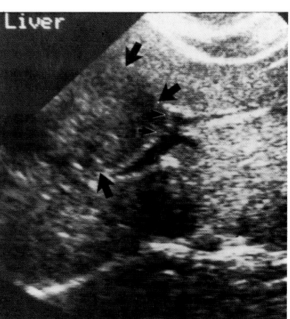

Fig. 6-115. Hilar cholangiocarcinoma. Case 1. **(A)** Polypoid hilar cholangiocarcinoma. Sonogram showing a polypoid mass (arrow) at the bifurcation area of biliary tree, anterior to the portal vein *(pv)*. The right intrahepatic bile ducts are dilated. Case 2. **(B)** Polypoid cholangiocarcinoma involving the common bile duct. Sonogram showing a polypoid mass (arrow) in the proximal common bile duct with meniscus. The distal tumor extent could not be determined sonographically. Case 3. **(C)** Bulky exophytic cholangiocarcinoma. Sonogram showing inhomogeneous, hypoechoic mass (large arrows) in the same region (as shown on CT scan). The normal left periportal fat plane is obliterated distally (small arrows), an indication of involvement. This was also considered sonographically unresectable because of similar portal venous involvement on right. (Fig. A from Choi et al,[358] with permission; Figs. B & C from Nesbit et al,[351] with permission.)

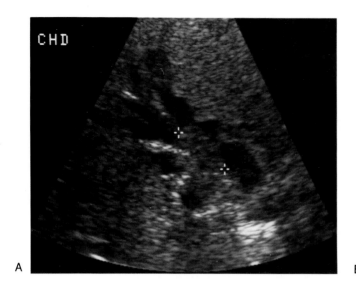
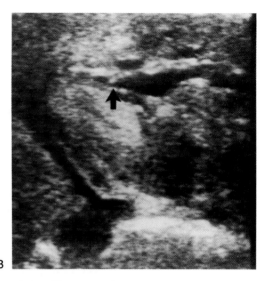

Fig. 6-116. Cholangiocarcinoma. Case 1. **(A)** Long-axis view of the dilated proximal common bile duct (23 mm). A solid mass (calipers) is seen within the duct. Case 2. **(B)** Infiltrating cholangiocarcinoma involving the left hepatic duct. Sonogram showing intrahepatic biliary ductal dilatation of only the left hepatic lobe with focal tapering (arrow); however, no definite mass was identified. This appearance suggests cholangiocarcinoma, and this mass was correctly identified as being localized to the left hepatic duct and therefore resectable. (Fig. B from Nesbit et al,[351] with permission.)

insidious in their development, with most presenting with right upper quadrant pain of acute onset, biliary colic, jaundice, weight loss, and nonspecific digestive disturbances.

Choledochal cysts have been described as being associated with biliary cancers.[354] Most of these cancers are adenocarcinomas. The frequency of these biliary malignant changes increases with age and is reported to be 23 to 39 percent.[354]

High-resolution real-time ultrasound can evaluate the extrahepatic biliary system in multiple planes, so if abrupt termination of the duct is seen on long-axis views, cancer should be considered.[355] The ultrasound features of cholangiocarcinoma may include (1) marked biliary obstruction in the presence of a normal pancreas, (2) focal biliary tract stricture or abrupt termination, (3) delineation of a mass involving the bile duct, (4) irregularly defined coarse acoustic shadowing arising from the obstructive mass, (5) contained intraluminal soft tissue echoes, and (6) echogenic bands across the lumen[352-357] (Figs. 6-115 to 6-117 and see Figs. 6-118 and 6-119). In most cases, a mass itself will not be identified.[356,357] When dilated ducts and a main pancreatic duct are demonstrated, a primary bile duct carcinoma should be suspected in the presence of a normal pancreatic head, although a small pancreatic or ampullary carcinoma cannot be excluded.[352,357] An intraductal neoplasm should be suggested if an intraluminal focus of low-level

echoes within the biliary tree, without a shadow is found.[357]

Three radiographic types of cholangiocarcinoma have been described, including infiltrating stenotic (69 percent), bulky exophytic (19 percent), and polypoid intraluminal (12 percent).[351] In the demonstration of masses in the extrahepatic bile ducts distal to the bifurcation,

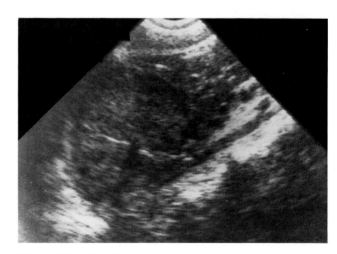

Fig. 6-117. Intrahepatic cholangiocarcinoma. Sonogram showing the hyperechoic appearance of intrahepatic cholangiocarcinoma in a 27-year-old woman with a large echogenic mass in the right lobe of liver (sagittal view). (From Ros et al,[359] with permission.)

ultrasound is superior to CT, depicting 50 percent in comparison with 28 percent by CT.[351] In detecting unresectability, the sensitivities of CT, ultrasound, and cholangiography are 44, 19 and 43 percent, respectively, with specificities of 78, 100, and 100 percent, respectively.[351]

Hilar. The patterns of hilar cholangiocarcinoma are classified as infiltrating (78 percent), exophytic (14 percent), and polypoid (8 percent)[358] (Figs. 6-115 and 6-116). The infiltrating pattern involves the bile duct wall and occludes the lumen, and is characteristically manifested as a focal biliary stricture, often without a mass[358] (Fig. 6-116B). With the exophytic type, there is more extensive spread into the surrounding hepatic parenchyma[358] (Fig. 6-115C). Although the polypoid pattern is rare, both ultrasound and CT depict polypoid intraluminal masses[358] (Fig. 6-115). Infiltrating and exophytic tumors were difficult to depict with ultrasound, whereas polypoid tumors were well identified.[358] In this series, CT was more accurate in the identification of tumor per se and in the evaluation of metastases. However, ultrasound should be the screening procedure in the evaluation of hilar cholangiocarcinoma because it is nonionizing, generally less expensive, and often more readily available.[358]

Intrahepatic. Intrahepatic cholangiocarcinoma arises from the peripheral intrahepatic bile ducts, appearing as a purely intrahepatic mass that requires differentiation from other, more common intrahepatic masses in adults such as metastatic lesions and hepatocellular carcinoma.[359] The appearance of this lesion is that of a predominantly homogeneous intrahepatic mass, frequently with satellite nodules.[359] On ultrasound, the most common appearance is that of a homogeneously hyperechoic mass, either single or multiple[359] (Fig. 6-117).

A discrepancy in the appearance of the intrahepatic bile ducts between CT and ultrasound imaging should be regarded with suspicion in the appropriate clinical setting.[360] With ultrasound the bile ducts are seen directly, so the possibility of a false-positive diagnosis by an infiltrating neoplasm along their course does not exist.[360] This may lead to a discrepancy between the two imaging modalities when neoplasm is seen to infiltrate up into the biliary ductal system.[360] When CT suggests intrahepatic biliary duct dilatation or when the appearance of the dilated ducts on CT is considerably more advanced than on the ultrasound study, the diagnosis of spread of the neoplasm through the biliary system should be suggested.[360]

Klatskin Tumor. Klatskin is the name given to the bile duct carcinoma or cholangiocarcinoma arising at the confluence of the right and left hepatic ducts is called Klatskin tumor.[361] It has the worst prognosis. There is an increased frequency in chronic ulcerative colitis, cystic diseases of the liver and biliary tree (such as Caroli's disease), and in patients infested with *Clonorchis sinensis*.[361]

The ultrasound features include (1) dilatation of the intrahepatic ducts but not the extrahepatic ducts; (2) nonunion of the right and left hepatic ducts; and (3)

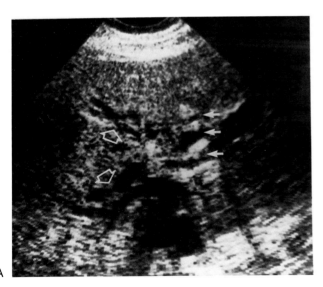
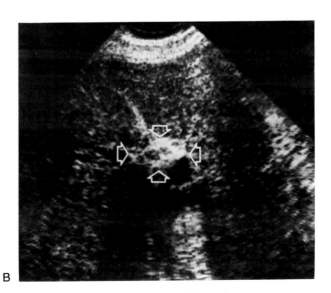

A   B

Fig. 6-118. Klatskin tumor. **(A)** Transverse scan of the liver demonstrating nonunion of the dilated right (open arrows) and left (solid arrows) hepatic ducts at the hilum. **(B)** Transverse scan at a slightly lower level, showing several small, solid masses in the region of the bifurcation (arrows). (From Meyer and Weinstein,[352] with permission.)

small, solid masses in the hepatic hilum[352] (Figs. 6-118 and 6-119). All patients in one series demonstrated dilated intrahepatic bile ducts with a normal-sized extrahepatic biliary tree.[361] Other abnormal findings included an apparent intraductal mass at the confluence of the right and left intrahepatic ducts, enlarged portal lymph nodes, and hepatic metastases.[361] In the face of intrahepatic duct dilatation without extrahepatic duct dilatation, a primary tumor should be suspected. The location of the tumor allows significant obstruction to occur before the primary tumor attains considerable size.[352]

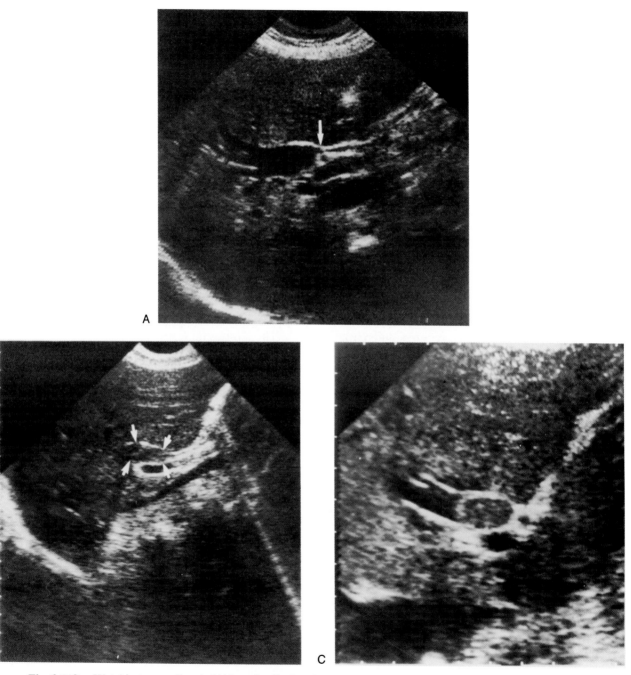

Fig. 6-119. Klatskin tumor. Case 1. **(A)** Longitudinal oblique scan through the porta hepatis showing dilatation of intrahepatic bile ducts abruptly tapering (arrow) at the porta hepatis to a normal-sized common hepatic duct. No mass was present. Case 2. **(B)** Longitudinal oblique sonogram through the porta hepatis demonstrating a mass (arrows) in the common hepatic duct. **(C)** Magnified view of the intraductal mass. (From Machan et al,[361] with permission.)

Differential Diagnosis. Bile duct narrowing in the portal region can have other etiologies, including sclerosing or suppurative cholangitis, benign strictures (idiopathic, postinflammatory, or postoperative), benign bile duct tumors, metastatic lesions, and proximal spread of carcinomas of the biliary tract arising more distally that may be mistaken for Klatskin tumors unless their full extent is appreciated.[361] It may not be possible to distinguish tumor from lymphadenopathy as a source of obstruction. Tumors of the gastrointestinal tract, breast, pancreas, and gallbladder show a propensity for spread to the porta hepatis. The possibility of Klatskin tumor should be raised when dilated intrahepatic ducts are visualized with a normal extrahepatic biliary tree.[361] Evidence suggestive of cancer can be demonstrated in at least 50 percent of patients by high-resolution real-time ultrasound.[361] Nonunion of the right and left intrahepatic ducts is identified in 90 percent by ultrasound and 94 percent by CT.[358] In 40 percent the tumor was detected by CT, whereas only in 21 percent was it detected by ultrasound.[358]

Accuracy. The accuracy of ultrasound detection depends on the location of the tumor. It is more accurate

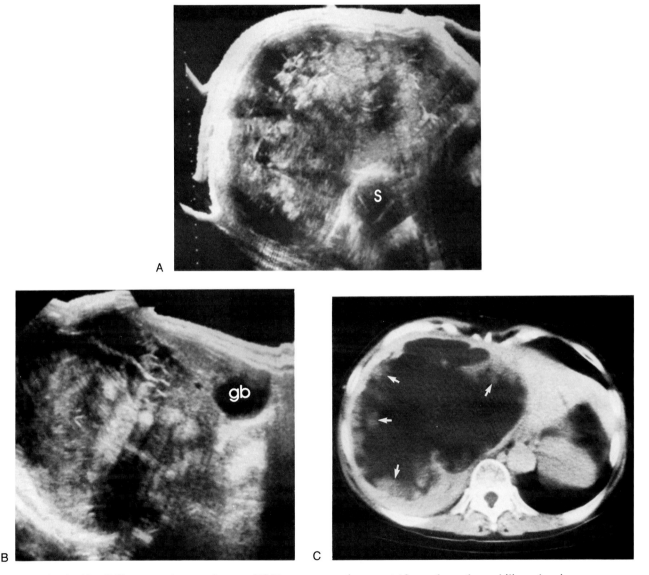

Fig. 6-120. Biliary cystadenocarcinoma. **(A)** Transverse static scan at 10 cm above the umbilicus showing an inhomogeneous pattern throughout the liver. There are echodense and anechoic areas. (*S*, spine.) **(B)** Longitudinal static scan at 1 cm to the right midline showing mixed echopattern. (*gb*, gallbladder.) **(C)** Enhanced CT scan showing a large low-density mass that contains multiple septations. There are small soft tissue density masses (arrows) within the mass.

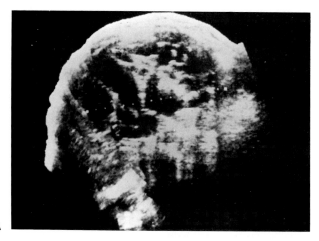
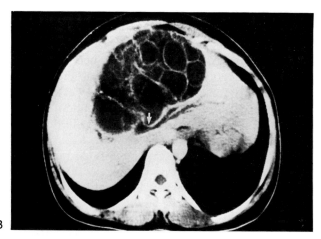

A   B

Fig. 6-121. Biliary cystadenoma. **(A)** Transverse sonogram of the upper abdomen showing a multiloculated mass in the liver. Internal septa show nodular thickening and papillary excrescences. **(B)** Contrast-enhanced CT scan showing prolapse of the cystic mass (arrow) into the dilated left intrahepatic bile duct. Contrast enhancement is seen along the wall and internal septa, which show papillary excrescences and nodular thickening. (From Choi et al,[365] with permission.)

for lesions involving the bifurcation and common hepatic duct than those involving the common bile duct.[353] Cholangiography is superior to ultrasound in determining the length of the involved segment, but ultrasound is superior in detecting hepatic invasion and lymphadenopathy.[353] At times, it is difficult to distinguish cholangiocarcinoma from hepatocellular carcinoma or hepatic metastases.[353]

Endoscopic Ultrasound. Endoscopic ultrasound may be performed to evaluate patients with proximal bile duct carcinoma.[362] This technique is accurate in assessing the depth of tumor infiltration, with an overall accuracy of 83.5 percent.[362] Other investigators have used endoscopic ultrasound to evaluate the extent of carcinoma of the papilla of Vater.[363] This technique is accurate in diagnosing carcinoma infiltration into the duodenal

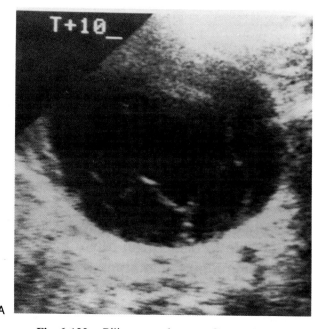
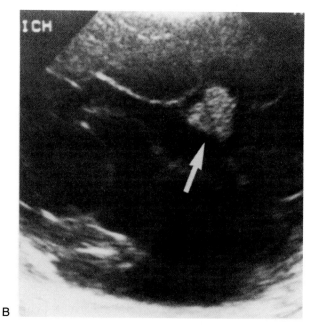

A   B

Fig. 6-122. Biliary cystadenoma. Case 1. **(A)** Sonogram showing a septated liver cyst. Case 2. **(B)** Sonogram showing an echogenic nodule (arrow) within a septated multilocular cyst. This was the only discrete nodule or mass seen in the eight benign cystadenomas in this series. (From Korobkin et al,[369] with permission.)

proper muscle layer (100 percent) and into the pancreas (75 percent).[363] Additionally, it can be helpful in diagnosing lymph node metastasis (accuracy, 92.9 percent) but is not as accurate in defining nonmetastatic lymph nodes (accuracy, 18.8 percent).[361] The overall accuracy in assessing local infiltration was 89.3 percent when compared with postoperative histologic findings.[363]

Cystadenoma and Cystadenocarcinoma

Biliary cystadenoma and cystadenocarcinoma are rare hepatic neoplasms, constituting 4.6 percent of the total intrahepatic cysts of bile duct origin.[364] These tumors resemble mucinous cystic neoplasms of the pancreas and are thought to originate from very slow growing bile ducts.[365] The incidence is greater in females, with a peak in the fifth decade; 80 percent of affected individuals are older than 30 years.[364,366] The right lobe is more commonly involved, with a tumor size that ranges from 1.5 to 30 cm; most are greater than 10 cm in diameter.[364] They may present as a painful epigastric mass, occasionally with intermittent jaundice.[367] They grow slowly, but a rapid increase in size may result from fluid accumulation.[367]

Other names given to these neoplasms include "mucin-hypersecreting" intrahepatic biliary neoplasms or papillary cholangiocarcinoma.[368] These cystadenomas appear well encapsulated and are composed of numerous cystic spaces lined with cuboidal or columnar epithelium of biliary tract origin.[367] The cyst wall contains biliary-type epithelium with a capsule of connective tissue, with mural cysts and polypoid cystic spaces that may communicate with the ducts.[367] The cysts con-

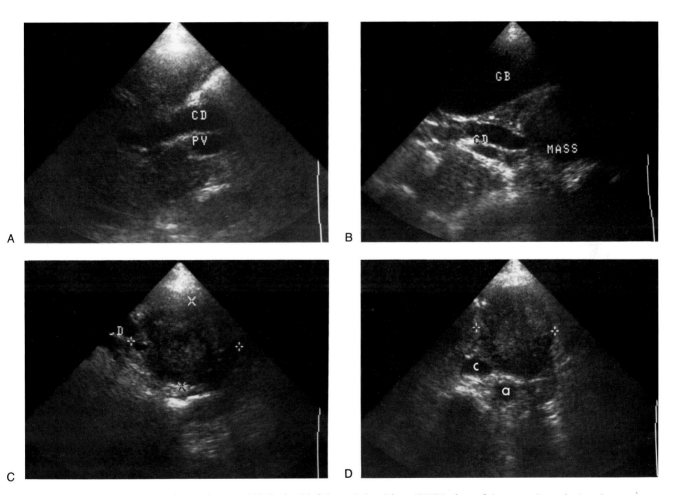

Fig. 6-123. Pancreatic carcinoma. **(A)** Sagittal left lateral decubitus (LLD) view of the porta hepatis showing that the proximal common bile duct *(CD)* is dilated. *(PV,* portal vein.) **(B)** Sagittal scan on the right showing the distended gallbladder *(GB)* along with the dilated duct *(CD)* and a mass *(MASS)* near the distal end of the duct. **(C)** Additional sagittal LLD view demonstrating the relationship of the mass (calipers) to the duct *(D).* **(D)** Transverse view showing the mass within the region of the uncinate process of the pancreas. *(a,* aorta; *c,* inferior vena cava.)

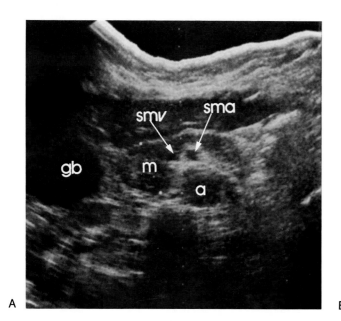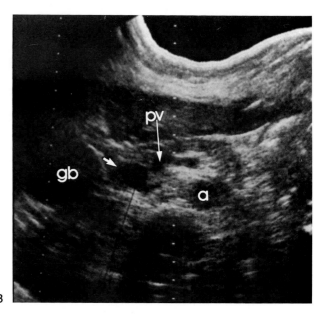

A   B

Fig. 6-124. Pancreatic carcinoma. **(A & B)** Transverse static scans with Fig. A 1 cm below Fig. B. The dilated common bile duct (arrow) is seen in Fig. B. The pancreatic head mass *(m)* is seen in Fig. A; (*a,* aorta; *sma,* superior mesenteric artery; *smv,* superior mesenteric vein; *pv,* main portal vein; *gb,* gallbladder.)

tain mucinous material, serous fluid, hemosiderin, cholesterol crystals, and necrotic or purulent material. Most biliary cystadenomas are multiloculated.[365]

Biliary cystadenomas and cystadenocarcinomas are characteristically cystic multiloculated intrahepatic masses with thick, highly echogenic internal septations and papillary projections[364-367] (Figs. 6-120 to 6-122). CT and ultrasound may demonstrate severe dilatation of the intrahepatic and/or extrahepatic bile ducts.[368] The findings indicating a mucin-hypersecreting intrahepatic biliary neoplasm include the presence of a liver tumor (mostly multilocular and cystic), marked biliary dilatation distal to the tumor, and filling defects in the dilated bile ducts.[368] On ultrasound, their appearance varies from unilocular cystic masses to multilocular cystic masses with multiple stellate tumors, although most tumors are single, multilocular, and cystic.[365] There may be ovoid, cystic masses with multiple septa and frequently papillary excrescences and/or fluid-fluid levels.[365] When there are mural or septal nodules, discrete soft tissue masses, and possibly thick and coarse calcifications, the likelihood of cystadenocarcinoma increases.[369] Calcifications have not been reported within these tumors.[365] These findings are similar to those in the pancreas and ovary. The differential diagnosis of such a lesion would include a complicated cyst, echinococcccal cyst, abscess, hematoma, and cystic metastases.[367] Aspiration may be performed in indeterminate cases, with mucinous bile-tinged or brownish cloudy fluid obtained. Resection of the lesion is usually curative, and since

cystadenocarcinomas are believed to arise from benign cystadenomas, complete surgical resection yields excellent results.[365]

Metastatic Disease

Pancreatic carcinoma is the most common cause of malignant obstruction of the biliary ductal system (Figs. 6-123 and 6-124). Less common causes are carcinoma of

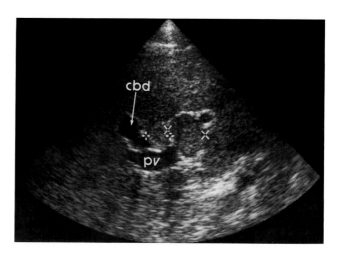

Fig. 6-125. Metastatic disease. Hepatoma. Transverse view of the porta hepatis showing multiple nodes (calipers) in this jaundiced patient. The proximal common bile duct *(cbd)* is dilated. (*pv,* portal vein.)

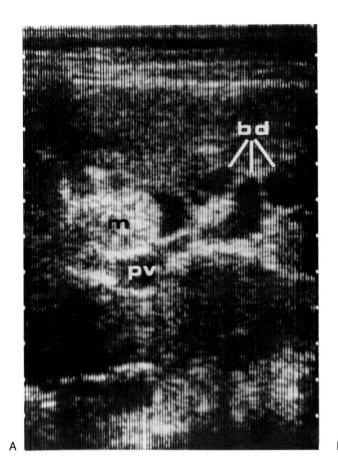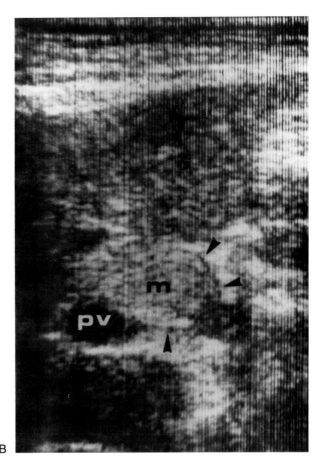

A

B

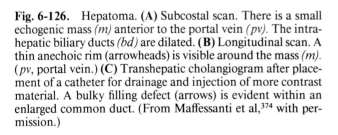

Fig. 6-126. Hepatoma. (A) Subcostal scan. There is a small echogenic mass *(m)* anterior to the portal vein *(pv)*. The intrahepatic biliary ducts *(bd)* are dilated. (B) Longitudinal scan. A thin anechoic rim (arrowheads) is visible around the mass *(m)*. *(pv*, portal vein.) (C) Transhepatic cholangiogram after placement of a catheter for drainage and injection of more contrast material. A bulky filling defect (arrows) is evident within an enlarged common duct. (From Maffessanti et al,[374] with permission.)

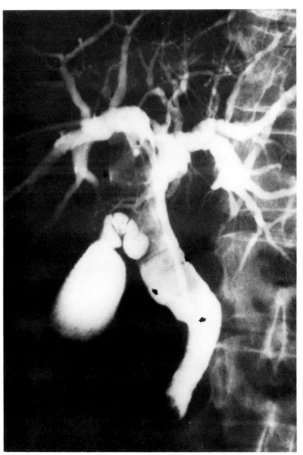

C

the ampulla of Vater, nodal masses due to either lymphoma (usually histiocytic) or other metastatic disease involving the liver hilum or peripancreatic lymph nodes, and primary biliary and gallbladder carcinoma[370] (Fig. 6-125). Lymphomatous involvement of the pancreas with extrahepatic bile duct obstruction is rare and represents an uncommon cause of obstructive jaundice.[371] Most patients develop jaundice as a result of nodes in the porta hepatis. With pancreatic involvement, the mass is a relatively hypoechoic lobulated area in the pancreatic

head.[371] Ultrasound of an intrinsic bile duct lesion can help in the differential diagnosis by demonstrating the presence or absence of shadowing.[372]

Hepatocellular carcinoma has also been shown to produce biliary obstruction. Hepatoma should be included in the differential diagnosis of filling defects in the proximal extrahepatic ducts.[373] The characteristic features include bulky obstructing intraluminal masses in the proximal extrahepatic ducts (Fig. 6-126). The location of the hepatoma is suggested to be intraductal rather

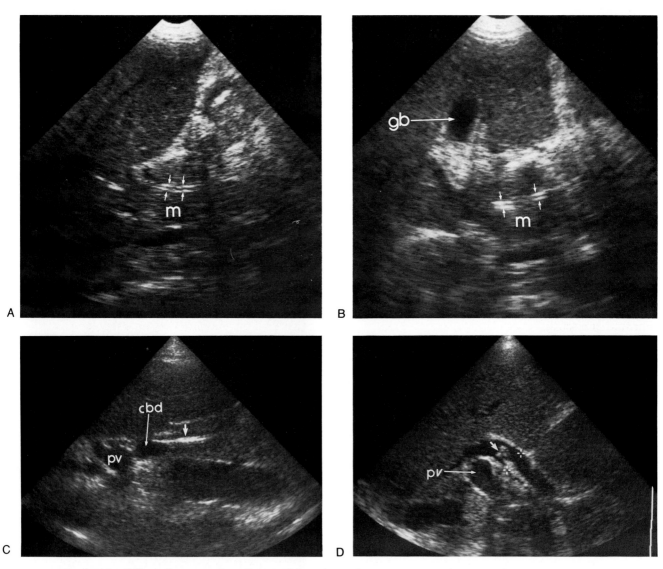

Fig. 6-127. Biliary decompression. Case 1. This patient with pancreatic carcinoma underwent percutaneous biliary decompression. The catheter (arrows) is seen within the common duct as two parallel echogenic lines on **(A)** longitudinal and **(B)** transverse scans. (*gb*, gallbladder; *m*, pancreatic head mass.) Case 2. Patient with obstruction secondary to metastatic prostatic carcinoma with an internal biliary stent. The ducts have not completely decompressed yet. **(C)** Sagittal view showing the stent (arrow) within the dilated (13-mm) proximal common bile duct *(cbd).* (*pv*, portal vein.) **(D)** Long-axis view showing the stent (arrow) and dilated proximal common bile (calipers). The distal common bile duct appears to be decompressed in Fig. C since no fluid is seen around the stent. (*pv*, portal vein.)

than extraductal because a thin anechoic rim representing the lumen nearly circumscribes the mass.[374] The distal common bile duct defects usually signify hematobilia and clots.

Postoperative/Interventional

Biliary Drainage Procedures

Percutaneous biliary drainage and transhepatic cholangiography may be performed with the guidance of real-time ultrasound. The merits of the procedure include the following: (1) it is a single-step procedure; (2) it uses no contrast material; (3) a left-sided approach is used, permitting longer intubation; and (4) there is no use of irradiation.[375] Ultrasound can detect catheters used for decompression of the biliary tree and is an appropriate method for determining the success of biliary decompression without instilling contrast material[376] (Fig. 6-127). (For further discussion, see Ch. 19.)

Ultrasound is indispensable as an aid in delineation of the left duct anatomy for directing needle puncture (Fig. 6-128). Accurate documentation and successful catheter drainage of the left duct obstruction are important contributions to total management of patients with high biliary obstruction.[377] A left hepatic duct approach is often selected because (1) it is the largest hepatic duct in most patients and is nearest to the body surface and (2) the entire biliary system can be opacified because contrast is heavier than bile and the left duct is located more anteriorly than the junction of the main hepatic duct.[378] (For further discussion, see Ch. 19.)

With ultrasound or CT, isolated intrahepatic ductal dilatation with or without calculi can be demonstrated.[379] Ultrasound can be used to direct the needle puncture for percutaneous transhepatic cholangiography and enable the differential diagnosis and appropriate therapy to be determined.[379]

Bilomas

Bilomas are localized collections of bile within the peritoneal cavity, which may occur after surgery or after blunt or penetrating trauma; they are readily detected by ultrasound or CT.[380-383] Spontaneous perforation of the common bile duct is a rare disorder in children, with the most common presenting complaints being jaundice and abdominal distention (due to ascites).[384] The symptoms occur as the biloma, formed by a bile leak, grows. As such, they are manifested at a variable delayed interval after the initial injury. Some patients are asymptomatic. Many bilomas present with unexpected clinical features such as pyogenic subhepatic abscess, localized biloma in the left upper quadrant despite surgery on the right side, and the presence of an active bile fistula.

The ultrasound features of bilomas include (1) a sharply defined echofree mass; (2) acoustic enhancement; (3) loculation; (4) location in the right, mid-upper, or left upper quadrant; and (5) contiguity with the liver or biliary structures[380-383,385] (Figs. 6-129 and 6-130). Ascites, loculated fluid collection around the gallbladder, or both may be found.[383] The loculation and size of the collection may be explained by the inflammatory reaction of the bile. Bile generates an intense inflammatory response that produces the sharply defined pseudocapsule.[382] The differential diagnosis should include hematoma and abscess, neither of which has pronounced acoustic enhancement.[385] With hepatobiliary scintigraphy it was demonstrated that the intraperitoneal fluid

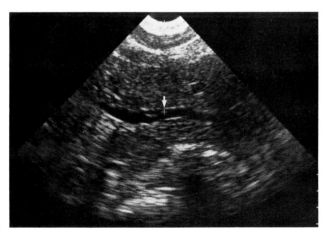
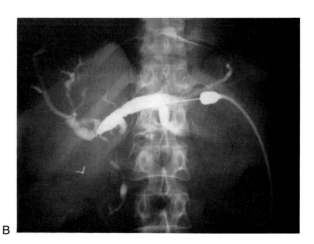

A   B

Fig. 6-128. Biliary decompression. Left duct approach. **(A)** Transverse scan localizing the depth (arrow) of a dilated left hepatic duct. **(B)** Transhepatic cholangiogram. There are dilated intrahepatic ducts with an area of stricture immediately distal to the right and left hepatic ducts. The common duct was normal in size.

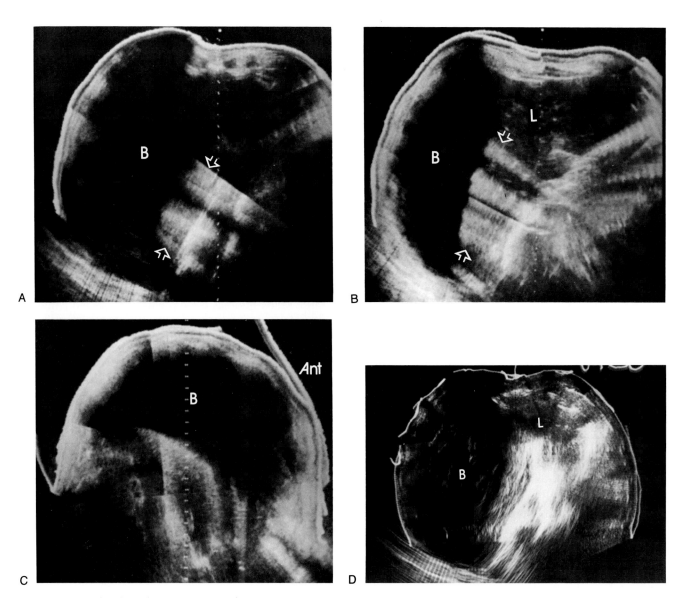

Fig. 6-129. Biloma. Postoperative cholecystectomy. Transverse scans at **(A)** 22 cm and **(B)** 16 cm above the umbilicus. A large fluid collection *(B)* is seen lateral to the liver *(L)*. It exhibits acoustic enhancement (open arrows). **(C)** Left lateral decubitus transverse scan at 15 cm above the iliac crest. The fluid *(B)* does not move. *(Ant,* anterior.) **(D)** Follow-up transverse scan at 20 cm above the umbilicus 1 month after Figs. A–C. The fluid collection *(B)* has developed internal septations. The fluid was aspirated and found to be bile. *(L,* liver.)

originated from the biliary tract.[384] It is important to recognize these findings to prevent delays in the diagnosis of a potentially fatal condition.[384]

A percutaneous aspiration may be guided by ultrasound to evaluate a gallbladder fossa fluid collection following biliary tract surgery.[386] Bile can be identified by visual inspection and an initial rapid dipstick (Multistix) technique, as well as by formal chemical analysis.[383] To confirm the diagnosis further and for drainage purposes, a catheter may be placed into the biloma. Percutaneous

radiologic catheter drainage provides adequate therapeutic drainage in most patients, except for those with a continuing active bile leak that eventually requires surgical correction.[383]

The diagnosis of biloma may be confirmed by a hepatobiliary nuclear medicine study.[385,387] Delayed views usually confirm the diagnosis.[385] Evidence for continued free bile leak includes a positive hepatobiliary nuclear medicine scan and copious amounts of bilious catheter drainage over a prolonged period.

Biliary Enteric Anastomoses

Cholecystocolic fistula may occur infrequently as a complication of long-standing cholelithiasis and cholecystitis in elderly patients. It is important to make the diagnosis because the patient is at increased risk for the development of cholangitis, gastrointestinal tract bleeding, malabsorption syndrome, and other medical problems, leading many physicians to advocate surgical intervention. Cholecystocolic fistulous tract formation constitutes 15 percent of the enterobiliary communications. It is second in frequency to the cholecystoduodenal fistula, which constitutes 70 percent of enterobiliary communications. The incidence in the general population of all enterobiliary fistula is 0.1 to 0.5 percent. Ninety percent occur in patients with cholelithiasis and chronic cholecystitis. Fibrous adhesions develop between the gallbladder and adjacent tissue, with necrosis of the gallbladder wall and perforation. The site of communication is usually the hepatic flexure or proximal transverse colon. In the absence of a stone, the fistula usually communicates with the common bile duct. Symptoms disappear after the gallbladder decompresses into the colon. The failure of ultrasound to demonstrate a previously revealed gallstone indicates passage. The fistula itself is usually obscured by biliary air[388] (similar to the case in Fig. 6-131).

For evaluation of the surgically established biliary-enteric anastomoses, hepatobiliary nuclear medicine is the preferred technique. Ultrasound is limited because of the gas within the anastomosis obscuring the bile ducts and the gas within the biliary tree producing confusing echoes that mimic intrahepatic biliary calculi. Ultrasound may be useful in measuring the bile duct caliber, but refluxed biliary air and persistent postoperative biliary dilatation are significant obstacles. Nuclear medicine is the best technique for this evaluation.[389]

Cholescintigraphy and percutaneous transhepatic cholangiography have been the favored procedures for determination of the patency of surgically created biliary-enteric anastomoses.[390] When evaluating 20 patients with patent anastomoses and no complication, ultrasound showed bile ducts ranging from 2 to 9 mm in diameter filled with bile, gas, or both.[390] With a normally functioning anastomosis, no patient was seen with evidence of a dilated bile-filled duct in the upright position.[390] With complete obstruction of the anastomosis in four patients, ultrasound showed dilated, bile-filled ducts ranging from 6 to 14 mm in diameter proximal to the anastomosis.[390] With partial obstruction, both gas and bile were seen in dilated bile ducts with superficial gas-filled ducts and dependent bile-filled ducts creating gas/fluid interfaces, which were persistent in the upright position.[390] This study suggested that ultrasound could be used accurately to assess surgically created biliary-enteric anastomoses for both anastomotic patency and other complications.[390]

When air is seen in the bile ducts, sonographic appearances range from small, bright, mobile, nondependent, echogenic densities to larger linear echogenicities producing either acoustic shadows or typical ring-down artifacts[390] (Fig. 6-131). When there is a large amount of air within the duct, assessment of the ductal diameter is difficult. Patients with complete obstruction usually do

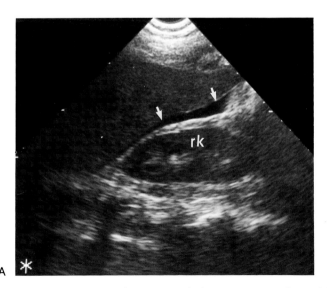
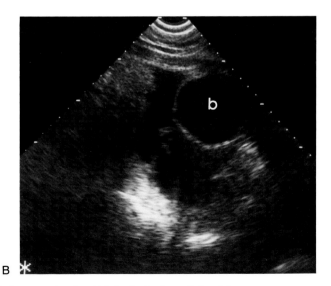

A   B

Fig. 6-130. Biloma. Postcholecystectomy patient with fever and pain. **(A)** Sagittal view of the right upper quadrant showing fluid (arrows) in a subhepatic location. (rk, right kidney.) **(B)** Sagittal view of the pelvis showing fluid. On a hepatobiliary nuclear medicine study, isotope was seen in the areas of the fluid demonstrated at ultrasound. This proved to be bile. (*b*, bladder.)

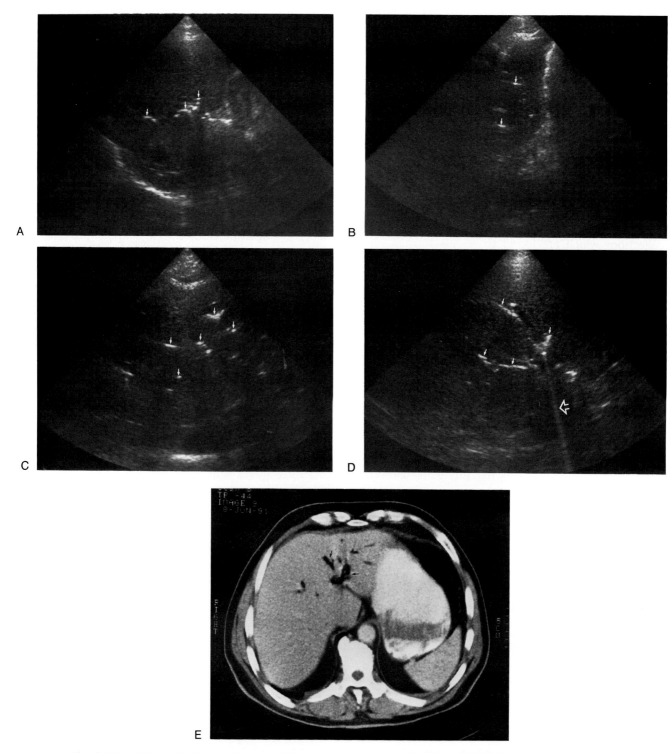

Fig. 6-131. Biliary air. Patient status post biliary-enteric anastomosis. Sagittal **(A)** right and **(B)** left scans and transverse **(C)** right and **(D)** left (left lateral decubitus) scans demonstrating multiple bright echogenic foci (arrows) in the region of the ducts. Note the associated ring-down artifact (open arrow) in Fig. D. **(E)** CT scan showing the biliary air (arrows).

not have large quantities of air.[390] Both gas and biliary calculi produce intraductal echogenicities with shadowing.[390] Experience with sonograms of upright patients suggests that ultrasound allows assessment of drainage of the bile ducts under gravity in postanastomotic patients; the surgically created anastomosis lacks a normal valvular mechanism.[390] As such, it is believed that ultrasound allows accurate assessment of patients with surgically created biliary-enteric anastomoses.[390]

Biliary Complications After Liver Transplantation

In 15 percent of cases in one series, there were biliary complications following liver transplants in pediatric patients.[391] Ultrasound is helpful in demonstrating bile duct dilatation that is often obscured with sludge or fluid collections which are found to be bile leakage when aspirated.[391]

In another series, biliary complications after liver transplantation were reviewed. The biliary abnormalities included bile duct stricture, occluded internal biliary obstruction, bile leak, choledocholithiasis, and an abscess in a cystic duct remnant.[392] In 86 percent of patients, bile duct dilatation was the positive ultrasound finding.[392] For the early detection of biliary abnormalities after liver transplantation, ultrasound is not a reliable test.[392]

REFERENCES

1. Foster SC, McLaughlin SM: Improvement in the ultrasonic evaluation of the gallbladder by using the left lateral decubitus position. J Clin Ultrasound 1977;5:253
2. Behan M, Kazam E: Sonography of the common bile duct: value of the right anterior oblique view. AJR 1978;130:701
3. Albarelli JN: Erect cholecystosonography. J Clin Ultrasound 1975;3:309
4. Parulekar SG: Evaluation of the prone view for cholecystosonography. J Ultrasound Med 1986;5:617
5. Parulekar SG: Sonography of the distal cystic duct. J Ultrasound Med 1989;8:367
6. Donald JJ, Fache JS, Buckley AR, Burhenne HJ: Gallbladder contractility: variation in normal subjects. AJR 1991;157:753
7. Dodds WJ, Groh WJ, Darweesh RMA et al: Sonographic measurement of gallbladder volume. AJR 1985;145:1009
8. Okulski TA, Eikman EA, Williams JW: Ultrasound measurement of contraction response of the gallbladder: comparison with the radionuclide test for cystic duct patency. Clin Nucl Med 1982;3:117
9. Davis GB, Berk RN, Scheible FW et al: Cholecystokinin cholecystography, sonography and scintigraphy:

10. Hopman WPM, Rosenbusch G, Jansen JBMJ et al: Gallbladder contraction: effects of fatty meals and cholecystokinin. Radiology 1985;157:37
11. Schlauch D, Gladisch R, Elfner R, Heene DL: A model for the comparison of pharmacologic agents influencing gallbladder contraction. J Ultrasound Med 1988;7:15
12. Parulekar SG: Ultrasound evaluation of common bile duct size. Radiology 1979;133:703
13. Laing FC, Jeffrey RB, Wing VW: Improved visualization of choledocholithiasis by sonography. AJR 1984;143:949
14. Dong B, Chen M: Improved sonographic visualization of choledocholithiasis. J Clin Ultrasound 1987;15:185
15. Simeone JF, Mueller PR, Ferrucci JT et al: Sonography of the bile ducts after a fatty meal: an aid in detection of obstruction. Radiology 1982;143:211
16. Darweesh RMA, Dodds WJ, Hogan WJ et al: Fatty-meal sonography for evaluating patients with suspected partial common duct obstruction. AJR 1988;151:63
17. Willson SA, Gosink BB, vanSonnenberg E: Unchanged size of a dilated common bile duct after a fatty meal: results and significance. Radiology 1986;160:29
18. Simeone JF, Butch RJ, Mueller PR et al: The bile ducts after a fatty meal: further sonographic observations. Radiology 1985;154:763
19. Maglinte DDT, Torres WE, Laufer I: Oral cholecystography in contemporary gallstone imaging: a review. Radiology 1991;178:49
20. O'Brien MJ, Gottlieb LS: The liver and biliary tract. p. 1071. In Robbins SL, Cotran RS (eds): Pathologic Basis of Disease. WB Saunders, Philadelphia, 1979
21. Kane RA: Ultrasonographic anatomy of the liver and biliary tree. Semin Ultrasound CT MR 1980;1:87
22. Cooperberg PL: Real-time ultrasonography of the gallbladder. p. 49. In Winsberg F, Cooperberg PL (eds): Clinics in Diagnostic Ultrasound: Real-Time Ultrasonography. Vol. 10. Churchill Livingstone, New York, 1982
23. Callen PW, Filly RA: Ultrasonographic localization of the gallbladder. Radiology 1979;133:687
24. Laing FC, Jeffrey RB: The pseudo-dilated common bile duct: ultrasonographic appearance created by the gallbladder neck. Radiology 1980;135:405
25. Birnholz JC: Population survey: ultrasonic cholecystography. Gastrointest Radiol 1982;7:165
26. Marchal G, deVoorde V, Dooren MV et al: Ultrasonic appearance of the filled and contracted normal gallbladder. J Clin Ultrasound 1980;8:439
27. McGahan JP, Phillips HE, Cox KL: Sonography of the normal pediatric gallbladder and biliary tree. Radiology 1982;144:873
28. Yeh H-C: Update on the gallbladder. p. 135. In Sanders RL (ed): Ultrasound Annual 1982. Raven Press, New York, 1982
29. Carroll BA, Oppenheimer DA, Muller HH: High-frequency real-time ultrasound of the neonatal biliary system. Radiology 1982;145:437
30. Sukov RJ, Sample WF, Sarti DA, Whitcomb MJ:

Cholecystosonography — the junctional fold. Radiology 1979;133:435

31. Bova JG: Gallstone simulated by gallbladder septation. AJR 1983;140:287

32. Sauerbrei E: Ultrasound of the common bile duct. p. 1. In Sanders RC, Hill MC (eds): Ultrasound Annual 1983. Raven Press, New York, 1983

33. Ralls PW, Quinn MF, Halls J: Biliary sonography: ventral bowing of the dilated common duct. AJR 1981;137:1127

34. Jacobson JB, Brodey PA: The transverse common duct. AJR 1981;136:91

35. Cooperberg P: High-resolution real-time ultrasound in the evaluation of the normal and obstructed biliary tract. Radiology 1978;129:477

36. Cooperberg PL, Li D, Wong P et al: Accuracy of common hepatic duct size in the evaluation of extrahepatic biliary obstruction. Radiology 1980;135:141

37. Sauerbrei EE, Cooperberg PL, Gordon P et al: The discrepancy between radiographic and sonographic bile-duct measurements. Radiology 1980;137:751

38. Mueller PR, Ferrucci JT, Simeone JF et al: Observations on the distensibility of the common bile duct. Radiology 1982;142:467

39. Glazer GM, Filly RA, Laing FC: Rapid change in the caliber of the nonobstructed common duct. Radiology 1981;140:161

40. Willi UV, Teele RL: Hepatic arteries and the parallel-channel sign. J Clin Ultrasound 1979;7:125

41. Berland LL, Lawson TL, Foley WD: Porta hepatis: sonographic discrimination of bile ducts from arteries with pulsed doppler with new anatomic criteria. AJR 1982;138:833

42. Bret PM, de Stempel JV, Atri M et al: Intrahepatic bile duct and portal vein anatomy revisited. Radiology 1988;169:405

43. Bressler EL, Rubin JM, McCracken S: Sonographic parallel channel sign: a reappraisal. Radiology 1987;164:343

44. Ralls RW, Mayekawa DS, Lee KP et al: The use of color Doppler sonography to distinguish dilated intrahepatic ducts from vascular structures. AJR 1989;152:291

45. Levy HM, Dobkin GR, Doubilet PM: The utility of image-directed Doppler ultrasound in the evaluation of the "parallel channel" sign. J Clin Ultrasound 1988;16:424

46. Bandai Y, Masatoshi M, Watanabe G et al: Sonographic differentiation between umbilical portion of the left portal vein and intrahepatic bile ducts. J Clin Ultrasound 1980;8:207

47. Durrell CA III, Vincent LM, Mittelstaedt CA: Gallbladder ultrasound in clinical context. Ultrasound CT MR 1984;5:315

48. Jackson RJ, McClelland D: Agenesis of the gallbladder: a cause of false-positive ultrasonography. Am Surg 1989;55:36

49. Taylor KJW, Rosenfield AT, DeGraaff CS: Anatomy and pathology of the biliary tree as demonstrated on ultrasound. p. 103. In Taylor KJW (ed): Clinics in Diagnostic Ultrasound: Diagnostic Ultrasound in Gastrointestinal Disease. Vol. 1. Churchill Livingstone, New York, 1979

50. McLoughlin MJ, Fanti JE, Kura ML: Ectopic gallbladder: sonographic and scintigraphic diagnosis. J Clin Ultrasound 1987;15:258

51. Murayama S, Mizushima A, Russell WJ, Higashi Y: Sonographic diagnosis of bicameral gallbladders: a report of three cases. J Ultrasound Med 1985;4:539

52. Garfield HD, Lyons EA, Levi CS: Sonographic findings in double gallbladder with cholelithiasis of both lobes. J Ultrasound Med 1988;7:589

53. Goiney RC, Schoenecker SA, Cyr DR et al: Sonography of gallbladder duplication and differential considerations. AJR 1985;145:241

54. Cunningham JJ: Empyema of a duplicated gallbladder: echographic findings. J Clin Ultrasound 1980;8:511

55. Lev-Toaff AS, Friedman AC, Rindsberg SN et al: Multiseptate gallbladder: incidental diagnosis on sonography. AJR 1987;148:1119

56. Pery M, Kaftori JK, Marvan H et al: Ultrasonographic appearance of multiseptate gallbladder: report of a case with coexisting choledochal cyst. J Clin Ultrasound 1985;13:570

57. Lawson TL: Gray scale cholecystosonography: diagnostic criteria and accuracy. Radiology 1977;122:247

58. Grossman M: Cholelithiasis and acoustic shadowing. J Clin Ultrasound 1978;6:182

59. Simeone JF, Ferrucci JT: New trends in gallbladder imaging. JAMA 1981;246:380

60. Crow HC, Bartrum RJ, Foote SR: Expanded criteria for the ultrasonic diagnosis of gallstones. J Clin Ultrasound 1976;4:289

61. Carroll BA: Gallstones: in vitro comparison of physical, radiographic and ultrasonic characteristics. AJR 1978;131:223

62. Good LI, Edell SL, Soloway RD et al: Ultrasonic properties of gallstones — effect of stone size and composition. Gastroenterology 1979;77:258

63. Simeone JF, Mueller PR, Ferrucci JT et al: Significance of nonshadowing focal opacities at cholecystosonography. Radiology 1980;137:181

64. Philbrick TH, Kaude JK, McInnis AN, Wright PG: Abdominal ultrasound in patients with acute right upper quadrant pain. Gastrointest Radiol 1981;6:251

65. Filly RA, Moss AA, Way LW: In vitro investigation of gallstone shadowing with ultrasound tomography. J Clin Ultrasound 1979;7:255

66. Gonzalez L, MacIntyre WJ: Acoustic shadow formation by gallstones. Radiology 1980;135:217

67. Taylor KJW, Jacobson P, Jaffee CC: Lack of an acoustic shadow on scans of gallstones: a possible artifact. Radiology 1979;131:463

68. Bartrum RJ Jr, Crow HC: Inflammation diseases of the biliary system. Semin Ultrasound CT MR 1980;1:102

69. Purdom RC, Thomas SR, Kereiakes JG et al: Ultrasonic properties of biliary calculi. Radiology 1980;136:729

70. Parulekar SG: Ultrasonic detection of calcification in gallstones: "the reverberation shadow." J Ultrasound Med 1984;3:123

71. Rubin JM, Adler RS, Bude RO et al: Clean and dirty shadowing at US: a reappraisal. Radiology 1991;181:231

72. Sommer FG, Taylor KJW: Differentiation of acoustic shadowing due to calculi and gas collections. Radiology 1980;135:399

73. Franquet T, Bescos JM, Barberena J, Montes M: Acoustic artifacts and reverberation shadows in gallbladder sonograms: their cause and clinical implications. Gastrointest Radiol 1990;15:223

74. Lafortune M, Gariepy G, Dumont A et al: The V-shaped artifact of the gallbladder wall. AJR 1986;147:505

75. Garel L, Lallemand D, Montagne JP et al: The changing aspects of cholelithiasis in children through a sonographic study. Pediatr Radiol 1981;11:75

76. Hessler PC, Hill DS, Detorie FM, Rocco AF: High accuracy sonographic recognition of gallstones. AJR 1981;136:517

77. Malet PF, Baker J, Kahn MJ, Soloway RD: Gallstone composition in relation to buoyancy at oral cholecystography. Radiology 1990;177:167

78. Scheske GA, Cooperberg PL, Cohen MM, Burhenne HJ: Floating gallstones: the role of contrast material. J Clin Ultrasound 1980;8:227

79. Lebensart PD, Bloom RA, Meretyk S et al: Oral cholecystosonography: a method of facilitating the diagnosis of cholesterol gallstones. Radiology 1984;153:255

80. Strijk SP, Boetes C, Rosenbusch G: Floating stones in nonopacified gallbladder: ultrasonographic sign of gas-containing gallstones. Gastrointest Radiol 1981;6:261

81. Mitchell DG, Needleman L, Frauenhoffer S et al: Gas-containing gallstones: the sonographic "double echo sign." J Ultrasound Med 1988;7:39

82. Gooding GAW: Food particles in the gallbladder mimic cholelithiasis in a patient with a cholecystojejunostomy. J Clin Ultrasound 1981;9:346

83. Klingensmith WC III, Eckhout GV: Cholelithiasis in the morbidly obese: diagnosis by US and oral cholecystography. Radiology 1986;160:27

84. Jequier S, Azouz EM: Calculus cholecystitis in an infant with aplastic anemia and graft-versus-host reaction. J Clin Ultrasound 1985;13:424

85. Buschi AJ, Brenbridge NAG: Sonographic diagnosis of cholelithiasis in childhood. Am J Dis Child 1980;134:575

86. Henschke CI, Teele RL: Cholelithiasis in children: recent observations. J Ultrasound Med 1983;2:481

87. Cunningham JJ: Sonographic diameter of the common hepatic duct in sickle cell anemia. AJR 1983;141:321

88. Sarnaik S, Slovis TL, Corbett DP et al: Incidence of cholelithiasis in sickle cell anemia using the ultrasonic gray-scale equipment. J Pediatr 1980;96:1005

89. Nzeh DA, Adedoyin MA: Sonographic pattern of gallbladder disease in children with sickle cell anaemia. Pediatr Radiol 1989;19:290

90. Borgna-Pignatti C, De Stefano P, Pajno D et al: Cholelithiasis in children with thalassemia major: an ultrasonographic study. J Pediatr 1981;99:243

91. Cunningham JJ, Houlihan SM, Altay C: Cholecystosonography in children with sickle cell disease: technical approach and clinical results. J Clin Ultrasound 1981;9:231

92. Callahan J, Haller JO, Cacciarelli AA et al: Cholelithiasis in infants: association with total parenteral nutrition and furosemide. Radiology 1982;143:437

93. Brill PW, Winchester P, Rosen MS: Neonatal cholelithiasis. Pediatr Radiol 1982;12:285

94. Keller MS, Markle BM, Jaffey PA et al: Spontaneous resolution of cholelithiasis in infants. Radiology 1985;157:345

95. Wagner LD, Weinberg B, Morrissey WJ et al: Cholelithiasis in a six-week-old asymptomatic neonate. J Clin Ultrasound 1989;17:692

96. Ramey SL, Williams JL: Nephrolithiasis and cholelithiasis in a premature infant. J Clin Ultrasound 1986;14:203

97. Matos C, Avni EF, Van Gansbeke D et al: Total parenteral nutrition (TPN) and gallbladder diseases in neonates: sonographic assessment. J Ultrasound Med 1987;6:243

98. Harbin WP, Ferrucci JT, Wittenberg J, Kirkpatrick RH: Nonvisualized gallbladder by cholecystosonography. AJR 1979;132:127

99. Raptopoulos V, D'Orsi C, Smith E et al: Dynamic cholecystosonography of the contracted gallbladder: the double-arc-shadow sign. AJR 1982;138:275

100. Laing FC, Gooding GAW, Herzog KA: Gallstones preventing ultrasonographic visualization of the gallbladder. Gastrointest Radiol 1977;1:301

101. MacDonald FR, Cooperberg PL, Cohen MM: The WES triad—a specific sonographic sign of gallstones in the contracted gallbladder. Gastrointest Radiol 1981;6:39

102. Conrad MR, Leonard J, Landay MJ: Left lateral decubitus sonography of gallstones in the contracted gallbladder. AJR 1980;134:141

103. Hammond DI: Unusual causes of sonographic nonvisualization or nonrecognition of the gallbladder: a review. J Clin Ultrasound 1988;16:77

104. Ferin P, Lerner RM: Contracted gallbladder: a finding in hepatic dysfunction. Radiology 1985;154:769

105. Kishk SMA, Darweesh RMA, Dodds WJ et al: Sonographic evaluation of resting gallbladder volume and postprandial emptying in patients with gallstones. AJR 1987;148:875

106. Giorgio A, Francica G, Amoroso P et al: Morphologic and motility changes of the gallbladder in response to acute liver injury: a prospective real-time sonographic study in 255 patients with acute viral hepatitis. J Ultrasound Med 1989;8:499

107. Kane RA, Jacobs R, Katz J, Costello P: Porcelain gallbladder: ultrasound and CT appearance. Radiology 1984;152:137

108. Shimizu M, Miura J, Tanaka et al: Porcelain gallbladder: relation between its type by ultrasound and incidence of cancer. J Clin Gastroenterol 1989;11:471

109. Laing FC, Jeffrey RB: Choledocholithiasis and cystic duct obstruction: difficult ultrasonographic diagnosis. Radiology 1983;146:475

110. Joseph S, Carvajal S, Odwin C: Sonographic diagnosis of Mirizzi's syndrome. J Clin Ultrasound 1985;13:199

111. Hilger DJ, VerSteeg KR, Beaty PJ: Mirizzi syndrome with common septum: ultrasound and computed tomography findings. J Ultrasound Med 1988;7:409

112. Jackson VP, Lappas JC: Sonography of the Mirizzi syndrome. J Ultrasound Med 1984;3:281

113. Becker CD, Hassler H, Terrier F: Preoperative diagnosis of the Mirizzi syndrome: limitations of sonography and computed tomography. AJR 1984;143:591

114. Koehler RE, Melson GL, Lee JKT, Long J: Common hepatic duct obstruction by cystic duct stone: Mirizzi syndrome. AJR 1979;132:1007

115. McIntosh DMF, Penney HF: Gray-scale ultrasonography as screening procedure in detection of gallbladder disease. Radiology 1980;136:725

116. Clair MR, Rosenberg ER, Ram PC, Bowie JD: Comparison of real-time and static-mode gray-scale ultrasonography in the diagnosis of cholelithiasis. J Ultrasound Med 1982;1:201

117. Raptopoulos V, Moss L, Reuter K, Kleinman P: Comparison of real-time and gray-scale static ultrasonic cholecystography. Radiology 1981;140:153

118. Crade M, Taylor KJW, Rosenfield AT et al: Surgical and pathologic correlation of cholecystosonography and cholecystography. AJR 1978;131:227

119. Bartrum RJ, Crow HC, Foote SR: Ultrasonic and radiographic cholecystography. N Engl J Med 1977;296:538

120. Arson S, Rosenquist CJ: Gray-scale cholecystosonography: an evaluation of accuracy. AJR 1976;127:817

121. Anderson JC, Harned RK: Gray-scale ultrasound of the gallbladder: an evaluation of accuracy and report of additional ultrasound signs. AJR 1977;129:975

122. Bartrum RJ, Crow HC, Foote SR: Ultrasound examination of the gallbladder—an alternate to "double-dose" oral cholecystography. JAMA 1979;236:1147

123. Leopold GR, Amberg J, Gosink BB, Mittelstaedt CA: Gray-scale ultrasonic cholecystography: a comparison with conventional radiographic techniques. Radiology 1976;121:445

124. Cooperberg PL, Burhenne HJ: Real-time ultrasonography: diagnostic technique of choice in calculous gallbladder disease. N Engl J Med 1980;302:1277

125. Crade M: Comparison of ultrasound and oral cholecystogram in the diagnosis of gallstones. p. 123. In Taylor KJW (ed): Clinics in Diagnostic Ultrasound: Diagnostic Ultrasound in Gastrointestinal Disease. Vol. 1. Churchill Livingstone, New York, 1979

126. McCluskey PL, Prinz RA, Guico R, Greenlee HB: Use of ultrasound to demonstrate gallstones in symptomatic patients with normal oral cholecystograms. Am J Surg 1979;138:655

127. Raskin MM: Hepatobiliary disease: a comparative evaluation by ultrasound and computed tomography. Gastrointest Radiol 1978;3:267

128. Brink JA, Simeone JF, Mueller PR: Routine sonographic techniques fail to quantify gallstone size and number: a retrospective study of 111 surgically proved cases. AJR 1989;153:503

129. Mathieson JR, So CB, Malone DE et al: Accuracy of sonography for determining the number and size of gallbladder stones before and after lithotripsy. AJR 1989;153:977

130. Filly RA, Allen B, Minton MJ et al: In vitro investigation of the origin of echoes within biliary sludge. J Clin Ultrasound 1980;8:193

131. Fakhry J: Sonography of tumefactive biliary sludge. AJR 1982;139:717

132. Ando H, Ito T: Ultrasonic characteristics of tumefactive biliary sludge: a thixotropic phenomenon. J Clin Ultrasound 1986;14:289

133. Conrad MR, Janes JO, Dietchy J: Significance of low level echoes within the gallbladder. AJR 1979;132:967

134. Fiske CE, Filly RA: Pseudo-sludge. A spurious ultrasound appearance within the gallbladder. Radiology 1982;144:631

135. Cover KL, Slasky BS, Skolnick ML: Sonography of cholesterol in the biliary system. J Ultrasound Med 1985;4:647

136. Grant EG, Smirniotopoulos JC: Intraluminal gallbladder hematoma: sonographic evidence of hemobilia. J Clin Ultrasound 1983;11:507

137. Sax SL, Athey PA, Lamki N, Cadavid GA: Sonographic findings in traumatic hemobilia: report of two cases and review of the literature. J Clin Ultrasound 1988;16:29

138. Kauzlaric D, Barmeir E: Sonography of intraluminal gallbladder hematoma. J Clin Ultrasound 1985;13:291

139. Buschi AJ, Brenbridge NAG, Cochrane JA, Teates CD: A further observation on gallbladder debris. J Clin Ultrasound 1979;7:152

140. Jeanty P, Ammann W, Cooperberg PL et al: Mobile intraluminal masses of the gallbladder. J Ultrasound Med 1983;2:65

141. Anastasi B, Sutherland GR: Biliary sludge—ultrasonic appearance simulating neoplasm. Br J Radiol 1981;54:679

142. Weeks LE, McCune BR, Martin JF, O'Brien TF: Unusual echographic appearance of a Courvoisier gallbladder. J Clin Ultrasound 1977;5:341

143. Britten JS, Golding RH, Cooperberg PL: Sludge balls to gallstones. J Ultrasound Med 1984;3:81

144. Love MB: Sonographic features of milk of calcium bile. J Ultrasound Med 1982;1:325

145. Chun GH, Deutsch AL, Scheible W: Sonographic findings in milk of calcium bile. Gastrointest Radiol 1982;7:371

146. Childress MH: Sonographic features of milk of calcium cholecystitis. J Clin Ultrasound 1986;14:312

147. Wales LR: Desquamated gallbladder mucosa: unusual sign of cholecystitis. AJR 1982;139:810

148. Elyaderani MK, Gabriele OF: Cholecystosonography in detection of acute cholecystitis: the halo sign—a significant sonographic finding. South Med J 1983;76:174

149. Worthen NJ, Uszler JM, Funamura JL: Cholecystitis: prospective evaluation of sonography and 99mTc-HIDA cholescintigraphy. AJR 1981;137:973

150. Raghavendka BN, Feiner HD, Subramanyam BR et al: Acute cholecystitis: sonographic-pathologic analysis. AJR 1981;137:327

151. Shuman WP, Mack LA, Rudd TG et al: Evaluation of acute right upper quadrant pain: sonography and ^{99m}Tc-PIPIDA cholescintigraphy. AJR 1982;139:61

152. Laing FC, Federle MP, Jeffrey RB, Brown TW: Ultrasonic evaluation of patients with acute right upper quadrant pain. Radiology 1981;140:449

153. Ralls PW, Halls J, Lapin SA et al: Prospective evaluation of the sonographic Murphy sign in suspected acute cholecystitis. J Clin Ultrasound 1982;10:113

154. Mindell HJ, Ring BA: Gallbladder wall thickening: ultrasonic finding. Radiology 1979;133:699

155. Marchal G, Crolla D, Baert AL et al: Gallbladder wall thickening: a new sign of gallbladder disease visualized by gray-scale cholecystosonography. J Clin Ultrasound 1978;6:177

156. Juttner H-U, Ralls PW, Quinn MF, Jenney JM: Thickening of the gallbladder wall in acute hepatitis: ultrasound demonstration. Radiology 1982;142:465

157. Fiske CE, Laing FC, Brown TW: Ultrasonographic evidence of gallbladder wall thickening in association with hypoalbuminemia. Radiology 1980;135:713

158. Handler SJ: Ultrasound of gallbladder wall thickening and its relation to cholecystitis. AJR 1979;132:581

159. Engel JM, Deitch EA, Sikkema W: Gallbladder wall thickness: sonographic accuracy and relation to disease. AJR 1980;134:907

160. Patriquin HB, DiPietro M, Barber FE, Teele RL: Sonography of thickened gallbladder wall: causes in children. AJR 1983;141:57

161. Finberg JH, Birnholtz JC: Ultrasound evaluation of the gallbladder wall. Radiology 1979;133:693

162. Cohan RH, Mahony BS, Bowie JD et al: Striated intramural gallbladder lucencies on US studies: predictors of acute cholecystitis. Radiology 1987;164:31

163. Lewandowski B, Winsberg F: Gallbladder wall thickness distortion by ascites. AJR 1981;137:519

164. Marchal GJF, Casaer M, Baert AL et al: Gallbladder wall sonolucency in acute cholecystitis. Radiology 1979;133:429

165. Teefey SA, Baron RL, Bigler SA: Sonography of the gallbladder: significance of striated (layered) thickening of the gallbladder wall. AJR 1991;156:945

166. Wegener M, Borsch G, Schneider J et al: Gallbladder wall thickening: a frequent finding in various nonbiliary disorders—a prospective ultrasonographic study. J Clin Ultrasound 1987;15:307

167. Shlaer WJ, Leopold GR, Scheible FW: Sonography of the thickened gallbladder wall: a nonspecific finding. AJR 1981;136:337

168. Sanders RC: The significance of sonographic gallbladder wall thickening. J Clin Ultrasound 1980;8:143

169. Ralls PW, Quinn MF, Juttner HU et al: Gallbladder wall thickening: patients without intrinsic gallbladder disease. AJR 1981;137:65

170. Kaftori JK, Pery M, Green J, Gaitini D: Thickness of the gallbladder wall in patients with hypoalbuminemia: a sonographic study of patients on peritoneal dialysis. AJR 1987;148:1117

171. Huang YS, Lee SD, Wu JC et al: Utility of sonographic gallbladder wall patterns in differentiating malignant from cirrhotic ascites. J Clin Ultrasound 1989;17:187

172. Saigh J, Williams S, Cawley K, Anderson JC: Varices: a cause of focal gallbladder wall thickening. J Ultrasound Med 1985;4:371

173. Ralls PW, Mayekawa DS, Lee KP et al: Gallbladder wall varices: diagnosis with color flow Doppler sonography. J Clin Ultrasound 1988;16:595

174. West MS, Garra BS, Horii SC et al: Gallbladder varices: imaging findings in patients with portal hypertension. Radiology 1991;179:179

175. Carroll BA: Gallbladder wall thickening secondary to focal lymphatic obstruction. J Ultrasound Med 1983;2:89

176. Brandt DJ, MacCarty RL, Charboneau JW et al: Gallbladder disease in patients with primary sclerosing cholangitis. AJR 1988;150:571

177. Becker CD, Burckhardt B, Terrier F: Ultrasound in postoperative acalculous cholecystitis. Gastrointest Radiol 1986;11:47

178. Deitch EA, Engel JM: Acute acalculous cholecystitis—ultrasonic diagnosis. Am J Surg 1981;142:290

179. Shuman WP, Rogers JV, Rudd TG et al: Low sensitivity of sonography and cholescintigraphy in acalculous cholecystitis. AJR 1984;124:541

180. Mirvis SE, Vainright JR, Nelson AW: The diagnosis of acute acalculous cholecystitis: a comparison of sonography, scintigraphy, and CT. AJR 1986;147:1171

181. Raduns K, McGahan JP, Beal S: Cholecystokinin sonography: lack of utility in diagnosis of acute acalculous cholecystitis. Radiology 1990;175:463

182. Raptopoulos V, Compton CC, Doherty P: Chronic acalculous gallbladder disease: multiimaging evaluation with clinical-pathologic correlation. AJR 1986;147:721

183. Jeffrey RB, Laing FC, Wong W, Callen PW: Gangrenous cholecystitis: diagnosis by ultrasound. Radiology 1983;148:219

184. Simeone JF, Brink JA, Mueller PR et al: The sonographic diagnosis of acute gangrenous cholecystitis: importance of the Murphy sign. AJR 1989;152:289

185. Kane RA: Ultrasonographic diagnosis of gangrenous cholecystitis and empyema of the gallbladder. Radiology 1980;134:191

186. Teefey SA, Baron RL, Radke HM, Bigler SA: Gangrenous cholecystitis: new observations on sonography. J Ultrasound Med 1991;10:603

187. Garcia OM, Kovac A, Plauche WE: Empyema of the gallbladder detected by gallium scan and abdominal ultrasonography. South Med J 1981;74:1020

188. Parulekar SG: Sonographic findings in acute emphysematous cholecystitis. Radiology 1982;145:117

189. Hunter ND, Macintosh PK: Acute emphysematous cholecystitis: an ultrasonic diagnosis. AJR 1980;134:592

190. Bloom RA, Libson E, Lebensart PD et al: The ultrasound spectrum of emphysematous cholecystitis. J Clin Ultrasound 1989;17:251

191. Nemcek AA Jr, Gore RM, Vogelzang RL, Grant M: The effervescent gallbladder: a sonographic sign of emphysematous cholecystitis. AJR 1988;150:575

192. Deitch EA, Engel JM: Ultrasonic detection of acute cholecystitis with pericholecystic abscesses. Am Surg 1981;47:211

193. Fleischer AC, Muhletaler CA, Jones TB: Sonographic detection of gallbladder perforation. South Med J 1982;75:606

194. Chau WK, Na AT, Feng TT, Li YB: Ultrasound diagnosis of perforation of the gallbladder: real-time application and the demonstration of a new sonographic sign. J Clin Ultrasound 1988;16:353

195. Takada T, Yasuda H, Uchiyama K et al: Pericholecystic abscess: classification of US findings to determine the proper therapy. Radiology 1989;172:693

196. Madrazo BL, Francis I, Hricak H et al: Sonographic findings in perforation of the gallbladder. AJR 1982;139:491

197. Bergman AB, Neiman HL, Kraut B: Ultrasonographic evaluation of pericholecystic abscesses. AJR 1979;132:201

198. Teefey SA, Wechter DG: Sonographic evaluation of pericholecystic abscess with intrahepatic extension. J Ultrasound Med 1987;6:659

199. Nyberg DA, Laing FC: Ultrasonographic findings in peptic ulcer disease and pancreatitis that simulate primary gallbladder disease. J Ultrasound Med 1983;2:303

200. Crade M, Taylor KJW, Rosenfield AT, Walsh JW: Ultrasonic imaging of pericholecystic inflammation. JAMA 1980;244:708

201. Hanada K, Nakata H, Nakayama T et al: Radiologic findings in xanthogranulomatous cholecystitis. AJR 1987;148:727

202. Bluth EI, Katz MM, Merritt CRB et al: Echographic findings in xanthogranulomatous cholecystitis. J Clin Ultrasound 1979;7:213

203. Chinn DH, Miller EI, Piper N: Hemorrhagic cholecystitis: sonographic appearance and clinical presentation. J Ultrasound Med 1987;6:313

204. Jenkins M, Golding RH, Cooperberg PL: Sonography and computed tomography of hemorrhagic cholecystitis. AJR 1983;140:1197

205. Greenberg M, Kangarloo H, Cochran ST, Sample WF: The ultrasonographic diagnosis of cholecystitis and cholelithiasis in children. Radiology 1980;137:745

206. Kumari S, Lee WJ, Baron MG: Hydrops of the gallbladder in a child: diagnosis by ultrasonography. Pediatrics 1979;63:295

207. Zeman RK, Burrell MI, Cahow CE, Caride V: Diagnostic utility of cholescintigraphy and ultrasonography in acute cholecystitis. Am J Surg 1981;141:446

208. Weissman HS, Frank M, Rosenblatt R et al: Cholescintigraphy, ultrasonography and computerized tomography in the evaluation of biliary tract disorders. Semin Nucl Med 1979;9:22

209. Sherman M, Ralls PW, Quinn M et al: Intravenous cholangiography and sonography in acute cholecystitis: prospective evaluation. AJR 1980;135:311

210. Weissman HS, Badin J, Sugarman LA et al: Spectrum of 99m-Tc-IDA cholescintigraphic patterns in acute cholecystitis. Radiology 1981;138:167

211. Massie JD, Moinuddin M, Phillips JC: Acute calculous cholecystitis in patient with patent cystic duct. AJR 1983;141:39

212. Reimer DE, Donald JW: Technetium-99-m-HIDA visualization of an obstructed gallbladder via an accessory hepatic duct. AJR 1981;137:610

213. Echevarria RA, Gleason JL: False-negative gallbladder scintigram in acute cholecystitis. J Nucl Med 1980;21:841

214. Ralls PW, Colletti PM, Halls JM, Siemsen JK: Prospective evaluation of ^{99m}Tc-IDA cholescintigraphy and gray-scale ultrasound in the diagnosis of acute cholecystitis. Radiology 1982;144:369

215. Freitas JE, Mirkes SH, Fink-Bennett DM, Bree RL: Suspected acute cholecystitis: comparison of hepatobiliary scintigraph versus ultrasonography. Clin Nucl Med 1982;7:364

216. Weissman HS, Frank MS, Bernstein LH, Freeman LM: Rapid and accurate diagnosis of acute cholecystitis with ^{99m}Tc-HIDA cholescintigraphy. AJR 1979;132:523

217. Samuels BI, Freitas JE, Bree RL et al: A comparison of radionuclide hepatobiliary imaging and real-time ultrasound for the detection of acute cholecystitis. Radiology 1983;147:207

218. Ralls PW, Colletti PM, Lapin SA: Real-time sonography in suspected acute cholecystitis: prospective evaluation of primary and secondary signs. Radiology 1985;155:767

219. Dillon E, Parkin GJS: The role of upper abdominal ultrasonography in suspected acute cholecystitis. Clin Radiol 1980;31:175

220. Gelfand DW, Wolfman NT, Ott DJ: Oral cholecystography vs gallbladder sonography: a prospective, blinded reappraisal. AJR 1988;151:69

221. McGahan JP, Lindfors KK: Acute cholecystitis: diagnostic accuracy of percutaneous aspiration of the gallbladder. Radiology 1988;167:669

222. Burth RA, Brasch RC, Filly RA: Abdominal pseudotumor in childhood: distended gallbladder with parenteral hyperalimentation. AJR 1981;136:341

223. Oppenheimer DA, Carroll BA: Spontaneous resolution of hyperalimentation-induced biliary dilatation: ultrasonic description. J Ultrasound Med 1982;1:213

224. Liechty EA, Cohen MD, Lemons JA et al: Normal gallbladder appearing as abdominal mass in neonates. Am J Dis Child 1982;136:468

225. Bradford BF, Reid BS, Weinstein BJ et al: Ultrasonographic evaluation of the gallbladder in mucocutaneous lymph node syndrome. Radiology 1982;142:381

226. Koss JC, Coleman BG, Mulhern CB et al: Mucocutaneous lymph node syndrome with hydrops of the gallbladder diagnosed by ultrasound. J Clin Ultrasound 1981;9:477

227. Sty JR, Starshak RJ, Gorenstein L: Gallbladder perforation in a case of Kawasaki disease: image correlation. J Clin Ultrasound 1983;11:381

228. Carter SJ, Rutledge J, Hirsch JH et al: Papillary adenoma of the gallbladder: ultrasonic demonstration. J Clin Ultrasound 1978;6:433

229. Hallgrimsson P, Skaane P: Hypoechoic solitary inflam-

matory polyp of the gallbladder. J Clin Ultrasound 1988;16:603

230. Price RJ, Stewart ET, Foley WD, Dodds WJ: Sonography of polypoid cholesterolosis. AJR 1982;139:1197

231. Berk RN, van der Vegt JH, Lichtenstein JE: The hyperplastic cholecysterolosis: cholesterolosis and adenomyomatosis. Radiology 1983;146:593

232. Ruhe AH, Zachman JP, Mulder BD, Rime AE: Cholesterol polyps of the gallbladder: ultrasound demonstration. J Clin Ultrasound 1979;7:386

233. Detweiler DG, Biddinger P, Staab EV et al: The appearance of adenomyomatosis with the newer imaging modalities: a case with pathologic correlation. J Ultrasound Med 1982;1:295

234. Costa-Greco MA: Adenomyomatosis of the gallbladder. J Clin Ultrasound 1987;15:198

235. Raghavendra BN, Subramanyam BR, Balthazar EJ et al: Sonography of adenomyomatosis of the gallbladder: radiologic-pathologic correlation. Radiology 1983; 146:747

236. Rice J, Sauerbrei EE, Semogas P et al: Sonographic appearance of adenomyomatosis of gallbladder. J Clin Ultrasound 1981;9:336

237. Schulman A, Loxton AJ, Heydenrych JJ, Abdurahman KE: Sonographic diagnosis of biliary ascariasis. AJR 1982;139:485

238. Cerri GG, Leite GJ, Simoes JB et al: Ultrasonographic evaluation of ascaris in the biliary tract. Radiology 1983;146:753

239. Schulman A, Roman T, Dalrymple R et al: Sonography of biliary worms (ascariasis). J Clin Ultrasound 1982;10:77

240. Allibone GW, Fagan CJ, Porter SC: Sonographic features of carcinoma of the gallbladder. Gastrointest Radiol 1981;6:169

241. Yeh H-C: Ultrasonography and computed tomography of carcinoma of gallbladder. Radiology 1979;133:167

242. Oken SM, Bledsoe R, Newmark H: The ultrasonic diagnosis of primary carcinoma of the gallbladder. Radiology 1978;129:481

243. Raghavendra BN: Ultrasonographic features of primary carcinoma of the gallbladder: report of five cases. Gastrointest Radiol 1980;5:239

244. Weiner SN, Koenigsberg M, Morehouse H, Hoffman J: Sonography and computed tomography in the diagnosis of carcinoma of the gallbladder. AJR 1984;142:735

245. Ruiz R, Teyssou H, Fernandez N et al: Ultrasonic diagnosis of primary carcinoma of the gallbladder: a review of 16 cases. J Clin Ultrasound 1980;8:489

246. Bondestam S: Sonographic diagnosis of primary carcinoma of the gallbladder. Diagn Imaging 1981;509:197

247. Tsuchiya Y: Early carcinoma of the gallbladder: macroscopic features and US findings. Radiology 1991; 179:171

248. Yum HY, Fink AH: Sonographic findings in primary carcinoma of the gallbladder. Radiology 1980;134:693

249. Harolds JA, Dennehy DC: Preoperative diagnosis of gallbladder carcinoma by ultrasonography. South Med J 1981;74;1024

250. Kumar A, Aggarwal S, Berry M et al: Ultrasonography of carcinoma of the gallbladder: an analysis of 80 cases. J Clin Ultrasound 1990;18:715

251. Franquet T, Montes M, Ruiz de Azua Y et al: Primary gallbladder carcinoma: imaging findings in 50 patients with pathologic correlation. Gastrointest Radiol 1991;16:143

252. Soiva M, Aro K, Pamilo M et al: Ultrasonography in carcinoma of the gallbladder. Acta Radiol 1987;28:711

253. Crade M, Taylor KJW, Rosenfield AT et al: The varied ultrasonic character of gallbladder tumor. JAMA 1979;241:2195

254. Suminski N, Johnson MB, Ralls PW: Color Doppler sonography in gallbladder carcinoma. J Clin Ultrasound 1991;19:183

255. Lane J, Buck JL, Zeman RK: Primary carcinoma of the gallbladder: a pictorial essay. RadioGraphics 1989;9:209

256. So CB, Gibney RG, Scudamore CH: Carcinoma of the gallbladder: a risk associated with gallbladder-preserving treatments for cholelithiasis. Radiology 1990;174:127

257. Kuo YC, Liu JY, Sheen IS et al: Ultrasonographic difficulties and pitfalls in diagnosing primary carcinoma of the gallbladder. J Clin Ultrasound 1990;18:639

258. Zargar SA, Khuroo MS, Mahajan R et al: US-guided fine-needle aspiration biopsy of gallbladder masses. Radiology 1991;179:275

259. Phillips G, Pochaczevsky R, Goodman J, Kumari S: Ultrasound patterns of metastatic tumors in the gallbladder. J Clin Ultrasound 1982;10:379

260. Bundy AL, Ritchie WGM: Ultrasonic diagnosis of metastatic melanoma of the gallbladder presenting as acute cholecystitis. J Clin Ultrasound 1982;10:285

261. Teixidor HS, Godwin TA, Ramirez EA: Cryptosporidiosis of the biliary tract in AIDS. Radiology 1991;180:51

262. Grumbach K, Coleman BG, Gal AA et al: Hepatic and biliary tract abnormalities in patients with AIDS: sonographic-pathologic correlation. J Ultrasound Med 1989;8:247

263. Romano AJ, vanSonnenberg E, Casola G et al: Gallbladder and bile duct abnormalities in AIDS: sonographic findings in eight patients. AJR 1988;150:123

264. Dolmatch BL, Laing FC, Federle MP et al: AIDS-related cholangitis: radiographic findings in nine patients. Radiology 1987;163:313

265. Stauffer RA, Adams A, Wygal J, Lavery JP: Gallbladder disease in pregnancy. Am J Obstet Gynecol 1982; 144:661

266. Williamson SL, Williamson MR: Cholecystosonography in pregnancy. J Ultrasound Med 1984;3:329

267. Yeh HC, Weiss MF, Gerson CD: Torsion of the gallbladder: the ultrasonographic features. J Clin Ultrasound 1989;17:123

268. Love L, Kucharski P, Pickleman J: Radiology of cholecystectomy complications. Gastrointest Radiol 1979; 4:33

269. Crowley SF, Hedvall SE: Cystic duct remnant: sonographic diagnosis. J Ultrasound Med 1985;4:261

270. Raptopoulos V: Ultrasonic pseudocalculus effect in postcholecystectomy patients. AJR 1980;134:145

271. Phillips G, Bank S, Kumari-Subaiya S, Kurtz LM: Percutaneous ultrasound-guided puncture of the gallbladder (PUPG). Radiology 1982;145:769

272. Salerno NR: Percutaneous aspiration and drainage of gallbladder. J Ultrasound Med 1982;1:129

273. Shaver RW, Hawkins IF, Soong J: Percutaneous cholecystostomy. AJR 1982;138:1133

274. Elyaderani MK, McDowel DE, Gabriele OF: A preliminary report of percutaneous cholecystostomy under ultrasonography and fluoroscopy guidance. J Clin Gastroenterol 1983;5:277

275. Radder RW: Ultrasonically guided percutaneous catheter drainage for gallbladder empyema. Diagn Imaging 1980;49:330

276. Weinberger E, Blumhagen JD, Odell JM: Gallbladder contraction in biliary atresia. JAR 1987;149:401

277. Abramson SJ, Treves S, Teele RL: The infant with possible biliary atresia: evaluation by ultrasound and nuclear medicine. Pediatr Radiol 1982;12:1

278. Kirks DR, Coleman RE, Filston HC et al: An imaging approach to persistent neonatal jaundice. AJR 1984;142:461

279. Majd M: ^{99m}Tc-IDA scintigraphy in the evaluation of neonatal jaundice. RadioGraphics 1983;3:88

280. Okasora T, Toyosaka A, Muraji T et al: The use of ultrasonography in the diagnosis of biliary atresia. Pediatr Surg Int 1987;2:231

281. Ikeda S, Sera Y, Akagi M: Serial ultrasonic examination to differentiate biliary atresia from neonatal hepatitis—special reference to changes in size of the gallbladder. Eur J Pediatr 1989;148:396

282. Green D, Carroll BA: Ultrasonography in the jaundiced infant: a new approach. J Ultrasound Med 1986;5:323

283. Toma P, Lucigrai G, Pelizza A: Sonographic patterns of Caroli's disease: report of 5 new cases. J Clin Ultrasound 1991;19:155

284. Marchal GJ, Desmet VJ, Proesmans WC et al: Caroli disease: high-frequency US and pathologic findings. Radiology 1986;158:507

285. Hussman KL, Friedwald JP, Gollub MJ, Melamed J: Caroli's disease associated with infantile polycystic kidney disease: prenatal sonographic appearance. J Ultrasound Med 1991;10:235

286. Mittelstaedt CA, Volberg FM, Fischer GJ, McCartney WH: Caroli's disease: sonographic findings. AJR 1980;134:585

287. Lucaya J, Gomez JL, Molino C, Atienza JG: Congenital dilatation of the intrahepatic bile ducts (Caroli's disease). Radiology 1978;127:746

288. Han BK, Babcock DS, Gelfand MH: Choledochal cyst with bile duct dilatation: sonography and ^{99m}Tc IDA cholescintigraphy. AJR 1981;136:1075

289. Reuter K, Raptopoulous VD, Cantelmo N et al: The diagnosis of choledochal cyst by ultrasound. Radiology 1980;136:437

290. Frank JL, Hill MC, Chirathivat S et al: Antenatal observation of a choledochal cyst by sonography. AJR 1981;137:166

291. Kangarloo H, Sarti DA, Sample WF, Amundson G: Ultrasonographic spectrum of choledochal cysts in children. Pediatr Radiol 1980;9:15

292. Torrisi JM, Haller JO, Velcek FT: Choledochal cyst and biliary atresia in the neonate: imaging findings in five cases. AJR 1990;155:1273

293. Markle BM, Potter BM, Majd M: The jaundiced infant and child. Semin Ultrasound CT MR 1980;1:123

294. Glass TA, Buschi AJ, Brenbridge NAG, Shaffer H: Choledochal cyst: sonographic evaluation of an unusual case. South Med J 1980;73:1391

295. Richardson JD, Grant EG, Barth KH et al: Type II choledochal cyst: diagnosis using real-time sonography. J Ultrasound Med 1984;3:37

296. Filly RA, Carlsen EN: Choledochal cyst: report of a case with specific ultrasonographic findings. J Clin Ultrasound 1976;4:7

297. Mettler FA, Wicks JD, Requard CK, Christie JH: Diagnostic imaging of choledochal cyst. Clin Nucl Med 1981;6:513

298. Zeman RK, Dorfman GS, Burrell MI et al: Disparate dilatation of the intrahepatic and extrahepatic bile ducts in surgical jaundice. Radiology 1981;138:129

299. Floyd JL, Collins TL: Discordance of sonography and cholescintigraphy in acute biliary obstruction. AJR 1983;140:501

300. Shawker TH, Jones BL, Girton ME: Distal common bile duct obstruction: an experimental study in monkeys. J Clin Ultrasound 1981;9:77

301. Gooding GAW: Acute bile duct dilatation with resolution in 43 hours: an ultrasonic demonstration. J Clin Ultrasound 1981;9:201

302. Scheske GA, Cooperberg PL, Cohen MM, Burhenne JH: Dynamic changes in the caliber of the major bile ducts, related to obstruction. Radiology 1980;135:215

303. Laing FC, London LA, Filly RA: Ultrasonographic identification of dilated intrahepatic bile ducts and their differentiation from portal venous structures. J Clin Ultrasound 1978;6:90

304. Conrad MR, Landay MJ, Janes JO: Sonographic "parallel channel" sign of biliary tree enlargement in mild to moderate obstructive jaundice. AJR 1978;130:279

305. Weill F, Eisencher A, Zeltner F: Ultrasonic study of the normal and dilated biliary tree: the "shotgun" sign. Radiology 1978;127:221

306. Weinstein BJ, Weinstein DP: Biliary tract dilatation in the nonjaundiced patient. AJR 1980;134:899

307. Zeman R, Taylor KJW, Burrell MI, Gold J: Ultrasound demonstration of anicteric dilatation of biliary tree. Radiology 1980;134:689

308. Weinstein DP, Weinstein BJ, Brodmerkel GJ: Ultrasonography of biliary tract dilatation without jaundice. AJR 1979;132:729

309. Zeman RK, Taylor KJW, Rosenfield AT et al: Acute experimental biliary obstruction in the dog: sonographic findings and clinical implications. AJR 1981;136:965

310. Thomas JL, Zornoza J: Obstructive jaundice in the absence of sonographic biliary dilatation. Gastrointest Radiol 1980;5:357

311. Ferrucci JT, Adson MA, Mueller PR et al: Advances in

the radiology of jaundice: a symposium and review. AJR 1983;141:1

312. Berk RN, Cooperberg PL, Gold RP et al: Radiology of the bile ducts: a symposium on the use of new modalities for diagnosis and treatment. Radiology 1982;145:1

313. Koenigsberg M, Weiner SN, Walzer A: The accuracy of sonography in the differential diagnosis of obstructive jaundice: a comparison with cholangiography. Radiology 1979;133:157

314. Haubek A, Pedersen JH, Burcharth F et al: Dynamic sonography in the evaluation of jaundice. AJR 1981;136:1071

315. Malini S, Sabel J: Ultrasonography in obstructive jaundice. Radiology 1977;123:429

316. Taylor KJW, Rosenfield AT, Spiro HM: Diagnostic accuracy of gray-scale ultrasonography for the jaundiced patient: a report of 275 cases. Arch Intern Med 1979;139:60

317. Hadidi A: Distinction between obstructive and nonobstructive jaundice by sonography. Clin Radiol 1980;31:181

318. Baron RL, Stanley RJ, Lee JKT et al: A prospective comparison of the evaluation of biliary obstruction using computed tomography and ultrasonography. Radiology 1982;145:91

319. Klingensmith WC, Johnson ML, Kuni CC et al: Complimentary role of Tc-99m-diethyl-IDA and ultrasound in large and small duct biliary tract obstruction. Radiology 1981;138:177

320. Raptopoulos V, Smith EH, Cummings T et al: Bile-duct dilatation after laparotomy: a potential effect of intestinal hypomotility. AJR 1986;147:729

321. Laing FC, Jeffrey RB, Wing VW, Nyberg DA: Biliary dilatation: defining the level and cause by real-time US. Radiology 1986;160:39

322. Honickman SP, Mueller PR, Wittenberg J et al: Ultrasound in obstructive jaundice—prospective evaluation of site and cause. Radiology 1983;147:511

323. Gibson RN, Yeung E, Thompson JN et al: Bile duct obstruction: radiologic evaluation of level, cause, and tumor resectability. Radiology 1986;160:43

324. Douillet P, Brunelle F, Chaumont P et al: Ultrasonography and percutaneous cholangiography in children with dilated bile ducts. Am J Dis Child 1981;135:131

325. Mueller PR, Ferrucci JT, Simeone JF et al: Postcholecystectomy bile duct dilatation: myth or reality. AJR 1981;136:355

326. Graham MF, Cooperberg PL, Cohen MM, Burhenne HJ: Ultrasonographic screening of the common hepatic duct in symptomatic patients after cholecystectomy. Radiology 1981;138:137

327. Graham MF, Cooperberg PL, Cohen MM, Burhenne HJ: The size of the normal common hepatic duct following cholecystectomy: an ultrasonographic study. Radiology 1980;135:137

328. Wedmann B, Borsch G, Coehen C, Paassen A: Effect of cholecystectomy on common bile duct diameters: a longitudinal prospective ultrasonographic study. J Clin Ultrasound 1988;16:619

329. Gross BH, Harter LP, Gore RM et al: Ultrasonic evaluation of common duct stones: prospective comparison with endoscopic retrograde cholangiopancreatography. Radiology 1983;146:471

330. Mintz MC, Grumbach K, Arger PH, Coleman BG: Sonographic evaluation of bile duct size during pregnancy. AJR 1985;145:575

331. Spinelli GD, Kleinclaus DH, Wenger JJ et al: Obstructive jaundice and abdominal aortic aneurysm: an ultrasonographic study. Radiology 1982;144:872

332. Einstein DM, Lapin SA, Ralls PW, Halls JM: The insensitivity of sonography in the detection of choledocholithiasis. AJR 1984;142:725

333. Parulekar SG, McNamara MP: Ultrasonography of choledocholithiasis. J Ultrasound Med 1983;2:395

334. Mueller PR, Cronan JJ, Simeone JF et al: Choledocholithiasis: ultrasonographic caveats. J Ultrasound Med 1983;2:13

335. Lewandowski B, French G, Winsberg F: The normal post-cholecystectomy sonogram: gas vs. clips. J Ultrasound Med 1985;4:7

336. Mitchell SE, Clark RA: A comparison of computed tomography and sonography in choledocholithiasis. AJR 1984;142:729

337. Cronan JJ: US diagnosis of choledocholithiasis: a reappraisal. Radiology 1986;161:133

338. Lim JH: Oriental cholangiohepatitis: pathologic, clinical, and radiologic features. AJR 1991;157:1

339. Lim JH, Ko YT, Lee DH, Hong KS: Oriental cholangiohepatitis: sonographic findings in 48 cases. AJR 1990;155:511

340. Lim JH, Ko YT, Lee DH, Kim SY: Clonorchiasis: sonographic findings in 59 proved cases. AJR 1989;152:761

341. Lim JH: Radiologic findings in clonorchiasis. AJR 1990;155:1001

342. Ralls PW, Colletti PM, Quinn MF et al: Sonography in recurrent oriental pyogenic cholangitis. AJR 1981;136:1010

343. Scheible FW, David GB: Oriental cholangiohepatitis: preoperative radiographic and ultrasonographic diagnosis. Gastrointest Radiol 1981;6:269

344. Federle MP, Cello JP, Laing FC, Jeffrey RB: Recurrent pyogenic cholangitis in Asian immigrants: use of ultrasonography, computed tomography and cholangiography. Radiology 1982;143:151

345. Ishida H, Yagisawa H, Nasu H et al: Ultrasonography of acute obstructive suppurative cholangitis: serial observation by ultrasound. J Clin Ultrasound 1987;15:51

346. Carroll BA, Oppenheimer DA: Sclerosing cholangitis: sonographic demonstration of bile duct wall thickening. AJR 1982;139:1016

347. Biggi E, Derchi L, Cicio GR, Valente M: Sonographic findings of hydatid cyst of the liver ruptured into the biliary duct. J Clin Ultrasound 1979;7:381

348. Subramanyam BR, Balthazar EJ, Naidich DP: Ruptured hydatid cyst with biliary obstruction: diagnosis by sonography and computed tomography. Gastrointest Radiol 1983;8:341

349. Gelin J, Marchal G, Vansteenbergen W et al: Sono-

graphic diagnosis of extrahepatic biliary echinococcosis. J Clin Ultrasound 1985;13:187

350. Barki Y, Charuzi I: Intrabiliary rupture of hydatid cyst of the liver: sonographic diagnosis. J Clin Ultrasound 1985;13:40

351. Nesbit GM, Johnson CD, James EM et al: Cholangiocarcinoma: diagnosis and evaluation of resectability by CT and sonography as procedures complementary to cholangiography. AJR 1988;151:933

352. Meyer DG, Weinstein BJ: Klatskin tumors of the bile ducts: sonographic appearance. Radiology 1983;148:803

353. Subramanyam BR, Raghavendra BN, Balthazar EJ et al: Ultrasonic features of cholangiocarcinoma. J Ultrasound Med 1984;3:405

354. Yoshida H, Itai Y, Minami M et al: Biliary malignancies occurring in choledochal cysts. Radiology 1989;173;389

355. Jones TB, Dubrisson RL, Hughes JJ, Robinson AE: Abrupt termination of the common bile duct: a sign of malignancy identified by high-resolution real-time sonography. J Ultrasound Med 1983;2:345

356. Levine E, Maklad NF, Wright CH, Lee KR: Computed tomographic and ultrasonic appearances of primary carcinoma of the common bile duct. Gastrointest Radiol 1979;4:147

357. Schnur MJ, Hoffman JC, Koenigsberg M: Ultrasonic demonstration of intraductal biliary neoplasms. J Clin Ultrasound 1982;10:246

358. Choi BI, Lee JH, Han MC et al: Hilar cholangiocarcinoma: comparative study with sonography and CT. Radiology 1989;172:689

359. Ros PR, Buck JL, Goodman ZD et al: Intrahepatic cholangiocarcinoma: radiologic-pathologic correlation. Radiology 1988;167:689

360. Pastakia B, Shawker TH, Horvath K: Biliary neoplasm simulating dilated bile ducts: role of computed tomography and ultrasound. J Ultrasound Med 1987;6:333

361. Machan L, Muller NL, Cooperberg PL: Sonographic diagnosis of Klatskin tumors. AJR 1986;147:509

362. Tio RL, Wijers OB, Sars PRA, Tytgat GNJ: Preoperative TNM classification of proximal extrahepatic bile duct carcinoma by endosonography. Semin Liver Dis 1990;10(2):114

363. Mitake M, Nakazawa S, Tsukamoto Y et al: Endoscopic ultrasonography in the diagnosis of depth invasion and lymph node metastasis of carcinoma of the papilla of vater. J Ultrasound Med 1990;9:645

364. Forrest ME, Cho KJ, Shields JJ et al: Biliary cystadenomas: sonographic-angiographic pathologic correlations. AJR 1980;135:723

365. Choi BI, Lim JH, Han MC et al: Biliary cystadenoma and cystadenocarcinoma: CT and sonography findings. Radiology 1989;171:57

366. Carroll BA: Biliary cystadenoma and cystadenocarcinoma: gray-scale ultrasound appearance. J Clin Ultrasound 1978;6:337

367. Frick MP, Feinberg SB: Biliary cystadenoma. AJR 1982;139:393

368. Kokubo T, Itai Y, Ohtomo K et al: Mucin-hypersecreting intrahepatic biliary neoplasms. Radiology 1988;168:609

369. Korobkin M, Stephens DH, Lee JKT et al: Biliary cystadenoma and cystadenocarcinoma: CT and sonographic findings. AJR 1989;153:507

370. Arger PH: Obstructive jaundice of malignant origin. Semin Ultrasound CT MR 1980;1:113

371. Swartz TR, Ritchie WGM: Bile duct obstruction secondary to lymphomatous involvement of the pancreas. J Clin Ultrasound 1983;11:391

372. Belta KS, Donnelly PB, Wexler JS: Sonographic demonstration of the intraluminal bile duct metastasis: a case report. Conn Med 1982;46:636

373. VanSonnenberg E, Ferrucci JT: Bile duct obstruction in hepatocellular carcinoma (hepatoma)—clinical and cholangiographic characteristics: report of 6 cases and review of the literature. Radiology 1979;130:7

374. Maffessanti MM, Bazzochi M, Melato M: Sonographic diagnosis of intraductal hepatoma. J Clin Ultrasound 1982;10:397

375. Makuuchi M, Bandai Y, Ito T et al: Ultrasonically guided percutaneous transhepatic bile drainage. Radiology 1980;136:165

376. Gooding GAW, Munyer TP: Ultrasonic localization of biliary decompression catheters. J Ultrasound Med 1983;2:325

377. Mueller PR, Ferrucci JT, vanSonnenberg E et al: Obstruction of the left hepatic duct: diagnosis and treatment by selective fine-needle cholangiography and percutaneous biliary drainage. Radiology 1982;145:297

378. Makuuchi M, Bandai Y, Ito T et al: Ultrasonically guided percutaneous transhepatic cholangiography and percutaneous pancreatography. Radiology 1980;134:767

379. Gibney RG, Cooperberg PL, Scudamore CH, Nagy AG: Segmental biliary obstruction: false-negative diagnosis with direct cholangiography without US guidance. Radiology 1987;164:27

380. Gould L, Patel A: Ultrasound detection of extrahepatic encapsulated bile: "biloma." AJR 1979;132:1014

381. Ralls PW, Eto R, Quinn M, Boger D: Gray-scale ultrasonography of a traumatic biliary cyst. J Trauma 1981;21:176

382. Zegal HG, Kurtz AB, Perlmutter GS, Goldberg BB: Ultrasonic characteristics of bilomas. J Clin Ultrasound 1981;9:21

383. Mueller PR, Ferrucci JT, Simeone JF et al: Detection and drainage of bilomas: special considerations AJR 1983;140:715

384. Haller JO, Condon VR, Berdon WE et al: Spontaneous perforation of the common bile duct in children. Radiology 1989;172:621

385. Esensten M, Ralls PW, Colletti P, Halls J: Posttraumatic intrahepatic biloma: sonographic diagnosis. AJR 1983;140:303

386. Hillman BJ, Smith EH, Holm HH: Ultrasound diagnosis and treatment of gallbladder fossa collections following biliary tract surgery. Br J Radiol 1979;52:390

387. Weissman HS, Chun KJ, Frank M et al: Demonstration

of traumatic bile leakage with cholescintigraphy and ultrasonography. AJR 1979;133:843

388. White M, Simeone JF, Muller PR: Imaging of cholecystocolic fistulas. J Ultrasound Med 1983;2:181

389. Zeman RK, Lee C, Stahl RS et al: Ultrasonography and hepatobiliary scintigraphy in the assessment of biliary-enteric anastomoses. Radiology 1982;145:109

390. Wilson SR, Toi A: Sonography accurately detects biliary obstruction in patients with surgically created biliary-enteric anastomosis. AJR 1990;155:794

391. Pariente D, Bihet MH, Tammam S et al: Biliary complications after transplantation in children: role of imaging modalities. Pediatr Radiol 1991;21:175

392. Zemel G, Zajko AB, Skolnick ML et al: The role of sonography and transhepatic cholangiography in the diagnosis of biliary complications after liver transplantation. AJR 1988;151:943

393. Mueller PR, Harbin WP, Ferrucci JT Jr et al: Fine needle transhepatic cholangiography: reflection after 450 cases. AJR 1981;136:85

394. Mittelstaedt CA: Ultrasound. p. 490. In Yamado T, Alpers OH, Owyang C et al (eds): Atlas of Gastroenterology. JB Lippincott, Philadelphia, 1992

Color Plates

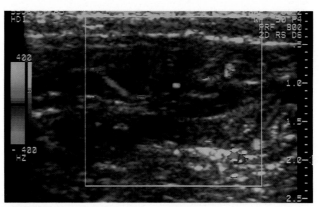
Plate 1-1

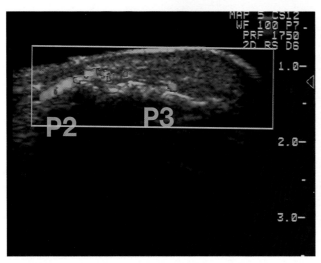
Plate 1-2

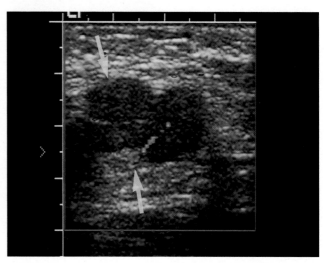
Plate 1-3

Plate 1-1. Color Doppler transverse scan of the anterior forearm in a normal subject showing blood flow distributed in the perimysium of the flexor digitorum superficialis muscle. Vessels are too small to be demonstrated on a gray-scale scan.

Plate 1-2. Normal anatomy of the fingers. Coronal oblique color Doppler scan of the tip of the third finger showing the distal branch of the proper palmar digital artery. (*P2*, second phalanx; *P3*, third phalanx.)

Plate 1-3. Metastatic axillary lymph node in a patient with breast carcinoma. Color Doppler scan showing increased vascularity inside the enlarged, deformed node (arrows).

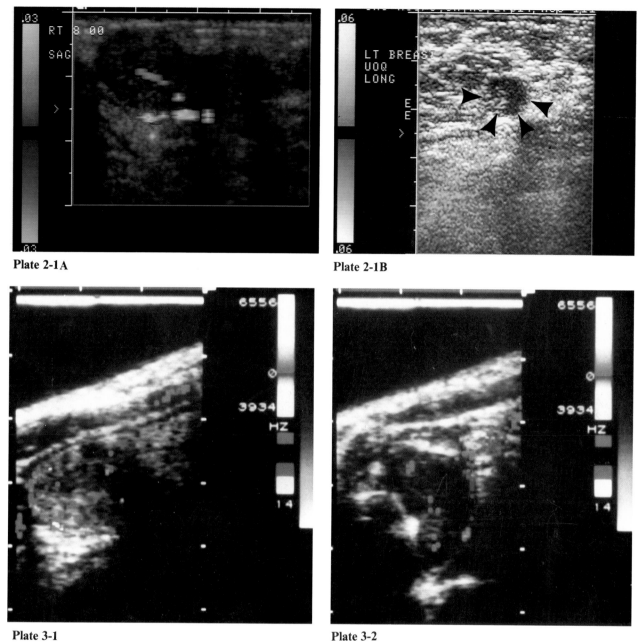

Plate 2-1A

Plate 2-1B

Plate 3-1

Plate 3-2

Plate 2-1. (A) Color Doppler signal from a fibroadenoma. Note the paucity of vessels with only a single feeding vessel evident and no tumor "blush" suggestive of malignancy. (B) Unfortunately, the same pattern is seen here (arrowheads), which proved to be infiltrating ductal carcinoma. (See also Fig. 2-41.) (Plate A courtesy of Leslie Scoutt, M.D., Yale University School of Medicine.)

Plate 3-1. A 7.5-MHz longitudinal sonogram of the same thyroid adenoma as in Fig. 3-49A that is vascular on color Doppler.

Plate 3-2. Color Doppler of the same parathyroid adenoma as in Fig. 3-49B shows both rim and central vascularity. (*T*, thyroid.)

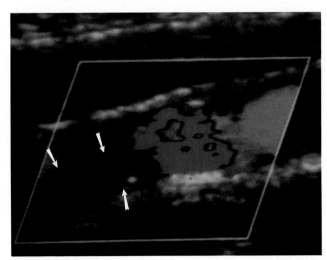

Plate 4-1

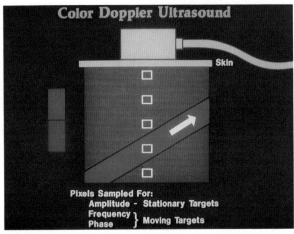

Plate 4-2A

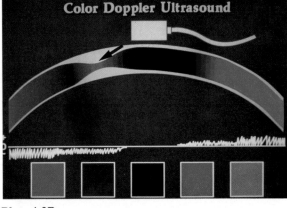

Plate 4-2B

Plate 4-1. Longitudinal scan at the origin of the right ICA (arrows) demonstrating absent ICA color Doppler flow. Abrupt reversal of flow just proximal to the total occlusion of the right ICA is indicated by a change from red to blue.

Plate 4-2. **(A)** Color diagram demonstrating the basic principles of color Doppler. **(B)** Diagram of a vessel with an area of narrowing (arrow), demonstrating the relative color changes produced by changing blood flow direction with respect to the Doppler transducer. The color assignments become less saturated at the opposite ends of the vessel where angle theta is smallest. Color saturation also decreases in the area of the stenosis (arrow). When angle theta is approximately 90 degrees, an absent color assignment or a black area is present.

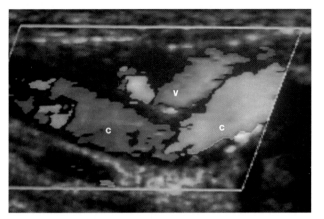

Plate 4-3

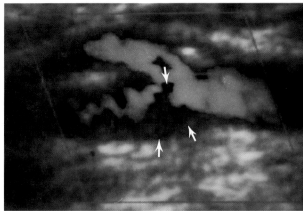

Plate 4-5

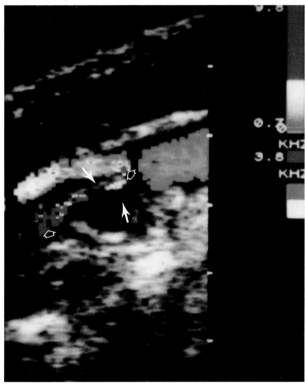

Plate 4-4

Plate 4-6

Plate 4-3. Longitudinal scan of a tortuous common carotid artery *(C)* and internal jugular vein *(V)* demonstrating reversal of the color assignment from red to blue within the CCA. This is due to a change in flow direction with respect to the Doppler transducer.

Plate 4-4. Longitudinal scan through the carotid bifurcation demonstrating a high-grade stenosis at the origin of the ICA (arrows). Color Doppler "green tagging" in the area of the high-grade stenosis is present (open arrows). This "green tagging" is consistent with a high-grade stenosis.

Plate 4-5. Longitudinal carotid bifurcation scan of the same patient as in Fig. 4-12, demonstrating a high-grade stenosis (arrows) at the origin of the right ICA. Although the degree of stenosis is quite high, the color assignments in the area of the stenosis are relatively homogeneous.

Plate 4-6. Normal color Doppler of the carotid bifurcation (arrows) demonstrating the normal flow separation seen at the origin of the ICA (open arrow). The relatively darker shades of blue are immediately adjacent to the darker shades of red (arrowhead). This configuration is consistent with flow separation as opposed to aliasing, which demonstrates contiguity of the less saturated forward and reverse flow colors. (Courtesy of Acoustic Technology Laboratories.)

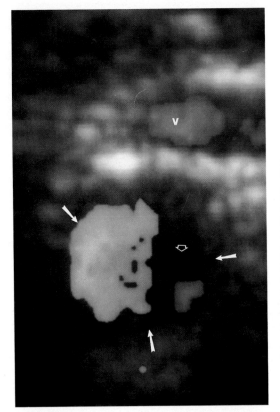

Plate 4-7A

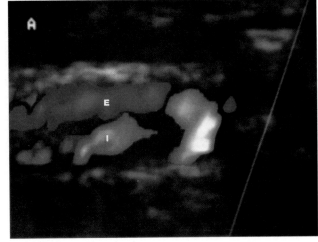

Plate 4-7B

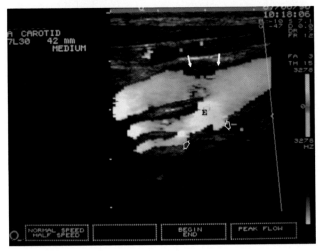

Plate 4-8

Plate 4-9

Plate 4-7. **(A)** Transverse scan through the left ICA bulb (arrows) demonstrating a hypoechoic plaque along the lateral aspect of the bulb (open arrow) and an area of retrograde (blue) eddying flow within areas of intraplaque ulceration. (*V,* internal jugular vein.) **(B)** Longitudinal scan in the region of the origin of a different left ICA (arrows) demonstrating a high-grade stenosis and an area of eddying flow projecting into the plaque (curved arrow), suggestive of intraplaque ulceration.

Plate 4-8. Color Doppler longitudinal image of the carotid bifurcation demonstrating moderate narrowing of the ICA origin (arrows). The external carotid artery *(E)* is clearly defined by the presence of branches (open arrows). (Courtesy of Acoustic Technology Laboratories.)

Plate 4-9. Longitudinal scan above the carotid bifurcation in a patient who has undergone Crutchfield clamp placement for a carotid artery aneurysm, demonstrating persistent antegrade ICA flow *(I)* supplied by retrograde ECA flow *(E).*

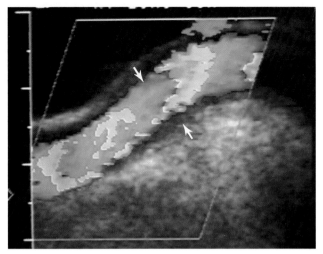

Plate 4-10

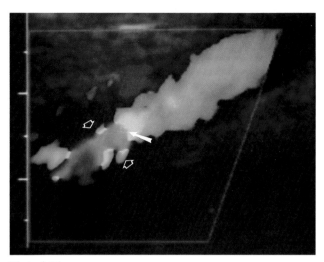

Plate 4-11

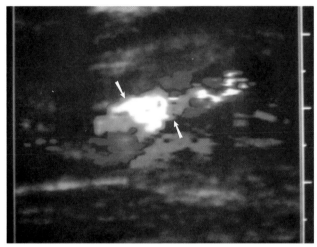

Plate 4-12

Plate 4-10. Longitudinal color Doppler image of the right CCA in the same hypertensive patient with spuriously increased velocities seen in Fig. 4-9, showing no significant stenosis (arrows). Color aliasing is also present.

Plate 4-11. Color Doppler scan in the region of the elevated ICA velocities in the same patient as in Fig. 4-21, demonstrating high-velocity color Doppler flow (arrow) but no significant narrowing of the ICA (open arrows). The spuriously increased velocity elevations are probably related to increased collateral flow secondary to the contralateral right ICA occlusion.

Plate 4-12. Longitudinal color Doppler scan in a patient with a history of an endarterectomy, demonstrating high-velocity disturbed flow (arrows) (heterogeneous color) in the proximal ICA in the region of the endarterectomy. These sorts of flow abnormalities are common for at least 6 months following endarterectomy. However, color Doppler clearly shows that there is no significant narrowing of the postendarterectomy site.

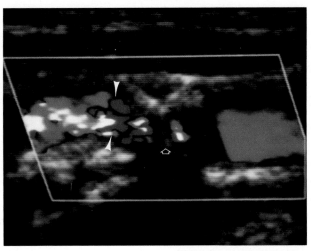

Plate 4-13

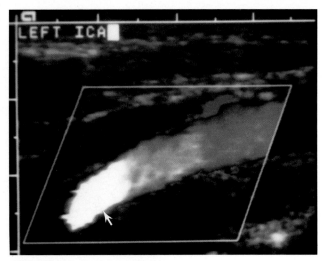

Plate 4-14

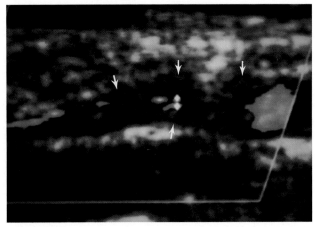

Plate 4-15

Plate 4-13. Longitudinal scan in the region of a calcified ICA origin plaque that is producing posterior acoustic shadowing (open arrow), which makes it impossible to directly evaluate the degree of stenosis produced by the plaque. The scan provides insights into the degree of stenosis via indirect assessment of its severity from the marked heterogeneity and increased velocity in the color Doppler flow just distal to the plaque (arrowheads).

Plate 4-14. Normal left ICA showing the dramatic change in color saturation as it dives deeply into the neck. At the more cephalic extent (arrow) there is desaturation, which is produced solely by a relatively decreased angle theta in this portion of the ICA compared with the more proximal portion of the vessel. The actual velocity in the ICA has not changed when corrected for angle theta. However, the color Doppler assignments are not corrected along all portions of the vessel.

Plate 4-15. Longitudinal scan through an ICA origin (arrows) demonstrating a long "string" of color flow (calipers) trickling through the high-grade long-segment stenosis.

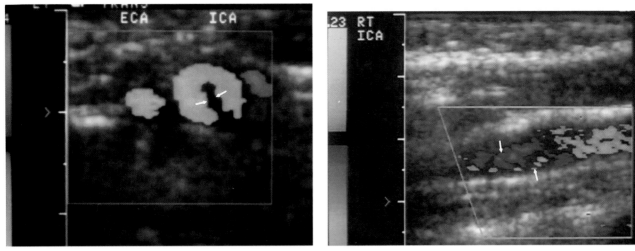

Plate 4-16　　　　　　　　　　　　　　　　**Plate 4-17**

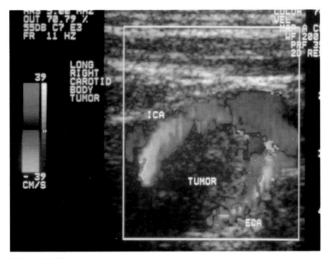

Plate 4-18

Plate 4-16. Transverse scan through the left carotid bifurcation demonstrating a linear, hypoechoic filling defect (arrows) projecting into the lumen of the proximal left ICA. This was proven to be a carotid web.

Plate 4-17. Longitudinal scan through the origin of the right ICA in a 35-year-old woman with left hemispheric symptoms, demonstrating abnormal flow patterns in the ICA, consistent with a dissection (arrows).

Plate 4-18. Longitudinal scan through the right carotid artery bifurcation demonstrating a carotid body tumor. (See also Fig. 4-24.) (Courtesy of Acoustic Technology Laboratories).

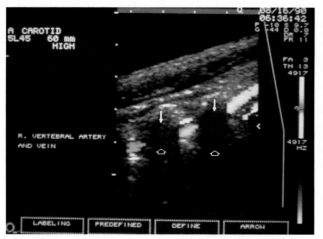

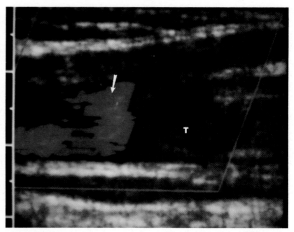

Plate 4-19

Plate 4-20

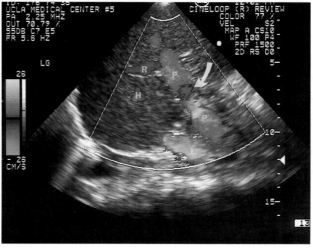

Plate 5-1

Plate 4-19. Longitudinal color Doppler image demonstrating the vertebral artery (red) and vertebral vein (blue). Transverse processes of the cervical spine (arrows) produce periodic shadowing (open arrows), which prevents visualization of segments of the vertebral vessels. (Courtesy of Acoustic Technology Laboratories.)

Plate 4-20. Color Doppler scans at a higher level in the same patient as in Fig. 4-34, demonstrating some preserved flow (arrow) above the level of the internal jugular vein thrombus *(T)*.

Plate 5-1. Normal portal venous anatomy. Flow in the main portal vein *(P)* is predominantly toward the transducer and is displayed in red. Areas of reversed flow (curved arrow) are encountered commonly and may represent normal helical flow or boundary separation layers. After the portal vein divides, flow in the posterior right branch *(R)* is away from the transducer and is displayed in blue. (*H*, right hepatic vein; *I*, IVC.)

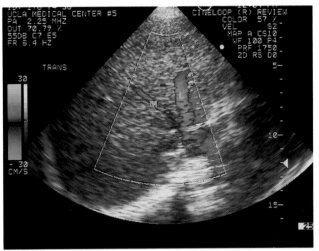

Plate 5-2A

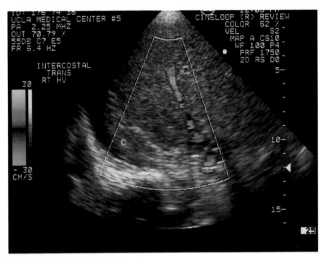

Plate 5-2B

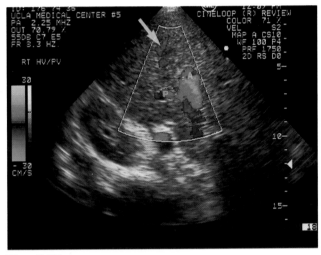

Plate 5-2C

Plate 5-2. Normal hepatic veins. **(A)** Middle *(M)* and left *(L)* hepatic veins are optimally visualized when scanned from a transverse subxiphoid approach. The right hepatic vein lies perpendicular to the Doppler beam when scanned from an anterior approach and may not return Doppler signals. **(B)** The right hepatic vein is optimally visualized by scanning from a lateral intercostal approach. (c, consolidated right lung.) **(C)** Color Doppler image illustrating the relationship between anterior *(A)* and posterior *(P)* branches of right portal vein and right hepatic vein (arrow). Portal veins tend to lie in the center of hepatic lobes or segments, while hepatic veins form the boundaries. (See also Fig. 5-12.)

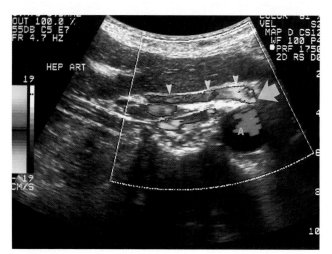

Plate 5-3

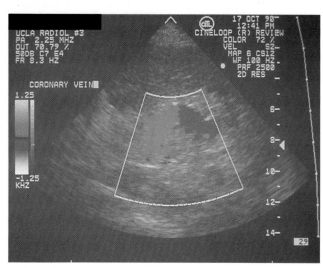

Plate 5-4

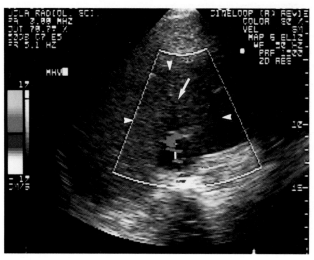

Plate 5-5

Plate 5-6

Plate 5-3. Hepatic artery. The celiac axis (arrow) arises from the abdominal aorta *(A)* and branches into the splenic artery (not shown) and hepatic artery (arrowheads). The hepatic artery courses along the anterior, superior border of the pancreas. (See also Fig. 5-13.)

Plate 5-4. Pseudo double-channel sign. Color Doppler easily confirms the vascular nature of both structures in Fig. 5-18 and excludes the possibility of ductal dilatation. Appropriately directed flow in the posterior tubule (blue) is that of the hepatic artery. The more anterior tubule (red) is a portal venous radical with reserved flow.

Plate 5-5. Budd-Chiari syndrome. The caudate lobe has a separate venous drainage from other portions of the liver. In this patient with Budd-Chiari syndrome secondary to polycythemia rubra vera, the only visible venous structure was found in the central liver (arrow) and emptied into the inferior vena cava *(I)*. The vessel was initially taken to be a patent middle hepatic vein. Closer examination determined that it was the large caudate vein. (arrowheads, caudate lobe.)

Plate 5-6. Dilated coronary vein. A large crescentic vessel thought to represent a dilated coronary vein is identified cephalic to a smaller, normal splenic vein (not shown). The patient has known portal hypertension. The vessel could be followed across the upper abdomen to the region of the stomach and esophagus.

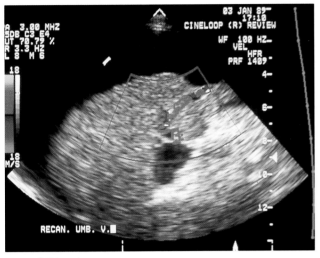

Plate 5-7A

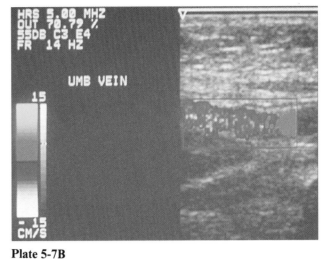

Plate 5-7B

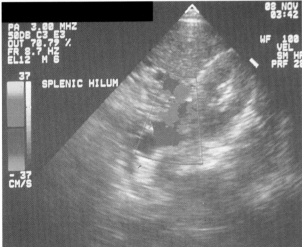

Plate 5-8

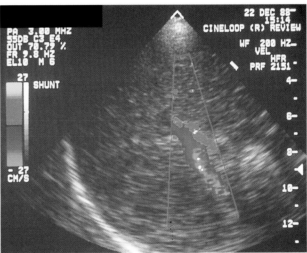

Plate 5-9

Plate 5-7. Umbilical vein collaterals. **(A)** The umbilical (or paraumbilical) vein serves as a common collateral pathway in patients with portal hypertension. Flow is displayed in red and is directed away from the liver. Recanalized umbilical vein serves as an intrahepatic shunt and may actually increase or normalize flow velocity in the main portal vein. **(B)** Scanning beneath the anterior abdominal wall, superficial portions of the umbilical vein can be followed as they course toward the umbilicus.

Plate 5-8. Splenorenal collaterals. An extensive network of left upper quadrant collaterals may be encountered as shown. These naturally occurring pathways serve a similar function to a surgically created splenorenal shunt and help to alleviate portal hypertension.

Plate 5-9. Reversed portal vein flow. Reversal of portal vein flow is indicated by blue in the vessel. Note the prominence of arterial flow, which is normally directed (displayed in red). (See also Fig. 5-34.)

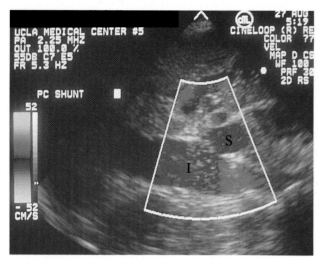

Plate 5-10A

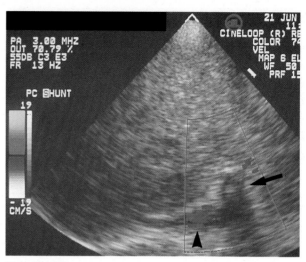

Plate 5-10B

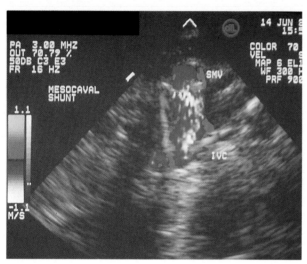

Plate 5-11

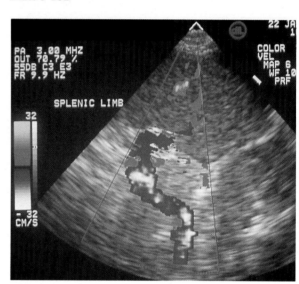

Plate 5-12

Plate 5-10. Portacaval shunt. **(A)** Patency is confirmed by demonstrating anastomosis. Note flow in the splenic/portal vein *(S)* and inferior vena cava *(I)*. **(B)** With thrombosis, flow is absent in the region of the shunt (arrow); flow in the inferior vena cava (arrowhead) persists. (See also Fig. 5-35.)

Plate 5-11. Mesocaval shunt. The shunt diverts blood from the mid/distal superior mesenteric vein *(SMV)* to the adjacent inferior vena cava *(IVC)* via Gore-Tex graft. Walls of such grafts are brightly echogenic; the color confirms patency. (See also Fig. 5-36.)

Plate 5-12. Splenorenal shunt. The splenic limb of the shunt is most optimally visualized from an anterior approach through the spleen. Note the large single vessel with flow running from the splenic hilus toward the left kidney. (See also Fig. 5-37.)

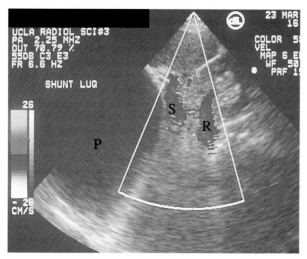

Plate 5-13A

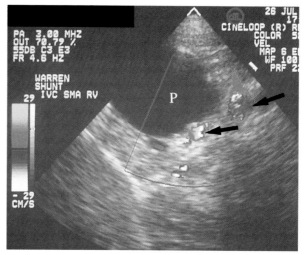

Plate 5-13B

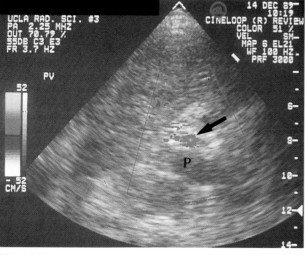

Plate 5-14

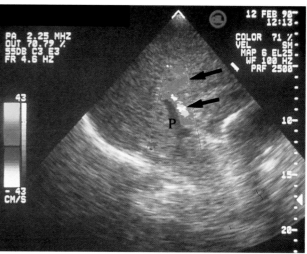

Plate 5-15

Plate 5-13. Abnormal splenorenal shunts. **(A)** This patient with a large left upper quadrant pseudocyst *(P)* has appropriately directed flow in splenic *(S)* and renal *(R)* limbs. Although anastomosis was difficult to visualize, normally directed flow in well-defined limbs is presumptive evidence of shunt patency. **(B)** A different patient with a pseudocyst *(P)* and recurrent esophageal hemorrhage has numerous venous structures in the left upper quadrant (arrows). Singular splenic and renal limbs were not identified; thrombosis was suspected. (See also Fig. 5-38.)

Plate 5-14. Portal vein thrombosis. Color Doppler sonogram in a patient with hepatoma showing the dilated thrombus-filled portal vein *(P)*. Note the accentuated hepatic arterial flow anteriorly (arrow). (See also Fig. 5-39.)

Plate 5-15. False-positive sonogram. Despite optimization of the scan technique, flow could not be demonstrated in the portal vein *(P)*. Hepatic artery flow was accentuated (arrows). The patient had a history of severe portal hypertension. (See also Fig. 5-40.)

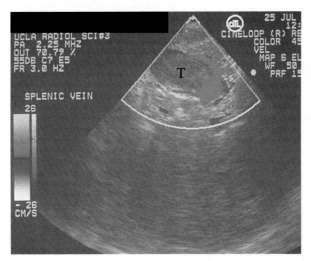

Plate 5-16

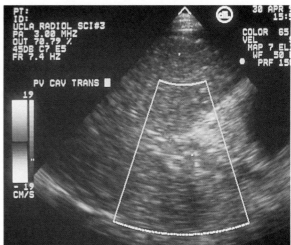

Plate 5-17

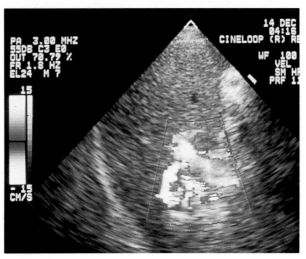

Plate 5-18

Plate 5-16. Splenic vein thrombosis. Patient with known cirrhosis and new onset of massive splenomegaly. The main portal vein was patent, but a large, nonocclusive thrombus *(T)* was found in the distal splenic vein.

Plate 5-17. Cavernous transformation of the portal vein. This patient with no history of liver disease presented with gastrointestinal bleeding. Color Doppler sonogram showing multiple serpiginous channels in the porta hepatis. A discrete single portal vein was not identified. (See also Fig. 5-41.)

Plate 5-18. Portal vein aneurysm. Pretransplant evaluation of a patient with cirrhosis and severe portal hypertension. Note the large, globular area of circular flow adjacent to the main portal vein, typical of portal vein aneurysm.

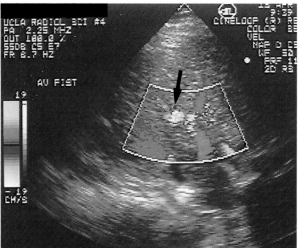

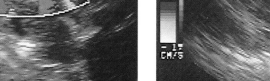

Plate 5-19A

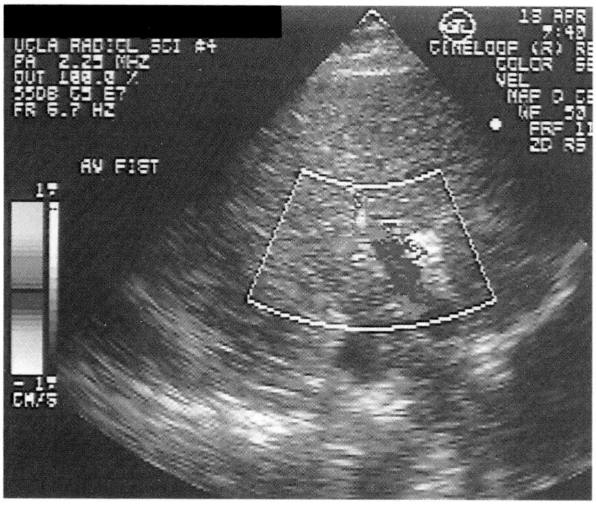

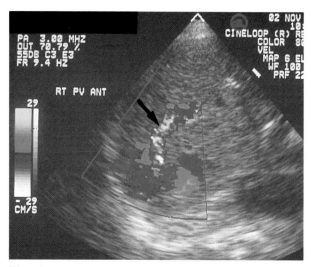

Plate 5-19B

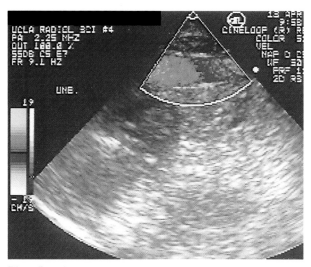

Plate 5-19C

Plate 5-20

Plate 5-19. Hepatic artery-to-portal vein fistula. **(A)** Color Doppler examination in a patient with a known fistula and multiple previous embolizations. The area of high flow velocity and marked turbulence (arrow) in the hepatic artery corresponds to the fistulous communication. **(B)** Portal vein flow is reversed (blue). **(C)** Large recanalized umbilical vein is present beneath the anterior abdominal wall. (See also Fig. 5-44.)

Plate 5-20. Hepatic vein-to-portal vein fistula. This patient was referred for biopsy of several "hypoechoic" masses beneath the dome of the liver. Color Doppler evaluation revealed swirling flow internally. Lesions could be easily connected to the portal vein (arrow) and hepatic veins. Findings are typical of hepatic vein-to-portal vein fistula. (See also Fig. 5-45.)

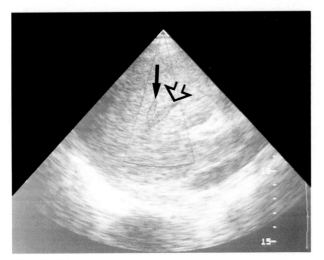

Plate 5-21A

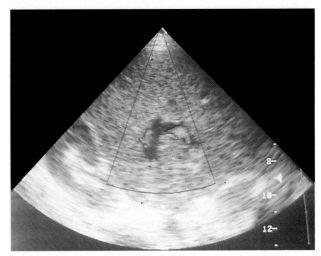

Plate 5-21B

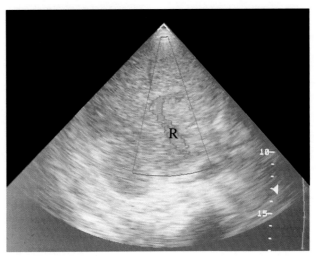

Plate 5-21C

Plate 5-21. Intrahepatic collaterals in Budd-Chiari syndrome. **(A)** Color Doppler evaluation showing "bicolor" hepatic vein bifurcation. Flow in one branch (arrow) was directed normally and displayed in blue. Flow in the adjacent branch (open arrow) was toward the periphery of the liver and displayed in red. **(B)** Another image from the same patient demonstrating a large intrahepatic collateral. **(C)** The patient had a large, patent right hepatic vein *(R)*. All three hepatic veins need not be involved in thrombotic process.

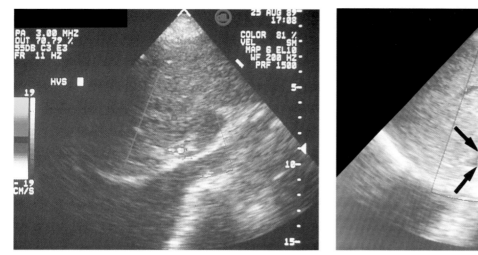

Plate 5-22

Plate 5-23

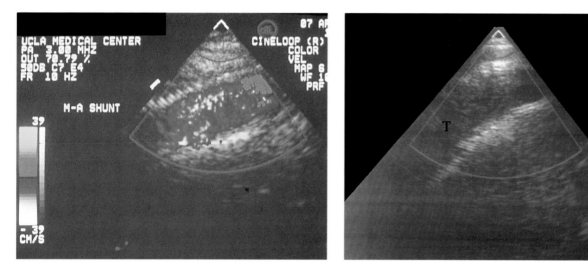

Plate 5-24A

Plate 5-24B

Plate 5-22. Budd-Chiari syndrome. Color Doppler evaluation in the expected region of hepatic veins showing several small vessels that do not appear to connect directly to the inferior vena cava. (See also Fig. 5-47.)

Plate 5-23. Budd-Chiari syndrome. Further evaluation of the patient shown in Fig. 5-47 and Plate 5-22 showing complete occlusion of the proximal inferior vena cava (arrows). The portal vein *(P)* is patent and appropriately directed. (See also Fig. 5-48.)

Plate 5-24. Mesoatrial shunt. **(A)** Longitudinal image from a color Doppler examination demonstrating a mesoatrial shunt in the right upper quadrant. Synthetic walls are brightly echogenic; color confirms patency. **(B)** A different patient with Budd-Chiari syndrome had minor pelvic surgery, and routine anticoagulant therapy was discontinued. The patient presented with recurrent ascites. Color Doppler imaging revealed thrombosis of the mesoatrial shunt *(T)*. (See also Fig. 5-49.)

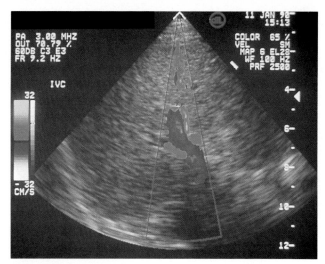

Plate 5-25

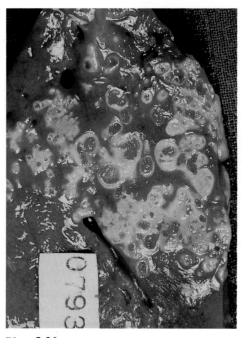

Plate 5-26

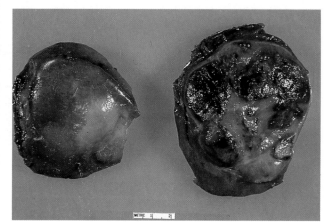

Plate 5-27

Plate 5-25. Hepatic veno-occlusive disease. This patient, who had undergone bone marrow transplantation, presented with right upper quadrant pain and abnormal liver function tests. Evaluation of hepatic *veins* was unremarkable. Reversal of portal vein flow, however, indicates hepatic veno-occlusive disease.

Plate 5-26. Echinococcus alveolaris disease. The pathologic specimen correlates well with the sonographic appearance in Fig. 5-59. (From Didier et al, [120] with permission.)

Plate 5-27. Infantile hemangioendothelioma. The lesion in Fig. 5-73 was found to be infantile hemangioendothelioma.

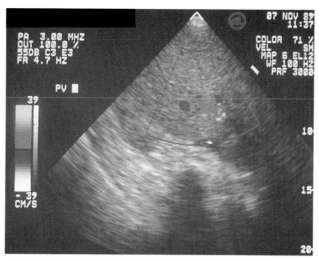

Plate 5-28

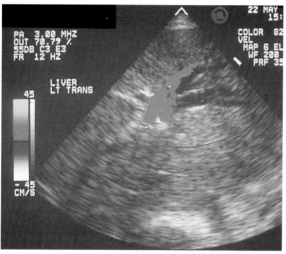

Plate 5-29

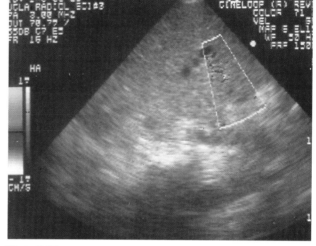

Plate 5-30

Plate 5-28. Hepatic artery thrombosis. Patient 3 weeks post-orthotopic liver transplantation with increasingly abnormal liver function tests. Color Doppler imaging showing normal flow in portal vein. Hepatic artery signals are not identified in the porta or elsewhere in the liver. (See also Fig. 5-106.)

Plate 5-29. Hepatic artery thrombosis with collateral formation. Patient 7 months status-post liver transplant with recurrent bouts of sepsis was found to have segmental intrahepatic biliary dilatation. (See also Fig. 5-107.)

Plate 5-30. Abnormal hepatic artery. Color Doppler evaluation identified a small, tortuous hepatic artery in the patient in Fig. 5-108 with some difficulty.

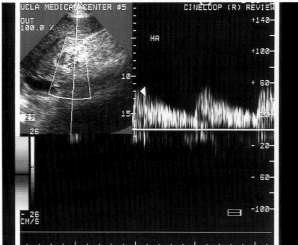

Plate 5-31

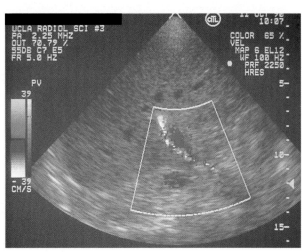

Plate 5-32

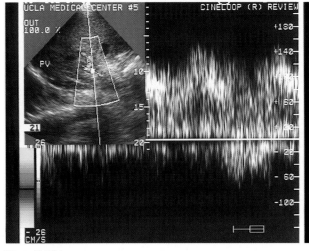

Plate 5-33A

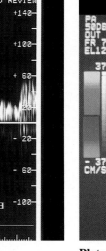

Plate 5-33B

Plate 5-31. Hepatic artery spectral patterns. Normal hepatic artery exhibits low-resistance waveform with flow throughout diastole. (See also Fig. 5-109.)

Plate 5-32. Portal vein. Color Doppler imaging showing a narrow waist in the region of the vascular anastomosis (arrows). Note the mild postanastomotic dilatation. (See also Fig. 5-110.)

Plate 5-33. Portal vein stenosis. **(A)** Color Doppler sonogram showing marked narrowing of the portal vein in region of anastomosis. Considerable post-stenotic turbulence is evidenced by a wide array of colors. **(B)** Spectral Doppler showing elevated portal vein velocity. The clinical significance of portal vein stenosis remains uncertain.

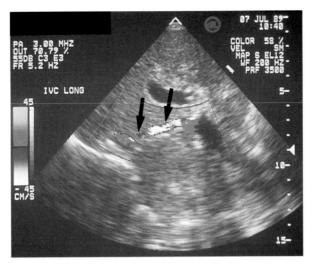

Plate 5-34

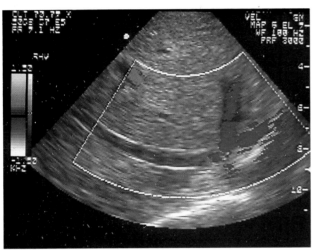

Plate 5-35A

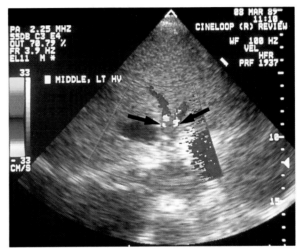

Plate 5-35B

Plate 5-34. Thrombosis of the inferior vena cava. Sonogram of a patient who has undergone a second transplant, showing marked narrowing of the proximal inferior vera cava (arrows). Note the large amount of thrombus posteriorly. (See also Fig. 5-111.)

Plate 5-35. Hepatic venous abnormalities. Hepatic vein thrombosis is unusual after transplantation. **(A)** The middle and left hepatic veins are normal. The right hepatic vein is thrombosed and contains echogenic clot. Thrombosis was confirmed by venography. **(B)** Another patient with mildly abnormal liver function tests post-transplant. Note the marked narrowing of the left and middle hepatic veins with high velocity of flow (arrows) at the junction with the inferior vena cava. The etiology of narrowing is probably mechanical; the significance is uncertain.

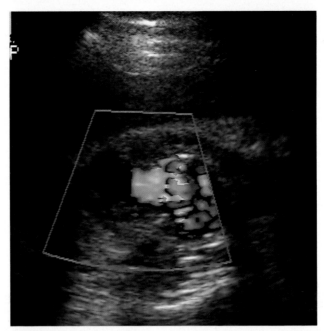

Plate 13-1

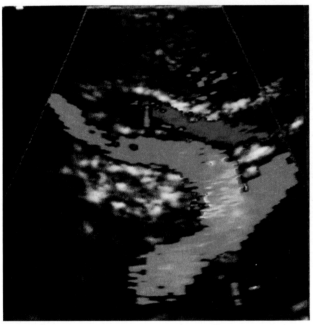

Plate 13-2A

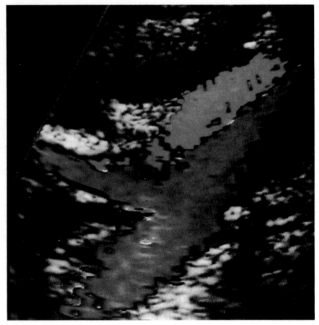

Plate 13-2B

Plate 13-1. Native kidney, arteriovenous malformation. With color Doppler, flow was demonstrated within the mass with mixing of colors. (See also Fig. 13-179.)

Plate 13-2. Normal renal transplant. **(A)** Color Doppler sonogram showing end-to-side anastomosis of main renal artery to external iliac artery. Flow within the artery (red areas) is toward the transducer. **(B)** Color Doppler sonogram showing end-to-side anastomosis of main renal vein to external iliac vein. Flow within the vein (blue areas) is away from the transducer. (See also Fig. 13-190.) (From Dodd et al,[433] with permission.)

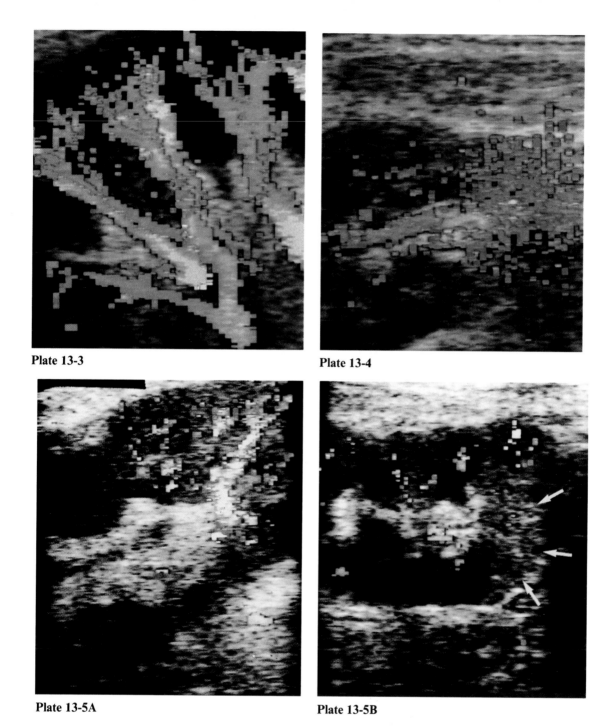

Plate 13-3

Plate 13-4

Plate 13-5A

Plate 13-5B

Plate 13-3. Normal renal transplant, color Doppler. Color Doppler image clearly showing arterial (red) and venous (blue) flow throughout the kidney. Color indicates the direction of flow relative to the transducer. Blood in the renal arteries flows toward the transducer and is red. Blood in the renal veins flows away from the transducer and is blue by convention. (From Surratt et al, [440] with permission.)

Plate 13-4. Renal transplant, renal artery stenosis. Color Doppler image, showing the soft tissue vibrations as a mixture of red and blue around the narrowed vessel. (See also Fig. 13-206.) (From Surratt et al,[440] with permission.)

Plate 13-5. Renal transplant, segmental vascular occlusion. **(A)** Case 1. Segmental infarct of the upper half of the allograft. Color Doppler image showing an absence of flow within the superior portion of the allograft and normal vasculature within the lower pole. On an angiogram (not shown), only the inferior main renal branch remained patent. The other arteries were thrombosed because of acute rejection. **(B)** Case 2. Small segmental infarction of the lower pole of the allograft. On the color Doppler image, an area of increased echogenicity is noted in the lower pole of the allograft, without flow. On the capillary phase of the angiogram (not shown), an infarction of the area in Plate B was shown. (See also Fig. 13-208.) (From Grenier et al,[457] with permission.)

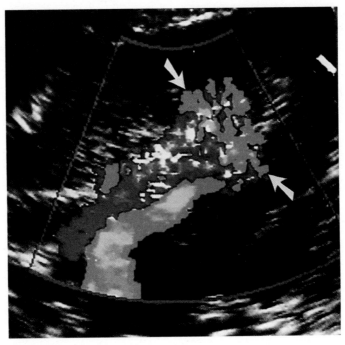

Plate 13-6

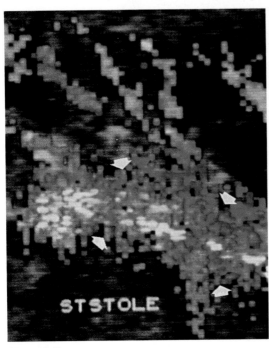

Plate 13-7

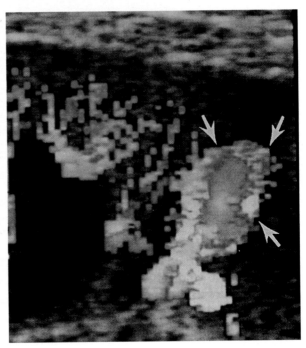

Plate 13-8

Plate 13-6. Renal transplant, intrarenal AVF. Color Doppler sonogram showing the prominent feeding artery (red areas), draining vein (blue areas), and region of the fistula (arrows). (See also Fig. 13-209.) (From Dodd et al,[433] with permission.)

Plate 13-7. Renal transplant, arteriovenous fistula. Color Doppler image demonstrating localized soft tissue vibrations (arrows) obscuring the segmental artery and vein of the fistula. (See also Fig. 13-210.) (From Surratt et al,[440] with permission.)

Plate 13-8. Renal transplant, intrarenal pseudoaneurysm. Color Doppler image showing the abnormality as a swirling mixture of red and blue within the lumen of the aneurysm (arrows). (See also Fig. 13-211.) (From Surratt et al,[440] with permission.)

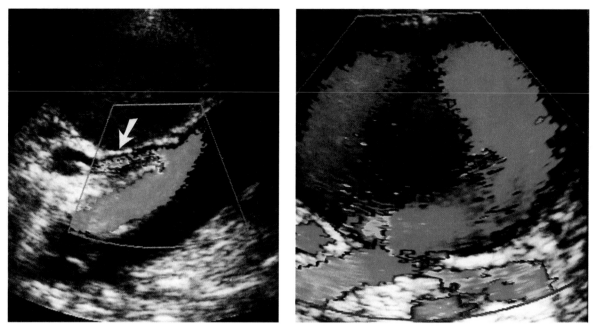

Plate 13-9   **Plate 13-10**

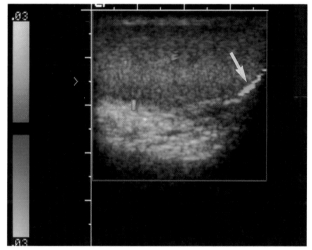

Plate 16-1

Plate 13-9. Renal transplant, extrarenal arteriovenous fistula. Color Doppler sonogram showing high-velocity color aliasing of the main renal artery (arrow). A duplex ultrasound spectrum obtained in the region of the fistula color aliasing (not shown) showed high-velocity, low-impedance arterial flow. A Doppler spectrum of the main renal vein (not shown) showed venous arterialization. (From Dodd et al,[433] with permission.)

Plate 13-10. Renal transplant, extrarenal pseudoaneurysm. Color Doppler sonogram of large anastomotic extrarenal pseudoaneurysm showing swirling flow. (From Dodd et al,[433] with permission.)

Plate 16-1. Color Doppler of the testicle demonstrating the capsular artery in red (arrow) and a few smaller intratesticular vessels as red and blue. (See also Fig. 16-3.)

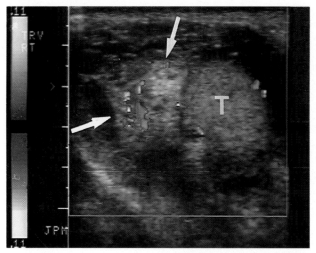

Plate 16-2

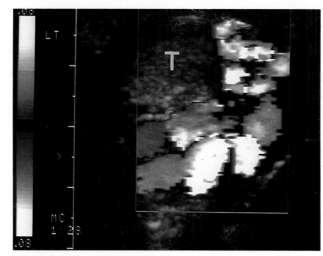

Plate 16-3

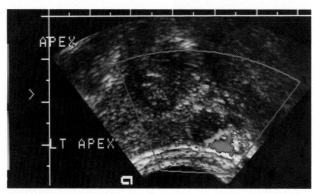

Plate 17-1

Plate 16-2. Color Doppler demonstrating increased blood flow in the thickened epididymis (arrows) adjacent to the testis *(T)*. (See also Fig. 16-11.)

Plate 16-3. Color Doppler during a Valsalva maneuver, demonstrating flow (red and blue) in a large varicocele around the testicle *(T)*. (See also Fig. 16-23.)

Plate 17-1. Color Doppler of another peripheral zone nodule. Note the increased blood flow at the periphery of the nodule. (See also Fig. 17-35.)

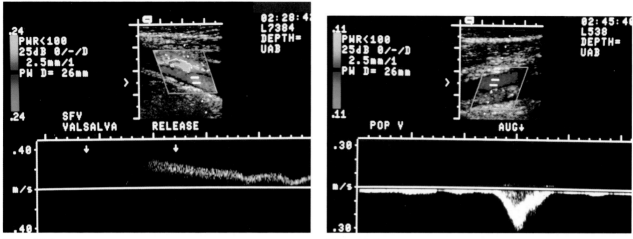

Plate 18-1

Plate 18-2

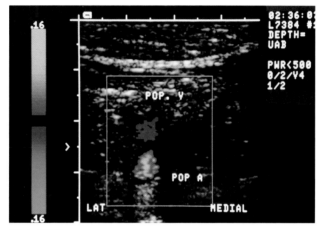

Plate 18-3

Plate 18-1.   Longitudinal color Doppler image shows normal response to Valsalva maneuver in the proximal superficial femoral vein *(SFV)* of this volunteer. During the Valsalva maneuver (arrow to left in spectral tracing), venous flow decreases in the leg resulting from increased abdominal pressure. After release of the Valsalva maneuver (rightward arrow), venous flow increases for several seconds, and then returns to baseline.

Plate 18-2.   Longitudinal color Doppler image shows normal response to augmentation of the calf. Venous flow directed cranially is encoded in blue; augmentation of flow occurs when gentle squeeze is applied to the calf muscles *(AUG)*. *(POP V,* popliteal vein.)

Plate 18-3.   Transverse color Doppler image in the popliteal fossa demonstrates the popliteal vein *(POP. V,* blue) posterior to the popliteal artery *(POP A,* red.)

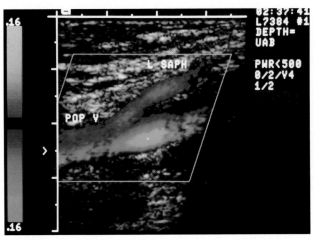

Plate 18-4

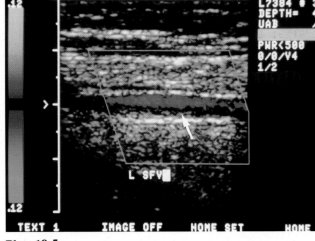

Plate 18-5

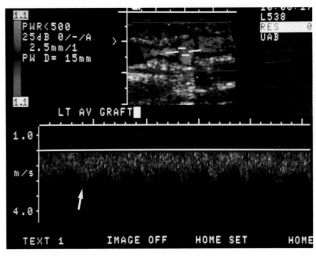

Plate 18-6

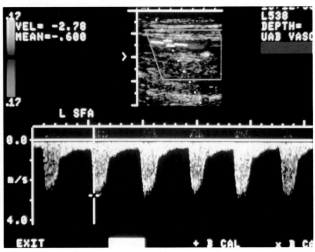

Plate 18-7

Plate 18-4. Longitudinal color Doppler image shows the lesser saphenous vein *(L SAPH)* entering the popliteal vein *(POP V)* behind the knee.

Plate 18-5. Longitudinal color Doppler image showing venous flow throughout this segment, outlining the region of intimal thickening (arrow). (*L SFV,* left superficial femoral vein.)

Plate 18-6. Longitudinal color Doppler image, evaluating a proximal forearm prosthetic loop graft for hemodialysis access. Spectral analysis shows typical high velocity venous flow with superimposed arterial pulsations (arrow).

Plate 18-7. Color Doppler image of the proximal left superficial femoral artery *(L SFA)* shows elevated peak systolic velocity of 2.78 m/s with moderate spectral broadening. The peak systolic velocity has more than doubled from baseline established more proximally; findings are consistent with 50 to 99 percent diameter reduction, confirmed by conventional angiography.

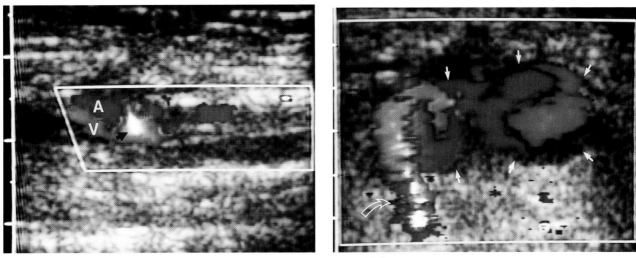

Plate 18-8   **Plate 18-9**

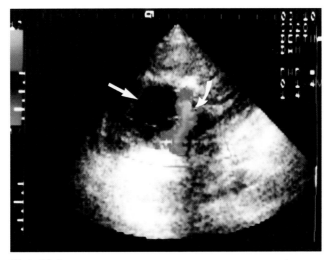

Plate 19-1

Plate 18-8.   Longitudinal color Doppler image of the brachial artery *(A)* and vein *(V)* demonstrates a high velocity jet (arrow), encoded in white; this marks the site of the arteriovenous fistula.

Plate 18-9.   Transverse color Doppler image of a lobulated pseudoaneurysm (arrows), which arises from the superficial femoral artery (open curved arrow). The swirl of colors in the pseudoaneurysm is typical.

Plate 19-1.   Color Doppler performed before needle puncture demonstrates a large vein (curved arrow) along the edge of the fluid collection (arrow).

7

Pancreas

Carol A. Mittelstaedt

It is only in recent years that the radiologist has been able to offer direct evaluation of the pancreas by computed tomography (CT) or ultrasound. Before that time, pancreatic disease was diagnosed by indirect changes seen on plain radiograph or upper gastrointestinal series. Now disease processes can be detected at an early stage, and follow-up studies provide greater insight into the correlation between clinical findings and morphologic changes in the gland. Pancreatic carcinoma can be diagnosed at an earlier stage, but it appears that long-term survival in these patients is not altered significantly. With the development of gray-scale imaging and high-resolution real-time, the role of ultrasound in pancreatic disease has improved significantly. However, of the abdominal organs, the pancreas is the most difficult to adequately visualize with ultrasound. To evaluate the pancreas successfully with ultrasound, the examiner must be meticulous with technique and familiar with normal and abnormal sonograms.

TECHNIQUE

Patient Preparation

It is best to perform an ultrasound examination of the pancreas after an overnight fast. If this is not possible, the patient should have been fasting for at least 6 to 8 hours. The purpose of the fasting is threefold. First, because the biliary system and pancreas are intimately related, they are usually examined together. If gallstones, dilated ducts, and/or choledocholithiasis is seen, an examina-tion of the pancreas is performed. If the pancreas is abnormal, the gallbladder and ducts are always evaluated. Fasting promotes greater dilatation of the gallbladder, thereby giving better evaluation of that structure. Second, fasting ensures that the stomach is empty. Because the stomach is directly anterior to the pancreas, its contents affect the sound beam transmission to the pancreas. Third, fasting tends to result in less bowel gas; this also improves the visualization of the pancreas.

Ultrasound System

The equipment of choice today for the most successful examination of the pancreas is a real-time system, preferably a sector format, because it requires a smaller contact surface. With this system, there is greater success in adequate visualization of the pancreas in more cases. This is due to the flexibility of the scanhead, which can be maneuvered easily, and to the ability to displace bowel gas by moving the scanhead. Also, the patient can be examined in almost any position and, very importantly, at the bedside or with a portable system. Besides being able to visualize the pancreas, the real-time system can easily identify bowel loops and the stomach by their peristalsis.

Transducers

As with any other ultrasound study, one should use the highest-frequency transducer possible to be able to adequately visualize the structure being examined.[1] In adults, the transducer frequency may vary from 3 to 5 MHz; in children, a 5- or 7.5-MHz transducer may be used routinely. The focal zone of the transducer should be matched to the depth of the pancreas.[2-4] Magnification of a specific area of interest may improve the fine detail. The time-gain-compensation (TGC) must be adjusted to optimize visualization of the entire gland.[5]

Scan Technique

To perform a complete examination of the pancreas, the examiner must identify and measure all portions of the pancreas (head, neck, body, and tail) in sagittal and transverse planes. The pancreatic contour, shape, and texture should be evaluated. The following structures must also be identified: superior mesenteric artery (SMA), superior mesenteric vein (SMV), portal vein, splenic vein, aorta, inferior vena cava (IVC), and common bile duct (CBD) (Fig. 7-1). In each study, the examiner should attempt to identify the gastroduodenal artery (GDA), common hepatic artery (CHA), pancreatic duct, left renal vein, duodenal bulb, and posterior wall of the stomach (Fig. 7-2). Often, however, the examiner is frustrated by bowel gas artifact and the inability to see the pancreas. The examiner must be prepared to improvise and to alter the standard routine as needed. All possible

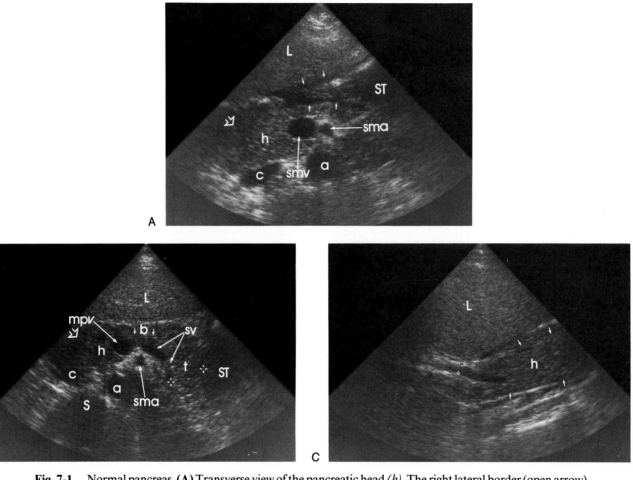

Fig. 7-1. Normal pancreas. **(A)** Transverse view of the pancreatic head *(h)*. The right lateral border (open arrow) of the pancreatic head is somewhat indistinct. The fluid-filled stomach *(ST)* is seen anterior and to the left. The anterior and posterior walls (arrows) of the stomach are seen a lucent stripes anterior to the pancreas. (*L,* liver; *c,* inferior vena cava; *a,* aorta; *sma,* superior mesenteric artery; *smv,* superior mesenteric vein.) **(B)** With the transducer angled to the left, a transverse scan visualizes the pancreatic head *(h)* (open arrow, right lateral border), body *(b)* and tail *(t,* calipers). The pancreatic duct (arrows) is faintly visualized as two echogenic lines within the body. The tail of the pancreas can be measured diagonally at the left lateral border of the aorta *(a)* and the splenic vein *(sv).* The splenic vein is seen extending along the posterior superior aspect of the pancreas. (*L,* liver; *c,* inferior vena cava; *S,* spine; *ST,* stomach; *mpv,* main portal vein; *sma,* superior mesenteric artery.) **(C)** Sagittal view of the pancreatic head *(h,* arrows) with a normal-sized common bile duct (calipers). The anteroposterior and craniocaudad measurements of the head can be made on this scan. The pancreas in all these views is isoechoic to liver *(L).*

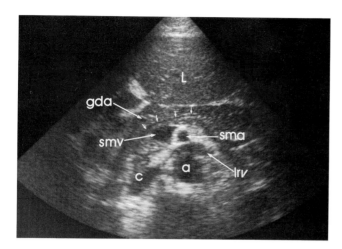

Fig. 7-2. Normal pancreatic texture and duct. Transverse scan. The pancreas and liver *(L)* are isoechoic. The pancreatic duct (arrows) is seen as a tubular lucency bordered by two echogenic lines (arrows). (*a,* aorta; *c,* inferior vena cava; *smv,* superior mesenteric vein; *sma,* superior mesenteric artery; *lrv,* left renal vein; *gda,* gastroduodenal artery.)

innovative techniques should be tried before concluding that the pancreas is impossible to visualize and referring the patient to CT. The success of visualization of the pancreas is directly linked to the persistence of the examiner.

The routine pancreatic examination begins with the patient supine. The lie and elevation of the pancreas must be identified for each patient to establish the correct scan plane and setting.[5] Scans should be taken along the long axis of the gland, as well as perpendicular to the long axis.[5] Sagittal and transverse scans of the head, neck, and body of the pancreas are taken. Measurements of the various portions of the pancreas are also noted. The echopattern of the pancreas is compared with that of the liver. Scans may be taken through the left kidney with the patient prone in order to evaluate the remainder of the tail of the pancreas. The prone position is particularly helpful when ascites interferes with pancreatic visualization.[6] Care should be taken not to mistake splenic flexure and distal transverse colon for the tail of the pancreas, because they cross anterior to the left kidney.[7] The colon is caudal to the tail of the pancreas. Coronal scans also improve the visibility of the pancreas and provide an additional view of the pancreas and peripancreatic region.[8]

As indicated, the goal of every pancreatic ultrasound examination is to successfully visualize the gland in its entirety. To do this in many cases, the examiner must find or produce a suitable acoustic window through which the pancreas can be visualized.[1] The stomach and colon are situated between the anterior abdominal wall and the pancreas. Many times, the left lobe of the liver

overlies the area of the pancreas. These structures can be used for possible acoustic windows in better visualizing the pancreas.

To improve the evaluation of the pancreas, especially if it is poorly seen with the patient supine, the water technique is also used.[9-11] To successfully apply this technique, the examiner must have an accurate conception of the positional changes of the stomach in various examining positions and of relative movements of air and fluid within the stomach.[1,10] The patient is asked to drink approximately 32 to 300 ml of water through a straw while upright or in the left lateral decubitus position.[9] The use of a straw keeps air intake minimal. Also, if the water is drawn up (tap water) and allowed to sit overnight, it will contain fewer microbubbles.[1]

Once the patient has completed the fluid intake, the examination can begin, with the patient either upright or in the left lateral decubitus position. In the upright position (with air in the gastric fundus) the pancreas is localized and scanned. The examiner may need to maneuver the patient and/or transducer positioning to maximize the stomach as an acoustic window. Once the stomach is positioned over the pancreas, the evaluation can begin. Again, by moving the patient and/or transducer, all portions of the pancreas can be identified (Fig. 7-3).

At times, the examination may be more successful if the patient is in the decubitus position, especially if the patient is unable to sit up. By moving the patient progressively from the left lateral decubitus to the right lateral decubitus position, portions of the pancreas may be selectively visualized as water distends the gut lumen.[9] In the right lateral decubitus position, fluid in the gastric antrum and duodenum can be seen, nicely outlining the pancreas (Fig. 7-4). The air in the stomach has moved to the fundus in this position. The pancreas may even be visualized well in the straight supine position. In the left decubitus position, by scanning far to the patient's left one may see portions of the tail of the pancreas.

Some authors in the past have advocated the use of glucagon to inhibit peristalsis. With real-time ultrasound, peristalsis is not a problem. In cases in which the water flows too quickly from the stomach to the small bowel to get an adequate examination of the pancreas, 0.5 to 1 U of glucagon may be given subcutaneously, followed by more fluids orally.[1] The use of glucagon produces gastric fundus dilatation, which provides a sonic window for the examination of the pancreas.[12]

More recent studies have also advocated the use of the water-filled stomach with glucagon for better visualization of the pancreas.[13] Injection of 0.3 mg of glucagon (to stop peristalsis) and administration of water to fill the stomach and duodenum almost always shows the pancreas to better advantage.[13] The disadvantage and cost of glucagon are offset by the great improvement in the quality of sonograms of the pancreas. Occasionally, a

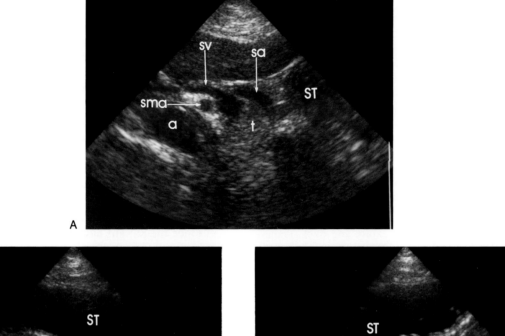

Fig. 7-3. Water technique, erect position. Pancreatic tail and splenic artery. **(A)** Transverse scan with the transducer angled upward and to the left. The fluid-filled stomach *(ST)* is seen anterior to the pancreatic tail *(t)*. (*a,* aorta; *sma,* superior mesenteric artery; *sv,* splenic vein, *sa,* splenic artery.) **(B)** Oblique transverse scan with the transducer angled more to the left than in Fig. A. The fluid-filled stomach *(ST)* is seen anterior to the pancreatic tail *(t)*. At this particular angle, the splenic artery is not visualized and the splenic vein *(sv)* is only faintly seen. (*a,* aorta; *sma,* superior mesenteric artery; *lra,* left renal artery; *lrv,* left renal vein.) **(C)** Sagittal view through the pancreatic tail (arrows) with the fluid-filled stomach *(ST)* anteriorly. (*sa,* splenic artery; *sv,* splenic vein.)

pancreatic pseudomass (caused by the first and second portions of the duodenum) is produced by this technique, but it is generally identified by careful monitoring with real-time.

Still another water technique used for visualization of the pancreas is tubeless hypotonic duodenography.[14] After an overnight fast, the patient drinks 500 ml of tap water (which has stood overnight) to which 2 ml of silicon antifoam emulsion (35 percent ICI, Silcolapse 5000) has been added. In the right lateral decubitus position, the patient is asked to belch. Once microbubbles in the duodenum are removed, 0.3 mg of glucagon is injected intravenously. Then the pancreatic head is scanned.

Good visualization of the fluid-filled distended duodenal loop outlining the pancreatic head is obtained in 90 percent of patients.[14]

Another technique to inhibit peristalsis is to give a fatty meal prior to the oral water.[1] Two to three ounces of fluid fat (Lipomul-oral) may be given, which not only decreases peristalsis but also is a potent inhibitor of gastric emptying.[1,10] One would not give a fatty meal to a patient with pancreatitis, or gallbladder disease.

Still other investigators promote the use of methylcellulose solution prior to fluids.[15] This is an aqueous suspension containing inert, viscid mucliages; it fills the stomach, allowing increased through transmission. Lit-

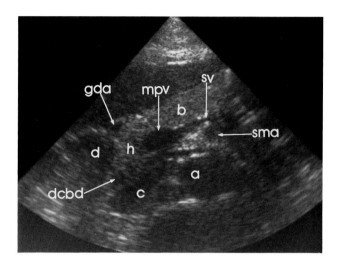

Fig. 7-4. Water technique, right lateral decubitus position. Transverse scan. In this position, the fluid-filled duodenum *(d)* facilitates the visualization of the head *(h)* and body *(b)* of the pancreas and distal common bile duct *(dcbd)*. *(a,* aorta; *c,* inferior vena cava; *mpv,* main portal vein; *sv,* splenic vein; *sma,* superior mesenteric artery; *gda,* gastroduodenal artery.)

tle air is swallowed with it. After administration of intravenous glucagon, the patient may be examined prone.

There has been a newer study that demonstrates the improvement in pancreatic visualization by the use of metoclopramide.[16] Visualization of the pancreas is improved in 44 percent of patients in whom gas obscured the pancreas. There is no improvement when fat is the primary deterrent. Metoclopramide hydrochloride (Reglan, AH Robbins) stimulates gastric and duodenal contractions by sensitizing tissues to acetylcholine, producing increased tone and amplitude of gastric contraction. There is no effect on motility of the colon or gallbladder and no stimulation of pancreatic, gastric, or biliary secretions. Originally, investigators gave the drug in its intravenous form, but the oral form is now available. There are several contraindications to the use of the drug, including (1) situations in which stimulation of gastrointestinal motility might be dangerous (as in gastrointestinal tract obstruction, hemorrhage, or perforation), (2) in patients with pheochromocytoma, and (3) in epileptics receiving medication that might cause extrapyramidal symptoms.[16] Because of its low cost, ready availability, ease of administration, and proven safety in widespread use, metoclopramide might be used more routinely as a premedication in patients in whom gas artifact is present since it appears to improve visualization of the pancreas.[16]

If the patient cannot drink fluid or is not allowed fluid orally, visualization of the pancreas is often significantly

improved by just moving the patient to the upright position.[1,10]

For complete evaluation of the pancreas, the region of the anterior pararenal space must be scanned in addition to the pancreas.[17] The initial examination is performed by using transverse and sagittal planes with the patient semiupright or sitting. If the body, head, or lesser sac region is not well visualized, a small amount (8 to 10 oz) of water is given orally. The patient is placed supine, in the right posterior oblique (RPO) decubitus position for 2 to 3 minutes and then rescanned semiupright slightly RPO. The region of the lesser sac is identified on both transverse and sagittal scans by identifying the posterior wall of the stomach and the pancreatic body (Fig. 7-5). To evaluate the transverse mesocolon region (which lies anterior to the SMA and SMV, beginning at the level of the head of the pancreas and extending caudally), scans are done sagittally along the long axis of the SMV. The region of the tail, lesser sac, and lateral aspect of the left anterior pararenal space is imaged in the coronal plane with the patient in the supine 30 to 45 degree RPO position. For an optimal examination of the lateral aspect of the anterior pararenal space, a coronal scan should be performed in each flank with the transducer over each kidney (Fig. 7-6). Gerota's fascia itself is not visualized, but fluid can be seen as a hypoechoic lesion adjacent to the echogenic fat in patients with anterior pararenal space inflammation (Fig. 7-6C–E). Since the pancreatic tail is adjacent to the splenic hilum, it can be seen in this area.

How often is the pancreas successfully visualized on

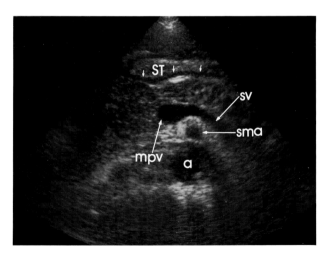

Fig. 7-5. Anterior pararenal space and lesser sac. Transverse view demonstrating the pancreas, with the posterior wall (arrows) of the stomach *(ST)* seen as a lucent stripe anterior to the pancreas. The lesser sac region would be between the posterior wall of the stomach and the pancreas. *(a,* aorta; *sma,* superior mesenteric artery; *mpv,* main portal vein; *sv,* splenic vein.)

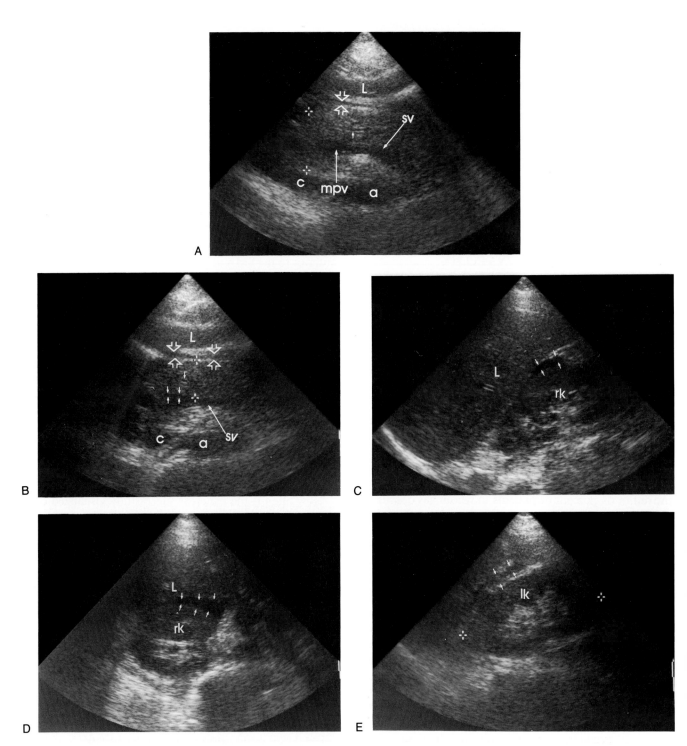

Fig. 7-6. Acute pancreatitis and anterior pararenal space fluid. Transverse views of the (**A**) enlarged head (calipers, 36 mm AP) and (**B**) body (calipers, 24 mm) in a patient with acute pancreatitis. The pancreas is diffusely enlarged but still isoechoic to the liver *(L)*. The portal vein *(mpv)* and splenic vein *(sv)* are poorly defined. There is perivascular inflammation with an indistinct area surrounding the portal and splenic veins as noted on Fig. B by the four small arrows. A normal-sized pancreatic duct (single arrow) is seen within the body. A small amount of fluid is seen anterior to the pancreatic body (open arrows). (*a*, aorta; *c*, inferior vena cava.) (**C**) Sagittal and (**D**) transverse views of the right upper quadrant demonstrating fluid (arrows) within the right anterior pararenal space between the liver *(L)* and right kidney *(rk)*. (**E**) Similarly, fluid (arrows) is seen within the left anterior pararenal space anterior to the left kidney *(lk)*.

an ultrasound examination? This depends on the patient as well as the persistence and thoroughness of the examiner. The head and body should be visualized 90 percent of the time.[18] For obvious reasons, ultrasound is most successful in thin patients.[19] When the water technique is not used, the reported nonvisualization rate is 19 percent.[10] With the water technique, this can be decreased to 1 percent.[10] As such, 93 percent of entire pancreases (head, neck, body, and tail) can be visualized by using all available techniques.[10] The upright position alone without the water technique may permit the visualization in 48 percent.[10]

NORMAL ANATOMY

The pancreas arises from two duodenal buds, dorsal and ventral, which fuse.[20] The ventral bud grows slowly and swings around the gut to join the dorsal bud. The entire body, the tail, and the cephalic portion of the head are from the dorsal anlage, while the caudal portion of the head (and uncinate process) are from the ventral bud. The ventral duct drains into the CBD; the dorsal duct grows from and maintains connection to the duodenum. Anastomoses of the pancreatic head duct system occur with fusion of the dorsal and ventral pancreas. The main pancreatic duct of Wirsung is formed by the anastomosis of the ventral duct with the dorsal duct. There are various degrees of regression of the proximal portion of the dorsal duct; it may completely disappear or remain as an accessory duct of Santorini. In 60 percent of adults, the main pancreatic duct does not empty directly into the duodenum but into the CBD just proximal to the ampulla of Vater.[20]

The normal pancreas in the adult is 15 cm in length and weighs 60 to 100 g.[20] It is usually located at the level of the first or second lumbar vertebra.[5] The pancreas is a nonencapsulated multilobular gland located in the retroperitoneal space extending from the second portion of the duodenum to the splenic hilum. Histologically, it is composed of two components, exocrine and endocrine. The exocrine portion is composed of numerous small glands (acini) aggregated into lobular acini separated by connective tissue. The ductal system begins with extremely fine radicles in secretor acini and, by progressive anastomosis, eventually drains into the duct of Wirsung. The endocrine portion of the pancreas is represented by the islets of Langerhans, which are groups of cells scattered throughout the pancreas.[4]

The regulation of pancreatic secretion is complex; it is related to humoral, vagal, and local neurogenic reflexes.[20] The most important humoral agent is secretin, which is produced in the duodenum. Fats and alcohol

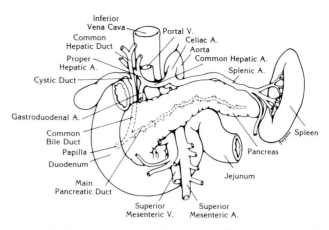

Fig. 7-7. Vascular and ductal landmarks. The relationship of the pancreas to associated vessels and ducts can be seen.

are particularly active stimulators of secretin. Pancreatic secretory activity is also correlated with the ingestion of food. The proteolytic enzymes trypsin and chymotrypsin are secreted as inactive precursors. They are most important in protein-digesting ferments. In addition to the proteases, amylase, lipase, phospholipase, and elastases are all elaborated by the pancreas and activated in the duodenum.[20] The main hormones produced by the endocrine portion of the gland are insulin (in beta cells) and glucagon (in alpha cells).

Examination of the pancreas takes not only persistence, but also an understanding of the normal anatomy of the pancreas and its anatomic landmarks (Fig. 7-7). When evaluating the pancreas, one must look at the parenchymal texture, contour, shape, and echopattern, as well as the sizes of the various portions of the gland and the pancreatic duct. Its blood supply is from the splenic artery, gastroduodenal artery, and SMA.[5] Its venous drainage is through tributaries of the splenic vein and SMV.

Vascular and Ductal Landmarks

Portal Vein and Tributaries

The portal vein is formed behind the neck of the pancreas by the junction of the SMV and the splenic vein (Figs. 7-1B, 7-4, 7-7, and 7-8). The splenic vein runs from the splenic hilum along the posterior superior aspect of the pancreas (Figs. 7-1B, 7-3A & C, and 7-5). The SMV runs posterior to the lower neck of the pancreas and anterior to the uncinate (Figs. 7-1A, 7-2, 7-7, and 7-8C). The portal vein courses superiorly at varying obliquity.[4]

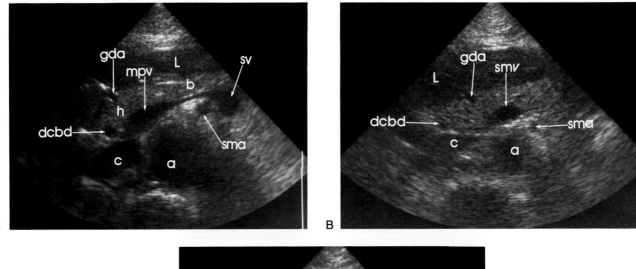

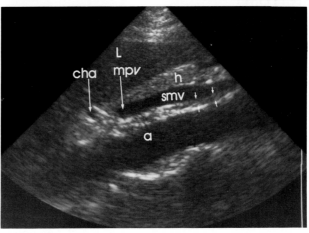

Fig. 7-8. Portal and splenic veins. **(A)** Transverse scan. The splenic vein *(sv)* joins the main portal vein *(mpv)* in the region of the neck of the pancreas. The body *(b)* is measured anterior to the aorta *(a)* and splenic vein. The pancreas is more echodense or hyperechoic than the liver *(L)*. *(gda,* gastroduodenal artery; *sma,* superior mesenteric artery; *c,* inferior vena cava; *dcbd,* distal common bile duct; *h,* pancreatic head.) **(B)** Transverse view of the pancreatic head slightly more inferior than in Fig. A. Anterolateral is the gastroduodenal artery *(gda)* with the distal common bile duct *(dcbd)* lateroinferior. The uncinate process is that portion of the pancreas posterior to the mesenteric vessels. *(smv,* superior mesenteric vein; *sma,* superior mesenteric artery; *a,* aorta; *c,* inferior vena cava; *L,* liver.) **(C)** Sagittal scan. The superior mesenteric vein *(smv)* is seen as a tubular structure paralleling the aorta *(a)* and draining into the main portal vein *(mpv)*. The head *(h)* of the pancreas can be seen inferior to the main portal vein and anterior to the superior mesenteric vein. The uncinate process (arrows) is seen between the aorta and the superior mesenteric vein. The anteroposterior and craniocaudal measurements of the head can be made on this scan. *(cha,* common hepatic artery; *L,* liver.)

Splenic Artery

The splenic artery arises from the celiac artery and runs along the superior margin of the gland, slightly anterior and superior, to follow its vein (Figs. 7-3A & C, 7-7, and 7-9A). As it approaches the lateral portion of the tail, it may run anterior to the pancreatic parenchyma[21] (Fig. 7-3C).

Common Hepatic Artery

The CHA arises from the celiac artery in 92 percent of patients (Fig. 7-9). It courses along the superior margin of the first portion of the duodenum and divides into the proper hepatic artery and GDA, usually when it crosses onto the front of the portal vein (Fig. 7-9). The proper hepatic artery is seen in 75 percent as it proceeds superi-

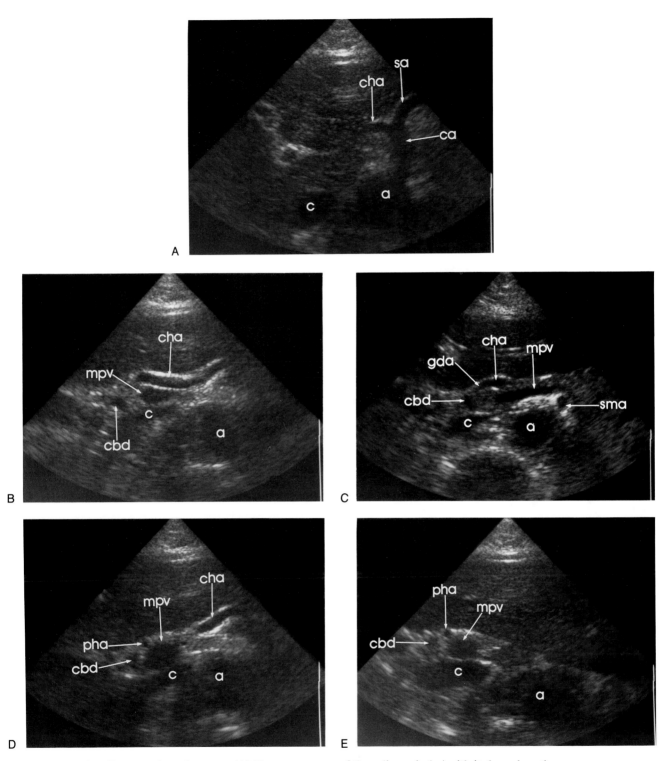

Fig. 7-9. Common hepatic artery. **(A)** Transverse scan of the celiac axis *(ca)* with its branches, the common hepatic artery *(cha)*, and the splenic artery *(sa)*. (*c*, inferior vena cava; *a*, aorta.) **(B)** Transverse oblique scan angled to the right from Fig. A). The common hepatic artery *(cha)* continues toward the porta hepatis. (*mpv*, main portal vein; *cbd*, common bile duct; *c*, inferior vena cava; *a*, aorta.) **(C)** Transverse scan angled more to the right than Fig. B, following the course of the common hepatic artery *(cha)* as it gives off the gastroduodenal artery *(gda)* branch. (*cbd*, common bile duct; *mpv*, main portal vein; *sma*, superior mesenteric artery; *c*, inferior vena cava; *a*, aorta.) **(D & E)** Transverse oblique scans with the transducer angled more toward the porta hepatis with visualization of the relationship of the common bile duct *(cbd)*, main portal vein *(mpv)*, and proper hepatic artery *(pha)*, (*c*, inferior vena cava; *a*, aorta; *cha*, common hepatic artery.)

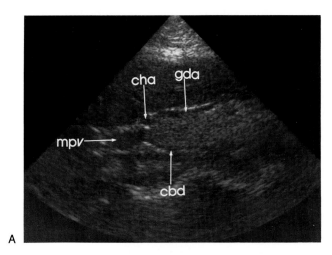 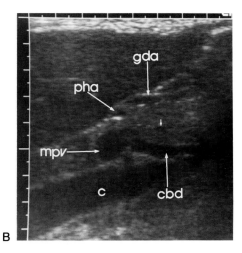

A   B

Fig. 7-10. Gastroduodenal artery and common bile duct. **(A & B)** Sagittal views of the pancreas demonstrating the relationship of the common bile duct *(cbd)*, gastroduodenal artery *(gda)*, and common hepatic artery *(cha)*. Fig. B is slightly to the right of Fig. A with the proper hepatic artery *(pha)* seen after the gastroduodenal artery branch in Fig. A. (arrow, pancreatic duct; *mpv,* main portal vein; *c,* inferior vena cava.)

orly along the anterior aspect of the portal vein with the CBD lateral to it (Fig. 7-9D & E). The GDA is less frequently seen (30 percent) (Figs. 7-2, 7-4, and 7-8 to 7-10) as it travels a short distance along the anterior aspect of the head just to the right of the neck before it divides into the superior pancreaticoduodenal branches (anterior and posterior). They join with their counterparts (inferior pancreaticoduodenal branches), which arise from the SMA. In some (14 percent), the right hepatic artery arises from the SMA, courses posterior to the medial portions of the splenic vein, and runs along the aspect of the portal vein.

Superior Mesenteric Artery

The SMA arises from the aorta behind the lower portion of the body and courses anterior to the third portion of the duodenum to enter the small bowel mesentery (Fig. 7-11). The SMA runs directly anterior to the aorta but may be tortuous (Figs. 7-1 to 7-3, 7-7, 7-8, and 7-11).

Common Bile Duct

The CBD crosses the anterior aspect of the portal vein to the right of the proper hepatic artery (Figs. 7-7 and 7-9). As the portal vein crosses anterior to the IVC, the duct passes off the front of the portal vein and goes behind the first portion of the duodenum to course inferior and somewhat posterior in the parenchyma of the head of the pancreas, where it is close to the second portion of the duodenum (Figs. 7-1C, 7-4, and 7-8 to 7-10). It joins the pancreatic duct close to the ampulla. In the head of

the pancreas, the internal diameter is not more than 4 mm (Figs. 7-4, 7-8, and 7-10).

Portions of the Pancreas

Head

The head of the pancreas is the portion of the pancreas to the right of the SMV (Figs. 7-1, 7-2, 7-4, 7-8, and 7-10). Its right lateral border is the second portion of the duodenum, which can often be identified by the air and/ or fluid within it (Fig. 7-4). The IVC is posterior to the

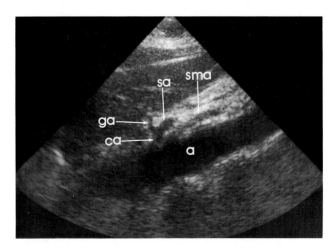

Fig. 7-11. Superior mesenteric artery. Sagittal scan. The superior mesenteric artery *(sma)* is seen to be the second branch of the abdominal aorta *(a),* with the celiac artery *(ca)* being the first branch. (*ga,* left gastric artery; *sa,* splenic artery.)

head of the pancreas.[5] Often, anteriorly the GDA (first branch of the CHA) can be identified (Fig. 7-8). The CBD can be seen anterior and lateral to the gastroduodenal artery (Figs. 7-8 and 7-10). The portal vein is cranial to the head[5] (Figs. 7-8C and 7-10). The uncinate process is usually included as the portion of the pancreatic head that is directly posterior to the SMV (Fig. 7-8C). The head of the pancreas is measured in the anteroposterior axis in the transverse plane, taking the maximum dimension (Figs. 7-1A and 7-8B). It is also measured in the sagittal plane, again taking the maximum anteroposterior axis (Figs. 7-1C, 7-8C, and 7-10). Normally, the head should measure 2.08 ± 0.40 cm transversely and 2.01 ± 0.39 cm longitudinally.[4,22,23]

Neck

The neck of the pancreas is the portion directly anterior to the SMV on a sagittal or transverse scan[5] (Figs. 7-1A, 7-2, and 7-8B). The portal vein is formed behind the neck of the pancreas by the junction of the SMV and the splenic vein[4] (Fig. 7-8C). It separates the body from the head of the pancreas. The neck is measured over the SMV. Its anteroposterior measurement is 1.00 ± 0.30 cm in the sagittal plane and 0.95 ± 0.26 cm in the transverse plane.[4,22]

Body

Although the anteroposterior dimensions of the body are small, it still represents the largest section of the pancreas. It can be seen anterior to the SMA (Figs. 7-1 to 7-4 and 7-8). Its anterior border is the posterior wall of the antrum of the stomach. Its right lateral border is the neck of the gland that is anterior to the SMV. Its left lateral border is not definite. The splenic vein courses along the posterior surface of the body[5] (Figs. 7-1B and 7-3). The tail of the pancreas begins at the left lateral margin of the vertebral body. The body measures 1.18 ± 0.36 cm in the longitudinal plane and 1.16 ± 0.29 cm in the transverse plane when measured over the SMA in the anteroposterior projection.[4,22]

Tail

The tail of the pancreas is the most difficult portion to visualize. It begins just to the left of the left lateral border of the vertebral body and extends to the splenic hilum[4] (Figs. 7-1B, 7-3, 7-5, and 7-8A). It may be at a higher level than the body (41 percent) or at the same level (51 percent), and it is infrequently (2 percent) at a lower level.[4] The splenic vein courses along the posterior surface of the body and tail (Fig. 7-3). The tail is seen ante-

rior to the left kidney, posterior to the stomach, and medial to the spleen (Fig. 7-3). It appears ovoid or elliptical and has the same echogenicity as on the supine view.[6] It should not be confused with the empty stomach; oral fluid may be given if there is a question.[24]

Size

Adult

A number of investigators have evaluated pancreatic size.[22,23,25] As expected, the size of the pancreas in adults normally decreases with age. All of the following measurements are made in the anteroposterior projection obtained at right angles to the true axis of the gland. They include the following: head, 2.01 ± 0.39 cm sagittally, 2.08 ± 0.40 cm transversely; body, 1.18 ± 0.36 cm sagittally, 1.16 ± 0.29 cm transversely; neck, 1.00 ± 0.30 cm sagittally, 0.95 ± 0.26 cm transversely; and tail, 0.7 to 2.8 cm.[4,22,23] The craniocaudal measurements include the following: head, 2.4 to 4.8 cm; body, 2.4 to 3.6 cm, and tail, 1.6 to 2.4 cm.[4] Taking a maximum dimension of 2.8 cm will embrace 96 percent of the normal population, but normal measurements do not exclude the presence of abnormalities.[22] Absolute measurements of pancreatic size may be misleading; symmetry and contour may be more important.[4]

Child

As expected, the pancreas is small in children and increases with age.[26] With advanced age, the gland again becomes smaller.[4] The head of the pancreas is measured in an anteroposterior projection including the uncinate process. The body is measured in an anteroposterior projection anterior to the aorta and splenic vein. The tail is measured in an anteroposterior projection diagonally at the left lateral border of the aorta and splenic vein. The measurements are given in Table 7-1.

TABLE 7-1. Measurements of Pancreatic Size in the Child

Age (yr)	Mean Size (cm) and Range[a]		
	Head	Body	Tail
0–6	1.6 (1.0–1.9)	0.7 (0.4–1.0)	1.2 (0.8–1.6)
7–12	1.9 (1.7–2.0)	0.9 (0.6–1.0)	1.4 (1.3–1.6)
13–18	2.0 (1.8–2.2)	1.0 (0.7–1.0)	1.6 (1.3–1.8)

[a] Measurements made in the anteroposterior axis on a transverse scan.
(From Coleman et al,[26] with permission.)

TABLE 7-2. Correlation of Pancreatic Size to the Transverse Lumbar Vertebral Body Measurement

Group	Range	Average	Standard Deviation
Control	0.24–0.41	0.3	0.06
Acute pancreatitis	0.21–1.0	0.58	0.24
Chronic pancreatitis	0.28–0.30	0.3	0.12

(From Fleischer et al,[27] with permission.)

Other investigators have correlated pancreatic size to the transverse lumbar vertebral body measurement.[27] The ratio of the greatest anteroposterior dimension of the body of the pancreas relative to the transverse vertebral body measurement (*P/V* ratio) was noted to be greater than 0.3 when associated with a hypoechoic parenchyma indicative of acute pancreatitis. The measurements are given in Table 7-2.

In a study that evaluated the normal and abnormal pancreas in children, the investigators found that correlation with age was as good as, or better than, correlation with other physical parameters.[28] These authors tabulated data for patients less than 1 month of age and those 1 month to 1 year of age. They noted that the pancreas grows substantially in the first year of life but much more slowly between 1 and 18 years.[28] The measurements are given in Table 7-3.

Other authors have found that pancreatic size correlated better with height; they found that it varied within each height group, especially in the short axis.[29]

Shape

Various shapes have been ascribed to the pancreas. They include sausage, dumbbell, and tadpole.[5,30] More commonly, the pancreas is described as comma-shaped with the larger portion being its head (Figs. 7-1, 7-2, and 7-8).

TABLE 7-3. Maximum Anteroposterior Dimensions of Pancreas

Age	No. of Patients	Mean Size (cm) ± 1 SD		
		Head	Body	Tail
<1 mo	15	1.0 ± 0.4	0.6 ± 0.2	1.0 ± 0.4
1 mo–1 yr	23	1.5 ± 0.5	0.8 ± 0.3	1.2 ± 0.4
1–5 yr	49	1.7 ± 0.3	1.0 ± 0.2	1.8 ± 0.4
5–10 yr	69	1.6 ± 0.4	1.0 ± 0.3	1.8 ± 0.4
10–19 yr	117	2.0 ± 0.5	1.1 ± 0.3	2.0 ± 0.4

(From Siegel et al,[28] with permission.)

Texture

A number of investigators have evaluated the normal echopattern or texture of the pancreas. The degree of echogenicity is determined to a greater extent by the amount of fat between the lobules and to a lesser extent by interlobular fibrous tissue.[4] The internal echoes of the pancreas consist of regularly and closely spaced elements of uniform intensity with uniformly distributed variation throughout the gland.[2]

Normally, when comparing the echopattern of the pancreas with that of the liver, the pancreas is either isosonic (as dense as the liver) (Figs. 7-1, 7-2, and 7-5) or hyperechoic (more dense than liver)[5,19,31–33] (Figs. 7-4, 7-8, and 7-10). Several studies have shown that the isosonic pattern represents 46 to 48 percent of normal individuals and the hyperechoic pattern represents 49 to 52 percent of normal individuals.[4,34] All agree that the normal pancreas is not less echodense than the liver.[34] This entire assignment of pattern is based on the assumption the liver is normal, using it as an internal standard. If there is significant hepatocellular disease and the liver is abnormally dense, the normal pancreas may appear less dense than the liver (Fig. 7-12).

It is known that with increasing age and body fat deposition, there are increased amounts of fat in the pancreas, accounting for an increased echodensity, and that these function independently.[35] The echodensity of the pancreas in adults is greater than that in children because the pancreas contains less fat in children.[4] In a histologic study, it was shown that after age 60, there is moderate to severe fat accumulation in the acinar cells of the pan-

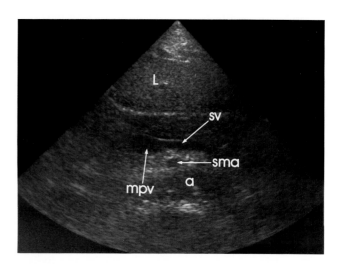

Fig. 7-12. Hypoechoic pancreatic texture. Transverse scan. This patient is known to have severe hepatocellular disease with a dense echopattern within the liver. The normal pancreas appears less dense than the liver *(L)*. (*a*, aorta; *sma*, superior mesenteric artery; *mpv*, main portal vein; *sv*, splenic vein.)

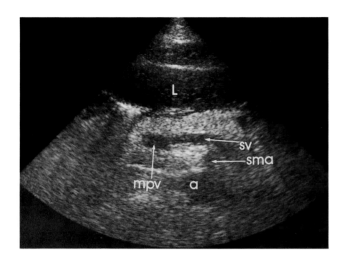

Fig. 7-13. Echodense pancreatic texture. Transverse scan. The pancreatic outline cannot be identified in this elderly obese patient. The pancreas is similar in density to retroperitoneal fat (more dense than the usual hyperechoic pancreas). Many of the normal vascular landmarks for the pancreas are seen. (*a*, aorta; *sma*, superior mesenteric artery; *mpv*, main portal vein; *sv*, splenic vein; *L*, liver.)

creas.[35] This may account for some of the problems in visualizing the pancreas. As the pancreas becomes more echodense, it tends to become less distinguishable from surrounding retroperitoneal fat (Fig. 7-13). The pancreas should normally be less echogenic than retroperitoneal fat.[5] However, the pancreatic echogenicity may not be entirely due to fat; fibrous tissue may account for a portion of the increased echogenicity.[31] When the pancreas is sufficiently dense that it cannot be distinguished from fat, it can be identified by the vascular anatomy.[4]

There have been few reports describing the echogenicity of the pancreas in premature and newborn infants. In one reported study, the normal pancreas usually appeared to be hyperechoic relative to the liver.[36] This pattern was found in 83 percent of premature infants and 60 percent of neonates. The cause of this pattern was not known but was postulated to be due to the prominent connective tissue septa between lobules, as well as supportive reticular tissue within lobules, in premature infants. By term, these tissues diminish and a prominent lobular pattern is seen with glandular elements closely packed together.

Prepancreatic Fat Deposition

At times, prepancreatic fat deposition may cause a problem in diagnosing pancreatic abnormalities.[37] This prepancreatic fat may vary from lucent relative to the echogenic pancreas to highly echogenic. The presence of

this fat is suggested if a less echogenic area is seen anterior to and delineated from the pancreas. The examiner must be aware of this prepancreatic fat and must differentiate it from fluid in the lesser sac, thickened gastric wall, and lymphadenopathy.[37]

Lipomatosis of the Pancreas

Lipomatosis of the pancreas, which is very common, is believed to be a paraphysiologic condition.[38] One group of authors reported a case with small nodular masses near each other in the region of the body and tail of the pancreas.[38] These masses had sharp, irregular contours with small echofree areas within; they were not homogeneously hypoechoic. It was postulated that the decreased echopattern associated with adipose tissue within the pancreas might be related to fibrosis, which makes the pancreas more echogenic and the adipose fat less echogenic. The possibility of lipomatosis of the pancreas should be kept in mind when masses are identified within the pancreas.

Other investigators describe a marked discrepancy between the anterior and posterior parts of the pancreas with ultrasound; this discrepancy is associated with uneven lipomatosis.[39] In the cases reported, the dorsal portion of the pancreatic head appeared less echogenic while the ventral part of the head, body, and tail appeared more echogenic (Fig. 7-14). The level of demarcation appeared to correspond to the expected fusion line of the embryologic dorsal and ventral pancreatic origin. This is

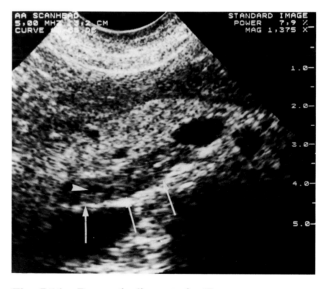

Fig. 7-14. Pancreatic lipomatosis. Transverse sonogram. There is a marked difference in echogenicity between the anterior and posterior parts (arrows) of the pancreatic head. (arrowhead, distal bile duct.) (From Marchal et al,[39] with permission.)

associated with uneven lipomatosis as demonstrated at pathologic examination.[39] This pattern may prove problematic since focal areas of hypoechogenicity are usually considered to be tumors. In this series ultrasound was considered more sensitive than CT in the detection of minor fat infiltration. The origin of the uneven pattern of lipomatosis is unclear.

Pancreatic insufficiency may be associated with complete replacement of the pancreas by fat.[40] Additionally, this condition may be associated with aging and increased body fat. It also occurs in patients with malabsorption syndrome, cystic fibrosis, obesity, diabetes mellitus, hereditary pancreatitis, and chronic pancreatitis.[40] In this condition, the pancreas may appear normal in size or may be massively enlarged, resulting in a condition known as lipomatous pseudohypertrophy. Although the pancreas may appear to have a normal echopattern on ultrasound, it may be seen to be replaced with fat on CT.

Other conditions appear to be associated with increased pancreatic echogenicity, including the ingestion of steroids.[41] As mentioned earlier, the normal pancreatic echogenicity appears to be related mainly to age and body fat. The retroperitoneal and pancreatic fat deposition is a normal phenomenon associated with aging and is seen to a greater extent in obese individuals. In one study, patients on doses of prednisone greater than 7.5 mg/day for longer than 6 months showed statistically significant changes in the pancreatic echogenicity when allowances were made for age and body fat. In a young person, a highly echogenic person may signify chronic pancreatitis. However, if that diagnosis is excluded, ingestion of steroids should be considered. There may be several reasons for the pattern associated with steroids. It may be related to abnormal fat metabolism and fat deposition due to an endocrine effect of the steroids, or the fatty infiltration may be secondary to a subacute pancreatitis.

Pancreatic Duct

Although it was once thought there was a high incidence of pancreatic disease associated with the visualization of the pancreatic duct, the normal pancreatic duct is commonly seen with the high-resolution real-time ultrasound systems currently available.[42-44] It is seen more frequently in the body (straightest portion) (82 to 86 percent) of the pancreas and least frequently in the tail.[4,5,42,45] The duct appears as an echogenic line or a lucency bordered by two echogenic lines[5,46,47] (Figs. 7-1B, 7-2, 7-10B, and 7-15). This duct is the duct of Wirsung or the main pancreatic duct and originates at the junction of the small ducts in the lobules of the tail as the conduit for pancreatic juice.[5] The accessory duct of

Santorini runs transversely in the upper anterior portion of the pancreatic head at a higher level than the main pancreatic duct.[4]

The main duct passes steeply cephalad from the papilla of Vater obliquely to the left, then transversely and upward across the midline to the left of the spine, and then upward more steeply in the tail[48] (Fig. 7-15). It can be easily seen in the standard ventral abdominal wall approach and axial plane.[43] The scanhead frequently has to be tilted or in an off-axis plane for optimal visualization. Visualization of the duct in the tail is more difficult; it is aided by changes in patient position or by oral ingestion of fluid. Failure to see the duct in the tail is presumed to be secondary to the small caliber as well as to technical difficulty. In the head, the duct has a dorsal-ventral course and is parallel to the ultrasound beam, so the right coronal view is usually needed for optimal visualization[43] (Fig. 7-15).

The mean internal diameter (measured in anteroposterior projection on a transverse scan) of the main duct is 3 mm in the area of the head and neck, 2.1 mm in the body proximal to the neck, and 1.6 mm in the body distal to the neck.[49] It then decreases toward the tail.[5,49] Normally, the duct should not measure more than 2 mm in internal diameter.[42,43,45,47] It is considered abnormal if it is greater than 2 mm or has nonparallel or convex walls (focal dilatation or beading).[42,43] Analysis of the pancreatic duct size and wall contour changes is not helpful in arriving at a specific histologic diagnosis.[43,47,50] In one series, 50 percent of patients with pancreatitis had a dilated duct.[43]

There is a discrepancy between ultrasound and endoscopic retrograde cholangiopancreatography (ERCP) in normal duct measurements.[46] The discrepancy may be due to the injection of contrast in the duct under pressure. The ultrasound measurement may be underestimated because the echoes of the wall of the duct are strong, causing apparent thickening of the walls, which results in underestimation of the inner diameter. There may also be difficulty in visualizing the duct in the head and tail, which is thought to be caused by a variable course of the duct and interfering echoes from neighboring organs, particularly the bowel (as a result of gas).[46]

Real-time ultrasound may be used to guide a thin-needle puncture of the duct. Percutaneous pancreatic ductography and percutaneous biopsy can be successfully performed as a single procedure without major complications.[46]

When identifying the pancreatic duct, the examiner should take care not to mistake the splenic vein, splenic artery, or posterior wall of the stomach for the duct[42,51,52] (Figs. 7-1B, 7-3, and 7-5). The splenic vein can be followed to its portal vein junction by real-time scanning if there is a question (Figs. 7-1B and 7-3A). The splenic artery is superior to the body and tail of the pancreas

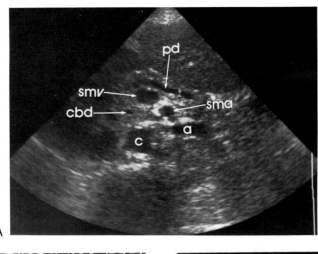

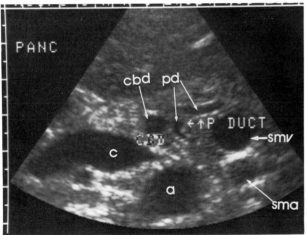

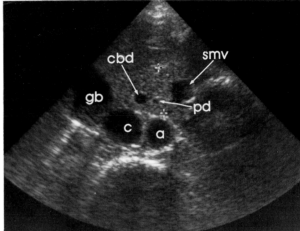

Fig. 7-15. Normal pancreatic duct. Transverse scans at (**A**) the level of the pancreatic body, (**B**) more inferior (magnified, more angled), and (**C**) at the level of the head demonstrating the relationship of the main pancreatic duct (*pd*, 2.5 mm in Fig. A) and common bile duct *(cbd)*. (*smv*, superior mesenteric vein; *sma*, superior mesenteric artery; *c*, inferior vena cava; *a*, aorta; *gb*, gallbladder.)

(Fig. 7-3A & C). It can be followed back to its origin in the celiac axis by real-time ultrasound.[51] The posterior wall of the antrum is directly anterior to the body of the pancreas (Figs. 7-1A, 7-5, and 7-15). It appears as an anechoic structure surrounded on both sides by an echogenic rim with the lumen of the stomach appearing dense.[5,52] It can easily be identified by having the patient drink fluid and by identifying the vascular landmarks.

Normal Variant

Left-Sided Pancreas

A left-sided pancreas is an unusual condition in which the pancreas lies wholly to the left of the aorta while maintaining the normal relationship to the SMA, SMV,

and splenic vein (although these vessels are displaced to the left).[53] It is possible that it is an acquired positional variation related to increasing laxity of retroperitoneal tissues with age.

CONGENITAL ABNORMALITIES

Congenital abnormalities of the pancreas other than cystic fibrosis are uncommon.[20] Agenesis or hypoplasia of the pancreas can occur; neither can be diagnosed by ultrasound. An annular pancreas represents persistence of the dorsal and ventral pancreas with the head encircling the duodenum.[20] Ultrasound may be able to identify a mass associated with the duodenal obstruction; there have been no case reports. Aberrant or ectopic pancreas is present in 2 percent of routine postmortem examinations.[20] The most favored sites are the stomach and duodenum, with jejunum, a Meckel's diverticulum, and ileum less common. The mass is usually 3 to 4 cm. There have been no ultrasound reports of this entity either.

Pancreas Divisum

Pancreas divisum is a common anomaly, which occurs when the dorsal and ventral pancreatic ducts fail to fuse during embryonic development.[54] It is present in up to 11 percent of necropsy specimens and up to 5.8 percent of asymptomatic patients undergoing ERCP.[54] Although most patients with this anomaly remain asymptomatic, recurrent acute pancreatitis and chronic pancreatic pain have both been reported. The ductal criteria for diagnosis is the failure to see union of the dorsal and ventral ducts and the ability to see the ventral duct directly joining the CBD.[54] ERCP remains the definitive diagnostic technique.

Cysts

Congenital cysts result from anomalous development of the pancreatic ducts.[20] They are usually multiple, ranging from microscopic to 3 to 5 cm in size.[20] Autopsy studies have shown pancreatic cysts to be one of the most common manifestations of von Hippel-Lindau syndrome, occurring in over 70 percent of patients with this condition.[55] These cysts can replace and enlarge the entire gland.[55] Exocrine and endocrine pancreatic insufficiency has been considered a result of the polycystic changes, although the cysts are usually asymptomatic.[55] These cysts appear as well-defined anechoic areas with acoustic enhancement (Fig. 7-16).

Less commonly are enteric cysts involving the pancreas.[56] These lesions more often involve the distal ileum, posterior mediastinum, and third part of the duodenum. The duodenal cysts can involve the pancreas and can be seen as a lobular or single cyst in the region of the pancreatic head.[56]

Cystic Fibrosis

Cystic fibrosis is the single most lethal genetic disease in the white population, with a conservative estimation of an incidence of 1 in 2,000; 1 in 20 individuals are genetic carriers.[57] Because of improvements in antimicrobial therapy, physical therapy, and general medical care, patients with cystic fibrosis are living longer and the disease is becoming recognized as a disease of adolescents and young adults.[57,58] The incidence of abdominal

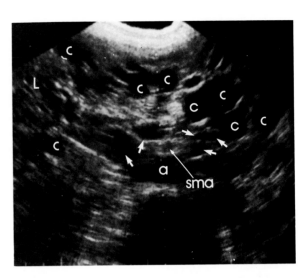

Fig. 7-16. Pancreatic cysts. Transverse scan. Several pancreatic cysts (arrows) are seen as well-defined anechoic areas within the pancreatic area in this patient with polycystic liver and kidney disease. (*c*, liver cysts; *sma*, superior mesenteric artery; *a* aorta; *L*, liver.)

problems specifically related to the liver, biliary tract, and pancreas increases with age.[58] Now more than 50 percent of newly diagnosed patients with cystic fibrosis survive to be 20 years old or older.[57]

The complications of cystic fibrosis are related to the increased secretion of abnormal mucus by the exocrine glands.[4,58] As such, the disease is variable. In the pancreas, there is precipitation or coagulation of secretions in the small pancreatic ducts; this forms obstructing eosinophilic concretions.[58] The proximal distension of the ductules and acini leads to their degeneration and replacement by small cysts. Atrophy of glandular elements

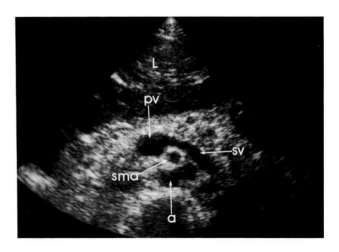

Fig. 7-17. Cystic fibrosis. Transverse scan of a child with cystic fibrosis. The pancreas is more echogenic than the liver, inhomogeneous, and poorly defined. (*a*, aorta; *sma*, superior mesenteric artery; *pv*, portal vein; *sv*, splenic vein; *L*, liver.)

and replacement of the altered architecture by fibrosis or fat are late changes. In 80 percent of patients, pancreatic achylia results, with attendant malabsorption.[58]

The identification of the pancreas in patients with cystic fibrosis is hampered by distension and redundancy of the gastrointestinal tract related to malabsorption and the lack of a scan window through the left lobe of the liver. The anteroposterior diameter of the abdomen is increased as a result of emphysema. In most patients, the pancreas appears echogenic, but often it is not appreciated as a defined homogeneous organ[57-59] (Figs. 7-17 and 7-18). A very common finding is a decrease in anteroposterior diameters of the pancreas and a pronounced age-independent increase in tissue echogenicity.[60] The increased echoes are thought to be due to fibrosis and fat infiltration.[4] The echodensity of the pancreas and the liver cannot be compared because the liver is often abnormal. Up to the stage at which there is total or near-total replacement of the pancreas by fat, there is no correlation between histologic findings and pancreatic function as judged by pancreatic function tests. The availability of ultrasound and CT to monitor the progression of cystic fibrosis is helpful in assessing the prognosis of a patient with this disease.[59,60]

The hepatic disease in patients with cystic fibrosis is an enigma. There is focal biliary cirrhosis (or fibrosis) with increasing frequency as patients age. This may be due to mechanical obstruction of the bile ductules by inspissated secretions. Progressive multinodular biliary cirrhosis occurs. Complications (specifically portal hypertension and sequelae) related to chronic hepatic disease occur in 2 percent of patients.[58] The liver is enlarged, with an increased echogenicity.[4]

The spleen is noted to be enlarged, with increased echogenicity assumed to be due to hemosiderin and/or fibrosis.[58]

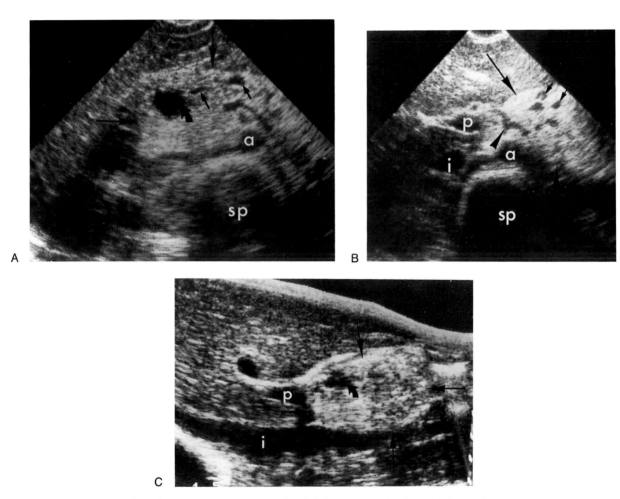

Fig. 7-18. Cystic fibrosis. Transverse scans showing **(A)** the head and body and **(B)** the tail. The pancreas (large arrows) is markedly enlarged and has increased echogenicity. The small hypoechoic areas probably represent small cysts (small arrows). The dilated common bile duct (curved arrow) is seen in transverse and **(C)** longitudinal scans. (*sp*, spine; *a*, aorta; *i*, inferior vena cava; *p*, portal vein; arrowhead, celiac bifurcation.) (From Daneman et al,[59] with permission.)

In the gastrointestinal tract, there are thickened irregular folds. Hyperplasia of Brunner's glands may account for the "donut" sign often seen in these patients.[58]

As far as the biliary tract is concerned, there is nonvisualization of the gallbladder in many patients. There may be obstruction of the cystic duct from mucosal hyperplasia, inspissated mucus, or actual atresia of the duct. The lumen is filled with thick bile, sludge, or defined concretions. The wall of the gallbladder is thickened or normal.[58]

ACUTE PANCREATITIS

The etiology and pathogenesis of acute pancreatitis are not clearly understood. The attack is related to biliary tract disease and alcoholism.[4,61] Gallstones are present in 40 to 60 percent of patients, and 5 percent of patients with gallstones present with acute pancreatitis.[20] Other rare causes include trauma, extension of inflammation from adjacent peptic ulcer disease or abdominal infection, blood-borne bacterial infection, viral infection (mumps), vascular thrombosis and embolism, polyarteritis nodosa, hypothermia, and drugs (corticosteroids, sulfonamides, oral contraceptives). Acute pancreatitis is also associated with hyperlipoproteinemia and hyperparathyroidism. It is idiopathic in 9 to 50 percent of patients.[20] Most cases occur in middle age.

The mechanism of acute pancreatitis is not firmly established. The anatomic changes in the pancreas are caused by the destructive lytic effects of the pancreatic enzymes proteases, lipase, and elastase, which are the keys to pancreatic destruction. There are several proposals to explain the production of acute pancreatitis: (1) bile reflux — important mechanism for activation of pancreatic enzymes; (2) hypersecretion and obstruction — rupture of ducts by pancreatic hypersecretion possibly potentiated by partial duct obstruction; (3) alcohol-induced changes — precise manner of the production of pancreatitis is unknown, but alcohol is a potent stimulator of pancreatic secretions; and (4) duodenal reflux — favored as the initiating mechanism by many authors.[20,62]

The morphologic changes in acute pancreatitis are many and varied.[61] The basic alterations include (1) proteolytic destruction of the pancreatic substance; (2) necrosis of blood vessels with subsequent hemorrhage; (3) necrosis of fat by lipolytic enzymes; and (4) accompanying inflammatory reaction.[20] The extent and predominance of each of these changes depends on the duration and severity of the process. It may be mild and self-limiting with transient edema. There may be interstitial edema that eventually leads to focal and frank necrosis.

Leukocyte reaction between areas of hemorrhage and necrosis and secondary bacterial invasion convert the areas into foci of suppurative necrosis or abscess. With time, the gland is replaced by diffuse or focal parenchymal or stromal fibrosis, calcifications, and irregular duct dilatation.[20]

The process may be severe, with damage to the acinar tissue and duct system producing damage by the exudation of pancreatic juice into the interstitium of the gland, leakage of secretions into the peripancreatic tissues, or both. After disruption of the acini or duct, the pancreatic secretions migrate to the surface of the gland. These secretions may take several pathways. The most common course is for the fluid to break through the pancreatic connective tissue layer and thin posterior layer of the peritoneum and enter the lesser sac. The pancreatic juice enters the anterior pararenal space by breaking through the thin layer of the fibrous connective tissue; alternatively, the fluid might migrate to the surface of the gland and remain within the confines of the fibrous connective tissue layer.[62]

The collections of fluid in the peripancreatic area generally retain communication with the pancreas. A dynamic equilibrium is established so that fluid is continuously absorbed from the collection and replaced by additional pancreatic secretions. Centrifugal drainage of the pancreatic juices may cease as the pancreatic inflammatory response subsides and the rate of pancreatic secretion returns to normal. Collections of extrapancreatic fluid should be reabsorbed or, if drained, should not recur with recovery of proper drainage through the duct.[62]

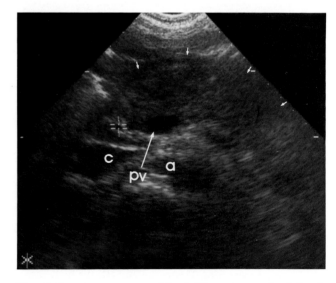

Fig. 7-19. Acute pancreatitis. Diffuse. A poorly defined, somewhat hypoechoic pancreas (arrows) is seen anterior to the poorly defined portal vein *(pv)*. (*c*, inferior vena cava; *a*, aorta; calipers, common bile duct.)

Because acute pancreatitis produces a combination of unfavorable and favorable consequences, the phenomenon of escape and pooling of pancreatic secretions occurs. The symptoms of this complication are prolonged, including persistent abdominal pain, fever, and leukocytosis beyond the 5 days of the usual attack of acute pancreatitis. Patients with these symptoms are at risk for abscess and hemorrhage. With expulsion of the pancreatic secretions, the pancreas itself appears to be spared, serving to decompress the gland. In complicated pancreatitis, there is an inverse relationship between the degree of autodigestion of the gland and the volume of peripancreatic fluid.[62]

The clinical course of acute pancreatitis usually begins with severe pain after a large meal or alcoholic binge. The pain is constant and intense. The serum amylase level increases within 24 hours, and the serum lipase level increases within 72 to 94 hours.[20] Five percent of these patients will die of the acute effects of the peripheral vascular collapse and shock during the first week of the clinical course.[20] Acute adult respiratory distress syndrome and acute tubular necrosis frequently accompany pancreatitis and are particularly ominous. Other complications include pseudocyst formation (10 percent), phlegmon (18 percent), abscess (1 to 9 percent), hemorrhage (5 percent), and duodenal obstruction.[20,63,64]

On ultrasound, there are several characteristic findings associated with acute pancreatitis.[4,26,62,65-69] The pancreas appears normal in 29 percent of cases.[4] There is a diffuse increase in the size of the gland in 52 percent of cases, with loss of the normal sonographic texture or focal enlargement in 28 percent of cases.[4] The affected gland has been described as hypoechoic to anechoic and less echogenic than liver (Fig. 7-19). However, with the high-resolution ultrasound now available, the echopattern appears to be isoechoic to liver in most cases (Figs. 7-6 and 7-20 to 7-22). The borders of the pancreas may

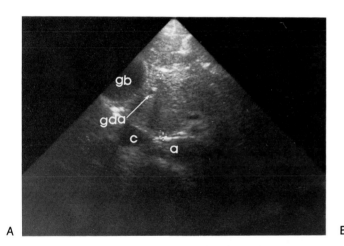

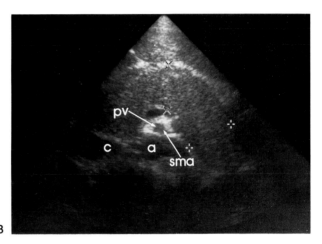

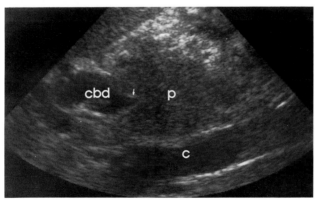

Fig. 7-20. Acute pancreatitis. Diffuse. The entire pancreas is enlarged, as seen on transverse scans, with **(A)** the head measuring 35 mm AP and **(B)** the body measuring 25 mm AP, and the tail measuring 27 mm AP, (*gb,* gallbladder; *gda,* gastroduodenal artery; *c,* inferior vena cava; *a,* aorta; *pv,* portal vein, *sma,* superior mesenteric artery.) **(C)** Oblique sagittal view through the pancreatic head *(p)* and distal common bile duct *(cbd)* demonstrating a narrowed distal end (arrow) to the duct. On ERCP, there was a stenosis at the distal end of the common bile duct. The pancreas is uniform in echopattern and isoechoic to liver.

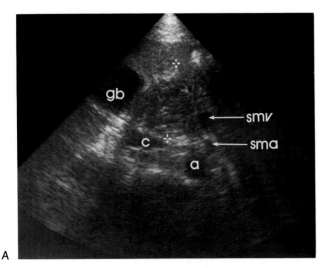 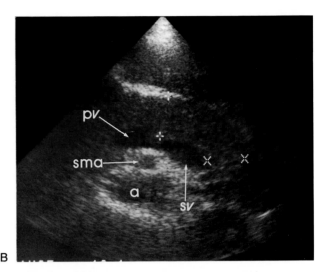

Fig. 7-21. Acute pancreatitis. Diffuse. Transverse scans of **(A)** the pancreatic head and **(B)** the body and tail demonstrate a diffusely enlarged isoechoic pancreas (head, 4.5 cm AP; body, 22 mm AP; tail, 22 mm AP). The borders of the pancreas are somewhat ill-defined, and the patient was focally tender during scanning over the pancreas. The borders of the splenic *(sv)* and portal *(pv)* veins are somewhat indistinct. (*a*, aorta; *sma,* superior mesenteric artery; *c,* inferior vena cava; *gb,* gallbladder; *smv,* superior mesenteric vein.)

be smooth, but they are usually indistinct. In addition, there may be loss of distinction of the splenic vein[65] (Fig. 7-6). The textural changes in acute pancreatitis, with the development of edema without overall enlargement of the pancreas may be seen at an earlier stage by ultrasound than by CT. Patients demonstrate an abnormal pancreatic ultrasonogram before an abnormal serum amylase level. Ultrasound usually does not reveal the peripancreatic thickening of the surrounding fascial planes as is seen on CT.[62]

CT appears to remain the primary imaging method in patients with moderate to severe pancreatitis.[17] In patients with milder forms of pancreatitis, real-time ultrasound may be a valuable screening tool for the diagnosis of gallstones and both intrapancreatic and extrapancreatic inflammatory lesions. The main limitation of real-time ultrasound in assessing extrapancreatic spread appears to be in defining abnormalities within the transverse mesocolon. Visualization of this area is limited by the high frequency of occurrence of bowel gas in the transverse colon and lack of a suitable acoustic window. By using semiupright patient positioning and coronal views, 77 percent of lesions in the anterior and pararenal space (Fig. 7-6) are visualized and 100 percent of lesions in the lesser sac are seen[17] (Figs. 7-6 and 7-23).

Hemorrhagic Pancreatitis

In acute hemorrhagic pancreatic necrosis or acute hemorrhagic pancreatitis, there is sudden more or less diffuse enzymatic destruction of the pancreatic sub-stance, caused presumably by sudden escape of the active lytic pancreatic enzymes into the glandular parenchyma. The enzymes cause focal areas of fat necrosis in and about the pancreas, which lead to rupture of pancreatic vessels and hemorrhage. Forty-five percent of patients have a sudden necrotizing destruction of the pancreas following an alcoholic debauch or excessively large meal.[20] Patients with acute hemorrhagic pancreatitis represent the severe form of the disease with decreased hematocrit and serum calcium level, hypotension despite volume replacement, metabolic acidosis, and adult respiratory distress syndrome.[20]

Hemorrhagic complications of pancreatitis include hemorrhagic necrosis of the pancreatic parenchyma, deposition of hemorrhagic fluid into the retroperitoneal tissue or peritoneal cavity, and hemorrhage into a pancreatic pseudocyst. The incidence of hemorrhage in patients with acute pancreatitis is 2 to 33 percent.[70] The hemorrhagic complication of pancreatitis is reported to have a poor prognosis, with a mortality of 25 to 100 percent.[70] With increasing awareness of the spectrum of the appearance of hemorrhagic pancreatic fluid collections, more clinically benign hemorrhagic events may be diagnosed. The presence of hemorrhagic fluid collections does not necessarily warrant drastic measures. The overall clinical setting should be a major factor in determining whether therapeutic intervention is warranted.[70]

The appearance of hemorrhagic pancreatic fluid collections on ultrasound depends on the age of the hemorrhage.[4,70] Acutely, a well-defined homogeneous mass (on CT, 45 to 65 Hounsfield units [HU]) is seen (Figs. 7-23 and 7-24). After 1 week the mass may appear cystic (on

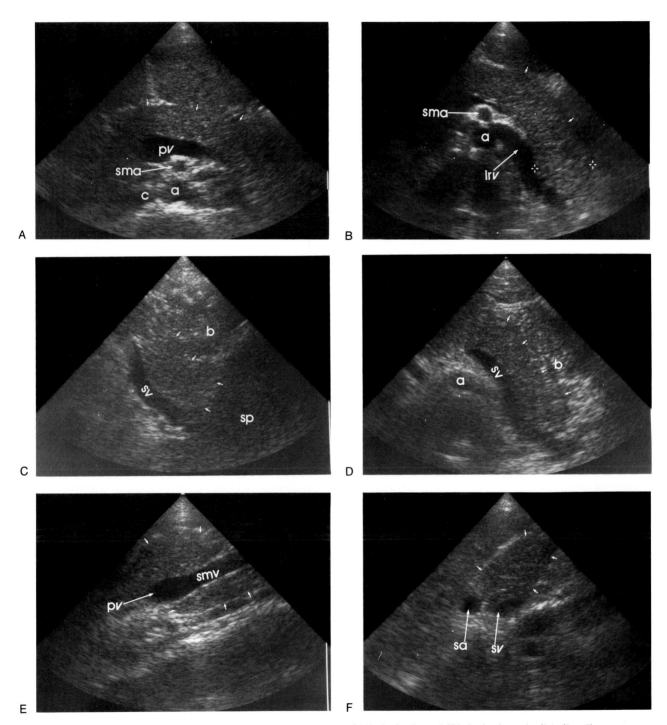

Fig. 7-22. Acute pancreatitis. Diffuse. Transverse scan of **(A)** the body and **(B)** the body and tail (tail, calipers, 31 mm AP). *(sma,* superior mesenteric artery; *pv,* portal vein; *c,* inferior vena cava; *a,* aorta; *lrv,* left renal vein; arrows, anterior border of pancreas.) **(C & D)** Relationship of the tail (arrows) to bowel *(b),* splenic vein *(sv),* and spleen *(sp).* **(E)** Sagittal view of the head (anterior, arrows) and uncinate process (posterior, arrows) with their relationship to the superior mesenteric vein *(smv).* *(pv,* portal vein.) **(F)** Sagittal view of the tail (arrows). *(sa,* splenic artery; *sv,* splenic vein.)

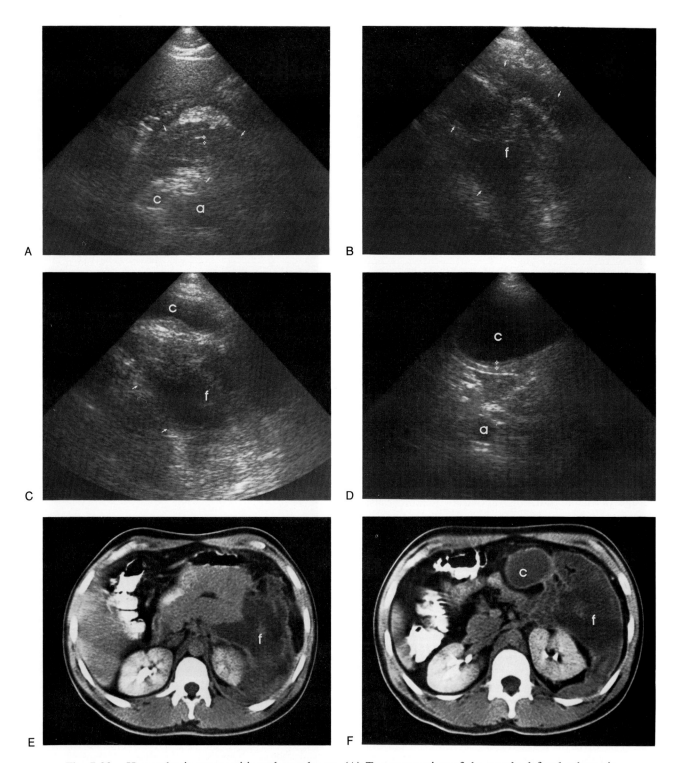

Fig. 7-23. Hemorrhagic pancreatitis and pseudocyst. **(A)** Transverse view of the poorly defined echogenic pancreas (arrows). The pancreatic duct (calipers) measured 3.3 mm. (*c*, inferior vena cava; *a*, aorta.) **(B & C)** Transverse views of the left pararenal area with poorly defined hypoechoic areas (*f*, arrows) in the region of the pancreatic tail. No anatomic landmarks are visualized. On Fig. C, which is more inferior than Fig. B, an anterior pseudocyst *(c)* is seen. **(D)** Transverse view more inferior than Fig. C with demonstration of the pseudocyst *(c)* in the anterior abdomen. (*a*, aorta.) **(E & F)** CT scans with Fig. E similar to Fig. B and Fig. F similar to Fig. C. Note the fluid in the left pararenal space corresponding to the poorly defined lucent areas *(f)* on Figs. B & C and the pseudocyst *(c)*. This is an example of how poorly pararenal fluid may be defined by ultrasound.

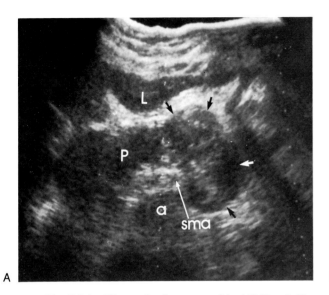

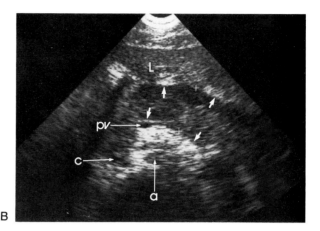

Fig. 7-24. Hemorrhagic pancreatitis. **(A)** Focal. Transverse scan through the pancreas *(P)*. A poorly defined mass (arrows), seen in the area of the pancreatic tail, has a similar echodensity to the liver *(L)*. The remainder of the pancreas was enlarged with a mass effect. On a CT scan this mass was shown to be very dense, consistent with hemorrhage. (*a*, aorta; *sma,* superior mesenteric artery.) **(B)** Diffuse. Transverse scan through the pancreatic body *(b)* and tail *(t)*. The pancreas is inhomogeneously echodense and diffusely enlarged. The pancreas was dense on CT scan. (*pv,* main portal vein; *L*, liver; *a*, aorta; *c*, inferior vena cava.)

CT, 14 to 25 HU) with solid elements or septation. After several weeks the hemorrhage may still appear cystic. In vitro studies have shown that hemorrhage and clotted blood appear either echogenic or lucent, depending on the age of the hemorrhage and the transducer used. Therefore, in the appropriate clinical setting ultrasound may demonstrate an echogenic well-defined pancreatic mass that suggests an acute hemorrhage (Fig. 7-24). Abscesses and pseudocysts appear similar but are not as homogeneous or as strongly echogenic.

Phlegmonous Pancreatitis

A phlegmon is a spreading diffuse inflammatory edema of soft tissues that may proceed to necrosis and even suppuration. It extends outside the gland in only 18 to 20 percent of patients with acute pancreatitis. A phlegmon appears hypoechoic with good through transmission. It does not represent extrapancreatic fluid. It usually involves the lesser sac, the left anterior pararenal space, and the transverse mesocolon (Fig. 7-25). Less commonly, it involves the small bowel mesentery, lower retroperitoneum, and pelvis.[4]

Liquefactive Necrosis

In unusual cases, a necrotic pancreas may become an excavated necrotic sac surrounded by a shell of tissue that conforms to the axis and contour of the pancreas.[4,62]

This debris-containing sac could be misinterpreted on ultrasound and CT and is often best defined by direct injection with contrast into the pancreatic duct.[63] On ultrasound, a debris-containing cystic structure is seen in

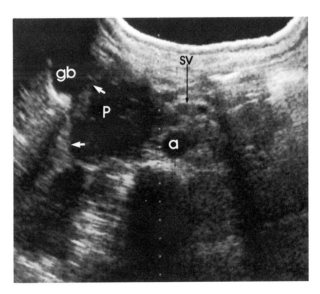

Fig. 7-25. Acute pancreatitis and phlegmonous extension. Focal. Transverse scan demonstrates focal enlargement of the pancreatic head *(P)*. The "mass effect" has poorly defined margins and is hypoechoic relative to the remainder of the gland. The inferior vena cava is not identified. There is phlegmonous extension into the area of the lesser sac (arrows). (*a*, aorta; *gb*, gallbladder; *sv*, splenic vein.)

the region of the pancreas without a definite extrapancreatic pseudocyst. It appears hypoechoic and resembles a diffusely edematous gland or cyst (Fig. 7-26). On ERCP, a ductal stricture and communication with the pancreatic sac are seen.[63] The lesion is usually treated with drainage like a pseudocyst.

Acute Pancreatitis in Children

The pancreas is more reliably seen in children than adults because children tend to be smaller with less body fat.[26] In young children, the liver normally lies lower in the abdomen and the left lobe is more prominent, which provides an excellent sonic window for improved visualization. As with adults, the normal pancreas is generally isosonic or hyperechoic with respect to the liver.[71] In children, the gland is isosonic more often than hyperechoic.[27] The most frequent indicators of pancreatitis in one study appeared to be a dilated duct (46 percent) and pancreatic enlargement (46 percent).[28] That study found evaluation of pancreatic size, echotexture, and contour less reliable.[28] The size, echogenicity, and contour must be assessed in the evaluation for acute pancreatitis. The gland is increased in size (generally in a diffuse fashion), hypoechoic (less dense than the liver), and indistinct in outline.[26]

Ultrasound is valuable in children with unexplained acute and chronic abdominal pain. In one series, the serum amylase level and/or amylase clearance ratio correlated poorly with the ultrasound and clinical evidence of pancreatitis.[71]

In children there are diverse causes of acute pancreatitis. These include trauma, drugs (steroids, L-asparaginase, hydrochlorothiazide, azothioprine, and salicylazosulfapyridine), infection (with measles, mumps, and rubella virus), congenital anomalies, and familial or idiopathic causes.[26]

Aspiration Biopsy

As a rule, biopsy and aspiration are unnecessary in cases of acute pancreatitis unless complications occur.

Clinical Considerations

On ultrasound 28 percent of patients with acute edematous pancreatitis have a normal-appearing pancreas, but there is usually focal or diffuse enlargement (61 percent) or phlegmonous changes (11 percent). Patients with a diagnosis of acute necrotizing pancreatitis never have a normal pancreas on ultrasound, and most (89 percent) have evidence of phlegmonous pancreatitis. The ultrasound appearance persists in phlegmonous pancreatitis for weeks to months after the patient has made a full clinical recovery.

In patients with a diagnosis of acute pancreatitis, the pancreas is visualized 62 percent of the time by ultrasound and 98 percent of the time by CT.[4] Ultrasound is useful in patients with pancreatitis to evaluate for biliary tract disease, which is often associated with stones and dilatation. A CT scan is performed if ultrasound is un-

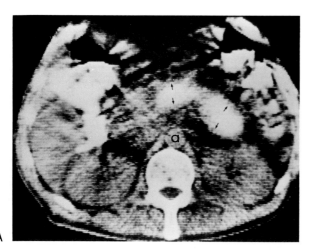
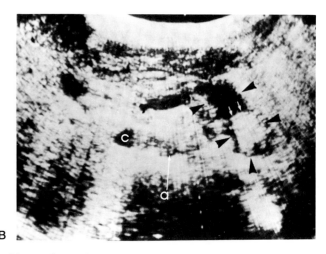

A   B

Fig. 7-26. Liquefactive necrosis. **(A)** CT scan performed immediately following an ERCP, demonstrating a central contrast-filled area (arrows) surrounded by a shell of pancreatic tissue, completely replacing the core and occupying the normal pancreatic axis. (*a*, aorta.) **(B)** Transverse scan showing a localized collection of solid material (necrotic tissue) layering out (white arrows) in the saclike fluid collection (arrowheads) in the area of the pancreatic tail. (*a*, aorta; *c*, inferior vena cava.) (From Burrell et al,[63] with permission.)

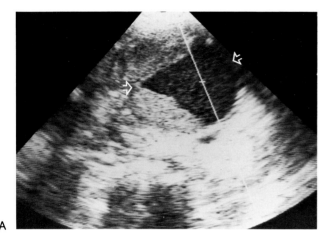
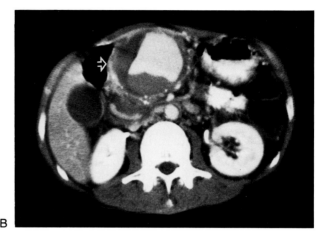

A   B

Fig. 7-27. Gastroduodenal artery aneurysm. **(A)** Transverse view through the region of the head of the pancreas with pancreatitis. A mass (arrows) containing a cystic area is seen. Flow was demonstrated by Doppler. **(B)** Enhanced CT scan demonstrating the contrast within the aneurysm (arrowhead).

successful and when complications of acute pancreatitis are suspected.

COMPLICATIONS OF PANCREATITIS

Aneurysms

Aneurysms secondary to acute pancreatitis are uncommon.[72] The splenic artery is the most often involved, but other splanchnic vessels, including the celiac artery, CHA, gastric artery, and gastroduodenal artery can be involved. The pancreatic arteries that are subject to aneurysm are the pancreaticoduodenal arcades and dorsal and transverse pancreatic arteries. A SMA aneurysm is an uncommon complication.

Because of the risk of aneurysm formation, the patient should be scanned carefully with real-time ultrasound (Figs. 7-27 and 7-28); not all lucent masses are pseudocysts.[72] Most aneurysms will demonstrate intrinsic pulsations of the arterial wall on real-time scanning. However, a splanchnic aneurysm need not show pulsation. It can be evaluated by Doppler. If a massive gastrointesti-

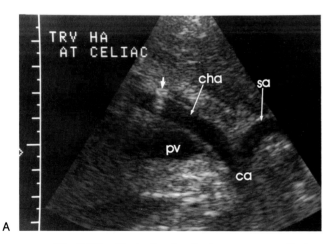
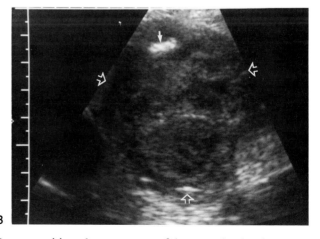

A   B

Fig. 7-28. Gastroduodenal artery aneurysm. Patient with pancreatitis and an aneurysm of the gastroduodenal artery. The scans were obtained following placement of a coil at the origin of the gastroduodenal artery. **(A)** Transverse scan demonstrating the common hepatic artery *(cha)* with a coil (arrow) at the origin of the gastroduodenal artery. (*pv*, portal vein; *sa*, splenic artery, *ca*, celiac artery.) **(B)** Transverse magnified view of the aneurysm (open arrows), which measured 57 by 77 mm. No flow was demonstrated by Doppler. The coil is seen as an echogenic area (arrow).

nal hemorrhage has occurred in association with acute pancreatitis, the examiner should look carefully for an aneurysm.[72] Some may be too small to identify. Ten percent of patients with chronic pancreatitis have pseudoaneurysms. Aneurysms occasionally do occur in the pancreatic bed secondary to pancreatitis.[72]

Venous Thromboses

Ultrasound demonstration of venous thrombosis subsequent to pancreatic benign inflammatory disease is less frequent than previously reported.[73] One series described the ultrasound findings of echogenic thrombi in the portal vein (acutely)—both thrombus and collaterals—and cavernous transformation in long-term calcifying pancreatitis. A failure to visualize the portal vein or its major tributaries should raise the possibility of venous thrombosis. This portal venous thrombosis may be secondary to extrinsic compression by a pseudocyst or by a local inflammatory phenomenon.

Abscess

The incidence of pancreatic abscess is 1 to 9 percent and is related to the severity of acute pancreatitis.[64] The likelihood of abscess development appears to be directly related to the degree of tissue necrosis.[62] Forty percent of abscesses are associated with postoperative pancreatitis, 4 percent with an alcoholic binge, and 7 percent with biliary disease.[64] There is an associated high mortality (32 to 65 percent) even with surgical drainage, and the untreated mortality in untreated patients is 100 percent.[27]

An abscess develops as a result of the superinfection of the necrotic pancreatic and retroperitoneal tissues and less commonly from superinfection of a pseudocyst. The infection is due to hematogenous, lymphatic, or transmural spread of enteric organisms from the adjacent gastrointestinal tract. The abscess may be unilocular or multilocular and can spread superiorly into the mediastinum, inferiorly into the transverse mesocolon, or down the retroperitoneum into the pelvis.

The clinical patterns are variable. The clinical diagnosis is difficult because a patient with acute necrotizing pancreatitis can have the signs and symptoms of an acute supportive process. If the patient with acute necrotic pancreatitis has a persistent fever and leukocytosis, an abscess should be considered.[4] With acute necrotizing pancreatitis, an abscess may develop 7 to 14 days after the onset of symptoms.[64] Most patients with acute pancreatitis improve in 1 to 10 days with conservative therapy, but 2 to 9 percent develop abscesses.[4,74,75] With acute interstitial pancreatitis, the patient may suffer a

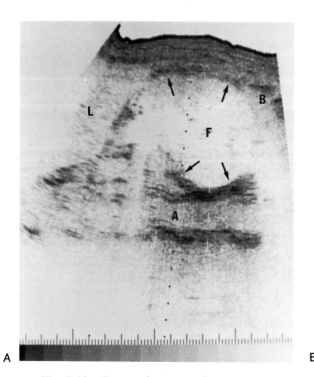

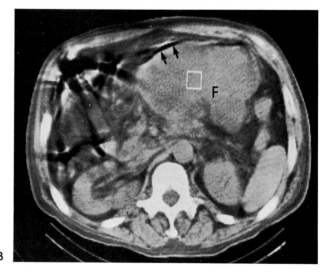

A   **B**

Fig. 7-29. Pancreatic abscess. Lesser sac abscess. **(A)** Longitudinal midline scan with a well-defined fluid collection *(F)* with smooth walls (arrows) and some internal echoes. (*L*, liver; *A*, aorta; *B*, bowel gas.) **(B)** CT scan. A well-defined, loculated lesser sac collection *(F)* is seen. (arrows, stomach.) (From Hill et al,[64] with permission.)

relapse, complicated by abscess, within 2 to 3 weeks.[64] The cardinal signs of abscess include fever, chills, hypotension, and a tender abdomen with a growing mass. Leukocytosis and bacteremia strengthen the diagnosis.[64]

The ultrasound appearance of an abscess may be very similar to that of acute pancreatitis or a pseudocyst. A hypoechoic mass that may have smooth walls with few to no internal echoes is present; some of these masses have irregular walls with increased internal echoes (Fig. 7-29). The mass may range from completely echofree to echodense.[4] If it is hidden by bowel gas, a gas-containing abscess can be missed by ultrasound. The only suggestive sign of an abscess on CT is gas, but the air may be present in the absence of abscess with sterile necrosis, phlegmon, or a pseudocyst that has ruptured into the gastrointestinal tract.[4,62,64] A positive diagnosis of an abscess cannot be made by ultrasound alone. If an abscess is clinically

suspected, an aspiration of the pancreatic/peripancreatic fluid should be performed.[4,62,64]

Aspiration/Biopsy

As described above, the ultrasound findings in pancreatic abscess are not greatly different from those in acute pancreatitis or, at times, pseudocyst. Because a patient with a pancreatic abscess is at significant risk, if an abscess is suspected an ultrasound-guided needle aspiration should be performed[64] and an immediate Gram stain performed to determine whether the fluid is sterile. An immediate diagnosis of abscess is made when nonsterile fluid is obtained and appropriate therapy may be instituted. With the addition of percutaneous aspiration, the high mortality rate associated with a pancreatic ab-

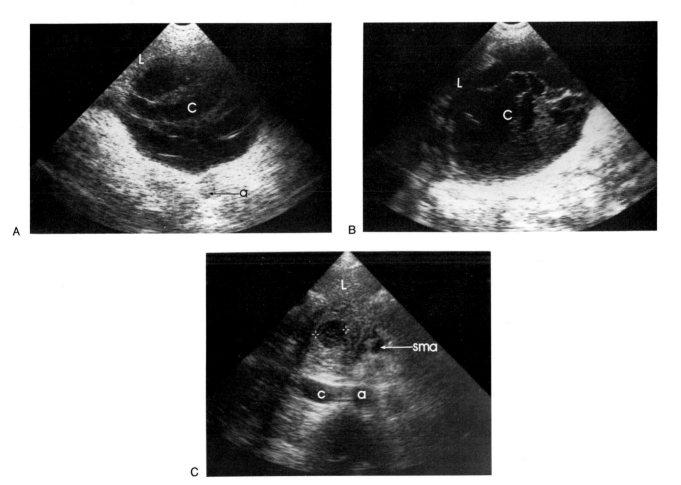

Fig. 7-30. Pseudocyst, septations. **(A)** Case 1. Transverse scan through the midline. A large cystic mass *(C)* is seen anterior to the aorta *(a)*. It contains many internal septations. (*L*, liver.) **(B)** Case 2. Transverse scan through a multiseptated pancreatic pseudocyst *(C)*. (*L*, liver.) **(C)** Case 3. Transverse view through a small pseudocyst (calipers, 19 mm) in the pancreatic head. The pseudocyst contained internal echoes consistent with hemorrhage. (*a*, aorta; *c*, inferior vena cava; *L*, liver; *sma,* superior mesenteric artery.)

scess may be reduced and surgery may be avoided in patients with sterile fluid collections.[64]

Pseudocyst

Pseudocysts represent collections of fluid that arise from a loculation of inflammatory processes, necrosis, or hemorrhage. The overwhelming majority are clinically important cysts and are almost always associated with pancreatitis. In 90 percent of cases they are due to acute pancreatitis or trauma.[20] Pseudocysts are said to occur in 10 to 50 percent of patients with acute pancreatitis.[4,63,76] They are usually single, are oval to round, and vary in size; they arise in any portion of the pancreas and can cause dilatation of the pancreatic duct. They are situated within or adjacent to the pancreas, particularly in the region of the tail. The wall may be thin or quite thick and fibrotic. There is no epithelial lining, no communication with the duct, and marked inflammatory reaction.[20] They are believed to occur because of obstruction followed by rupture of the pancreatic duct, which allows pancreatic juice to escape into the intersti-

tium of the gland. Because there is no capsule, the fluid may rupture into and accumulate in the lesser sac or extend down into the retroperitoneal soft tissue planes in any direction.[4]

On ultrasound, a pseudocyst has a typical appearance. It usually has sharply defined smooth walls and demonstrates acoustic enhancement[2,62,69,77,78] (Fig. 7-23C). At times the lesion may demonstrate multiple septations or multiple internal echoes, and may even fail to exhibit acoustic enhancement[77] (Figs. 7-30 and 7-31). The success rate of ultrasound in detecting pseudocysts varies from 50 to 92 percent.[4] Those in the head and body are usually seen, whereas those in the tail are often hidden by the stomach. The wall of the cyst is usually smooth, although some walls are irregular. The fluid is often echofree, but is sometimes filled with internal echoes; if a fluid-debris level is superimposed, abscess or hemorrhage should be considered.

One group of investigators evaluated the ultrasound features of pseudocysts to determine whether ultrasound could predict infected ones—there was no statistically significant difference between the infected and noninfected ones in size, wall characteristics, multiplicity, or

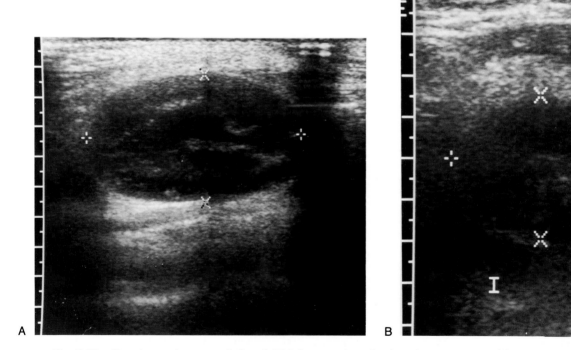

Fig. 7-31. Pseudocyst, lesser sac, infected. This burn patient developed acute pancreatitis and a pseudocyst containing many internal echoes or septations as seen on **(A)** the sagittal view of the pseudocyst (calipers, 76 mm long, 43 mm AP). **(B)** Transverse view of the pancreatic head and uncinate process with a poorly defined mass effect (35 mm AP, 43 mm transverse) secondary to pancreatitis anterior to the inferior vena cava *(I)*.

air content.[79] The most important feature is the presence of internal echoes within the pseudocyst, with more intense internal echoes associated with infection (Fig. 7-31). This lesion can mimic cystadenoma or cystadenocarcinoma by its ultrasound appearance.

There are various locations for these pseudocysts.[43,62,63,74] The most common site is the lesser sac because it is directly anterior to the pancreas and posterior to the body of the stomach[62,69] (Figs. 7-30 to 7-33). The second most common location of the extrapancreatic fluid collection is the anterior pararenal space[62] (Figs. 7-32 and 7-34 to 7-37). This is directly posterior to the lesser sac and is bounded by the anterior layer of Gerota's fascia. The spleen represents the lateral border of the anterior pararenal space on the left. Fluid occurs more commonly in the left pararenal space than the right. Sometimes the posterior pararenal space is also fluid-

filled as fluid spreads from the anterior pararenal space to the posterior pararenal space on the same side. In addition, fluid may enter the peritoneal cavity either via the foramen of Winslow or by disrupting the peritoneum in the anterior surface of the lesser sac.[62]

At times, the location of a pseudocyst may be confusing. One can be located in the mediastinum by extending through the esophageal (T10) or aortic (T12) hiatus[80,81] (Figs. 7-38 and 7-39). A mediastinal pseudocyst may be commonly associated with a pleural effusion rich in protein and amylase.[80] It is important to locate the pseudocyst and identify it as such because the operative procedure entails internal drainage below the xyphoid.[80] Besides extending into the mediastinum, a pseudocyst may extend into the small bowel mesentery or down into the retroperitoneum into the pelvis and even the groin.[4] A pseudocyst may also be confused with renal abnor-

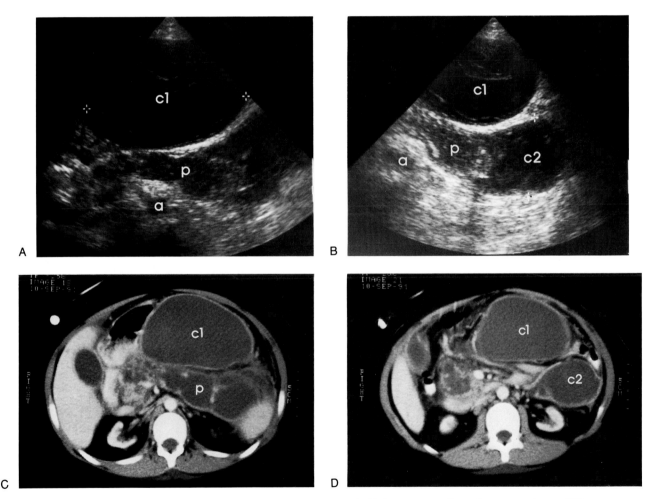

Fig. 7-32. Pseudocysts, lesser sac and left pararenal. **(A & B)** Transverse views demonstrate two different pseudocysts (calipers), one in the lesser sac area (*c1*, 71 × 110 mm) and one anterior to the pancreatic tail area (*c2*, 6 cm). The pseudocyst in the lesser sac contains septations, while the other contains internal echoes. The pancreas *(p)* itself is very lucent. (*a*, aorta.) **(C & D)** CT scans with Fig. C corresponding to Fig. A and Fig. D to Fig. B, with both pseudocysts seen, as is the lucent pancreas *(p)*.

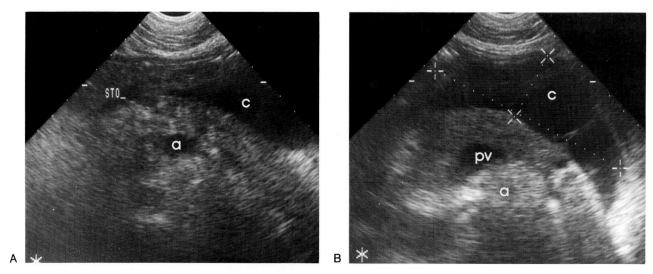

Fig. 7-33. Pseudocyst, lesser sac and left pararenal area. **(A & B)** Transverse views demonstrating a pseudocyst *(c)* in the lesser sac area posterior to the stomach *(STO)* and anterior to the pancreas. (*pv,* portal vein; *a,* aorta.)

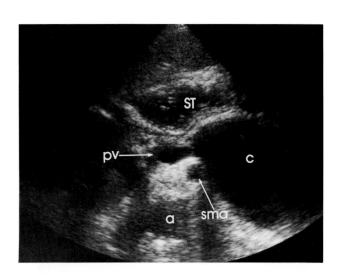

Fig. 7-34. Pseudocyst, left anterior pararenal space. Transverse view showing a cystic mass *(c)* in the region of the tail of the pancreas and posterior to the fluid-filled stomach *(ST)*. It is compressing the splenic vein (not visualized). (*a,* aorta; *sma,* superior mesenteric artery; *pv,* portal vein.)

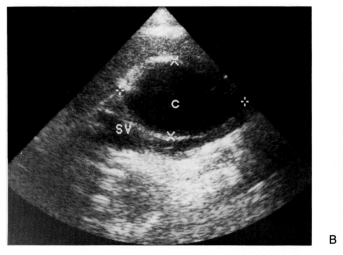

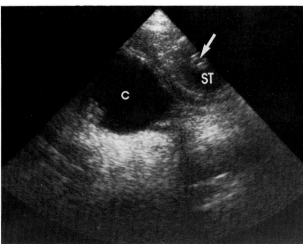

Fig. 7-35. Pseudocyst, left anterior pararenal space. **(A)** Transverse and **(B)** sagittal views with a pseudocyst (*c,* 28 × 50 mm) noted compressing the splenic view *(sv)* on Fig. A and posterior and superior to the fluid-filled stomach *(ST)* on Fig. B. (arrow, nasogastric tube.)

400

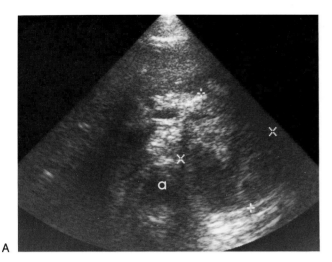
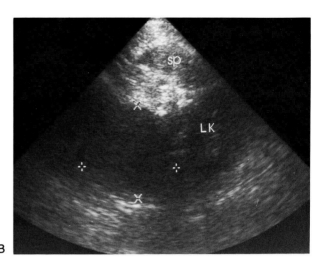

A

B

Fig. 7-36. Hemorrhagic pseudocyst, pancreatic tail. **(A)** Transverse scan demonstrating an echogenic mass (calipers, 56 × 71 mm) in the region of the pancreatic tail in the left anterior pararenal area. It was noted to be separate from the stomach and kidney. (*a*, aorta.) **(B)** Coronal transverse scan showing the relationship of the mass (calipers, 52 × 56 mm) to the left kidney *(LK)* and the spleen *(sp)*. On a CT scan, there was increased density within the mass, consistent with hemorrhage.

mality when it is located in the transverse mesocolon or anterior pararenal space adjacent to the left kidney[82] (Fig. 7-37). Since a renal cyst cannot always be distinguished from a pseudocyst by imaging alone, fine-needle aspiration may be performed to obtain fluid for amylase evaluation.[83]

At times, the pseudocyst may be in the region of the spleen[84,85] (Fig. 7-40). There may be release of proteo-

lytic active enzymes with erosion of the splenic hilum and further extension into the splenic parenchyma as a known complication of pancreatitis.[84,86] If an intrasplenic pseudocyst is suspected, this must be confirmed. Once confirmed, surgical intervention is mandatory because of the danger of secondary hemorrhage.[85] Nuclear medicine and angiography may be used in conjunction with ultrasound to verify the diagnosis.[85]

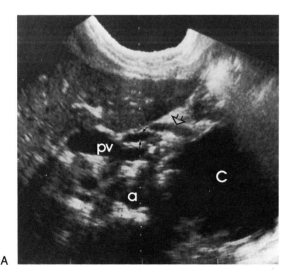
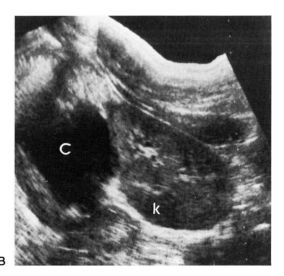

A

B

Fig. 7-37. Pseudocyst, pararenal. Transverse cone-down scan 1 cm below the xyphoid **(A)**. A cystic mass *(C)* is seen in the left upper quadrant. (*a*, aorta; *pv*, main portal vein; solid arrows, pancreatic duct; open arrow, splenic artery.) **(B)** Longitudinal prone scan. A cystic mass *(C)* that appears to involve the left kidney *(k)* is seen. By using the vascular landmarks, the pancreatic origin of the mass could be established.

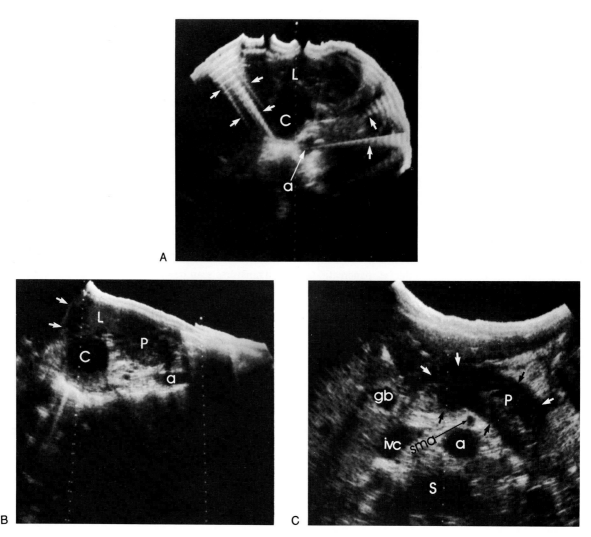

Fig. 7-38. Pseudocyst, mediastinal. Patient with acute pancreatitis and a pseudocyst extending up to the chest through the lesser sac. **(A)** High transverse scan. The pseudocyst *(C)* is seen in the midline extending up from the lesser sac. (*a*, aorta; *L*, liver; arrows, reflective pattern due to air from the lung.) **(B)** Longitudinal midline scan. The pseudocyst *(C)* is seen next to the diaphragm (arrows) extending upward. The pancreas *(P)* itself is enlarged and hypoechoic. (*L*, liver; *a*, aorta.) **(C)** Transverse cone-down scan through the pancreas *(P)*. The body and tail are enlarged (arrows) and hypoechoic, consistent with acute pancreatitis. (*a*, aorta; *ivc*, inferior vena cava; *sma*, superior mesenteric artery; *gb*, gallbladder; *S*, spine.)

Besides simulating splenic, renal, and mediastinal abnormalities, a pseudocyst may also involve the duodenum.[87] Duodenal involvement may occur because the nonperitonealized posterior surface of the duodenum is in direct contact with the head of the pancreas, with no effective barrier to the anatomically disruptive effect of the secretions. Whether these appear intramural or as severe extrinsic compressive lesions depends on the variable interplay between the depth of penetration and extent of infiltration. With accumulation of secretions and increased pressure, extension may occur within the wall of the duodenum or it may rupture from the cyst cavity into the bowel lumen. The second portion of the duodenum is the most frequently involved, with the site of involvement usually on its lateral or posterolateral surface[87] (Fig. 7-41).

Many pseudocysts regress; a 20 percent rate of spontaneous regression has been reported.[4,87] Some decompress into the pancreatic duct, others into the gastrointestinal tract.[4] From 5 to 15 percent of the cysts rupture.[77,88,89] Fifty percent of those that resolve rupture into the gastrointestinal tract and 50 percent rupture into the peritoneal cavity.[77] The stomach is most commonly involved with drainage into the duodenum rare.[90]

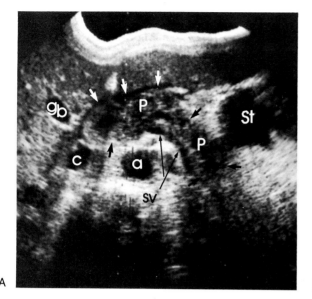

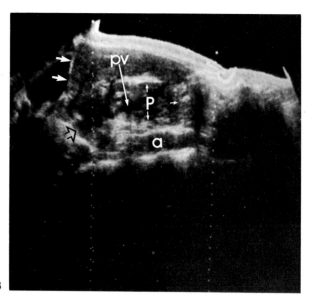

Fig. 7-39. Pseudocyst, mediastinal — followup. These scans were performed 2 weeks after those in Fig. 7-38. **(A)** Transverse scan, similar to Fig. 7-38A. The pancreas (*P*, arrows) is smaller and more echogenic. Now the splenic vein *(sv)* can be identified. (*gb,* gallbladder; *c,* inferior vena cava; *a,* aorta; *St,* fluid-filled stomach.) **(B)** Longitudinal midline scan similar to Fig. 7-38B. No pseudocyst is seen where the previous lesion was seen (open arrow.) (*P,* small arrows, pancreas; large solid arrows, diaphragm; *pv,* portal vein; *a,* aorta.)

These cysts rupture from the tryptic digestion of the wall; in cases in which erosion into an adjacent hollow viscus occurs, digestion of the visceral wall and pressure necrosis are produced by the expanded cyst.[89] There is a 70 percent mortality associated with rupture into the peritoneal cavity.[88] There is an operative mortality of 25 percent for surgical excision, with 6 percent mortality for external drainage of an acute immature pseudocyst.[91] There is a 7 percent mortality for internal drainage.[91]

The introduction of CT and ultrasound has enhanced the rational management of patients with pseudocysts.[62] The availability of ultrasound monitoring has led the

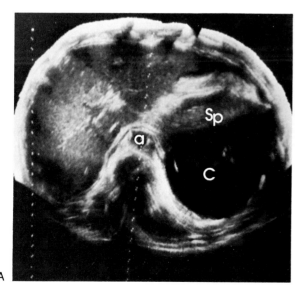

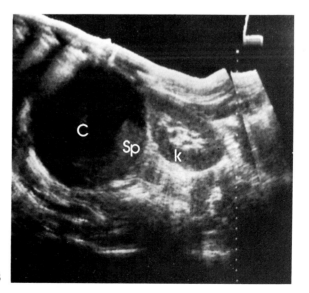

Fig. 7-40. Pseudocyst, splenic. **(A)** Transverse static scan. An anechoic mass *(C)* is seen posterior to the spleen *(Sp).* (*a,* aorta.) **(B)** Prone longitudinal static scan. The same pseudocyst *(C)* is seen superior and posterior to the spleen *(Sp).* (*k,* left kidney.) (Fig. A from Mittelstaedt et al,[198] with permission; Fig. B from Mittelstaedt,[199] with permission.)

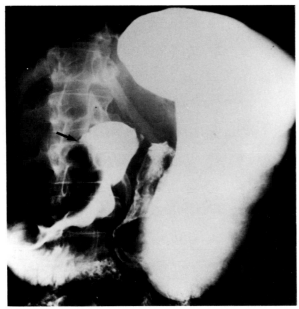

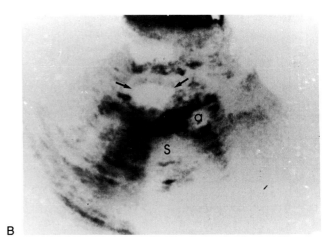

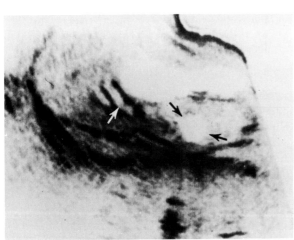

Fig. 7-41. Pseudocyst, duodenal. **(A)** Upper gastrointestinal series, right anterior oblique view. A smooth, lobulated filling defect is seen within the lumen of the distal first and second parts of the duodenum. The lumen is severely narrowed. An acute angle is formed at the junction of the filling defect and the duodenal wall (arrow). **(B)** Transverse and **(C)** longitudinal static scans at the level of the pancreas. A 5-cm mass is seen in the region of the head of the pancreas. It has an anechoic center (black arrows). The common bile duct (white arrow) measures 7 mm. (*a*, aorta; *S*, spine.) (From Bellon et al,[87] with permission.)

surgeon to advocate a more conservative approach. A patient who is stable or improving is treated conservatively for 3 to 4 weeks. This delay eliminates the use of surgery on patients whose condition resolves and provides time for formation of a firm fibrous wall that holds suture for internal anastomosis.[62] Cyst wall maturation generally takes 4 to 6 weeks.[88]

In the past, a persistent pseudocyst was an indication for surgery. Now these lesions can be successfully drained percutaneously. The success rate with no recurrence is 16 to 18 percent.[4] Pseudocysts in the lesser sac tend to reaccumulate, so aspiration is more successful in those not contiguous with the pancreas. The amylase level in the fluid from cysts successfully treated with drainage is lower than in those unsuccessfully treated. Successful drainage is more likely if the cyst is mature, although it can be used to relieve symptoms.[4]

Several structures may be confused with a pseudocyst. One might be a fluid-filled stomach. This diagnosis should be made by using real-time ultrasound and by identifying the characteristic appearance of the stomach with peristalsis. A pancreatic pseudocyst may also mimic a dilated pancreatic duct, which may have an unusual configuration at times[88,92] (Fig. 7-42). Because there is no capsule, the unusual configuration of the cyst conforms to the borders of the surrounding tissue.[92] With careful scanning, the examiner should try to identify whether the cystic structure in question is in the middle of the gland and whether it connects with the duct on real-time scanning. Several transverse sections along the pancreatic axis with various degrees of angulation may be necessary to show the interconnection between the cystic structure and the duct.[86] Lastly, a left renal vein varix has been reported to simulate a pseudocyst.[93] It can

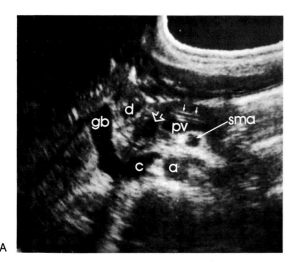 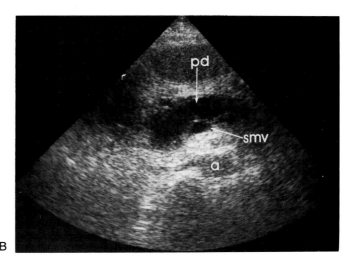

A B

Fig. 7-42. Dilated duct versus pseudocyst. **(A)** Case 1. Pseudocyst. Transverse scan. A round cystic area (open arrow) representing a pseudocyst is seen in the region of the head of the pancreas. With careful real-time scanning, the pancreatic duct (small arrows) was seen as a separate structure. (*gb,* gallbladder; *d,* duodenum; *c,* inferior vena cava; *pv,* portal vein; *sma,* superior mesenteric artery; *a,* aorta.) **(B)** Case 2. Dilated pancreatic duct. Transverse scan showing interconnecting cystic structures *(pd)* within the body and head of the pancreas. There was little identifiable pancreatic parenchyma. This patient had chronic pancreatitis. (*a,* aorta; *smv,* superior mesenteric vein.)

appear as a hypoechoic, well-circumscribed mass anterior to the left kidney. Venous dilatation should be considered in a patient with known portal hypertension because it is in a location where portosystemic shunting is known to occur.[93]

In children, blunt trauma to the abdomen is the main cause of pseudocysts.[94-96] Child abuse is one of the most common causes of this injury.[94] Pancreatitis, cyst, and loculated peripancreatic effusion are sequelae of trauma.[94] The patients present with pain, fullness, nausea and vomiting, anorexia, and weight loss.[96] The cyst may occur rapidly and is seen as an echofree, unilocular ellipsoid mass.[94] A significant number of cysts resolve spontaneously, and so the cysts should be monitored by ultrasound. Size alone should not be an absolute criterion in determining surgical intervention.[95] Ultrasound can be used to establish the diagnosis of cyst and for follow-up evaluation.[97]

Aspiration/Biopsy

Some investigators advocate the percutaneous drainage of pancreatic pseudocysts to verify the diagnosis and to treat patients in whom surgery is contraindicated.[98,99] Ultrasound can be used to guide the percutaneous puncture of a pseudocyst; it is an easy and simple procedure with little risk and discomfort to the patient. It can be used for verification of the diagnosis, for definitive therapy, for decompression in case of threatening rupture,

and for gaining time for maturation of the cyst membrane before surgical intervention.[98,100] In one series, four cysts were treated this way without any recurrence or surgical intervention by 6 to 12 months.[101]

Nowadays, percutaneous catheter drainage of pancreatic pseudocysts have become more common. This technique has been used for drainage of traumatic pseudocysts in children[102] and for mediastinal pseudocysts,[103] as well as in a transgastric drainage approach in adults.[104-108] The transgastric approach mimics the benefits of surgical cystogastrostomy while avoiding the disadvantages of external drainage.[105] Since most pseudocysts lie adjacent to the stomach, the transgastric route is often selected.[106] Drainage is maintained for a minimum of 6 weeks to allow a mature fistula to develop between the stomach and pancreas.[105] This technique is safe and effective and offers a low risk of recurrence and fistula formation.[106]

Successful percutaneous catheter drainage is associated with lower morbidity and mortality, and cure is expected in 67 to 77 percent of cases.[106-108] Percutaneous drainage is an effective frontline treatment for most pancreatic pseudocysts; cure is likely if fluid collections are drained adequately and if sufficient time is allowed for closure of fistulas with pancreatic duct.[109] Various routes can be used: transperitoneal, retroperitoneal, transhepatic, transgastric, and transduodenal.[109] Surgery for acute pseudocysts may be postponed or eliminated by this technique.[101] It permits relief of pain and

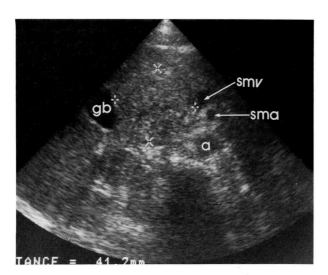

Fig. 7-43. Chronic pancreatitis. Focal mass. Transverse scan of the pancreatic head demonstrating a focal mass (calipers, 42 × 48 mm) in the region of the pancreatic head. This proved to be secondary to chronic pancreatitis. (*gb,* gallbladder; *a,* aorta; *sma,* superior mesenteric artery; *smv,* superior mesenteric vein.)

obstructive symptoms and provides extra time when necessary for maturation of the cyst wall. Surgical management of pseudocysts consists of internal drainage into an adjacent viscus. This is a safe, reliable procedure once the cyst wall has thickened to facilitate satisfactory anastomosis. Ten percent of cysts resolve while waiting for maturation.[101]

CHRONIC PANCREATITIS

Chronic relapsing pancreatitis is a better term for this disease process. It often represents progressive destruction of the pancreas by repeated flare-ups of a mild or subclinical type of acute pancreatitis. The same type of patient gets chronic pancreatitis as acute pancreatitis, but it most commonly affects alcoholics and, less frequently, patients with biliary tract disease. Hypercalcemia and hyperlipidemia predispose individuals to chronic pancreatitis. Chronic pancreatitis is not usually preceded by an attack of classic hemorrhagic pancreatitis. It is much more common in men than women. Up to 40 percent of patients have no recognizable predisposing factors. The pathogenesis of chronic pancreatitis is obscure.[20]

Many morphologic changes are associated with chronic pancreatitis. Most commonly, there are chronic calcifying changes. These morphologic changes include atrophy of the acini, increase in the interlobular fibrous tissue, and chronic inflammatory infiltration. Stones made of calcium carbonate are located inside the ductal system, and pseudocysts are common. Another type of chronic pancreatitis is a chronic obstructive pancreatitis. The lesions are in the lobules, and the ductal epithelium is less involved. The most common cause of this type of pancreatitis is stenosis of the sphincter of Oddi with associated cholelithiasis.[20]

Pancreatic lithiasis is associated with alcoholic pancreatitis. Pancreatic ductal calculi are the result rather than the cause of chronic pancreatic disease, and they

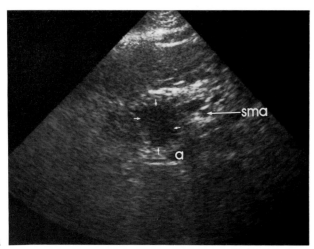

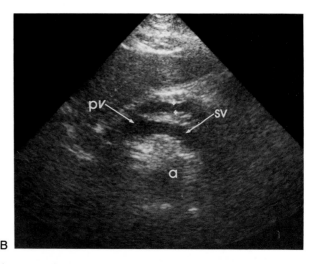

A   B

Fig. 7-44. Chronic pancreatitis. Focal mass and pancreatic ductal dilatation. **(A)** Transverse scan demonstrating a hypoechoic mass (chronic pancreatitis, arrows) in the pancreatic head. By ultrasound alone, this mass cannot be distinguished from tumor. (*a,* aorta; *sma,* superior mesenteric artery.) **(B)** Transverse view of the dilated pancreatic duct (calipers, 5.7 mm) within the body of the pancreas. (*pv,* portal vein; *a,* aorta; *sv,* splenic vein.)

have no significance over and above that of ordinary pancreatic calculi.[110] From 20 to 40 percent of patients with chronic pancreatitis develop lithiasis.[111] The incidence is greater in men than women, and there is a strong association with alcoholic pancreatitis. In chronic pancreatitis, the calcifications seen are almost always true stones lying free in the pancreatic duct rather than the parenchyma.[46] The stones consist of a protein matrix and various amounts of calcium carbonate. Initially the lesion probably consists of a protein plug that precipitates into the small ducts, causing obstruction with secondary dilatation.[111] Calcium carbonate salts are subsequently deposited onto the protein matrix forming the stone. The stone extrudes into the duct as the disease progresses and obstructs the main pancreatic duct or even the ampulla of Vater. The progression of the disease can be seen on follow-up examinations. In 92 percent of patients there is ductal dilatation and in 54 percent there is lithiasis involving the main pancreatic duct.[111]

Patients with chronic pancreatitis experience recurrent episodes of pain at intervals of months to years. Over time, the intervals between episodes decrease. The

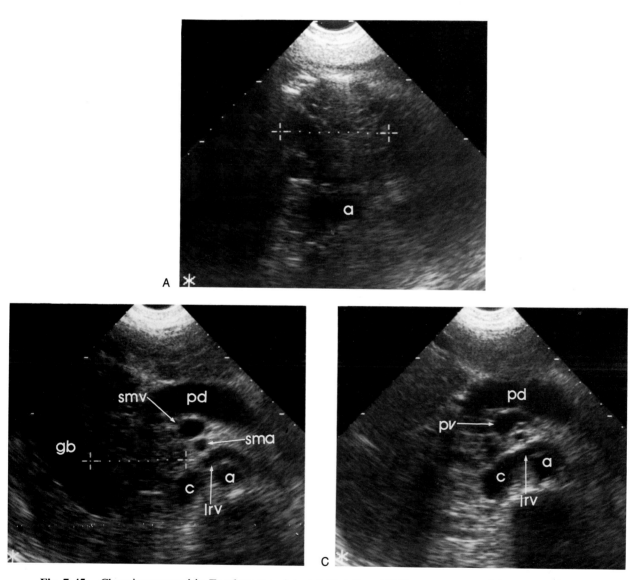

Fig. 7-45. Chronic pancreatitis. Focal mass and ductal dilatation. **(A)** Transverse scan of the pancreatic head (calipers, 6.8 cm AP) with mass effect. The pancreatic head is somewhat inhomogeneous. (*a*, aorta.) **(B)** Transverse scan more superior than Fig. A with the dilated pancreatic duct *(pd)* seen, as well as the pancreatic head mass (calipers, 19 mm). (*smv,* superior mesenteric vein; *sma,* superior mesenteric artery; *a*, aorta; *c*, inferior vena cava; *lrv,* left renal vein; *gb,* gallbladder.) **(C)** Transverse scan more superior than Fig. B with the dilated pancreatic duct *(pd)* visualized. (*a*, aorta; *c*, inferior vena cava; *lrv,* left renal vein; *pv,* portal vein.)

precipitating factor appears to be alcohol, overeating, or the use of opiates. Diabetes, steatorrhea, and pancreatic pseudocysts occur frequently. Frank diabetes occurs in 14 to 90 percent and steatorrhea in 25 to 35 percent. Duodenal obstruction and jaundice occur in one-third of patients.[20]

With chronic pancreatitis, there are several changes on ultrasound.[47,50,62,69] There is increased echogenicity of the pancreas beyond the normal amount due to fibrotic changes, fatty changes, or both.[4,112] At times it may be difficult to even identify the pancreas on ultrasound if its density blends in with that of the surrounding retroperitoneal fat.[69] Focal or diffuse enlargement of the gland (seen in 27 percent of patients) may be associated with an irregular outline of the gland in 45 percent[69] (Figs. 7-43 to 7-45).

Calcification, ductal dilatation, and an irregular outline to the gland are also seen with chronic pancreatitis[50,62,64] (Figs. 7-44 to 7-48). There may be strictures, stenoses, irregularities, and dilatation of the pancreatic duct.[47] Pancreatic duct dilatation is present in 41 percent of patients and is most probably present when there is pancreatic calcification (92 percent of patients)[4] (Figs. 7-44 to 7-48). The calcifications on ultrasound appear as small, highly reflective particles that give the gland a stippled appearance[111] (Figs. 7-47 and 7-48). Shadowing is sometimes associated with the stones, which may have a focal or diffuse distribution. Intraductal stones can be located accurately by ultrasound. Stones in the duct are identified because they are surrounded by the echofree structure of the duct.[111] The significance of ductal stones is unclear.[110]

Although a radiograph may be sufficient to establish the presence of pancreatic calcifications, ultrasound

often provides additional information concerning the duct dilatation and lithiasis in the main duct. The duct may be dilated secondary to stricture or as a result of an extrinsic stone from a smaller pancreatic duct into a major duct.[4] Ultrasound can be used to determine the distribution of the calculi and the characteristics of the peripheral or ductal calculi. The exact site and cause of an obstruction cannot be seen as well by ultrasound as by ERCP.[110] The most common site of obstruction is at the papilla and the site of origin of the main duct[47] (Fig. 7-49). ERCP is the most accurate method of investigating duct dilatation and intraductal lithiasis.[111] The ultrasound finding of ductal dilatation and calculi can forewarn the endoscopist to expect difficulty.

A recent ultrasound series demonstrated the following findings associated with chronic pancreatitis: inhomogeneously increased echogenicity (53 percent), focal dense echoes (40 percent), pseudocyst formation (21 percent), abnormal pancreatic ducts (20 percent), extrahepatic biliary dilatation (19 percent), and a hypoechoic head mass (7 percent).[113] Thirteen percent of patients had normal sonograms. There did not appear to be a direct relationship between the presence of focal high-intensity echoes within the pancreatic parenchyma and radiographic calcification. This study suggested that there were varied ultrasound findings with chronic pancreatitis. In a recent CT series, main pancreatic duct dilatation (68 percent), parenchymal atrophy, and pancreatic calcification (50 percent) were the most common findings in chronic pancreatitis, along with fluid collections (30 percent), focal pancreatic enlargement (30 percent), and biliary ductal dilatation (29 percent).[114]

There are several complications of chronic pancreatitis. Pseudocysts develop in 20 percent of patients[4] (Fig. 7-48). Thrombosis of the splenic vein and/or portal vein can be seen. When a focal mass is seen with chronic pancreatitis, carcinoma should be considered because it occurs in 4 to 25 percent of such patients.[4,111] The symptoms of carcinoma and chronic pancreatitis are so similar that they are not helpful in differentiating between the two conditions. Ultrasound cannot distinguish a benign from a malignant mass unless secondary signs of carcinoma are present (adjacent nodes or liver metastases) (Fig. 7-50). The accuracy rate in the absence of metastases varies but can be as high as 100 percent.[4] The presence of calcification in the mass makes tumor unlikely. CT has the same difficulty as ultrasound in the diagnosis of pancreatic carcinoma in the presence of chronic pancreatitis, and in such patients, ERCP or percutaneous biopsy may be necessary. False-negative results may still be obtained.

Chronic pancreatitis may require palliative surgery, generally pancreatojejunostomy with or without pancreatic resection, to relieve pain. Recurrence of symptoms postoperatively may lead to an attempt at retro-

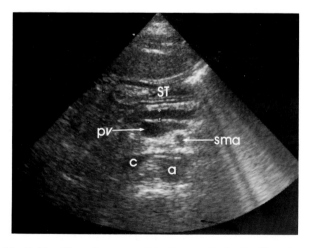

Fig. 7-46. Chronic pancreatitis. Pancreatic ductal dilatation. Transverse scan demonstrating a dilated pancreatic duct (calipers, 5.8 mm) within the pancreatic body. There is little parenchyma around the duct. (*ST,* stomach; *pv,* portal vein; *sma,* superior mesenteric artery; *c,* inferior vena cava; *a,* aorta.)

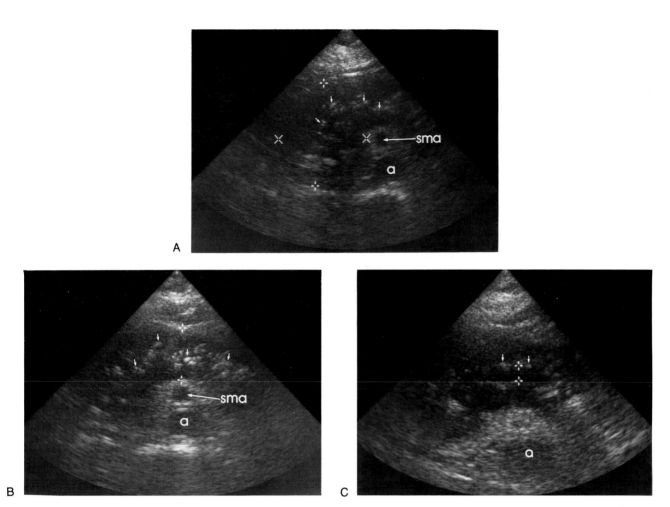

Fig. 7-47. Pancreatic lithiasis and dilated pancreatic duct. Transverse views (**A**) inferior, (**B**) more superior, and (**C**) superior. Multiple calculi (echogenic foci, arrows) are seen within the midportion of the pancreas. The pancreatic duct (calipers, 66 mm) is dilated in Fig. C. The pancreas is diffusely enlarged, with the head measuring 55 mm AP. (*a*, aorta; *sma,* superior mesenteric artery.)

grade opacification of the anastomosis by endoscopy to establish patency. With real-time guidance, a 22-gauge needle can be inserted with injection of 5 ml of water-soluble iodinated contrast diluted with gentamycin into the pancreatojejunostomy, jejunal loop, and biliary tree.[115] Percutaneous pancreatography can be used in selected cases of pancreatic duct dilatation not opacified by endoscopy.

Chronic Renal Failure

Pancreatic findings associated with chronic renal failure have been reported.[116] In up to one-fifth of patients with chronic renal failure, there are morphologic changes of chronic pancreatitis. There appear to be several factors that may be responsible for these findings, including biliary tract disease (which is more frequent in

patients with chronic renal failure), duration of long-term hemodialysis, and hyperparathyroidism.[116] The most obvious etiologic factor appears to be the duration of chronic renal failure. As many as 72 percent of patients with long-standing chronic renal failure demonstrate secretory dysfunction. Patients suffering from renal failure for less than 8 years do not appear to have any evidence of pancreatic disease.

Hereditary Pancreatitis

Hereditary pancreatitis is a recurrent inflammation of the pancreas from childhood with an unusual prevalence among blood relatives in accordance with Mendel's law —autosomal dominant. The sex distribution is equal, and the condition occurs exclusively in white people. The patients present with recurrent attacks of severe

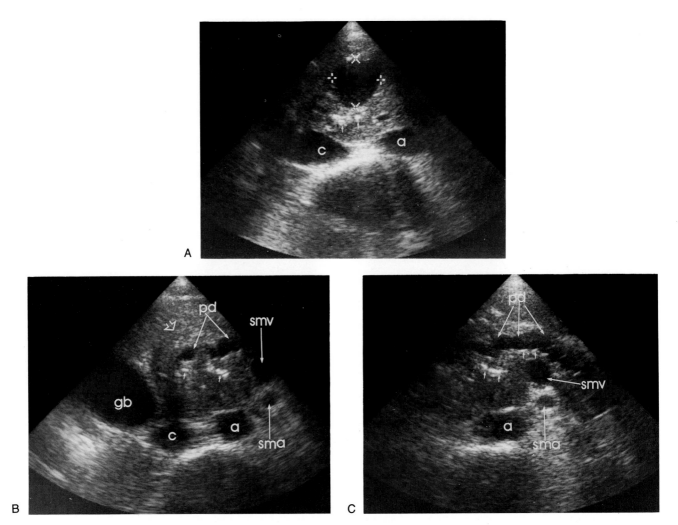

Fig. 7-48. Chronic pancreatitis. Enlargement, ductal dilatation, calculi, and pseudocyst. **(A)** Transverse view of the pancreatic head with a pseudocyst (calipers) in the head. There are echogenic foci (arrows) within the head, representing calculi. (*c*, inferior vena cava; *a*, aorta.) **(B)** Transverse scan at a higher level than Fig. A with an enlarged pancreas (open arrow, border) and a dilated pancreatic duct *(pd)* with calculi (arrows). (*smv*, superior mesenteric vein; *sma*, superior mesenteric artery; *a*, aorta; *c*, inferior vena cava; *gb*, gallbladder.) **(C)** Transverse scan of the body and tail region with the dilated pancreatic duct (*pd*, 6.6 mm) visualized along with calculi (arrows). (*a*, aorta; *smv*, superior mesenteric vein; *sma*, superior mesenteric artery.)

pain in childhood. There are pancreatic calcifications in 30 to 50 percent and a dilated pancreatic duct. Pseudocysts develop in 10 percent of patients.[117]

Pancreatography

A good pancreatogram provides valuable information for planning surgery.[118] Although a preoperative pancreatogram may be obtained by endoscopic retrograde cannulation of the duct, it can also be obtained percutaneously. A needle placed in the obstructed duct may cause pancreatitis, and, as in transhepatic cholangiogra-phy in the obstructed biliary tree, it should be followed by surgical decompression within 24 to 48 hours.[118] The pancreatic duct can be demonstrated in 84 percent of normal individuals by this technique.[46]

With real-time guidance, a percutaneous pancreatic ductogram and a percutaneous aspiration biopsy can be successfully performed as a single procedure without major complications.[46] Because chronic pancreatitis and carcinoma cannot always be distinguished by ultrasound alone, this combination technique is especially helpful.[46] When there is abrupt obstruction of the pancreatic duct with extensive dilatation proximal to the obstruction, a carcinoma should be suspected.[46]

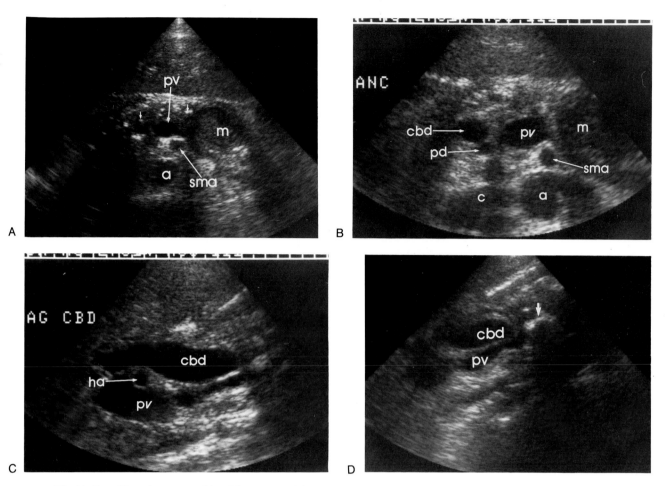

Fig. 7-49. Chronic pancreatitis with common bile duct obstruction. Transverse scans of **(A)** the body and tail region (not magnified) and **(B)** head (magnified). An echogenic mass (*m*, 29 × 36 mm) is seen within the tail; this was believed to represent a hemorrhagic pseudocyst or possibly neoplasm. The common bile duct *(cbd)* is dilated as well as the pancreatic duct *(pd)*. There are multiple calculi (arrows), seen as echogenic foci on Fig. A. (*pv*, portal vein; *sma*, superior mesenteric artery; *a*, aorta; *c*, inferior vena cava.) **(C & D)** Sagittal views of the dilated common bile duct *(cbd,* 15 mm) with Fig. D through the distal common bile duct. A large, echodense structure (arrow) representing a calculus is seen within the region of the pancreatic head on Fig. D. Rather than being obstructed by a stone, a stenotic distal duct was found at ERCP. (*pv*, portal vein; *ha*, hepatic artery.)

Ultrasound-guided percutaneous pancreatography can be performed successfully without complications.[119,120] It is easy to perform, and it (1) assists localization of pancreatic masses at fine-needle biopsy, (2) demonstrates pancreatic duct morphology when ERCP has failed or is nondiagnostic, (3) enables mapping of the ductal system prior to pancreatic surgery, and (4) provides an assessment of duct appearance that may be more accurate than in ECRP in differentiating carcinoma from chronic pancreatitis.[119] The three main indicators for the procedure are (1) the need for improved guidance during fine-needle aspiration biopsy in patients with suspected malignancy, (2) a failed or inadequate ERCP when a pancreatogram is required prior to

pancreatic surgery or for diagnostic purposes, and (3) the need for further delineation of duct morphology and identification of the full extent of ducts in patients with chronic pancreatitis and a pancreatic mass.

TRAUMA

Pancreatic injury from nonpenetrating abdominal trauma is uncommon, and the diagnosis is made difficult by the absence of specific signs during physical examination. In children, blunt trauma is a common cause of pseudocyst. Acute traumatic injury to the pancreas

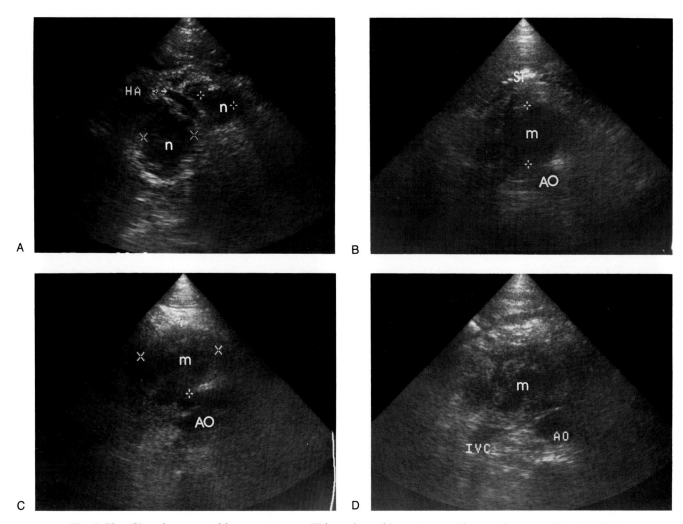

Fig. 7-50. Chronic pancreatitis versus tumor. This patient did not have a history of pancreatitis. **(A)** High transverse scan demonstrating nodal masses (hypoechoic areas, *n*) surrounding the hepatic artery *(HA)*. **(B–D)** Transverse views through the body (Figs. B & C, 40 mm) and head (Figs. C & D, 4 × 5 cm) of the pancreas. The pancreas is very inhomogeneous and suspicious for tumor *(m)*. At surgery, there were inflammatory nodes and chronic pancreatitis. *(AO,* aorta, *IVC,* inferior vena cava; *ST,* stomach.)

includes contusion with edema, laceration, hemorrhage, and transection, which almost always occurs in the body of the pancreas since it is compressed against the spine.[121,122] The pancreas and duodenum are fixed in position, so they absorb the total force of the abdominal blow. Their relation to the spine and ribs causes them to be damaged in such situations.[122] Clinically, these patients present with epigastric pain with or without radiation, as well as with nausea and vomiting. In one series in children, there were isolated pancreatic injuries in 3 percent and isolated duodenal injuries in 8 percent.[122]

The ultrasound findings with pancreatic trauma, which are often more subtle than those on CT, depend on the extent of the trauma. With contusion, a focal hypoechoic mass or a diffuse hypoechoic enlargement of the gland may be seen. A fracture line in the body of the pancreas along with fluid in the pararenal spaces may be seen with a transection[123] (Fig. 7-51). A well-defined anechoic mass with associated acoustic enhancement may be seen with a traumatic pseudocyst. With rupture, fluid may be demonstrated in the retroperitoneum and/or peritoneum.

Usually, abdominal CT is performed in all patients with acute blunt abdominal trauma with symptoms of peritoneal irritation and/or hyperamylasemia on initial evaluation or during an observation period.[123,124] Even CT findings are subtle, but CT appears to be superior to ultrasound in the evaluation of pancreatic trauma.[124]

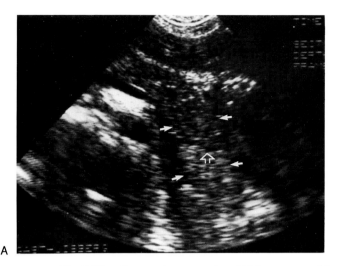 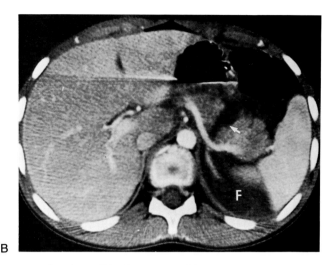

A   B

Fig. 7-51. Pancreatic transection. **(A)** Sonogram of the pancreas showing mild enlargement of the body and tail (arrows) and a lucency between the body and tail (open arrow), compatible with transection of the pancreas. **(B)** The pancreatic injury is dramatically demonstrated on CT scan. A through-and-through fracture line separating the body and tail of the pancreas (arrow) is seen. Note the presence of fluid *(F)* around the pancreas and spleen. (From Van Steenbergen et al,[123] with permission.)

Perhaps the echogenicity of pancreatic hemorrhage obscures the fracture within the pancreas.[124] The demonstration of pancreatic transection or of severe inflammatory changes might select patients who should immediately undergo surgical exploration. The late effects of pancreatic trauma (pseudocyst, chronic pancreatitis, and pancreatic fistula) can easily be detected on ultrasound and ERCP.

PANCREATIC NEOPLASM

Pancreatic Cyst

True cysts are lined with a mucous epithelium and may be congenital or acquired.[20] Congenital cysts are believed to be the result of anomalous development of the pancreatic duct.[4,20] They may be single but are usu-

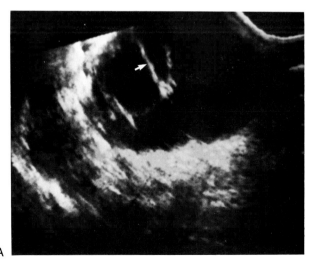 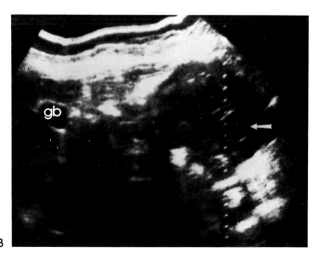

A   B

Fig. 7-52. Macrocystic adenoma. **(A)** Longitudinal static scan. A large cystic lesion in the tail of the pancreas is seen with thin septations (arrow) in the superior part of the mass. **(B)** Transverse static scan. A mass is seen in the tail of the pancreas containing cysts (arrow) that are larger than 2 cm. Acoustic enhancement is seen. (*gb*, gallbladder.) (From Wolfman et al,[126] with permission.)

ally multiple and without septation, and they vary in size from microscopic to 3 to 5 cm.[20] Acquired cysts are retention cysts (cystic dilatation of the pancreatic duct from any cause), parasitic cysts, and neoplastic cysts. Besides true cysts, there are pseudocysts that are not lined by epithelium but have a fibrous wall when mature. They are postinflammatory or post-traumatic in origin.[4]

Cystadenoma and Cystadenocarcinoma

Cystic pancreatic neoplasms are rare tumors, accounting for only 10 to 15 percent of all pancreatic cysts and 1 percent of pancreatic cancers.[125] These tumors have been subclassified pathologically into microcystic (serous) adenomas and mucinous cystic neoplasms; the latter are subdivided into mucinous (macrocystic) cystadenoma and mucinous (macrocystic) cystadenocarcinoma.[125,126] These subtypes are clinically important since microcystic adenomas are benign, do not have malignant potential, and, if asymptomatic, do not require surgical removal.[125] Mucinous cystadenomas are believed to either coexist with or develop into mucinous cystadenocarcinomas.[125] All these mucinous cystic neoplasms should be surgically removed.[125] In a recent study, 12 percent of patients with cystic pancreatic tumors had a clinical history of pancreatitis; all but one had either mucinous cystadenoma or cystadenocarcinoma.[125] There is a known association of von Hippel-Lindau syndrome with microcystic adenoma.[125]

The macrocystic adenoma is an uncommon, slow-growing tumor that is thought to arise as a cystic neoplasm from the ducts.[20] It is composed primarily of one (but less than six cysts) large cyst (2 to 20 cm), with or without septations, that is lined with mucin-producing cells.[4,20,125] There is significant malignant potential. Patients generally present with epigastric pain and/or a palpable mass. Several concurrent diseases are reported with this neoplasm, including diabetes, calculous disease of the biliary tract, and arterial hypertension.[4,127] Macrocystic adenomas occur most frequently in middle-aged women, with 60 percent appearing in the tail and 5 percent in the head of the pancreas.[126] The body and tail, then, are the most frequent sites.[4,128,129] There are frequently foci of calcification (reported in 26 percent of patients).[125] The therapy of choice is surgical excision.

The microcystic adenoma (formally called serous cystadenoma or glucagon-rich cystadenoma) is a benign neoplasm typically seen in elderly women with presenting symptoms and signs such as pain, weight loss, jaundice, and palpable mass.[130] One-half of cystic pancreatic neoplasms are microcystic adenomas. The microcystic adenoma is composed of tiny cysts (more than 6 cysts, <2 cm) lined with flattened or cuboidal cells that contain glycogen and little to no mucin. These lesions are totally benign. Microcystic adenomas also occur more frequently in women than in men and involve mainly the body and tail of the pancreas (60 percent) but may arise in the head (30 percent) or may be diffuse (10 percent).[4,126]

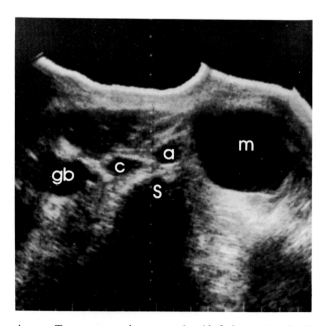

Fig. 7-53. Cystadenocarcinoma. Transverse static scan at a level inferior to the tail of the pancreas. An anechoic mass *(m)* is seen. (*a*, aorta; *c*, inferior vena cava; *gb*, gallbladder.)

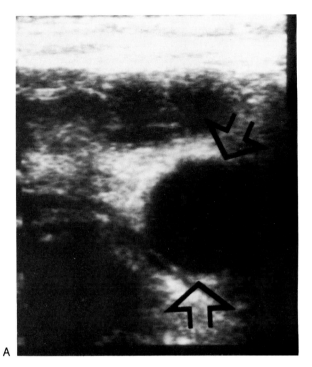

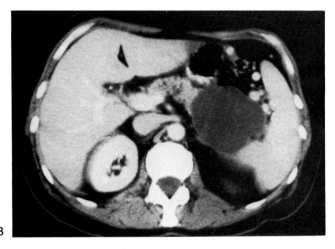

A   B

Fig. 7-54. Typical mucinous (macrocystic) cystadenoma. **(A)** Sonogram showing unilocular cyst (open arrows) within the pancreatic tail. The mass was proved surgically to be mucinous cystadenoma. Sonographically, findings are indistinguishable from those of pancreatic pseudocyst. **(B)** CT scan of a large cystic mass in the pancreatic tail. Cysts are more than 2 cm in diameter and few in number. Mucinous cystadenoma was proved surgically. (From Johnson et al,[125] with permission.)

On ultrasound, these cystic neoplasms appear similar to pseudocysts.[6,62,126–129,131–133] The macrocystic adenomas contain cysts greater than 2 cm in diameter. They are classic anechoic cysts with acoustic enhancement and internal septations[4,126,129,132,133] (Figs. 7-52 to 7-55). The internal septations usually are thin, and as the gain is increased, the cystic areas fill in with echoes.[4] In 10 to 18 percent of these adenomas, calcification is present within the wall and is seen as focal echogenic areas with shadowing; these cysts cannot be distinguished as benign or malignant.[4] Other investigators have identified four ultrasound patterns associated with cystadenocarcinoma: (1) anechoic mass with posterior enhancement and irregular margins; (2) anechoic mass with internal homogeneous echoes that are stratified in the supine position and mobile in the decubitus position; (3) anechoic mass with irregular internal vegetations protruding into the lumen and showing no movement; and (4) completely echogenic mass with nonhomogeneous pattern.[131]

The microcystic adenomas contain cysts less than 2 cm in diameter, with a central, stellate scar that may be calcified with radiating bands of connective tissue[4] (Figs. 7-56 and 7-57). This tumor is usually well circumscribed and oval. It occasionally contains calcifications; these

are seen as focal echogenic areas with or without shadowing within the central scar.[4,130] On ultrasound, there are small cysts with central calcification.[126] When the cysts are small, the tumor appears echogenic.[4] Ultrasound may demonstrate a totally echogenic mass as a result of the myriad of interfaces produced by microscopic cysts.[130] A preoperative biopsy with pathologic examination aids in making a definitive diagnosis and directs appropriate therapy. The following signs can help distinguish microcystic adenoma from pancreatic carcinoma: large size, sharply defined tumor margins, honeycomb appearance, increased echogenicity, and central scar (with or without calcifications).[130]

The sizes of most of the cysts within the mass and the total number of cysts are the two most important criteria in separating microcystic from mucinous subtypes.[125] When these criteria are used, 50 percent of microcystic adenomas and 90 percent of mucinous cystadenomas and carcinomas fit the criteria so that the correct tumor subtype can be suggested in 78 to 93 percent of microcystic tumors and 93 to 95 percent of mucinous tumors.[125] Differentiation of cystadenoma from cystadenocarcinoma is impossible unless there is evidence of local invasion or distant metastases.[125] Despite the difficulties in separating mucinous cystadenoma from cyst-

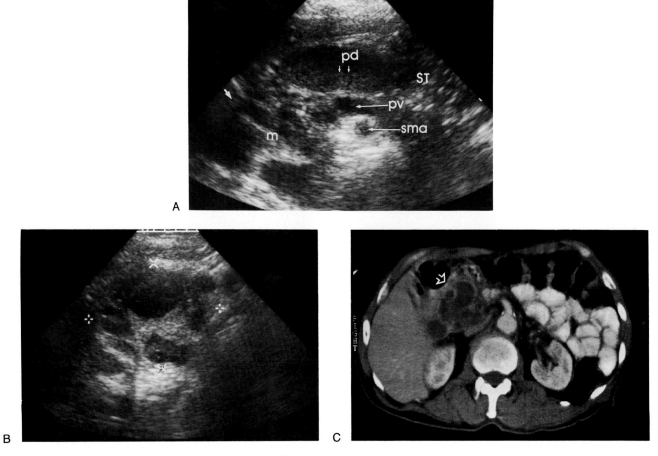

A

B

C

Fig. 7-55. Mucinous cystadenocarcinoma. **(A)** Transverse scan through the body demonstrating a markedly dilated pancreatic duct *(pd)* containing a fluid-fluid level (arrows). There is a mass *(m)* with indistinct borders in the pancreatic head region. (arrow, mass; *ST*, stomach; *sma,* superior mesenteric artery; *pv,* main portal vein.) **(B)** Transverse view of the pancreatic head region, where a large multicystic mass *(m*, calipers, 50 × 61 mm) is seen. **(C)** CT scan, similar to Fig. B, with a multicystic mass (arrow).

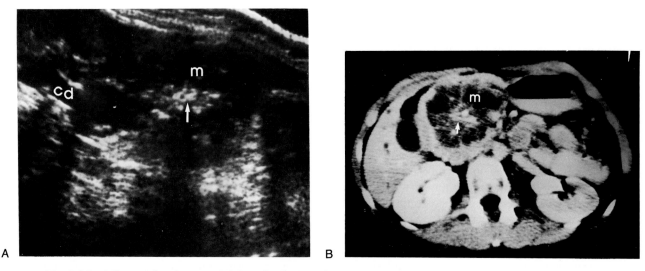

A

B

Fig. 7-56. Microcystic adenoma. **(A)** Longitudinal static scan to the right of midline. A dilated common bile duct *(cd)* is seen obstructed by a large mass *(m)* in the head of the pancreas. Centrally located calcifications are seen within the mass (arrow). Tiny cysts are barely visible. **(B)** Enhanced CT scan. A mass *(m)* is seen in the head of the pancreas with central calcification (arrow), and numerous cysts are separated by radiating bands of fibrosis. (From Wolfman et al,[126] with permission.)

416

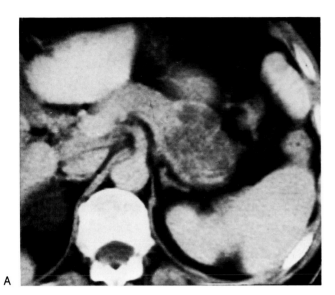
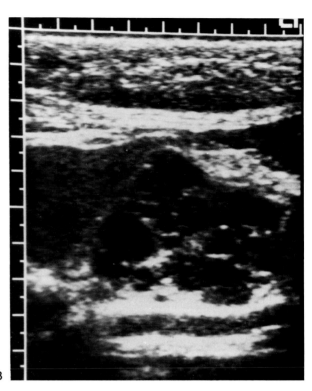

A   B

Fig. 7-57. Typical microcystic adenoma. **(A)** CT scan of adenoma within the pancreatic tail. Multiple small, well-defined cysts are visible within the mass. **(B)** Sonogram in another patient showing multiple small cysts within the mass in the pancreatic head. Microcystic adenoma was removed at surgery. (From Johnson et al,[125] with permission.)

adenocarcinoma, in this reported study the authors were able to correctly classify more than 90 percent of tumors as mucinous.[125]

Ductectatic Mucinous Cystadenoma/ Cystadenocarcinoma

A new type of mucinous cystadenoma/cystadenocarcinoma has been reported, termed *ductectatic*.[134] There is no preponderance of women with this type, and the patients tend to be much older. This tumor is characterized by localized cystic dilatation of a side branch of the main pancreatic duct. The dilated duct is covered with atypical papillary hyperplastic epithelium that is difficult to distinguish from mucinous cystadenoma or cystadenocarcinoma. These lesions appear typically in the uncinate process and are a conglomeration of communicating cysts 1 to 2 cm in diameter that are covered with a thin, fibrous capsule. On ultrasound, these lesions are difficult to distinguish from a simple cyst unless the lesion is lobulated or has irregular margins.[134] The location of the cyst in the uncinate process is an important key to the correct diagnosis. ERCP is valuable in making

the diagnosis by demonstrating the cystic lesion communicating with the pancreatic duct. The characteristic ERCP findings include localized, prominent cystic dilatation of a side branch of the main pancreatic duct with grapelike clusters or pear-shaped pools of contrast material associated with filling defects of various sizes. The differential diagnosis for this lesion includes retention cyst, true cyst, pseudocyst, and mucin-producing ductal cancer.

Adenocarcinoma

Carcinoma of the pancreas is a usually fatal tumor involving the exocrine portion of the gland, with its beginning in the ductal epithelium. It is one of the leading causes of cancer death in the United States,[135] representing 6 percent of all neoplastic deaths in the United States and 95 percent of all malignant pancreatic tumors.[4] Cures by surgical resection are rare. If the disease is confined to the pancreas or there is limited extension outside the pancreas, it is stage I disease.[135] At this stage, the tumor can be removed en bloc.[135] In stage II disease, the tumor has extended into the surrounding tissue and may

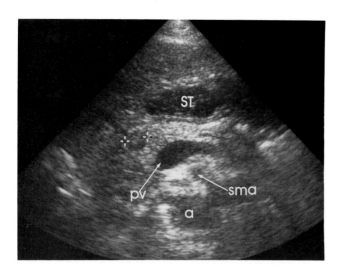

Fig. 7-58. Adenocarcinoma of the pancreatic head. Transverse scan. A small (10.6-mm), somewhat inhomogeneous, well-defined mass (calipers) is seen within the head of the pancreas. The borders of the superior mesenteric artery *(sma)* are indistinct. The patient had multiple metastatic liver lesions as well. *(ST,* fluid-filled stomach; *pv,* portal vein; *a,* aorta.)

preclude complete surgical resection.[135] In stage III disease, there is involvement of regional lymph nodes, and in stage IV disease there is spread to the liver or elsewhere.[135] The only resectable tumor is the one that has not directly invaded the neighboring organs, has not me-

tastasized to the lymph nodes, does not involve the major extrapancreatic vessels, and has no liver metastases.[135]

Pancreatic carcinoma occurs in the sixth, seventh, and eighth decades of life with a male preponderance. There have been rare reports of this lesion in children.[136] There is an increased risk of carcinoma of the pancreas in patients who smoke. There is an unexplained correlation between mortality from cancer of the pancreas and per capita consumption of fats and possibly calories. In 60 to 70 percent of cases, the tumor is in the head of the pancreas, in 20 to 30 percent it is in the body, and in 5 to 10 percent it is in the tail; in 21 percent it is diffuse.[4,20] The tumors in the head become symptomatic earlier than those in the body or tail.[4,20] The detection rate depends on an adequately visualized gland and varies from 81 to 94 percent.[4] When there is adequate visualization of the pancreas, the likelihood of missing a pancreatic neoplasm is extremely low, with a negative predictive value of 99 percent.[4,18] The sensitivity of ultrasound detection of the lesion has been reported to be 69 to 94 percent, and the specificity is reported to be 82 to 99 percent.[135]

The clinical course of carcinoma of the pancreas is insidious. Some of the symptoms include weight loss (70 percent of cases), abdominal pain (50 percent), back pain (25 percent), anorexia, nausea and vomiting, generalized malaise, and weakness.[4,20] The average time from onset of symptoms to diagnosis is 4 months, and that from onset of symptoms to death is 8.3 months to

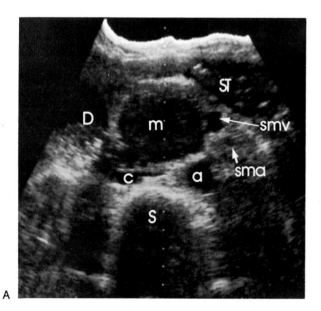

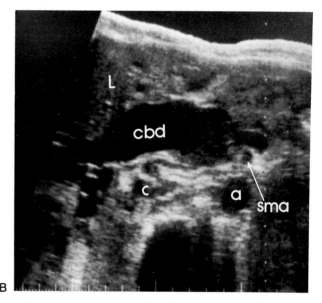

A   B

Fig. 7-59. Adenocarcinoma of the pancreatic head. Common bile duct obstruction. **(A)** Transverse scan demonstrating a hypoechoic mass *(m)* compressing the inferior vena cava *(c)* and displacing the superior mesenteric artery *(sma)* and vein *(smv)* to the left. *(a,* aorta; *ST,* fluid-filled stomach; *D,* fluid-filled duodenum.) **(B)** Oblique transverse scan higher than Fig. A demonstrating a dilated common bile duct *(cbd).* *(a,* aorta; *c,* inferior vena cava; *sma,* superior mesenteric artery; *L,* liver.)

1.6 years.[4,20,137] The 5-year survival rate is only 0.9 to 2 percent.[4,20,136,137] Poor survival is a reflection that 80 to 85 percent of patients with carcinoma of the pancreas have local spread or distant metastases when first seen clinically.[137]

A spectrum of ultrasound findings associated with pancreatic carcinoma have been described.[2,19-21,67,68,135,138,139] The findings can be grouped into two categories: intrapancreatic and extrapancreatic. Intrapancreatic findings include the appearance of the primary tumor and the pancreatic duct. Extrapancreatic findings include biliary obstruction, hepatic metastases, regional lymph node involvement, ascites, spleen enlargement and invasion, and alteration of the upper abdominal vessels.[21,50,135,138,140]

The primary tumor represents a localized change in the echodensity of the pancreas. The echopattern is hypoechoic, less dense than normal pancreas and liver (Figs. 7-58 to 7-63). From 95 to 100 percent of these tumors have been reported to be hypoechoic.[21,135] In one series, 3 percent were reported to be echogenic.[4] The borders of the mass are irregular, and the mass is usually quite distinct from the rest of the gland.[4,78] As a result of tumor necrosis, fluid collections may be associated with pancreatic cancer; these fluid collections may be the result of a localized distension of part of an obstructed pancreatic duct. There may or may not be pancreatic enlargement. Masses in the head of the pancreas tend to be smaller than those in the tail, as a result of compression of the common bile duct[4] (Figs. 7-58 to 7-61). One

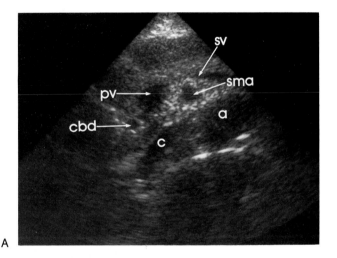

A

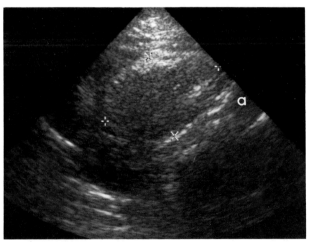

B

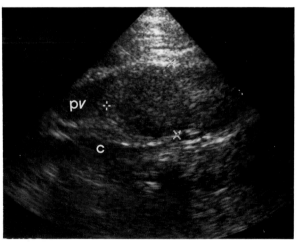

C

Fig. 7-60. Adenocarcinoma of the uncinate process. **(A)** Transverse scan at the level of the distal common bile duct *(cbd)* demonstrating a normal sized duct. *(sma,* superior mesenteric artery; *a,* aorta; *pv,* portal vein; *sv,* splenic vein; *c,* inferior vena cava.) **(B)** Transverse scan just inferior to Fig. A in the region of the uncinate process demonstrating a mass (calipers, 52 × 32 mm) that is isoechoic to the liver and pancreas. *(a,* aorta.) **(C)** Sagittal scan through the mass (calipers) that is compressing the superior mesenteric vein and inferior vena cava *(c).* *(pv,* portal vein.)

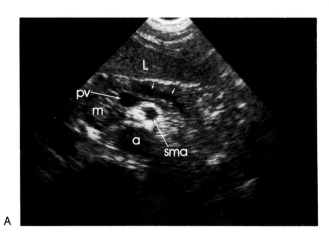 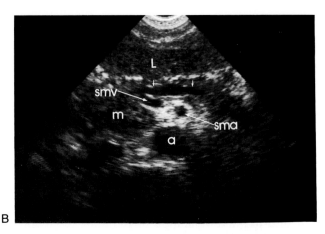

Fig. 7-61. Adenocarcinoma of the pancreatic head. Pancreatic duct obstruction. **(A & B)** Transverse scans with Fig. A more superior than Fig. B. An inhomogeneous mass *(m)* is seen in the pancreatic head. The pancreatic duct (arrows) is dilated within the pancreatic body. (*sma,* superior mesenteric artery; *smv,* superior mesenteric vein; *pv,* portal vein; *a,* aorta; *L,* liver.)

series has reported a tumor of 1.5 cm to be the smallest size detected by ultrasound, although smaller intrapancreatic lesions may be detected[135] (Fig. 7-58). Most patients have larger tumors at the time of presentation. In patients with large tumors, lack of visualization of any adjacent normal pancreas is a common finding.[135] This may be the result of tumor extension, a desmoplastic response to the tumor, or pancreatic atrophy.[135]

When pancreatic duct dilatation is visualized, this does not necessarily indicate unresectability and may even be a sign of a small, potentially resectable tumor.[135] A dilated pancreatic duct was visualized in 41 percent of patients in one series[135] (Figs. 7-61 and 7-62). The duct is

usually dilated with tumors of 3.4 cm; larger tumors, 4.9 cm, are not associated with a visibly dilated duct. The pancreatic ductal dilatation shows either a smooth pattern or irregular duct dilatation that closely corresponds to the dilatation patterns on ERCP.[46] Abrupt obstruction of the pancreatic duct and extensive dilatation proximal to the dilatation suggest carcinoma.

Since most patients with carcinoma of the head of the pancreas also have obstructive jaundice, one should search for a mass whenever an obstructive biliary tree is noted. Obstruction of the CBD can be produced by a direct effect of the mass in the head of the pancreas or adenopathy in the porta hepatis[4] (Fig. 7-59). In some

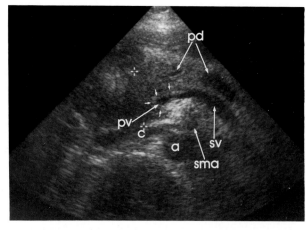 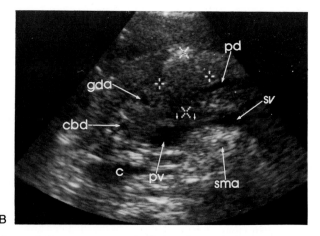

Fig. 7-62. **(A & B)** Adenocarcinoma. On transverse views of the pancreas, an indistinct hypoechoic area (calipers) is noted within the region of the head and body of the pancreas. The pancreatic duct *(pd)* is dilated, and its margins are poorly defined. There is involvement (arrows) of the portal vein *(pv).* The outline of the superior mesenteric artery *(sma)* is lost with perivascular thickening. The common bile duct *(cbd)* was not obstructed. (*c,* inferior vena cava; *a,* aorta; *gda,* gastroduodenal artery; *sv,* splenic vein.)

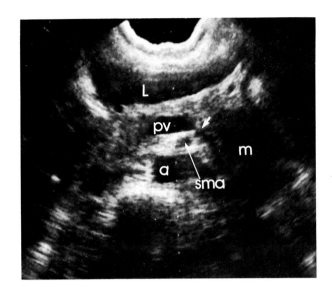

Fig. 7-63. Adenocarcinoma of the pancreatic tail. Splenic vein compression. Transverse scan. The splenic vein (arrow) is compressed by the hypoechoic pancreatic tail mass *(m)*. (*a*, aorta; *L*, liver; *sma,* superior mesenteric artery; *pv*, main portal vein.)

cases ductal dilatation is the only sign of carcinoma. This can be seen with carcinoma of the ampulla, cholangio-carcinoma near the ampulla, Crohn's disease of the duodenum, and stenosis of the ampulla. ERCP may be needed for the diagnosis. If the mass is very hypoechoic with extensive adenopathy, lymphoma should be considered.

Metastases to the liver associated with pancreatic carcinoma tend to be small and hypoechoic.[135] Detection of liver metastases indicates stage IV disease.[135] The associated lymph node involvement may be significantly more difficult to detect than the large, homogeneous, very low echo amplitude nodes of lymphoma.[135] Ultrasound may underestimate the extent of disease in evaluating lymph node involvement. Ascites is not a common finding.

A number of alterations in the upper abdominal vasculature may be produced by a pancreatic carcinoma. In 36 percent of the tumors involving the pancreatic head and body, there may be compression of the adjacent posteriorly situated IVC.[135] A mass in the head of the pancreas may compress the anterior wall of the IVC (50 percent of cases)[4,141] (Fig. 7-59A). Other vessels affected include the superior mesenteric vessels, splenic vein, and portal vein (Figs. 7-59 to 7-63).

The superior mesenteric vessels may be displaced posteriorly by a pancreatic mass.[21] The amount of the displacement depends on the site of the tumor.[4] The vessels are displaced anteriorly when carcinoma is in the unci-

nate process and posteriorly to the left and often to the right when carcinoma is in the head or body of the pancreas (Fig. 7-59A). Soft tissue thickening caused by neoplastic infiltration of the perivascular lymphatics may be seen surrounding the celiac axis or SMA (Figs. 7-61 and 7-62). This occurs more commonly with carcinoma of the body and tail (52 percent) than with carcinoma of the head (25 percent). In some patients (11 percent), this may be the only sign of carcinoma.

One of the crucial determinants for surgical resectability of carcinoma of the pancreas is vascular involvement.[142] Since resection of the SMA entails considerable risk, involvement by locally advanced tumor growth is a determinant for unresectability.[142] With involvement of the SMA, there is prominent thickening of the area around the SMA (called the *cuff sign*) with or without decreased echogenicity compared with adjacent retro-pancreatic connective tissue (Figs. 7-61 and 7-62). The mean thickness of the periarterial area in cancer patients with involvement of the SMA has been reported to be 8.5 mm.[142] With no involvement, the thickness is 4 mm (it is 2 mm in the control group). By using an upper limit of normal of 7 mm for the thickness of the SMA, the sensitivity is 91 percent with a specificity of 100 percent and an overall accuracy of 96 percent.[142]

Involvement of the portal venous system is of more prognostic significance than IVC compression.[135] There may be mild compression to complete occlusion with or without demonstrable collateral vessels. Collateral venous channels that develop may be visualized in the periportal area and along the wall of the stomach. If there is nonvisualization of a major portal vessel (such as the portal vein, splenic vein, or SMV) in association with pancreatic tumor, vascular involvement is suggested. A pancreatic mass can compress the splenic vein, producing secondary splenic enlargement (Fig. 7-63). Tumor may displace or invade the splenic or portal vein or produce thrombosis (12 to 48 percent)[4] (Figs. 7-62 and 7-63). The SMV and portal vein are affected by pancreatic head lesions, while the splenic vein is involved by lesions in the body and tail.[135] The splenic vein was most frequently involved by both proximal and distal tumors.[135]

One group of investigators has compared the evaluation of the portal venous system in pancreatic carcinoma by ultrasound with that by angiography.[143] The main tributaries of the portal system were evaluated for evidence of compression, displacement, or occlusion.[143] Ultrasound demonstrated a sensitivity of 90 percent and a specificity of 95 percent for splenic vein abnormalities when compared with angiography. The sensitivity and specificity were 75 and 100 percent, respectively, for portal vein evaluation and 100 and 94 percent, respectively, for SMV evaluation.[143] Preoperative angiography may be unnecessary if a thorough ultrasound evaluation of the portal venous system is performed.[143] It is generally accepted that the major criterion for surgical unresectability is local spread of tumor causing occlusion or encasement of the major veins in the portal system.[143] Palliative surgery rather than total resection may be planned when ultrasound shows occlusion of the portal vein or occlusion of both the SMV and splenic vein, and angiography may be avoided.

Hepaticopancreatic Ampullary Tumor

Tumors located in the hepaticopancreatic ampullary region are called such since they are located at the confluence of the bile duct, pancreatic duct, and duodenum.[144] It is usually diagnosed early since jaundice occurs at an early stage. The ultrasound findings described include intraluminal polypoid mass within the distal common bile duct and a sharply delineated (intraluminal) mass producing abrupt termination of the distal duct.[144] Other tumors cannot be differentiated without histologic study, but ampullary carcinoma should be suspected in patients in whom the bile duct dilatation extends down to the distal common bile duct and is associated with a small mass with a sharply delineated outline. In retrospect, the sensitivity of ultrasound in this series was 75 percent, and the prospective diagnostic sensitivity was 50 percent.[144] Improved detection and prompt treatment of these tumors may occur with improved ultrasound resolution, more experience with this modality, and accurate diagnosis of these tumors by ultrasound.[144]

Solid Papillary Epithelial Neoplasm

Most pancreatic carcinomas are ductal cell adenocarcinomas.[145] There is a solid and papillary epithelial neoplasm located within the tail; it is frequently seen in young females (mean age, 24 years).[145,146] It is an uncommon, low-grade malignant tumor amenable to cure by surgical excision.[146] Usually the patient does not have symptoms until the tumor is large. Multiple areas of hemorrhage and cystic degeneration are frequently found within this tumor, but mitotic figures are rarely seen. After surgical resection, the prognosis is remarkably good, although hepatic invasion, duodenal invasion, and distant metastasis have been reported.[145]

The lesion may appear similar to cystadenoma or cystadenocarcinoma on ultrasound, since there are septations in the cystic portions, possibly as a result of prominent papillae projecting into the large space of cystic degeneration[145,146] (Fig. 7-64). On ultrasound and CT, a mass that can be solid, mixed cystic and solid, or

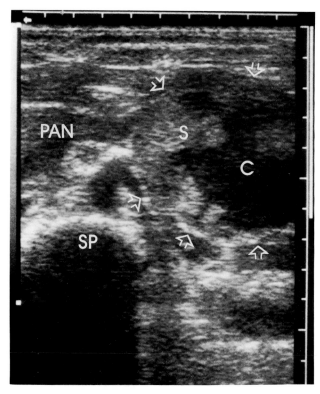

Fig. 7-64. Solid and papillary pancreatic neoplasm. Sonographic features of a solid and papillary neoplasm of the pancreas. Transverse scan. The tumor (arrows) is located in pancreatic tail; it is composed of cystic *(C)* and solid *(S)* components. (*PAN,* pancreas; *SP,* spine.) (From Lin et al,[145] with permission.)

largely cystic may be demonstrated.[146] Calcification within the mass is not common. Even though its ultrasound features are indistinguishable from those of cystadenoma and cystadenocarcinoma, the occurrence in young females without remarkable clinical symptoms, in association with a hemorrhagic component, should lead to the suspicion of a solid papillary tumor.[145]

Pleomorphic Carcinoma

Pleomorphic carcinoma of the pancreas (representing 2 to 7 percent of pancreatic carcinomas) is an uncommon lesion that contains bizarre giant cells and resembles sarcoma histologically.[147] The associated masses are large, lobular, and hypoechoic and contain variable amounts of coarse echoes, with the main tumor mass more often located in the body or tail rather than the head of the pancreas (Fig. 7-65). The most striking finding with this tumor is the demonstration of widespread lymphadenopathy in the peripancreatic region (often mimicking lymphoma), which extends caudally to the

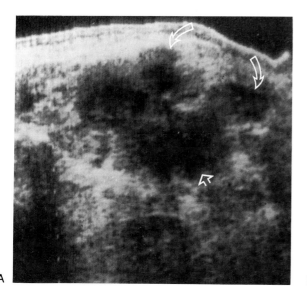
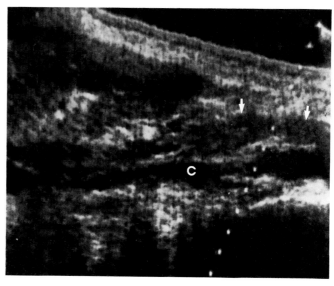

A   B

Fig. 7-65. Pleomorphic carcinoma. **(A)** Transverse ultrasound image of pleomorphic carcinoma involving the body and tail of the pancreas. The mass is large, irregular, and lobular (open arrowhead). It is essentially hypoechoic with heterogeneous echotexture. No cystic areas are seen. Mesenteric lymphadenopathy is also noted (open arrows) and was seen on multiple sections. **(B)** Longitudinal ultrasound image along the inferior vena cava *(c)* in the same patient. Metastatic involvement of the pericaval lymph nodes is noted (arrows). Involvement extends caudally along the entire length of the vena cava. (From Wolfman et al,[147] with permission.)

pancreas toward the aortic bifurcation and superiorly to the level of the esophageal hiatus. The extensive nodal involvement associated with this tumor is not typical for ductal adenocarcinoma. At the time of initial workup, widespread metastases are evident. The incidence of pulmonary metastases is much higher with this tumor than with ductal carcinoma. The clinical course of this tumor is fulminant, and death usually occurs within 2 to 3 months of the onset of symptoms.

Mucin-Hypersecreting Carcinoma

A mucin-hypersecreting carcinoma of the pancreas associated with diffuse dilatation of the main pancreatic duct has been described.[148] This particular lesion is associated with a good prognosis. It is characterized by marked dilatation of the entire or segmental main duct associated with filling defects on ERCP and by excretion of mucin through the patulous orifice of the enlarged papilla of Vater at endoscopy. Pathologic examination shows that this adenocarcinoma, secreting excessive mucin, is found mainly in the main duct.

On ultrasound a number of findings may be demonstrated: (1) smooth, diffuse dilatation of the main duct; (2) a polypoid lesion within the main duct; (3) a solid-appearing mass secondary to the varying degree of mucin; and (4) atrophy of pancreatic parenchyma.[148] Main-duct dilatation can be seen associated with pan-

creatic carcinoma, papillary carcinoma, and chronic pancreatitis. Dilatation of the pancreatic duct is seen in 56 percent of patients with this pancreatic carcinoma (mean diameter, 8.7 mm) and in 58 percent of patients with chronic pancreatitis (mean diameter, 6.7 mm).[148] In patients with chronic pancreatitis the duct is usually irregular in its dilatation, whereas in patients with carcinoma it is smooth or beaded. Pancreatography is mandatory to confirm or rule out mucin-hypersecreting carcinoma of the pancreas when there is diffuse dilatation of the main duct without findings of invasive cancer or chronic pancreatitis at ultrasound.[148]

Differential Diagnosis

At times it may be difficult to differentiate between pancreatic neoplasm and acute or chronic pancreatitis since all can produce a focal mass.[149] In acute pancreatitis, the mass is usually uniformly hypoechoic with good through transmission unless there is hemorrhage or gas caused by necrosis and/or suppuration. A focal mass confined to the pancreas directly anterior to the aorta is not likely to be inflammation. The presence of adenopathy silhouetting the wall of the aorta by a contiguous pancreas process is most probably caused by tumor. Differentiation from chronic pancreatitis is difficult.[4]

One group of investigators performed serum CA 19-9 assessment, ultrasound, CT, and CT-guided fine-needle aspiration biopsy of pancreatic lesions. The accuracy of all diagnostic and nondiagnostic studies was 81 percent for CA 19-9 assessment, 72 percent for ultrasound, 77 percent for CT, and 94 percent for fine-needle aspiration biopsy. It appeared from the study that CT-guided fine-needle aspiration biopsy is the most reliable examination for differentiating between carcinoma and chronic pancreatitis.[149]

Conclusion

The primary imaging methods for the detection of pancreatic masses are CT and ultrasound since they are noninvasive.[150] With advances in equipment, scanning techniques, and interpretive skills, the success rate in detecting pancreatic carcinoma has continued to improve.[150] There has been little emphasis on the use of ultrasound to resolve inconclusive findings on CT. A finding of fullness of the pancreatic head unaccompanied by a low-density area or secondary signs of tumor on CT is an indication for ultrasound. Ultrasound can often confirm the presence of a solid hypoechoic lesion within the pancreatic head, but it cannot distinguish between pancreatic carcinoma and chronic focal pancreatitis. Ultrasound is valuable in excluding or confirming a mass when the CT findings are inconclusive. In about 85 percent of patients, ultrasound allows visualization of the pancreas, and it will confirm or exclude a pancreatic lesion in most but not all of these.[150]

The accuracy of ultrasound in evaluating patients for pancreatic neoplasm is operator dependent; its specificity and sensitivity for tumor detection often exceed 90 percent when state-of-the-art equipment is used.[151] Patients with no evidence of liver metastases, lymphadenopathy, or vascular involvement are thought to have resectable disease.[151]

Islet Cell Tumor

There are several types of islet cell tumors; some are functional (85 percent), and others are nonfunctional (15 percent).[4] They represent either benign adenomas or malignant tumors. Although these tumors may be malignant or benign, 92 percent of the nonfunctional tumors are malignant.[4] The nonfunctioning islet cell tumors constitute one-third of all islet cell tumors.[152] There is a 1.6 percent incidence of these tumors in an autopsy series.[153] They are slow-growing tumors with a 5-year survival of 44 percent.[4] An association (17 percent) between von Hippel-Lindau syndrome (a rare autosomal-dominant disorder characterized by central nervous system [CNS] hemangioblastoma, retinal angiomas, renal cell carcinomas, pheochromocytomas, and visceral cysts) and islet cell tumors has been shown.[55]

The diagnosis of these tumors is based on clinical and endocrinology features. Angiography the single most effective method for localizing small insulinomas.[154] Ultrasound can detect 51 percent of the tumors. The presence of cancer is difficult to determine at the cellular level; it can be diagnosed when there is invasion of surrounding structures or liver metastases.[4]

The most common functional islet cell tumor is the insulinoma (60 percent), followed by the gastrinoma (18 percent) and the tumors producing watery diarrhea, hypokalemia, and achlorhydria (WDHA syndrome).[4,155] Functional tumors are more difficult to detect than nonfunctional ones because functional tumors produce symptoms when small as a consequence of their hormonal activity. The rate of malignancy is higher in gastrinomas (25 to 60 percent) than in insulinomas (10 percent).[4] The diabetes-producing tumors (glucagonomas and somatostatinomas) are usually malignant and several centimeters in diameter. Of the non-beta islet cell tumors responsible for WDHA syndrome, 50 percent are malignant. Accurate preoperative localization allows a simple curative enucleation, which carries a lower morbidity and mortality risk than pancreatic resection.[154]

Clinically, patients with insulinomas experience fasting hypoglycemia and inappropriate elevated plasma insulin levels.[155] In 70 percent of cases there is a solitary adenoma, in 10 percent there are multiple adenomas, and in 10 percent there are metastases. The lesions may be minute to 1,500 g. Some 90 percent of insulinomas are less than 2 cm in diameter, and their small size makes them difficult to palpate during surgery.[154] They occur most frequently in the body and tail of the pancreas, where the concentration of islets of Langerhans is greatest.[153]

In patients with Zollinger-Ellison syndrome, the lesions are gastrinomas. These pancreatic lesions are associated with gastric hypersecretion and peptic ulcer disease. Most of the lesions are in the pancreas, with 13 percent in the duodenum; more than 60 percent are malignant.

Each functioning tumor, with the exception of somatostatinoma, is described in association with multiple endocrine neoplasia type I (MEN I) syndrome. In MEN syndrome, there are adenomas in the pituitary, pancreas, and parathyroid. In MEN I syndrome (autosomal dominant, multiglandular), there are tumors or hyperplasia of the parathyroid, pituitary, adrenal cortex, and pancreas with peptic ulcer disease and gastric hypersecretion. In MEN II syndrome (Sipple syndrome), there are multiple pheochromocytomas, medullary carcinoma of the thyroid, parathyroid hyperplasia or adenoma, and no pancreatic islet cell tumor.[4]

Nonfunctional islet cell tumors represent 15 to 33 per-

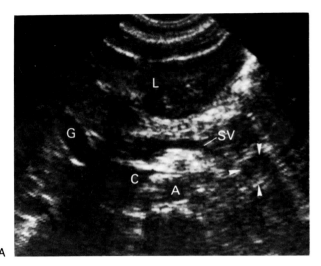

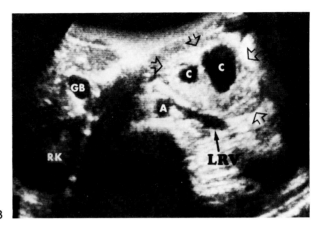

A   B

Fig. 7-66. Islet cell tumors. **(A)** Case 1. Insulinoma (10 × 20 mm). Transverse scan with hypoechoic tumor (arrowheads) in the tail of the pancreas. (*G*, gallbladder; *SV*, splenic vein; *C*, inferior vena cava; *A*, aorta; *L*, liver.) **(B)** Case 2. Cystic degeneration. Transverse scan 3 cm caudal to the xyphoid. A mass in the tail of the pancreas (open arrows) is seen containing two cystic cavities *(C)*. (*A*, aorta; *LRV*, left renal vein; *GB*, gallbladder; *RK*, right kidney.) (Fig. A from Gunther et al,[157] with permission; Fig. B from Raghavendra and Glickstein,[153] with permission.)

cent of all pancreatic islet cell tumors.[156] The nonfunctional tumors are easier to detect because they reach a larger size before they cause symptoms. They usually range in size from 1 to 20 cm; they often are not diagnosed until they reach a larger size.[156] They are usually solitary, and they cause abdominal pain (36 percent), jaundice (28 percent), or a palpable mass (8 percent).[4] Most of these tumors (60 to 92 percent) are malignant.[156] Cancer is diagnosed when either peripancreatic vascular invasion or distant metastases are found or when histologic examination reveals perineural or perivascular invasion.[156] There are certain characteristics that appear to pertain to this tumor: large size (more than 10 cm in diameter), evenness of margins, intratumoral calcification, and hypoechogenicity with more or less large necrotic areas.[156] The associated liver lesions are hyperechogenic or "targetlike" lesions.[156]

Ultrasound is very effective in evaluating the non-beta cell tumors by looking for a primary pancreatic mass and hepatic metastases in patients with glucagonomas, somatostinoma, nonfunctioning tumors, and WDHA syndrome.[155] In general, the islet cell tumors appear homogeneous, solid, and frequently hypoechoic, whereas some larger ones are moderately echogenic[153,155,157] (Figs. 7-66 to 7-70). Calcification and fluid spaces may be seen in the larger lesions (Figs. 7-66B and 7-70). The tumors are spherical, well marginated, homogeneous, and slow growing. The solid masses are more likely to be functional, and those containing necrotic cystic areas are

more likely to be nonfunctional.[152] In 31 percent of patients there are liver metastases. Those from functional tumors tend to be echogenic,[4] whereas those from the nonfunctional tumors run the gamut from high-level to low-level echoes with target lesions present[4,155] (Fig. 7-71). Others describe the liver metastases in functioning islet cell tumors to be characteristically isodense.[155] The

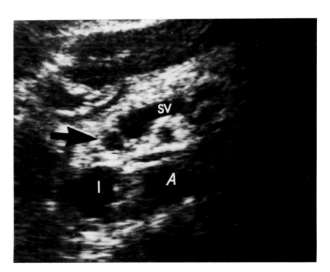

Fig. 7-67. Insulinoma. Transverse preoperative sonogram showing a typical hypoechoic insulinoma (arrow) within the echogenic parenchyma of the pancreatic head. (*A*, aorta; *I*, inferior vena cava; *sv*, splenic vein.) (From Galiber et al,[160] with permission.)

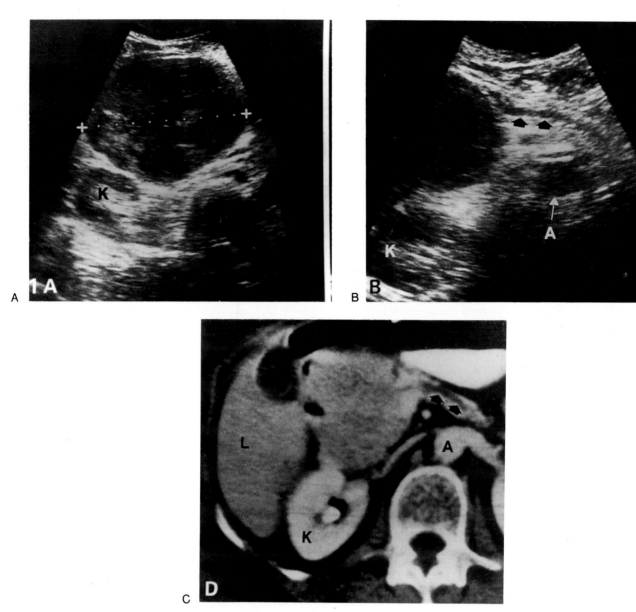

Fig. 7-68. Nonfunctional islet cell tumor of the pancreatic head. **(A & B)** Ultrasonography (contiguous axial scans) showing a large hypoechoic mass with even margins, causing mild dilation of the pancreatic duct (arrows, Fig. B) anterior to the aorta *(A).* (*K,* kidney.) **(C)** CT scan. The large mass turns focally hyperdense after fast intravenous contrast material administration; in a more cranial scan the slightly dilated pancreatic duct can be seen (arrows). (*L,* liver; *K,* kidney, *A,* aorta.) (From Fugazzola et al,[156] with permission.)

role of ultrasound varies with the type of pancreatic islet cell tumor.

In detection of Zollinger-Ellison syndrome, ultrasound compares favorably with detection of gastrinomas by angiography and CT. On ultrasound, these lesions are homogeneously hypoechoic.[155] Ultrasound has been reported to identify lesions smaller than 1 cm.[158] Insulinomas are homogeneously solid with no cavitation or calcification.[155]

The overall detection rate of islet cell tumors by ultrasound is 51 percent, with the lowest rate for the insulinomas (30 percent) because of their small size and the patient's obesity. Ultrasound has been reported to have a sensitivity of 63 percent in the detection of hepatic gastrinomas with a specificity of 100 percent, a positive predictive value of 100 percent, and a negative predictive value of 89 percent.[159] Ultrasound has a sensitivity of 30 percent for detection of extrahepatic gastrinomas, with a

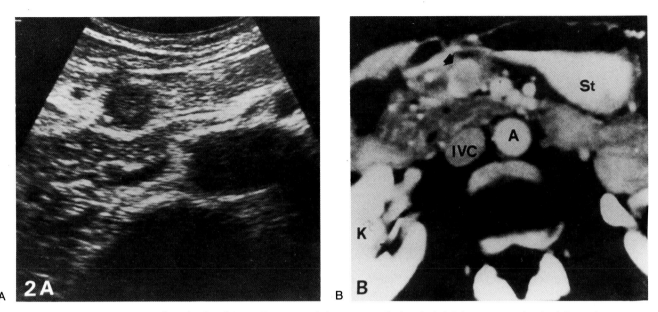

Fig. 7-69. Small nonfunctioning islet cell tumor of the pancreatic head. **(A)** Ultrasonography (axial scan) showing a hypoechoic mass with even margins, about 1.5 cm in diameter (incidental finding). **(B)** CT scan. The small mass turns evenly hyperdense after intravenous contrast material administration (arrow). (*K*, kidney; *St*, stomach; *IVC*, inferior vena cava; *A*, aorta.) (From Fugazzola et al,[156] with permission.)

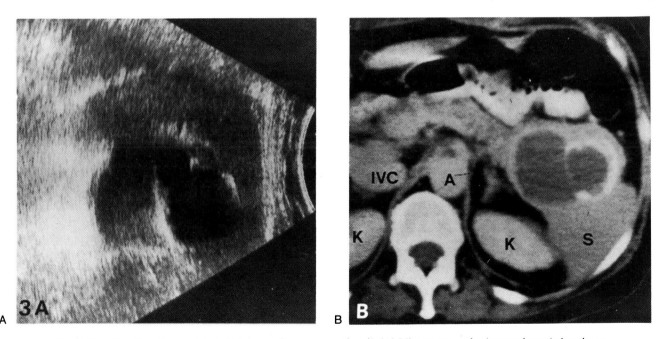

Fig. 7-70. Nonfunctioning islet cell tumor of the pancreatic tail. **(A)** Ultrasonography (coronal scan) showing a cystic multiseptated mass with partly calcified walls. **(B)** CT scan. Its information is superimposable over that provided by ultrasonography. (*K*, kidney; *S*, spleen; *IVC*, inferior vena cava; *A*, aorta.) (From Fugazzola et al,[156] with permission.)

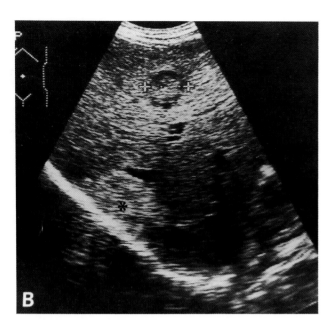

Fig. 7-71. Liver metastases. Ultrasonography (longitudinal scan) showing two metastases, one hyperechogenic (asterisk) and the other hyperechogenic with a peripheral hypoechoic rim, at the right lobe. (From Fugazzola et al,[156] with permission.)

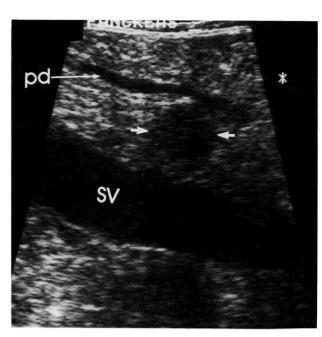

Fig. 7-72. Insulinoma. Transverse intraoperative sonogram of the pancreatic tail demonstrating a 1.2-cm insulinoma (arrows) sandwiched between the main pancreatic duct *(pd)* and splenic vein *(SV)*. (From Galiber et al,[160] with permission.)

specificity of 94 percent, a positive predictive value of 100 percent, and a negative predictive value of 25 percent.[159]

Investigators have evaluated pre- and intraoperative ultrasound, CT, and angiography in the localization of pancreatic insulinomas.[160,161] About 90 percent of these tumors are benign, solitary, and small (<2 cm). Up to 27 percent of patients have occult lesions at time of surgery. The typical lesion appears as a well-circumscribed mass that is hypoechoic, although 10 percent of the tumors in this series[161] were either isoechoic or hyperechoic (Fig. 7-72). The presence of a halo around the tumor may allow detection. A sensitivity of 100 percent is achieved by a combination of surgical palpation and intraoperative ultrasound.[160] Removal of the tumor is facilitated and the long-term prognosis is excellent for tumors that could be localized either preoperatively or during surgery. The sensitivity for detection of multiple masses within one patient is low. The prospective sensitivities in this series were 84 percent for intraoperative ultrasound, 61 percent for ultrasound, 54 percent for angiography, and 30 percent for CT.[160]

Another group of investigators have also evaluated the value of intraoperative ultrasound in localizing islet cell tumors.[162] In 11 percent of their cases, the surgical management was changed by intraoperative ultrasound. Several patients had tumors that would not have been found without intraoperative ultrasound. This study concluded that palpation and intraoperative ultrasound are complementary because intraoperative ultrasound can image tumors that are not palpable and can provide additional information about malignant potential that was not detected by palpation.[162] Additionally, intraoperative ultrasound appears to be able to differentiate between malignant islet cell tumors and benign tumors.[162]

Metastatic Neoplasm

Lymph Nodes

The pancreatic head and body are ringed along their lateral and posterior margins by anterior and posterior pancreaticoduodenal, anterior paracaval, and superior mesenteric lymph nodes.[163] The anterior chain of nodes follows the distribution of the gastroduodenal artery, while the posterior chain lies predominantly anterolateral to the IVC. These nodes receive efferent drainage from the head of the pancreas and duodenum and communicate with the gastric, hepatic, and mesenteric nodes. These are the nodes that lie between the duodenal sweep and the pancreatic head. Metastatic tumors may involve both the anterior and the posterior pancreaticoduodenal lymph nodes (Fig. 7-73). The tumors that in-

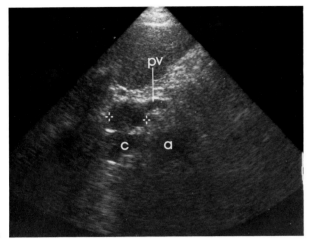

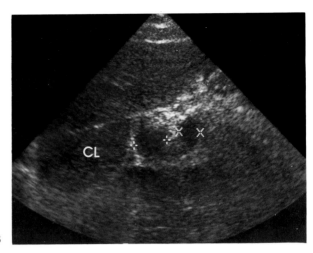

A   B

Fig. 7-73. Peripancreatic nodes in a patient with metastatic testicular carcinoma. **(A)** Transverse scan in the region of the pancreatic head with a hypoechoic mass (calipers) representing metastatic nodes. (*pv*, portal vein; *c*, inferior vena cava; *a*, aorta.) **(B)** Sagittal scan in the region of the porta hepatis with nodes (calipers). (*CL*, caudate lobe of the liver.)

volve these nodes most frequently include lymphoma of gastrointestinal origin, lung carcinoma, and breast carcinoma.[164] These nodes may be associated with biliary and duodenal obstruction. At times, pancreaticoduodenal lymph node enlargement mimics pancreatic cancer, creating confusion[164] (Figs. 7-73 and 7-74). The most helpful sign for differentiation is demonstration of intact tissue planes separating adenopathy from the pancreas and the extrapancreatic vascular displacement.[164]

These pancreaticoduodenal, anterior paracaval, and

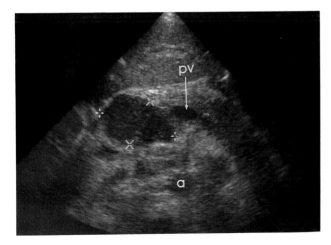

Fig. 7-74. Peripancreatic nodes in a patient with tuberculosis and AIDS. There is a hypoechoic mass (calipers, 33 × 55 mm) in the region of the head of the pancreas that is difficult to differentiate from pancreatic carcinoma. This was a nodal mass secondary to tuberculosis. (*a*, aorta; *pv*, portal vein.)

superior mesenteric lymph nodes can be involved with metastatic disease and can be a source of a false-positive diagnosis for pancreatic carcinoma. They may appear as well-defined, echopoor, ovoid or rounded masses in the retropancreatic location or may surround and silhouette the region of the pancreatic head and body[163] (Figs. 7-73 to 7-75). With a confluent mass of peripancreatic nodes, they may be impossible to distinguish from pancreatic disease (Figs. 7-73 to 7-75). The nodes are usually retropancreatic, lying posterior to the splenic vein and splenic-portal confluence, anterior to the IVC, and lateral to the SMA (Figs. 7-73 to 7-75). As a rule, masses arising anterior to the splenic vein are thought to be pancreatic in origin and those posterior to the splenic vein are thought to be extrapancreatic.[165] Occasionally, a pancreatic lesion can project posteriorly.[165] Needle biopsy may help in the differential diagnosis.

Metastatic Disease to the Pancreas

Direct invasion by tumors from surrounding organs may also appear as a primary pancreatic mass with a hypoechoic echopattern.[166] This can occur with gastric, colonic, duodenal, and biliary tumors. Because the mass cannot be distinguished from a primary carcinoma, the diagnosis is made by a percutaneous needle biopsy. The pancreas is rarely involved by metastatic disease from other primary tumors[4]; when secondarily involved, most often it is from direct extension.

Owing to their small size and the paucity of clinical symptoms, pancreatic metastases are diagnosed infre-

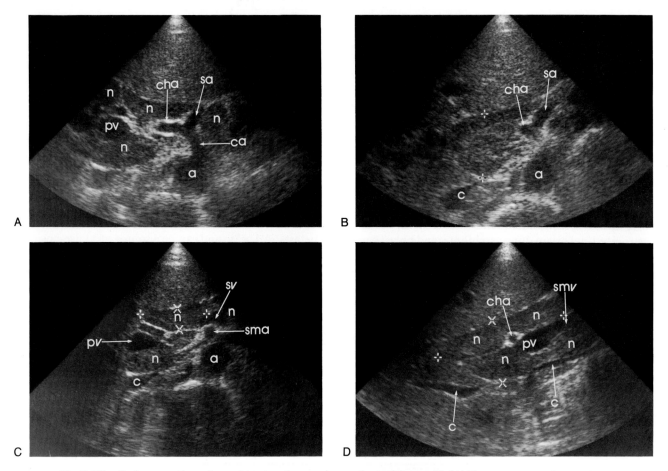

Fig. 7-75. Peripancreatic nodes and pancreatic mass in a patient with sarcoid. **(A)** Transverse scan demonstrating multiple nodes *(n)* surrounding the celiac artery *(ca)* and its branches. (*a,* aorta; *pv,* portal vein; *cha,* common hepatic artery; *sa,* splenic artery.) **(B)** Transverse view slightly lower than Fig. A showing a large mass (calipers) in the area of the pancreatic head. (*cha,* common hepatic artery; *sa,* splenic artery; *a,* aorta.) **(C)** Transverse view more inferior than Figs. A & B with multiple nodes *(n).* (*pv,* portal vein; *sv,* splenic vein; *sma,* superior mesenteric artery; *a,* aorta; *c,* inferior vena cava.) **(D)** Sagittal view with the nodal masses compressing the superior mesenteric vein *(smv),* portal vein *(pv),* and inferior vena cava *(c).* (*cha,* common hepatic artery; *n,* nodes.)

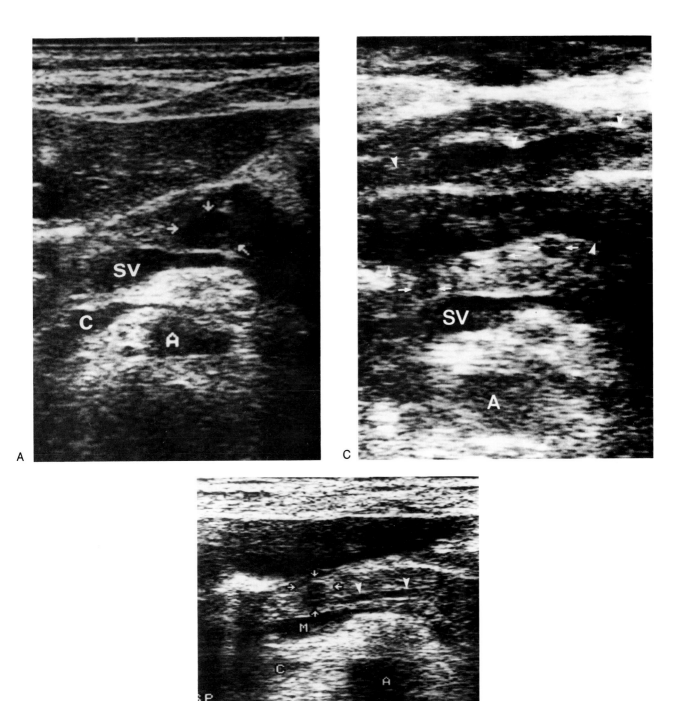

Fig. 7-76. Pancreatic metastases. **(A)** Multiple metastases to the pancreas from bronchial carcinoma. Transverse section showing a hypoechoic focus 1.5 cm in diameter (arrows) in the body of the pancreas. (*SV,* splenic vein; *A,* aorta; *C,* inferior vena cava.) **(B)** Solitary metastasis to the pancreas from bronchial carcinoma. Transverse section of the upper abdomen showing a hypoechoic focus (arrows) 1 cm in diameter at the transition between the head and body of the pancreas. The pancreatic duct (arrowheads) is dilated to 4 mm in diameter distal to the space-occupying lesion. (*M,* splenic vein; *A,* aorta; *C,* inferior vena cava.) **(C)** Multiple metastases to the pancreas from gastric carcinoma. Cross-sectional view of the upper abdomen showing multiple hypoechoic foci 0.5 to 1.0 cm in diameter (arrows) in the body of the pancreas. Ventral to the pancreas, the carcinomatous thickened stomach wall (arrowheads) of the antrum, sectioned longitudinally, can be discerned. (*SV,* splenic vein; *A,* aorta.) (From Wernecke et al,[167] with permission.)

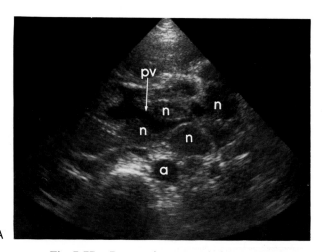
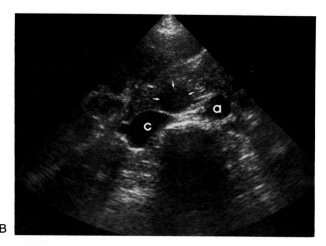

Fig. 7-77. Pancreatic metastasis from gallbladder carcinoma. **(A)** Transverse scan showing multiple nodes *(n)* surrounding the portal vein *(pv)*. (*a*, aorta.) **(B)** At the level of the pancreatic head, there is a hypoechoic mass (arrows). By ultrasound alone, this could not be distinguished from a primary neoplasm. (*a*, aorta; *c*, inferior vena cava.)

quently.[167] They generally appear as homogeneous, solid, space-occupying lesions with a more hypoechoic internal structure (Figs. 7-76 and 7-77). The diagnosis of metastases should be considered if multiple masses are found within the pancreas in a patient with a known primary tumor. Of primary consideration would be pancreatic carcinoma, acute pancreatitis, and focal infiltrates with Hodgkin's disease and non-Hodgkin's lymphoma. Some investigators have reported an incidence of pancreatic metastases in 8.4 percent of patients with carcinoma of the lung, 19 percent with breast carcinoma, and up to 37.5 percent with malignant melanoma.[167] As such, primary tumors include melanoma; bronchial, ovarian, mammary, prostate, renal, and hepatocellular carcinoma; and various sarcomas.

Intra-abdominal lymphomas may also involve the pancreas, producing a large, lumpy mass that is hypoechoic (Figs. 7-78 and 7-79). The superior mesenteric vessels should be displaced anteriorly instead of posteriorly as seen with a primary pancreatic mass. Again, the definitive diagnosis is made by percutaneous needle biopsy.[19]

Extramedullary plasmacytomas of the gastrointestinal tract (10 to 13 percent) are rare; extramedullary plasmocytomas are found in 71 percent of patients with multiple myelomas at autopsy with the vast majority involving the head and neck of the pancreas.[168] Pancreatic involvement is usually microscopic. There has been a report of a plasmacytoma involving the pancreas appearing as a multilobular mass with fine low-level echoes and moderate acoustic enhancement that suggest lymphoma. The definitive diagnosis is made by percutaneous needle biopsy.[168]

Sarcoidosis

Other entities besides tumor should be considered when a hypoechoic mass is demonstrated within the pancreas.[169] Sarcoidosis may produce a hypoechoic mass within the pancreas as well as peripancreatic nodes (Fig. 7-75). This disease process may be associated with multisystem involvement such as involvement of the lung, liver, spleen, skin, parotid, bone, muscle, heart, and nervous system. Any lymph node group may be involved. This disease process can produce bulky mass-like granulomatous tissue, which may mimic neoplastic disease. This diagnosis should be kept in mind in the proper clinical setting.

Aspiration/Biopsy

The diagnosis of pancreatic carcinoma is difficult, and in most patients it is made only at the stage of the disease at which the lesion is not resectable. Several investigators have described the use of the aspiration/biopsy procedure in evaluating patients for pancreatic carcinoma.[137,170-181] The indications for a fine-needle biopsy include the following: (1) to avoid surgery by obtaining a histologic diagnosis; (2) to determine staging of a neoplastic disease process; and (3) to facilitate treatment planning.[170] The essential indication is to obtain pathologic evidence of cancer without exploratory laparotomy.

With the recent improvements in localizing methods, the availability of thin needles for aspiration, and the

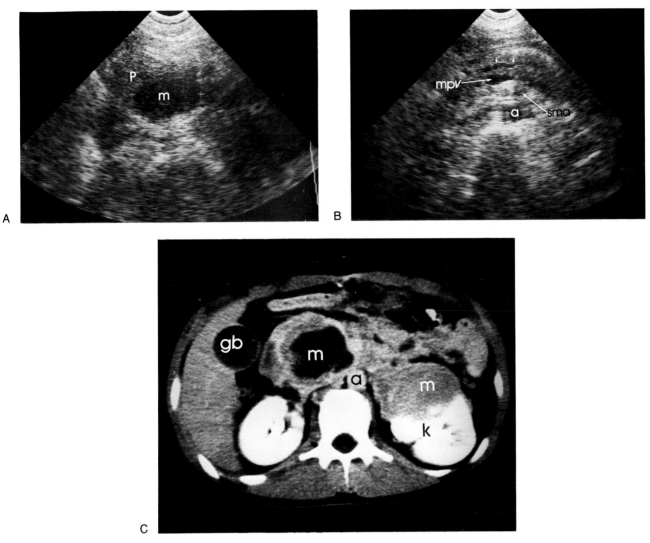

Fig. 7-78. Pancreatic lymphoma. Histiocytic lymphoma. **(A)** Transverse scan through the pancreatic head *(P).* A hypoechoic mass *(m)* is seen. The usual vascular landmarks are not identified. **(B)** Transverse scan at a higher level than Fig. A. The pancreatic duct (arrows) is noted to be dilated within the pancreatic body. (*mpv,* main portal vein; *a,* aorta; *sma,* superior mesenteric artery.) **(C)** Enhanced CT scan. The pancreatic head lymphomatous mass *(m)* appears to be of low density. There is also a similar mass *(m)* in the left kidney *(k).* (*a,* aorta; *gb,* gallbladder.)

increased sophistication of cytologic techniques, the use of aspiration/biopsy has extended to investigation of the mass lesions of the pancreas and other abdominal structures. With fine-needle biopsy, a diagnosis can be made in 78 to 88.7 percent of pancreatic carcinomas.[137,170,173,178,180] The positive cytologic diagnosis is not influenced by the location of the tumor, but positive results are more frequent in patients with distant metastases than in those with localized tumor or locally invasive carcinoma.[173] The main reasons for failure to obtain a positive cytologic diagnosis are small tumor size and sampling errors.[181] Tumors are frequently masked by associated pancreatitis. The composition of the pancreatic tumor is variable, often yielding necrotic material and inflammatory cells. The sensitivity of the procedure has been reported to be 66 to 86 percent with a specificity of 100 percent.[137,181] This corresponds to a rate of over 75 percent correct results with percutaneous aspiration biopsy of the pancreas.[170] There are no false-positive diagnoses. A negative cytologic result does not exclude cancer. By combining cytologic investigation with carcinoembryonic antigen (CEA) assay on the specimen obtained by percutaneous biopsy, the diagnostic rate has increased to 100 percent.[173] Success with the fine-needle aspiration/biopsy technique requires experienced and skilled cytopathologists.[170]

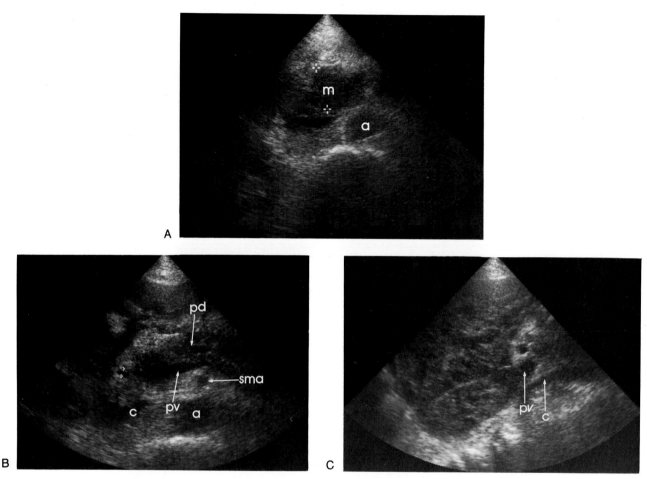

Fig. 7-79. Pancreatic lymphoma. Poorly differentiated lymphocytic lymphoma. (A) Transverse scan in the region of the pancreatic head showing a hypoechoic mass (*m*, calipers) in the region of the uncinate process. (*a*, aorta.) (B) Transverse scan at a higher level than Fig. A with a dilated pancreatic duct *(pd)* and an inhomogeneous hypoechoic pancreas. The distal common bile duct (calipers) was not dilated. (*c*, inferior vena cava; *a*, aorta; *pv*, portal vein; *sma*, superior mesenteric artery.) (C) Sagittal scan of the liver with diffuse involvement. (*pv*, portal vein; *c*, inferior vena cava.)

The risk of pancreatitis following percutaneous biopsy appears to be small.[182] In a series of 184 biopsies in 178 patients, the incidence of severe pancreatitis was 3 percent, and it usually developed within 24 to 48 hours. All five patients had masses of 3 cm or smaller. Perhaps larger masses (3 to 4 cm in diameter) are surrounded by more fibrotic tissue. The increased incidence of pancreatitis in this series may be due to an increasing tendency to perform biopsy on smaller lesions as technology, experience, and technique improve.[182]

One group of investigators use 18-gauge cutting needles and the Biopty gun.[183] They report a correct diagnosis in 94 percent of patients. There were no cases of postbiopsy pancreatitis; 4 percent of patients had a vasovagal reaction and experienced mild pain. The advantage of the cutting-needle biopsy technique over the fine-needle technique is that it minimizes the risk of poor sampling technique and sample handling because of the automated performance of the Biopty gun and easy formalin fixation technique. The larger amount of tissue obtained and the better preservation of that tissue improve pathologic evaluation.[183]

ENDOSCOPIC ULTRASOUND

Conventional ultrasound is often compromised by intervening bowel gas. Endoscopic ultrasound (EUS) represents a relatively new method for visualization of the

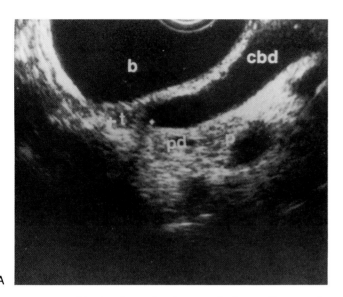 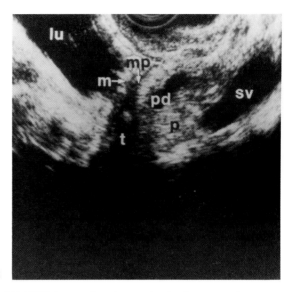

A

B

Fig. 7-80. Endoscopic ultrasound of ampullary carcinoma. **(A)** EUS image showing a clearly demarcated hypoechoic ampullary carcinoma *(t)* with penetration into the adjacent dilated common bile duct *(cbd)* but with no evidence of infiltration into the adjacent pancreas *(p)* or pancreatic duct *(pd)*. (*b*, water-filled balloon.) **(B)** EUS image showing a hypoechoic ampullary tumor *(t)* penetrating through the muscularis propria *(mp)* with no evidence of involvement of the adjacent pancreas *(p)*. (*pd*, pancreatic duct; *sv*, splenic vein; *lu*, duodenal lumen; *m*, mucosa.) (From Tio et al,[187] with permission.)

pancreas. It is a useful adjunct to standard imaging methods in the evaluation of pancreatic tumors.[184] Further improvements in technique and instrumentation are needed to broaden the clinical application of EUS in the evaluation of pancreatic disease.[184]

With this technique, a high-frequency transducer (7.5 to 12 MHz) coupled to an endoscope is placed close to the pancreas, providing images of pancreatic parenchyma and adjacent retroperitoneal structures.[184-187] On the newer systems, the transducer frequency is switchable and there is a channel for EUS-guided cytologic puncture.[187]

Since the endoscopic visualization of the gastrointestinal mucosa and the ultrasound examination of the extraluminal organs are obtained during a single procedure, mucosal and intramural disease of the hollow gut can be rapidly differentiated from disease of extraluminal organs. The examiner is able to visualize the heart, aorta, spleen, pancreas, liver, gallbladder, kidney, and gastrointestinal mucosa and can detect moderate-sized pancreatic tumors and hepatic metastases less than 1 cm in diameter.[185] However, the topographic anatomic orientation is difficult because the scan plane is strictly determined by the endoscope and the pancreas cannot be examined in two planes.[186] Refinements in our knowledge of anatomy as visualized by EUS are needed before the technique can be put to widespread use.[154]

Currently, EUS has a limited role in the diagnosis of pancreatic disease.[184]

The diagnosis of carcinoma is made by EUS when a hypoechoic inhomogeneous pancreatic tumor is noted obstructing the pancreatic duct[187] (Fig. 7-80). The diagnosis of ampullary carcinoma is made when a hypoechoic tumor is imaged in the region of the papilla of Vater with destruction or alteration of the normal ampullary anatomy, with or without penetration into adjacent structures (Fig. 7-80). Penetration is defined as continuation of the main hypoechoic tumor mass within surrounding structures.[187] Lymph nodes with a hypoechoic pattern and clearly delineated boundaries are considered to be suggestive of cancer.[187] By contrast, lymph nodes with a hyperechoic (echogenic) pattern and indistinctly demarcated boundaries are indicative of a benign condition.[187] There appears to be a close correlation between the size and extent of pancreatic carcinoma and the long-term prognosis.

One group of investigators has evaluated the preoperative classification of ampullopancreatic carcinoma by EUS.[187] The overall accuracy of EUS in assessment of tumor classification in pancreatic and ampullary carcinomas is 92 and 88 percent, respectively.[187] EUS has an accuracy of 74 and 54 percent, respectively, in the diagnosis of regional lymph nodes. It is believed that early-stage tumors can be distinguished from advanced stages

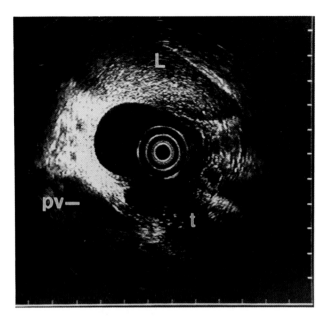

Fig. 7-81. Endoscopic ultrasound scan. Pancreatic carcinoma. Scan showing pancreatic carcinoma involving the portal vein *(pv)*. (*t*, tumor; *L*, liver.) (From Boyce and Sivak,[184] with permission.)

by EUS. The detailed images of ductular and parenchymal abnormalities allow distinction between pancreatic and ampullary carcinomas on the basis of anatomic location.[187]

There appears to be a close correlation between EUS and the histologic findings.[187] The extent of the tumor may be difficult to diagnose by ERCP, although this technique is highly accurate in staging the ductular abnormalities of pancreatic and ampullary carcinomas.[187] The origin and extent of the primary tumor can be seen by EUS, in contrast to ERCP. When there is deep penetration by extensive ampullary carcinoma into adjacent pancreatic parenchyma, it may not be distinguished from pancreatic carcinoma solely on the basis of the echopattern.[187] Partial or total destruction of the normal anatomy of the papilla is compatible with an ampullary carcinoma.[187]

EUS can also evaluate the invasion of carcinomatous infiltration into adjacent major blood vessels, such as the splenoportal confluence, portal vein, splenic vein, or aorta; this can be clearly imaged using the real-time technique[187] (Fig. 7-81). By using only the echopattern of the vascular abnormalities, vascular compression by tumor may be difficult to distinguish from carcinomatous invasion.[187]

Besides evaluating patients for pancreatic carcinoma, EUS can be used for evaluation of pancreatic islet cell tumors[188] (Figs. 7-82 and 7-83). EUS is superior to transabdominal ultrasound for accurately determining localization and tumor delineation.[188] These tumors are visualized as hypoechoic masses with central echogenic portions; their margins are clear, with a smooth contour.

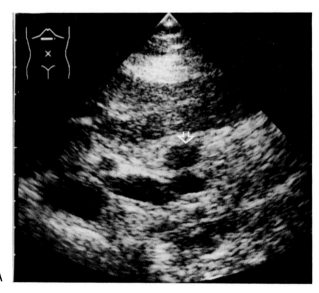

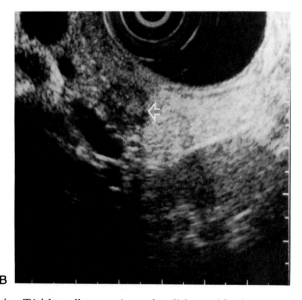

A   B

Fig. 7-82. Islet cell tumor. **(A)** Ultrasound visualized a benign T1 islet cell tumor (arrowhead) located in the body of the pancreas as a hypoechoic mass with distinct margin (3.75 MHz). **(B)** Endoscopic ultrasound scan of the same tumor (arrowhead) clearly showing an irregular central echogenic portion. Microcysts and lateral shadowing are also visible (7.5 MHz). (From Yamada et al,[188] with permission.)

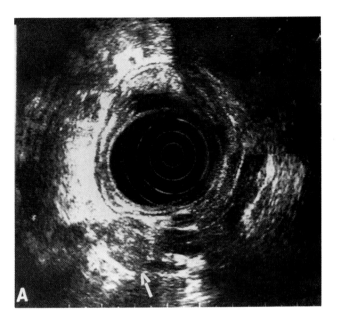

Fig. 7-83. Endoscopic ultrasound scan of pancreas showing a 9-mm gastrinoma (arrow) in the head of the pancreas. (From Boyce and Sivak,[184] with permission.)

It may be difficult to discriminate an islet cell tumor from cancer on the basis of visualizing irregular central echogenic portions. Intratumourous cysts may arise from hemorrhage or liquefactive necrosis, and these cysts increase in number and size as the tumor enlarges.[188] EUS is especially useful in the analysis of tumor margins and contours and in identifying the internal echopattern, in addition to showing delineation of lateral shadowing, all of which offer new possibilities for the diagnosis of pancreatic islet cell tumors.[188] The lateral shadowing occurs when smooth interfaces that are higher or lower in acoustic velocity become refracted and reflected.

EUS may eventually become a standard diagnostic procedure in the preoperative TNM (tumor, node, metastasis) classification of pancreatic and ampullary carcinomas and may help select the appropriate patients for surgery.[187] EUS is more invasive than endoscopy but less invasive than ERCP. To be successful, the operator must have extensive experience with both ultrasound and endoscopy, particularly since this is a side-viewing endoscope. There are disadvantages to this technique: difficulties in achieving topographic anatomic orientation as a result of a small field of image and in maneuvering the transducer to obtain the most adequate section of the target lesion.[187] In the near future, a biopsy may be performed by using the biopsy channel. Perhaps in the future there may be small catheter echoprobes, which

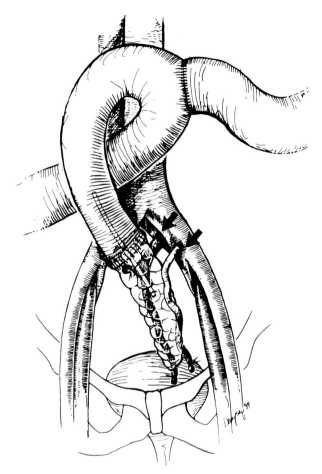

Fig. 7-84. Pancreatic transplant. Drawing shows the technique of segmental pancreas graft transplantation. The pancreatic segment is obtained from a liver donor or cadaveric donor from whom the liver is also harvested. The pancreas is divided at the level of donor portal vein. The body and tail of the graft are harvested with the splenic artery and vein, which are anastomosed to the recipient iliac vessels (arrows). The cut end of the graft is intussuscepted into the Roux-en-Y limb of the recipient jejunum. A pancreatic stent is placed in the duct and eventually will pass through the intestine. (From Low et al,[189] with permission.)

could be used immediately after routine ERCP or even duodenoscopy.[187]

PANCREATIC TRANSPLANTATION

Selected patients are undergoing pancreatic transplantation in an attempt to prevent, arrest, or reverse progression of the complications associated with diabetes: retinopathy, nephropathy, or neuropathy.[189-191]

Continuous improvement in the function of pancreatic grafts and survival rates has been associated with improved surgical techniques combined with increasingly efficacious immunosuppresion.[189] A 1-year graft survival rate of 40 percent has been reported for pancreatic grafts.[190,192]

There has been an evolution in the surgical techniques related to pancreatic transplantation.[189] The graft may be segmental or whole; all live donor grafts are segmental[189] (Figs. 7-84 to 7-86). There is a lower risk of thrombosis in whole grafts, which have a higher blood flow and larger beta-cell mass.[187] In most cases, the revascularization may be accomplished by using the iliac vessels; occasionally, it is done by using the recipient splenic or inferior mesenteric vessels.[189]

Early on, the post-transplant appearance of the graft does not correlate well with endocrine function.[189] In the immediate postoperative period, an anechoic or hypoechoic graft may be seen. Within several weeks after transplantation, if no complications intervene, the appearance of the graft normalizes[189] (Fig. 7-87). The pancreas displays a normal parenchymal pattern on ultrasound, similar to that of muscle, once function stabilizes.[193] If a uniform pattern is demonstrated on ultrasound, the graft is believed to be normal,[193] and the pancreatic dimension should not exceed 3, 2.5, and 2.5 cm, respectively, for the head, body, and tail.[193] Included in the examination is the Doppler evaluation of the graft vasculature.[189] Both within the pancreatic parenchyma and throughout the length of the extraparenchymal vascular pedicle, arterial and venous Doppler signals should be obtained[189] (Fig. 7-88).

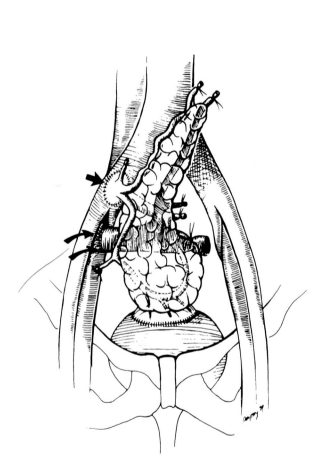

Fig. 7-85. Pancreatic transplant. Drawing shows the whole pancreas graft from a cadaveric nonliver donor. A Carrel aortic patch (straight arrow), including origins of the celiac axis and superior mesenteric artery, is anastomosed to the recipient iliac artery; the native pancreatic arterial supply is left intact. The portal vein (curved arrows) drains to the recipient iliac vein. A patch of donor duodenum is anastomosed to the bladder. (From Low et al,[189] with permission.)

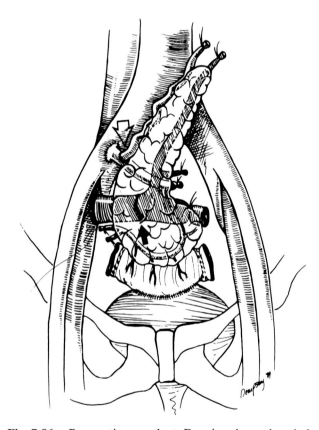

Fig. 7-86. Pancreatic transplant. Drawing shows the whole pancreas graft from a cadaveric liver donor. A small patch of aorta containing the superior mesenteric artery is anastomosed to the recipient iliac artery. The donor splenic artery is anastomosed to the donor superior mesenteric artery (open arrow). The gastroduodenal artery is ligated at its origin. The portal vein is sectioned just beyond the termination of the splenic vein. A segment of the donor iliac vein is anastomosed to the donor portal vein stump (solid arrow) to provide a venous conduit of sufficient length for anastomosis to the recipient iliac vein. The whole segment of donor duodenum is anastomosed to the bladder. (From Low et al,[189] with permission.)

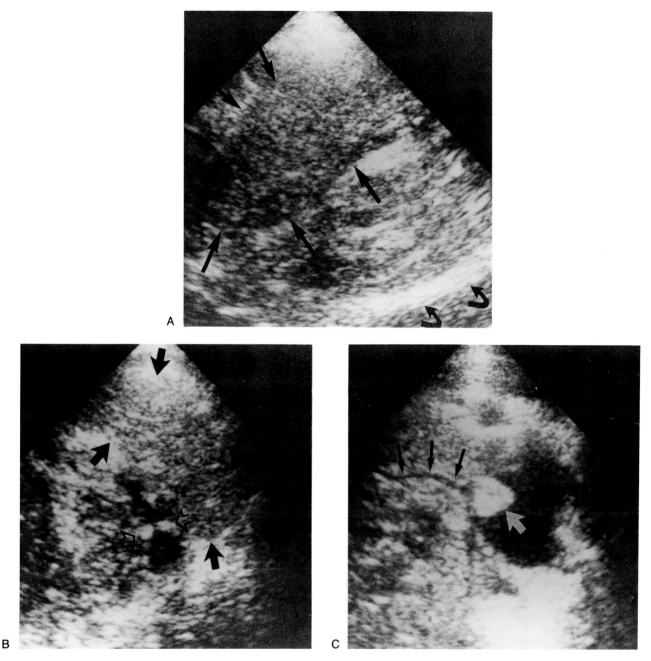

Fig. 7-87. Pancreatic transplant. Sonograms of normal pancreas transplant with bladder drainage. **(A)** Longitudinal sonogram of graft lying medial and anterior to the iliopsoas muscle showing homogeneous texture (straight arrows), the iliac wing (curved arrows) is posterior. **(B)** Transverse sonogram showing similar sonographic features (solid arrows). Venous anastomosis is marginated by bright echoes (open arrows) representing surgical sutures. **(C)** Longitudinal sonogram showing the papilla of Vater (white arrow) projecting into the distended donor duodenum. The pancreatic duct (black arrows) courses superiorly from the papilla. (From Low et al,[189] with permission.)

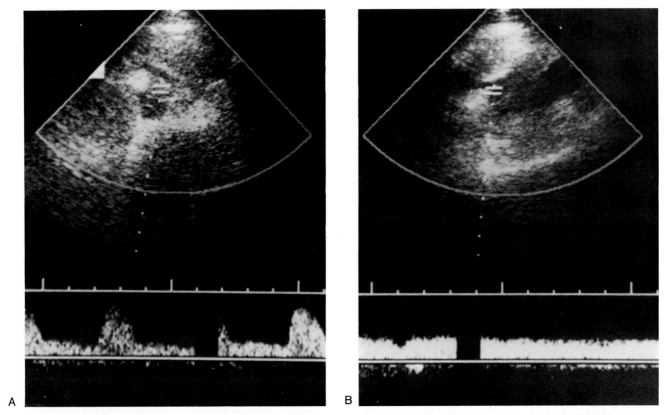

Fig. 7-88. Pancreatic transplant. Normal Doppler findings of pancreas graft vasculature. **(A)** The arterial waveform is typical of a low-impedance system with continuous diastolic flow. **(B)** Venous flow within the vascular pedicle of the graft is continuous. (From Low et al,[189] with permission.)

In evaluating these patients, the goal is to characterize any complications and possibly to guide the percutaneous aspiration or drainage of associated fluid collections.[189] When performing the ultrasound evaluation, it is helpful to have a full urinary bladder, which elevates bowel loops out of the pelvis and distends the donor duodenal loop, if one is used.[189] Bowel loops may completely surround the graft when enteric drainage is used; this may result in nonvisualization of the graft.[189] Both the pelvis and peripancreatic area should be examined to detect the presence of free or loculated fluid.[189] Ultrasound may also detect post-transplant fluid collections, which are usually peripancreatic.[189]

Complications are frequently associated with pancreatic transplantation.[189] Rejection, which is the most common cause of endocrine failure, occurs in up to 35 percent.[189] The early signs of acute and chronic rejection may be subtle, and pancreatic damage may occur before evidence of rejection is detected and treatment is undertaken.[193] When patchy or diffuse areas of decreased echogenicity are seen or the graft is enlarged, acute rejection is diagnosed.[193] The abnormalities demonstrated within the parenchyma include inhomogeneity, poor margination, dilated pancreatic duct, intrapancreatic fluid, and relative change in attenuation, echogenicity, or size.[191] More specific ultrasound features include inhomogeneous parenchymal echotexture (seen in rejection) and ductal dilatation (seen in pancreatitis).[189] In acute rejection, impaired diastolic flow may be demonstrated with Doppler[189] (Fig. 7-89).

Since most physical and laboratory abnormalities, including fever, abdominal pain, graft tenderness, leukocytosis, hyperglycemia, changes in insulin requirement, and elevated serum amylase and decreased urine amylase levels, are relatively nonspecific, clinical surveillance of pancreatic allografts is difficult.[191] The primary means of detecting graft rejection include monitoring of serum glucose, amylase, and lipase levels.[193] Since there is a high risk of complication, pancreatic biopsy is seldom performed.[193] Ultrasound has been reported to have a sensitivity of 82 percent for the diagnosis of acute rejection.[189]

One series has reported the Doppler evaluation of the diagnosis of acute rejection.[194] The authors found that

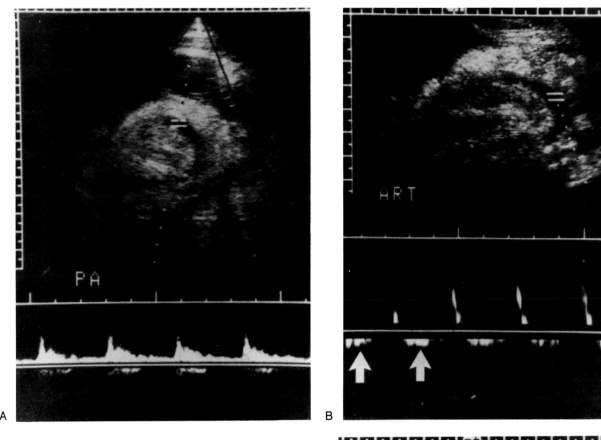

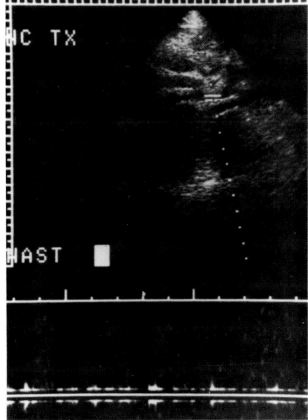

Fig. 7-89. Pancreatic transplant. Progressive loss of intra-pancreatic blood flow in a graft removed for necrosis. **(A)** Intrapancreatic arterial flow is easily demonstrated by duplex sonography in a large vessel. Venous flow was also present. **(B)** Three days later the arterial waveform is abnormal, with reversal of flow in diastole (arrows). The graft is also inhomogeneous. The venous flow was unchanged. **(C)** After an additional 4 days, arterial flow is undetectable in the major vessel supplying the graft. This Doppler finding was accompanied by an overall decrease in echogenicity of the graft. (From Snider et al,[191] with permission.)

the Doppler arterial resistive indices correlated with clinical events after transplantation.[194] In the parenchymal vessels in all instances of normal transplant function, a resistive index (RI) of 0.70 or less was found.[194] In 87.5 percent of patients with rejection, a RI of greater than 0.70 was demonstrated.[194] The positive predictive value of an RI of greater than 0.70 in predicting rejection was 90 percent.[194]

Chronic rejection is associated with increased parenchymal echogenicity and decreased graft size.[189] It is suspected if the graft is small, demonstrates increased echogenicity, or cannot be visualized.[193] During rejection the pancreas is mildly enlarged and has multiple foci of anechogenicity giving a patchy pattern; the pancreatic duct is normal.[192] An enlarged edematous pancreas with a dilated duct and peripancreatic fluid may be demonstrated by ultrasound.[192]

Other complications are associated with pancreatic transplantation. In 8 to 22 percent of patients, pancreatic or peripancreatic abscess may be seen; this is a life-threatening problem.[189] Other associated complications include pancreatitis, fluid collections (such as hematoma), lymphocele, urinoma, pseudocyst, diffuse pancreatic ascites, and leaks at the exocrine anastomoses.[189-191]

Vascular complications associated with transplantation may be detected by Doppler.[189] These complications include vascular thrombosis, anastomotic strictures, and pseudoaneurysms[189] (Fig. 7-90). In 12 to 20 percent of pancreatic grafts, thrombosis may lead to graft failure.[189,191] Other authors have found acute thrombosis the second most common cause of graft failure, usually occurring within the first week after transplantation.[190] If arterial and venous flow is demonstrated within the graft parenchyma by Doppler, graft vasculature is believed to be patent. Inability to demonstrate arterial or venous flow by Doppler may be secondary to vascular thrombosis, rejection, or pancreatitis or even to technical difficulties such as obesity.[189] The inability to detect venous flow and/or visualization of thrombosis within a distended splenic or portal vein is diagnostic of venous thrombosis of the pancreatic transplant.[190] Acute venous thrombosis is indicated if there is absence of detectable venous flow on duplex ultrasound together with nonvisualization of pancreatic allograft on the radioisotopic angiogram.[190]

CONCLUSION

Some investigators recommend ultrasound as the method of choice in evaluating patients for pancreatic abnormalities.[19] It is a rapid and economical tool, allowing a scan in 15 to 30 minutes, as opposed to CT, which takes 30 to 60 minutes, and the equipment costs one-fifth as much as CT equipment. Ultrasound is able to define pancreatic anatomy in detail and has a high degree of accuracy in evaluating for gallstones and biliary dilatation, and in helping to identify patients with gallstone pancreatitis. It is reported to have an accuracy of 90 percent in detecting pancreatic disease.[195] Small defects in the parenchyma may be seen by ultrasound before there are any changes in the size or contour of the gland.[18] By performing a physical examination at the time of the ultrasound, a tender mass can be correlated with the examination. In addition, the ultrasound equipment is mobile and as such can be performed in conjunction with special procedures or in the intensive care unit. An initial ultrasound does not preclude other studies.

Both ultrasound and ERCP provide accurate information in evaluation of pancreatic disease.[196] A combination of ultrasound and ERCP constitutes a comprehensive complementary diagnostic approach to the patient with upper abdominal problems. Ultrasound shows the size, outline, and consistency of the gland, and ERCP outlines the duct. Both techniques require considerable expertise, and the results depend on the expertise of the individuals who obtain and interpret the images. ERCP is an invasive procedure and carries the possibility of complication. Each technique fails to provide information in fewer than 10 percent of cases, and each has a sensitivity and specificity in excess of 90 percent. Together they provide a powerful diagnostic combination.[196]

Although CT is a little more accurate than ultrasound, ultrasound, because of its noninvasive nature, lack of ionizing radiation, and lower cost per examination, has not been replaced by CT for the pancreatic examination as predicted by some authors years ago. In considering the modality of choice, the body habitus is one of the most important factors. Thin patients do better with ultrasound; obese patients do better with CT.[4] Patients may be screened by ultrasound except those suspected of having complications of acute pancreatitis (i.e., phlegmon, abscess, and hemorrhage). If the ultrasound screening test is normal, CT is performed only if there is a high index of suspicion of pancreatic disease or the ultrasound was a suboptimal examination.[4]

Ultrasound was the first cross-sectional modality that permitted direct imaging of the pancreas followed by CT.[197] The findings associated with acute pancreatitis can be imaged by both CT and ultrasound; these include gland enlargement, indistinct gland contour, changes in parenchymal texture or attenuation, phlegmon or fluid collection formation, and thickening of the peripancre-

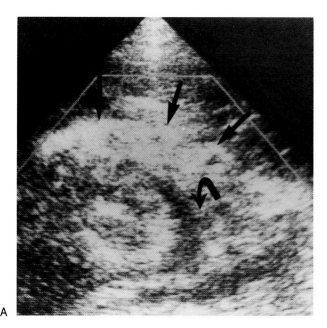
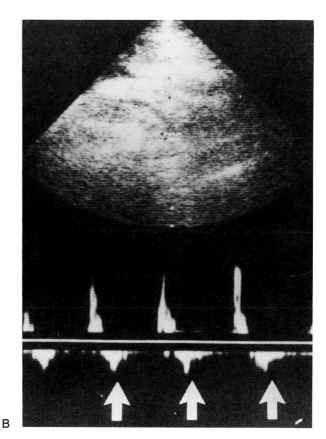

A

B

Fig. 7-90. Pancreatic transplant. Arterial and venous thrombosis. (A) Sonogram showing that the graft is markedly echogenic and inhomogeneous (straight arrows). The artery supplying the graft (curved arrow) is anastomosed to the recipient iliac artery. (B) Doppler signal in the graft artery showing sharp systolic peaks and reversal of diastolic flow (arrows) seen 3 days earlier. No Doppler signal could be obtained from the graft vasculature 4 days later. Pancreatectomy revealed arterial and venous thrombosis with hemorrhagic necrosis. (From Low et al,[189] with permission.)

atic fascial planes.[197] Patients with acute pancreatitis who do not improve within 24 to 36 hours should have a CT scan to assess the severity of the inflammatory process and to identify any complications such as gland necrosis, abscess or fluid collection, vascular involvement, and involvement of contiguous organs or the gastrointestinal tract.[197] The complications of chronic pancreatitis can also be assessed by ultrasound and CT.

Great strides have been made in the detection, diagnosis, and treatment of complications of pancreatic inflammatory disease over the past decades. The ability to assess and formulate the different types of surgical, endoscopic, and radiologic treatments will improve as our knowledge increases. Despite the improved accuracy of diagnosis, ductal carcinoma survival rates are virtually unchanged over the last decade. An accurate, low-cost screening examination must be found before the survival rate can be improved.

REFERENCES

1. Bowie JD, MacMahon H: Improved techniques in pancreatic sonography. Semin Ultrasound CT MR 1980; 1:170

2. Kunzman A, Bowie JD, Rochester D: Texture patterns in pancreatic sonograms. Gastrointest Radiol 1979; 4:353

3. Kwa A, Bowie JD: Transducer selection for pancreatic ultrasound based on skin to pancreas distance in the supine and upright position. Radiology 1980;134:541

4. Hill MC: Pancreatic sonography: an update. p. 1. In Sanders RC (ed): Ultrasound Annual 1982. Raven Press, New York, 1982

5. Weinstein BJ, Weinstein DP: Sonographic anatomy of the pancreas. Semin Ultrasound CT MR 1980;1:156

6. Goldstein HM, Katragadda CS: Prone view ultrasonography for pancreatic tail neoplasm. AJR 1978;131:231

7. Berger M, Smith EH, Bartrum RJ Jr et al: False-positive

diagnosis of pancreatic tail lesions caused by colon. J Clin Ultrasound 1977;5:343

8. Lawson TL, Berland LL, Foley WD: Coronal upper abdominal anatomy: technique and gastrointestinal applications. Gastrointest Radiol 1981;6:115

9. Crade M, Taylor KJW, Rosenfield AT: Water distention of the gut in the evaluation of the pancreas by ultrasound. AJR 1978;131:348

10. MacMahon H, Bowie JD, Beezhold C: Erect scanning of pancreas using a gastric window. AJR 1979;132:587

11. Jacobson P, Crade M, Taylor KJW: The upright position while giving water for the evaluation of the pancreas. J Clin Ultrasound 1978;6:353

12. Weighall SL, Wolfman NT, Watson N: The fluid-filled stomach: a new sonic window. J Clin Ultrasound 1979;7:353

13. Op den Orth JO: Sonography of the pancreatic head aided by water and glucagon. RadioGraphics 1987;7:85

14. Op den Orth JO: Tubeless hypotonic duodenography with water: a simple aid in sonography of the pancreatic head. Radiology 1985;154:826

15. Warren PS, Garrett WJ, Kossoff G: The liquid-filled stomach: an ultrasonic window to the upper abdomen. J Clin Ultrasound 1979;6:315

16. DeCret RP, Jackson VP, Rees C et al: Pancreatic sonography: enhancement by metoclopramide. AJR 1986; 146:341

17. Jeffrey RB, Laing FC, Wing VW: Extrapancreatic spread of acute pancreatitis: new observations with real-time US. Radiology 1986;159:707

18. Taylor KJW, Buchin PJ, Viscomi GN, Rosenfield AT: Ultrasonographic scanning of the pancreas: prospective study of clinical results. Radiology 1981;138:211

19. Crade M, Taylor KJW: Ultrasound diagnosis of pancreatic pathology. J Clin Gastroenterol 1979;1:171

20. Robbins SL, Cotran RS (eds): The pancreas. p. 1092. In Pathologic Basis of Disease. WB Saunders, Philadelphia, 1979

21. Weinstein DP, Weinstein BJ: Pancreas. p. 35. In Goldberg BB (ed): Clinics in Diagnostic Ultrasound: Ultrasound in Cancer. Vol. 6. Churchill Livingstone, New York, 1981

22. deGraaff CS, Taylor KJW, Simonds BD, Rosenfield AJ: Gray-scale echography of the pancreas. Radiology 1978;129:157

23. Niederau C, Sonnenberg A, Muller JE et al: Sonographic measurements of the normal liver, spleen, pancreas and portal vein. Radiology 1983;149:537

24. Gooding GAW, Laing FC: Rapid water infusion: a technique in the ultrasonic discrimination of gas-free stomach from a mass in pancreatic tail. Gastrointest Radiol 1979;4:139

25. Haber K, Freimanis AK, Asher WM: Demonstration and dimensional analysis of the normal pancreas with gray-scale echography. AJR 1976;126:624

26. Coleman BG, Arger PH, Rosenberg HK et al: Gray-scale sonographic assessment of pancreatitis in children. Radiology 1983;146:145

27. Fleischer AC, Parker P, Kirchner SG, James AE Jr: So-

nographic findings of pancreatitis in children. Radiology 1983;146:151

28. Siegel MJ, Martin KW, Worthington JL: Normal and abnormal pancreas in children: US studies. Radiology 1987;165:15

29. Ueda D: Sonographic measurement of the pancreas in children. J Clin Ultrasound 1989;17:417

30. Weill F, Schraub A, Eisenscher A, Bourgoin A: Ultrasonography of the normal pancreas: success rate and criteria for normality. Radiology 1977;123:417

31. Marks WM, Filly RA, Callen PW: Ultrasonic evaluation of normal pancreatic echogenicity and its relationship to fat deposition. Radiology 1980;137:475

32. Ghorashi B, Rector WR: Gray scale sonographic anatomy of the pancreas. J Clin Ultrasound 1977;5:25

33. Taylor KJW: Anatomy of pancreas by gray-scale ultrasonography. J Clin Gastroenterol 1979;1:67

34. Filly RA, London SS: The normal pancreas: acoustic characteristics and frequency of imaging. J Clin Ultrasound 1979;7:121

35. Worthen NJ, Beabeau D: Normal pancreatic echogenicity: relation to age and body fat. AJR 1982;139:1095

36. Walsh E, Cramer B, Pushpanathan C: Pancreatic echogenicity in premature and newborn infants. Pediatr Radiol 1990;20:323

37. Op den Orth JO: Prepancreatic fat deposition: a possible pitfall in pancreatic sonography. AJR 1986;146:1017

38. Bock E, Grandinetti F, Corcioni E, Solivetti FM: Lipomatosis of the pancreas: mistake in diagnostic imaging. J Clin Ultrasound 1986;14:398

39. Marchal G, Verbeken E, VanSteenbergen WV et al: Uneven lipomatosis: a pitfall in pancreatic sonography. Gastrointest Radiol 1989;14:233

40. So CB, Cooperberg PL, Gibney RG, Bogoch A: Sonographic findings in pancreatic lipomatosis. AJR 1987; 149:67

41. Gupta AK, Arenson AM, McKee JD: Effect of steroid ingestion on pancreatic echogenicity. J Clin Ultrasound 1987;15:171

42. Parulekar SG: Ultrasonic evaluation of the pancreatic duct. J Clin Ultrasound 1980;8:457

43. Lawson TL, Berland L, Foley WD et al: Ultrasonic visualization of the pancreatic duct. Radiology 1982; 144:865

44. Eisenscher A, Weill F: Ultrasonic visualization of Wirsung's duct: dream or reality? J Clin Ultrasound 1979;7:41

45. Bryan PJ: Appearance of normal pancreatic duct: a study using real-time ultrasound. J Clin Ultrasound 1982; 10:63

46. Ohto M, Saotome N, Saisho H et al: Real-time sonography of the pancreatic duct: application to percutaneous pancreatic ductography. AJR 1980;134:647

47. Weinstein DP, Weinstein BJ: Ultrasonic demonstration of the pancreatic duct: an analysis of 41 cases. Radiology 1979;130:729

48. Porter A, Warren G: The morphology of the main pancreatic duct at E.R.C.P. as a guide to its demonstration by ultrasound. Australas Radiol 1982;26:149

49. Hadidi A: Pancreatic duct diameter: sonographic measurement in normal subjects. J Clin Ultrasound 1983;11:17

50. Kaude JV, Wood MB, Cerda JJ, Nelson EW: Ultrasonographic demonstration of the pancreatic duct. Gastrointest Radiol 1979;4:239

51. Sanders RC, Chang R: A variant position of splenic artery mimicking the pancreatic duct. J Clin Ultrasound 1982;10:391

52. McGahan JP: The posterior gastric wall: a possible source of confusion in the identification of the pancreatic duct. J Clin Ultrasound 1984;12:366

53. Dunn GD, Gibson RN: The left-sided pancreas. Radiology 1986;159:713

54. Zeman RK, McVay LV, Silverman PM: Pancreas divisum: thin-section CT. Radiology 1988;169:395

55. Binkivitz LA, Johnson CD, Stephens DH: Islet cell tumors in von Hippel-Lindau disease: increased prevalence and relationship to the multiple endocrine neoplasias. AJR 1990;155:501

56. Martin DF, Haboubi NY, Tweedle DEF: Enteric cyst of the pancreas. Gastrointest Radiol 1987;12:35

57. Phillips HE, Cox KL, Reid MH, McGahan JP: Pancreatic sonography in cystic fibrosis. AJR 1981;137:69

58. Willi UV, Reddish JM, Teele RL: Cystic fibrosis: its characteristic appearance on abdominal sonography. AJR 1980;134:1005

59. Daneman A, Gaskin K, Martin DJ, Cutz E: Pancreatic changes in cystic fibrosis: CT and sonographic appearances. AJR 1983;141:653

60. Swobodnik W, Wolf A, Wechsler JG et al: Ultrasound characteristics of the pancreas in children with cystic fibrosis. J Clin Ultrasound 1985;13:469

61. Mack E: Clinical aspects of pancreatic disease. Semin Ultrasound CT MR 1980;1:166

62. Donovan PJ, Sanders RC, Siegelman SS: Collections of fluid after pancreatitis: evaluation of computed tomography and ultrasonography. Radiol Clin N Am 1982;20:653

63. Burrell M, Gold JA, Simeone J et al: Liquefactive necrosis of the pancreas: the pancreatic sac. Radiology 1980;135:157

64. Hill MC, Dach JL, Barkin J et al: The role of percutaneous aspiration in the diagnosis of pancreatic abscess. AJR 1983;141:1035

65. Doust BD, Pearce JD: Gray-scale ultrasonic properties of normal and inflamed pancreas. Radiology 1976;120:653

66. Foley WD, Stewart ET, Lawson TL et al: Computed tomography, ultrasonography and endoscopic retrograde cholangiopancreatography in the diagnosis of pancreatic disease: a comparative study. Gastrointest Radiol 1980;5:29

67. Johnson ML, Mack LA: Ultrasonic evaluation of the pancreas. Gastrointest Radiol 1978;3:257

68. Lee JKT, Stanley RJ, Melson GL, Sagel SS: Pancreatic imaging by ultrasound and computed tomography: a general review. Radiol Clin N Am 1979;14:105

69. Sarti DA, King W: The ultrasonic findings in inflammatory pancreatic disease. Semin Ultrasound CT MR 1980;1:178

70. Hashimoto BE, Laing FC, Jeffrey RB, Jr, Federle MP: Hemorrhagic pancreatic fluid collections examined by ultrasound. Radiology 1984;150:803

71. Cox KL, Ament ME, Sample WF et al: The ultrasonic and biochemical diagnosis of pancreatitis in children. J Pediatr 1980;96:407

72. Gooding GAW: Ultrasound of superior mesenteric artery aneurysm secondary to pancreatitis: a plea for real-time ultrasound of sonolucent masses in pancreatitis. J Clin Ultrasound 1981;9:255

73. Zalcman M, Gansbeke DV, Matos C: Sonographic demonstration of portal venous system thromboses secondary to inflammatory diseases of the pancreas. Gastrointest Radiol 1987;12:114

74. Woodard S, Kelvin FM, Rice RP, Thompson WM: Pancreatic abscess: importance of conventional radiology. AJR 1981;136:871

75. Ranson JHC, Spencer FC: Prevention, diagnosis and treatment of pancreatic abscess. Surgery 1977;82:99

76. Gonzalez AC, Bradley EL, Clements JL Jr: Pseudocyst formation in acute pancreatitis: ultrasonographic evaluation of 99 cases. AJR 1976;127:315

77. Laing FC, Gooding GAW, Brown T, Leopold GR: Atypical pseudocysts of the pancreas: an ultrasonographic evaluation. J Clin Ultrasound 1979;7:27

78. Stuber JL, Templeton AW, Bishop K: Sonographic diagnosis of pancreatic lesion. AJR 1972;11:406

79. Lee CM, Chang-Chein CS, Lin DY et al: The real-time ultrasonography of pancreatic pseudocyst: comparison of infected and noninfected pseudocysts. J Clin Ultrasound 1988;16:393

80. Gooding GAW: Pseudocyst of the pancreas with mediastinal extension: an ultrasonographic demonstration. J Clin Ultrasound 1977;2:121

81. Asokan S, Alagratnam D, Eftaha M et al: Ultrasonography of a mediastinal pseudocyst. AJR 1977;129:923

82. deGraff CS, Taylor KJW, Rosenfield AT, Kinder B: Gray-scale ultrasonography in the diagnosis of pseudocyst of pancreas simulating renal pathology. J Urol 1978;120:751

83. Baker MK, Kopecky KK, Wass JL: Perirenal pancreatic pseudocysts: diagnostic management. AJR 1983;140:729

84. Conrad MR, Landay MJ, Khoury M: Pancreatic pseudocysts: unusual ultrasound features. AJR 1978;130:265

85. Farman J, Dallemand S, Schneider M et al: Pancreatic pseudocysts involving the spleen. Gastrointest Radiol 1977;1:339

86. Kuligowska E, Miller K, Birkett D, Burakoff R: Cystic dilatation of the pancreatic duct simulating pseudocyst on sonography. AJR 1981;136:409

87. Bellon EM, George CR, Schreiber H, Marshall JB: Pancreatic pseudocysts of the duodenum. AJR 1979;133:827

88. Sarti DA: Rapid development and spontaneous regression of pancreatic pseudocysts documented by ultrasound. Radiology 1977;125:789

89. Clements JL Jr, Bradley EL III, Eaton SB Jr: Spontaneous internal drainage of pancreatic pseudocysts. AJR 1976;236:985

90. Leopold GR, Berk RN, Reinke RT: Echographic radiological documentation of spontaneous rupture of a pancreatic pseudocyst into the duodenum. Radiology 1972;120:699

91. Czaja AJ, Fisher M, Marin GA: Spontaneous resolution of pancreatic masses (pseudocysts?): development and disappearance after acute alcoholic pancreatitis. Arch Intern Med 1975;135:558

92. Semogas P, Cooperberg PL: Atypical pseudocyst of pancreas mimicking a diluted pancreatic duct. J Assoc Can Radiol 1980;31:258

93. Spira R, Kwan E, Gerzof SG, Widrich WC: Left renal vein varix simulating a pancreatic pseudocyst by sonography. AJR 1982;138:149

94. Slovis TL, VonBerg VJ, Mikelic V: Sonography in the diagnosis and management of pancreatic pseudocysts and effusion in children. Radiology 1980;135:153

95. Bloom RA, Abu-Dalu K, Pollak D: Spontaneous resolution of a large pancreatic pseudocyst in a child. J Clin Ultrasound 1983;11:37

96. Kagan RJ, Reyes HM, Asokan S: Pseudocyst of the pancreas in childhood. Arch Surg 1981;116:1200

97. Harkanyi Z, Vegh M, Hittner I, Popik E: Gray-scale echography of traumatic pancreatic cysts in children. Pediatr Radiol 1981;11:81

98. Hancke S, Pedersen JF: Percutaneous puncture of pancreatic cysts guided by ultrasound. Surg Gynecol Obstet 1976;142:551

99. Andersen BN, Hancke S, Nielsen SAD, Schmidt A: The diagnosis of pancreatic cyst by endoscopic retrograde pancreatography and ultrasonic scanning. Ann Surg 1977;185:286

100. Gronvall J, Gronvall S, Hegedus V: Ultrasound-guided drainage of fluid-containing masses using angiographic catheterization techniques. AJR 1977;129:997

101. MacErlean DP, Bryan PJ, Murphy JJ: Pancreatic pseudocyst: management by ultrasonically guided aspiration. Gastrointest Radiol 1980;5:255

102. Jaffe RB, Arata JA, Matlak ME: Percutaneous drainage of traumatic pancreatic pseudocysts in children. AJR 1989;152:591

103. Wittich GR, Karnel F, Schurawitzki H, Jantsch H: Percutaneous drainage of mediastinal pseudocysts. Radiology 1988;167:51

104. Kuligowska E, Olsen WL: Pancreatic pseudocysts drained through a percutaneous transgastric approach. Radiology 1985;154:79

105. Sacks D, Robinson ML: Transgastric percutaneous drainage of pancreatic pseudocysts. AJR 1988;151:303

106. Matzinger FRK, Ho CS, Yee AC, Gray RR: Pancreatic pseudocysts drained through a percutaneous transgastric approach: further experience. Radiology 1988;167:431

107. Freeny PC, Lewis GP, Traverso LW, Ryan JA: Infected pancreatic fluid collections: percutaneous catheter drainage. Radiology 1988;167:435

108. Torres WE, Evert MB, Baumgartner BR, Bernardino ME: Percutaneous aspiration and drainage of pancreatic pseudocysts. AJR 1986;147:1007

109. VanSonnenberg E, Wittich GR, Casola G et al: Percutaneous drainage of infected and noninfected pancreatic pseudocysts: experience in 101 cases. Radiology 1989;170:757

110. Isikoff MB, Hill MC: Ultrasonic demonstration of intraductal pancreatic calculi: a report of 2 cases. J Clin Ultrasound 1980;8:449

111. Weinstein BJ, Weinstein DP, Brodmerkel GJ Jr: Ultrasonography of pancreatic lithiasis. Radiology 1980;134:185

112. Shawker TH, Linzer M, Hubbard VS: Pancreatic size and echo amplitude in chronic pancreatitis. Proceedings from Twenty-eighth American Institute of Ultrasound in Medicine. J Ultrasound Med 1983;2:2

113. Alpern MB, Sandler MA, Kellman GM et al: Chronic pancreatitis: ultrasound features. Radiology 1985;155:215

114. Luetmer PH, Stephens DH, Ward EM: Chronic pancreatitis: reassessment with current CT. Radiology 1989;171:353

115. Matter D, Adloff M, Warter P: Ultrasonically guided percutaneous opacification of a pancreatojejunostomy. Radiology 1983;148:218

116. Lerch MM, Riehl J, Mann H et al: Sonographic changes of the pancreas in chronic renal failure. Gastrointest Radiol 1989;14:311

117. Fried AM, Selke AC: Pseudocyst formation in hereditary pancreatitis. J Pediatr 1978;93:950

118. Cooperberg PL, Cohen MM, Graham M: Ultrasonographically guided percutaneous pancreatography: report of two cases. AJR 1979;132:662

119. Lees WR, Heron CW: US-guided percutaneous pancreatography: experience in 75 patients. Radiology 1987;165:809

120. Matter D, Bret PM, Bretgnolle M: Pancreatic duct: US-guided percutaneous opacification. Radiology 1987;163:635

121. Kaude JV, McInnis AN: Pancreatic ultrasound following blunt abdominal trauma. Gastrointest Radiol 1982;7:53.

122. Foley LC, Teele RL: Ultrasound of epigastric injuries after blunt trauma. AJR 1979;132:593

123. VanSteenbergen W, Samain H, Pauillon M et al: Transection of the pancreas demonstrated by ultrasound and computed tomography. Gastrointest Radiol 1987;12:128

124. Jeffrey RB, Laing FC, Wing VW: Ultrasound in acute pancreatic trauma. Gastrointest Radiol 1986;11:44

125. Johnson CD, Stephens DH, Charboneau JW et al: Cystic pancreatic tumors: CT and sonographic assessment. AJR 1988;151:1133

126. Wolfman NT, Ramquist NA, Karstaedt N, Hopkins MB: Cystic neoplasms of the pancreas: CT and sonography. AJR 1982;138:37

127. Herrera L, Glassman CI, Komins JI: Mucinous cystic neoplasm of the pancreas demonstrated by ultrasound and endoscopic retrograde pancreatography. Am J Gastroenterol 1980;73:512

128. Lloyd TV, Antonmattei S, Freimanis AK: Gray-scale sonography of cystadenoma of pancreas: report of two cases. J Clin Ultrasound 1979;7:149

129. Carroll B, Sample F: Pancreatic cystadenocarcinoma: CT body scan and gray-scale ultrasound appearance. AJR 1978;131:339

130. Moser RP: From the archives of the AFIP: microcystic adenoma of the pancreas. RadioGraphics 1990;10:313

131. Busilacchi P, Rizzatto G, Bazzocchi M et al: Pancreatic cystadenocarcinoma: diagnostic problem. Br J Radiol 1982;55:558

132. Wolson AH, Walls WJ: Ultrasonic characteristics of cystadenoma of the pancreas. Radiology 1976;119:203

133. Freeny PC, Weinstein CJ, Taft DA, Allen FH: Cystic neoplasms of the pancreas: new angiographic and ultrasonographic findings. AJR 1978;131:795

134. Itai Y, Ohhashi K, Nagai H et al: "Ductectatic" mucinous cystadenoma and cystadenocarcinoma of the pancreas. Radiology 1986;161:697

135. Shawker TH, Garra BS, Hill MC: The spectrum of sonographic findings in pancreatic carcinoma. J Ultrasound Med 1986;5:169

136. Masterson JB, Bowie JD, Port RB et al: Carcinoma of the pancreas occurring in a child: a case report with description of gray-scale ultrasound findings. J Clin Ultrasound 1978;6:189

137. Mitty HA, Efremidis SC, Yeh H-C: Impact of fine-needle biopsy on management of patients with carcinoma of the pancreas. AJR 1981;137:1119

138. Weinstein DP, Wolfman NT, Weinstein BJ: Ultrasonic characteristics of pancreatic tumors. Gastrointest Radiol 1979;4:245

139. Arger PH, Mulhern CB, Bonavita JA et al: An analysis of pancreatic sonography in suspected pancreatic disease. J Clin Ultrasound 1979;7:91

140. Gosink BB, Leopold GR: The dilated pancreatic duct: ultrasonic evaluation. Radiology 1978;126:475

141. Walls WJ, Templeton AW: The ultrasonic demonstration of inferior vena caval compression: a guide to pancreatic head enlargement with emphasis on neoplasm. Radiology 1977;123:165

142. Kosuge T, Makuuchi M, Takayama T et al: Thickening of the root of the superior mesenteric artery on sonography: evidence of vascular involvement in patients with cancer of the pancreas. AJR 1991;156:69

143. Garra BS, Shawker TH, Doppman JL: Comparison of angiography and ultrasound in the evaluation of the portal venous system in pancreatic carcinoma. J Clin Ultrasound 1987;15:83

144. Robledo R, Prieto ML, Perez M et al: Carcinoma of the hepaticopancreatic ampullar region: role of US. Radiology 1988;166:409

145. Lin JT, Wang TH, Wei TC: Sonographic features of solid and papillary neoplasm of the pancreas. J Clin Ultrasound 1985;13:339

146. Friedman AC, Lichtenstein JE, Fishman EK et al: Solid and papillary epithelial neoplasm of the pancreas. Radiology 1985;154:333

147. Wolfman NT, Karstaedt N, Kawomoto EH: Pleomorphic carcinoma of the pancreas: computed-tomographic, sonographic, and pathologic findings. Radiology 1985; 154:329

148. Itai Y, Kokubo T, Atomi Y et al: Mucin-hypersecreting carcinoma of the pancreas. Radiology 1987;165:51

149. DelMaschio A, Vanzulli A, Sironi S et al: Pancreatic cancer versus chronic pancreatitis: diagnosis with CA 19-9 assessment, US, CT, and CT-guided fine-needle biopsy. Radiology 1991;178:95

150. Ormson MJ, Charboneau JW, Stephens DH: Sonography in patients with a possible pancreatic mass on CT. AJR 1987;148:551

151. Campbell JP, Wilson SR: Pancreatic neoplasms: how useful is evaluation with US? Radiology 1988;167:341

152. Gold J, Rosenfield AT, Sostman D et al: Nonfunctioning islet cell tumors of the pancreas: radiographic and ultrasonographic appearances of two cases. AJR 1978; 131:715

153. Raghavendra BN, Glickstein ML: Sonography of islet cell tumor of the pancreas: report of two cases. J Clin Ultrasound 1981;9:331

154. Fink IJ, Krudy AG, Shawker TH: Demonstration of an angiographically hypovascular insulinoma with intraarterial dynamic CT. AJR 1985;144:555

155. Shawker TH, Doppman JL, Dunnick NR, McCarthy DM: Ultrasonic investigation of pancreatic islet cell tumors. J Ultrasound Med 1982;1:193

156. Fugazzola C, Procacci C, Andreis ICB et al: The contribution of ultrasonography and computed tomography in the diagnosis of nonfunctioning islet cell tumors of the pancreas. Gastrointest Radiol 1990;15:139

157. Gunther RW, Klose KJ, Ruckert K et al: Islet-cell tumors: detection of small lesions with computed tomography and ultrasound. Radiology 1983;148:485

158. Kuhn F-P, Gunther R, Ruckert K, Beyer J: Ultrasonic demonstration of small pancreatic islet cell tumors. J Clin Ultrasound 1982;10:173

159. London JF, Shawker TH, Doppman JL et al: Zollinger-Ellison syndrome: prospective assessment of abdominal US in the localization of gastrinomas. Radiology 1991;178:763

160. Galiber AK, Reading CC, Charboneau JW: Localization of pancreatic insulinoma: comparison of pre- and intraoperative US with CT and angiography. Radiology 1988;166:405

161. Gorman G, Charboneau JW, James EM et al: Benign pancreatic insulinoma: preoperative and intraoperative sonographic localization. AJR 1986;147:929

162. Norton JA, Cromack DR, Shawker TH et al: Intraoperative ultrasonographic localization of islet cell tumors. Ann Surg 1988;207:160

163. Schnur MJ, Hoffman JC, Koenigsberg M: Gray-scale ultrasonic demonstration of peripancreatic adenopathy. J Ultrasound Med 1982;1:139

164. Zeman RK, Schiebler M, Clark LR et al. The clinical and imaging spectrum of pancreaticoduodenal lymph node enlargement. AJR 1985;144:1223

165. Abiri MM, Kirpekar M: An unusual anatomic location of pancreatic masses. J Ultrasound Med 1986;5:703

166. Simeone JF, Dembner AG, Mueller PR: Invasion of the pancreas by gastric carcinoma: ultrasonic appearance. J Clin Ultrasound 1980;8:501

167. Wernecke K, Peters PE, Galanski M: Pancreatic metastases: US evaluation. Radiology 1986;160:399

168. Rice NT, Woodring JH, Mostowycz L, Purcell M: Pancreatic plasmacytoma: sonographic and computerized tomographic findings. J Clin Ultrasound 1981;9:46

169. Sagalow BR, Miller CL, Wechsler RJ: Pancreatic sarcoidosis mimicking pancreatic cancer. J Clin Ultrasound 1988;16:131

170. Goldstein HM, Zornoza J, Wallace S et al: Percutaneous fine needle aspiration biopsy of pancreatic and other abdominal masses. Radiology 1977;123:319

171. Itoh K, Yamanaka T, Kasahara K et al: Definitive diagnosis of pancreatic carcinoma with percutaneous fine needle aspiration biopsy under ultrasound guidance. Am J Gastroenterol 1979;71:469

172. Cohen MM: Early diagnosis of pancreatic cancer using ultrasound and fine needle aspiration cytology. Am Surg 1979;45:715

173. Tatsuta M, Yamamoto R, Yamamura H et al: Cytologic examination and CEA measurement in aspirated pancreatic material collected by percutaneous fine-needle aspiration biopsy under ultrasonic guidance for the diagnosis of pancreatic carcinoma. Cancer 1983;52:693

174. Goldman ML, Naib ZM, Galambos JT et al: Preoperative diagnosis of pancreatic carcinoma by percutaneous aspiration biopsy. Dig Dis 1977;22:1076

175. Ho C-S, McLoughlin MJ, McHattie JD, Laing-Che T: Percutaneous fine-needle aspiration biopsy of the pancreas following endoscopic retrograde cholangiopancreatography. Radiology 1977;125:351

176. Smith EH, Bartrum RJ, Chang YC: Ultrasonically guided percutaneous aspiration biopsy of the pancreas. Radiology 1974;112:737

177. Phillips G, Schneider M: Ultrasonically guided percutaneous fine-needle aspiration biopsy of solid masses. Cardiovasc Interventional Radiol 1981;4:33

178. Ohto M, Karasawa E, Tsuchiya Y et al: Ultrasonically guided percutaneous contrast medium injection and aspiration biopsy using a real-time puncture transducer. Radiology 1980;136:171

179. Taylor KJW, Brand MH: Ultrasonic biopsy guidance in the management of patients with pancreatic cancer. J Clin Gastroenterol 1979;1:267

180. Lieberman RP, Crummy AB, Matallana RH: Invasive procedures in pancreatic disease. Semin Ultrasound CT MR 1980;1:192

181. Hall-Craggs MA, Lees WR: Fine-needle aspiration biopsy: pancreatic and biliary tumors. AJR 1986;147:399

182. Mueller PR, Miketic LM, Simeone JF et al: Severe acute pancreatitis after percutaneous biopsy of the pancreas. AJR 1988;151:493

183. Elvin A, Andersson T, Scheibenpflug L, Lindgren PG: Biopsy of the pancreas with a biopsy gun. Radiology 1990;176:677

184. Boyce GA, Sivak MV Jr: Endoscopic ultrasonography in the diagnosis of pancreatic tumors. Gastrointest Endosc 1990;36:S28

185. Dimagno EP, Regan PT, Clain JE et al: Human endoscopic ultrasonography. Gastroenterology 1982;83:824

186. Lutz H, Lux G, Heyder N: Transgastric ultrasonography of the pancreas. Ultrasound Med Biol 1983;9:503

187. Tio TL, Tytgat GNJ, Cikot RLJM et al: Ampullopancreatic carcinoma: preoperative TNM classification with endosonography. Radiology 1990;175:455

188. Yamada M, Komoto E, Naito Y et al: Endoscopic ultrasonography in the diagnosis of pancreatic islet cell tumors. J Ultrasound Med 1991;10:271

189. Low RA, Kuni CC, Letourneau JG: Pancreas transplant imaging: an overview. AJR 1990;155:13

190. Boiskin I, Sandler MP, Fleischer AC, Nylander WA: Acute venous thrombosis after pancreas transplantation: diagnosis with duplex doppler sonography and scintigraphy. AJR 1990;154:529

191. Snider JF, Hunter DW, Kuni CC et al: Pancreatic transplantation: radiologic evaluation of vascular complications. Radiology 1991;178:749

192. Patel B, Markivee CR, Mahanta B et al: Pancreatic transplantation: scintigraphy, US, and CT. Radiology 1988;167:685

193. Yuh WTC, Wiese JA, Abu-Yousef MM et al: Pancreatic transplant imaging. Radiology 1988;167:679

194. Patel B, Wolverson MK, Mahanta B: Pancreatic transplant rejection: assessment with duplex US. Radiology 1989;173:131

195. Whalen JP: Radiology of the abdomen: impact of new imaging methods. AJR 1979;133:585

196. Cotton PB, Lees WR, Vallon AG et al: Gray-scale ultrasonography and endoscopic pancreatography in pancreatic disease. Radiology 1980;134:453

197. Freecy PC: Radiology of the pancreas: two decades of progress in imaging and intervention. AJR 1988;150:975

198. Mittelstaedt CA, McCartney WH, Mauro M et al: Spleen. p. 235. In Simeone J (ed): Clinics in Diagnostic Ultrasound: Coordinated Diagnostic Imaging. Vol. 14. Churchill Livingstone, New York, 1984

199. Mittelstaedt CA: Ultrasound of the spleen. Semin Ultrasound CT MR 1981;2:233

8

Gastrointestinal Tract

Carol A. Mittelstaedt

For years, the gastrointestinal (GI) tract has created problems for ultrasound. If it is not full of fluid simulating a cyst, then it is full of stool causing a pseudotumor or gas that creates artifacts and prevents visualization of many of the abdominal anatomic structures. The development of real-time ultrasound has greatly improved this situation by making it easier to identify the GI tract, especially by observing peristalsis. Today, evaluation of the GI tract is the "last frontier" for the sonologist/sonographer who really enjoys a challenge.

TECHNIQUE

Preparation

Ultrasonographic evaluation of the GI tract is tailored to the portion of the tract being examined, as is the preparation. If the upper GI tract (UGI, consisting of the stomach and duodenum) is being examined, the patient is scanned prior to the oral ingestion of tap water. Patients may drink 10 to 40 oz of water through a straw, providing they are not scheduled for an UGI series the same day or are not prohibited from taking fluids by mouth. For evaluation of the lower GI tract (LGI, consisting of the small bowel and colon), there is usually no preparation. Occasionally a water enema is needed when evaluating a pelvic mass.

Scan Technique

Real-time ultrasound adds significantly to the recognition and evaluation of the GI tract by displaying characteristic changes in configuration of the tract produced by peristaltic contraction or motion of the intraluminal contents. As a rule, patients are not referred for ultrasound of the GI tract; they are referred because of nonspecific complaints or an abdominal mass. Usually, they have not had barium studies. As such, it is important for the sonographer and sonologist to recognize a GI tract lesion when visualized and to evaluate it as completely as possible.

Stomach

Sometimes a cystic mass is identified in the left upper quadrant (Fig. 8-1). Is this the stomach or a cystic mass of other origin? In the past, without real-time ultrasound, the examiner may have given such a patient a substance to drink that produced carbonation and would have scanned before and after drinking to evaluate the mass for change. As a rule, a dramatic change would occur once air had entered the "mass." It is easier to observe air within the stomach than to try and denote a change in fluid amount, such as would be seen after drinking large amounts of fluid or after nasogastric (NG) tube suction. Also, prior to real-time ultrasound, the examiner could scan the patient on another day to look for a change in the mass.

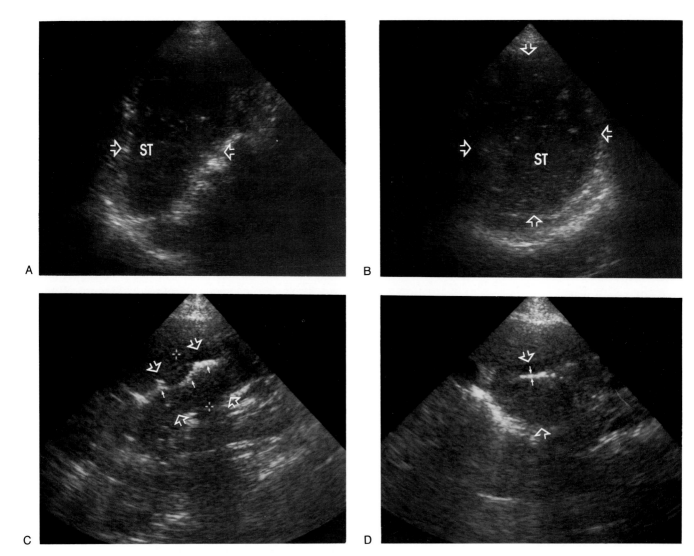

Fig. 8-1. Fluid-filled stomach—mass. On **(A)** sagittal and **(B)** transverse scans of the left upper quadrant, a cystic mass (*ST,* open arrows) is seen containing tiny echogenic areas (microbubbles). This proved to be a distended fluid-filled stomach even though the patient had not eaten. On **(C)** sagittal and **(D)** transverse views of the pylorus (open arrows), there appeared to be wall thickening. The diameter of the pylorus was 28 mm, with a wall thickness of 14 mm. The air in the pyloric lumen is seen as an echogenic area (small arrows). These findings were suspicious for neoplasm. At endoscopy, the patient was found to have a large (2 cm) duodenal ulcer with pylorospasm.

The entire study now is greatly simplified with real-time ultrasound. By viewing the cystic "mass" by real-time scanning, one can observe characteristic peristalsis. If no motion is visible, the patient can be asked to drink 10 to 40 oz of tap water while upright, which permits the examiner to monitor the change on real-time ultrasound. If the "mass" is indeed fluid-filled stomach, real-time ultrasound will determine it as such, since a swirling motion and many microbubbles of air will be seen. (Fig. 8-2).

Although the most common evaluation of the stomach is performed to differentiate it from a cystic mass, there is occasionally a solid mass in the left upper quadrant and a question concerning its relationship to the stomach. Once again, the patient is scanned by real-time ultrasound prior to water ingestion. Then the patient drinks 10 to 40 oz of tap water through a straw. The straw is used to diminish the amount of air ingested. The scanning begins with the patient upright and continues in the left lateral decubitus, supine, and right lateral decubitus positions, much like a barium UGI series. By moving patients through these various maneuvers, the examiner takes advantage of the fluid in the stomach as an acoustic window, which displaces the air to the nondependent location. With transverse, sagittal, and sometimes oblique scans, it is usually easy to identify the stomach and its relationship to the mass in question.[1] The only real limitation of this entire technique is an uncooperative patient or one unable to move, which is infrequent.

To specifically scan the stomach for intraluminal mass or masses, a different method must be used.[2] Some investigators give 1 mg of hyoscin-N-butyl bromide (Buscopan), a smooth muscle relaxant, intramuscularly before giving fluid. Then the patient drinks 1,000 ml of tea over 3 to 5 minutes, using a straw. The patient is scanned in a half-sitting or shallow left posterior position.[2] Others recommend 1 mg of intravenous glucagon before oral water for gastric distension.[3] This method produces gastric dilatation for 30 to 60 minutes.

For a very thorough examination of the gastric wall, the fluid-filled stomach may be evaluated in various positions, thus permitting visualization of the gastric wall in all sections.[4] This can be performed by giving a fasting patient 500 ml to a maximum of 1,000 ml of orange juice to drink.[4] At the same time, the patient is given 20 mg of Buscopan intravenously.[4] By using a curved array transducer, the stomach may be examined with the patient in five different positions, including (1) head-down (angle of inclination 20 degrees, left lateral position); (2) head-up (angle of inclination 30 to 40 degrees); (3) head-up, supine; (4) head-up, right lateral position; and (5) standing.[4] When this technique is carefully carried out, visualization of the distal portions of the stomach is better than that of the proximal part.[4] Eighty-two percent of lesions can be correctly identified and, in

94.9 percent of cases with no gastric disease, the sonogram appears normal.[4] However, this technique cannot totally exclude gastric disease but may appear suitable as a supplementary diagnostic procedure to gastroscopy and radiologic investigation of the stomach.[4]

When specifically examining for hypertrophic pyloric stenosis, the procedure is begun with the patient supine. No fluid may be needed, since the stomach is often already filled with fluid owing to the obstructive effect of the stenosis. The examination by real-time ultrasound evaluates the stomach and identifies the region of the pylorus (Fig. 8-3). This region should be scanned in the sagittal and transverse planes to obtain views of the wall from which measurements can be taken. The transverse plane should be 90 degrees to the long axis of this channel for the most accurate measurement. By obtaining long-axis views, the examiner can often see the radiologic "string sign" characteristic of pyloric stenosis. With the patient drinking fluid (such as Pedilyte), the lumen is often nicely outlined and peristalsis (or no peristalsis) through the pyloric channel may be observed.

Duodenum

The duodenum may cause problems either because its air interferes with visualization of the head of the pancreas or its fluid content simulates a mass (Fig. 8-4). The duodenum can be evaluated by the same techniques used in gastric scanning: a scan is made before the patient ingests water, and then another is made with the patient upright after ingesting 10 to 40 oz of tap water. By placing the patient in the right lateral decubitus position, the duodenum is nicely outlined with fluid. This entire technique of fluid distension of the stomach and duode-

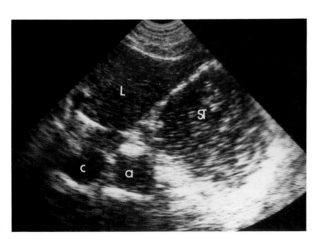
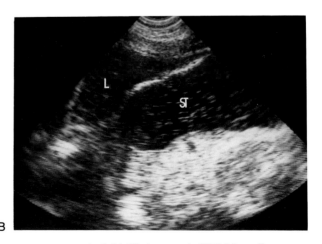

A   B

Fig. 8-2. Microbubbles in stomach. **(A)** Transverse and **(B)** sagittal scans of a fluid-filled stomach *(ST)*. Note all the small linear echodensities representing microbubbles of air within the ingested fluid. (*L*, liver; *a*, aorta; *c*, inferior vena cava.)

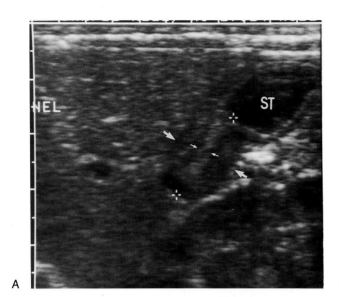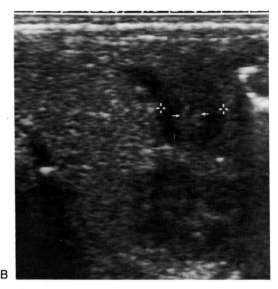

Fig. 8-3. Hypertrophic pyloric stenosis. **(A)** On long-axis view of the pylorus, the channel length (calipers) measured 18 mm. **(B)** In cross-section, the pyloric diameter (calipers) measured 13 mm. The pyloric wall thickness (large arrows) measured 5 mm. This was obtained by measuring between the echogenic pyloric lumen (small arrows) and the outer margin of the pylorus (large arrows). (*ST*, stomach lumen.)

num can be used to evaluate the pancreas and other prevertebral structures.

When evaluating the duodenum, such as in cases of suspected midgut volvulus or pain radiographic evidence of complete obstruction, fluid is placed into the patient's stomach via an NG tube, ideally with the tip at the antrum.[5] Once the stomach is filled, the NG tube may be removed. Transverse and sagittal images may be obtained from the level of the epigastrium at the midline and to the right of midline to examine the antropyloric region and the duodenum with the patient in the supine and right lateral decubitus positions.[5] Transverse views with the patient in the supine and right lateral decubitus positions may allow examination of fluid coursing through the transverse duodenum once the duodenal C-loop is examined, and the fluid may be followed to the area of the ligament of Treitz.[5] A determination of normal small bowel rotation may be made by seeing fluid coursing through the transverse duodenum and crossing the vertebral body from the right to the left side of the abdomen.[5] Once the study is completed, the NG tube is reinserted and the fluid is removed to prevent gastrointestinal reflux and possible aspiration.

This method of fluid distension of the duodenum can facilitate the diagnosis of abnormalities in the duodenum as well as in the antropyloric region. Ultrasound may prove to be a fine tool for triage and may help tailor the UGI series.[5]

Small Bowel

For evaluation of the small bowel, no special water technique is used. If fluid-filled structures are seen and their bowel origin is in question, the examiner simply scans with real-time ultrasound, looking for peristalsis, air movement, or movement of the intraluminal fluid contents. In most cases, some peristalsis is seen. If not, bowel can usually be identified by its characteristic appearance; it is tubular in the long axis and round in the transverse axis. Often the valvulae conniventes are seen within the small bowel that is distended with fluid.

Appendix

The right lower quadrant is examined with the bladder empty; a high-resolution linear array transducer is used.[6] With graded compression, the area of maximum tenderness is scanned. The compression serves several purposes: (1) the anterior and posterior abdominal walls are approximated with displacement of the bowel contents and compressing fat and soft tissues, bringing the appendix and bowel loops into the focal zone of the transducer; (2) visualization of the retrocecal and paracecal areas is improved by the displacement of gas and other bowel loop contents out of the scan field; and (3) the pliability of the appendix and other bowel loops in the right lower quadrant may be assessed.[6]

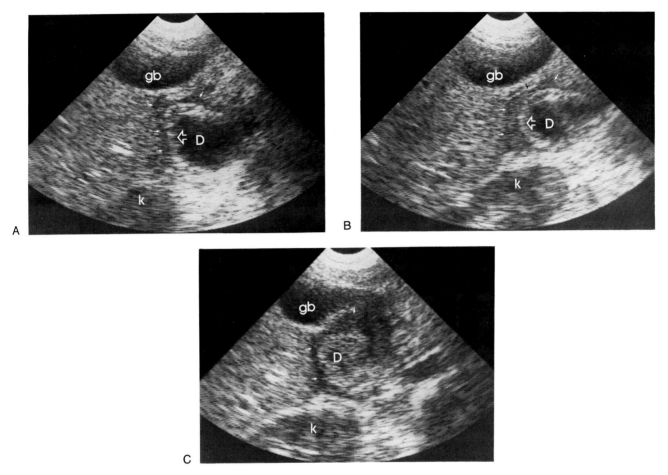

Fig. 8-4. Fluid-filled duodenum. Sagittal scans through **(A)** a distended, **(B)** a partially contracted, and **(C)** a contracted second portion of the duodenum *(D)*. The duodenal wall (hypoechoic areas, arrows) is thickened. The patient had pancreatitis with inflammation of the bowel wall. The duodenum was identified on real-time scans by its location and peristalsis. *(gb,* gallbladder; *k,* right kidney.)

Colon

Ultrasound is usually not used to evaluate the colon. Occasionally, the colon is fluid-filled (usually in diarrhea or obstruction) and is present as a mass. In such cases, ultrasound scanning visualizes a fluid-filled tubular structure in the characteristic location of colon and often the haustral markings in the ascending and transverse colon are seen. When a solid mass is present, it may be difficult to identify its colonic origin unless the bowel wall can be seen as well as the echogenic air-filled lumen.

The water enema technique has generally been reserved for evaluation of pelvic masses in the past.[7] When there was a question of whether a mass was colonic or pelvic, a water enema was used (Fig. 8-5). In this procedure the patient is first scanned with the bladder full. Then a barium enema bag is half filled with lukewarm water or isotonic saline. A Bortex enema tip is inserted into the rectum, and instillation of the water is controlled, with the patient initially in the left lateral decubitus position. The examiner can follow the rectum and rectosigmoid colon by real-time scanning, similarly to how fluoroscopy is used in a barium enema. As a rule, this technique was used only for evaluation of the rectum and rectosigmoid colon to differentiate a questioned pelvic mass. The well-defined fluid-filled bowel provides a soft tissue interface and establishes a boundary between various pelvic structures, which permits assessment of tumor extension.[7] It also defines the relationship to the sacrum. This technique is not routinely used, since the patient often experiences discomfort with distension and the pelvic mass origin can usually be evaluated by the high-resolution endovaginal ultrasound technique.

Some investigators are using the water enema tech-

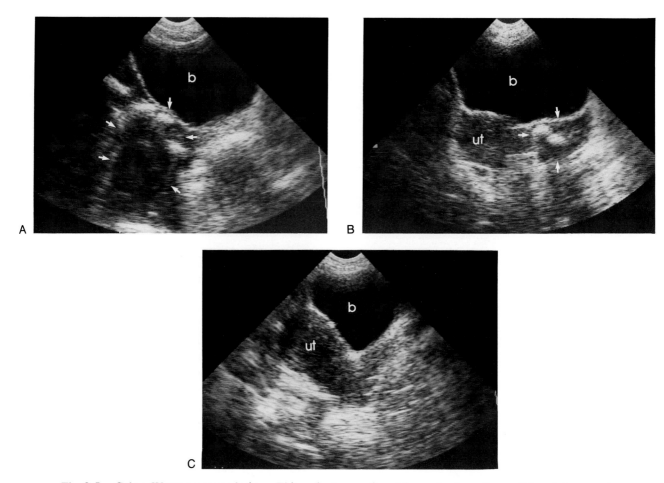

Fig. 8-5. Colon. Water enema technique. This patient was referred for evaluation of a possible pelvic mass. A mass effect (arrows) was seen within the left pelvis on **(A)** sagittal and **(B)** transverse scans. The uterus *(ut)* was noted to be separate from the "mass" on transverse (Fig. B) and **(C)** right sagittal scans. (*b*, bladder.) To differentiate the "mass" from colon, a water enema was performed under real-time visualization. *(Figure continues.)*

nique to evaluate the entire colon.[8,9] By utilizing retrograde water instillation into the colon, the entire length of the colon starting at the rectosigmoid borderline and ending at the cecum can be visualized by ultrasound in 90 percent of patients after the instillation of water.[9] This technique improves the ultrasound visualization of the colon and enables a detailed examination. Not only the colonic lumen but also the colonic wall and connective tissue surrounding the colon can be evaluated[8] (Fig. 8-6). Normally, the colon wall has a thickness of 4 mm and five layers of different echopatterns can be seen as follows: layers 1 and 2, mucosa; layer 3, submucosa; layer 4, muscularis propria; and layer 5, serosa and subserous fatty tissue.[8]

Several groups of investigators have modified the water enema technique for examination of the colon.[9-11] For bowel preparation, the patient is given either three

10-g magnesium sulfate laxative tablets 24 hours before the examination or a laxative intestinal lavage on the morning of the examination.[9-11] Up to 1,500 ml of water is instilled into the colon following the injection of 20 mg of Buscopan.[9-11] The patient is examined in various body positions. Compression on the abdomen by the transducer quickly and lightly causes stool particles or gas bubble to move, facilitating differentiation between artifacts and real abnormalities of the bowel wall. By using this technique, the entire colon between the rectosigmoidal transition and the cecum can be visualized in approximately 15 minutes in 96 percent of patients.[10]

Other techniques for ultrasound examination of the colon have been described, including filling of the colon with fluid by oral ingestion.[12] All patients to be studied are prohibited from taking remnant-rich food on the day

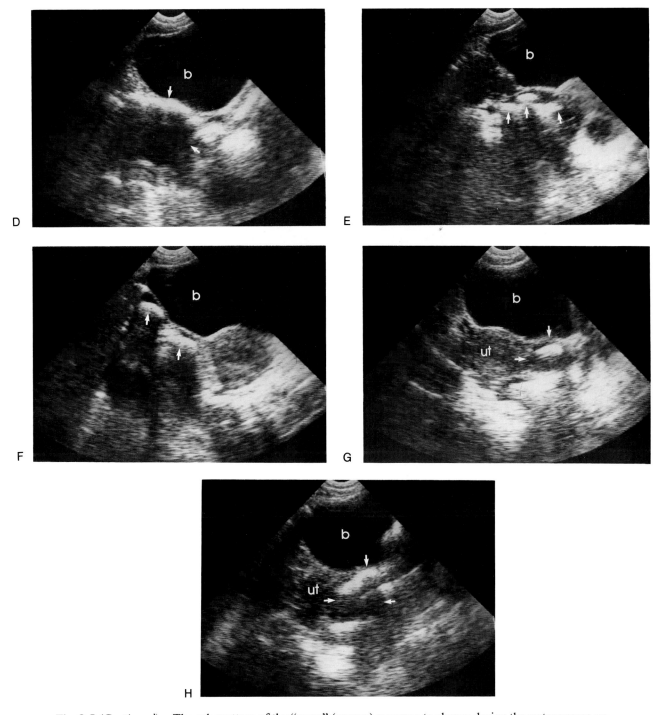

Fig. 8-5 *(Continued).* The echopattern of the "mass" (arrows) was seen to change during the water enema on sequential (**D–F**) sagittal and (**G & H**) transverse scans. The dense echoes (arrows), due to the air, were seen to move. The "mass" seen on ultrasound was colon. (*ut*, uterus; *b*, bladder.)

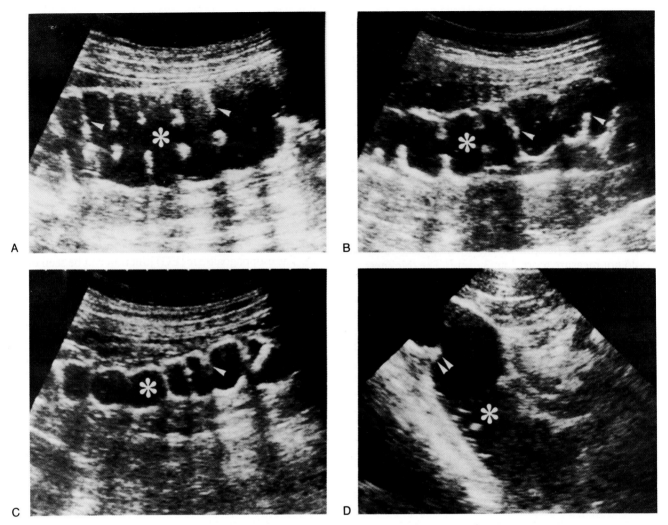

Fig. 8-6. Sonoenterocolonography. **(A)** Sonogram of the ascending colon of a normal control (longitudinal scan). **(B)** Sonogram of the descending colon of a normal control (longitudinal scan). **(C)** Sonogram of the transverse colon of a normal control (longitudinal scan). **(D)** Sonogram of the rectosigmoid colon of a normal control (longitudinal scan). (asterisk, lumen of colon; arrowheads, Haustral fold.) (From Hirooka et al,[12] with permission.)

before the examination and are given laxatives such as magnesium citrate (Magcorol) on the preceding night.[12] The patients abstain from eating on the day of the examination but are allowed some morning coffee or tea with sugar.[12] Over a period of 30 minutes, 90 ml D-sorbitol with 900 ml of boiled gas-free water or diluted tea is given orally.[12] Almost all patients defecate watery stools within 60 to 90 minutes after the water intake.[12] Once the defecation begins, the ultrasound examination is started.

The water-filled colon is examined in both sagittal and transverse projections.[12] In the left anterior oblique position, the ascending colon and hepatic flexure of the transverse colon are visualized. In the semiupright or sitting position, the transverse and rectosigmoid colon is relatively well visualized.[12] Between 90 and 150 minutes after water administration, the colon is sufficiently filled with water for optimal visualization.[12]

By using the technique of the water-filled colon via oral ingestion of fluid, all the colon walls except for the rectosigmoid are satisfactorily visualized.[12] The ileocecal area and ascending colon are sometimes examined insufficiently with barium enema and colonoscopy, whereas sonocolonography visualizes these areas well.[12] This technique may also be valuable in following up patients with inflammatory bowel disease.

NORMAL ANATOMY

There are certain patterns that help identify the GI tract on ultrasound; they are related to gas, mucus, and fluid within the tract. Intraluminal air is echogenic and is usually associated with an incomplete or mottled distal acoustic shadow produced by the scattering effect of gas contained within the tract.[13-17] This shadow may appear similar to that produced by stones.[17] The mucus pattern is an intraluminal echogenicity but is not associated with an acoustic shadow.[13-20] The rim of lucency represents the wall (intima, media, and serosa), and its periserosal fat produces the outer echogenic border of the tract wall[18,19] (Fig. 8-7). This rim should not measure more than 5 mm even when that portion of the tract is contracted.[17] If that portion of the tract is distended, it should not measure more than 3 mm.[21] The thickness is measured from the edge of the echogenic core (intraluminal gas) to the outer border of the anechoic halo (bowel wall)[21] (Fig. 8-7). If the segment is dilated, the measurement is taken from the fluid to the outside of the wall. Distension is considered adequate if the stomach is greater than 8 cm, the small bowel is greater than 3 cm, and the lower bowel is greater than 5 cm.[21] The entire halo should measure less than 2 cm.[16] When this abnormal pattern is present, it is pathologically significant in more than 90 percent of patients.[20] However, it is seen in benign disease in more than 50 percent of cases.[20] As such, the GI tract in cross-section looks much like a target, whereas in long axis it looks much like a kidney.[15,17,20]

When fluid is present within the tract, it gives intraluminal transonicity, with motion of tiny particles seen within the fluid in a linear pattern.[16,17] These particles represent trapped intraluminal gas and/or food particles. The direction of the bubbly motion characteristically depends on the segment of the tract being scanned.[17]

Stomach

On the usual sonogram of the upper abdomen, the stomach as a whole is not visualized. However, portions can be frequently identified even without gastric distension. The esophagogastric (EG) junction can be seen on a sagittal scan to the left of midline as a "bull's-eye" or "target" structure anterior to the aorta and posterior to the left lobe of the liver, next to the hemidiaphragm (Fig. 8-8). Visualization of the EG junction depends on the left lobe of the liver being large enough to project anterior to it. Without the left lobe in this location, the EG junction is not usually identified. It is important to be familiar with this structure, because at times it can be misinterpreted as an abnormality.

The gastric antrum can also be seen as a "target" sign in the midline (Fig. 8-7). This configuration can be seen on sagittal scanning just inferior to the liver. Air is often seen within the lumen.

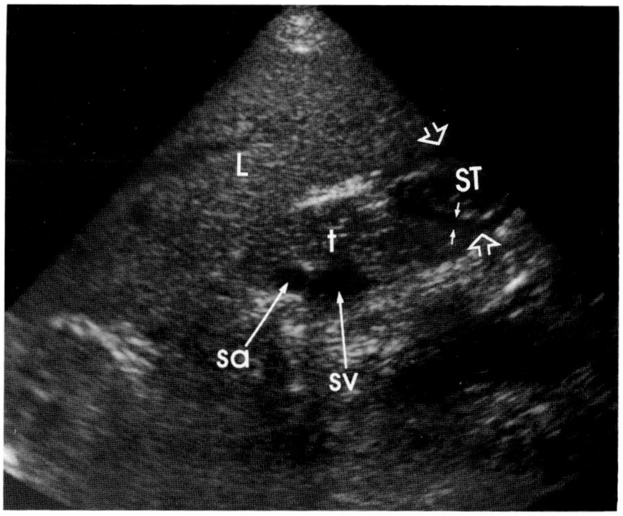

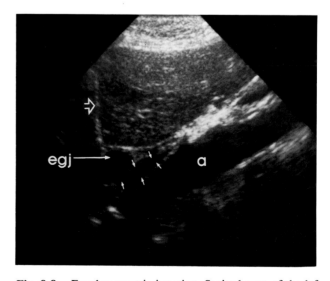

Fig. 8-7. Target pattern. Sagittal scan to the left of midline through the tail *(t)* of the pancreas and contracted stomach (seen as a target, open arrows). The wall is the hypoechoic area (small arrows) around the lumen *(ST)*, the echogenic center. The thickness of the wall is determined by measuring from the edge of the echogenic center to the outer border of the halo. (*L,* liver; *sa,* splenic artery; *sv,* splenic vein.)

Fig. 8-8. Esophagogastric junction. Sagittal scan of the left upper quadrant. The esophagogastric junction *(egj)* is seen as a target lesion anterior to the aorta *(a),* inferior to the diaphragm (open arrow), anterior to the right crus (small arrows), and posterior to the left lobe of the liver.

The remainder of the stomach is not usually visualized without water distension. With distension, most of the stomach can usually be visualized, provided the patient drinks at least 40 oz and the stomach contents do not rapidly empty into the duodenum and small bowel (Figs. 8-2 and 8-9). To promote nonemptying, the patient may be asked to drink while in the left lateral decubitus position. The patient is then scanned, first in this position and then in the supine and right lateral decubitus positions. The wall of the stomach is thin and uniform. There should be no intraluminal masses, provided the patient has not eaten and there is no gastric outlet obstruction. Peristalsis occurs with a swirling fashion, much like a tornado.

When the water technique is used, the various layers of the stomach can often be delineated (Fig. 8-10). The mucosa is relatively hypoechoic, and the luminal surface is highlighted by echogenic gas and mucus.[22] The submucosal layer is more echogenic, with the muscularis hypoechoic. The serosa and periserosal fat (the outer layer) are usually echogenic.

When a lesion is present, the fluid-filled stomach ultrasound technique may identify the layer of origin. The ultrasound finding of a serosal layer of normal gastric wall running toward the serous side of a tumor allows differentiation of intramural from extraserosal tumors.[23] If a serosal "bridging layer" (three layers seen on the mucosal side of the tumor and at least two of them continuous with layers 1 and 2 of the normal gastric wall) is present, the tumor lies within the gastric wall as compared with those external to the gastric wall.[23] If mucosal bridging continuous with mucosal layers of normal gastric wall is present, intramucosal or deeply infiltrated carcinoma can be excluded.[23] It is important when scanning to orient the transducer vertically to the area of transition between the lesion and the stomach wall.[23]

Duodenum

As a rule, only the gas-filled duodenal cap is seen in its characteristic location to the right of the pancreas (Fig. 8-11). Sometimes fluid is seen within the second portion of the duodenum (Figs. 8-4 and 8-12). In either case, the duodenum is identified by its characteristic location and contiguity with the stomach.

The duodenum may be divided into four portions.[24] The first portion is superior and courses anteroposteriorly from the pylorus to the level of the neck of the gallbladder. At the level of the gallbladder, the duodenum takes a sharp bend into the second or descending portion, which runs along the right side of the inferior vena cava approximately at the level of L4 (Figs. 8-4 and 8-12). The transverse portion passes right to left with slight inclination upward in front of the great vessels and crura (Fig. 8-12B). The fourth or ascending portion rises to the right of the aorta and reaches the upper border of L2, where at the duodenojejunal flexure it turns forward to become the jejunum (Fig. 8-12C). This portion is usually not seen by ultrasound.

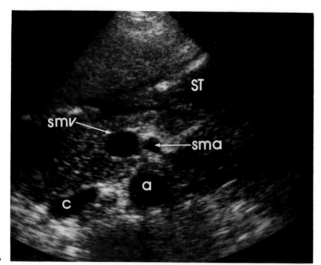
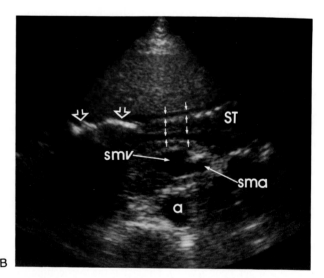

Fig. 8-9. Gastric antrum. **(A & B)** Transverse scans demonstrating the gastric antrum in the midline anterior to the pancreas, aorta *(a)*, and inferior vena cava *(c)*. In Fig. A there is fluid within the lumen *(ST)* of the stomach; in Fig. B there is more air (open arrows) than fluid *(ST)*. The anterior and posterior walls (small arrows) of the stomach, which are seen as lucent areas surrounding the echodense lumen, are best demonstrated in Fig. B. (*a,* aorta; *c,* inferior vena cava; *sma,* superior mesenteric artery; *smv,* superior mesenteric vein.)

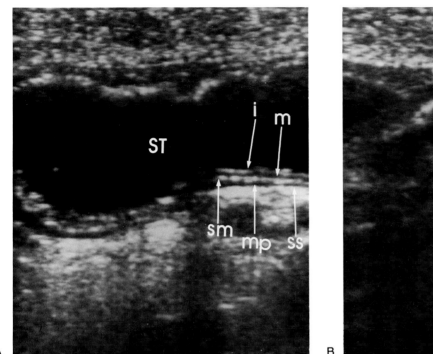
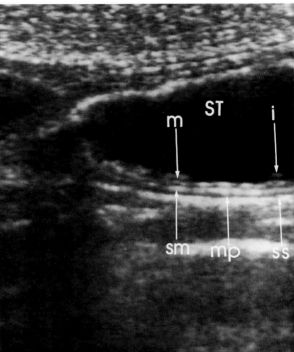

A   B

Fig. 8-10. Normal gastric wall. On **(A)** sagittal and **(B)** transverse views of the fluid-filled gastric antrum using a 5-MHz linear array transducer and magnification, the normal structure of the gastric wall can be visualized. The five layers include *i*, interface echo (echodense); *m*, mucosa (hypoechoic); *sm*, submucosa (echodense); *mp*, muscularis proprius (hypoechoic); and *ss*, subserosa, serosa, and interface echo (echodense). (ST, fluid-filled stomach.)

Small Bowel

Most of the small bowel, other than the duodenum, normally cannot be visualized by ultrasound. One might see air moving within the abdomen on real-time ultrasound and not be able to identify the structure. Occasionally, there is fluid within the lumen. If there is adequate fluid, the valvulae conniventes may be seen as linear echodensities spaced 3 to 5 mm apart, a configuration referred to as the "keyboard" sign[16,25] (Fig. 8-13). The valvulae conniventes are seen in the duodenum and jejunum. The ileum appears with smooth, featureless walls. The small bowel wall is less than 3 mm thick.[26]

Appendix

The terminal ileum may be visualized by its medial location to the cecum, its tubular appearance, its small caliber, its thin (1 to 2 mm) hypoechoic muscular wall, active peristalsis, and fluid content mixed with air bubbles.[6] As a rule, the normal appendix is not routinely visualized.[6] If it is seen, it appears as a thin (≤6 mm in caliber), 8- to 10-cm long, filiform, blind-ended structure without peristalsis[6] (Fig. 8-14).

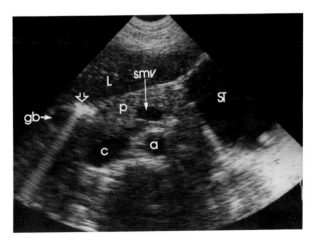

Fig. 8-11. Duodenum cap. On this transverse scan through the pancreas, the gas-filled second portion of the duodenum (open arrow) is identified by its location lateral to the head of the pancreas *(p)* and its reflective pattern (reverberation artifacts). Often on real-time ultrasound, peristalsis is seen. (*ST*, fluid-filled stomach; *smv*, superior mesenteric vein; *a*, aorta; *c*, inferior vena cava; *gb*, gallbladder; *L*, liver.)

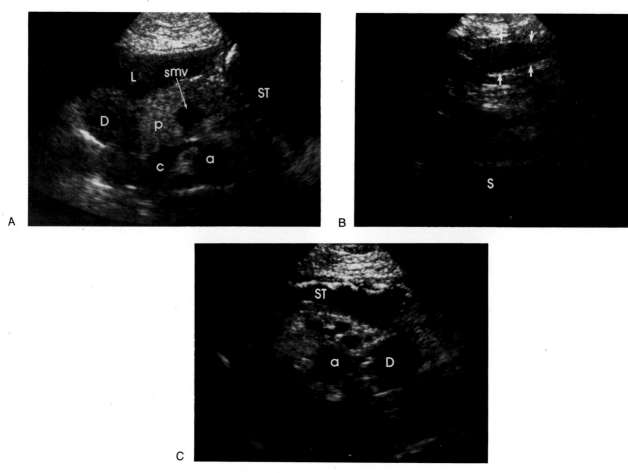

Fig. 8-12. Duodenum. **(A)** Second portion of the duodenum. The fluid-filled second portion of the duodenum *(D)* is seen lateral to the head of the pancreas *(p)*. (*ST,* fluid-filled stomach; *a,* aorta; *c,* inferior vena cava; *smv,* superior mesenteric vein; *L,* liver.) **(B)** Third portion of the duodenum. This portion of the duodenum (arrows) is anterior to the area of the aorta, inferior vena cava, and spine *(S)*. Peristalsis within the loop could be seen on real-time ultrasound. **(C)** Fourth portion of the duodenum at a higher level than Fig. B. This portion of the duodenum *(D)* is often confused with a mass in the pancreas. It is located just to the left of the aorta *(a)*. (*ST,* fluid-filled stomach.)

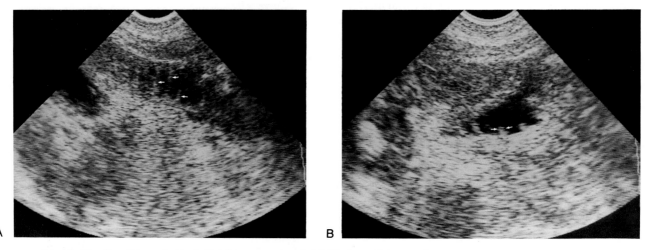

Fig. 8-13. Small bowel. **(A & B)** This represents fluid-filled small bowel since the valvulae conniventes are identified as linear echogenic structures (arrows) approximately 3 to 5 mm apart within the fluid-filled bowel lumen.

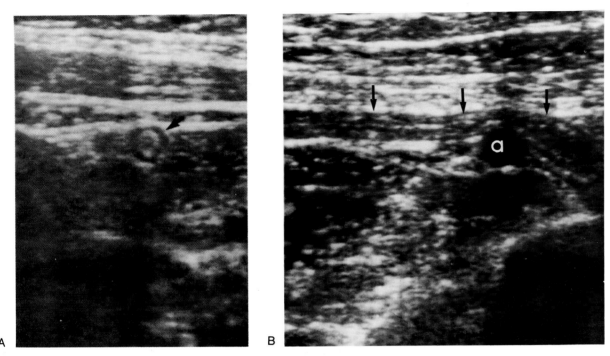

Fig. 8-14. Normal appendix. Examples of visualized appendices with diameters less than 6 mm. **(A)** Transverse view of appendix (arrow). Patient had benign clinical follow-up without surgery. **(B)** Longitudinal scan of normal appendix (arrows). The diagnosis was confirmed at surgery. (*a*, external iliac artery.) (From Jeffrey et al,[156] with permission.)

Colon

Much like the small bowel, the colon is not usually visualized well enough on real-time ultrasound to be identified as such. Occasionally, when filled with fluid, the colon can be identified by its haustral markings, which are 3 to 5 cm apart[16,25] (Fig. 8-15). Whereas the ascending and transverse colons have haustral markings, the descending colon is seen as a tubular structure with an echogenic border.[16] At times, it may appear as a mass but can be identified as a tubular structure in its characteristic location.

GASTRIC ABNORMALITIES

Gastroesophageal Reflux

Since gastroesophageal reflux is so common in newborns, it is often considered a normal variation.[27-29] It is a problem for the clinician to determine which cases of gastroesophageal reflux are physiologic and which are pathologic.[27]

Several groups of authors have reported the noninvasive use of real-time ultrasound to evaluate for this abnormality.[27-29] With ultrasound, neonates may be evaluated in the nursery and do not have to be removed from nursery life-support systems or exposed to radiation.[27] The patient is examined in the supine position 45 minutes after a gavage feeding, using the standard echocardiographic suprasternal and right subclavicular approaches with counterclockwise rotation of the transducer.[27] Alternatively, the patient may be examined after a meal consisting of formula in young infants and only drinks and semisolids in older children.[28] In this plane, angulation of the transducer allows visualization of the length of the esophagus between the diaphragm and larynx.[27] The children are examined in the supine position, and apart from rolling the child from side to side, no reflux-provoking measures are applied.[28]

By using this ultrasound technique, the amount and level of the refluxed material, duration and effectiveness of the esophageal clearance activity, and association between successive episodes of abnormal esophageal transport can be documented and related to movement, gagging, apnea, and bradycardia[27] (Fig. 8-16). The anatomy and pathophysiology of the EG junction can be evaluated, and the mechanisms known to prevent reflux can be studied in detail[28] (Figs. 8-16 to 8-18). The morphologic findings associated with significant reflux are (1) a

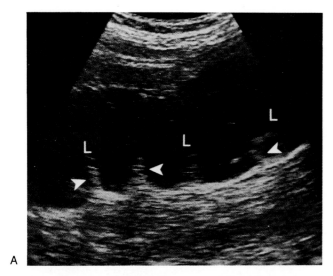

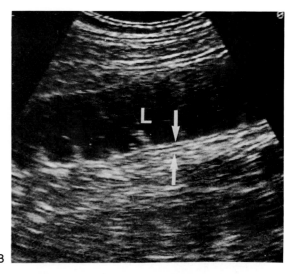

Fig. 8-15. Normal colon. **(A)** The fluid-filled lumen *(L)* appears as an echofree ribbon-shaped structure. The haustra (arrowheads) project as echogenic indentations into the lumen. **(B)** Normal colon with typical wall stratification (arrows). (*L*, lumen.) (From Limberg,[11] with permission.)

short intra-abdominal part of the esophagus; (2) rounded gastroesophageal angle; and (3) a "beak" at the EG junction.[28] The competency of the lower esophageal sphincter (LES) depends mainly on its intra-abdominal location. The length of the intra-abdominal part of the esophagus and the angle of the HIS result in a check-valve mechanism when the gastric fundus is distended.[28] The ability of the diaphragmatic crura to hold the distal

esophagus in place in the esophageal hiatus prevents it from sliding upward[28] (Figs. 8-17 and 8-18). A sliding hiatal hernia of distal esophagus leading to LES incompetency can be identified (Fig. 8-18) and a causal relationship between reflux and ensuing symptoms can be suspected.[28]

Ultrasound can be recommended as a first-line screening test in symptomatic children because it is rela-

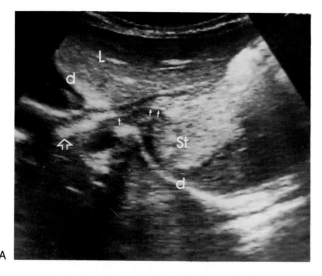

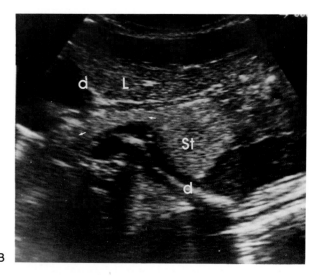

Fig. 8-16. Gastroesophageal reflux. **(A)** Longitudinal plane, showing the retrocardiac part (open arrowhead) but essentially the abdominal tubular structure between the diaphragm *(d)* and stomach *(St)*, which represents the abdominal esophagus plus additional transdiaphragmatic esophagus (single arrow) and small part of the collapsed gastric mucosa (two arrows). (*L*, liver.) **(B)** Reflux is easily shown as bright echoes (arrows) flowing back from the stomach *(St)*, during a very short period (<25 s). (*d*, diaphragm; *L*, liver.) (From Gomes and Menanteau,[29] with permission.)

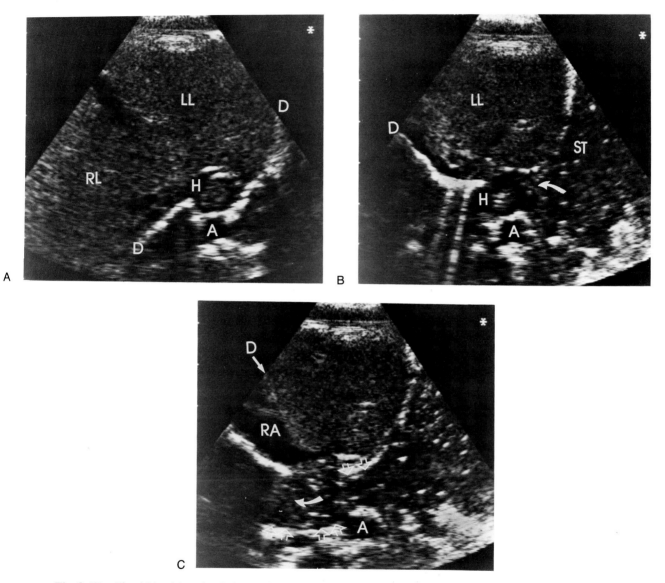

Fig. 8-17.   Fixed hiatal hernia of distal esophagus with pathologic reflux. **(A)** Transverse section through high upper abdomen showing a large "hernia" *(H)* penetrating the diaphragm *(D)*. *(LL,* left lobe of liver; *RL,* right lobe of liver; *A,* aorta.) **(B)** Longitudinal section through the intra-abdominal part of the esophagus showing the "hernia" *(H)* in the diaphragmatic hiatus and the beak at the gastroesophageal junction (curved arrow). *(D,* diaphragm; *LL,,* left lobe of liver; *ST,* fluid-filled stomach; *A,* aorta.) **(C)** Same sectioning plane showing massive reflux (curved arrow) with ballooning of distal esophagus (open arrows). *(D,* diaphragm; *RA,* right atrium; *A,* aorta.) (From Westra et al,[28] with permission.)

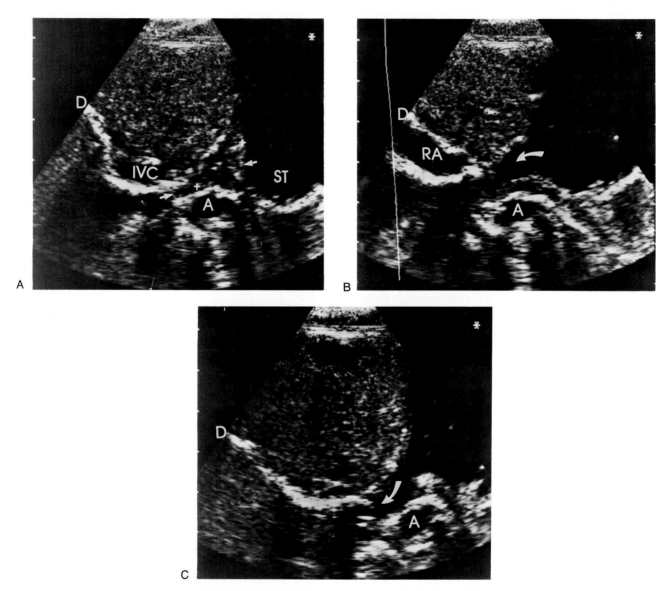

Fig. 8-18. Nonfixed sliding hiatal hernia of distal esophagus with reflux. **(A)** Long intra-abdominal part of the esophagus. The esophageal length is 2.4 cm (arrows), and the gastroesophageal angle is slightly rounded. (*D*, diaphragm; *IVC*, inferior vena cava; *ST*, fluid-filled stomach; *A*, aorta.) **(B)** After upward sliding of the distal esophagus, a prominent beak (curved arrow) is noted at the gastroesophageal junction, just preceding **(C)** reflux (curved arrow on Fig. C). (*D*, diaphragm; *RA*, right atrium; *A*, aorta.) (From Westra et al,[28] with permission.)

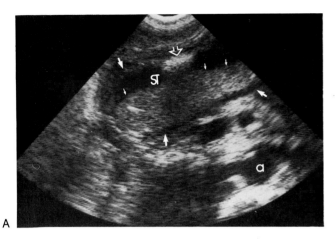
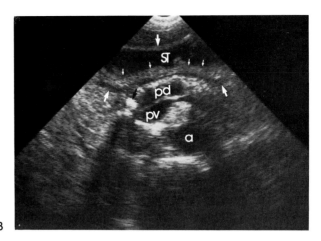

A   B

Fig. 8-19. Gastric dilatation. This patient had a history of chronic pancreatitis. **(A & B)** Transverse images displaying a fluid-filled gastric antrum *(ST)* with a fluid-fluid level (small white arrows) and a reflective pattern (open arrow). The pancreatic duct *(pd)* is noted to be dilated in Fig. B with an internal calculus (black arrow). (*a,* aorta; *pv,* main portal vein.)

tively inexpensive, noninvasive, physiologic, and widely available and does not involve ionizing radiation.[28] It can be used to demonstrate clinical significant reflux and a predisposing hiatal hernia of the esophagus in symptomatic patient.[28] One group of authors show this technique to be 95 percent sensitive for gastroesophageal reflux, with a specificity of 58 percent.[28]

Dilatation

At times, a large fluid-filled stomach may present as an abdominal mass (Figs. 8-1 and 8-19). The fluid-filled stomach may be secondary to pylorospasm, inflammation, intrinsic or extrinsic tumor, electrolyte imbalance, diabetes, amyloidosis, neurologic disease, or medication.[30] Such a stomach is seen as a pear-shaped cystic structure that may fill the left upper quadrant and sometimes even extends into the pelvis. The stomach is easily recognized on real-time ultrasound by its characteristic configuration, discrete thin walls, movement of strong echoes (food particles) when light pressure is applied, gas-fluid-food level, and compressibility.[26]

Bouveret Syndrome

Bouveret syndrome is gastric outlet obstruction secondary to a gallstone impacted within the duodenal bulb.[31] Stones larger than 2.5 cm may produce obstruction in the intestine, particularly the distal ileum, and so may occur proximally or distally in the colon or rectum.[31] The eroding stone will pass spontaneously in 80

to 90 percent of cases.[31] A preoperative diagnosis of Bouveret syndrome is made in only one-third of cases.

The gallstone within the duodenum may produce the double-arc sign on ultrasound with the duodenal wall producing the anterior arc, similar to what is commonly seen with gallbladder disease (Fig. 8-20). A careful search should be made for pneumobilia. In the proper clinical setting, the ultrasound demonstration of a large calculus

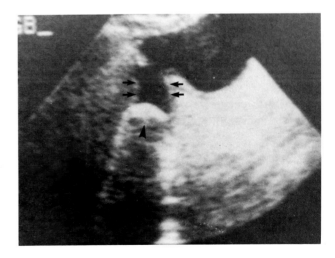

Fig. 8-20. Bouveret syndrome. Transverse sonogram of upper abdomen showing distended fluid-filled stomach proximal to a single arcuate reflector. Examination in different obliquities did not show the gallbladder or calculus separate from the distal stomach nor the double-arc-shadow sign. Real-time evaluation shows a deformed, dilated, fluid-filled pylorus (arrows) in continuity with the large calculus (arrowhead) in the duodenal bulb. (From Maglinte et al,[31] with permission.)

in the right upper quadrant without demonstration of the gallbladder and its persistent contiguity with a dilated fluid-filled stomach in multiple scan planes should suggest the diagnosis.[31]

Duplication

Duplication cysts are embryologic mistakes and may or may not cause symptoms, depending on their location, size, and histology.[32] The criteria for the diagnosis of gastric duplication include (1) cyst lined with alimentary tract epithelium; (2) well-developed muscular wall; and (3) contiguity with the stomach. Gastric duplication is rare and may arise from the duodenum or pancreas; occasionally it arises without communication with the gastrointestinal tract.[33] These cysts occur more frequently in females than males (2:1) and are usually on the greater curvature of the stomach.[32,34]

Once cysts are identified, a search should be made for other duplications along the alimentary tract. Although duplications are usually epigastric, intrathoracic occurrences have been reported. Such a patient usually presents in infancy with symptoms of high intestinal obstruction including distension, vomiting, and abdominal pain. Duplications may also be associated with complications such as abdominal pain, vomiting, hemorrhage, and fistula formation.[33] The solid component of the mass is apparently caused by hemorrhage and inspissated material within the cyst.[34]

On ultrasound, such a cyst appears as an anechoic mass with a thin inner echogenic rim (mucosa) and a wider outer hypoechoic rim (muscle layer) (Figs. 8-21 and 8-22). This pattern should suggest an enteric cyst.[33,34] On ultrasound, the differential diagnosis for such a lesion should include mesenteric or omental cyst, pancreatic cyst or pseudocyst, enteric cyst, renal cyst, splenic cyst, congenital cyst of the left lobe of the liver, and gastric distension.[35]

Hypertrophic Pyloric Stenosis

Hypertrophic pyloric stenosis (HPS) is familial, with a 4:1 male/female ratio. There is a 5.9 percent occurrence in children whose parents had HPS. If a mother has HPS, she has a four times greater chance of having affected offspring than does a father.[36] There is a random occurrence of 3:1,000 infants, with a male/female ratio of 5:1.[36]

The typical patient presents with projectile vomiting in the second or third week of life. HPS may occur as projectile, bile-free emesis in a previously healthy 6-week-old infant.[36] It is rarely seen with symptoms at birth or as late as 5 months.[36] The abdominal mass that is detected by palpation in 40 to 100 percent of cases is the hypertrophied muscle.[37,38]

Pyloric stenosis is characterized by hypertrophy and hyperplasia of the circular muscle, which results in elongation of the pylorus and constriction of the canal.[39] The narrowing may lead to edema or inflammatory changes. Several factors have been proposed as the cause of this disease.[36] Some investigators have postulated that there is a decreased number of ganglion cells and neurofibrils in the pylorus; others have pointed to immaturity of ganglion cells.[36]

The diagnosis of pyloric stenosis is usually based on medical history.[40] In the hands of an experienced clinician, the diagnosis is usually straightforward. With a patient of the appropriate age, a history of projectile vomiting, observation of peristaltic wave crossing the anterior abdominal wall, and palpation of the pyloric "olive," there is sufficient indication for surgery. When some of the clinical findings are unclear, imaging studies are necessary for the diagnosis. If there is a question, the UGI series is often the diagnostic imaging procedure of choice, although there is a reported error rate of 4.5 to 11.1 percent. Such a series also involves ionizing radiation and introduces additional fluid into an obstructed stomach.[37,40]

Many investigators have evaluated the use of ultrasound in the evaluation of HPS. A number of factors and/or measurements have been identified, including (1) volumetric measurement of NG aspirate; (2) pyloric diameter; (3) pyloric muscle thickness; (4) pyloric length; (5) "cervix sign"; (6) "double-track" sign; (7) antropyloric muscle thickness; and (8) pyloric volume. These are discussed below along with the accuracy of ultrasound in making this diagnosis. Ultrasound has the advantage of visualizing the hypertrophied muscle directly.[40–42]

Volumetric Measurement

The volumetric measurement of the NG aspirate may be evaluated in patients with suspected HPS.[43] Of the patients with a NG aspirate of 10 ml or more, 91.7 percent have pyloric stenosis.[43] It is postulated that patients with a NG aspirate of 10 ml or greater should be referred for further ultrasound evaluation while those with less should be referred for fluoroscopic confirmation of gastroesophageal reflux.

Pyloric Diameter

The pyloric diameter, imaged in cross-section, is seen as a target medial to the gallbladder, anterior and caudal to the portal vein, anterior to the kidney, and lateral to

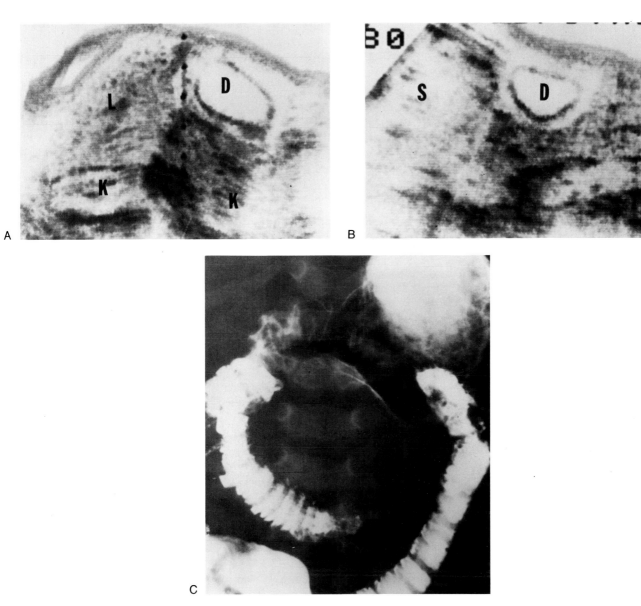

Fig. 8-21. Gastric duplication. A mass *(D)* is seen anteriorly within the left upper quadrant on **(A)** transverse and **(B)** longitudinal scans. It is anechoic with a thin echogenic inner lining. The outer anechoic wall is about 10 mm wide. (*L*, liver; *K*, kidney; *S*, stomach.) **(C)** UGI series. The epigastric mass compresses and displaces the antrum, duodenum and transverse colon. (From Moccia et al,[33] with permission.)

the head of the pancreas (Figs. 8-3, 8-23, and 8-24). The target lesion associated with HPS is usually located by orienting the transducer in a sagittal plane. The long axis of the pyloric channel, which may be in a sagittal or transverse plane, is identified, and then the pylorus is imaged at a 90 degree plane to the long axis to obtain the pyloric diameter.

A measurement of 15 mm or more for the pyloric diameter is considered abnormal; normal is usually less than 10 mm.[36,39,40-42] Some investigators use a maxi-

mum measurement of 13 to 13.4 mm for a positive diagnosis.[26,39,41,42,44] A 72 percent accuracy has been reported in diagnosing HPS by using an anteroposterior diameter of 15 mm or greater, with no normal pyloruses found greater than 15 mm.[45] With a range of 20 mm or greater for target lesion size, an accuracy of 100 percent has been reported.[45] At times, there is a problem in using the transverse diameter since there may be a wide variation among the normal and hypertrophied pyloruses, producing a distinct overlap.[36]

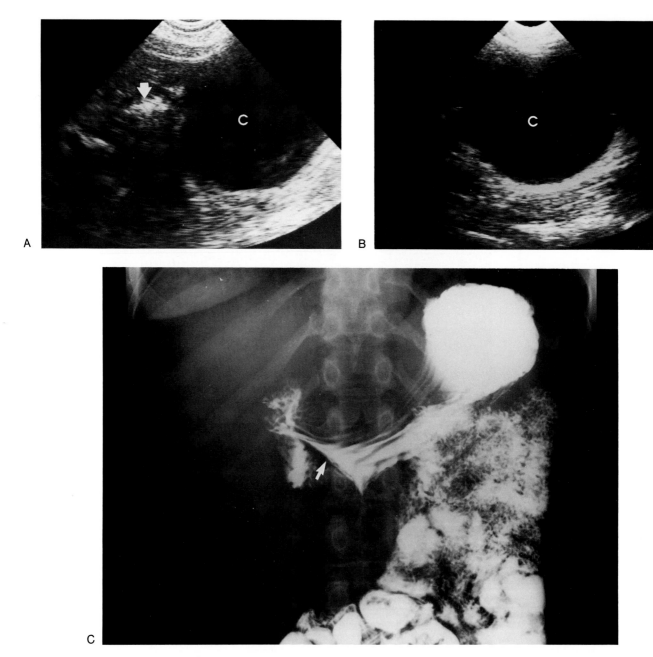

Fig. 8-22. Gastric duplication. **(A)** Sagittal and **(B)** transverse scans of an asymptomatic adolescent girl demonstrating a large cystic mass (*C*, 9.6 cm long) in the midabdomen, which contains some internal echoes. It is inferior to the stomach (arrowhead). **(C)** UGI series demonstrating a mass effect (arrow) on the lesser curvature of the stomach.

Pyloric Muscle Thickness

The wall or hypoechoic rim of the target represents the hypertrophied muscle[46,47] (Fig. 8-3B). Normally, it is less than 4 mm thick.[39-42] This muscle thickness can be measured from the longitudinal and/or cross-sectional views. Some authors consider a rim measurement greater than 4 to 4.5 mm to be diagnostic for HPS.[26,39,41,42,44] A muscle thickness of 4 mm has been found to be diagnostic but with a false-positive rate of 9 percent.[48] A 92 percent accuracy is achieved by using a wall thickness of 4 mm or greater.[45] The most significant and discriminating measurement in the diagnosis of HPS appears to be 4.8 ± 0.5 mm, with the normal

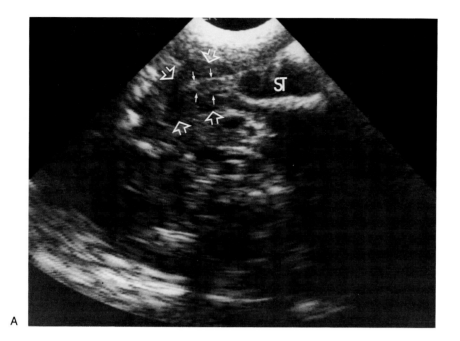

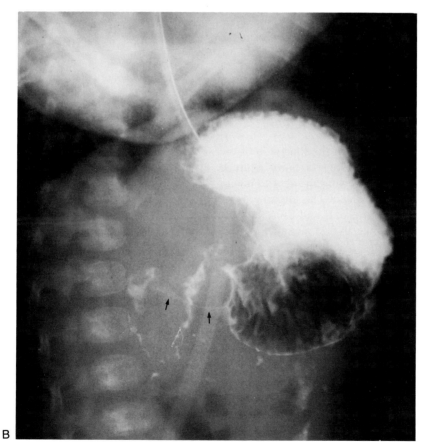

Fig. 8-23. Hypertrophic pyloric stenosis. **(A)** Oblique transverse view demonstrating the pyloric channel (small arrows) in the long axis. The contracted echogenic lumen is seen, as well as the thickened wall (open arrows). (*ST,* fluid-filled stomach.) **(B)** UGI series showing the typical narrowing (arrows) of the pyloric channel.

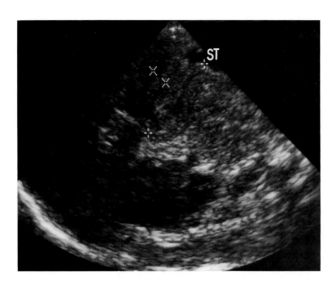

Fig. 8-24. Hypertrophic pyloric stenosis. This 19-day-old male infant with a positive family history of pyloric stenosis presented with projectile vomiting. The pyloric length (+ calipers) was 21 mm, with a wall width (× calipers) of 4.5 mm and a diameter of 18 mm. (*ST*, stomach lumen.)

thickness usually averaging 1.8 ± 0.4 mm.[49] As such, a wall thickness of 4 mm or more is a key positive finding, and it is confirmed at surgery more easily if obtained on a longitudinal view.[36]

Pyloric Length or Channel

By aligning the transducer with the long axis of the pyloric channel, the most diagnostic images are obtained (Figs. 8-3, 8-23, and 8-24). An echogenic central line of mucosa indicates the pyloric length. This alignment displays the continuity of the mucosal and muscle layers between the stomach and pylorus and depicts the characteristic elongated pyloric channel as a mucosal double-track sign, such as described on barium studies[41,42,45] (Figs. 8-3, 8-23, and 8-24). There is variability in the literature with regard to the measurement used for the channel length. Most investigators use a measurement of 18 mm or more; some use 19 to 20 mm.[36,39,48,49] In most normal individuals the length never exceeds 14 to 15 mm.[36-39] The abnormal muscle length may be 2.1 ± 0.3 cm.[49]

"Cervix" Sign

Another sign associated with HPS is the "cervix" sign. This refers to the extension of the hypertrophied muscle into the antrum; the elongated narrow pyloric channel forms an image that looks somewhat like a cervix[36] (Fig. 8-24).

"Double-Track" Sign

A new sign associated with pyloric stenosis is the "double-track" sign.[50] This sign is produced with fluid-aided real-time ultrasound. It is seen as a result of pyloric fluid compressed into smaller tracks as it is impinged on circumferentially by thickened circular muscle (Fig. 8-23A). When this sign is combined with the previously noted measurements, it may aid in making the clinical diagnosis in cases of HPS.

Antropyloric Muscle Thickness

Other authors have evaluated the antropyloric muscle thickness as a criterion for the diagnosis of pyloric stenosis.[51] This thickness is measured in the midlongitudinal plane of the fully distended, fluid-filled antrum. The normal thickness is found to be 2 mm or less, with 3 mm or greater being abnormal and diagnostic for HPS; a muscle from 2 to less than 3 mm is considered abnormal but not diagnostic specifically for HPS.[51]

Pyloric Volume

One group of investigators has not been able to confidently diagnose HPS by ultrasound in 45 percent of patients undergoing surgery because all three (diameter *[PD]*, length *[PL]*, thickness) criteria were not fulfilled.[52] Pyloric volume *(PV)* measurements were found to be helpful: $PV = 0.25 \times PD^2 \times PL$.[52] In patients less than 4 weeks of age, the criterion of pyloric volume of 1.4 ml or greater aided in the identification of early pyloric stenosis more accurately than any existing criteria.[52] It was found that a criterion of a pyloric volume 1.5 ml or more helped identify early HPS more accurately than any of the existing criteria, especially in young infants with a short history of vomiting and a small pyloric muscle mass.[52]

General

Ultrasound is particularly helpful in evaluating patients who do not have the classic "olive," and it can play an important role in the medical decision process.[52] Indirect signs of HPS on ultrasound include obstructed fluid-filled stomach, exaggerated peristaltic waves, failure of fluid to pass from the stomach into the duodenum, and failure to image the descending duodenum.[37,40] Known morphologic changes associated with pyloric stenosis include impingement on the fluid-filled antrum, prepyloric antral thickening, extensive fluid in the proximal portion of the pyloric canal, and the angle formed between the antral peristaltic wave and the pyloric mass.[44]

Since ultrasound scanning results in no false-positive diagnoses of HPS, it is recommended as the initial diagnostic imaging procedure in a patient suspected of having this disease. If the sonogram is positive, no other examination is needed. If it is negative or equivocal, UGI series may be performed.[40] Some investigators believe that nonvisualization of the pylorus is strong evidence against HPS.[45]

Evolving HPS

HPS is an evolving disease, which may make diagnosis difficult on the basis of a single examination.[53] Using a criterion of 18 mm or greater for channel length in one series, the investigators found 2 false-negative results.[53] This may be because the disease was at an early stage when minimal hypertrophy may mimic the upper range of normal. As such, ultrasound is a simple noninvasive examination that can be used to monitor patients when there is a high index of suspicion for HPS.

Postoperative HPS

Besides evaluating patients for HPS, ultrasound can be used to monitor patients after surgery. In one series, the pyloric wall was found to return to normal (4 mm) within 6 weeks of surgery.[39]

Adult HPS

One group of authors have described the entity of adult HPS.[54] It can be diagnosed by ultrasound in a similar way to infant HPS. The normal adult pylorus ranges in thickness from 3.8 to 8.5 mm (average, 5.8 mm). If the muscle is longer than 9 mm and there is persistent channel elongation of more than 1 cm, it is abnormal.[54]

Gastritis and Ulcer Disease

The use of fluid-aided ultrasound in patients with peptic ulcer disease has been evaluated by a number of investigators.[4,55,56] The patient is examined in various positions, especially upright, with good distention of the gastric wall. The signs seen on ultrasound include (1) gastric wall edema associated with an ulcer crater, (2) gastric wall edema, (3) increased wall thickness (mean, 12.88 mm), (4) asymmetric thickening of the mucosa and muscularis, and (5) spasm and deformity.[56]

Benign gastric ulcers are associated with gastric wall thickening and loss of the five-layer structure of the gastric wall.[56] The ulcer crater may not be evident, and the

thickness of the gastric wall may be reduced. An ulcer with an elevated margin may be seen as a sharply circumscribed widening of the wall of the stomach with a central dish-shaped niche[4] (Fig. 8-25). With ulcer penetration, there may be a circumscribed widening of the stomach wall with poorly defined outside contours that are relatively hypoechoic; in some cases, the echopattern is homogeneous and in others it is inhomogeneous.[4]

In patients with severe inflammation and active disease, the wall is thicker on ultrasound.[55] Chronic gastritis may cause diffuse or localized thickening of the gastric wall, whereas localized thickening is seen with benign gastric ulcer disease. This thickening cannot be distinguished from tumor by ultrasound alone.[26] In those with duodenal ulcer, duodenitis, or antral gastritis, the distal gastric antrum is abnormally thickened on ultrasound; this may prove a valuable indicator to the presence of inflammation[55] (Fig. 8-1C and D). Ultrasound is not routinely used to evaluate ulcer disease, and there have been no reports of ulcer craters identified by this modality.

Ultrasound can prove useful in detecting benign ulcerations and can be used to supplement follow-up examinations but cannot replace endoscopy and contrast radiography. A large portion of the stomach is relatively inaccessible to ultrasound. Ultrasound of the stomach and duodenum is sensitive (91 percent) and specific (89 percent) in detecting or excluding wall abnormalities that are indicative of inflammation associated with peptic ulcer disorders.[55] Wall abnormalities can be detected in 91 percent of patients with abnormal UGI series and endoscopy results in antropyloric and duodenal regions, although none of the documented ulcers may be visible by ultrasound.[55] Eighty-nine percent of those considered normal on ultrasound were normal on UGI series and endoscopy.[55] Ultrasound may be useful in monitoring disease activity in patients already diagnosed by endoscopy or UGI series; its potential may be improved with higher-resolution equipment.[55]

Complications

Ultrasound may be helpful in evaluating complications of peptic ulcer disease[57] (Fig. 8-26; see also Fig. 8-59). The most common complications of peptic ulcer disease in decreasing order of frequency are obstruction, hemorrhage, penetration, and perforation.[39] Perforation occurs in 3 to 13 percent of patients with benign peptic ulcer disease. Thirty percent of patients with perforation do not exhibit air on a radiograph. In addition, penetration into adjacent structures may not be apparent on an abdominal radiograph or contrast study. The passage of food and digestive juices through the perforation incites a peritoneal response and production of an exudate. On

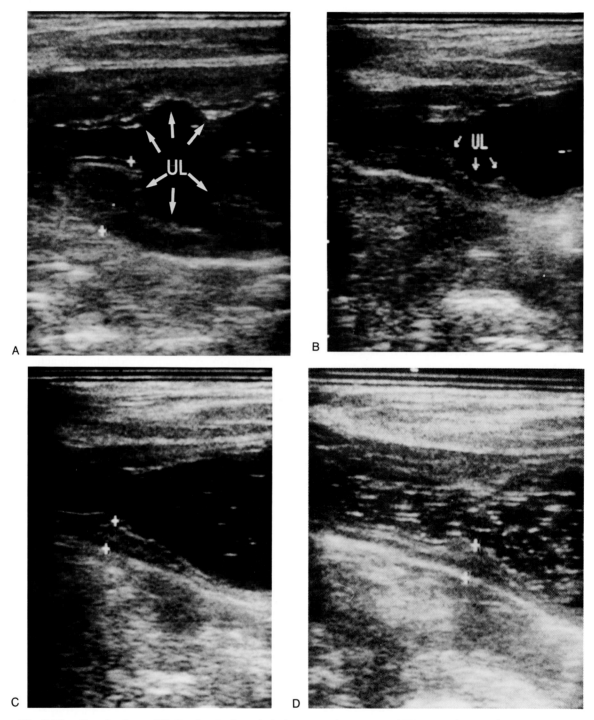

Fig. 8-25. Gastric ulcers. **(A)** On day 2 after admission, two ulcer craters (*UL,* arrows) were observed on the anterior and posterior walls of the gastric antrum. The gastric wall is 16 mm thick and edematous. The five-layer structure is poorly identified. **(B)** On day 9 after admission, one of the ulcer craters (*UL,* arrows) is still seen and the gastric wall is 8 mm thick. **(C)** On day 16 after admission, there is no evidence of ulcer and the gastric wall is 6 mm thick. **(D)** On day 23 after admission, the gastric wall is still 6 mm thick and its five-layer structure is partially identified. (From Tomooka et al,[56] with permission.)

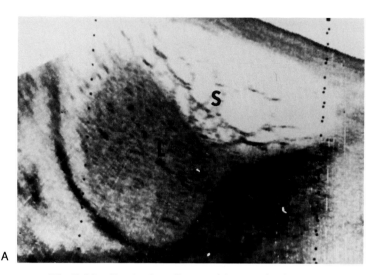
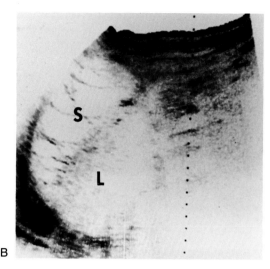

Fig. 8-26. Peptic ulcer disease with complications. Scans 1 week after an episode of right upper quadrant pain. **(A)** Longitudinal scan demonstrating a large predominantly anechoic fluid collection along the anterior and diaphragmatic surfaces of the liver *(L)*, which displaces it posteriorly. There are septa *(S)* within the fluid. **(B)** Transverse scan with the septa *(S)* seen within the fluid as well as the separation of the liver *(L)* from the rib cage. The patient had an UGI series, demonstrating an 8-mm ulcer that was projecting from the anterosuperior aspect of the pylorus. (From Madrazo et al,[57] with permission.)

ultrasound the exudate may appear fluid-filled, mixed, or solid (Fig. 8-26).

Ultrasound can demonstrate free air in perforated peptic ulcers.[58] Visualization of an interference echo with a shifting phenomenon is a very strong indication of the presence of free air in the abdominal cavity. This interference echo can be defined as the interruption of echo transmission when the space between the parietal peritoneum and the surface of the liver is filled with air (Fig. 8-27). The underlying structures cannot be visualized when there is an interference echopattern. This free air within the abdominal cavity can be shifted by changing the patient's position; detecting a shift in the echopattern is strong ultrasound evidence to support the presence of free air.[58] In one series, ultrasound was able to detect free intraperitoneal air (associated with perforated peptic ulcer) in 9 of 10 patients whereas it was visualized in only 8 of 10 by abdominal and chest radiography.[58] The differential diagnosis should include Chilaiditi syndrome, in which the colon is interposed between the right hemidiaphragm and the liver, producing the typical interference echopattern.[58] This pattern might also be detected in the presence of gas-producing subphrenic abscess or subphrenic accumulation of blood clot.

Since the distal stomach and proximal duodenum are the most frequent sites of peptic ulcer disease, focal peritonitis due to perforation usually is located in the right upper quadrant, which is accessible to ultrasound scanning. This characteristic peritoneal exudate surrounds

the perforated ulcer and can vary depending on the elapsed time between the perforation and surgery. The exudate is fibrinous in its early stage and becomes viscous in its later stage. Unlike free peritoneal fluid, this localized exudate does not change shape or location when the patient's position is altered.[57] A number of findings are described in association with acute perforated peptic ulcer; these include subphrenic and/or subhepatic fluid collections, thickening of the gallbladder wall (more than 4 mm), and the presence of an inflammatory mass in the upper abdomen.[58]

Gastric Ulcer Disease in Infants

The cause of gastric ulcers in infants is unknown. Factors such as stress and hyperacidity (the same as in adults) are often incriminated. It can also be seen with food allergy, especially milk allergy.[59] Gastric ulcer disease may be present in a number of patients with chronic regurgitation and vomiting that might not be explained by conventional imaging modalities.[59]

A number of ultrasound findings have been associated with gastric ulcer disease in infants.[59] These include thickening of the mucosa (>4 mm) in the antropyloric region, elongation of the antropyloric canal, persistent spasm, and delayed gastric emptying[59] (Fig. 8-28). The thickening of the gastric wall is rather uniform, although it may be asymmetric and lumpy. The appearance of mucosal thickening may result from a longitudinal cut

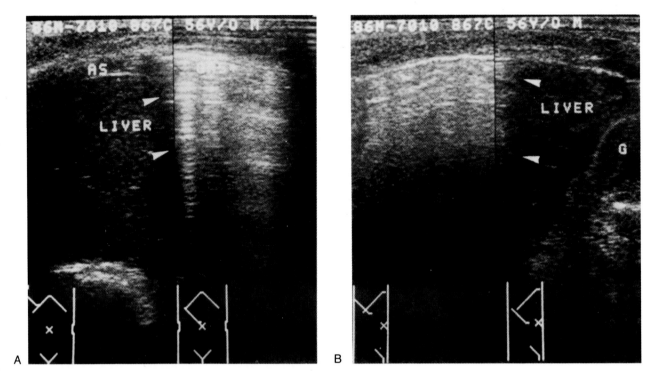

Fig. 8-27. Free air in perforated peptic ulcers. **(A)** The lower portion of the liver is obscured by an interference echopattern (arrowheads) in the supine position. The upper portion of the liver *(LIVER)* and ascites *(AS)* can be identified. **(B)** The interference echopattern is moved to the upper portion of the liver (arrowheads) by shifting the patient's position from supine to left decubitus. The lower portion of the liver *(LIVER)* and gallbladder *(G)* appear. (From Chang-Chien et al,[58] with permission.)

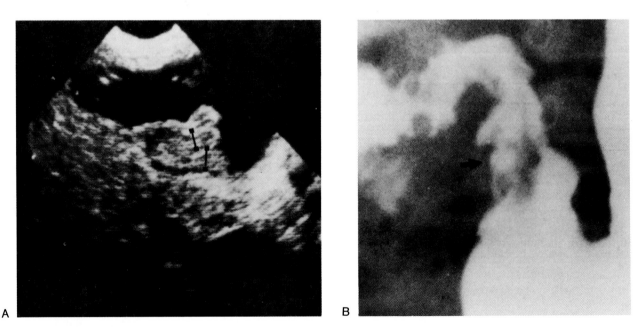

Fig. 8-28. Gastric ulcer disease in infants. **(A)** Marked thickening of echogenic gastric antrum (dots connected by lines). In this patient the mucosa measured 5.0 mm. The antropyloric region also is elongated (2.1 mm) and fixed in spasm. The circular muscle (black line around mucosa) is minimally thickened (2 mm). **(B)** UGI series in the same patient showing deformity of the antrum and a gastric ulcer (arrow). (From Hayden et al,[59] with permission.)

obtained tangential to midline of the long axis of the stomach. As such, a true midline longitudinal axis should be obtained. The transducer can be rocked side to side to judge accurately where the midline of the antrum is.

Specific measurements are taken at three sites in the antrum, and the average is obtained (Fig. 8-28). The spastic antropyloric canal is measured for length by noting the distance from the distal end of the antrum to a point where the gastric lumen becomes normal.[59] The normal range is 2.5 to 3.5 mm; the abnormal range is 4 to 7.5 mm with a mean of 5.5 ± 1.41 mm.[59]

Chronic Granulomatous Disease

Chronic granulomatous disease is an X-linked recessive disorder that results from a defect in the bactericidal activity of the polymorphonuclear leukocytes.[60] Stomach involvement is not common but may be underdiagnosed owing to incomplete obstruction and spontaneous resolution. On ultrasound, circumferential antral thickening causes a target lesion.[60] Ultrasound cannot differentiate such thickening from cancer, inflammation such as Crohn's disease, peptic ulcer disease, and postradiation changes.

Gastric Phytobezoar

Bezoars may be divided into three categories depending on their composition: trichobezoars, phytobezoars, and concretions.[61] Trichobezoars are composed of hair balls and are typically seen in young women.[61] Phytobe-zoars are composed of vegetable matter, with the most common cause (in the normal stomach) being the ingestion of unripe persimmons. In postoperative patients or those with gastric atony, the fibrous components of a variety of fruits and vegetable matter are often the cause.[61] A variety of inorganic materials including sand, asphalt, and shellac produce concretions.[61]

Gastric bezoars are movable intraluminal masses of congealed ingested materials that can be demonstrated in a UGI series by typical coating with barium.[61] These patients may present with nausea, vomiting, pain, or early satiety, although bezoars may cause no specific symptoms. Initial signs and symptoms may simulate those of an abdominal tumor, including a firm epigastric mass (87 percent), tenderness to palpation, vomiting, and weight loss.[62] More than 90 percent of trichobezoars occur in females, with 80 percent in people under age 30; they are also seen in mentally retarded adults and patients having undergone gastrectomy.[62] Patients with vagotomy are predisposed to phytobezoar formation.[61]

The ultrasound findings of gastric bezoars includes a complex mass with internal mobile echogenic components in a fasting patient[61] (Fig. 8-29). With a gastric trichobezoar, a broad band of high-amplitude echoes or a hyperechoic curvilinear dense strip at the anterior margin may be seen superficially with a complete sonic shadowing posteriorly.[62,63] The densely packed food bound tightly together by fine meshwork of hair, and molded by gastric mobility over a long period into a compact mass of many tiny interfaces, might explain the clean shadow of the trichobezoar.[63] The "clean" nature of the acoustic shadow should suggest either foreign material or tissue rather than gas, which characteristically produces a "dirty" shadow.[62,63] The specificity of the

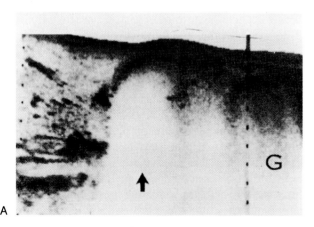
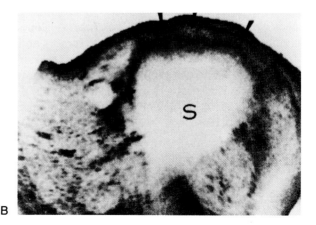

Fig. 8-29. Gastric trichobezoar. **(A)** Parasagittal scan 1 cm to the left of midline showing a broad band of high-amplitude echoes along the anterior wall of the mass, with a sharp, clean shadow posteriorly (arrow). Compare with the "dirty" shadow produced by bowel gas *(G)*. **(B)** Transverse scan 4 cm caudal to the xiphoid process showing the echogenic border of the mass (arrows) and the complete sonic shadow *(S)* cast by the echogenic mass. (From McCracken et al,[62] with permission.)

examination may be increased by having the patient drink water during the study.[61]

Gastric Clearing in Infants

Ultrasound can be used to evaluate gastric emptying in infants. Gastric volume can be calculated from the anteroposterior, craniocaudal, and laterolateral antral diameters.[64] There has been a significant correlation between the half-time of gastric emptying derived by scintigraphy and the half-time measured by ultrasound. The gastric filling index (GFI) is the mean of the product of diameters in parasagittal cross-section and the product of diameters in transverse cross-section, which is considered an index of gastric volume.

A highly accurate volume determination by ultrasound may not be possible because of the presence of air within the stomach, the variable shape and location of the organ, and the fluid content in the antrum. Ultrasound may be useful in identifying patients in whom further investigation is needed.[64]

Miscellaneous Gastric Wall Abnormalities

Gastric Wall Abnormalities in Children

Other abnormalities of the stomach can be evaluated by ultrasound.[65] One group of investigators found a normal gastric wall thickness of less than 3 mm in children, with an abnormal wall thickness of 5 to 15 mm.[65] This abnormal wall thickness was seen in a variety of conditions including varioliform gastritis, gastric ulcer, lymphoid hyperplasia, and gastric hamartoma.[65] Gastric abnormalities can be seen in children with chronic granulomatous disease, Crohn's disease, eosinophilic gastroenteritis, gastritis, lymphoid hyperplasia, Henoch-Schönlein purpura, pernicious anemia, tumors and as late complications of ingestion of iron, acid, or (rarely) alkali.[65] Ultrasound can be helpful in the detection of clinically unsuspected gastric lesions and helpful in identifying other lesions.[65] Confidence in making a diagnosis can be increased with water ingestion.

Focal Foveolar Hyperplasia

Focal foveolar hyperplasia is the most common cause of a gastric polypoid mass in adults and is rare in children.[66] It may represent a hyperregeneration of gastric mucosa still under injurious influence, whereas a hyperplastic polyp represents response to a subsiding or prior injury. It may be seen in association with adjacent gastric inflammation, Billroth II operations, bile reflux into the stomach, and Ménétrier's disease.[66] Ultrasound can identify the origin of a polypoid mass as being superficial to muscle, excluding many diagnoses (Fig. 8-30). A similar appearance on ultrasound may be seen with anything that produces mucosal enlargement, such as Ménétrier's disease or inflammatory swelling, including peptic disease.[66]

Ménétrier's Disease

Ménétrier's disease is a rare disorder characterized by giant hypertrophy of the gastric mucosa.[67] It is also known as transient protein-losing gastropathy, hypertrophic gastropathy, and giant rugal hypertrophy.[67] It occurs predominantly in middle-aged men, and there is a 10 percent risk of complicating carcinoma.[67] The disease is even rarer in children than in adults, with boys more frequently affected than girls.[67]

The clinical symptoms include edema occasionally associated with ascites, pleural effusions, anorexia, vomiting, abdominal pain, and diarrhea.[67] The clinical picture may include generalized edema, hypoproteinemia, and the characteristic thickening and hypertrophy of the gastric folds, especially in the fundus and corpus.[67] Frequently concomitant with Ménétrier's disease are viral infections specifically with cytomegalovirus (CMV).[67]

In the fasting state, sonograms of the empty stomach display a polypoid mucosal hypertrophy especially in the fundus and the corpus[67] (Fig. 8-31). The entire stomach wall may be thickened and poorly echogenic; the rugae may be flattened after ingestion of fluid, but the wall remains thickened.[67] The gastric rugae are best demonstrated by ultrasound after ingestion of a small amount of water. When hypertrophied rugae are demonstrated by ultrasound, the differential diagnosis must include lymphoma, eosinophilic gastritis, multiple polyps (i.e., Peutz-Jeghers syndrome), gastric varices, Zollinger-Ellison syndrome, and lymphangiectasia.[67]

Gastric Amyloidosis

Although gastrointestinal amyloidosis is often asymptomatic, widespread dysfunction may occur.[68] This disease process may be defined as an extracellular deposition of the fibrous protein amyloid in one or more sites of the body.[68] On the basis of the protein deposit in the amyloid fibrils, amyloidosis may be classified into two major groups: one in which the fibrils consist mainly of amyloid light-chain (AL) protein originating from the light chains of immunoglobulins, and another in which fibrils consist primarily of amyloid protein A, originating from serum amyloid A protein.[68] The latter is seen in secondary amyloidosis and the former in primary amyloidosis.[68]

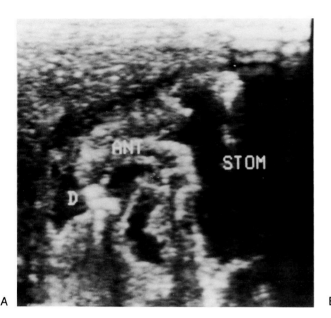 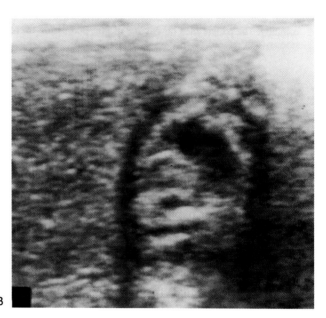

A B

Fig. 8-30. Focal foveolar hyperplasia. **(A)** Longitudinal sonogram demonstrating the mass in the distal stomach. The proximal stomach *(STOM)*, antral mass *(ANT)*, and duodenum *(D)* are labeled. **(B)** Transverse scan showing the lobular mass on the lumen side of the normal muscle layers. (From McAlister et al,[66] with permission.)

The gastrointestinal tract is usually involved in AL amyloidosis.[68] However, widespread involvement of the stomach is not common.[69] This condition can produce concentric narrowing of the gastric antrum. There have been reports of prepyloric obstruction due to amyloidosis.

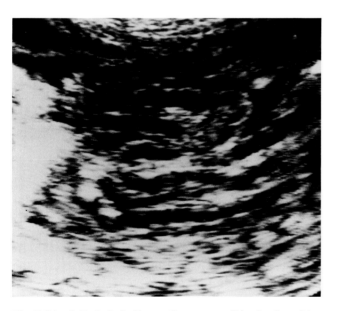

Fig. 8-31. Ménétrier's disease. Sonogram of the fundus of the empty stomach showing thickened gastric mucosa with hypertrophic rugae. (From Gassner et al,[67] with permission.)

The ultrasound findings associated with this disease process may appear similar to those of antral cancer. On ultrasound, the homogeneous hypoechogenicity of the thickened gastric wall cannot be distinguished from that of malignant etiologies and from other benign causes of gastric wall thickening[69] (Fig. 8-32). The walls of the stomach as well as the colon may be markedly thickened.[68] Additionally, decreased intestinal motility occasionally leading to pseudo-obstruction is frequently found with gastrointestinal amyloidosis.[68]

Hematoma

Intramural hemorrhage into the GI tract is a rare complication in hemophiliacs and can be due to other causes including bleeding diathesis, anticoagulant therapy, blunt trauma, leukemia, Henoch-Schönlein anaphylactoid purpura, and thrombocytopenic purpura.[70] It may be associated with signs and symptoms of obstruction and may present as a left upper quadrant mass.

On ultrasound, an intramural gastric hematoma may appear as a large complex mass consisting of coagula and blood when the symptoms of obstruction appear[70] (Figs. 8-33 and 8-34). After several weeks, the uneven and nonhomogeneous mass will change into an anechoic mass as a result of liquefaction of the hematoma. The fluid-filled stomach technique would be helpful in the assessment of the origin of the mass. This helps to identify the relationship of the mass to the stomach.

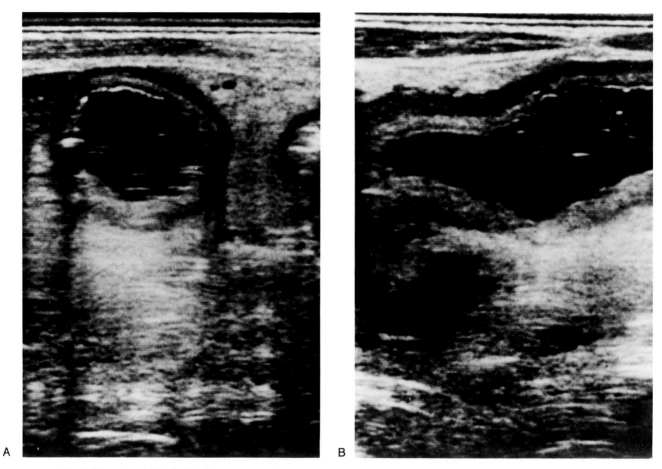

Fig. 8-32. Amyloidosis. **(A)** Transverse and **(B)** longitudinal sonograms through the gastric antrum after water ingestion demonstrating diffuse thickening with the multiple-layer appearance. (From Shirahama et al,[68] with permission.)

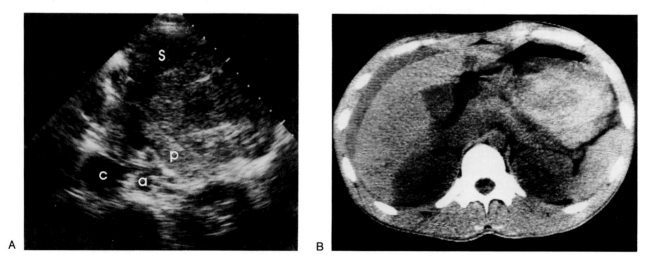

Fig. 8-33. Gastric hematoma. **(A)** Sonogram showing an echogenic mass in the posterior wall of the stomach and lesser sac. (*a*, aorta; *c*, inferior vena cava; *p*, pancreas; *S*, stomach.) **(B)** CT scan showing a high-density mass behind the stomach. (From Morimoto et al,[70] with permission.)

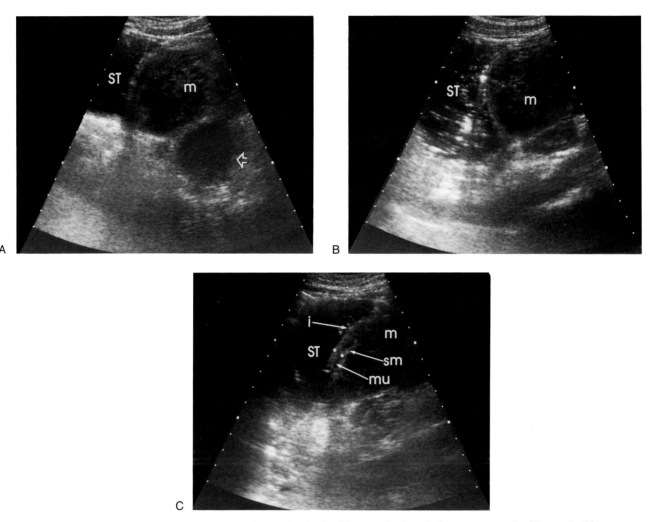

Fig. 8-34. Gastric hematoma. This patient, who had a history of ethanol abuse, presented with a palpable abdominal mass and a decreased hematocrit. A complex cystic mass (*m*, 81 × 95 × 80 mm) was seen in the left upper quadrant on (**A**) transverse and (**B**) sagittal views. It was located to the right of the spleen and to the left of the stomach *(ST)* with extension (open arrow, Fig. A) toward the pancreatic area. To evaluate the relationship of the stomach to the mass, the patient had been given water to drink. As demonstrated, the mass was inferior to the stomach in Fig. B and lateral in Fig. A. (**C**) On a sagittal view, the layers of the inferior gastric wall (calipers) can be identified. The mass appeared to be distorting the muscularis propria layer and, to some extent, the submucosa (*sm*, echodense.) At angiography, the mass was shown to be avascular. (*i*, interface echo [echodense]; *mu*, mucosa [hypoechoic]; see Fig. 8-10.)

Benign Tumors

Polyps

The fluid-filled stomach technique may be used in evaluation of benign gastric lesions.[4] Small benign polypoid lesions are usually not seen by ultrasound; however, one study reports identification of polypoid gastric lesions.[2] These lesions could be seen only with fluid distension of the stomach and appeared as solid masses adherent to the gastric wall[2] (Fig. 8-35). A polyp may be seen as a polypoid formation with variable echogenicity. In addition, large polyps may be inhomogeneous; contours may be sharply or not sharply delimited depending on the nature of the surface; and detection of the pedicle may be possible.[4] The differential diagnosis of such polypoid lesions should include hyperplastic polyps, pseudopolypoid lesions, polypoid infiltration, or gastric mucosal lymphoma.[2]

Leiomyomas

Leiomyoma, the most common tumor of the stomach, can be seen as a mass similar to carcinoma and is usually small and asymptomatic.[26,71] It is four times more frequent than sarcoma; the patient population has a mean age of 41 years. Gastric leiomyomas represent 2.5 percent of gastric tumors, and 10 percent are located in the cardia.[22] These lesions are often associated with other GI abnormalities such as cholelithiasis, peptic

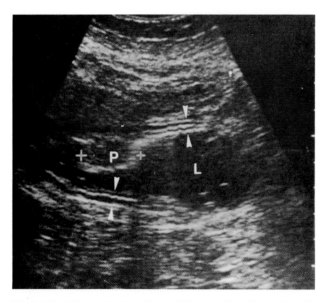

Fig 8-35. Hyperplastic polyps of the antral wall. A polypoid mass (*P*, 25 mm) is seen in the anterior wall of the antrum. (arrowheads, layers of the antral wall; *L*, gastric lumen.) (From Worlicek et al,[4] with permission.)

ulcer disease, adenocarcinoma, and leiomyosarcoma. As the size of the mass increases, the incidence of malignant transformation also increases.[22] Even when the leiomyoma is large and symptomatic, it is rarely palpable.[71]

On ultrasound, this lesion may be seen as a hypoechoic mass continuous with the muscular layer of the stomach.[22] It may be visualized as a circular or oval space-occupying lesion with a homogeneous echopattern and hemispheric bulging into the lumen, frequently separated from the lumen by two or three layers continuous with those of normal wall.[4] It may appear as a solid mass with cystic areas that represent necrosis[71] (Figs. 8-36 and 8-37). An exogastric pedunculated configuration, although sometimes seen, is uncommon. Endosonography may yield better information than conventional ultrasound, but an anatomic location in the cardia would make for a difficult examination.[22]

Malignant Tumors

Gastric Carcinoma

From 90 to 95 percent of malignant tumors of the stomach are carcinomas, with 3 percent being lymphomas and 2 percent being leiomyosarcomas. Gastric carcinoma is the sixth leading cause of cancer death in the United States and occurs more frequently in males (2:1). Half of these tumors occur in the pylorus, and one-fourth occur in the body and fundus. The lesions may be fungating, ulcerated, diffuse, polypoid, and/or superficial. Three-fourths of these tumors occur in patients over 50 years old. The clinical manifestations are nonspecific, with 25 percent of patients presenting with a palpable mass.[38]

On ultrasound, the examiner looks for the typical target or pseudokidney ascribed to GI lesions[26,30,72] (Figs. 8-38 and 8-39). Although the target lesion may be seen with tumor, it also may be secondary to lymphoma, metastatic disease, caustic gastritis, pancreatitis involving the stomach, and chronic granulomatous disease of childhood[73] (Fig. 8-40). Identification depends on the type, location, and extent of the tumor. It may be seen as a large mass in the left upper quadrant or as gastric wall thickening; the latter is due to tumor infiltration of the wall and may or may not exhibit surrounding inflammatory changes.[74] This wall thickening may be localized or diffuse.[26,72,75] With localized thickening, the wall is eccentrically thickened (Figs. 8-38, 8-39, 8-41, and 8-42). The wall may have a C-shaped appearance when only the involved wall is delineated.[26,74] When a mass is demonstrated on ultrasound, it usually indicates significant infiltration of the mucosa and muscularis and/or

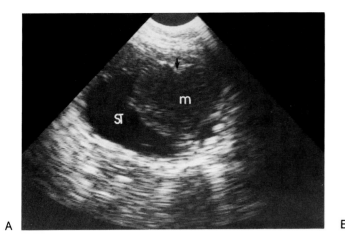

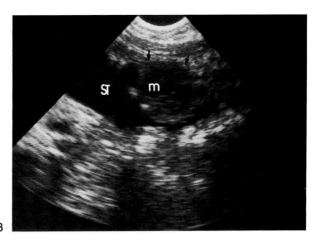

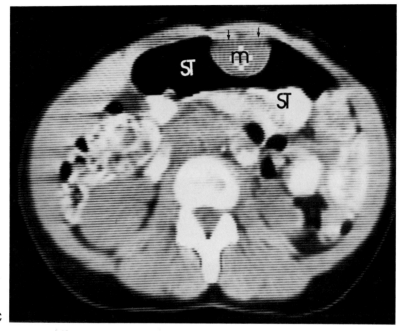

Fig. 8-36. Gastric leiomyoma. **(A)** Transverse and **(B)** longitudinal real-time scans of the fluid-filled stomach *(ST)*. An echodense mass *(m),* the leiomyoma, is seen projecting from the anterior surface of the stomach (arrows). **(C)** CT image further confirming the presence of a soft tissue-density intraluminal gastric (ST) mass (m).

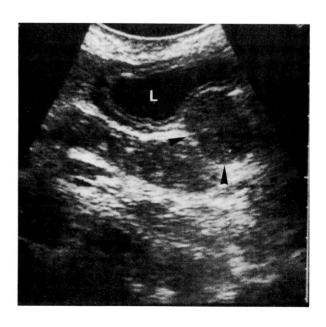

Fig. 8-37. Leiomyoma. Longitudinal section showing a submucosal leiomyoma (25 × 18 mm) of the posterior wall of the antrum, with three preserved wall layers over the lesion (arrowheads). (*L*, lumen.) (From Worlicek et al,[4] with permission.)

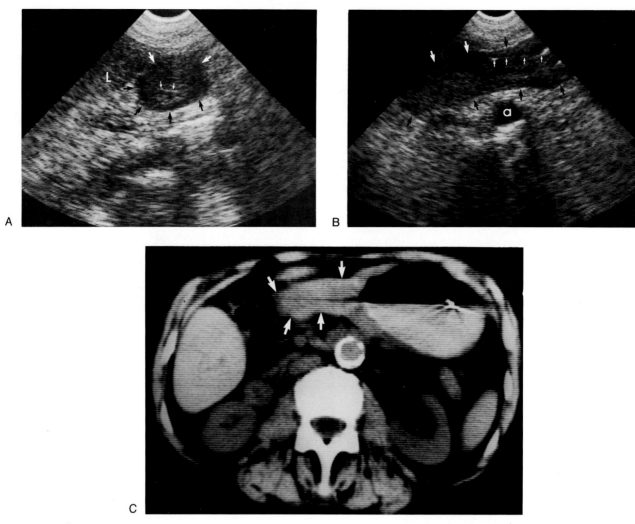

Fig. 8-38. Gastric carcinoma (pyloric). **(A)** Sagittal scan showing a target pattern (arrows). The echodense center (small arrows) or lumen is eccentrically located. (*L*, liver.) **(B)** Transverse scan, with an appearance similar to cases of pyloric stenosis, showing thickening of the wall (arrows). The lumen (small arrows) is eccentrically located. (*a*, aorta.) **(C)** CT scan confirming thickening of the pyloric wall (arrows). The lumen is not identified.

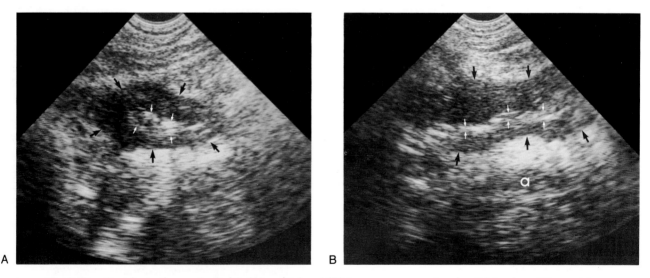

Fig. 8-39. Gastric carcinoma (pyloric). **(A)** sagittal and **(B)** transverse scans showing thickening of the gastric wall (black arrows). The lumen is echogenic (white arrows). (*a*, aorta.)

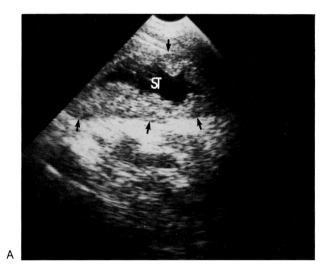

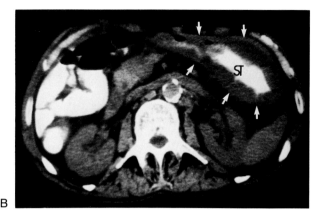

Fig. 8-40. Gastric wall thickening in pancreatitis. This patient had pancreatitis and pseudocysts within the tail of the pancreas. The gastric wall (arrows) is noted to be thickened on **(A)** a transverse real-time scan and **(B)** a CT scan. (*ST,* fluid-filled stomach.)

exogastric extension. An antral carcinoma may present with gastric dilatation due to obstruction. This gastric dilatation may also be secondary to pylorospasm, inflammation, intrinsic or extrinsic tumor, electrolyte imbalance, diabetes, neurologic disease, or medication.[30]

Using the fluid-filled stomach technique and examining the stomach in various positions, a number of lesions may be identified.[4] In contrast to endoscopic ultrasound, this technique can visualize all portions of the stomach.[4] When there is circumscribed irregular thickening of the gastric wall, a malignant process is suspected, although ulcer penetration may appear similar.[4] Scirrhous carcinoma, leiomyosarcoma, and lymphoma, which cause malignant infiltration of the stomach, can be largely

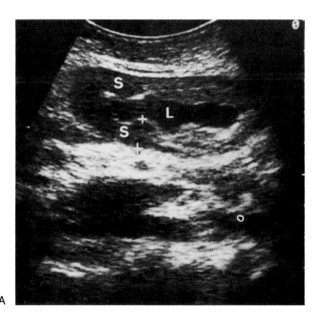

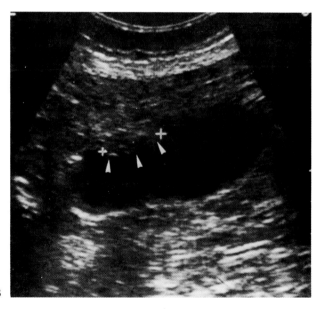

Fig 8-41. Gastric carcinoma. **(A)** Longitudinal section through the proximal antrum showing a scirrhous carcinoma *(S)* of the stomach with circumferential infiltration of the wall. The thickness of the wall (calipers) was 9 mm, and the lumen *(L)* was narrowed. **(B)** Carcinoma (arrowheads) of the anterior wall of the antrum (diameter, 21 mm). (From Worlicek et al,[4] with permission.)

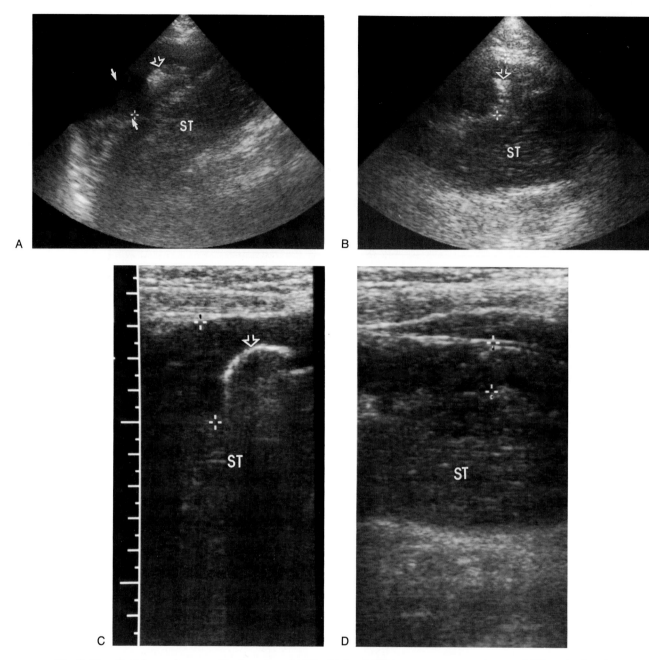

Fig. 8-42. Gastric carcinoma with ulceration. **(A)** Sagittal and **(B)** transverse sector views and **(C)** sagittal and **(D)** transverse linear-array views of the gastric wall demonstrating wall thickening (arrows, calipers, 12.8 mm), anteriorly and loss of the normal wall delineation. There is air (open arrow) within an ulcer crater in Figs. A–C. (*ST,* gastric lumen.) *(Figure continues.)*

proven by the appearance of circumferential, possibly stenosing, thickening of considerable parts of the stomach wall associated with rigidity of the wall.[4]

The fluid-filled stomach technique may be helpful in evaluating gastric cancers. By using this method, an early cancer may be seen as a flat polypoid formation, moderately hypoechoic with preserved wall layering[4] (Fig.

8-41B). A localized carcinoma may be seen as a hypoechoic or moderately echoic circumscribed wall thickening with irregular contours and interrupted wall layering, possibly dish-shaped.[4] A scirrhous carcinoma may be visualized as an extensive, predominantly hypoechoic mural infiltration; partly uniform, partly irregular or polypoidlike thickening of the wall; and/or lack of dis-

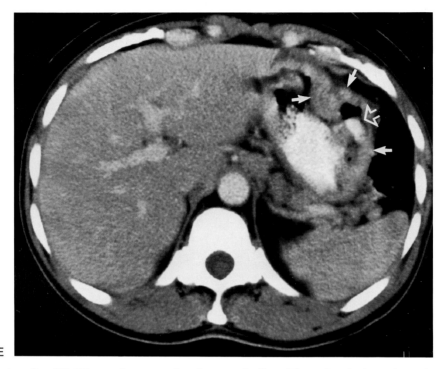

Fig. 8-42 *(Continued).* **(E)** CT scan demonstrating the same findings. The patient had gastric carcinoma with ulceration.

tensibility of the stomach wall with narrowing of the lumen or stenosis[4] (Fig. 8-41A).

One group of investigators has reported a calcified target lesion associated with mucinous carcinoma of the stomach.[76] The calcifications associated with gastric carcinoma are generally small (1 to 3 mm) and granular.[76] They are homogeneously distributed in the gastric wall, partially or completely occupying the circumference of the organ.[76] This particular pattern—a target lesion in the gastric area with calcifications in the wall—is a specific sign of mucinous carcinoma.[76]

Besides identifying the gastric primary tumor, ultrasound may be used for staging.[77] When such a patient is referred for evaluation of liver metastases (Fig. 8-43), it is worthwhile to gather additional information about the extent of the tumor. This is done by performing a complete sonographic examination of the abdomen and pelvis and by attempting to visualize the primary neoplasm and its relationship to surrounding organs (Fig. 8-43). Ultrasound has a sensitivity of 71.4 percent and a specificity of 85.7 percent for evaluation of lymph node metastases.[77] For direct invasion, it has a sensitivity of 75 percent and a specificity of 100 percent.[77] This carcinoma may spread to the surrounding gastric wall and adjacent organs and structures directly or to perigastric lymph nodes via the lymphatics. There is hematogenous spread to the liver and distant organs. In addition, there

is peritoneal seeding to the omentum, parietal peritoneum, ovaries, and pelvic cul-de-sac (Fig. 8-43). Preoperative knowledge of the local and distant extent of the tumor greatly help the surgeon to plan the therapeutic approach more accurately. Such knowledge may even obviate a laparotomy in patients with far-advanced disease. Such patients may instead receive other types of treatment and undergo surgery only if palliative procedures for relief of obstruction and/or hemorrhage are needed.[77]

Lymphoma

Lymphoma can occur as a primary tumor of the GI tract. As a primary tumor, it most often affects the stomach and ileum; the colon and rectum are affected less frequently. Presumably, gastric lymphoma arises within lymphoid aggregates; it represents 1 to 5 percent of gastric neoplasms.[78,79] In the small bowel and colon, lymphoma originates in normal mucosal lymphoid aggregates. In disseminated lymphoma, the primary tumor occurs as multifocal lesions in the GI tract.

Gastric lymphoma has a number of gross anatomic findings including enlarged and thickened mucosal folds; multiple submucosal nodules, ulceration; a large, predominately extraluminal mass; or a combination of two or more of these features.[78] As a tumor arising from

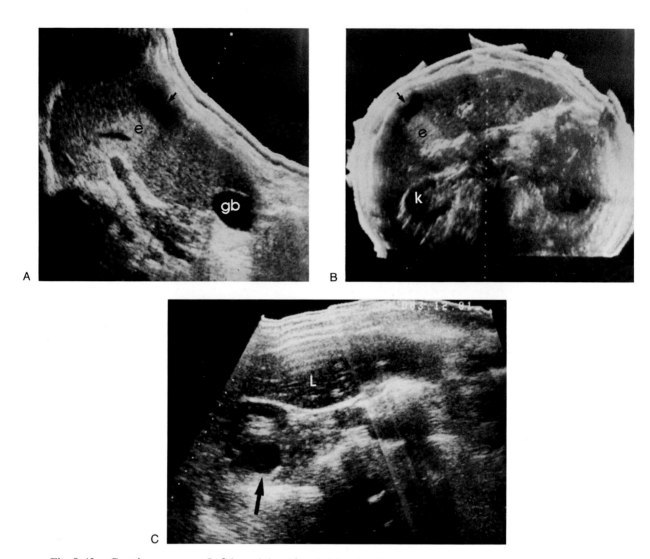

Fig. 8-43. Gastric metastases. Left lateral decubitus **(A)** longitudinal and **(B)** transverse scans of the liver in a patient with gastric carcinoma. An anechoic lesion (arrow) proved to be a metastasis. Note the posterior acoustic enhancement *(e)*. (*k*, right kidney; *gb*, gallbladder.) **(C)** Transverse scan of the right kidney in a patient with tumor recurrence. A rounded 2-cm hypoechoic metastasis is seen in the posterior kidney (arrow). (*L*, liver.) *(Figure continues.)*

lymphoid tissue of the lamina propria of the gastric mucosa, primary gastric non-Hodgkin's lymphoma may spread into the deep mucosa and infiltrate the muscularis propria serosa and perigastric lymph nodes at late stages.[79]

Patients with gastric lymphoma present with similar symptoms to those with gastric carcinoma. The associated symptoms are nonspecific (nausea, vomiting, weight loss) and cannot be distinguished from those caused by gastric tumors of epithelial origin.[79] Ninety percent of lymphoma patients complain of pain,[38] and 25 percent have an abdominal mass.[78]

On ultrasound, gastric lymphoma is usually seen as a relatively large and poorly echogenic (hypoechoic)

mass[26,74,78,80,81] (Figs. 8-44 and 8-45). There may be marked thickening of the gastric walls as a result of tumor infiltration.[26] One group of investigators have reported two features helpful in the diagnosis of gastric lymphoma: (1) the spoke-wheel pattern within the targetlike lymphomatous mass; and (2) thickened hypoechoic gastric wall.[78] The spoke-wheel pattern is produced by the marked increase in thickness and height of the mucosal folds. The echogenic spokes are produced by the mucosal surfaces dividing the folds. The thickened hypoechoic wall pattern is homogeneous, with an absence of induced fibroblastic reaction within the infiltrated wall. When an exophytic lesion is present, it may be difficult to differentiate lymphoma and leiomyosar-

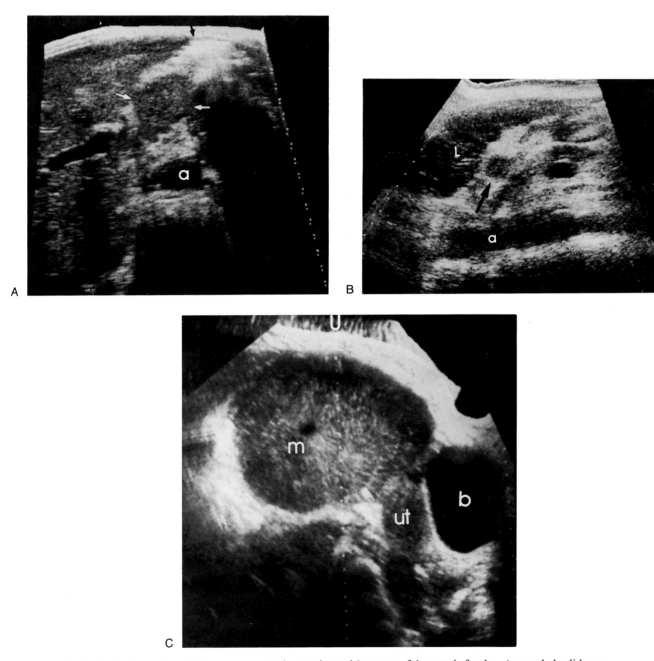

Fig. 8-43 *(Continued).* **(D)** Transverse scan in a patient with tumor of the gastric fundus. A rounded solid mass, which has medium-level echoes (white arrows) due to lymph node metastasis, is seen along the lesser curvature, medial to the acoustic shadow that is caused by air within the body of the stomach (black arrow). (*a*, aorta.) **(E)** Longitudinal scan along the aorta *(a)* in a patient with an ulcerated tumor of the lesser curvature. In the celiac region, an enlarged lymph node is seen as a relatively small (1.5-cm) rounded solid mass with medium-level echoes (arrow). (*L*, liver.) **(F)** Longitudinal scan demonstrating an echodense mass *(m)* that is separate from the uterus *(ut)*. This represents metastatic disease to the ovary or Kruckenberg tumor. (*b*, bladder; *U*, level of the umbilicus.) (Figs. C–E from Derchi et al,[77] with permission.)

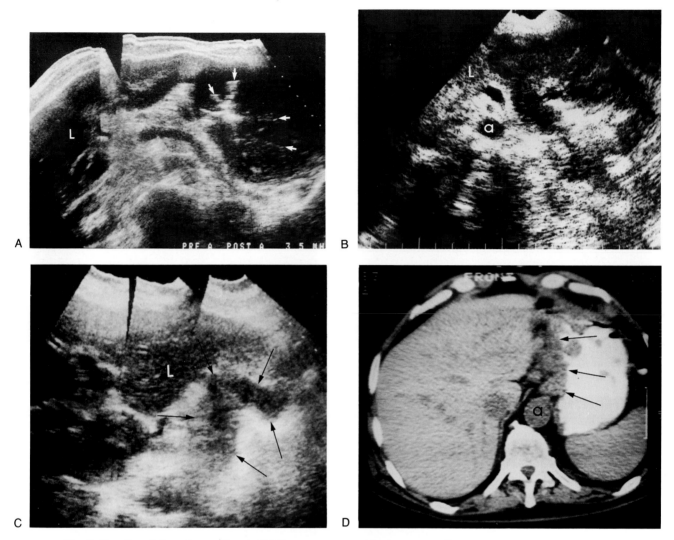

Fig. 8-44. Gastric lymphoma. Case 1. **(A)** Transverse scan with a large targetlike mass occupying most of the left epigastrium. The thickened gastric wall has a hypoechoic, almost echofree structure. High and thick mucosal folds may be seen within the mass, outlined by the strong luminal echoes (arrows) that radiate from an echogenic core toward the periphery like the spokes of the wheel. (*L*, liver.) Case 2. **(B)** Transverse scan with a large gastric mass. The thickened gastric wall is less echogenic than the liver *(L)* parenchyma; the luminal echoes are distorted and irregular without a radial pattern. (*a*, aorta.) Case 3. **(C)** Transverse scan demonstrating thickening of only the lesser curvature and anterior wall of the stomach (arrows). (*L*, liver.) **(D)** CT scan showing both thickening (arrows) of the gastric wall and polypoid gastric lesions. (*a*, aorta.) (From Derchi et al,[78] with permission.)

coma. Leiomyosarcoma is usually a complex mass with both solid hyperechoic tissue and areas of liquefactive necrosis.[78]

By using the fluid-filled stomach technique, the gastric wall may be evaluated for lymphoma. Lymphomatous infiltration may be seen as circumscribed or extensive circumferential wall thickening of variable echodensity; the wall may be regularly delimited or have infiltrated polypoid folds.[4]

Additional studies have identified further patterns as-

sociated with lymphoma.[82] The additional ultrasound patterns identified are circumferential involvement of the bowel wall and the presence of bulky tumors and nodular extraluminal spread. The classic (and most common) target pattern indicates advanced circumferential intestinal infiltration with tumor. At times, giant gastric folds with a central starlike configuration of echogenicity are visible on ultrasound. Seventy-two percent of patients with gastric lymphoma have ultrasound findings consisting of a space-occupying mass with

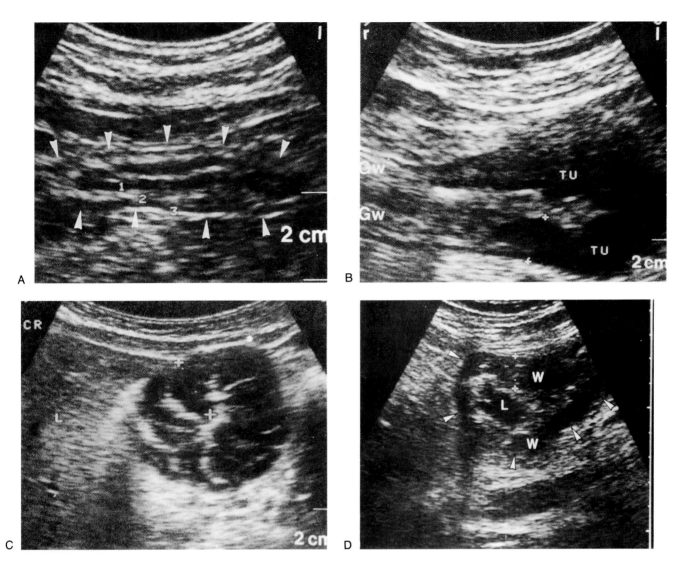

Fig. 8-45. Gastric lymphoma. **(A)** Histologically confirmed lymphoma of the stomach confined to the mucosa. Longitudinal sonogram through the antrum (arrowheads) showing isolated thickening of the mucosa *(1)* with individual layers of gastric wall *(2,* submucosa; *3,* muscularis). **(B)** Transverse sonogram of a 73-year-old man with primary gastric non-Hodgkin's lymphoma of low-grade malignancy showing histologically confirmed transmural segmental lymphoma involvement *(TU).* *(Gw,* normal gastric wall.) **(C)** Generalized non-Hodgkin's lymphoma and secondary gastric involvement. Sonogram through the body of the stomach showing transmural-circumferential lymphoma involvement, with giant folds presenting a starlike configuration. *(L,* liver.) **(D)** Chronic lymphatic leukemia. Oblique section showing lymphoma infiltration of the antrum (arrowheads) with irregular circumferential thickening of the wall *(W,* anterior wall; 13 mm) and a narrowed lumen *(L).* (Figs. A–C from Goerg et al,[82] with permission; Fig. D from Worlicek et al,[4] with permission.)

bright central echoes and uniformly hypoechoic wall thickening of various extents.

Leiomyosarcoma

Leiomyosarcoma, the second most common gastric sarcoma, is usually a large bulky intramural or subserosal mass and represents 1 to 5 percent of gastric tumors.[38,83–85] These lesions occur in the fifth and sixth decades of life.[84] They are generally globular or irregular and may become huge, outstripping their blood supply, with subsequent central necrosis leading to cystic degeneration and cavitation. This cavity may connect with the GI tract.[84]

On ultrasound, a typical target lesion may be identified, but the pattern is variable. If there is necrosis with-

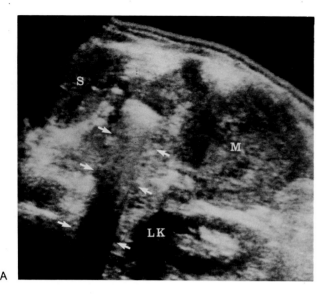

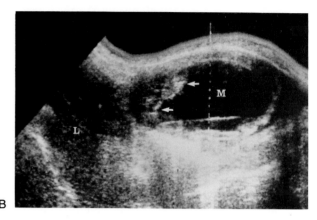

Fig. 8-46. Gastric leiomyosarcoma. Case 1. **(A)** Longitudinal scan in the right lateral decubitus position showing a leiomyosarcoma along the greater curvature. A hyperechoic mass *(M)* is seen in the left upper quadrant, separate from the spleen *(S)* and anterior to the left kidney *(LK)*. There is acoustic shadowing (arrows) from air in the gastric lumen following ingestion of water. Case 2. **(B)** Longitudinal scan with leiomyosarcoma within the anterior wall of the body of the stomach. A large mass *(M)* is seen that is hyperechoic at the periphery (arrows) and has a central fluid level due to liquefaction necrosis. (*L*, liver.) (From Subramanyam et al,[83] with permission.)

out liquefaction, the mass may appear without enhancement as an echofree zone.[83] With liquefactive necrosis, there are fluid-containing spaces.[83] Hemorrhage and necrosis may occur, causing irregular echoes or a cystic cavity.[74] A pattern of a solid mass anteriorly located outside a solid viscus, the presence of necrosis, and intestinal lumen and/or air in close relation to the mass are highly suggestive of a leiomyosarcoma[83] (Figs. 8-46 and 8-47).

By using the fluid-filled stomach technique, certain patterns may be identified with leiomyosarcoma. With this lesion, a circumferential, eccentrically growing tumor mass or, in the initial stage, a localized submucosal roundish or oval space-occupying lesion of variable echodensity is characteristic.[4]

Metastatic Disease

Metastatic carcinoma to the stomach is rare. There is a reported incidence of metastatic neoplasms of the stomach of 2 percent in patients with known cancers.[86] The most common form is generalized lymphoma or leukemia, with most multiple growths affecting primarily the submucosa and muscularis.[38] The most frequently encountered primary tumor is melanoma (especially class IV), followed by lung and breast cancer.[86] Other less common sources include testis, thyroid, cervix, uterus, ovary, and pancreas.[86] Most often, metastatic lesions are found within the submucosal layer, forming circum-

scribed nodules or plaques.[86] If the lesion is aggressive, such as with anaplastic bronchogenic carcinoma, the mass may infiltrate the wall.[26]

On ultrasound a target pattern may again be identified.[72] The resultant localized mass within the stomach

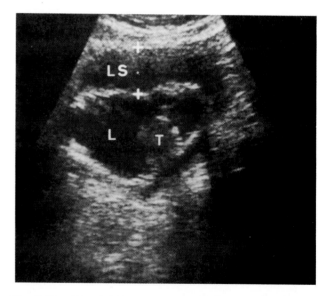

Fig. 8-47. Gastric leiomyosarcoma. Oblique section through the antrum showing a leiomyosarcoma *(LS)* with irregular thickening of the wall up to 18 mm, a tumor "finger" *(T)* arising in the less-thickened posterior wall, and a fluid-filled lumen *(L)*. (From Worlicek et al,[4] with permission.)

usually is poorly echogenic but sometimes is irregularly echogenic or has an echofree necrotic cavity.[86] These lesions are usually globular.

By using the fluid-filled stomach technique, metastatic gastric disease may be discovered. With metastatic infiltration, there is circumscribed thickening or uniform widening of the wall, with absence of layering.[4] It is helpful to perform ultrasound on patients at risk for metastatic lesions to recognize secondary gastric tumors at an early stage.[86]

SMALL BOWEL ABNORMALITIES

Obstruction and/or Dilatation

Small bowel obstruction is associated with dilatation of the bowel loops proximal to the site of the obstruction; radiography is usually more useful in this situation than ultrasound. The dilated loops are usually filled with gas, which impedes the transmission of the sound beam. In 6 percent of cases, though, the dilated loops are filled with fluid and can easily be mistaken for a soft tissue mass on radiographs.[26]

The hallmark of intestinal obstruction on ultrasound, whether due to mechanical cause or absence of peristalsis, is intraluminal accumulation of fluid.[87] The dilated fluid-filled loops can be identified by their tubular (long axis) and oval or round (cross-section) echofree appearance[17,26,87–89] (Figs. 8-48 and 8-49). In adynamic ileus, dilated bowel loops have normal to somewhat in-creased peristaltic activity.[90] There is generally less distension than with dynamic ileus. In dynamic (obstructive) ileus, the fluid-filled loops are almost perfectly round with minimal deformity at the interfaces with adjacent loops of distended bowel.[90] Often the valvulae conniventes can be seen, as well as peristalsis.[25,26,87,89] Peristaltic motion is demonstrated by a "bubblelike" pattern.[25] The level of the obstruction may be judged by the distribution of the distended fluid-filled loops.[17] If fluid-filled loops are only in the upper abdomen, obstruction of the distal small bowel should be suspected.

Ultrasound can be helpful in differentiating fluid-filled bowel loops from cystic abdominal masses. Sausage-shaped cystic structures with uneven margins representing mucosal folds are distributed throughout the abdomen and sometimes are accompanied by peristalsis.[91] Ultrasound can detect intestinal obstruction by fluid-filled bowel loops instead of air-distended loops; subtle elongated masses representing these bowel loops may be missed on plain radiography. Ultrasound can easily distinguish fluid-filled loops of bowel from normal bowel in ascites.[91] On sonograms, normal bowel is located in the central part of the peritoneal cavity with free fluid distributed in the flanks as well as the cul-de-sac, whereas fluid-filled bowel is distributed across the entire abdomen.[91]

Fluid-filled loops of bowel are not always associated with obstruction.[87] They occur with gastroenteritis and with paralytic ileus. If no peristalsis is seen, pressure applied with the transducer can often demonstrate pliability and compressibility of the bowel wall, as well as induce the movement of echoes.[26]

Closed-Loop Obstruction or Volvulus

Sometimes a single dilated aperistaltic loop of bowel is observed, such as with a closed-loop obstruction or volvulus.[26,88] With this problem, air cannot enter the involved bowel loop, and ultrasound provides important information.[87] With volvulus, the involved loop is doubled back on itself abruptly, so that a U appearance is seen on a sagittal scan and a C-shaped anechoic area with a dense center is seen on transverse scan[90] (Fig. 8-49). The dense center represents the medial bowel wall and mesentery.

Duodenal Obstruction and/or Dilatation

Many abnormalities of the duodenum may be diagnosed by ultrasound in neonates.[5] These abnormalities include duodenal obstruction, malrotation with or without associated volvulus, incomplete rotation, and duodenal stenosis.[5] These neonates and infants are often

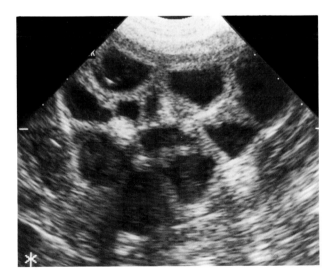

Fig. 8-48. Small bowel obstruction. Sagittal scan of the lower abdomen demonstrating multiple round cystic structures. These represent dilated fluid-filled bowel loops in cross-section.

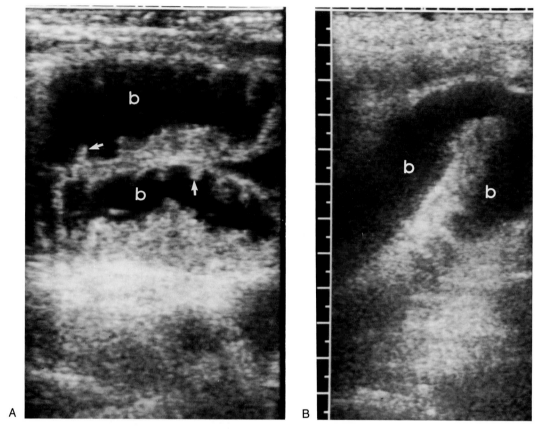

Fig. 8-49. Small bowel obstruction, closed loop. **(A)** Transverse and **(B)** sagittal scans of the right lower quadrant demonstrating a dilated fluid-filled small bowel *(b)* loop. It is C-shaped in Fig. B. In Fig. A the valvulae conniventes (arrows) are identified. The patient had a strangulated femoral hernia.

evaluated with ultrasound since they had been vomiting. The use of fluid distention of the stomach and duodenum provides a dynamic view of the duodenal rotation and anatomy and, at the very least, provides a method of triaging infants who may require surgery, UGI series, or follow-up ultrasound to make the definitive diagnosis.[5] The overall sensitivity and specificity of fluid-aided ultrasound evaluation of these duodenal abnormalities are 100 and 99 percent, respectively.[5]

Midgut Volvulus. Midgut volvulus is an acute medical emergency that often occurs during the neonatal period.[92] The infant usually presents with an acute onset of vomiting in which the vomitus contains bile. The radiograph may be normal or have the classic signs of intestinal obstruction; only when a distended descending duodenum is seen is the diagnosis made with certainty. Once duodenal obstruction is demonstrated, a presumptive diagnosis of duodenal bands, malrotation, and potential midgut volvulus can be made. Ultrasound may suggest the diagnosis if to-and-fro hyperperistaltic mo-

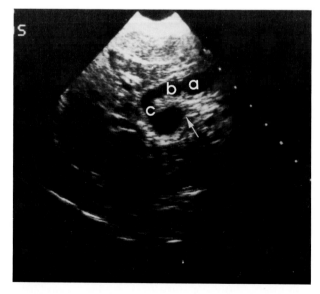

Fig. 8-50. Duodenal obstruction. Midgut volvulus. Longitudinal real-time scan showing distension of the fluid-filled antropylorus *(a)*, duodenal bulb *(b)*, and duodenal C-loop *(c)*. Tapering of the distal obstructed duodenum (arrow) is seen. (From Hayden et al,[92] with permission.)

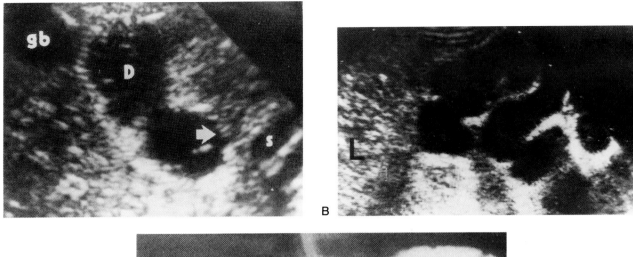

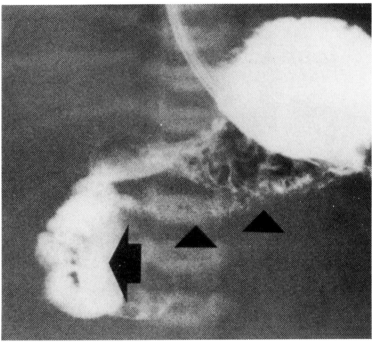

Fig. 8-51. Midgut volvulus. **(A)** Transverse upper abdominal sonogram showing the distended descending duodenum *(D)*, which is abruptly cut off as it comes in front (arrow) of the spine *(s)*. *(gb,* gallbladder.) **(B)** Right parasagittal sonogram showing the distended fluid-filled bowel with thick hyperechoic walls. At surgery, midgut malrotation with volvulus and extensive bowel necrosis were found. *(L,* liver.) **(C)** Bedside UGI radiograph with water-soluble diatrizoate meglumine (30 percent Hypaque; Winthrop-Breon Laboratories) immediately followed by barium enema examination showing both the abnormally positioned duodenojejunal junction and the distended duodenum (arrow). The right colon is superimposed on the duodenum. No gas is present in the intestine. (arrowheads, transverse colon.) (From Leonidas et al,[93] with permission.)

tion is observed in an obstructed duodenal loop[92] (Figs. 8-50 and 8-51).

Midgut volvulus may be diagnosed by seeing the fluid-filled proximal duodenum ending in a twist or "arrowhead" configuration.[5] The duodenum does not cross the midline, and the more distal duodenum is not seen to fill with fluid.[5] By following the fluid in the duodenum from the antrum to the ligament of Treitz, normal rota-tion can be seen as well as malrotation without volvulus, and subtle abnormalities in the course of the duodenum can be seen even when it crosses from right to left.[5]

Midgut Malrotation. Incomplete rotation and fixation of the gut in a fetus is called midgut malrotation.[93] The symptoms are often produced by obstructing peritoneal bands that cross over the descending duodenum or occasionally, the cecum, which may lie on top of the duodenum.[93] Midgut volvulus, a common complication of midgut malrotation, may become life-threatening; it may also produce ischemic bowel necrosis, which may be fatal.[93] With midgut volvulus, there is usually vomiting, abdominal distension, and occasionally bloody stools.[93]

Although a fluid-filled, distended duodenum seen at ultrasound in infants may be nonspecific, it may be seen with midgut rotation.[93] Additional findings may include dilated, thick-walled bowel loops mainly to the right of the spine and peritoneal fluid (Figs. 8-52 and 8-53). A number of findings are associated with midgut malrotation: distended proximal duodenum; extrinsic,

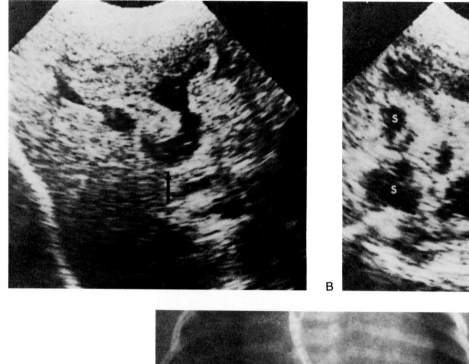

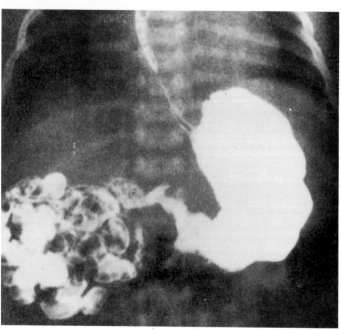

Fig. 8-52. Malrotation without volvulus. **(A)** Transverse-oblique view showing that the distal portion of the second part of the duodenum (arrow) taking a sharp turn to the right rather than the leftward sweep of a normal duodenal C-loop. This is indicative of malrotation. **(B)** Longitudinal view of the infrahepatic region showing fluid filling the small bowel loops *(s)* on the right side of the abdomen. **(C)** UGI series showing the small bowel on the right side of the abdomen. (From Cohen et al,[5] with permission.)

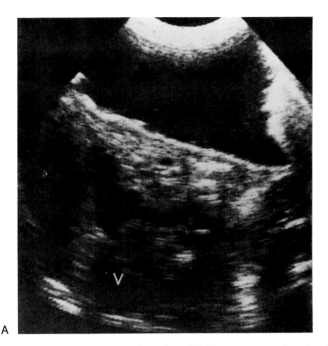

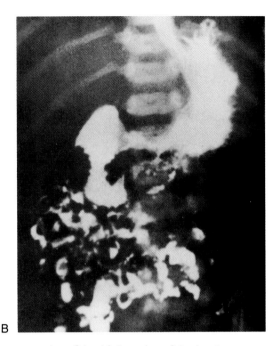

A   B

Fig. 8-53. Z-type malrotation. **(A)** Transverse section showing narrowing of the third portion of the duodenum as it crosses the vertebral body *(V)*. The fluid follows an unusual course distally. **(B)** UGI series showing narrowing of the third portion of the duodenum. Contrast material continued distally in a zigzag fashion. A Z-type malrotation was found during surgery. (From Cohen et al,[5] with permission.)

arrowhead-type compression of the duodenum over the spine; abnormal relationship of the superior mesenteric artery and vein, with the latter to the left of the former; and the presence of distended, thick-walled loops of bowel below the duodenum and to the right of the spine, in association with peritoneal fluid[93] (Figs. 8-52 and 8-53). The ultrasound findings of duodenal obstruction associated with thickened bowel loops to the right of the spine and peritoneal fluid should lead the examiner to suspect midgut malrotation complicated by volvulus, a potentially fatal condition, and a UGI series should be performed for further evaluation.[93]

Duodenal Stenosis. Ultrasound can be helpful in the evaluation of patients with duodenal stenosis.[94] Abnormalities such as multiple duodenal polyps, duodenal wall cysts, and annular pancreas may be evaluated by ultrasound.[94] Duodenal wall cysts are uncommon causes of duodenal stenosis. Obstruction or relative stenosis may cause dilatation of the more proximal duodenal bulb and pyloric channel. Duodenal atresia may be associated with dilatation. Nausea and vomiting may occur with duodenal stenosis.

Fluid-filled bowel can aid in the ultrasound evaluation of stenotic processes in the duodenum[94] (Fig. 8-54). Duodenal lesions might be identified on ultrasound by knowledge of their sonographic location.[95] Polyps ap-

pear similar to those in the gallbladder when surrounded with fluid. Narrowing of the duodenal may also be demonstrated by ultrasound.[5] Duodenal lesions are described as an epigastric mass that is solid or has a heterogeneous pattern or a targetlike structure.[95] Most duodenal lesions have high-level central echoes and a hypoechoic periphery, which is consistent with a GI origin. In one series, the authors were able to identify the duodenal origin of a lesion in 16 of 18 abnormalities.[95] Careful analysis of the relationships of the lesion to abdominal vessels and all surrounding structures and demonstrating the mass continuing into the normal duodenum may be of help for proper localization.[95]

Superior Mesenteric Artery Syndrome. In superior mesenteric artery syndrome, the stomach and duodenum may be dilated to the point in the third portion of the duodenum where the superior mesenteric vessels indent the duodenum. The pathogenesis of the syndrome is controversial, but mechanical factors appear to be important in its production. As a rule, these findings are seen with the patient supine and disappear when the patient is prone. This condition is more common in extremely thin patients (especially females with anorexia nervosa) and in patients with extensive burns, rapid weight loss, acute pancreatitis, severe trauma, or a body cast.

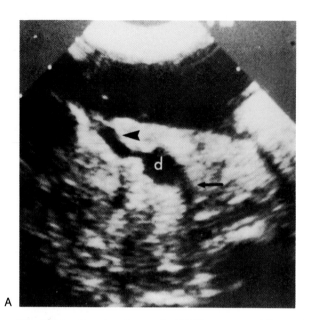
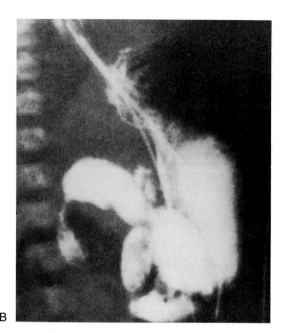

A   B

Fig. 8-54. Duodenal stenosis. **(A)** Transverse-oblique view of the pylorus and proximal duodenum showing a dilated duodenal bulb *(d)* proximal to a point of narrowing (arrow). The pyloric channel (arrowhead) is dilated and fluid filled proximal to the point of stenosis. **(B)** UGI series. Contrast-enhanced examination showing narrowing of the most proximal aspect of the second portion of the duodenum as the cause of the pyloric dilatation seen on ultrasound. At surgery, duodenal stenosis without an annular pancreas was found. (From Cohen et al,[5] with permission.)

In most cases of superior mesenteric artery syndrome, no findings are seen on ultrasound. However, one may see a dilated fluid-filled second portion of the duodenum that exhibits a to-and-fro peristaltic motion on real-time ultrasound (Fig. 8-55). On a sagittal scan, the dilated duodenum can be followed to the point where the superior mesenteric artery crosses the duodenum and the duodenum becomes nondilated (Fig. 8-55).

Miscellaneous Obstruction/Dilatation

Matted Bowel Loops. At times, matted loops of bowel may present a confusing picture on ultrasound (Fig. 8-56). Matted loops may be caused by adhesions, peritoneal implants, or intraperitoneal inflammatory processes. These loops assume a variety of appearances such as a group of tortuous, echofree tubular structures; a complex of masslike lesions with echofree areas and areas with weak or strong echoes; and an irregular lesion with weak echoes similar to a solid mass[26] (Fig. 8-56).

Afferent Loop Obstruction. Afferent loop obstruction usually occurs after a subtotal gastrectomy in which a Billroth II anastomosis is performed for ulcer disease. It is an uncommon complication caused by obstruction of

the duodenum and jejunum at any site proximal to the gastrojejunal anastomosis.[96] Its prevalence varies between 0.2 and 20 percent.

There are many causes of afferent loop syndrome, including internal hernia, kinking of the anastomosis, adhesive band, stomal stenosis, recurrent carcinoma or metastasis, and marginal ulcer. In these instances, the obstruction most often is due to internal herniation or a kink of the afferent loop.[97] Less often the afferent loop is obstructed secondary to recurrent pancreatic tumor after a Whipple operation or to recurrent gastric carcinoma.[97] Internal hernia is the most common cause, with an occurrence rate of 0.5 to 1.0 percent; it is highest in the immediate postoperative period.[96]

Patients with afferent loop obstruction may present with an abdominal emergency that mimics acute pancreatitis, both chemically and biochemically. Those with the more chronic or intermittent form present with bouts of abdominal pain due to distension of the loop from pancreatic and biliary secretions. The symptoms are alleviated by copious bilious emesis, which relieves distension.[97] Perforation of the afferent loop may occur; therefore, prompt recognition is important.[97]

Afferent loop obstruction is difficult to diagnose confidently before surgery. Barium studies show nonfilling of the loops, which is not helpful in making the diagno-

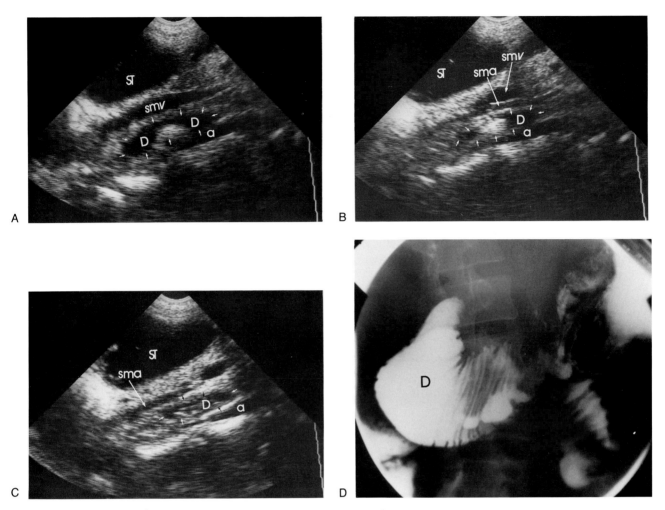

Fig. 8-55. Superior mesenteric artery syndrome. **(A–C)** Sequential sagittal right lateral decubitus scans from the long axis of the superior mesenteric vein *(smv)* to that of the superior mesenteric artery *(sma).* The fluid-filled stomach *(ST)* is seen anteriorly. The dilated third portion of the duodenum (*D*, arrows) is seen posterior to the superior mesenteric vein in Fig. A. By scanning from the superior mesenteric vein to the superior mesenteric artery, the duodenal lumen is greatly decreased in size posterior to the superior mesenteric artery (Figs. B & C). (*a*, aorta.) **(D)** Cone-down view from an UGI study. The dilated duodenum *(D)* is seen to be compressed in its third portion.

sis. On endoscopy, the afferent loop is successfully visualized in only 75 to 80 percent of patients.[97]

Ultrasound may be helpful in the recognition of large and dilated bowel loop at the midabdomen, lying anterior to the abdominal aorta.[96] When visualized on ultrasound, this entity typically appears as a large cystic structure in the upper abdomen and may have echogenic debris in its dependent part[98] (Fig. 8-57). In the coronal plane, the presence of a U-shaped configuration of an obstructed afferent duodenal loop is helpful in making a diagnosis. Some peristalsis may be seen within the loop.[97]

At times it is difficult to differentiate afferent loop obstruction from a pancreatic pseudocyst. This differen-

tiation may be possible by locating the afferent loop behind the superior mesenteric artery and vein. The dilated afferent loop is seen on ultrasound as a tubular structure in the upper abdomen crossing transversely over the midline. The distal end of the afferent loop should be traced toward the anastomosis. It is thought that the afferent loop syndrome can be diagnosed by ultrasound on the basis of the detection, location, and shape of the dilated loop.[96]

Ileovesical Anastomosis. Occasionally a dilated ileal loop associated with an ileovesical anastomosis is mistaken for an abscess.[99] The curved tubular nature of the ileal loop becomes apparent on serial scans. Peristalsis

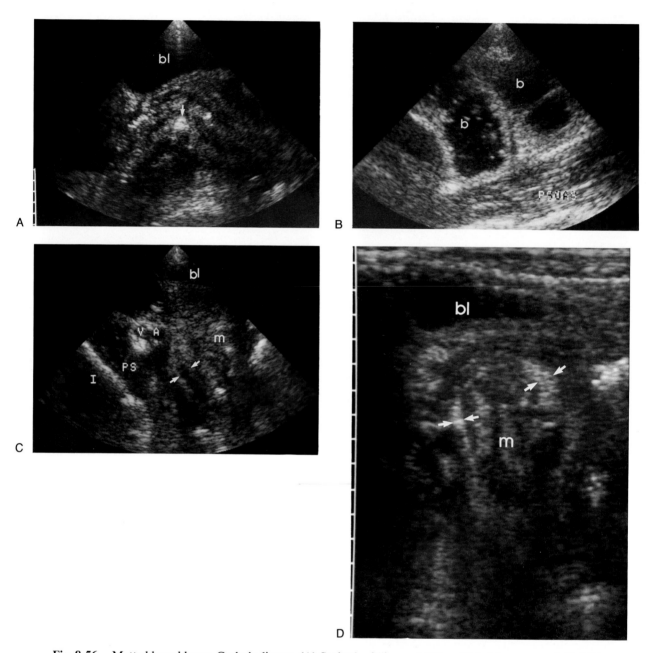

Fig. 8-56. Matted bowel loops, Crohn's disease. **(A)** Sagittal midline and **(B)** sagittal right scans and **(C & D)** transverse views of the pelvis demonstrating a poorly defined mass effect *(m)* in the pelvis. Peristalsing bowel loops *(b)* could be seen on some views. Air within the bowel lumen is denoted by the echogenic areas (arrows) in Figs. A & D, with fluid (arrows) seen within a bowel segment on Fig. C. (*bl,* bladder; *I,* ilium, *PS, PSOAS,* psoas muscle; *V,* iliac vein; *A,* iliac artery.) *(Figure continues.)*

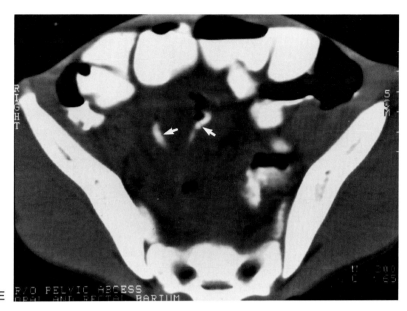

E

Fig. 8-56 *(Continued).*   **(E)** CT scan showing thickening of the bowel wall, narrowing of the bowel lumen, and matting of the loops.

may or may not be seen on real-time ultrasound; it is sometimes absent owing to marked long-standing dilatation.[99]

Ulcer Disease

Investigators have studied the amount of gastric fluid identified on ultrasound with the presence of duodenal ulcer disease and gastric outlet obstruction.[100] When evaluating these patients, the patient is placed in the right lateral decubitus position to allow gastric fluid to accumulate in the antrum; the fluid can be quantified by measuring the maximal cross-sectional area of the antral fluid in square centimeters. No fluid or a small amount (<5 cm²) is seen in 61 percent, whereas a large amount of fluid (>5 cm²) is seen in 39 percent.[100] An ulcer may be detected in 46 percent of those with a large amount of fluid and in 10 percent of those with a small amount of fluid. Excessive gastric fluid detected on ultrasound can be associated with gastric hypersecretion, which can accompany duodenal ulcer or of a gastric outlet obstruction. From 30 to 40 percent of patients with duodenal ulcer disease are true hypersecretors and have acid and volume secretion rates above the upper limits of normal, with the highest output of basal gastric secretion in the morning. As such, the ultrasound detection of a large amount of gastric fluid may be associated with a signifi-

cantly higher prevalence of duodenal ulcer and gastric outlet obstruction[100] (Fig. 8-1).

Duodenal ulcers have been evaluated by ultrasound.[101] A hyperechoic area in various shapes and sizes corresponding to ulcers on radiographs is identified adjacent to the gallbladder and the head of the pancreas[101] (Fig. 8-58). The surrounding hypoechoic halo of various thicknesses represents the duodenal wall edema, and infiltration with the hyperechoic center represents the ulcer crater.[101] The echogenicity of the crater may be due to necrotic fibrinoid debris covering the surface of the niche as a thin layer.[101] Although ultrasound is not the primary modality for evaluation for peptic ulcer disease, the sonographer/sonologist should be aware of the findings on ultrasound so that an UGI series may be performed as the next diagnostic study.

The most common complications associated with peptic ulcer disease are obstruction, hemorrhage, penetration, and perforation.[102] There is penetration to adjacent organs in up to 26 percent of cases of peptic ulcer of the duodenum.[100] The most common sites of penetration include (in decreasing order of frequency) the pancreas, gastrohepatic omentum, biliary tract, liver, and greater omentum[31] (Fig. 8-59). When the sonographic demonstration of a connection between a gas-filled liver mass suggestive of an abscess and duodenum is seen in a patient with known peptic ulcer disease, the diagnosis of penetration should be considered.

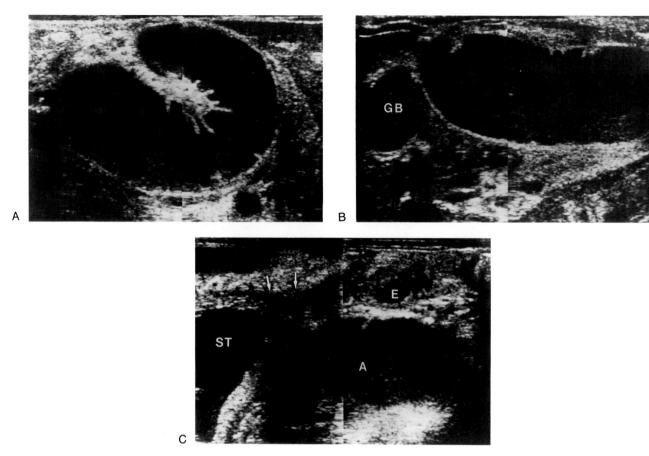

Fig. 8-57. Afferent loop syndrome. This 60-year-old man had afferent loop syndrome caused by internal hernia. **(A)** Longitudinal sonogram of the midabdomen showing a U-shaped and dilated duodenum. **(B)** Transverse sonogram of the midabdomen showing a dilated afferent loop crossing transversely over the midline. (*GB,* gallbladder.) **(C)** Sonogram showing that the distal end of the dilated afferent loop can be traced toward the anastomosis site of gastrojejunostomy (arrows). The efferent loop is not dilated. (*ST,* remnant stomach; *A,* afferent loop; *E,* efferent loop.) (From Lee et al,[96] with permission.)

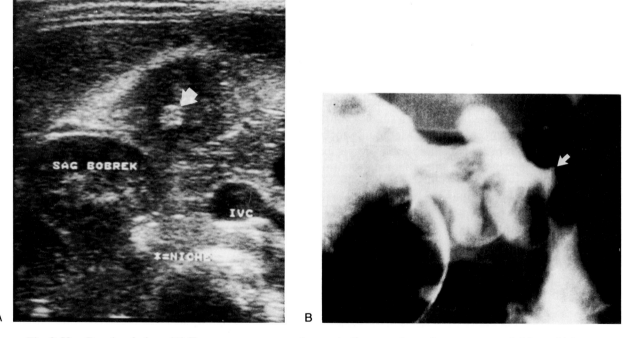

Fig. 8-58. Duodenal ulcer. **(A)** Transverse sonogram demonstrating an echogenic core surrounded by a thick hypoechoic halo lateral to the head of the pancreas (arrow). (*IVC,* inferior vena cava.) **(B)** UGI. Ulcer and spasm at the apex of the duodenal bulb (arrow). (From Tuncel,[101] with permission.)

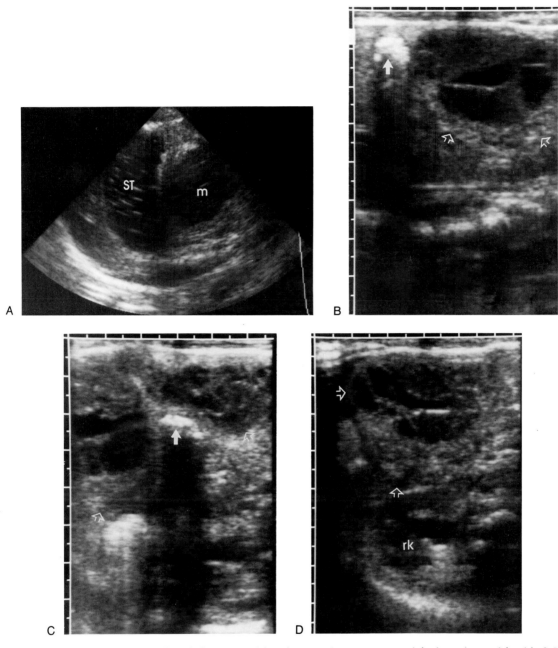

Fig. 8-59. Duodenal perforation, infant. A multicystic mass (*m*, open arrows) is demonstrated in this 2.5-month-old child with a decreased hematocrit. It is inferior to the fluid-filled stomach *(ST)* on sagittal views **(A)** to the left and **(B)** to the right. The mass has a multicystic appearance as it extends across the midline on **(C)** the transverse view and on **(D)** the transverse view on the right. The relationship of the fluid-filled stomach to the mass could be seen in Fig. A. Air (arrow) could be visualized within the lumen of the second portion of the duodenum in Fig. B and in the third portion in Fig. C. (*rk,* hydronephrotic right kidney.)

Hematoma

Recognition of an intestinal hematoma is important to the therapy and prognosis. Intramural hemorrhage may occur from complex causes, with or without trauma. Such causes include bleeding diatheses, hemophilia, anticoagulant therapy, blunt trauma, leukemia, lymphoma, Henoch-Schönlein anaphylactoid purpura, and thrombocytopenic purpura.[70,103,104] Intramural hematoma, specifically injuries to the duodenum and proximal jejenum, are the most frequent visceral injuries

to be documented radiologically in abused children.[105] Intramural hemorrhage in the GI tract is a rare complication in hemophiliacs and can be associated with signs and symptoms of obstruction.[70] With Henoch-Schönlein purpura, the major symptoms are skin eruption, abdominal pain, and hematuria.[106] Abdominal pain usually precedes the onset of skin lesions.

Hematomas may occur at any portion of the intestinal tract but are most common in areas adjacent to relatively fixed portions of the intestine.[104] When the duodenum is affected, there may be secondary effects of gastric outlet

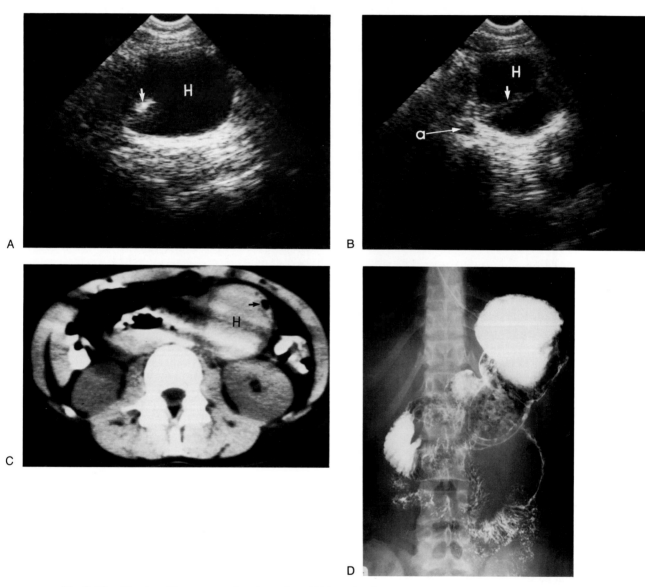

Fig. 8-60. Duodenal hematoma, fourth portion. **(A)** Longitudinal real-time scan to the left of midline showing an anechoic mass *(H)* with an echodense area (arrow) at its apex. This represented duodenal lumen. **(B)** Transverse real-time scan, again showing the duodenal lumen as an echodense area (arrow) more medial with the anechoic area *(H)* being the hematoma. (*a*, aorta.) **(C)** CT scan similar to Fig. B. The hematoma *(H)* appears dense, with air (arrow) in the bowel lumen. **(D)** UGI series showing displacement of bowel loops (arrows) by the mass.

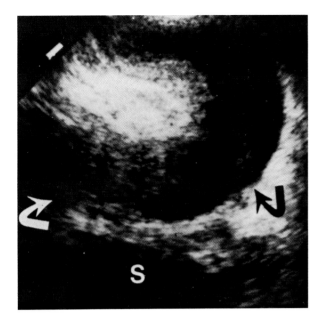

Fig. 8-61. Duodenal hematoma. Transverse sonogram of the left upper quadrant in a 2-year-old boy with vomiting and abdominal tenderness. A large mass (arrows) is anterior to the spine *(S)* and has an echogenic center and a hypoechoic, asymmetrically thickened bowel wall. Marked gastric distension from obstruction and moderate ascites were also present. (From Orel et al,[105] with permission.)

obstruction, obstruction of the biliary tree, and extrinsic compression on the inferior vena cava.[107] Since the duodenum is fixed in position, it is more often affected by trauma than is the remainder of the GI tract. Because a lesion in the duodenum produces thickening of the wall,

the target sign or possibly an echogenic mass (extramural and intramural) will be visible[90,103,107] (Figs. 8-60 and 8-61). A hematoma usually produces eccentric thickening of the bowel wall.[90]

With an intramural hematoma of the duodenum, a solid mass may be demonstrated at the level of the junction of the second and third portions of the duodenum.[108] This mass may extend into the retroperitoneum, indenting the viscus inferiorly and posteriorly[108] (Fig. 8-62). The first and second portions of the duodenum may be distended with fluid, with near obliteration of its lumen in the third portion by a bilobed, solid intraluminal mass[108] (Fig. 8-63). Ultrasound may be the first examination done on patients with epigastric abdominal pain or with a palpable mass.

Ultrasound can delineate the normal and abnormal bowel by the visualization of its typical configuration and peristalsis. On ultrasound, hematomas often show a strong internal echoes due to thrombi, as may an abscess, but in the proper clinical setting intramural intestinal hematoma can be diagnosed by ultrasound[104] (Figs. 8-60 to 8-64). On ultrasound, a long, transverse, hourglass-shaped fluid collection in the left abdomen extending across the midline may be seen with fine internal irregular echoes. The compressed and narrowed lumen of the intestine displays a layer of parallel echogenic lines inside the hematoma.[104] An intramural intestinal hematoma may be seen as a tubular anechoic or hypoechoic mass containing a core of strong echoes.[70]

Ultrasound may support or establish the diagnosis of duodenal hematoma in cases of suspected child abuse. The ultrasound examination may reveal findings consistent with hematoma involving the second through the

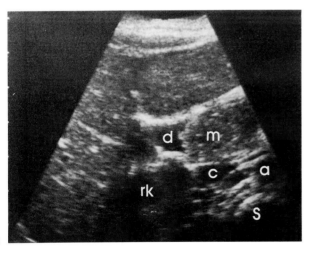

A

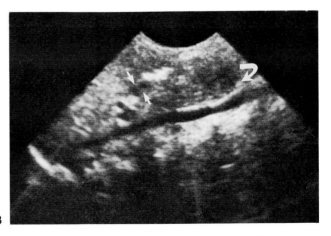

B

Fig. 8-62. Duodenal hematoma. **(A)** Transverse section demonstrating a heterogeneous mass *(m)* protruding extrinsically into the medial and posterior aspects of the dilated duodenal lumen *(d)*. (*rk,* right kidney; *c,* inferior vena cava; *a,* aorta; *S,* spine.) **(B)** Longitudinal sonogram demonstrating a mass (curved arrow) compressing the inferior vena cava and indenting the inferior and posterior aspects of the dilated duodenal lumen (arrows). (From Hernanz-Schulman et al,[108] with permission.)

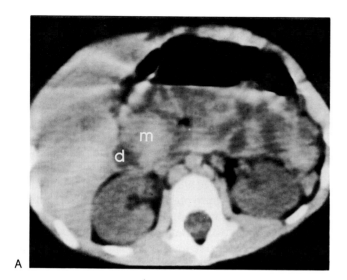

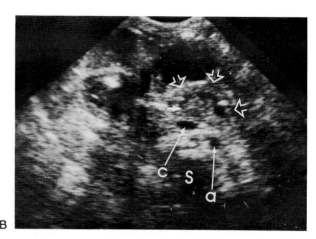

Fig. 8-63. Duodenal hematoma. **(A)** CT scan without contrast showing an antecaval mass of high attenuation *(m)* adjacent to a distended, fluid-filled duodenum *(d)*. **(B)** Transverse scan at the level of the third portion of the duodenum showing a bilobed mass (short arrow) projecting into the duodenal lumen, lying anterior to the inferior vena cava *(c)* and aorta *(a)*. (*S*, spine; open arrows, anterior duodenal wall). (From Hernanz-Schulman et al,[108] with permission.)

fourth portions of the duodenum. Additionally, a mildly enlarged pancreas compatible with pancreatitis and a moderate amount of hemorrhagic ascites may be demonstrated.[105] The bowel-related abnormality is suggested by the central echogenic core representing the compressed mucosa and a thick, sonolucent halo representing a thickened bowel wall infiltrated by edema, hemorrhage, or neoplasm. The appearance may be variable depending on the age of the process.[105] Other pathologic processes of the bowel may appear similar and must be differentiated. Ultrasound can prove helpful in screening for visceral injury when child abuse is suspected.[105]

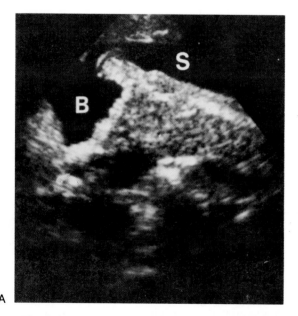

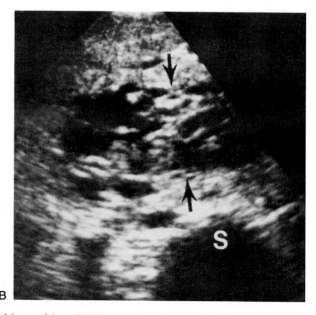

Fig. 8-64. Duodenal hematoma in a 4½-year-old girl with vomiting. **(A)** Transverse sonogram of the upper abdomen showing a distended, fluid-filled stomach *(S)* and duodenal bulb *(B)*. The pancreas is normal. **(B)** Transverse sonogram at a slightly lower level showing a complex mass (arrows) that is contiguous with duodenal bulb and anterior to the spine *(S)*. (From Orel et al,[105] with permission.)

Duplication

The etiology of duplication cysts is most commonly thought to involve errors of canalization. The solid GI tract at 6 weeks of intrauterine life becomes a hollow tube by week 8, as multiple vacuoles coalesce. If there are two channels rather than one running through part of the solid cord, a duplication cyst occurs parallel to the normal lumen. Duodenal duplication cysts are rare in adults.[109] This accounts for 4 to 12 percent of all duplications of the GI tract, with an incidence of less than 1 per 100,000 births.[109] This abnormality is more likely to occur in neonates than in adults.

An abdominal mass is the most common clinical finding, accompanied by various degrees of nausea, vomiting, and high intestinal obstruction. Obstruction is the most common symptom, with the ileum being the most common site. Diagnosis of such a lesion is usually made in the first year of life, often within the first week. The radiographic diagnosis is limited to the extrinsic pressure defect produced by the cyst, since only 10 to 20 percent of duplications communicate with the duodenal lumen.

Ultrasound evaluation of a suspected abdominal mass in children has become routine. Identifying this rare congenital anomaly can aid in diagnosis and obviate extensive workup. Lesions can have different appearances, ranging from an anechoic cyst to an echogenic mass[46,110] (Fig. 8-65). Ultrasound can define the cyst and its location. An echogenic inner rim is highly suggestive of this diagnosis.[34] If the cyst contains clear fluid, the lucent mass will have strong posterior wall echoes and acoustic enhancement. When hemorrhage occurs within the cyst, echogenic debris may form.[109] An echogenic mass may be seen, which is the result of hemorrhage and inspissated material.[34] The site of the cyst cannot be predicted from the location of the cyst on ultrasound.[32] The differential diagnosis would include gallbladder, choledochal cyst, and pseudocyst.

Enterolith formation may occur in duodenal duplication cysts as well as in a diverticulum (especially Meckel's diverticulum), as can "milk of calcium" and

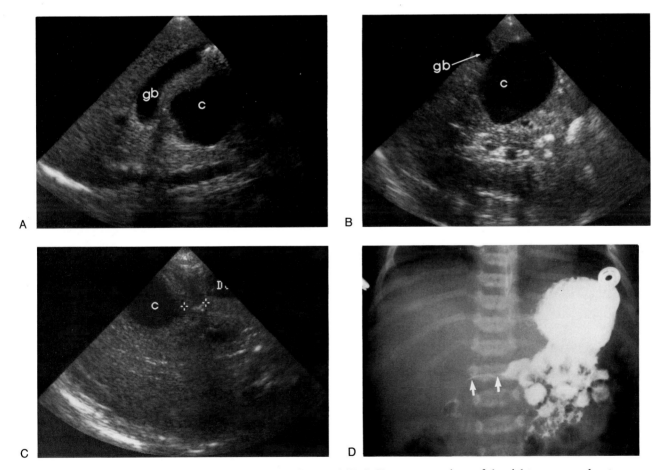

Fig. 8-65. Duodenal duplication cyst. **(A)** Sagittal and **(B & C)** transverse views of the right upper quadrant demonstrating a cystic mass (*c*, 34 mm) that is inferior and medial to the gallbladder *(gb)*. The duodenum *(D)* is seen medially in Fig. C. **(D)** UGI series showing the mass effect (arrows) produced by the cyst.

hemorrhage.[109] Hemorrhage results in the formation of echogenic debris with the cyst. The formation of the enteroliths is thought to be secondary to chronic stasis and alkalinity of the intestinal chyme, both of which exist in duodenal duplication cysts.[109]

Intussusception

Intussusception is the most common cause of obstruction in children, but it is fairly uncommon in adults.[26,111] In 75 to 85 percent of adult cases, there is an identifiable bowel lesion at the leading point.[26,113] When located in the colon, 50 percent of such lesions prove to be malignant, whereas most lesions in the small bowel are benign.[112] Most cases of intussusception are ileocolic, and most present between the ages of 6 months and 2 years.[113]

The clinical presentation of intussusception is varied and nonspecific. It may have a protracted course, with symptoms present for 3 or more months. If it is chronic, which is the more common variety in adults, the patient may have minimal pain, diarrhea, and, less frequently, vomiting. If it is acute, the patient may present with abdominal pain, vomiting, and rectal passage of blood and mucus or "currant jelly" stools.[114] An abdominal mass is present in 63 to 85 percent of cases.[111]

There are various categories of enterocolic intussusception: (1) enteric (the small bowel invaginates into the small bowel); (2) ileocolic (the ileum invaginates through the stationary ileocecal valve); (3) ileocecal (the ileocecal valve itself leads to the intussusception); and (4) colocolic (the colon invaginates into the colon).[115] With the ileocecal type, the constricting effect of the ileocecal

valve may lead to early ischemic gangrene of the intussuscepted ileum.[115] These are often idiopathic and resemble the childhood variety, especially in younger adults.[115]

As the intussusceptum progresses into the intussuscipiens, the bowel wall becomes edematous.[112] The intussusceptum is telescoped into the intussuscipiens until it can go no farther owing to traction on the mesentery, which is dragged between the entering and returning walls of the intussusceptum. Venous obstruction ensues, with exudation of fluid and resultant wall edema. The edema is greatest at the apex of the intussusceptum, but extends to involve the entering and returning intussusceptum walls.[116]

A barium enema is indicated to confirm the diagnosis and, in acute cases, to reduce it hydrostatically.[114] When the presentation is atypical, ultrasound can be helpful. Ultrasound is being used more frequently as the primary screening procedure for the evaluation of abdominal complaints. The two main ultrasound patterns described with intussusception are (1) targetlike, bull's eye, doughnut, or pseudokidney; and (2) concentric ring signs. Two additional patterns described with intussusception are (1) a highly reflective intussusceptum and (2) an unstructured pattern corresponding to a solid tumor.[117] With the proper clinical setting, the visualization of a doughnut or pseudokidney should strongly suggest intussusception and lead to a contrast enema.[112]

Doughnut, Target, Pseudokidney Pattern

A variation in the typical targetlike or bull's-eye pattern seen with GI lesions may occur[72] (Fig. 8-66 to 8-69). The doughnut configuration is seen on cross-section imaging of the mass, with a pseudokidney demonstrated

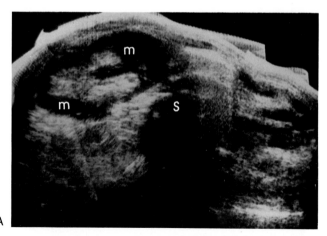

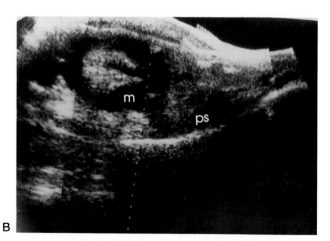

Fig. 8-66. Intussusception. **(A)** Transverse scan 4 cm above the umbilicus showing a large intra-abdominal mass *(m),* having a target pattern, to the right of midline. The hypoechoic rim represents the edematous intussuscipiens that surrounds the hyperechoic center; this is due to multiple interfaces of compressed mucosal and serosal surfaces of the intussusceptum. *(S,* spine.) **(B)** Longitudinal scan to the right of midline showing a mass *(m)* sitting on the anterior margin of the psoas muscle *(ps).* (From Weissberg et al,[112] with permission.)

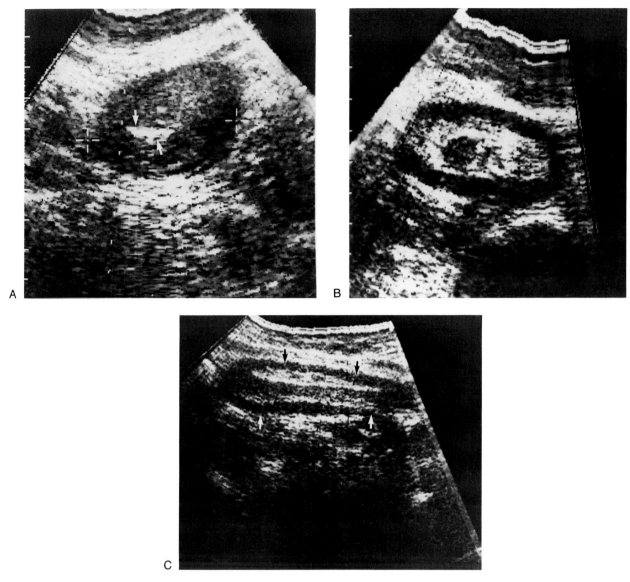

Fig. 8-67. Intussusception. **(A)** Transverse scan of the intussusception at the level of the apex of the intussusceptum, showing a targetlike pattern; the central echogenic lumen (arrows) is surrounded by a very thick hypoechoic rim. The thick hypoechoic rim is due to severe edema of the entering and returning intussusceptum walls and the resultant obliteration of interface between them. **(B)** Cross-section of the intussusception at a more proximal level showing a hypoechoic outer ring surrounding a highly reflective area with an echopoor center. The outer and inner hypoechoic areas represent the returning and entering walls of the intussusceptum, respectively. The echogenic area is the interface between the walls. **(C)** Longitudinal view of the intussusception (arrows) obtained by a scan through its long axis, showing three hypoechoic stripes delineating two echogenic areas. (From Montali et al,[118] with permission.)

on longitudinal section.[113] The thickened hypoechoic rim represents the edematous intussuscipiens that surrounds the hyperechoic center (due to multiple interfaces of compressed mucosal and serosal surfaces of the intussusceptum).[114] The belief that the central echogenic area represents the intussusceptum or the donor component may be inaccurate. Instead, the sonolucent rim may represent the edematous limbs of the infolded loop of the intussusceptum.[113] In advanced cases with marked edema, the various intervening layers of mucosa and serosa are so stretched that they are not echogenic. Instead, only the mucosa in the center of the inner loop, compressed from all sides, is seen as the echogenic center of the doughnut and pseudokidney.

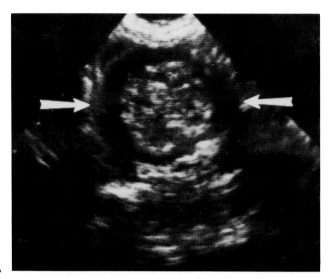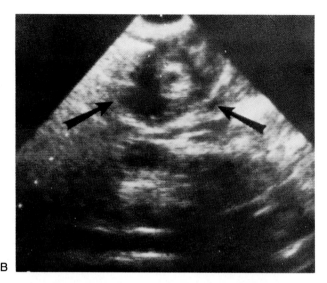

Fig. 8-68. Intussusception. Variations of classic findings. **(A)** Note the thin, sonolucent doughnut (arrows) with large center of echogenicity. **(B)** Concentric rings and target sign. Note the outer echofree rim, the inner echogenic circle, and the innermost anechoic area (arrows). The latter area is believed to represent fluid in the lumen of the proximal end of the intussusception. (From Swischuk et al,[113] with permission.)

Concentric Ring Sign

The multiple concentric ring sign is thought to be a characteristic pattern associated with this entity.[115] When there are lesser degrees of edema, the various layers of mucosa and serosa are less stretched and thinned, becoming echogenic; this probably results in the formation of concentric rings or layering.[113] When concentric rings are visualized and a sonolucent center is also present, the findings represent fluid in the proximal end of the incompletely compressed lumen of the inner loop (Figs. 8-67 to 8-69).

The ultrasound findings of two mixed hypoechoic-echogenic oval structures within the large hyperechoic center suggest the presence of an ileocecal type of intussusception[115] (Fig. 8-69). The ileocecal type of intussusception is best treated by right hemicolectomy because of the strangulation at an early stage as a result of the constricting effect of the ileocecal valve.

Differential Diagnosis

The target lesion seen on ultrasound is nonspecific and can appear after primary or secondary cancer, lymphoma, Crohn's disease, inflammation due to pancreatitis, bowel infarction, radiation ileitis, and hematoma. It can also be seen with other causes of segmental intestinal edema and has been described with necrotizing enterocolitis.[113] An ultrasound scan of the long axis helps to make a more definite diagnosis of intussusception (Figs. 8-67 and 8-69). On a cross-section through the apex of the intussusceptum, the more common target lesion is seen with a very thick hypoechoic rim that is due to the severe edema of the entering and returning intussusceptum walls and resultant obliteration of the interface between them[118] (Fig. 8-67). When scanning through the more proximal portion where the parietal edema is less severe, an image of two concentric rings and an inner circular area is seen.[116,118,119] The outer and inner rings represent the returning and entering walls of the intussusceptum, respectively; the intermediate hyperreflective ring separates the walls as a result of changes in the interface between them. When the long axis is scanned, three parallel stripes of low echogenicity are delineated, as well as two reflective areas.[118]

Reduction

One group of investigators found ultrasound helpful in predicting the likelihood of reducing the intussusception with a contrast enema.[113] Reduction with contrast enema is less likely, if not impossible, if a classic, thick, doughnut and/or pseudokidney configuration with tightly compressed central echoes is present.[114] Reduction is much more likely if layering or concentric rings were seen or when the sonolucent doughnut and pseudokidney signs consisted of a thin outer sonolucent rim.[113]

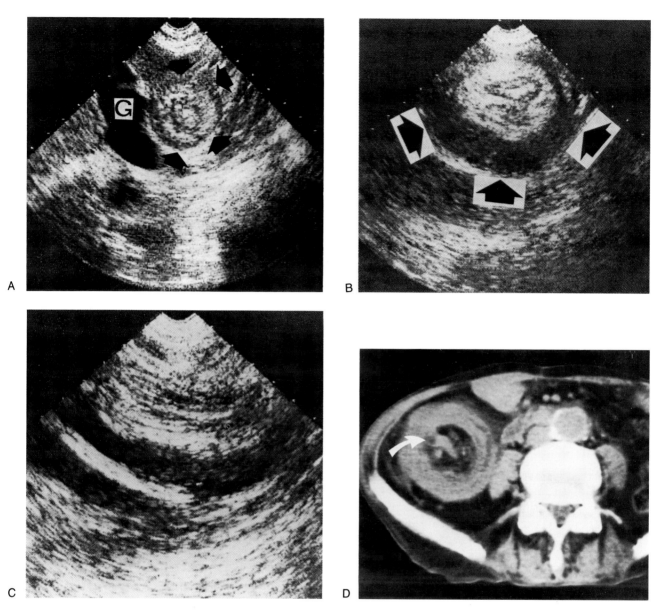

Fig. 8-69. Ileocecal intussusception. **(A)** Sagittal ultrasonogram at the hepatic flexure showing a typical "multiple concentric ring sign" (arrows). (*G*, gallbladder.) **(B)** Ultrasonogram of the right midabdomen. Transverse scan showing two mixed hypoechoic-echogenic oval structures within the large hyperechoic center of the mass. The large hyperechoic center is surrounded by a thick hypoechoic rim (arrows). **(C)** Longitudinal ultrasonogram of the right midabdomen demonstrating multiple thin, parallel hypoechoic and echogenic stripes within the large hyperechoic center corresponding to the two oval structures seen in cross-section. **(D)** CT scan of the lower midabdomen showing a small tubular structure (arrow) consistent with the invaginated vermiform appendix within the core of fatty tissue representing intussuscepted mesentery. (From Skaane and Skjennald,[115] with permission.)

Jejunoileal Bypass

Intussusception may be a complication in jejunoileal bypass surgery to correct obesity; it occurs secondary to inadequate fixation of the free end of the defunctionalized loop. Intussusception is thus difficult to diagnose and is confused with colonic pseudo-obstruction because it has the same symptoms of crampy abdominal pain.[120] It is a potentially catastrophic complication and occurs in 0.5 to 3.5 percent of bypass patients.[121] After surgical bypass, a large percentage of the small bowel cannot be visualized by conventional radiographic techniques.[120] As with the usual type of intussusception, the ultrasound pattern is that of a large target: a hypoechoic or anechoic mass with a hyperechoic center is seen.[121]

Cystic Fibrosis

Intussusception is a known complication in patients with cystic fibrosis, but its presentation may be atypical in these patients.[122] Abdominal pain is often a complaint in patients with cystic fibrosis; it may be secondary to fecal impaction, meconium ileus equivalent, gallbladder disease, pancreatitis, and appendicitis.[122] The average age of onset in these patients is 9 years, with a range of 4 to 16 years.

On ultrasound, targetlike masses are seen on cross-sectional imaging as has been previously described. With cystic fibrosis, the adherent abnormal stool is considered to be the lead point in the intussusception. This complication of meconium ileus equivalent should be pursued in refractory cases by ultrasound or barium enema.[122]

Miscellaneous

Ultrasound should be the first imaging modality in cases of suspected intussusception. It can not only diagnose the abnormality but also predict the reducibility of

the lesion. Ultrasound evaluation is most important in patients with atypical or confusing clinical findings and those in whom contrast studies are contraindicated.[112]

Meckel's Diverticulitis

Meckel's diverticulum is located on the antimesenteric border of the ileum approximately 2 ft (61 cm) from the ileocecal valve.[123] Present in 2 percent of the population, it is usually discovered incidentally during laparotomy. The most common childhood presentation is that of maroon stools due to ectopic gastric mucosa that can lead to ileal ulceration and hemorrhage. Adult patients may present with intestinal obstruction. There may also be rectal bleeding and diverticular inflammation. Acute appendicitis and acute Meckel's diverticulitis may not be distinguished clinically.[123]

Unlike other bowel diverticula, the wall of Meckel's diverticulum is composed of mucosal, muscular, and serosal layers.[123] When the orifice of the diverticulum becomes occluded, the diverticulum becomes inflamed. The normal mucosal secretions then collect in the lumen, causing increased intraluminal pressure. The noncompressibility of the obstructed inflamed diverticulum indicates that the intraluminal fluid is trapped.[123]

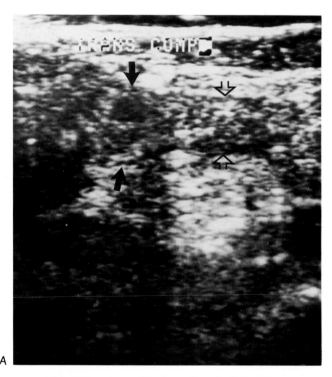 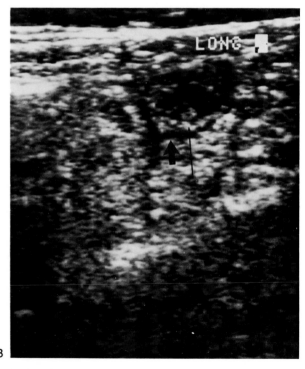

A   B

Fig. 8-70. Acute Meckel's diverticulitis. **(A)** Transverse abdominal image obtained through the longitudinal plane of a noncompressible inflamed Meckel's diverticulum (solid arrows) and compressed normal ileum (open arrows). **(B)** Sagittal abdominal image obtained through a transverse plane of an inflamed Meckel's diverticulum. Mucosal and submucosal (thin arrow) as well as muscular (thick arrow) layers are seen. (From Larson et al,[123] with permission.)

When evaluating a patient for acute appendicitis by using ultrasound, it is important to consider the diagnosis of Meckel's diverticulitis.[123] The area of maximum tenderness should be evaluated along with its distance from the cecum (Fig. 8-70). Its persistent location adjacent to the ileum should indicate its origin.[123]

Intestinal Lymphangiectasia

Intestinal lymphangiectasia reflects a disorder of the development of the lymphatic channels that affects segments of the bowel to various extents, with the congenital form often involving not only the intestines but also one or more extremities.[124] Patients may present in childhood or adulthood. With the severe congenital forms, there is early onset of massive peripheral edema, frequently asymmetric in distribution.[124] Most patients exhibit diarrhea, often associated with nausea, vomiting, abdominal pain, and the symptoms of malabsorption.[124] Pathologically, lymphangiectasia is characterized by telangiectasia of the lymphatic vessels of the lamina propria, submucosa, serosa and/or mesentery.[124]

Usually the radiographic findings include thickened jejunal and ileal folds; dilution of the barium column, distally; and absent or minimal dilatation of the bowel lumen.[124] Several causes of the thickened bowel wall have been hypothesized, including dilatation of bowel lymphatics or mucosal and submucosal edema secondary to hypoproteinemia.[124]

The ultrasound findings with this entity include demonstration of diffuse, grossly thickened bowel walls, ascites, marked mesenteric edema, and dilated mesenteric lymphatics all of which are highly suggestive of intestinal lymphangiectasia[124] (Fig. 8-71). The amount of peristalsis is usually diminished.

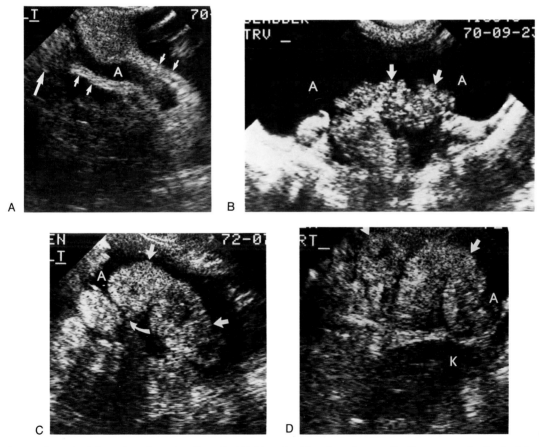

Fig. 8-71. Intestinal lymphangiectasia. Case 1. **(A)** Bowel with edematous walls (large arrow) attached to thickened mesentery (small arrows) and floating in ascites *(A)*. **(B)** Transverse view, just above the bladder, showing multiple dilated mesenteric lymphatics (arrows) appearing as a cluster of small, round, echogenic densities surrounded by ascites *(A)*. They were differentiated from the bowel by their much smaller size and different sonographic appearance. Case 2. **(C)** Thickened bowel walls (arrows) and mesentery (curved arrow) surrounded by ascites *(A)*. **(D)** Thickened bowel walls (arrows). *(A*, ascites; *K*, kidney.) (From Dorne and Jequier,[124] with permission.)

Pneumatosis Intestinalis

A number of abnormalities have been associated with pneumatosis intestinalis, including bowel infarction, collagen vascular disease, chronic bronchitis and asthma, ulcer disease, and diverticulitis.[125] On ultrasound, air may be seen within the edematous walls of an affected bowel loop[125] (Fig. 8-72). The air may be seen as a central bright line. To differentiate air within the bowel wall from air within the bowel lumen, the patient may be scanned in the decubitus position. In this position, with the air in the bowel lumen there may be bubbling because of mixing of air and fluid in the lumen of the dilated loop.

Small Bowel Bezoar

Bezoars are more commonly found within the stomach but frequently pass into the small bowel after nonoperative treatment of gastric bezoars, including enzy-

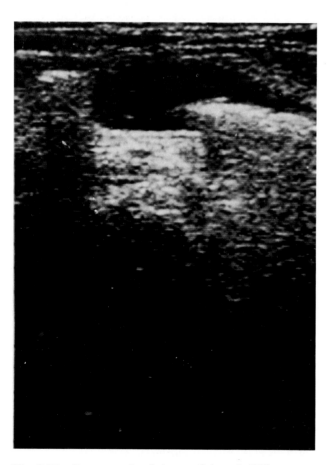

Fig. 8-72. Pneumatosis of the small bowel. Oblique scan tracing the bright echo line into the echopoor mass representing the edematous bowel wall. (From Vijayaraghavean,[125] with permission.)

matic digestion and endoscopic fragmentation.[126] These procedures may cause fragments that pass into the small bowel, where they may result in small bowel obstruction. Although the normal stomach can usually digest this material, people with impaired gastric emptying seem to be at increased risk for bezoar formation, accounting for its increased occurrence in patients with previous gastric surgery (especially with associated vagotomy) and also in diabetics with gastroparesis.[126] These patients may develop vague abdominal discomfort, gastric outlet obstruction, or even ulceration or perforation.[126]

On ultrasound, there may be a large, echogenic intraluminal mass with complete acoustic shadowing so that it mimics a heavily calcified lesion[126] (Fig. 8-73). Correlation with plain films may reveal no calcification. As such, small bowel bezoars should be included in the differential diagnosis of small bowel obstruction in any patient with a history of gastric surgery or medical therapy of gastric bezoars.[126]

Intestinal Ascaris

Approximately one-fourth the world's population is infected with the large roundworm *Ascaris lumbricoides.*[127] On ultrasound, these worms may be visualized within fluid-filled small bowel loops (Fig. 8-74). On cross-section, two circles are seen; the outer lines represent the outer wall of the *Ascaris* worm, and the two inner lines are the wall of its gut.[127]

Malabsorption

Malabsorption may be secondary to several causes such as impaired liver function or intolerance to cows' milk. One group of authors has described an associated ultrasound pattern of small bowel loops filled with hyperechoic content, which may constitute a new indicator of impaired intestinal absorption in neonates[128] (Fig. 8-75).

Crohn's Disease

Crohn's disease (regional enteritis) is a recurrent granulomatous inflammatory disease that affects the terminal ileum and/or colon at any level. This granulomatous inflammatory reaction involves the entire thickness of the bowel wall. Patients present with diarrhea, fever, and right lower quadrant pain. The complications of this disease include fibrosing strictures and fistulas to another loop of bowel, bladder, perineum, or peritoneal abscess.[38]

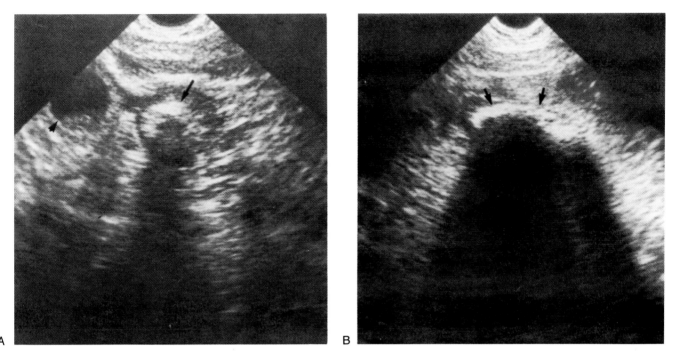

A

B

Fig. 8-73. Small bowel bezoar. **(A)** Sagittal ultrasound of the patient's left lower quadrant demonstrating the fluid-filled bowel loop (arrowhead) and a second loop containing an intraluminal, bright, echogenic, shadowing focus (arrow). **(B)** Transverse scan demonstrating the same echogenic focus in long axis (arrows). (From Tennenhouse and Wilson,[126] with permission.)

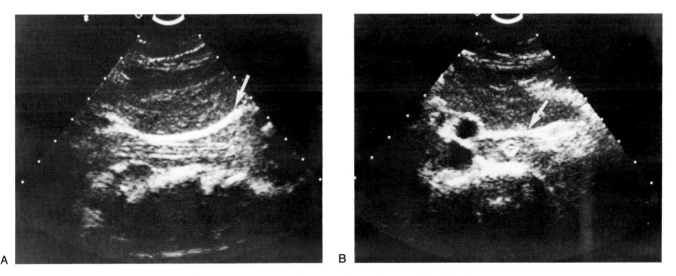

A

B

Fig. 8-74. Intestinal ascaris. **(A)** Transverse ultrasound scan in the right iliac fossa showing a longitudinal section of the worm within the bowel lumen (arrow). **(B)** Longitudinal ultrasound scan in the right iliac fossa showing a cross-section of the small bowel with a cross-section of the worm within it. (arrow, bowel wall.) (From Peck,[127] with permission.)

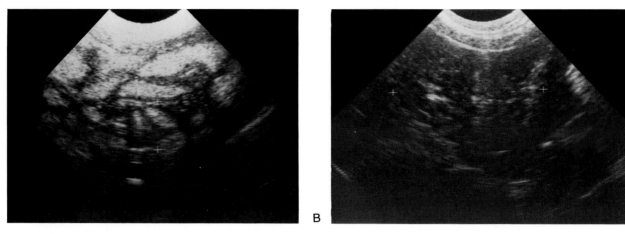

Fig. 8-75. Malabsorption. Supine sagittal scan of the left flank. **(A)** Patient on cows' milk diet. Diffuse hyperechoic round and tubular masses are seen. The distance between the two calipers is 12 mm. **(B)** Patient on soya milk diet. The pattern is no longer present. (From Avni et al,[128] with permission.)

The following characteristics of Crohn's disease may be identified on ultrasound: (1) symmetrically swollen bowel; (2) target pattern (bowel in cross-section) with the preserved parietal layers around the stenotic and hyperdense lumen; (3) findings most prominent in ileocolonic disease, with uniformity increased wall thickness involving all the layers but especially the mucosa and submucosa (barely distinguishable); (4) "matted-loop" pattern found in the late stages, especially in patients who have undergone a simple intestinal bypass operation in which the diseased tract, left in situ, is eventually affected by the disease progression; (5) rigidity to pressure exerted with the transducer (advanced stages); (6) absent or sluggish peristalsis; (7) and dilatation with hyperperistalsis and water and air stasis[129] (Figs. 8-56, 8-76, and 8-77). The target lesion seen with Crohn's disease is due to the

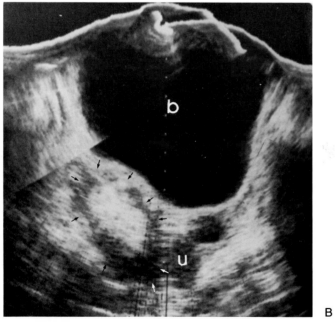

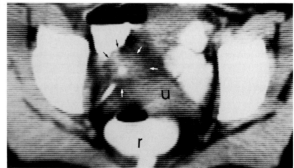

Fig. 8-76. Crohn's disease, pelvic mass. **(A)** Transverse scan of the pelvis demonstrating a target lesion (arrows) within the right pelvis. The dense center is bowel lumen. (*u*, uterus; *b*, bladder.) **(B)** CT scan with oral and rectal barium showing a soft tissue-density mass (arrows) in the right pelvis. Barium is seen within the center lumen of the mass. (*u*, uterus; *r*, rectum.)

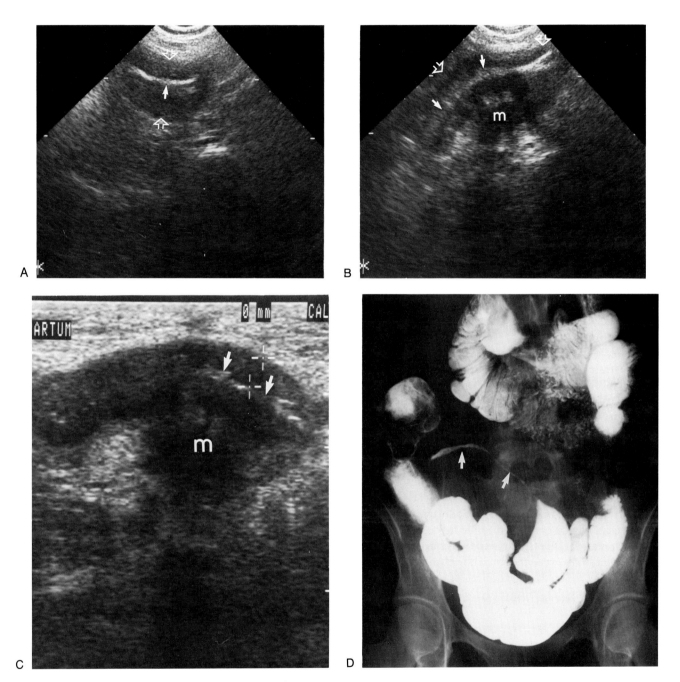

Fig. 8-77. Crohn's disease, abscess. **(A)** Sagittal and **(B & C)** transverse views showing bowel wall thickening as well as an associated hypoechoic mass *(m)*. The lumen of the affected bowel loop is echogenic (arrows). The thick wall (calipers, open arrows) can be measured between the lumen and outer surface. By using the linear array transducer (Fig. C), there is more optimal evaluation of the soft tissues of the abdominal wall for fistula formation. **(D)** GI series demonstrating the affected bowel loop with a narrowed lumen (arrows).

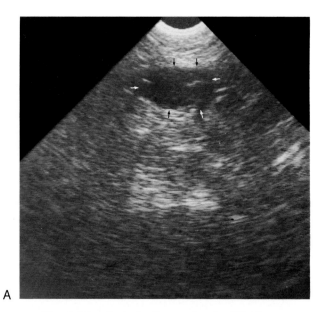
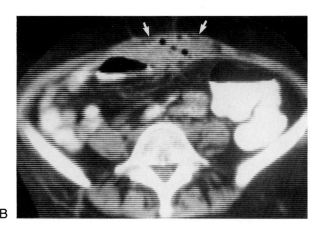

Fig. 8-78. Crohn's disease, fistula. **(A)** Transverse real-time scan showing a hypoechoic superficial mass (arrows) anteriorly within the abdomen. **(B)** CT scan showing a soft tissue-density mass (arrows) within the abdominal wall, having internal air consistent with abdominal wall abscess and fistula formation.

thickened bowel wall[26] (Fig. 8-76). Ultrasound may demonstrate pathologic thickenings of the intestinal wall and enable the examiner to diagnose the nature of the swelling. Ultrasound is rapidly becoming the first study performed in cases of abdominal colic and swelling; it is indispensable in recognizing and evaluating Crohn's disease.[129]

When a "reniform" mass is seen on ultrasound, there are two entities to be considered — inflammatory bowel disease and tumors.[129] If the ileocolonic wall is thickened over 5 mm, it is considered to be abnormal. The ultrasound scan can be correlated to the degree of intestinal distension and to the type of endoluminal content. The differentiation between the small bowel and colon can be made by the different appearances of the two: recognition of the valvular conniventes of the small intestine versus constant presence of air within the colon and haustral markings.

Disease Progression/Abscess

Serial ultrasound is ideal for demonstrating progression or regression of the inflamed bowel loops as well as abscesses; the bowel is identified by visualizing peristalsis[130] (Figs. 8-77 to 8-79). Real-time ultrasound helps to differentiate fluid-filled or matted, inflamed bowel loops from abscesses (Figs. 8-56 and 8-77). Linear real-time scanning is better suited for delineation of the abdominal

wall abscess, which is the most common abscess associated with this disease (Fig. 8-77C). Endovaginal or transrectal ultrasound may be helpful in evaluating the pelvic bowel loops and searching for abscesses (Fig. 8-79). Intraperitoneal abscesses frequently surround matted, inflamed bowel. The incidence of external fistula is 8.7 to 21 percent.[130]

Abscess formation may produce irregular or ill-defined, poorly echogenic masses on ultrasound. They can extend into the iliopsoas muscle or anteriorly into the rectus muscle; they may even compress the bladder.[26] An associated abscess may contain gas bubbles if bowel gas enters these fistulae or if gas-containing bacteria are present. These may be difficult to see on ultrasound.[130] On ultrasound, matted bowel loops produce a large mass with irregular internal echoes; these conditions may simulate a large abscess[130] (Fig. 8-56).

Postsurgical Recurrence

Ultrasound can be used to evaluate patients for postsurgical recurrence of Crohn's disease[129] (Figs. 8-80 and 8-81). One group of investigators studied these patients and found the sensitivity of ultrasound to be 82 percent, with a specificity of 100 percent and overall accuracy of 93.7 percent.[129] Ultrasound is able to distinguish between inflammatory and neoplastic lesions by identifying the specific bowel wall layers.[129]

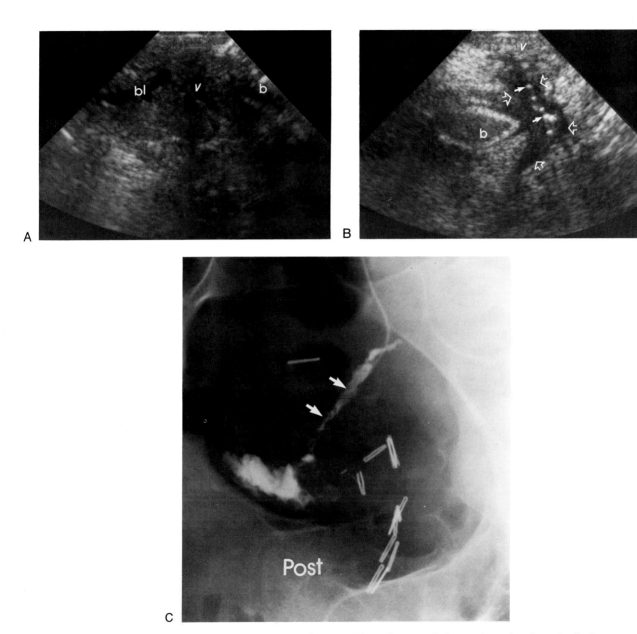

Fig. 8-79.   Vaginal-enteric fistula and Crohn's disease. This patient was being evaluated endovaginally for a pelvic abscess associated with her known vaginal-enteric fistula. **(A)** Sagittal view showing the relationship of bladder *(bl)*, vagina *(v)*, and bowel *(b)*. **(B)** Transverse view showing the air within the fistulous tract as bright, linear, echogenic foci (arrows). The hypoechoic tract (open arrows) is angled to the right. (*b*, bowel; *v*, vagina.) **(C)** Sinogram (projected similar to Fig. B) demonstrating the tract (arrows). (*Post,* posterior.)

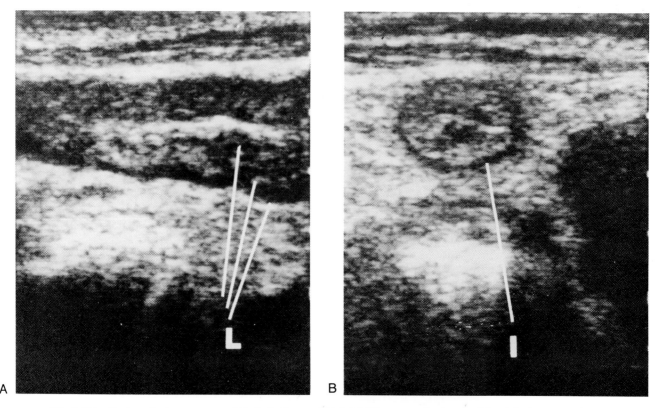

Fig. 8-80. Postsurgical recurrence of Crohn's disease. **(A)** A 5-MHz parasagittal scan of the right lower quadrant showing the bowel wall thickness with a regular rim and layers *(L)*. **(B)** Transverse sonogram showing inflammatory *(I)* reniform mass (thickened but undamaged layers). (From DiCandio et al,[129] with permission.)

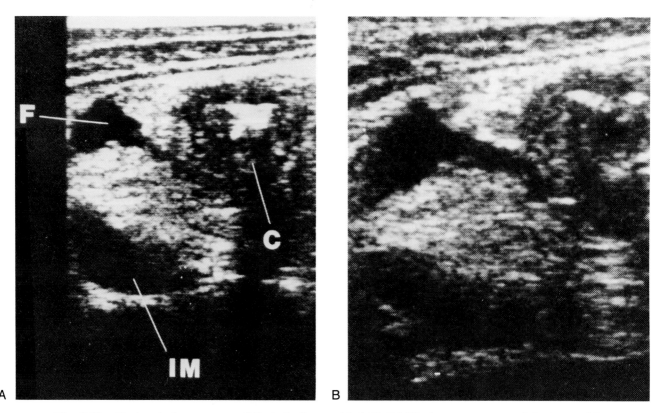

Fig. 8-81. Postsurgical recurrence of Crohn's disease. **(A & B)** 5-MHz transverse scans of the lower right quadrant showing a thickened small bowel loop *(C)* with perivisceral fistula *(F)* confirmed at surgery. (*IM,* right iliac muscle.) (From DiCandio et al,[129] with permission.)

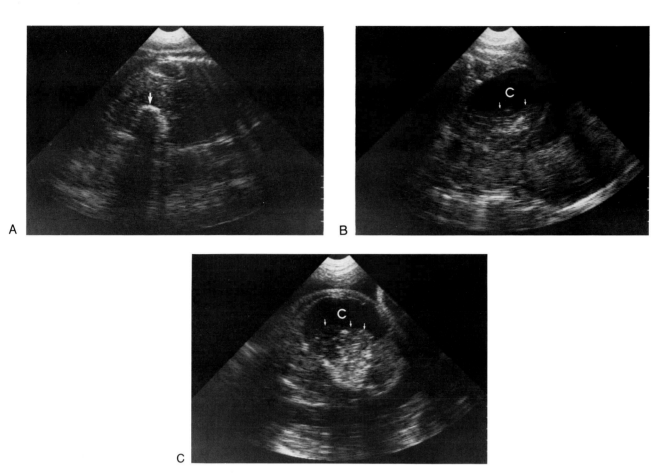

Fig 8-82. Meconium cyst in utero. **(A)** Longitudinal scan of the fetal abdomen showing several echogenic areas (arrow), which represent calcifications, within the fetal abdomen. Transverse scans with the patient **(B)** supine and **(C)** in the right lateral decubitus position, showing a rounded cystic mass *(C)* containing a fluid-filled level (arrows), which shifted with change in maternal position.

Meconium Cyst and Peritonitis

Meconium peritonitis is a sterile chemical peritonitis resulting from extrusion of meconium from the fetal gut into the peritoneal cavity.[130,131] In utero, it is possible to see polyhydramnios, fetal ascites, and echogenic calcific foci with shadowing[132] (Fig. 8-82). The causes of these conditions include bowel perforation proximal to obstruction, meconium ileus, volvulus, hernia, and atresia (Figs. 8-82 to 8-85). Intestinal stenosis or atresia and meconium ileus accompany 65 percent of cases.[131] This irritant meconium causes peritonitis, which frequently localizes and results in formation of a sterile abscess (Fig. 8-84). With healing, calcification takes place and scattered plaques form on the peritoneal surface.[134]

Meconium Cyst

There are three clinical forms of meconium peritonitis: cystic, fibroadhesive, and generalized.[135] A meconium cyst is formed when bowel perforates in utero (occurring in 17 to 60 percent of patients with meconium peritonitis) and meconium is extruded into the peritoneal cavity, which becomes walled off by fibrous adhesions (Figs. 8-82 and 8-85). Ultimately, a well-defined capsule of fibrous granulomatous tissue is formed. The cyst may contain only spilled meconium or may encase bowel loops. If the perforation remains open, the meconium cyst is in communication with the bowel at the site of perforation. This cyst is relatively uncommon and is lined with a thick membrane that contains thick plaque

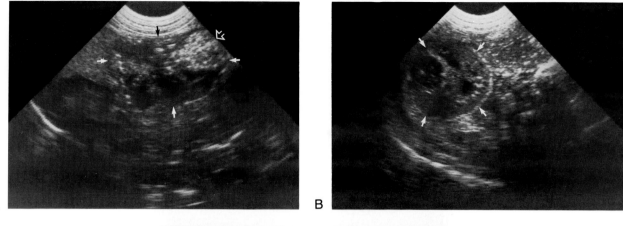

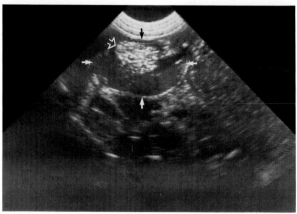

Fig. 8-83. Meconium ileus. Ileoatresia. A complex mass (arrows) is seen on **(A)** longitudinal and transverse scans from **(B)** superior to **(C)** inferior. There is one large, dense area (open arrow) with multiple lucent areas in a radial pattern. At surgery, these were found to be necrotic bowel loops arranged in a spiral fashion, with a large proximal ileal segment. *(Figure continues.)*

and scattered calcific deposits. On ultrasound, the following pattern has been described: an inhomogeneous mass with several central areas of increased echogenicity, faint posterior shadowing, and a highly echogenic, thick peripheral rim[135-137] (Figs. 8-82 to 8-85). Such a mass could represent an omental or mesenteric cyst, GI tract duplication cyst, choledochal cyst, or ovarian cyst; the thick, well-circumscribed echogenic cyst wall, which contains areas of focal calcification, should be compatible with meconium cyst associated with meconium peritonitis.[137]

Inspissated Meconium

Other findings have been reported with meconium abnormalities.[138] A soft tissue mass may be seen on plain films, with the ultrasound revealing the mass to be homogeneously echogenic and surrounded by fluid-filled dilated bowel loops (Fig. 8-86). This appearance is most consistent with a bowel loop filled with meconium. The appearance is not consistent with pseudocyst since the borders are relatively ill-defined and lobulated and there is no thick, highly echogenic rim (corresponding to calcification).[138] This finding helps to identify an obstructed meconium-filled small bowel loop and to differentiate between meconium ileus and ileal atresia.

Meconium Peritonitis

There are a number of causes of neonatal ascites, including hematologic disease, bowel perforation, obstructive uropathy, cardiovascular disease, chylous ascites, intrauterine infection, and biliary peritonitis.[139] An additional etiology may be meconium peritonitis.[139] Meconium peritonitis may be characterized by a chemical peritonitis that has an intense fibroplastic reaction to

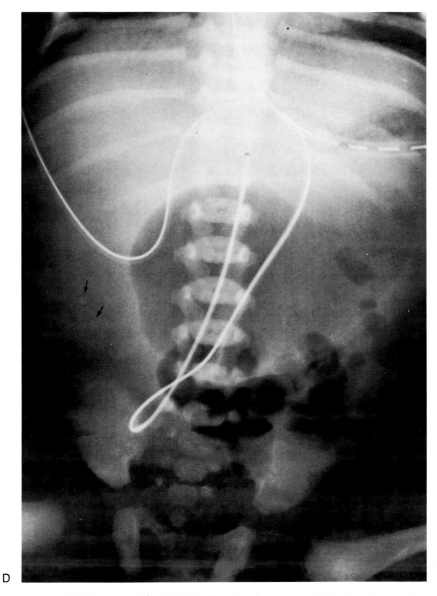

Fig. 8-83 *(Continued).* **(D)** Plain film showing some calcifications (arrows).

digestive enzymes contained in the meconium. Bowel obstruction does not have to be present, although it is usually combined with perforation as the most frequent cause of meconium peritonitis. If the bowel perforation closes before birth, fibroadhesion occurs and meconium peritonitis usually results. Perforation may persist post-natally, or a dense adherent membrane may be formed on the peritoneal surface, which effectively seals off the site of perforation and leads to fibroadhesive meconium

peritonitis. If perforation occurs late during the perinatal period, bowel contents escape freely into the peritoneal cavity and a generalized pattern is produced.

On ultrasound, echogenic ascites may be visualized, with meconium peritonitis mimicking liver paren-chyma[139] (Fig. 8-87). Ascites associated with echogenic densities along the peritoneal surface can denote calcification and has been seen with meconium peritonitis. The pattern associated with generalized meconium peri-

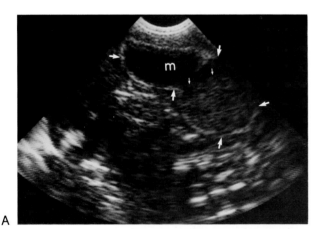

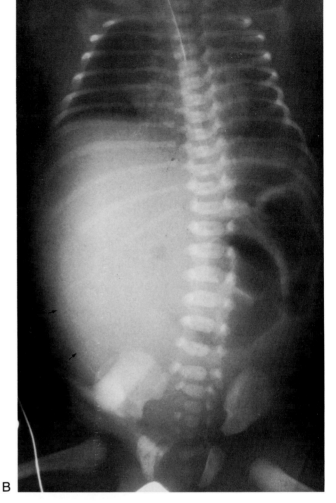

A   B

Fig. 8-84. Meconium ileus. Cystic fibrosis with a sterile abscess. **(A)** A "figure-eight" configuration mass (*m*, arrows) representing the abscess is seen within the right abdomen with a fluid-fluid level (small arrows). **(B)** Plain film showing a mass effect within the right abdomen with meconium (arrows).

tonitis has been described as a "snowstorm" pattern.[139] The echoes within the fluid have low amplitude and a homogeneous distribution.

Tumors

Lymphoma

Neoplastic disease, except for lymphoma, is rare in the small bowel.[26] Lymphoma of the GI tract most frequently occurs around age 65, but it is the most common tumor of the GI tract in children, especially younger than 10 years of age.[140] This lymphoma is usually part of a systemic involvement and presents with multiple nodules, although it originates in the GI tract in 10 to 20 percent.[140] Intraperitoneal masses frequently involve the mesenteric vessels that encase them.[26]

Patients with small bowel lymphoma may present with intestinal blood loss, weight loss, and anorexia. Abdominal pain is frequent, with a spruelike syndrome. There is a variable degree of intestinal obstruction, which may be related to encroachment on the bowel lumen. More than 50 percent of children have a palpable mass.[140]

The most frequent histologic type that involves the bowel is non-Hodgkin's lymphoma, which includes Burkitt's undifferentiated, and histiocytic lymphomas. Burkitt's lymphoma has a particular tendency to involve loops of the bowel in a rapidly growing mass[46] (Figs. 8-88 to 8-90). Hodgkin's disease almost never presents as an isolated GI process, although it eventually involves the

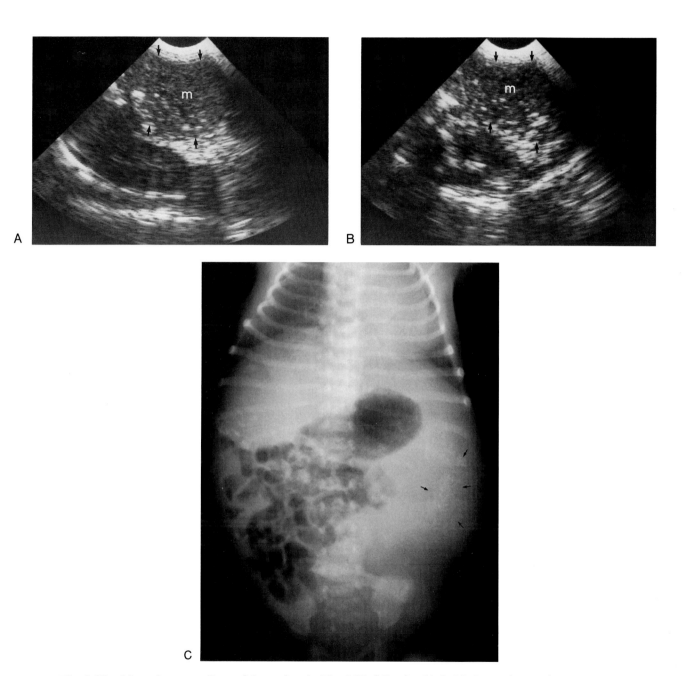

Fig. 8-85. Meconium cyst. Scan of the patient in Fig. 8-82, following birth. No longer is a cystic mass seen. Instead, a poorly defined echogenic mass (arrows, *m*) is seen on **(A)** longitudinal and **(B)** transverse scans. The mass contained many internal echoes and exhibited acoustic enhancement. Its borders were difficult to discern. **(C)** Plain radiograph showing a mass effect in the left abdomen containing meconium (arrows). At surgery, a large cyst filled with meconium-stained fluid was found in the left upper quadrant. Calcification was seen within the cyst and the right upper quadrant.

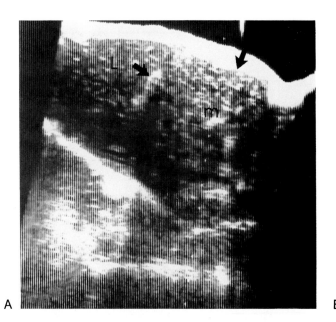
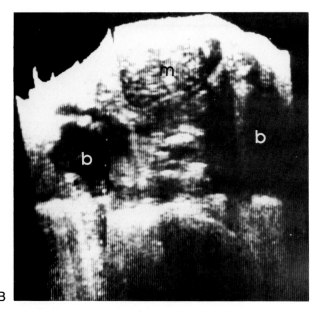

Fig. 8-86. Meconium ileus. **(A)** Midline longitudinal abdominal sonogram showing a solid mass below the liver and stomach (arrows). (*m,* mass *L,* liver.) **(B)** Transverse section through the same mass as in Fig. A showing continuity of the mass *(m)* with similar material below it. Dilated bowel loops *(b)* surrounding the meconium-filled masses are seen. (From Barki Y and Bar-Ziv,[138] with permission.)

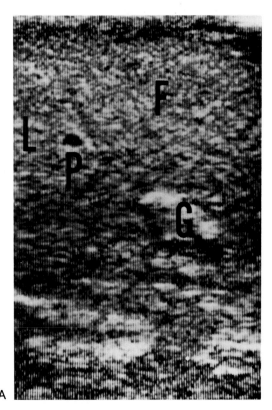
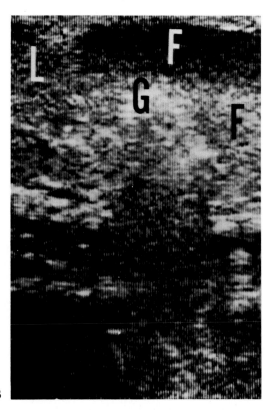

Fig. 8-87. Meconium peritonitis. **(A)** Coronal scan of the left abdomen in the right decubitus position showing massive ascitic fluid *(F)* mimicking liver parenchyma *(L).* A branch of the portal vein *(P)* and posteriorly located bowel gas *(G)* are also demonstrated. **(B)** Sagittal scan of the epigastrium showing the tendency toward sedimentation of the ascitic fluid contents *(F),* which represents sedimented small meconium particles. (From Wu,[139] with permission.)

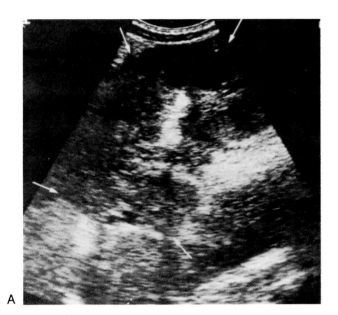

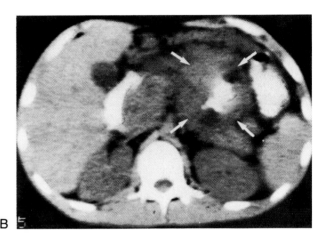

A

B

Fig. 8-88. Lymphoma of the ascending portion of the duodenum and proximal jejunum. (A) Longitudinal scan of the left hypochondrium showing a large mass with strong central echoes and hypoechoic periphery (arrows). The lesion was located posterointerior to the stomach, and its duodenal nature could not be demonstrated by sonography. (B) CT scan demonstrating the presence of contrast material within the mass (arrows), indicating its gastrointestinal nature; the duodenal origin of the lesion could be identified by following, on different slices, the course of the duodenum from its origin to the lesion itself. (From Derchi et al,[95] with permission.)

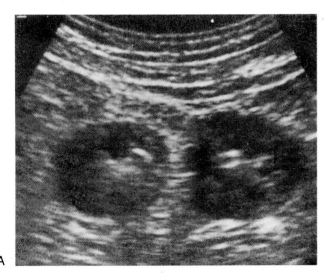

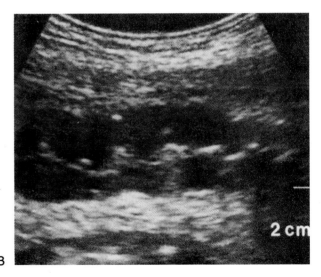

A

B

Fig. 8-89. Non-Hodgkin's lymphoma of low-grade malignancy and histologically proven lymphoma involvement of the small bowel. (A) Transverse sonogram showing two bowel loops with typical target lesions due to transmural circumferential infiltration. (B) Longitudinal sonogram of a small-bowel loop showing its tubular appearance. (From Goerg et al,[82] with permission.)

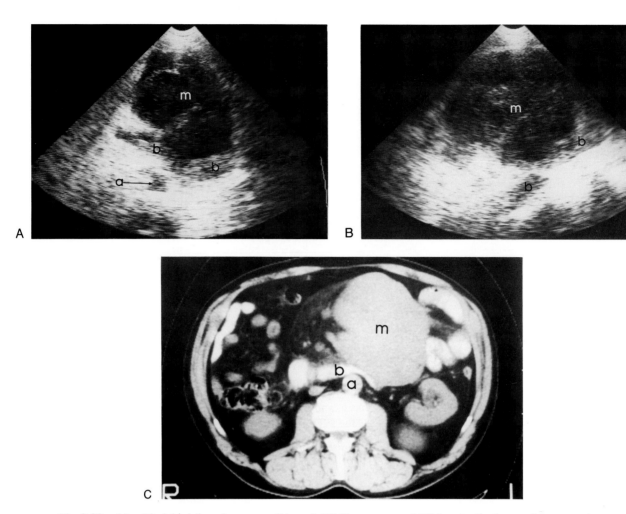

Fig. 8-90. Non-Hodgkin's lymphoma, small bowel. **(A)** Transverse and **(B)** longitudinal scans demonstrating a mass *(m)* of mixed density involving the small bowel *(b)* and extending into the mesentery. (*a*, aorta.) **(C)** CT scan similarly showing a soft tissue-density mass *(m)* and bowel *(b)* involvement. (*a*, aorta.)

GI tract in 50 percent of cases. Lymphoma in children starts as a unifocal lesion, usually in the terminal ileum in the lymphoid follicles, and spreads circumferentially throughout the submucosa, gradually involving the muscular coat to present as a subserosal tumor.

Primary lymphoma of the small bowel usually presents as a large irregular mass that has internal echoes due to necrosis. In most cases, the lymphoma mass is complex, with completely anechoic areas and central densely reflective areas indicative of GI mucosa and/or mucus[140] (Figs. 8-88 to 8-90). This pattern reflects the thickening of the bowel wall. The polypoid type of lymphoma tends to extend into the mesentery in a predominantly exoenteric manner. Ultrasound is able to detect a mass that has either an eccentric or exoenteric growth

pattern.[140] The patterns that have been described include (1) a large discrete mass (5 to 11 cm in diameter) with a target pattern, (2) an exoenteric pattern with a large mass on the mesenteric surface of bowel, and (3) a small anechoic mass (1 to 2 cm) representing subserosal nodes or mesenteric nodal involvement.

Lymphomatous involvement of the intestinal wall may lead to a "pseudokidney" or "hydronephrotic-pseudokidney" appearance of the involved bowel.[141] (Fig. 8-90). The lumen may be dilated with fluid, probably because of the lack of peristalsis of the diseased segment. The bowel wall is uniformly thickened with homogeneous low echogenicity between the well-defined mucosal and serosal surfaces that contain a persistent, echofree, wide and long lumen.

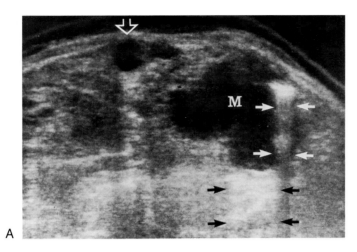

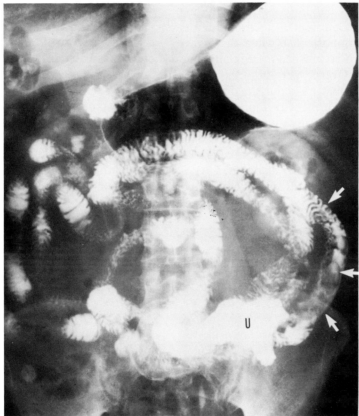

Fig. 8-91. Small bowel leiomyosarcoma. **(A)** Transverse scan of the lower abdomen showing a hypoechoic mass *(M)* with enhanced transmission (black arrows), suggesting liquefaction necrosis. Note the eccentric location of the acoustic shadow (white arrows) adjacent to the mass *(M)*. Omental metastasis (open arrow) has a similar appearance. **(B)** Small bowel series showing extrinsic pressure (arrows) on the jejunal loops and an ulceration *(U)*. (From Subramanyam et al,[83] with permission.)

Leiomyosarcoma

Leiomyosarcoma represents 10 percent of the primary small bowel tumors.[83,84] From 10 to 30 percent of these occur in the duodenum, 30 to 45 percent in the jejunum, and 35 to 55 percent in the ileum. Most occur in the fifth and sixth decades of life.[83,84] On ultrasound, the diagnosis may be suggested if a large, solid mass containing necrotic areas is seen anterior to a solid viscus and if intestinal lumen and/or air is in close relation to the mass[83] (Figs. 8-91 and 8-92).

Carcinoid

Carcinoids (argentaffinomas) can arise anywhere in the GI tract, bronchi, biliary tree, or pancreas or wherever enterochromaffin cells are normally found.[38] In decreasing order of frequency, they are found in the appendix (35 to 45 percent), small bowel (20 to 25 percent), rectum (15 percent), and lower bowel (excluding the rectum, 10 percent). Detection of carcinoid tumors at a resectable stage is important, because the 5-year survival rate is up to 90 percent when there is complete excision of the lesion.[142] Over 73 percent of the lesions are less than 1.5 cm in diameter and thus are difficult to see. The intraluminal component of a symptomatic malignant carcinoid tumor is typically small in relation to the extension into the mesentery, and the barium enema is occasionally normal.[142] On ultrasound, a carcinoid tumor has been described as a sharply marginated hypoechoic mass with a strong back wall and as a lobulated

contour with a lack of acoustic enhancement; both of these patterns are nonspecific.

Peutz-Jeghers Syndrome

Peutz-Jeghers syndrome is characterized by polyps throughout the GI tract, particularly the small bowel, and is associated with melanin pigmentation of the buccal mucosa, lips, and digits.[38] These polyps represent hamartomatous overgrowths rather than true neoplasms but have a slightly (3 percent) increased incidence of malignancy in the GI tract.[143] If the patient presents with symptoms of intussusception, and a UGI series with barium is temporarily contraindicated, ultrasound may be helpful. If there is distension of the small bowel loops, large intraluminal oval structures (polyps) may be seen.

Associated Mesentery Abnormalities

The ultrasound appearance of the normal and abnormal mesentery has been evaluated.[144] The normal mesentery has an elongated shape with an echogenic surface and small vessels in the center[144] (Fig. 8-93). The small bowel mesentery is a fan-shaped structure that connects the convolutions of the jejunum and ileum to the posterior wall of the abdomen. It consists of two layers of peritoneum containing blood vessels, nerves, lacteals, lymphatic glands, and a variable amount of fat. It is approximately 0.5 to 1 cm thick with a maximum breadth of 0.7 to 1.2 cm.[144]

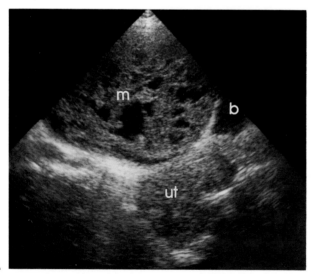
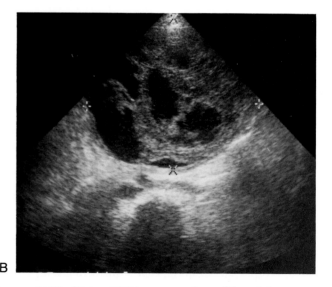

A   B

Fig. 8-92.   Smooth muscle (spindle cell) tumor of the jejunum. **(A)** Sagittal and **(B)** transverse views of the pelvis demonstrating a large (12-cm) multicystic mass (*m*, calipers). The mass was thought to be adnexal in origin at ultrasound. At surgery, a smooth muscle tumor of the jejunum was found. (*b*, bladder; *ut*, uterus.)

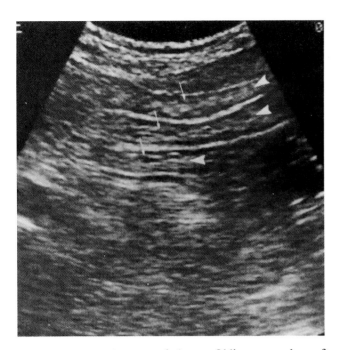

Fig. 8-93. Normal mesenteric leaves. Oblique scan plane of the left inferior abdominal quadrant demonstrating normal mesenteric leaves in vivo (arrowheads). The leaves have the same structural pattern seen in vitro and are divided from each other by specular reflections corresponding to their peritoneal surfaces. Small vascular structures (arrows) are seen in their center. (From Derchi et al,[144] with permission.)

A number of abnormalities affecting the mesentery can be detected by ultrasound. At times, it may be difficult to identify the mesentery as the source of origin of a large abdominal mass. Enlarged lymph nodes are seen as solid, hypoechoic, well-circumscribed masses (Figs. 8-94 and 8-95). With mesenteric lymphoma and mesenteric desmoid tumors, the mesenteric vessels may be encased within enlarged lymph nodes. The key factor is the proper location of the mass itself within the mesentery. This is helped by the identification of mesenteric vessels and analysis of their relationships with any space-occupying abdominal lesions.[144]

Retractile Mesenteritis

Retractile mesenteritis is caused by chronic inflammation and fibrosis; it is a rare disorder characterized by either focal or diffuse thickening of the mesentery.[145] It represents the final stage of a series of inflammatory changes affecting the mesentery. It more commonly affects males and occurs at various ages; it is not usually found in children younger than 8 years. Pathologically, the lesions are composed of fibrous tissue, lipophages,

lymphocytes, plasma cells, and eosinophils.[145] The abnormality involves mesenteric and subserosal fat.

There has been little in the literature describing the ultrasound findings of this entity. The ultrasound findings are similar to those in patients with liposarcoma, leiomyosarcoma, teratoma, abscess, and hematoma.[145] On radiography, the findings include (1) separation of intestinal loops, (2) kinking or angulation of the small intestine, and (3) narrowing of the colon.

Mesenteric Adenitis and Terminal Ileitis or Bacterial Ileocecitis

The most frequent clinical diagnosis in patients with acute appendicitis undergoing surgery is mesenteric adenitis.[146] A combination of mesenteric adenitis and an edematous, thickened terminal ileum has been found in some of these patients.[146] In the past, this disease process was thought to be secondary to the acute phase of Crohn's disease, but now it has been determined to be secondary to bacterial infection caused by *Yersinia enterocolitica, Campylobacter jejuni, Salmonella enteritidis,* and, rarely, *Yersinia pseudotuberculous.*[146,147] This infection is confined to the terminal ileum, cecum, and mesenteric lymph node.[147] Ultrasound may be helpful in differentiating between this disease process and appendicitis.[146]

The main ultrasound findings in bacterial ileocecitis include mural thickening of the terminal ileum, cecum, and part of the ascending colon; enlargement of the mesenteric lymph nodes; and nonvisualization of an inflamed appendix.[147] The three bacterial groups demonstrate a slightly different ultrasound pattern, but there is considerable overlap[147] (Fig. 8-96). In *Campylobacter* and *Salmonella* ileocecitis, the mesenteric lymph nodes are moderately enlarged, whereas those in *Yersinia* ileocecitis are markedly enlarged, but, again, there is considerable overlap[147] (Fig. 8-96 to 8-100).

Without exception, the mural thickening of the terminal ileum is symmetric.[147] The layer structure observed on ultrasound is presumed. In most cases, the anteroposterior diameter of the ileum greatly exceeds 5 mm and is moderately compressible.[147]

When the ileum is followed by ultrasound toward the ileocecal valve, the characteristic ovoid, concentric, predominantly hyperechoic configuration is seen in the sagittal and axial planes.[147] On real-time ultrasound the axial configuration of the ileocecal valve may change from time to time when peristalsis causes a slight protrusion of the ileum into the cecum, which may coincide with the colicky attacks[147] (Fig. 8-101).

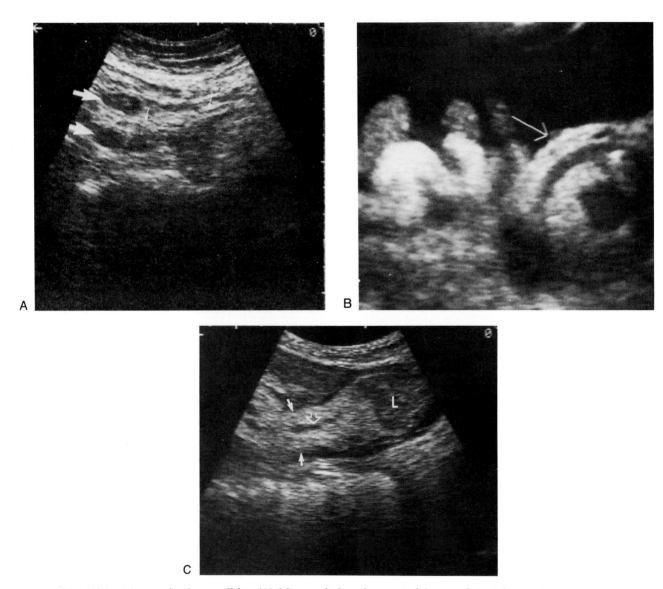

Fig. 8-94. Mesenteric abnormalities. **(A)** Mesenteric lymphoma. Axial scan of the left superior abdominal quadrant showing two enlarged mesenteric nodes (large arrows) surrounding a peripheral mesenteric vessel (small arrows). **(B)** Metastatic nodule on the peritoneal surface of the mesentery (arrow) in a patient with metastatic peritoneal disease from an ovarian primary tumor. **(C)** Mesenteric edema. Oblique scan of the left inferior abdominal quadrant showing that the mesentery (solid arrows) is thickened and diffusely hyperechoic. The mesenteric veins (open arrow) are dilated. There is also mild thickening of the wall of the small bowel loop *(L)*. (From Derchi et al,[144] with permission.)

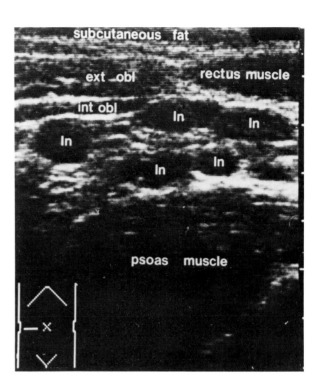

Fig. 8-95. Ultrasound image of various enlarged mesenteric lymph nodes *(ln)*. Note the centimeter scale (the markers are 1-cm apart) and the scanning plane. The echopoor nodes are well demarcated from the echogenic surroundings and are easily perceptible. Even when the nodes are slightly echogenic, the peripheral zone is always echopoor. At interval appendectomy, a biopsy was performed on one of the nodes (histologic findings included specific reactive changes), and a normal appendix, without any remnants of inflammation, was removed. (*ext obl,* external oblique muscle; *int obl,* internal oblique muscle.) (From Puylaert,[146] with permission.)

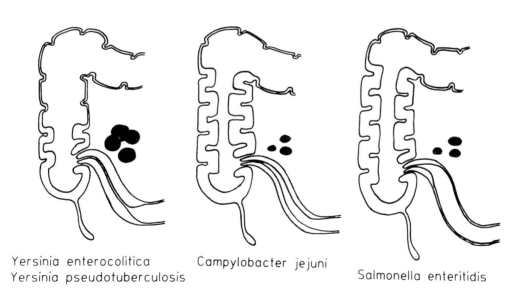

Yersinia enterocolitica
Yersinia pseudotuberculosis

Campylobacter jejuni

Salmonella enteritidis

Fig. 8-96. Schematic presentation of relative involvement of the terminal ileum, cecum, ascending colon, and mesenteric lymph nodes in bacterial ileocaecitis caused by different bacteria. However, there is considerable overlap. (From Puylaert,[147] with permission.)

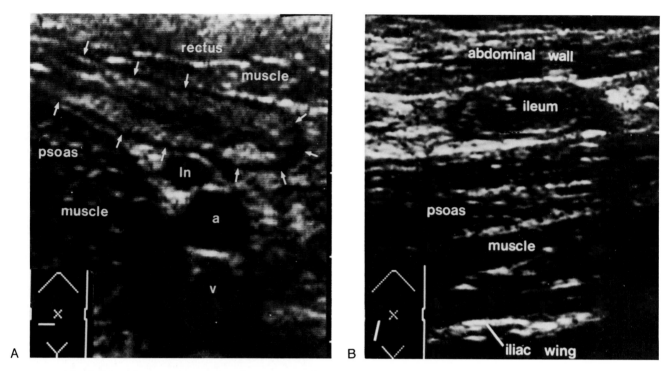

Fig. 8-97. Ultrasound scans showing acute terminal ileitis. Note the different centimeter scales (markers are 1 cm apart) and the scanning plane in each image. **(A)** In the longitudinal view, the tubular nature (arrows) becomes clear. **(B)** In the axial view, a somewhat flattened bull's eye is seen. Regional enlarged nodes *(ln)* are seen. (*a*, right iliac artery; *v*, right iliac vein.) (From Puylaert,[146] with permission.)

Ultrasound may show a typical haustral pattern in the sagittal view if the wall thickening extends from the cecum to the ascending colon[147] (Fig. 8-102). A diagnosis of bacterial ileocolitis should be made if the wall thickening and prominent haustration pattern are demonstrated throughout the colon.[147]

Yersinia Ileitis. The ultrasound findings of *Yersinia* terminal ileitis have been investigated.[146,148] In those patients studied, the only ultrasound findings consisted of enlarged mesenteric lymph nodes in combination with mural thickening of the terminal ileum[146,148] (Fig. 8-99). The wall of the bowel was always hypoechoic and was 7 to 10 mm thick.[148] The nodes visualized are sharply demarcated round or oval hypoechoic masses 7 to 21 mm in diameter. The best parameter for differentiating pathologic from normal lymph nodes is the anteroposterior diameter of the node, which must exceed 4 mm before the node can be considered abnormal.[146] Additionally, the pathologic nodes are more numerous, more lucent, more spherical, and more sharply delineated from the surrounding structures than are normal nodes.[146] The

number of nodes varies from 3 to 6 per patient. The conclusion from this study was that ultrasound could be helpful in the detection of acute terminal ileitis caused by *Yersinia.*[148]

Campylobacter Ileocolitis. *Campylobacter jejuni* is one of the leading causes of bacterial enteritis in the Western world and represents the second pathogenic agent after *Yersinia.*[149] The symptoms may vary from a mild, short-term complaint resembling common viral gastroenteritis to severe symptoms that may mimic those of explosive ulcerative colitis or even surgical conditions.[149] Similar to those described with *Yersinia* ileitis, the ultrasound findings include enlarged mesenteric lymph nodes, mural thickening of the terminal ileum, and nonvisualization of the appendix[149] (Fig. 8-100). Although the ultrasound findings may not be able to identify the etiologic pathogen, it is not relevant from the therapeutic standpoint since both conditions are treated conservatively without surgery.[149] The most important role of ultrasound is in differentiating the surgical and nonsurgical conditions in patients with clinical symptoms of appendicitis.[149]

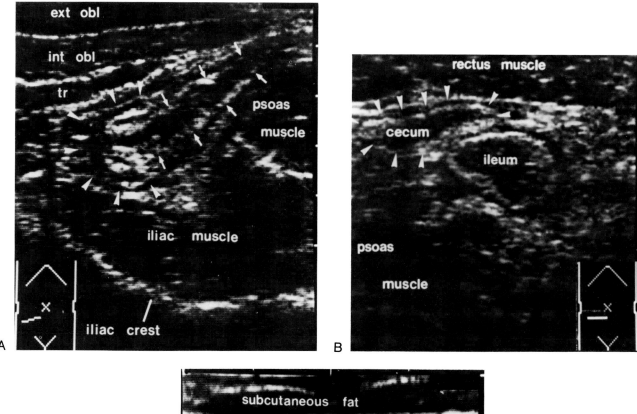

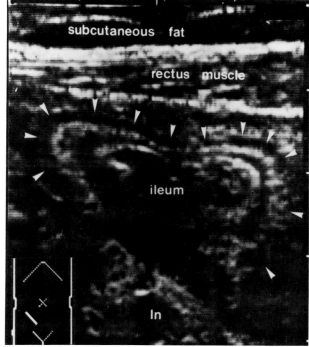

Fig. 8-98. Various ultrasound appearances of cecal wall thickening and of the ileocecal valve in acute terminal ileitis. Arrowheads point to the thickened cecal wall. **(A)** Arrows point to the terminal ileum, actually discharging into the cecum. (*ext obl,* external oblique muscle; *int obl,* internal oblique muscle; *tr,* transverse abdominis muscle.) **(B)** The ileum is seen just prior to its discharging into the cecum. **(C)** Axial view of the ileocecal valve showing multiple concentric rings; the real-time image somewhat resembles bowel invagination. (*ln,* lymph node.) (From Puylaert,[146] with permission.)

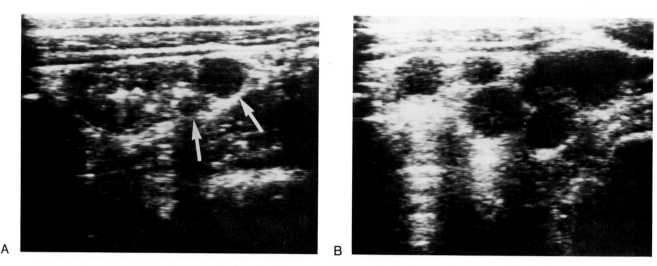

Fig. 8-99. *Yersinia* terminal ileitis in an 11-year-old girl with pain in the right lower quadrant and diarrhea. **(A)** Longitudinal sonogram showing mural thickening of the terminal ileum with a strong echogenic center surrounded by an anechoic rim. Note the enlarged lymph nodes (arrows). **(B)** Transverse sonogram showing distinct, enlarged lymph nodes. (From Matsumoto et al,[148] with permission.)

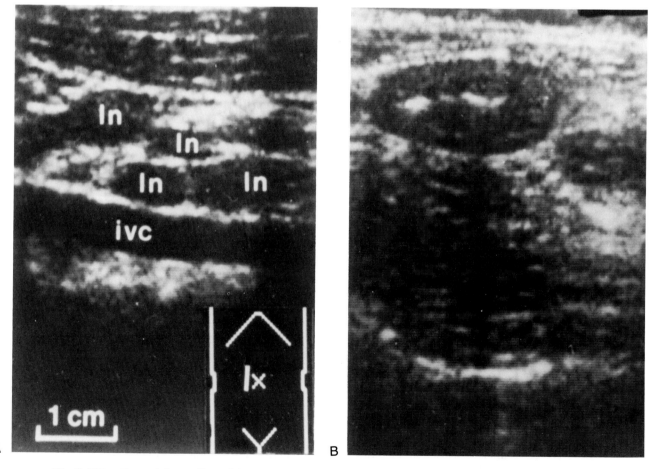

Fig. 8-100. *Campylobacter* ileocolitis. **(A)** Ultrasound scan showing moderately enlarged mesenteric lymph nodes *(ln)* anterior to inferior vena cava *(ivc)* during compression of abdomen. **(B)** Axial section through the inflamed ileum demonstrating bull's eye pattern. (From Puylaert et al,[149] with permission.)

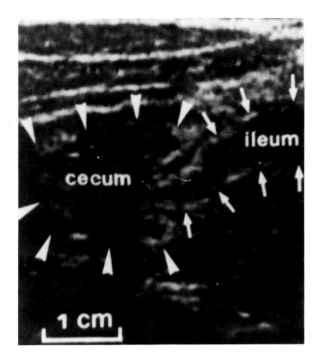

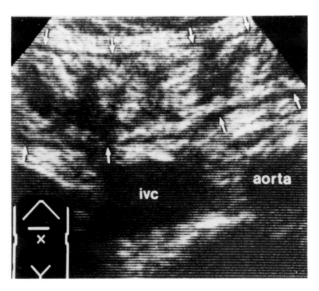

Fig. 8-102. Prominent haustra. Scan demonstrating prominent haustra (arrows) due to mural thickening. (*ivc,* inferior vena cava.) (From Puylaert et al,[149] with permission.)

Fig. 8-101. Longitudinal view of an abnormal ileocecal valve. The ileum (arrows) discharges into the cecum (arrowheads). (From Puylaert et al,[149] with permission.)

Salmonella Ileitis (Typhoid Fever). The mortality rate from typhoid fever in the Western world is about 2 percent, even though the disease is curable.[150] This may be due to a delay in diagnosis, which may occur if the disease is not considered, or to the time taken for the blood cultures to show positive results (at least 18 to 36 hours and sometimes over a week).[150] The ultrasound features, which include enlarged mesenteric lymph nodes and mural thickening of the terminal ileum and cecum, may also be seen with bacterial enteritis caused by other microorganisms such as *Yersinia enterocolitica* and *Campylobacter jejuni*[150] (Fig. 8-103). Also included in the differential diagnosis would be Crohn's disease, tuberculous ileitis, and lymphoma. The abnormality would be seen in the ileocecal region.[150]

Differential Diagnosis. In about 40 percent of appendicitis patients, there are enlarged mesenteric lymph nodes, but generally these nodes are not as numerous or as large as the nodes in patients with mesenteric adenitis.[146] Care should be taken to not confuse the inflamed appendix with an inflamed terminal ileum. None of the patients with the ultrasound findings of bacterial ileocecitis have been found to have acute appendicitis. As such, in patients with acute right lower quadrant pain whose appendix is nonvisualized on ultrasound and

whose ultrasound findings consist of enlarged mesenteric lymph nodes with mural thickening of the terminal ileum, the diagnosis of mesenteric adenitis and acute terminal ileitis (bacterial ileocecitis) should be considered.[146]

APPENDICEAL ABNORMALITIES

Acute Appendicitis

In the Western world, acute appendicitis is still the most common cause of emergency surgery of the abdomen.[151] Most investigators agree that 20 to 25 percent of the appendices removed are normal.[151,152] Acute appendicitis can occur at any age but is more prevalent in young adults.[38] In men, the negative appendectomy rate is usually below 20 percent, with rates of 10 to 15 percent reported.[153] By contrast, women often have acute gynecologic problems with symptoms that mimic those of appendicitis, resulting in a negative appendectomy rate of 34 to 46 percent[152,153] (Figs. 8-104 and 8-105). The complications of this disease include peritonitis, localized periappendiceal abscess, pylephlebitis with thrombosis of the portal venous drainage, liver abscess, and septicemia.[26]

The ultrasound findings associated with acute appendicitis have been investigated.[151–159] In the past, there were no findings associated with appendicitis that could be seen on ultrasound[26]; however, the typical target le-

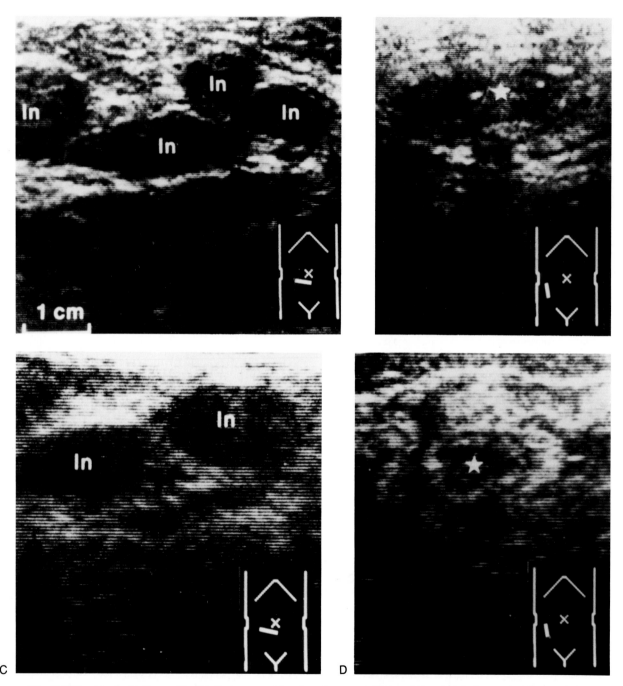

Fig. 8-103. Typhoid fever. **(A–D)** Sonograms showing features of bacterial enteritis in two patients with typhoid fever. Enlarged mesenteric lymph nodes *(ln)* (Figs. A & C), in combination with mural thickening of the terminal ileum and cecum, give rise to a characteristic axial image of the ileocecal valve (star) (Figs. B & D). (From Puylaert et al,[150] with permission.)

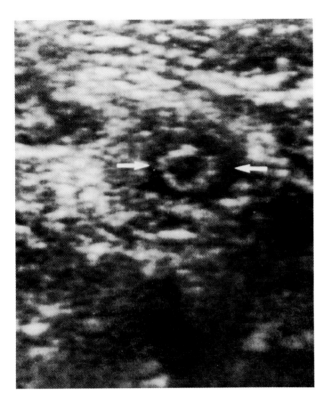

Fig. 8-104. Acute appendicitis. Typical example of acute appendicitis. Transverse sonogram of an appendix 9 mm in maximal diameter (arrows). (From Jeffrey et al,[156] with permission.)

sion had been reported in the right lower quadrant with this disease[154,155] (Figs. 8-104 and 8-105). Thickening of the bowel wall in this instance was due to edema, and the echogenic core was due to the necrotic appendix or appendiceal lumen.[154] The normal appendix may now be visualized by ultrasound[156] (Fig. 8-14). Also, an appendicolith can be seen as an intraluminal focus of high-amplitude echoes with acoustic shadowing[157] (Figs. 8-106 and 8-107). Ultrasound has several advantages over other techniques: (1) the structure being evaluated — the appendix — is close to the surface of the abdomen; (2) the bowel can be displaced or compressed, eliminating the disturbing gas artifacts; and (3) the area of maximum tenderness indicated by the patient can be directly examined.[151]

Noncompressible Appendix

The primary criterion for the diagnosis of acute appendicitis on ultrasound is visualization of a noncompressible appendix.[153] When the appendix is examined by ultrasound, the inflamed appendix is most often visualized at the base of the cecal tip during maximum graded compression (Figs. 8-104 and 8-105). The area of the psoas and iliacus muscles and external iliac artery and vein should be scrutinized. The inflamed appendix is seen as a sausage-shaped, blind-ending structure on a sagittal scan or as a target lesion on transverse section[158]

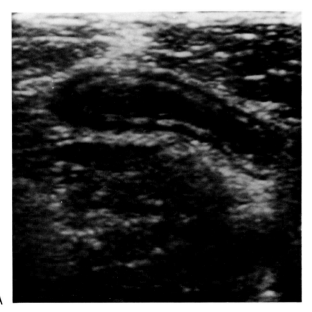
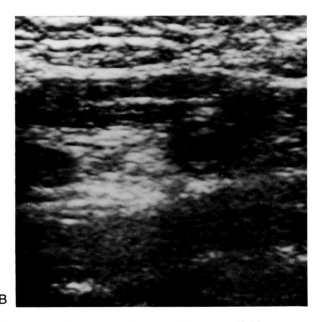

A   B

Fig. 8-105. Acute suppurative appendicitis. **(A & B)** Sonograms of proven acute suppurative appendicitis without perforation. The inflamed appendix appears as a blind-ending tubular structure in its longitudinal plane (Fig. A) and as a target lesion in its transverse plane (Fig. B). The lumen is filled with hypoechoic material, and the mucosa is relatively intact. (From Kao et al,[163] with permission.)

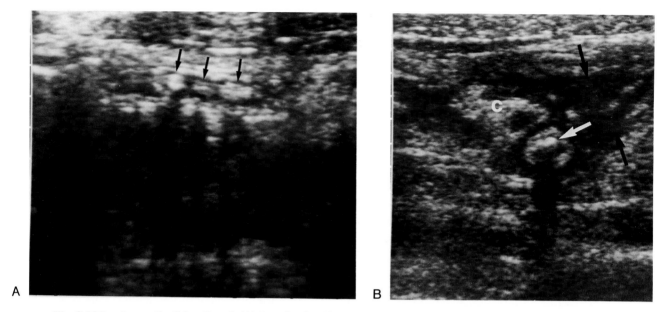

Fig. 8-106. Appendicoliths. Case 1. **(A)** Longitudinal image of an appendix showing multiple appendicoliths (arrows) and a diameter of 6 mm. Despite the relatively small diameter of the appendix, the patient had pathologically proved acute appendicitis. Case 2. **(B)** Transverse sonogram demonstrating an appendicolith with acoustic shadowing (white arrow). Note the marked edema of the adjacent mesentery (black arrows) and cecum *(C).* (Fig. A from Jeffrey et al,[156] with permission; Fig. B from Jeffrey et al,[153] with permission.)

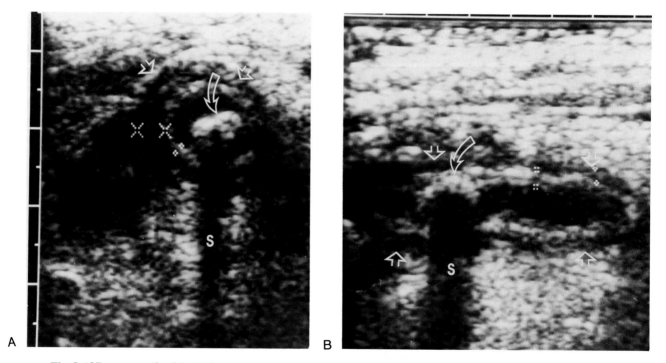

Fig. 8-107. Appendicolith. **(A)** Transverse and **(B)** longitudinal views of a gangrenous appendix (open arrows) showing an intraluminal, hyperechoic, rounded structure (open curved arrow) with shadowing that proved to be an appendicolith. (*S,* shadowing.) (From Abu-Yousef,[6] with permission.)

(Fig. 8-105). It can be characterized by lack of peristalsis and compressibility and by demonstration of its blind-ending tip.[157] The overall sensitivity of this criterion have been reported to be 89 percent, with a specificity of 95 percent and an accuracy of 93 percent.[153] The accuracy in women is 96 percent.[153] Eighty-nine percent of inflamed appendices have been identified by ultrasound.[151]

Appendiceal Wall Thickness

The mural thickness of the appendix is assessed by measuring the distance from the echogenic mucosa to the outer anechoic wall.[153] The hypoechoic wall is thickened to more than 2 mm.[152] The lumen may be seen as an echogenic area or as an anechoic area if there is fluid distension of the lumen, depending on the presence and degree of obstruction of the appendix[152] (Figs. 8-104 and 8-105). The mucosa/submucosa appears as a thin echogenic line surrounding the lumen.[152,157] The outer hypoechoic ring represents the muscularis externa.[157]

Appendiceal Diameter

Besides the identification of a noncompressible appendix by ultrasound in a patient suspected of having acute appendicitis, an additional finding should be sought—the dimensions of the visualized appendix.[156,157] Appendicitis is diagnosed if the maximal outer diameter of the appendix in transverse section along the short axis of the appendix is greater than 6 to 7 mm.[156,157] In patients with appendiceal diameters of 6 mm or less, there is a benign clinical follow-up or a histologically normal appendix is removed at surgery.[156] If the maximum outer appendiceal diameter is 6 mm or less, a period of close clinical observation is probably warranted rather than early surgery, with two exceptions: (1) when there is compelling clinical evidence of appendicitis and (2) when multiple appendicoliths are identified by ultrasound.[156] In one series, 78 of 84 patients who had surgery (with appendiceal diameters greater than 6 mm) were found to have acute appendicitis.[152] The accuracy of ultrasound has been reported to be 95.7 percent, with a specificity of 98 percent.[157]

Appendiceal Calculus

An appendiceal calculus can be recognized as a hyperechoic structure that has an acoustic shadow[154] (Figs. 8-106 and 8-107). These calculi or fecaliths result from accumulation and inspissation of fecal material around vegetable fiber. When present, they may obstruct the appendiceal lumen, frequently resulting in acute appendicitis. They are also associated with a high incidence of

acute complications such as perforation. In 10 to 14 percent of cases of acute appendicitis, appendiceal calculi are present; they are associated with perforation in 50 percent.[152]

Gas-Containing Appendix

The gas-containing appendix can be a potential pitfall in the sonographic diagnosis of acute appendicitis.[160] On plain film, the presence of gas within the appendix may or may not be associated with acute appendicitis. On ultrasound, gas is seen within the appendix as high-amplitude echogenic foci causing either distal reverberation artifacts (comet tails) or "dirty" acoustic shadowing.[160] This finding is important because it may be assumed to be secondary to either a normal bowel loop or a gas-containing periappendical abscess.[160] Gas within the appendix should not preclude the diagnosis of acute appendicitis if other diagnostic criteria are met.[160]

Diagnostic Criteria

The ultrasound findings of acute appendicitis may be expanded to include the following: (1) appendiceal diameter greater than 6 mm; (2) muscular wall thickness greater than 3 mm; and (3) visualization of a complex mass.[159] The most useful diagnostic test (sensitivity, 68 percent; specificity, 98 percent) is the combined criteria of an appendix with a muscular wall thickness of greater than 3 mm and visualization of a complex mass separate from the adnexa in females.[159] While ultrasound is not recommended as a screening test, it is recommended in a diagnostic role after initial clinical screening.[159]

Accuracy

Various published reported have described the accuracy of ultrasound in the diagnosis of appendicitis. In the diagnosis of acute appendicitis it has a specificity of 95 percent, a sensitivity of 80 percent, and an accuracy of 90 percent.[152] The predictive value of a positive test is 91 percent, and that of a negative test is 89 percent.[152] In women of childbearing years, the overall accuracy is 96.7 percent, with a sensitivity of 82.6 percent and a specificity of 100 percent.[159] With the use of ultrasound, the negative laparotomy rate may be reduced from 22.9 to 13.2 percent.[159]

Differential Diagnosis

Besides helping to make the diagnosis of acute appendicitis, ultrasound has value in establishing alternative diagnoses.[158] It is recommended for evaluation of all patients in whom the clinical diagnosis of acute appendicitis is equivocal, especially in women of childbearing age since it is sometimes difficult to differentiate clinically between acute appendicitis and pelvic inflammatory disease and the complications of pregnancy that are prevalent in this population.[152] Acute gynecologic disease is the most common disease to be confused clinically with acute appendicitis.[158] Often an alternative diagnosis is made by ultrasound.[158] As is well known, the rate of misdiagnosis of appendicitis in women 20 to 40 years old is high, approximately 40 percent.[158] As such, when the sonogram is negative for acute appendicitis, the abdomen and pelvis should be examined.[158] Of those without appendicitis, 53 percent are ultimately discharged with abdominal pain of unknown origin.[158] In the cases in which no specific diagnosis is established, ultrasound suggests the correct diagnosis in 70 percent.[158]

Acute Appendicitis in Children

Acute appendicitis is the most common cause of an acute abdomen in children.[161] It is particularly difficult to diagnose in some children.[162] The younger the child, the more difficult it will be to make an accurate diagno-

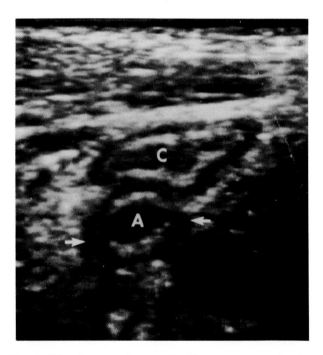

Fig. 8-108. Retrocecal appendix. Transverse scan showing an inflamed retrocecal appendix. Asymmetric thickening of the appendiceal wall is noted, with a focus of inflammation (arrows). (*A*, appendix; *C*, cecum.) (From Jeffrey et al,[153] with permission.)

sis.[162] In this younger age group, perforations of the appendix tend to occur earlier.[163]

As described above, the noncompressible appendix can be used as the primary criterion for establishing a diagnosis of acute appendicitis in children.[163] The target pattern found has a hypoechoic center correlating with a small amount of fluid or pus, with the echogenic line representing the submucosa and the hyperechogenic surrounding rim representing the muscular layer.[162] The maximal transverse diameters vary from 1 to 2 cm in children.[163] The appendiceal diameter is 4 to 5 mm in 4-month-old children and between 3.5 and 4.5 mm in other normal individuals.[162] As such, the diameter limit of 6 mm described in adults can be used in children as well.[162]

Two other patterns have been described with appendicitis in children. One pattern is that of diffuse hypoechogenicity, which correlates with a more advanced stage of inflammation; this is associated with a higher degree of perforation (75 percent).[162] The other pattern is that of diffuse hypoechogenicity with posterior enhancement. This is seen with appendices filled with pus under pressure at the time of surgery.[162]

Retrocecal Appendicitis

Retrocecal appendicitis in children has been investigated.[164] No bowel loops are interposed between the appendix and the lateral wall of the abdomen in the retrocecal appendix.[164] As usual, the inflamed appendix can be seen as a target image on cross-section and as a tubular structure in the sagittal plane (Fig. 8-108). The incidence of complex masses is greater in retrocecal appendicitis, reflecting a higher incidence of perforation.[164] Ultrasound is highly specific (100 percent) for retrocecal appendicitis, with a sensitivity of 94.5 percent, similar to that of normal appendicitis.[164] As such, ultrasound can be helpful in establishing the correct diagnosis in doubtful cases in which avoiding delay or unnecessary surgery is important.[164]

Complications

A number of complications have been found in children with appendiceal inflammatory disease.[161] The more frequent sequelae include peritonitis and subsequent pelvic and abdominal abscesses, but others include pylephlebitis and liver abscesses.[161] Pylephlebitis may lead to thrombosis and secondary cavernous transformation of the portal and splenic veins and/or may cause the portal vein to act as a conduit for spread of bacteria to the liver, resulting in liver abscess.[161]

Management

The management of appendiceal masses in children is controversial.[161] Many investigators recommend conservative treatment and interval appendectomy as the treatment of choice; others favor immediate appendectomy in every case of appendicitis.[165] In the series reported, 87.5 percent of those initially treated conservatively had an uneventful resolution of the appendiceal mass, with a mean hospital stay of 10.5 days.[165] Of the 12.5 percent who failed to respond to conservative management, 7 percent showed worsening of their symptoms during hospitalization and required drainage of an appendiceal abscess and 3 percent were readmitted with recurrence of symptoms.[165] These authors concluded that conservative management of appendiceal masses is a safe and effective method of treatment.[165]

Perforation with Acute Appendicitis/ Abscess

A strong inverse correlation between the incidence of rupture and age has been found, ranging from 93 percent in children younger than 1 year to 33 percent in those older than 10 years, possibly because of lack of early recognition and treatment.[157] The rate of appendiceal perforation ranges from 13 to 31 percent, with rates as high as 65 percent in the elderly.[166] In a review of the current series, the perforation rate was 21 percent before ultrasound and 22 percent after ultrasound.[166]

A number of ultrasound findings have been reported with perforation associated with acute appendicitis; these include loculated pericecal fluid, prominent peri-

cecal fat, and circumferential loss of the submucosal layer of the appendix[166] (Figs. 8-109 to 8-112). The overall sensitivity of these findings was 86 percent when one or more findings were combined.[166] With appendiceal perforation, there may be asymmetric appendiceal wall thickening, periappendiceal mass or abscess, and lack of significant tenderness during the examination in the presence of positive findings, probably as a result of relief of the intrappendiceal pressure after rupture.[152] The most specific ultrasound feature of appendiceal perforation is the presence of loculated pericecal fluid indicating abscess.[166] Ultrasound is less accurate in diagnosing perforation (56 percent) than in diagnosing acute appendicitis.[166]

With an abscess, ultrasound may demonstrate an echofree or poorly echogenic lesion in which irregular or ill-defined borders are restricted to the right lower quadrant[154] (Figs. 8-109 to 8-112). An abscess may range from almost echofree to a heterogeneous mass to gas-containing lesions with high internal echogenicity and acoustic shadowing.[155] This abscess may extend.[26] A retrocecal appendiceal abscess may be seen as a complex cystic mass posterior to the kidney[131] (Fig. 8-111). Periappendiceal abscess or peritonitis does not necessarily mean perforation, because the organism may permeate the wall.[38] In women it may be difficult to differentiate an appendiceal abscess from a tubo-ovarian abscess, twisted ovarian cyst, ruptured tubal pregnancy, or ruptured follicular or luteal ovarian cyst.[154]

The need for immediate surgery is controversial in the surgical literature for those with perforating appendicitis and larger periappendiceal inflammatory masses.[166] Antibiotic therapy followed by interval appendectomy in patients with large periappendiceal phlegmons is an ac-

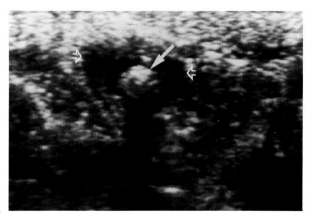
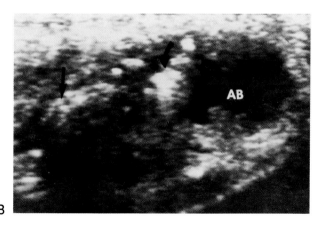

Fig. 8-109. Ruptured appendix with periappendiceal abscess and appendicolith. **(A)** Marked thickening of the appendiceal wall and appendicolith (closed arrow) is seen. **(B)** Longitudinal scan demonstrating a complex periappendiceal abscess *(AB)* with fluid and gas bubbles (curved arrow) caudad to the appendix. (straight arrow, level of the appendicolith). (From Jeffrey et al,[153] with permission.)

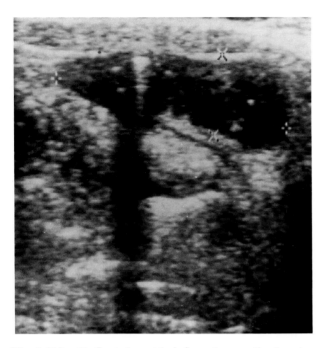

Fig. 8-110. Perforated acutely inflamed appendix. Longitudinal sonogram of a perforated, acutely inflamed appendix showing marked distension of the lumen at the distal tip with intramural echogenic foci due to gas. (From Kao et al,[163] with permission.)

ceptable alternative to immediate surgery.[166] Percutaneous catheter drainage followed by interval appendectomy in patients with well-defined and well-localized periappendiceal abscesses can be performed with a low morbidity.[166]

Postappendectomy Fluid Collections

In approximately 5 percent of children who have undergone appendectomy for acute appendicitis, clinically symptomatic fluid collections may develop within the pelvis and can be followed for size and course by ultrasound.[167] Although these fluid collections may take up to 2 months to resolve, they can be treated conservatively and nonoperatively.[167]

In patients with appendiceal perforation, the frequency of postoperative fluid collections is 14 percent, which is greater than the 3 percent in those with uncomplicated appendicitis.[167] Although ultrasound may demonstrate the presence of septations, debris, and/or a fluid level within an anechoic mass, it is not specific for the nature of the fluid[167] (Fig. 8-113). At times, a postoperative abscess is found by ultrasound (Fig. 8-114). Care should be taken not to mistake colon for abscess. Hematomas, necrotic tumors, and abscesses may all have this appearance. There must be periodic clinical and ultrasound monitoring during the postoperative period and treatment with a broad-spectrum antibiotic regimen de-

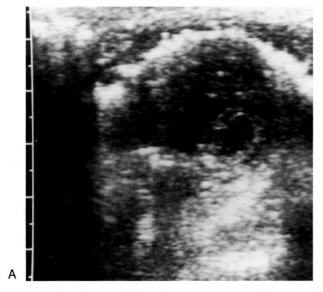

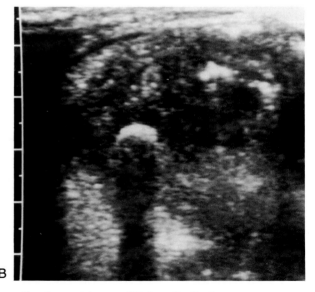

A   B

Fig. 8-111. Perforated retrocecal appendix with periappendiceal mass/abscess. **(A)** Longitudinal sonogram showing the acutely inflamed appendix surrounded by a hypoechoic mass displacing the cecum anteriorly. **(B)** Transverse sonogram showing a hyperechoic structure with distal acoustic shadowing due to appendicolith and foci of gas within the abscess. (From Kao et al,[163] with permission.)

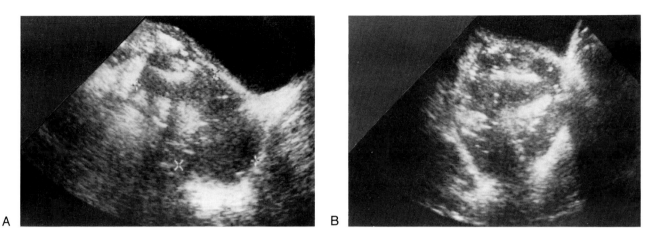

Fig. 8-112. Acute suppurative appendicitis with perforation. **(A)** Longitudinal and **(B)** transverse sonograms of the pelvis showing a large hypoechoic collection with foci of hyperechogenicity due to gas inside and outside the bowel loops. This patient had proved acute suppurative appendicitis with perforation. (From Kao et al,[163] with permission.)

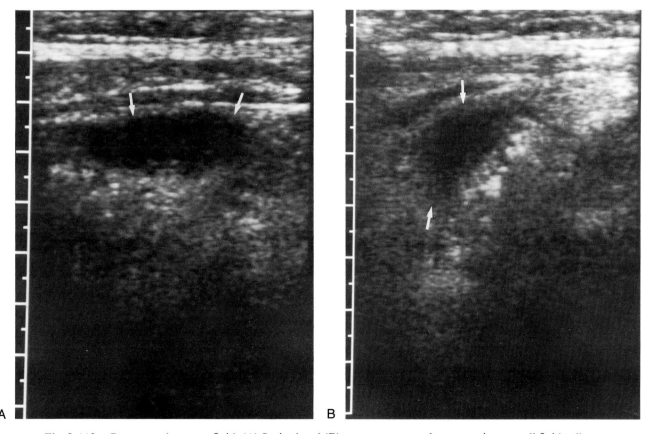

Fig. 8-113. Postappendectomy, fluid. **(A)** Sagittal and **(B)** transverse scans demonstrating a small fluid collection (arrows) in the region of the removed appendix.

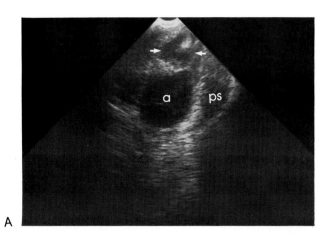

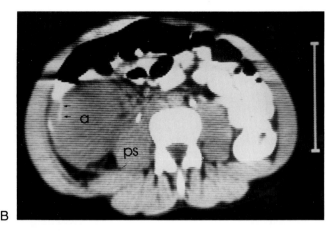

A   B

Fig. 8-114. Appendicitis, postoperative abscess. **(A)** Longitudinal real-time scan showing a hypoechoic mass *(a)* anterior to the psoas *(ps)* muscle. A target pattern with a thickened wall and dense center was seen anterior to the mass, representing the cecum (arrows). **(B)** CT scan at a similar level to Fig. A showing a soft tissue-density mass *(a)* anterior to the psoas *(ps)* muscle. Contrast (arrows) can be seen entering the mass. This mass represented a postoperative abscess.

signed to cover gram-negative and anaerobic bacteria for conservative treatment of such patients.[167]

Radiation Appendicitis

Ultrasound may demonstrate an inflamed appendix in patients who have received radiation therapy for extensive rectal carcinoma.[168] These patients may have no clinical signs of acute appendicitis.[168] In patients undergoing subsequent surgery for resection for rectal carcinoma, the appendix was found to be abnormal and was resected, demonstrating radiation enteritis of the appendix.[168] This diagnosis — radiation appendicitis — is another diagnosis to be considered when an inflamed appendix is demonstrated by ultrasound in patients without clinical signs of appendicitis.[168]

Crohn's Appendicitis

In 25 percent of cases of Crohn's ileocolitis, the appendix may be involved, with appendicitis being the initial manifestation of this disease.[6,152] The appendix may become involved secondary to cecal or terminal ileal granulomatous disease and local extension. In these patients, the right lower quadrant pain may last longer and be less severe than in patients with acute nongranulomatous appendicitis.[6] The Crohn's disease may be limited to the appendix without involvement of the colon or small bowel, but this is much rarer. In isolated cases in which Crohn's disease involves only the appendix, the patient presents with clinical manifestations of acute ap-

pendicitis. These two entities may not be differentiated by ultrasound.[154]

In the presence of excessive muscular wall thickening in the absence of fluid distension of the appendix and the presence of inflammatory changes in the cecum and terminal part of the ileum, the diagnosis of Crohn's disease should be suggested[152] (Fig. 8-115). After appendectomy, the rate of recurrence of Crohn's disease in the colon or small bowel is low (14 percent), and fistula formation has not been reported.[152]

Mucocele

Mucoceles are relatively rare lesions, occurring in 0.25 to 0.3 percent of a series of 43,000 appendectomies.[169-171] These mucoceles may be incidental at surgery in 23 to 50 percent of cases.[171] Patients are generally older than 50 years of age, with a mean age of presentation of 55 years and with a female/male ratio of 4:1.[172,173] From 23 to 25 percent of patients may be asymptomatic.[171,173] If the patients are symptomatic, they present with vague abdominal distress, acute or chronic pain, and, rarely, intermittent colicky pain caused by intussusception of the mucocele into the cecum.[171] In 64 percent of patients, there is acute or chronic right lower quadrant pain.[170,173]

Mucocele is usually a benign condition that obliterates the lumen of the appendix as a result of inflammatory scarring or fecaliths, with accumulation of sterile mucus in the isolated segment. The term *mucocele* implies a distension of the appendix by mucus and does not convey its true pathologic nature.[170,171,174] Postappendiceal

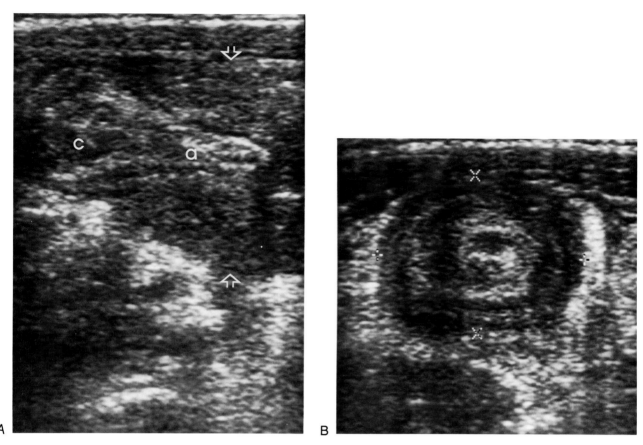

Fig. 8-115. Crohn's appendicitis. Child with chronic right lower quadrant pain. **(A)** Sagittal and **(B)** transverse views of the appendix showing massive (29 × 40 mm) thickening of the appendiceal wall (open arrows, calipers). The appendiceal lumen *(a)* is surrounded by thickened wall. There was no small bowel involvement with Crohn's disease at surgery. (*c*, cecum.)

scarring is the most common cause of mucocele, with others including fecaliths, appendiceal polyps, cecal carcinoma, cecal diaphragm, carcinoma of the ascending colon, and appendiceal valve. There is progressive cystic dilatation up to 4 to 6 cm.[38]

There are two principal theories for the formation of mucoceles.[154,175] The obstruction theory asserts that the distal mucosa of the appendix is stimulated to produce excessive secretion of mucin as a result of proximal obstruction of the lumen by feces, inflammatory fibrosis, or a neoplasm. The second theory suggests that the mucosa of the obstructed appendix undergoes an ill-defined neoplastic change. Either way, the appendix progressively distends owing to the accumulation of mucus. Other authors identify four patterns that are related to the causative mechanisms: (1) retention cysts, (2) mucosal hyperplasia, (3) mucinous cystadenomas, and (4) mucinous cystadenocarcinoma.[174]

There are several classifications of mucoceles. If the tumor remains encapsulated and there are no malignant cells, the lesion should be called a mucocele.[172] This is classified as benign, representing a mucocele caused by obstruction of the appendiceal lumen.[171] The malignant type represents the mucin-secreting adenocarcinoma.[171] If the mucus spreads through the abdominal cavity without evidence of malignant cells, the condition is called pseudomyxoma peritonei. If the pseudomyxoma peritonei results from rupture of a benign mucocele, the procedure is to simply remove the mucocele and the collection of fluid; it carries a good prognosis. If the pseudomyxoma peritonei is due to a primary mucinous cystadenocarcinoma of the appendix in which mucus containing malignant cells has spread diffusely throughout the abdominal cavity, the prognosis is worse, since the mucocele behaves like an invasive neoplasm. One-fourth of these mucoceles rupture, causing peritoneal seeding.[38]

The clinical significance of this disease lies in its complications: rupture, leakage of the mucocele with development of pseudomyxoma peritonei, torsion with gan-

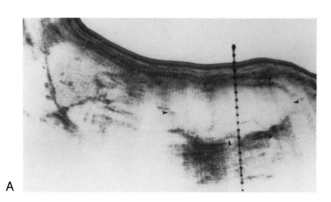
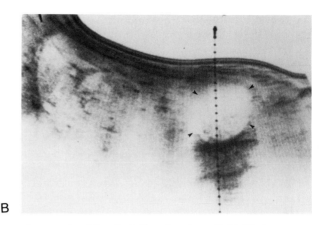

A   B

Fig. 8-116. Mucocele of the appendix. **(A)** Longitudinal scan 3 cm to the right of midline showing a fluid-filled right lower quadrant mass (arrowheads) containing thin septae. **(B)** Scan farther to the right of the mass (arrowheads) showing some dependent layering of internal echoes. (From Athey et al,[172] with permission.)

grene, hemorrhage, and herniation into the cecum, which causes various degrees of bowel obstruction. The pseudomyxoma peritonei assumes a malignant potential only when epithelial cells occur within the gelatinous peritoneal fluid in association with carcinoma.[171]

On ultrasound, a mucocele may be seen as a predominantly cystic mass or a well-defined hypoechoic mass, which may contain an echogenic solid area, in the right lower quadrant[154,169–173,175] (Figs. 8-116 and 8-117). This mass has an irregular inner wall caused by mucinous debris with various degrees of epithelial hyperplasia.[171] The mass may contain septations and may be echogenic.[174] Calcification may be indicated if the walls of the mass are highly echogenic[171] (Fig. 8-117). Additionally, there may be polypoid excrescences projecting intraluminally from the wall, possibly representing proliferation of the appendiceal mucosa.[171] In some incidences,

dependent echoes are seen within the mucocele; these may represent protein macroaggregates layering within the mucocele.[171] The most diagnostic features on ultrasound appear to be the echogenic (calcified) wall and the lining epithelium or papillary processes demonstrated within a cystic right lower quadrant mass.[174] In some instances, the mass projects within the pelvis and presents as an adnexal mass.[173]

Tumor

Primary adenocarcinoma of the appendix is very uncommon. Carcinoid accounts for 88.2 percent of carcinomas of the appendix and mucinous adenocarcinoma for 8.3 percent.[176] Most patients with primary appendiceal carcinoma present clinically as having acute appen-

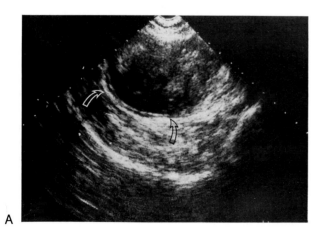
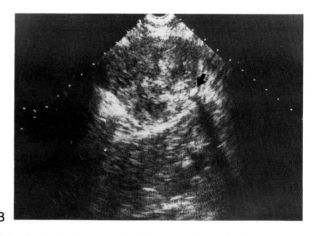

A   B

Fig. 8-117. Mucocele of the appendix. **(A)** Sonogram of the right midabdomen showing a mixed anechoic and echogenic mass. A thin inner echogenic rim (arrows) is consistent with the presence of a lining epithelium. **(B)** Lower sonogram showing a highly echogenic focus with acoustic shadowing (arrow) consistent with calcification of the wall. (From Skaane et al,[174] with permission.)

dicitis. Because of the obstruction of the appendix by carcinoma, appendicitis or perforation results. Ultrasound visualizes the condition as an asymmetric central echogenic core originating from the collapsed lumen and having an irregular and lobulated anatomy with a wall thickness greater than 2 cm secondary to tumor.[176]

COLONIC ABNORMALITIES

Normally, the colon is not usually identified as a structure as such on ultrasound, since it usually contains gas bubbles that produce acoustic shadows[26] (Fig. 8-118).

Imperforate Anus

Real-time ultrasound provides a noninvasive method to determine the level of obstruction in a patient with an imperforate anus. This is a common congenital anomaly that requires rapid evaluation and possibly early surgery. The appropriate surgery depends on the position of the distal rectal pouch and its relationship to the puborectalis portion of the levator sling. If the pouch is less than 1.5 cm from the perineum, it is consistent with a low lesion that can be passed through the puborectalis portion of the levator sling.[177,178] If the pouch terminates above the base of the bladder, it is indicative of a high lesion.[177]

To evaluate the rectal pouch, the patient, with a full bladder, is scanned supinely in the lithotomy position by either an anterior or sagittal midline transperineal approach.[178] The examiner places a finger in the pouch to measure the distance from the perineum[177] (Figs. 8-119 and 8-120).

Fecal Masses

Fecal impactions are caused by incomplete evacuation of feces over an extended length of time and may lead to the formation of a fecaloma (a large, firm mass of stool).[179] Most fecal masses are located in the area of the rectum, but they can also appear in the sigmoid or at times all segments of the colon. Although fecalomas are most commonly seen in elderly and debilitated patients, when they occur in psychiatric patients and in children with undiagnosed megacolon and psychogenic problems they can be associated with other predisposing factors such as drug intake (anticholinergics, narcotics), previous abdominal surgery, and painful anal disease.[179] Associated complications include stercoral ulcerations, intestinal obstruction, spontaneous perforation of the colon, and obstruction of the urinary tract.[179] A fecaloma may be visualized on ultrasound as a highly echogenic mass with a posterior acoustic shadow, and it should be considered in the differential diagnosis of a highly reflective and shadowing abdominal and/or pelvic mass[179] (Fig. 8-121).

Crohn's Disease and Ulcerative Colitis

Patients with Crohn's disease and ulcerative colitis have been evaluated by ultrasound with the water-filled colon technique.[9] The criteria used for detection and differentiation of inflammatory large bowel disease in-

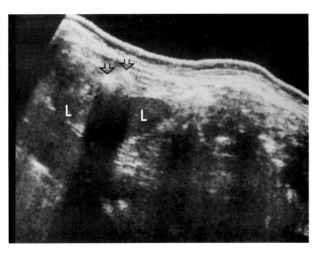

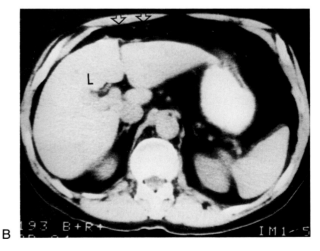

Fig. 8-118. Colon interposition. This patient presented with vague abdominal pain. **(A)** Longitudinal scan demonstrating a reflective pattern (open arrows) with shadowing produced by air in the bowel anterior to the liver. *(L)*. Peristalsis was seen within this area on real-time ultrasound. **(B)** CT scan demonstrating an air-filled transverse colon (open arrows) anterior to the liver *(L)*.

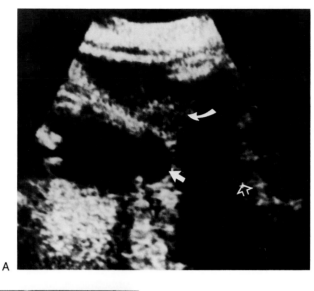

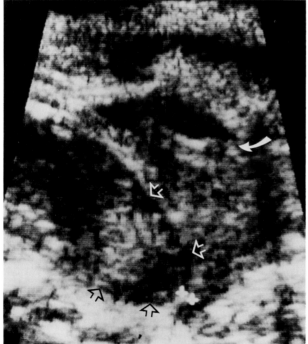

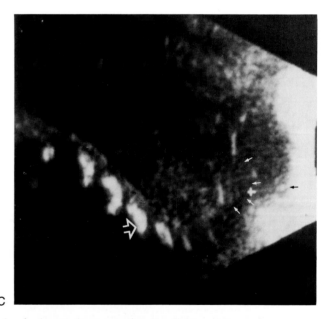

Fig. 8-119. Imperforate anus. **(A)** Longitudinal transabdominal scan demonstrating the distal rectal pouch (arrow) terminating above the base of the bladder (curved arrow). The examiner's finger, which is echogenic, is seen at the anal dimple (open arrow). **(B)** Longitudinal transabdominal scan demonstrating the distal rectal pouch (calipers, open arrows) terminating cephalic to the base of the bladder (curved arrow) in an infant with a high imperforate anus. **(C)** Longitudinal transperineal scan showing the distal rectal pouch (white caliper, arrows) and the perineal surface (black arrow). The pouch-skin distance (caliper to black arrow) was less than 1.1 cm. (open arrow, sacrum.) (From Oppenheimer et al,[177] with permission.)

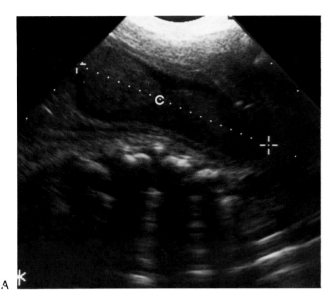 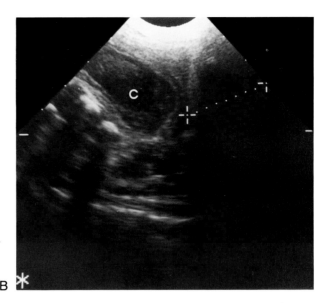

Fig. 8-120. Imperforate anus, high lesion. **(A)** Sagittal view of the pelvis showing a distended distal colon *(c)*. **(B)** Sagittal view showing that the end of the pouch was 2.7 cm (calipers) from the anal dimple. (*c*, distended distal colon.)

clude (1) the width of the intestinal lumen, (2) the appearance of haustration, (3) the thickness of the bowel wall, and (4) the presence of the typical bowel stratification.[9] The ultrasound results have been compared with those of the colonoscopic and histologic examinations.[9]

The following characteristics have been described for the diagnosis of Crohn's disease: (1) clearly thickened hypoechoic bowel wall, (2) loss of typical wall stratification, (3) loss of haustration, (4) diminished compressibility, and (5) no peristaltic motion[9] (Figs. 8-122 and 8-123). In cases of Crohn's disease, hypoechoic wall thickening of 1.1 ± 0.3 cm up to 1.5 cm may be found[8,9] (Fig. 8-122). The wall thickness increases as the inflammation becomes transmural. As the disease becomes more advanced, visualization of wall stratification is no longer possible.[8]

With ulcerative colitis, the following are found: (1) moderately thickened hypoechoic bowel wall; (2) typical wall stratification; (3) loss of haustration; (4) diminished compressibility; and (5) no peristaltic motion[9] (Figs. 8-124 and 8-125). With ulcerative colitis, the wall thickness is increased only moderately (0.6 ± 0.2 cm).[9] Without extensive inflammatory pseudopolyposis in patients with active ulcerative colitis but with multiple ulcers and the appearance of spontaneous bleeding, the ultrasound examination shows that the stratification of the bowel wall remains.[9]

Although ultrasound may not be able to make a clear differentiation between active Crohn's disease and acute ulcerative colitis, it should be able to identify the pres-

ence of inflammatory bowel disease. The inflammation in ulcerative colitis is diffuse and solely mucosal, whereas that in severe Crohn's disease is focal, submucosal, and transmural.[9] Severe active colonic Crohn's disease and ulcerative colitis can be detected by ultrasound with a sensitivity of 91 and 89 percent, respectively, since these two disease processes demonstrate different ultrasound patterns.[9] Colonic ultrasound can be 100 percent specific for detection of inflammatory bowel disease caused by active Crohn's disease and 97 percent specific for ulcerative colitis.[9]

Ultrasound will never replace contrast radiography in diagnosing acute inflammatory large bowel disease; it may serve to reduce the need for repeated abdominal radiographs and hence diminish radiation exposure. Additionally, with acute severe inflammatory large bowel disease, there is an increased risk of perforation when colonoscopy is performed.[9] Ultrasound may be seen as a safe and useful alternative diagnostic method with high sensitivity for the detection and differentiation of inflammatory colonic disease.[9]

Miscellaneous Colitis

Neutropenic Colitis

Several names have been applied to this entity, including typhlitis, neutropenic enterocolitis, necrotizing enteropathy, and ileocecal syndrome.[180] Whatever the

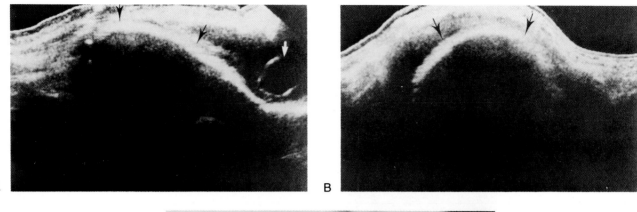

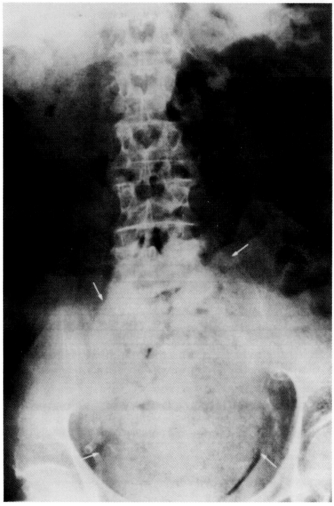

Fig. 8-121. Fecal masses. **(A)** Longitudinal and **(B)** transverse scans of the pelvis of a 74-year-old woman showing a large mass with a highly echogenic surface and posterior acoustic shadow (black arrows). The urinary bladder is displaced anteriorly, and the pelvic organs cannot be identified. The Foley catheter is visible within the urinary bladder (white arrow). **(C)** Plain abdominal film of the pelvis showing a soft tissue pelvic mass with a "soap bubble" appearance suggesting stool (arrows). (From Derchi et al,[179] with permission.)

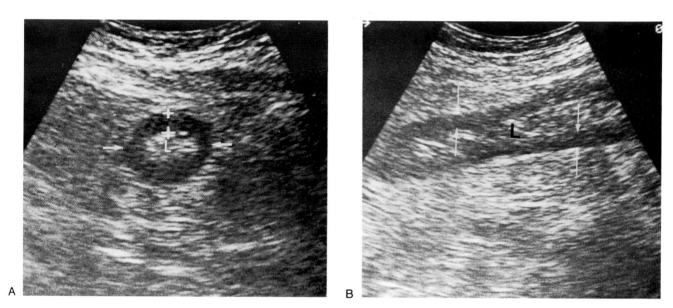

A
B

Fig. 8-122. Acute Crohn's disease. **(A)** Transverse and **(B)** longitudinal scans of an inflamed bowel segment showing the typical target configuration in Fig. A and pseudokidney pattern in Fig. B. The echogenic lumen *(L)* is surrounded by a concentric thickened echopoor gastrointestinal wall (arrows). (From Limberg,[11] with permission.)

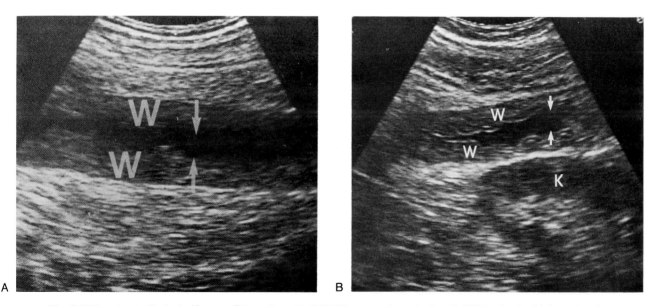

A
B

Fig. 8-123. Acute Crohn's disease of the colon. **(A & B)** The gastrointestinal wall *(W)* is clearly thickened and appears echopoor. The typical wall stratification and the haustra are no longer demonstrable. The intestinal lumen is narrow (arrows). (*K*, left kidney.) (From Limberg,[11] with permission.)

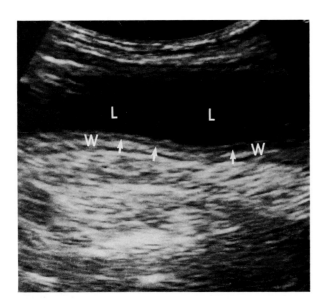

Fig. 8-124. Acute ulcerative colitis of the descending colon. The gastrointestinal wall *(W)* is only moderately thickened. The typical wall stratification remains. The quality with which colonic sonography reveals the two layers (arrows) representing the mucosa is remarkable. The gastrointestinal wall appears echopoor. (*L,* gastrointestinal lumen.) (From Limberg,[11] with permission.)

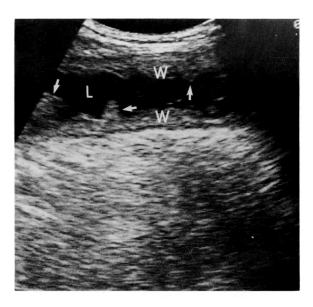

Fig. 8-125. Acute ulcerative colitis with extensive inflammatory pseudopolyposis. The gastrointestinal wall *(W)* is clearly thickened. The typical wall stratification is no longer demonstrable. The inflammatory pseudopolyps (arrows) project as echogenic small tumors into the intestinal lumen *(L).* (From Limberg,[11] with permission.)

name, this disease is an infection of the bowel that develops in patients with profound neutropenia, which occurs commonly in patients receiving chemotherapy for leukemia, lymphoma, or aplastic anemia and in immunosuppressed patients with organ transplants.[180,181] This disease rapidly progresses to sepsis and eventually death if left untreated. Patients with this abnormality generally present with right-sided abdominal pain, bloody diarrhea, and fever.[180,181] Occasionally a mass is demonstrated on clinical examination.

The right colon is most frequently involved by neutropenic colitis.[180] This portion of the colon may be at increased risk since there are areas of relative stasis and distensibility. These properties, in conjunction with the effects of antimetabolites, may lead to regional mucosal damage, allowing bacterial invasion of the bowel wall by the native flora. The colonic bacteria multiply unchecked in the tissue in the neutropenic state, leading to edema, thickening, and often perforation.[180]

On ultrasound, marked thickening of the wall of the colon may be seen[180] (Figs. 8-126 and 8-127). The lumen may be anechoic, indicating fluid content. The right and transverse colons are affected, and loculated ascites may be present.[180] Although the ultrasound findings may not be specific, in the proper clinical setting the diagnosis should be considered.

Amebic Colitis

Endemic in the tropics, amebic colitis is not uncommon among visitors to these areas.[182] The offending trophozoite form of the parasite burrows into the intestinal wall, giving rise to flask-shaped mucosal ulcers, crypt abscesses, and inflammatory thickening of the colonic wall. The cecum and ascending colon are the most common sites of involvement. With chronic infection, the formation of a mass of granulation tissues (ameboma) may occur.

On ultrasound, the colonic wall is asymmetrically thickened. The thickened bowel wall (ranging from 8 to 17 mm) appears to be hypoechoic, surrounding a strongly echogenic gas-containing lumen[182] (Fig. 8-128). With a concomitant hepatic abscess, the diagnosis of amebic colitis is strongly suggested. It is not possible to differentiate this cause of bowel wall thickening from others by ultrasound alone.

Pseudomembranous Colitis

A sporadic, frequently severe and sometimes fatal iatrogenic disease, pseudomembranous colitis occurs almost exclusively in patients with antibiotic-related diarrhea.[183] It has been associated with a number of

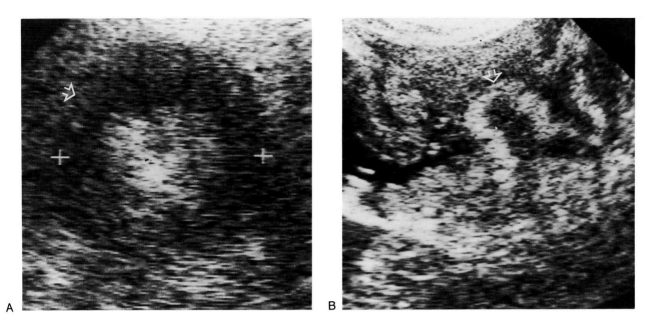

Fig. 8-126. Neutropenic typhlitis. **(A)** A 55-year-old man with a myelodysplastic syndrome developed typhlitis while undergoing systemic chemotherapy. Transverse sonographic scan showing thick-walled (2.5-cm) hypoechoic cecum (arrow). **(B)** A 36-year-old man with acute lymphoblastic leukemia developed typhlitis 5 days after completion of induction therapy in preparation for bone marrow transplantation. Sagittal sonographic scan showing thick-walled (1.2-cm) hyperechoic cecum and ascending colon (arrow). (From Teefey et al,[181] with permission.)

antibiotics including ampicillin, tetracycline, chloramphenicol, lincomycin, and clindamycin.[184] The microflora of the colon is altered by the antibiotics, facilitating colonization of the colon by *Clostridium difficile,* whose enterotoxin is cytotoxic and causes this disease.[183]

The most common clinical features of pseudomembranous colitis include watery diarrhea, colicky abdominal pain, pyrexia, leukocytosis, hypoalbuminemia, and hypovolemia.[183,184] This inflammatory, necrotizing bowel disorder usually involves the mucosa, although submucosal changes have been reported.[184]

This disease is diagnosed either by the endoscopic demonstration of characteristic pseudomembranes on the rectal or colonic mucosa or by finding the entero-

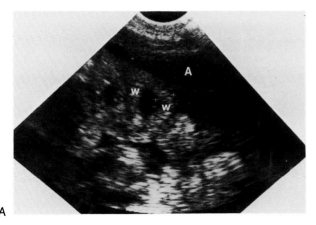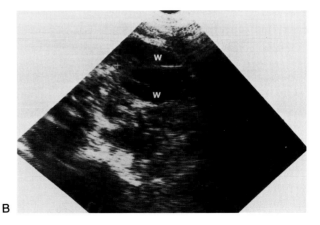

Fig. 8-127. Neutropenic colitis. Sonographic demonstration of neutropenic colitis. **(A)** Transverse image demonstrating a thickened colonic wall *(w)* measuring 8 mm. The lumen contains fluid. Loculated ascites *(A)* is present. **(B)** Longitudinal image demonstrating a thickened wall *(w).* The lumen is fluid-filled. (From Glass-Royal et al,[180] with permission.)

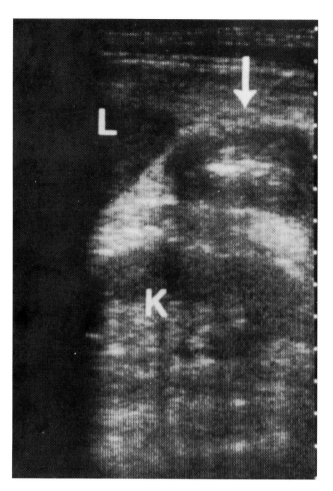

Fig. 8-128. Amebic colitis. Thickened wall of ascending colon in amebic colitis (arrow). (*K*, kidney; *L*, liver.) (From Hussain and Dinshaw,[182] with permission.)

toxin of *C. difficile* in the feces.[183] The disease usually responds to active conservative management once it is diagnosed. This includes the maintenance of fluid and electrolyte balance, the institution of appropriate antibiotic therapy, and the cessation of treatment with the implicated antibiotic.[183]

On ultrasound, the most striking feature includes moderate to marked thickening of the colon wall (range, 6 to 28 mm)[183,184] (Figs. 8-129 and 8-130). The thickened wall appears predominantly hypoechoic, and an irregular echogenic layer may be visible on its inner side, occluding the lumen.[184] Ultrasound may localize the bowel wall thickening to the area of the submucosal and mucosal layers. The colic lumen may be barely visible as a result of the marked thickening of the wall extending from the epigastrium to the left hypochondrium up to the left iliac fossa.[184] Marked distension of bowel loops full of gas at the level of the cecum and ascending colon

may also be visualized.[184] On plain radiograph, indirect evidence of colon wall thickening may be seen, including thumbprinting or thickened haustral bands.[183] Ascites may be found in addition to the bowel wall thickening.[183] As such, the constellation of findings — gross thickening of the colon wall, ascites, and the dearth of intraluminal contents, principally gas — are the key findings for this diagnosis.[183] The marked bowel wall thickening results from the associated gross submucosal edema.

In all patients with nonspecific clinical features, especially postoperative and intensive care patients who are likely to have received antibiotics, the bowel may be evaluated by ultrasound. In patients with a supporting clinical history and gross colonic wall thickening, ascites, and pancolitis, the diagnosis of pseudomembranous colitis should be considered. These findings should lead to a differential diagnoses of inflammatory bowel disease, tuberculosis, lymphangiectasia, intramural hemorrhage, ischemic colitis, and leukemic infiltration.[183,184] Although ultrasound may not be able to make the specific diagnosis, it should draw attention to it and lead to a recommendation for endoscopy and fecal *C. difficile* assay for a confirmatory diagnosis.[183]

Necrotizing Enterocolitis

Necrotizing enterocolitis (NEC) is an inflammatory process of the bowel seen in newborns and premature infants and characterized by the clinical findings of gastric retention, bilious vomiting, abdominal distension, bloody stools, diarrhea, and sometimes erythema of the abdominal wall.[185] It is among the most serious abdominal emergencies in newborns and young infants.[186] Complications include bowel perforation in 12 to 31 percent, which is an absolute indication for surgical intervention since the mortality in untreated patients is almost 100 percent.[187]

On plain film, there is bowel distension, pneumatosis of the bowel wall, portal venous gas, pneumoperitoneum, signs of intraperitoneal fluid, and the so-called fixed loop.[185] It may be difficult to define the free intraperitoneal air on plain film.[187]

On ultrasound, a tubular structure with a well-defined wall is seen across the left upper abdomen and in the left flank; it has the course and configuration of the transverse and descending colon.[185] The degree of damage to the bowel wall will depend on the extent of ischemia to which a segment of bowel is subjected. The finding of thickened bowel wall reflects the earliest pathologic process (i.e., transmural inflammation), which is the stage prior to the formation of intramural air[186] (Fig. 8-131). Portal venous system gas associated with this entity is an

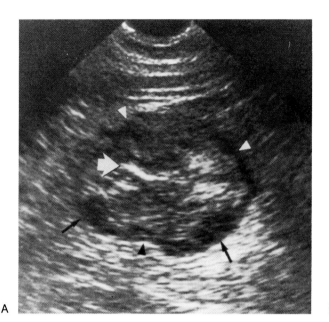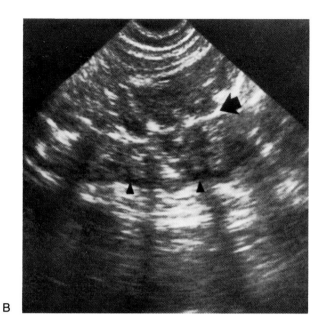

A   B

Fig. 8-129. Pseudomembranous colitis. A 54-year-old man with severe pseudomembranous colitis who underwent colectomy because of severe fluid and electrolyte imbalances. **(A)** Transverse and **(B)** sagittal sonographic images of the ascending colon demonstrating gross thickening of the bowel wall with effacement of the lumen (thick arrow). The pseudomembranous plaque, mucosal, and submucosal layers are not individually resolved but are collectively represented by a heterogeneous zone of medium echogenicity. The muscularis propria is shown as an outer hypoechoic layer (arrowheads). The focal expansions in this layer (thin arrows) are the taeniae coli muscles. (From Downey and Wilson,[183] with permission.)

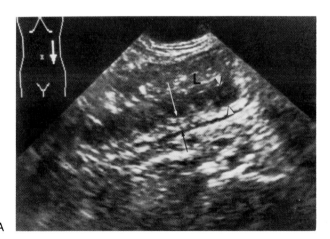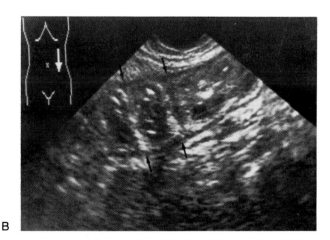

A   B

Fig. 8-130. Pseudomembranous colitis. **(A)** Coronal sonographic image of a 44-year-old man with mild pseudomembranous colitis and inflammatory changes mainly in the mucosal layer, showing a thickened, hypoechoic area (arrowheads) adjacent to the lumen *(L)* that represents the edematous mucosa. Surrounding this is a slightly thickened echogenic layer (arrows) representing the submucosa. The normal muscularis propria is shown as an outer, thin, hypoechoic layer. **(B)** Coronal sonographic scan of the descending colon of a 29-year-old woman with less severe pseudomembranous colitis showing thickened haustral bands (arrows). (From Downey and Wilson,[183] with permission.)

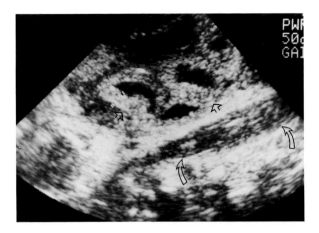

Fig. 8-131. Necrotizing enterocolitis. Longitudinal sonogram of the left flank, just below the tip of the left kidney, showing thick-walled, fluid-filled loops of bowel (open arrows). They were interpreted as being caused by nonspecific transmural inflammation; the age and presenting symptoms were consistent with necrotizing enterocolitis. The left psoas muscle is also seen (curved arrows). (From Patel et al,[186] with permission.)

uncommon and inconsistent finding and cannot be relied on for early diagnosis of this disease[186] (Fig. 8-132). If these findings are present on a sonogram of a neonate with a compatible clinical history, the diagnosis of necrotizing enterocolitis is almost certain.[186]

Late complications of this disease may include stenoses and acquired atresias in both large and small bowels, enteric fistulae, malabsorption, and the formation of enterocysts. On ultrasound, the enterocyst can be visualized with its mixed fluid and solid debris content, its well-defined wall, and its tubular form[185] (Fig. 8-133).

Air confined to Morison's pouch has been identified as an early sign of pneumoperitoneum[187] (Figs. 8-133 and 8-134). Morison's pouch is an intraperitoneal recess bounded anteriorly by the liver, posteriorly by the right kidney, and inferiorly by the coronary ligament, which forms the roof of the pouch.[187] This space corresponds to a loose areolar connective tissue space rich in lymphatics and veins connected to the portal system. This pericholecystic hyperechogenicity may correspond to an exten-

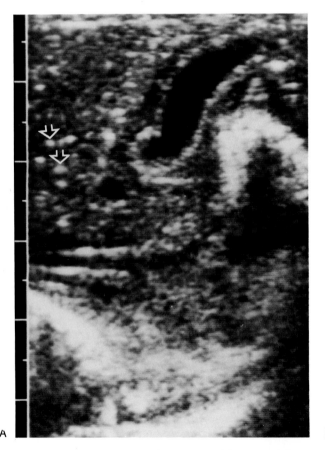

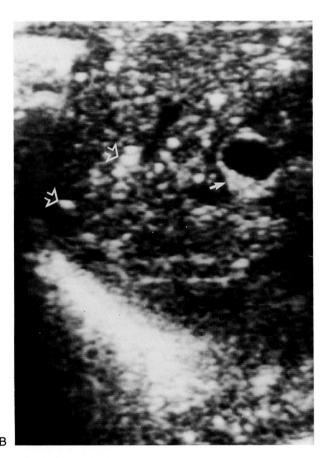

Fig. 8-132. Necrotizing enterocolitis. Necrotizing enterocolitis with gas in the portal system in a 10-day-old infant with hyaline membrane disease and hypoproteinemia. **(A)** Sagittal scan of the gallbladder. Hyperechogenicities are present but less diffuse. A hypoechoic rim can be seen around the gallbladder. (open arrows, portal gas.) **(B)** Oblique scan through the gallbladder neck. Hyperechogenicities are better visualized (arrow). (open arrow, portal gas.) (From Avni et al,[188] with permission.)

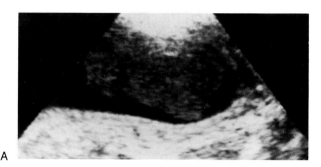

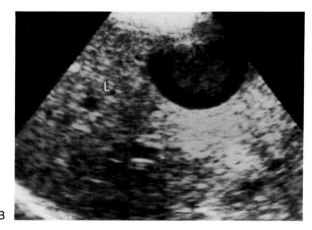

A

B

Fig. 8-133. Necrotizing enterocolitis, enterocyst formation. (**A**) Coronal sonogram of the left lateral abdomen showing a well-defined enterocyst with intraluminal fluid and solid debris. (**B**) Longitudinal sonogram of the left upper quadrant, 90-degree angle from the view in Fig. A, showing the enterocyst as a mass inferior to the left lobe of the liver (L). (From Ball and Wyly,[185] with permission.)

sion of the disease from the bowel up to the pericholecystic area[188] (Fig. 8-134). It may result from diffusion by contiguity through the lesser sac and/or the right gutter.[188] It could be related to the foamy infiltrate typical of NEC. Another explanation could be air within the pericholecystic vascular system similar to portal air.[188] This air can be seen as a triangular lucency in the right upper quadrant (Fig. 8-134). It may be difficult to differentiate this air from that in a bowel loop.

Pneumatosis Intestinalis

As with pneumatosis intestinalis affecting the small bowel, that involving the colon may be associated with a wide variety of abnormalities such as bowel infarction,

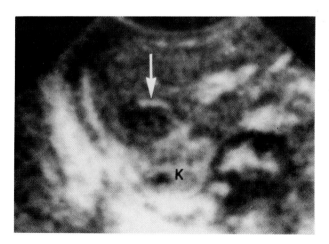

Fig. 8-134. Necrotizing enterocolitis. Transverse sonogram showing an abscess collection in Morison's pouch (arrow). (*K*, kidney.) (From Brill et al,[187] with permission.)

collagen vascular disease, chronic bronchitis and asthma, ulcer disease, and diverticulitis.[125,189] In rare cases, it has been found in association with inflammatory bowel disease, including ulcerative colitis.[189] On ultrasound, intramural gas (high-amplitude echoes with acoustic shadowing) may be demonstrated along with bowel wall thickening[189] (Fig. 8-135). Ultrasound may be more sensitive in the detection of intramural air than plain film. The true value of recognizing this sign on ultrasound is in the early diagnosis of bowel ischemia.

Diverticular Disease

The term *diverticular disease* includes both diverticulosis and diverticulitis, both of which are characterized by numerous saccular outpouchings in the colon.[38] Diverticular disease is quite common in Western societies, occurring in about one-third of people over the age of 60.[38] Most often diverticulosis is asymptomatic, but at times it can produce symptoms. Both forms of diverticular disease can produce generalized lower abdominal discomfort with intermittent or continuous pain.[38] Constipation, which is frequent, sometimes alternates with diarrhea. In most cases, the condition is found incidently during a barium enema examination. The sigmoid colon is the most often involved segment of colon (in 95 percent of cases), but the descending colon and entire colon may be affected.[38]

Diverticula represent herniations of the mucosa through the muscle coat at points of weakness, such as between the longitudinal taeniae and where the circular muscle is weakened by the segmental blood vessels that pierce it in two rows on each side of the colon. The

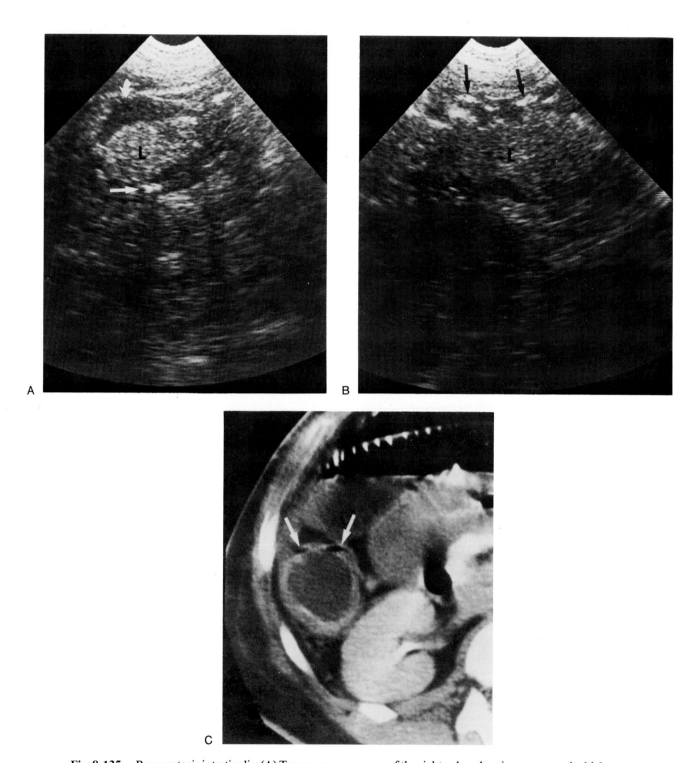

Fig. 8-135. Pneumatosis intestinalis. **(A)** Transverse sonogram of the right colon showing asymmetric thickening of right colonic wall (curved arrow) with areas of intramural gas with acoustic shadowing (arrow). (*L*, fluid-filled lumen.) **(B)** Longitudinal sonogram showing intramural gas (arrows). Acoustic shadowing is less apparent on this view. (*L*, fluid-filled lumen.) **(C)** CT scan confirming the presence of intramural gas (arrows) and colonic wall thickening. (From Vernacchia et al,[189] with permission.)

mechanical force creating these herniations at points of weakness is provided by elevated intracolonic pressure. The increased pressure is attributed to changes in the quantity and character of the stools, which in turn alter the force and mechanical characteristics of the peristaltic contractions.[38]

Colon can be distinguished from small bowel by the following: its location (especially immediately posterior to the urinary bladder), its lack of valvulae conniventes, and its lack of typical small bowel peristalsis.[190] In asymptomatic patients, diverticula are rarely noticeable on ultrasound, even though diverticula of the colon occur in about 50 percent of adults.[191] With spasm, edema, and inflammation of the gut wall, there is improved visualization of the thickened gut segment; inflammation of the diverticular wall accentuates the diverticulum. Inflamed diverticuli are seen on ultrasound as outpouchings protruding beyond the lumen of the gut into or beyond the thickened wall[191] (Figs. 8-136 and 8-137). Ultrasound may be helpful in the preliminary evaluation of patients with a classic presentation of acute diverticulitis.[191] It is important to be able to differentiate acute diverticulitis from other causes of acute right lower quadrant pain such as acute appendicitis.

Ultrasound has been used to evaluate patients for acute diverticulitis.[191] To make the diagnosis on the basis

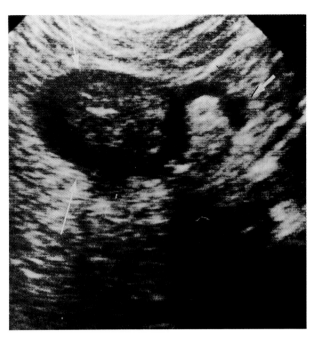

Fig. 8-137. Diverticulitis in a 52-year-old man with left lower quadrant pain, fever, and elevated white blood cell count. Cross-sectional sonogram showing a thickened loop of gut (long arrows) with a large, inflamed diverticulum (short arrow) that has thickened wall protruding beyond the margin of the gut wall. Contrast enema confirmed acute diverticulitis. (From Wilson and Toi,[191] with permission.)

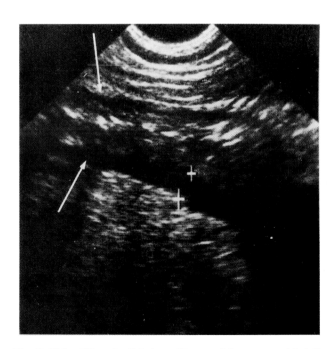

Fig. 8-136. Diverticulitis in a 63-year-old woman with left lower quadrant pain. Sagittal sonogram showing a thick loop of gut (arrows) with typical thick muscularis propria (calipers). An inflamed diverticulum was seen on other views. Contrast enema confirmed acute diverticulitis. (From Wilson and Toi,[191] with permission.)

of ultrasound, two of the following must be present: (1) focal gut wall thickening (greater than 4 mm with a range of 5 to 15 mm); (2) inflamed diverticula (echogenic shadowing foci seen in outpouches of thickened colon wall or beyond pericolonic soft tissues); (3) inflammatory changes in the pericolic fat (poorly defined zones of hypoechogenicity in pericolic fat); (4) intramural or pericolic inflammatory mass (presence of fluid or air in mass/abscess); and (5) intramural fistulae[190,191] (Figs. 8-136 to 8-140). Additional findings include a round or oval focus of various echogenicity that protrudes from a segmentally thickened colonic wall and is surrounded by hypoechoic foci with internal strong echoes, and echogenic shadowing foci with surrounding hypoechoic bands.[192] Long segments of the colon may be involved; the maximum length is 2 to 9 cm with the maximum thickness 5 to 17 mm.[190,192] The thickening of the colon may be secondary to inflammation rather than smooth muscle hypertrophy.[190] In some patients, extraluminal gas and thickening of the lateroconal fascia are seen.[192] One of the major ultrasound findings in uncomplicated acute diverticulitis appears to be the hypoechoic round or oval focus protruding from segmentally thickened colonic wall.

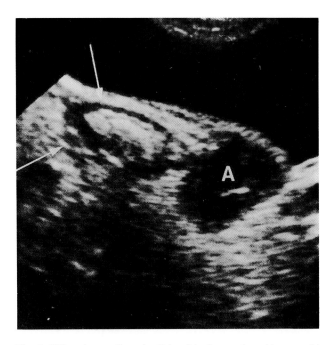

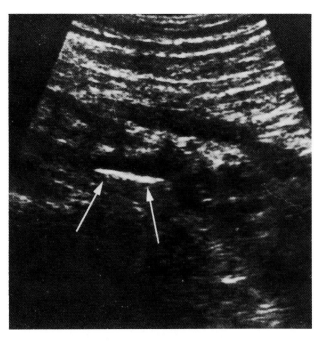

Fig. 8-138. Acute diverticulitis with abscess in a 41-year-old man with recurrent severe pelvic pain, fever, and elevated white blood cell count. Oblique sonogram showing an abscess *(A)* adjacent to a mildly thickened loop of gut (arrows). CT scan and surgery confirmed acute diverticulitis with abscess formation. (From Wilson and Toi,[191] with permission.)

Fig. 8-139. Acute diverticulitis in a 35-year-old man with recurrent left lower quadrant pain and fever. Sagittal sonogram showing a loop of thickened gut with an intramural sinus tract seen as an echogenic line (arrows) deep to the muscularis propria. Surgery confirmed acute diverticulitis. (From Wilson and Toi,[191] with permission.)

If perforation of an inflammatory diverticulum or spread of a peridiverticulitis gives rise to a paracolic abscess, a hypoechoic to anechoic mass may be identified within the pelvis (Fig. 8-138). Intramural abscesses may be seen as well-circumscribed anechoic masses within the thickened colonic wall (Fig. 8-139). Abscesses appear as poorly delineated pericolonic cystic masses containing echogenic debris. The associated peritoneal cavity abscesses usually appear as predominantly cystic masses containing echogenic debris.[190] If a hypoechoic mass is seen, and the patient is known to have diverticular disease and is symptomatic, an abscess should be suspected. If an abscess is highly suspected, computed tomography (CT) is recommended, as it would be if the ultrasound were nondiagnostic.[191]

Not only might ultrasound prove helpful in establishing the diagnosis of acute diverticulitis, but also it might be helpful in monitoring the patient while on therapy.[190,191] Patients who have exhibited bowel wall thickening on initial scans have been noted to have improvement (less bowel wall thickening) on scans obtained 4 to 7 days after presentation.[191] The rapid change may be more likely be secondary to relief of spasm and resolu-

tion of edema and inflammation than to decreased smooth muscle hypertrophy.[191]

The accuracy of the ultrasound evaluation of acute diverticulitis has been assessed.[193] A sensitivity of 84.6 percent is found, with a specificity of 80.3 percent, a positive predictive value of 76 percent, and a negative predictive value of 87.7 percent.[193] The ultrasound diagnosis is most likely if the bowel wall thickening is diffuse and hypoechoic and is more than 4 mm or at least a 5-cm segment is involved.[193] In many patients (28.8 percent), fluid-filled bowel loops are seen. In 5.7 percent, air-containing diverticula are seen within the poorly echoic enlarged bowel wall. Pericolonic abscesses or colovesical fistulas may be missed by ultrasound. It can be concluded that ultrasound may be used as a screening method in patients with the clinical signs of acute diverticulitis.[193]

Colovesical Fistula

With colovesical fistulas, the patient presents with the typical symptoms of pneumaturia or fecaluria.[194] The most common cause is diverticular disease, but it may

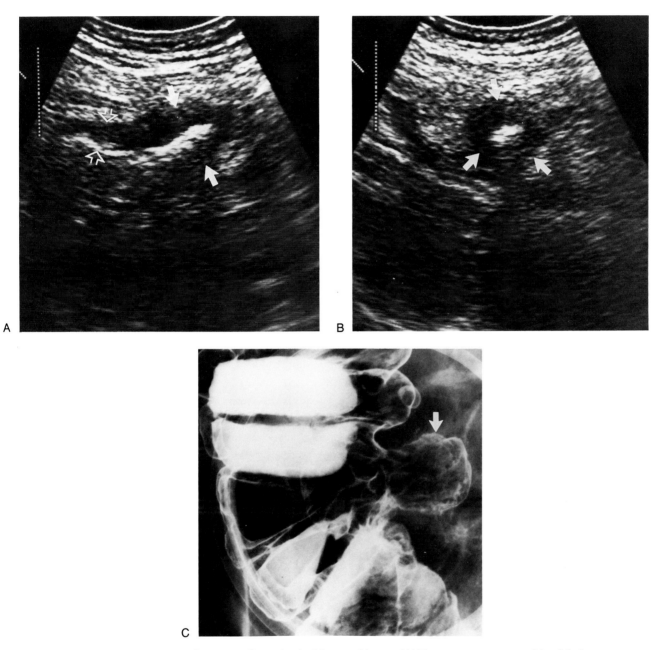

Fig. 8-140. Diverticulitis of the ascending colon in 56-year-old man. **(A)** Transverse sonogram of the right lower quadrant showing an echogenic focus with surrounding hypoechoic band (solid arrows), which is protruding medially from the slightly thickened colonic wall (open arrows). **(B)** Longitudinal sonogram showing a round echogenic shadowing focus with a surrounding hypoechoic band (arrows). **(C)** Follow-up double-contrast barium enema showing a large diverticulum (arrow) protruding medially from the ascending colon immediately above the ileocecal valve. A few small diverticula also are seen in ascending colon. (From Wada et al,[192] with permission.)

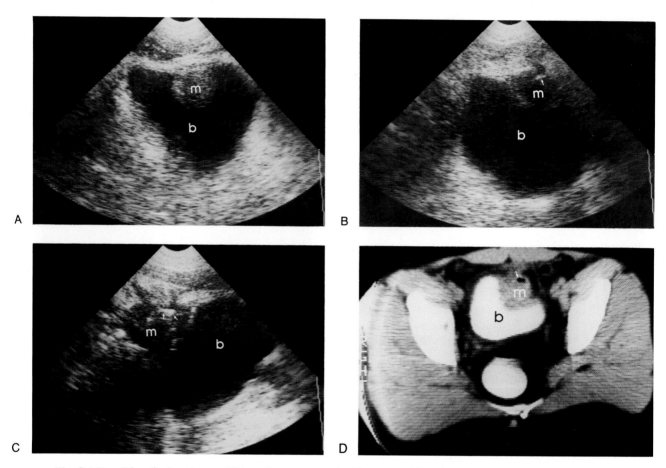

Fig. 8-141.   Diverticular abscess. This patient presented with suprapubic pain. At cystoscopy, a bladder wall mass was visualized; biopsy revealed inflammation. **(A & B)** Transverse scans through the bladder *(b)*, from inferior to superior views, showing an echodense mass *(m)* projecting into the bladder. In Fig. B there was a linear echodensity (arrow) within the mass. Peristalsis was seen there with real-time scanning. **(C)** Longitudinal scan demonstrating a mass *(m)* superior to the bladder *(b)*. As in Fig. B, peristalsis was seen in the area of the linear echodensity (arrows). As such, this mass was believed to be related to the bowel. **(D)** CT scan similar to Fig. B, showing a soft tissue-density mass *(m)* projecting into the bladder *(b)*. Air (arrow) is seen within the mass. On a CT scan at a higher level than in Fig. D, air was seen within many diverticuli. At surgery, the patient was found to have a diverticular abscess involving the bladder wall.

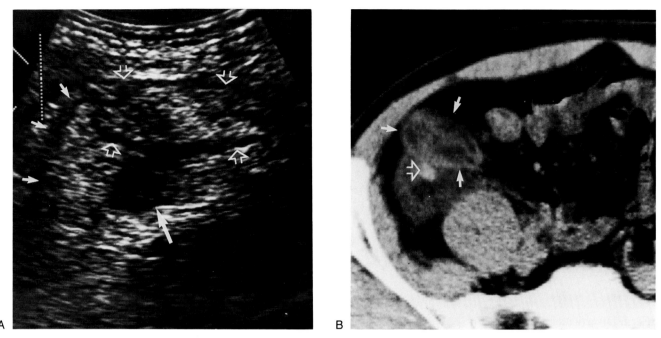

A   B

Fig. 8-142. Cecal diverticulitis in a 41-year-old man. **(A)** Initial transverse sonogram of the right lower quadrant showing a round hypoechoic focus (large white arrow) protruding from thickened cecal wall (open arrows). Thickened lateroconal fascia (small arrows) is also seen. **(B)** CT scan obtained immediately after sonography showing a small area of slightly increased density (open arrow) adjacent to the thickened cecal wall (solid arrows). This small high-density area corresponds to the hypoechoic focus on the sonogram. A soft tissue density indicative of pericecal inflammatory change is seen behind the cecum. (From Wada et al,[192] with permission.)

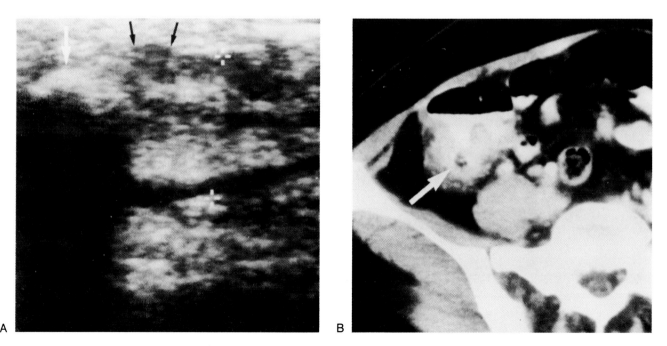

A   B

Fig. 8-143. Cecal diverticulitis. **(A)** Compression sonogram in a patient with surgically proved cecal diverticulitis showing an echogenic shadowing focus (white arrow) at the right margin of the cecum, with adjacent thickening of cecal wall (black arrows). Calipers mark the anterior and posterior margins of the cecum. Gas normally present within the cecal lumen is displaced by the compression maneuver and is not visualized. **(B)** CT scan showing marked cecal wall thickening around a stool-filled diverticulum (arrow). Probable identification of a normal appendix was made on a more caudal image. (From Townsend et al,[195] with permission.)

also be secondary to neoplasm.[194] The fluid within the bladder provides a good contrast background to compression of the bowel. With ultrasound, an echogenic beak may be seen connecting the peristaltic bowel lumen and urinary bladder (Fig. 8-141). Echogenic material may be forced from the beak into the bladder lumen by manual compression of the lower abdomen.[194] The size of the "jet" is related to the size of the fistula, the condition of the bowel, and the nature of the feces. Additional findings include movable echogenic material without acoustic shadowing in the urinary bladder, reverberation artifacts from the superficial portion of the bladder indicative of gas, and bowel adhering to the dome of the bladder that has an echogenic beak connecting the peristaltic lumen of the bowel and urinary bladder[194] (Fig. 8-141). The strong echogenicity of the fistula may be due to its hyperreflective lumen or its contents.

Cecal Diverticulitis

As with *Campylobacter* enteritis or Crohn's disease, cecal diverticulitis may mimic acute appendicitis.[195] It is a relatively uncommon cause of right lower quadrant pain. It is important to make the correct diagnosis because this entity is treated initially with antibiotics.

This diagnosis should be suggested if, on compression ultrasound examination of the right lower quadrant, diverticulum or diverticula are seen with a thickened noncompressible cecal wall and focal tenderness.[195] Discrete outpouchings that contain shadowing echogenic material are noted emanating from the wall of an abnormally thickened noncompressible cecum[195] (Figs. 8-142 and 8-143). Fecaliths may be present, as may a pericolic abscess. Without the presence of a diverticulum, a pericecal inflammatory mass would be nonspecific.[195]

Tumor

Colonic Polyp

It may be difficult to identify colonic polyps by ultrasound because of the presence of mucus, feces, and gas within the colon, which, in the supine position, collects anteriorly, causing more or less complete distal acoustic shadowing.[196] The colon may be examined by ultrasound using a warm isotonic saline enema with the patient in the supine position.[196] By using this technique, better identification of the rectosigmoid colon may be accomplished. A polyp head may be seen during the real-time examination as a lobular surface area (Figs. 8-144 and 8-145), although an adequate assessment of the bowel wall thickness at the base of the polyp may not be possible. Under optimal conditions, real-time ultrasound may provide detailed information about polypoid lesions.[196] Still, the ultrasound examination cannot replace the barium enema or colonoscopy in the primary evaluation of the large bowel.

By using a retrograde instillation of fluid into the colon, polyps larger than 7 mm can be identified in 91 percent of patients, whereas those smaller than 7 mm are not always visualized.[10] These colonic polyps appear as hyperechoic structures projecting into the colonic lumen.[10]

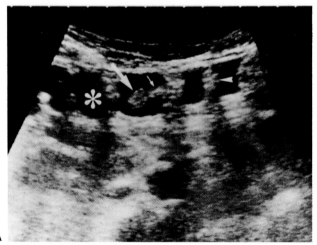
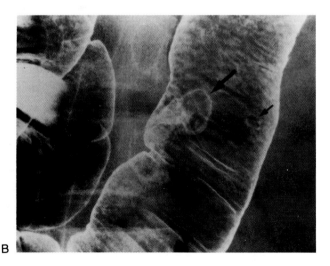

Fig. 8-144. Colonic polyp. **(A)** Sonogram showing a pedunculated polyp less than 20 mm in size. The shaft (short arrow) and the head (long arrow) of the polyp are clearly noted in this figure. (asterisk, bowel lumen; arrowhead, haustral fold). **(B)** Radiograph of the polyp. The sessile polyp, smaller than 10 mm (short arrow), near the large pedunculated polyp (long arrow) was overlooked. (From Hirooka et al,[12] with permission.)

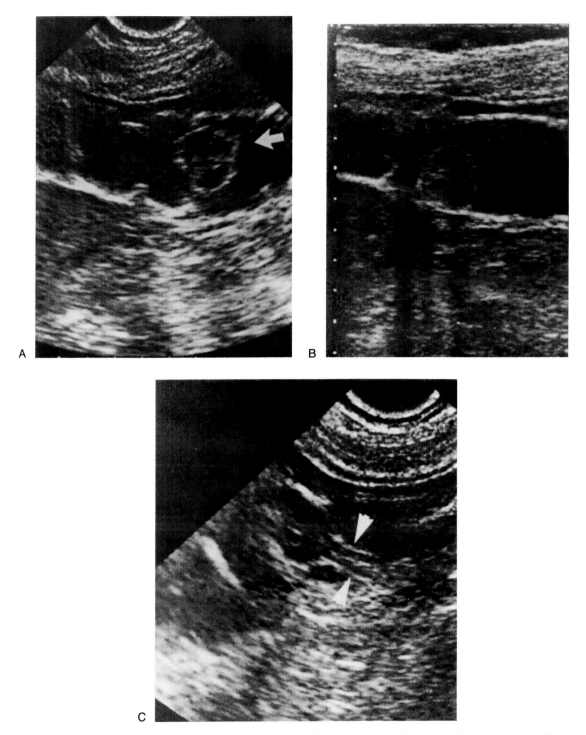

Fig. 8-145. Colonic polyp. **(A)** Half of the polyp head in the fluid-filled descending colon shows a lobular surface (arrow). **(B)** The other part of the polyp head has a smooth surface contour. **(C)** A long, smooth stalk (arrowheads) with central vessels is clearly identified. (From Skaane,[196] with permission.)

Carcinoma

It is a prime challenge for the medical profession to identify cancer of the colon, since this lesion produces symptoms early and is potentially curable by resection. Colon carcinoma is the second commonest cancer in the United States, with a 5-year survival rate of approximately 50 percent.[196] The peak incidence occurs in the seventh decade, with fewer than 20 percent occurring in patients under 50 years of age. Eighty percent of cases occur in the rectum, rectosigmoid, or sigmoid colon, with 2.6 to 5 percent being multiple.[14,38] Lesions of the left colon tend to grow in an annular encircling fash-

ion, whereas those on the right tend to be polypoid and fungating masses. The patient most commonly presents with rectal bleeding and/or a change in bowel habit.[38] With increased use of screening along with endoscopic polypectomy, the mortality rate may be lowered.[197]

A number of factors lead to an increased risk for colorectal carcinoma.[197] The most common of these is a prior adenoma or a family history of colon carcinoma.[197] If a prophylactic colectomy is not performed in patients with familial polyposis coli or Gardner syndrome, colon carcinoma will develop.[197] At additional risk are patients who have had extensive ulcerative colitis for 7 years or

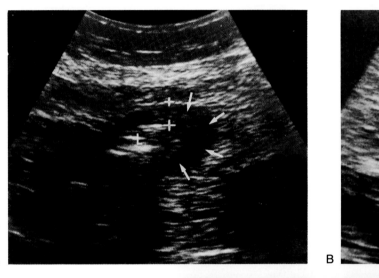

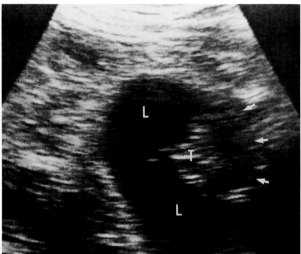

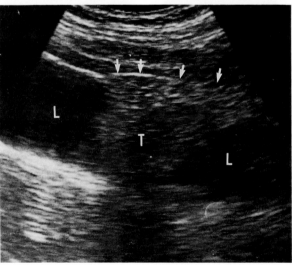

Fig. 8-146. Colon carcinoma. **(A)** Carcinoma of the transverse colon. A target lesion with an eccentric thickened anechoic gastrointestinal wall (arrows) and an echogenic lumen *(L)* is seen. **(B)** Carcinoma of the rectosigmoid colon. The tumor *(T)* appears as an echogenic structure projecting into the fluid-filled echofree intestinal lumen *(L)*. The base of the tumor has infiltrated the surrounding tissue (arrows). **(C)** Carcinoma of the descending colon almost completely occluding the intestinal lumen *(L)*. The tumor *(T)* has penetrated into the surrounding tissue (arrows), and the normal structure of the intestinal wall has been destroyed. (From Limberg,[11] with permission.)

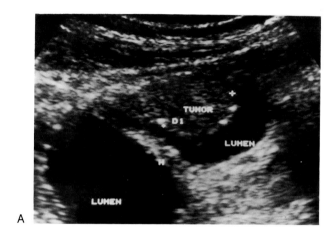
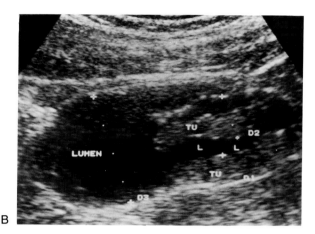

Fig. 8-147. Colon carcinoma. **(A)** A 2.5-cm carcinoma of the sigmoid. **(B)** Stenosing carcinoma of the descending colon. (*Tu,* tumor; *L,* lumen.) (From Limberg,[10] with permission.)

more; the same is true for patients with Crohn's disease, but to a lesser extent.[197] Also at risk are patients who have had breast or uterine carcinoma, those who have had pelvic radiation, and those with ureterosigmoidostomy.[197]

It is recommended that patients at average risk — those aged 40 and over without a known predisposing factor — undergo a periodic digital rectal examination involving testing for fecal occult blood and sigmoidoscopy.[197] The fecal occult blood test is the cornerstone in this screening approach because it has a positive rate of 2 to 6 percent. Colon cancer is seen in approximately 10 percent of patients over age 40 who present with recent onset of rectal bleeding.[197] Up to 72 percent of colonic polyps and up to 55 percent of colonic carcinoma cannot be detected by the fecal occult blood test.[10]

The primary method of detecting colorectal carcinoma is not CT or ultrasound, but these modalities may reveal the cancer as an incidental finding. Bowel wall thickening may be visualized by ultrasound, resulting in a target or pseudokidney configuration (Figs. 8-146 and 8-147). This bowel wall thickening may be asymmetric, resulting in variations of the target pattern. Preoperative assessment should be directed first toward an examination of the large bowel for synchronous neoplasms and then secondarily for a search for possible metastatic disease.[197] There is synchronous carcinoma in approximately 5 percent of patients.[197]

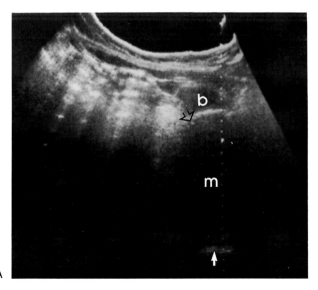
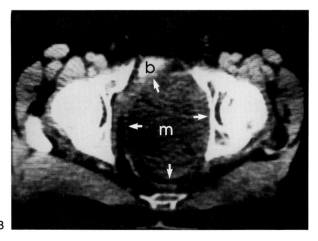

Fig. 8-148. Colon carcinoma. Rectal carcinoma. **(A)** Longitudinal scan showing hypoechoic mass (*m*, arrows) posterior to the bladder *(b)*. **(B)** CT scan showing a large soft tissue mass (*m*, arrows) posterior to the bladder *(b)* in the area of the rectum.

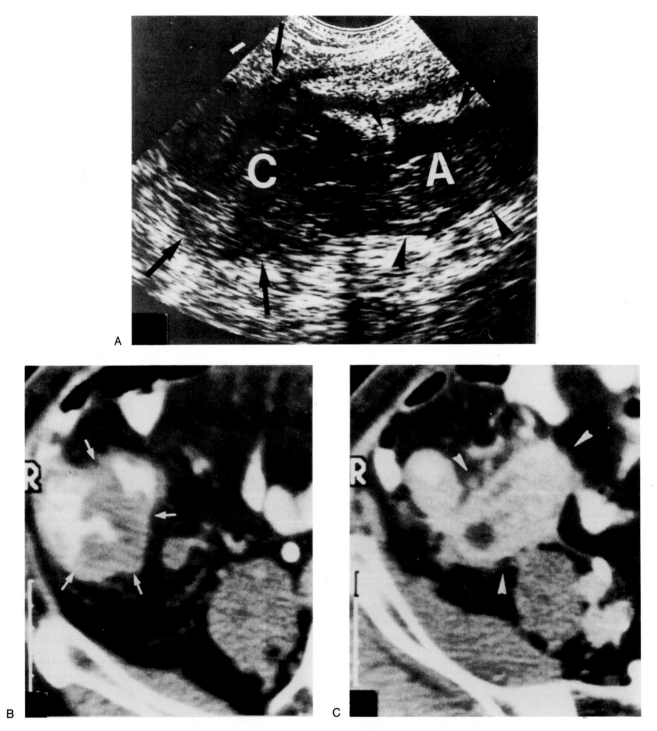

Fig. 8-149. Appendiceal involvement in cecal carcinoma. **(A)** Oblique sonogram of the right lower quadrant showing the markedly thickened appendix (*A*, arrowheads) contiguous with a hypoechoic mass, representing the cecal carcinoma (*C*, arrows). **(B & C)** CT scans confirming the sonographic diagnosis of cecal carcinoma (arrows) associated with appendicitis (arrowheads). (From Becking et al,[201] with permission.)

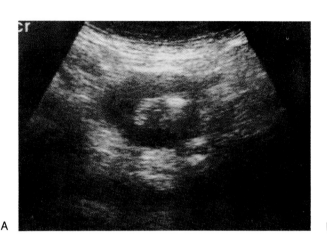

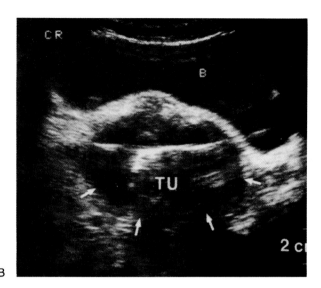

Fig. 8-150. Lymphoma. **(A)** An 83-year-old man with generalized non-Hodgkin's lymphoma of low-grade malignancy. Sonogram showing a target lesion in the transverse colon. Pathologic examination showed transmural circumferential infiltration by non-Hodgkin's lymphoma. **(B)** Primary high-grade malignant non-Hodgkin's lymphoma of the sigmoid colon with transmural involvement and bulky disease. Midline sonogram of lower abdomen showing a well-defined hypoechoic mass lesion (*TU*, arrows) with echogenic gas collections behind the urinary bladder *(B)*, mimicking abscess formation of the pouch of Douglas. (From Goerg et al,[82] with permission.)

Although these lesions are usually diagnosed by barium enema, rectal examinations, or sigmoidoscopy, they are sometimes detected by ultrasound. Because it is limited by intraluminal gas, ultrasound only occasionally is able to see either mural or intramural lesions (Fig. 8-147). With a high degree of obstruction and a fluid-filled proximal bowel, the obstructive lesion may be visible, as in hypertrophic pyloric stenosis.[198] If the bowel wall is thickened and compressed or obliterated, a tumor should be suspected.[198] A bull's-eye pattern is generally seen, with wall thickening producing the hypoechoic oval mass and a central echogenic area produced by luminal air.[26,199,200] The more the wall is infiltrated, the broader the hypoechoic area[200] (Figs. 8-146 and 8-148). If this mass is in the right lower quadrant, the examiner should suspect a cecal origin; if it is in the right upper

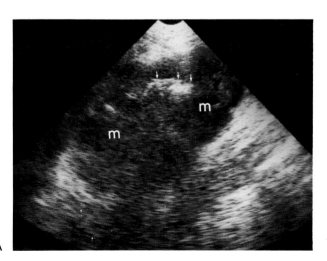

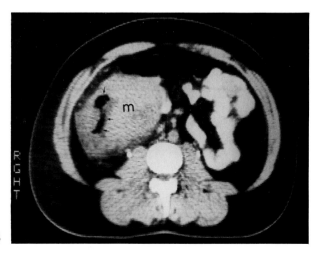

Fig. 8-151. Colon, non-Hodgkin's lymphoma. **(A)** Sagittal real-time scan demonstrating a large, lobulated hypoechoic mass *(m)*. A reflective pattern (arrows), which represents air in the bowel lumen, is seen. **(B)** CT scan demonstrating a soft tissue-density mass *(m)* that encases the colon. Air (arrows) is seen within the bowel lumen.

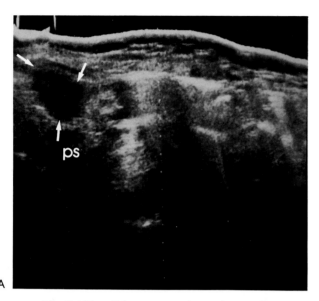 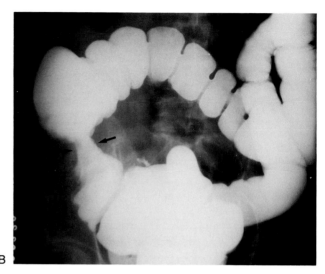

Fig. 8-152. Colon, metastatic ovarian carcinoma. **(A)** Transverse scan at 7 cm above the umbilicus showing a hypoechoic mass (arrows) in the right abdomen anterior to the psoas muscle *(ps).* **(B)** Barium enema showing an apple-core-type lesion (arrows) involving the ascending colon in the region of the mass on ultrasound.

quadrant, hepatic flexure tumor should be suspected. The differential diagnosis for the target pattern should include tuberculosis and amebiasis as well as tumor.[200]

By using retrograde instillation of fluid into the colon, the diagnostic value of ultrasound is improved in assessing neoplastic disease of the colon examined by colonic ultrasound.[10] Tumor on ultrasound is evaluated by the diameter of the intestinal lumen, thickness of the GI wall, evidence of local wall thickening, and presence of intraluminal echogenic structures fixed to the wall[10] (Figs. 8-146 and 8-147). This technique has a sensitivity of 94 percent in detecting colonic carcinoma, with a specificity of 100 percent.[10] These results suggest that colonic ultrasound might be an effective screening procedure for neoplastic diseases of the colon.[10]

It may be difficult to distinguish between primary appendicitis with inflammatory mass formation and secondary appendicitis due to cecal cancer.[201] Both entities may have identical symptoms. A cecal neoplasm may cause appendicitis and may mimic the clinical symptoms of acute appendicitis.[201] With cecal cancer, ultrasound may demonstrate a hypoechoic cecal mass, contiguous with a clearly visible thickened appendix[201] (Fig. 8-149). This diagnosis should be considered in middle-aged or elderly patients with clinical signs of appendicitis.[201]

Lymphoma

Representing only 0.5 percent of all malignant tumors of the colon, primary colonic lymphoma accounts for 4 percent of all extranodal lymphoma and represents 5 to 9.4 percent of primary GI tract lymphomas.[202] Colonic lymphomas are infrequent relative to their occurrence in the stomach and small intestine. These tumors have the same morphologic and clinical characteristics as those in the upper segments of the bowel, which were described above.

Ultrasound shows a target pattern or simply a hypoechoic mass (Figs. 8-150 and 8-151). This lesion may be seen as a complex lobulated mass with a hypoechoic periphery and a central echogenic area. If on real-time scanning a reflective pattern (due to bowel gas) or peristalsis is seen within the mass, the examiner should suspect bowel involvement. Colonic involvement is suspected if such a mass is in the area of the colon.

Metastatic Disease

Metastatic disease to the colon is uncommon. Such lesions could produce a target pattern or a solid mass (Fig. 8-152).

TRANSRECTAL ULTRASOUND

TECHNIQUE

Transrectal ultrasound is a technique in which a 4- to 7-MHz radial (axial) transducer or a 5- to 7-MHz longitudinally oriented transducer is inserted into the rectum[203-205] (Fig. 8-153). These transducers are covered with a fluid-filled disposable shear latex rubber sheath to avoid contamination of the transducer and probe with the rectal mucosa and rectal contents.[204] A cleansing enema may be given prior to the study. The examination may be performed in the dorsal lithotomy position or left lateral decubitus position. Images may be obtained at 1-cm intervals from the level of 2 cm superior to the anus to the level of 15 cm from the anus or the maximum depth of the transducer.[205] The examination takes from 10 to 15 minutes. Patients tolerate the procedure well, and no complications usually occur.[204]

NORMAL ANATOMY

On transrectal ultrasound, the normal rectal wall appears as two dark hypoechoic and three white hyperechoic lines when a 7-MHz transducer is used[203,205,206] (Fig. 8-153). The inner white line represents the water balloon, together with an interface of water and mucosa. The middle white line is the interface between the mucosa and muscularis. The outer hyperechoic white line represents the interface of the muscularis and fat. The inner hypoechoic dark line is the mucosa, with the outermost hypoechoic dark line the muscularis.[203] As such, the following hyperechoic layers are seen: the balloon-

mucosa interface, the submucosa, and the muscularis propria-perirectal fat interface.[205,206] The two hypoechoic layers are the muscularis mucosa and the muscularis propria.[205]

Although transrectal ultrasound was initially developed for evaluation of the prostate, it has more recently been adapted for evaluation of rectal and perirectal disease.[206,207] It can detect all masses situated within 12 cm of the anus.[207] A number of abnormalities have been identified by this technique, including primary and secondary rectal carcinoma, metastases, villous adenoma, leiomyosarcoma, endometriosis, sacrococcygeal teratoma, chordoma, retroperitoneal cystic hamartoma, pelvic lipomatosis, diverticulitis, and perirectal abscess.[206] Additionally, it may be helpful in the localization of perirectal abscesses and in the sonographically guided biopsy of perirectal masses.[206]

APPLICATIONS

Rectal Tumor

The purpose of transrectal ultrasound with regard to rectal carcinoma is threefold: (1) to improve surgical planning; (2) to provide a prognosis in nonsurgical candidates, and (3) to indicate which patients are suitable for local excision.[205] Transrectal ultrasound has been used in the assessment of the depth of tumor invasion in patients with rectal carcinoma.[197,203-205,207] Rectal carcinoma appears as a low-echogenicity lesion that abruptly interrupts the normal sequence of the layers[206] (Figs. 8-154 and 8-155). The tumor may be smooth or lobulated.[207] Involvement of only the mucosa cannot be distinguished from lesions involving both the mucosa and submucosa.[207] If there is extension into the perirectal area, there is a break in the hyperechoic line of acoustic reflectors of the submucosal-fascial layer.[207] Transrectal ultrasound is the only imaging technique that differentiates individual layers of the rectal wall (assessing the depth of invasion) and characterizes the lymph nodes.[203]

Lymph Node Disease

In both the assessment of the depth of invasion and lymph node disease, transrectal ultrasound is an accurate method of staging rectal tumors.[208] With nonspe-

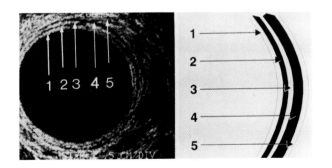

Fig. 8-153. Transrectal ultrasound. Sonogram and drawing show five layers of normal rectum: *(1)* interface between balloon and mucosa, *(2)* deep mucosa and muscularis mucosa, *(3)* interface between submucosa and muscularis propria, *(4)* muscularis propria, and *(5)* interface between muscularis propria and perirectal fat. (From St Ville et al,[206] with permission.)

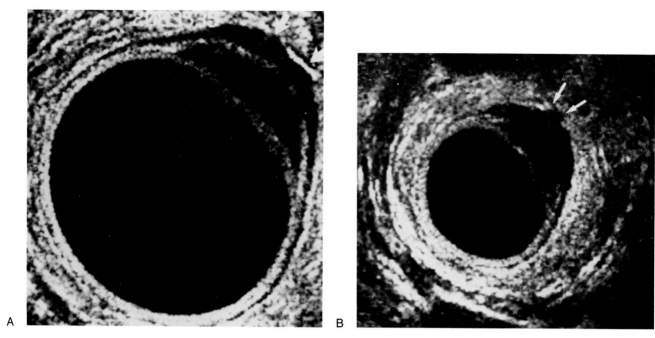

Fig. 8-154.   Transrectal ultrasound of primary rectal carcinoma with local invasion. **(A)** Sonogram showing soft-tissue mass with the muscularis propria in the left anterolateral wall of the rectum (arrows). **(B)** Sonogram obtained at a higher level showing a mass, which appears to disrupt the muscularis propria (arrows) and invade the perirectal fat planes. (From St Ville et al,[206] with permission.)

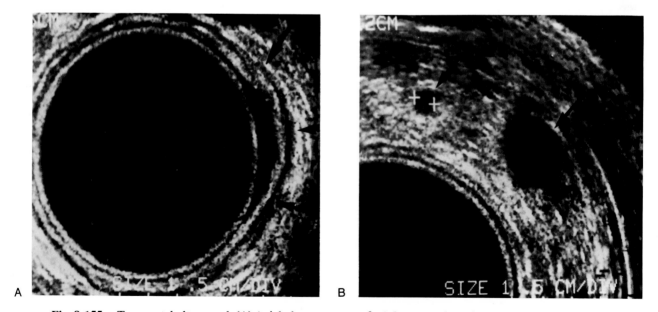

Fig. 8-155.   Transrectal ultrasound. **(A)** Axial ultrasonogram of a 1.5-cm rectal carcinoma depicted within the muscularis propria (arrows). **(B)** Axial ultrasonogram cephalic to the carcinoma, demonstrating 1-cm and 3-mm perirectal lymph nodes (arrows) that were found to be malignant at operation. Because of the ultrasonographic findings, the surgical procedure was changed from local excision to abdominoperineal resection. (From Jochem et al,[205] with permission.)

cific inflammatory change, enlarged hyperechoic lymph nodes may be seen[206] (Fig. 8-155). Metastases are most likely when lymph nodes are hypoechoic.[206]

Recurrent Rectal Tumor

As a rule, local recurrence usually occurs early (70 to 80 percent of recurrences appear within 2 years of surgery) and with a variable but high incidence (6 to 32 percent).[209] Transrectal ultrasound can confirm and more accurately define the extent of neoplastic infiltration with recurrence.[209] On ultrasound, such a lesion can be seen as a round, hypoechoic, nonhomogeneous perirectal mass that is completely extramural in the early stages with later infiltration of the rectal wall[209] (Fig. 8-156). This technique is 97 percent accurate, 94 percent sensitive, and 98 percent specific, with a positive predictive value of 85 percent and a negative predictive value of 99 percent.[209] As such, transrectal ultrasound may have a place in the postoperative evaluation of patients with rectal carcinoma.[209]

Abscess

Besides evaluation for neoplastic disease, transrectal ultrasound may be used to evaluate for abscesses, partic-

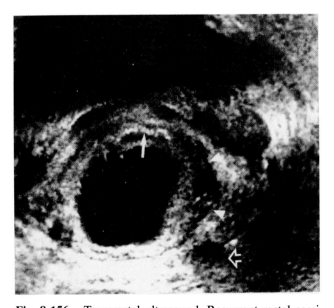

Fig. 8-156. Transrectal ultrasound. Recurrent rectal carcinoma. Sonogram obtained after abdominoperineal resection showing diffuse thickening of the rectal wall and disruption of the muscularis propria (arrowhead). Enlarged perirectal lymph nodes also were identified (open arrow). A surgical suture is present in the anterior rectal wall (solid arrow). Biopsy revealed recurrent rectal carcinoma. (From St Ville et al,[206] with permission.)

ularly supralevator abscess.[210] There are a number of causes of perirectal abscesses (usually cryptoglandular in origin), including foreign body, trauma, cancer, Crohn's disease, hemorrhoids, anal fissures, or surgery.[210] These abscesses may be classified into four types on the basis of their associated physical findings: perianal, ischirectal, intersphincteric, and supralevator.[210] As a rule, they are diagnosed by physical examination. They may be seen on ultrasound as a thick-walled, relatively echofree mass posterior to the rectum[210] (Fig. 8-157).

Transrectal ultrasound can be helpful in guiding needle aspiration by using the biopsy guide attachment and can help differentiate between abscesses and noninfected perirectal fluid collections. Not only can the fluid be aspirated with ultrasound guidance, but also a catheter may be placed.

Accuracy

Transrectal ultrasound may prove to be a relatively inexpensive examination that could provide important diagnostic information, including the extent of benign and malignant intramural and extrarectal tumors.[207] This method appears to be accurate for detecting perirectal tumor spread, with a reported sensitivity of 83 to 94 percent.[197] In the detection of tumor extension into fat this method is 67 percent sensitive, with a specificity of 77 percent, a positive predictive value of 73 percent, and a negative predictive value of 72 percent.[204] In the same series, CT was shown to be 53 percent sensitive and 53 percent specific, with a positive predictive value of 56 percent and a negative predictive value of 50 percent.[204] Its sensitivity in the detection of lymph node infiltration was 50 percent, with a specificity of 92 percent, a positive predictive value of 68 percent, and a negative predictive value of 84 percent.[204] CT demonstrated a sensitivity of 27 percent, a specificity of 88 percent, a positive predictive value of 46 percent, and a negative predictive value of 76 percent.[204] As such, this study suggests that transrectal ultrasound may be as accurate as CT or more so in the preoperative staging of rectal carcinoma.[204]

Other authors have evaluated the accuracy of transrectal ultrasound. In 75 percent of cases the depth of invasion of the tumor is accurately predicted, with 22 percent overstaged and 3 percent understaged.[208] In 88 percent of cases lymph nodes are properly classified into positive and negative groups, with a specificity of 90 percent and a sensitivity of 88 percent.[208] As such, this method is considered an accurate preoperative staging modality.[208]

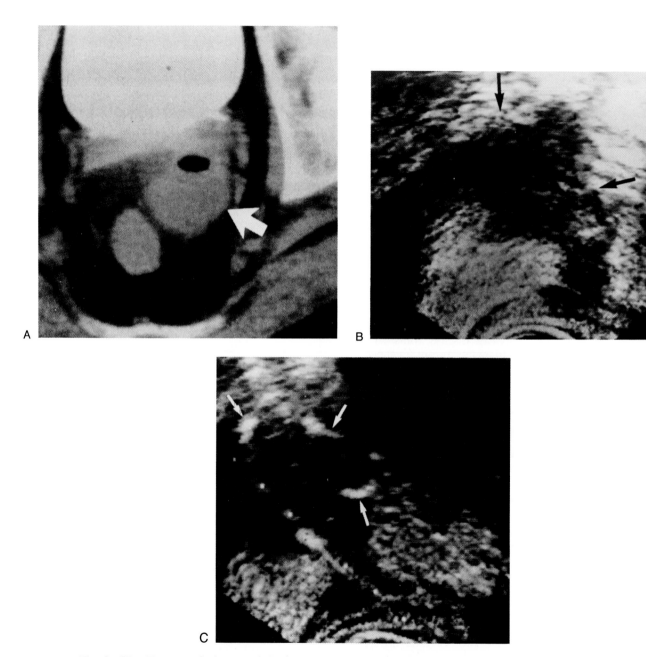

Fig. 8-157. Transrectal ultrasound. Perirectal abscess. **(A)** CT scan in a patient with inflammatory bowel disease showing a perirectal abscess anterior to the rectum (arrow) that could not be found during surgery. **(B)** Transrectal sonogram obtained after surgery showing a poorly defined hypoechoic area anterior to the rectum (arrows). **(C)** Under sonographic guidance, a guidewire (arrows) was inserted and secured to the skin. Surgery was repeated, and the guidewire was used successfully to locate the abscess cavity. (From St Ville et al,[206] with permission.)

ENDOSCOPIC ULTRASOUND

Endoscopic ultrasound is a relatively new technique that combines a high-frequency transducer (for evaluation of the bowel wall layers and surrounding tissues) with an endoscope, which allows direct visualization. The problem caused by the air in the gut lumen is circumvented by direct contact of the transducer with the bowel wall via a water-filled balloon in the esophagus or water filling the stomach.[211] This technique allows detailed imaging of the GI tract wall and the surrounding structures. Endosonography of the colon is an even newer application of this technique.

TECHNIQUE

Most models of endoscopes are side-viewing and measure 13 mm in diameter with a radial transducer at the tip. The frequencies of the transducers used vary from 7.5 to 12 MHz (some are switchable), with a field of view varying from 180 to 360 degrees to the plane of the endoscope. The maximum resolution with the 12-MHz transducer is less than 0.5 mm, with 1.0 mm for the 7.5

transducer.[212] The scanning radius is a maximum of 7 cm at 7.5 MHz and 3 cm at 12 MHz.[212]

There are certain problems encountered with this technique. When this particular endoscope is used, the procedure is more technically difficult than with the "traditional" endoscope since the tip is larger and more rigid.[213] The procedure requires a longer time and more sedation.[213] The main limitation of the ultrasound is the inability to move the endoscope past the stenosis in the case of esophageal carcinoma.[214]

For evaluation of the colon, a side-viewing echoduodenoscope is used.[215] The frequency of the ultrasound transducer is 7.5 MHz with a penetration depth of approximately 10 cm and an axial resolution of 0.2 mm.[215] For the study, the patient is placed in the left lateral decubitus position after administration of phosphate or water enema.[215] Polypoid or exophytic configurations of tumors can be clearly visualized by filling the rectal lumen with water.[215] Mural and nodal abnormalities can be clearly visualized by filling the balloon attached to the transducer and/or colorectal lumen with water.[215]

NORMAL ANATOMY

When the lumen is distended with a 3-cm-diameter water-filled balloon, the normal thickness of the esophageal wall is approximately 3 mm and is uniform throughout.[211] Within the normal esophagus, five layers

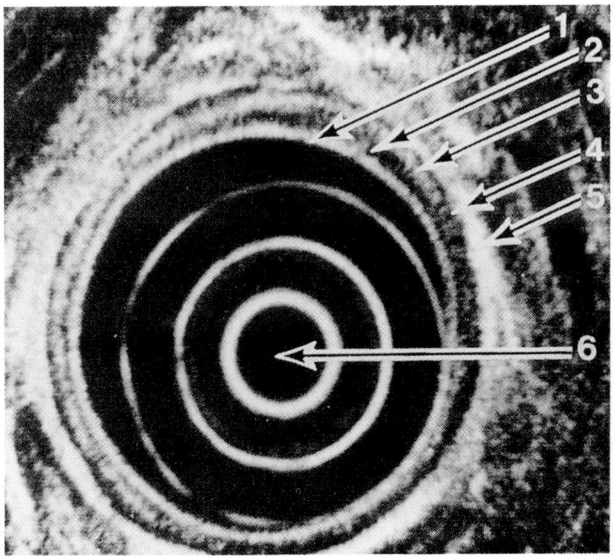

Fig. 8-158. Endoscopic sonography of esophageal wall. Actual cross-sectional image of the esophagus as visualized by endoscopic sonography (12-MHz transducer). (*1*, mucosal interface, highly echogenic; *2*, muscularis mucosa, hypoechoic; *3*, submucosa, highly echogenic; *4*, lamina propria, hypoechoic; *5*, adventitial interface, highly echogenic; *6*, transducer with inflated balloon.) (From Botet and Lightdale,[211] with permission.)

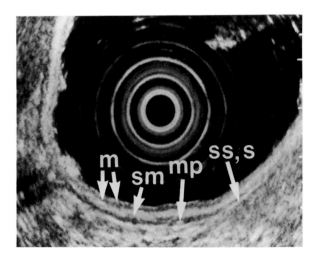

Fig. 8-159. Endoscopic ultrasound image showing the normal gastric wall with the five-layer structure. (*m*, mucosa; *sm*, submucosa; *mp*, muscularis propria; *ss, s*, subserosa and serosa) (From Fujishima et al,[220] with permission.)

may be demonstrated by ultrasound: (1) hyperechoic interface between the probe and the balloon; (2) hypoechoic layer corresponding to the mucosa and the inner part of the submucosa; (3) hyperechoic layer representing the outer part of the submucosa; (4) hypoechoic layer representing the muscularis propria; and (5) hyperechoic layer corresponding to the adventitia and the periesophageal fat[214] (Fig. 8-158).

The esophagus may be divided into upper, middle, and lower segments by ultrasound. By using the landmarks of the vertebral column posteriorly and the tracheal air column anteriorly, the upper esophagus is seen to extend from the oropharynx to the superior aspect of the aortic arch.[211] Extending from the aortic arch to the subcarinal region, the middle portion of the esophagus is noted by its relationships to the aortic arch and descending aorta posteriorly and the trachea and carina anteriorly.[211] With the descending aorta posteriorly and the left atrium anteriorly, the lower portion of the esophagus extends from the subcarinal region to the cardia.[211]

As with the esophagus, five layers may be defined within the stomach wall (Fig. 8-159). The stomach wall thickness varies according to the degree of gastric distension. When the stomach is fully distended, the wall thickness is approximately 3 mm.

The stomach may be divided into the fundus, the body, and the antrum. The fundus is noted by the aorta with the celiac axis posteriorly, the left hepatic lobe to the right, and the spleen to the left.[211] When visualizing the body of the stomach, the left hepatic lobe is to the right and anteriorly with the body and tail of the pancreas to the left and posteriorly.[211] The left hepatic lobe is noted anteriorly when the antrum is visualized, with the pancreas, splenic vein, and portal vein posteriorly.[211]

ESOPHAGEAL ABNORMALITIES

A number of abnormalities can be identified within the esophagus by this technique; they include carcinoma, leiomyomas, duplication cysts, and varices[211] (Figs. 8-160 to 8-162). Additionally, the esophagus may be evaluated for recurrence of esophageal carcinoma following resection.[216]

Carcinomas are characterized by disruption of the layers of the esophageal wall, beginning with the mucosa and possibly extending to involve all layers and invading the surrounding structures[211] (Fig. 8-160). A number of criteria have been used to define esophageal involvement: (1) involvement is present when the esophageal wall is thickened with a width of at least 5 mm; (2) tracheal or bronchial involvement is certain when an intraluminal mass or thickened wall is present or when tumoral extension is seen between the trachea and the aortic arch or between the left main bronchus and the descending aorta; (3) aortic infiltration is diagnosed when tumor develops intimate contact with the aorta

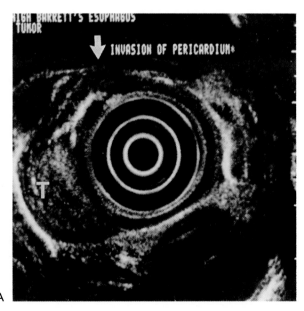

A

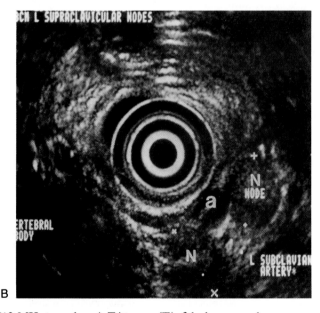

B

Fig. 8-160. Esophageal malignant process. **(A)** Tumor (12-MHz transducer). T4 tumor *(T)* of the lower esophagus has invaded the pericardium. A discontinuity in the pericardial fat (arrow) was confirmed at surgery. **(B)** Nodes (7.5-MHz transducer). Two 1.4-cm nodes *(N)* surround the left subclavian artery *(a)*. Although larger than 1 cm, they appear hyperechoic; they were found to be reactive at surgery. (From Botet and Lightdale,[211] with permission.)

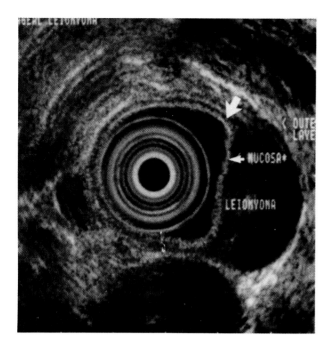

Fig. 8-161. Esophageal leiomyoma. Endoscopic sonography with a 7.5-MHz transducer showing a characteristic hypoechoic lesion arising from muscularis mucosa (large arrow). The overlying mucosa (small arrow) is intact. (From Botet and Lightdale,[211] with permission.)

that is more than 90 degrees of the aortic circumference associated with deformation of the aortic lumen; (4) amputation of the vessel lumen and lack of opacification are signs of tumoral spread to pulmonary veins; (5) pericardial effusion is synonymous with pericardial tumoral infiltration; and (6) pleural involvement is judged to be present when pleural thickening adjacent to tumor or pleural effusion is present.[214,217]

Lymph nodes containing metastatic disease as small as 2 mm in diameter may be visualized. The following criteria suggest nodal involvement; (1) round nodes are more likely to be malignant than those that appear elongated; (2) nodes that are hypoechoic or isoechoic are more likely to be malignant; and (3) nodes that are hyperechoic are more commonly benign.[211] Recurrent disease may be suspected when a nodular hypoechoic thickening at the anastomosis is seen.[216]

Endoscopic ultrasound is significantly more accurate (92 percent) than CT (60 percent) in staging the depth of tumor growth.[213] It is more accurate (88 percent) than CT (74 percent) in staging regional lymph nodes, but this is not statistically significant.[213] CT is more accurate (90 percent) than endoscopic ultrasound (70 percent) in staging distant metastases.[213] With the combined use of CT and endoscopic ultrasound, the highest concordance with surgical and pathologic findings in overall staging (86 percent) was significantly more accurate than that of

CT alone (64 percent).[213] As such, endoscopic ultrasound represents a significant advance in the accuracy of evaluating tumor invasion and an improvement in evaluation of esophageal regional node involvement.

GASTRIC ABNORMALITIES

A number of gastric abnormalities may be defined by endoscopic ultrasound, including gastritis, ulcer, polyps, varices, and carcinoma (Figs. 8-162 to 8-164). Additionally, the stomach may be evaluated for the possibility of recurrence after resection of a gastric carcinoma.[216] It may be helpful in the staging of gastric lymphoma.[216]

Esophagogastric varices may be visualized by endoscopic ultrasound (Fig. 8-162). It may be possible not only to identify these lesions but also to evaluate the devascularity after sclerosing therapy or surgery and to evaluate for portal hypertension.[218]

Gastric myogenic tumors may also be investigated by endoscopic ultrasound.[219] Frequently there is evidence of necrosis within these tumors; this area is larger in leiomyosarcoma than in leiomyoma.[219] An irregularly shaped lucent area is seen within the tumor, corresponding to the area of liquefaction necrosis[219] (similar to Fig. 8-161). With endoscopic ultrasound, these lesions can be seen as hypoechoic tumors arising from the proper muscle layer with irregularly shaped lucent areas.[219]

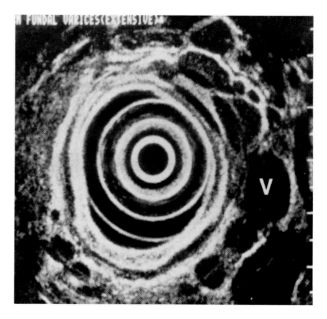

Fig. 8-162. Gastric varices (12-MHz transducer). These large varices *(V)* are characterized as hypoechoic rounded or elongated structures with a strong posterior wall enhancement when imaged with a higher-frequency transducer. (From Botet and Lightdale,[211] with permission.)

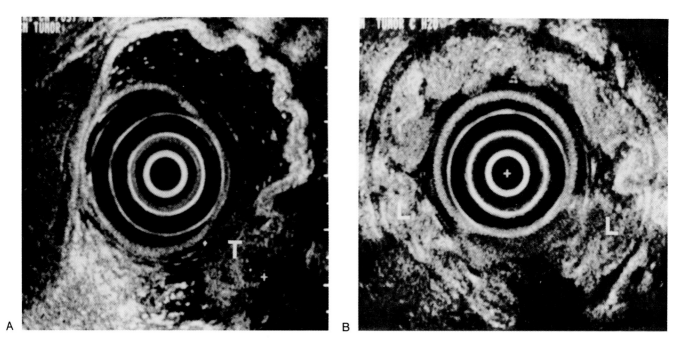

A   B

Fig. 8-163. Malignant gastric processes with a 12-MHz transducer. **(A)** Adenocarcinoma. Tumor *(T)* involves all layers of the gastric wall, extending beyond the serosa but not involving any adjacent structure. **(B)** Gastric lymphoma. Folds *(L)* are thickened and prominent, and there is circumferential involvement. (From Botet and Lightdale,[211] with permission.)

With gastric carcinoma, there is disruption of the wall beginning with the mucosa[211] (Figs. 8-163 and 8-164). Additional findings may include nodal involvement of the gastric drainage. The endoscopic ultrasound differentiation of scirrhous carcinoma of the stomach from hypertrophic gastritis has been evaluated.[220] As a gastric carcinoma in which the tumor spreads predominantly in the submucosa, scirrhous carcinoma of the stomach (representing 5 to 15 percent of all gastric cancers) produces a marked desmoplastic response in the gastric wall.[220] It is often difficult to diagnose this tumor at an early stage. The characteristic features of scirrhous carcinoma include an irregular hypoechoic enlargement of the third (submucosa) and fourth (muscularis propria) layers.[220] Compared with the thickness in healthy subjects, the mean thickness of the third and fourth layers is increased sixfold and threefold, respectively.[220] The mucosal layer appears normal at ultrasound in patients with scirrhous carcinoma, and it is possible to discern the five-layer structure of the gastric wall.[220] In cases of hypertrophic gastritis, only the mucosal layer is thickened.[220] Recognizing these patterns can aid in the differential diagnosis of scirrhous carcinoma and such benign disease as hypertrophic gastritis with thickened gastric wall.[220]

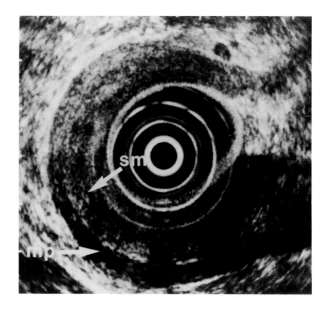

Fig. 8-164. Endoscopic ultrasound image accurately depicting submucosal invasion by carcinoma as hypoechoic thickened submucosa *(sm)* and muscularis propria *(mp)*. Multiple endoscopic biopsies and cytologic examinations had failed to reveal the carcinoma in this case. (From Fujishima et al,[220] with permission.)

Gastric lymphoma has been investigated by endoscopic ultrasound.[79] The stomach may be involved by lymphoma, particularly of the non-Hodgkin's type, arising from the lamina propria of the mucosa.[211] As a tumor arising from lymphoid tissue of the lamina propria of the gastric mucosa, primary gastric non-Hodgkin's lymphoma may spread in the deep mucosa and infiltrate the muscularis propria serosa and perigastric lymph nodes.[79] Gastric lymphomas have been described as having the following endoscopic appearance: (1) giant rigid gastric folds, which sometimes produce a polypoid appearance; (2) stellate ulcers, which are often multiple and interconnected by long fissures; (3) localized or extended hypoechoic infiltration; and (4) thickening with superficial ulcerations.[79] When comparing gastric carcinoma and lymphoma, carcinoma appears to have a more echogenic pattern and a different trend of diffusion, with no extended longitudinal hypoechoic filtration of superficial layers or extended hypoechoic transmural infiltration.[79]

The findings at endoscopic ultrasound and those at pathologic examination are concordant (92 percent) when the depth of tumor penetration is evaluated with those at CT and pathologic examination (42 percent).[221] There is a concordance of 78 percent with evaluation of regional lymph node metastasis and 48 percent with dynamic CT.[221] There is a concordance of 73 percent in overall determination of stage with both dynamic CT

and endoscopic ultrasound compared with a concordance of 45 percent for dynamic CT alone.[221]

Ampulla and Pancreas

Since survival in patients with ampullary neoplasms is correlated with the stage of the tumor, accurate staging is essential.[213] The entire pancreas may be examined by endoscopic ultrasound in a staged drawback from the second portion of the duodenum to the proximal body of the stomach.[213] Even with this technique, there appear to be difficulties in distinguishing focal chronic pancreatitis from pancreatic carcinoma[213] (Fig. 8-165). This technique may be helpful in the identification of small neoplasms of islet cells such as insulinomas and gastrinomas.[213]

COLONIC ABNORMALITIES

Endosonography of the colon is a relatively new application of this technique. This technique may be more accurate in the preoperative staging of rectal carcinoma than CT.[222] Evaluation of the colon with the transrectal transducer is limited by the length of the transducer.[222] With this technique, metastatic involvement of lymph

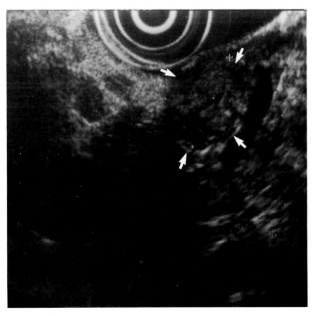

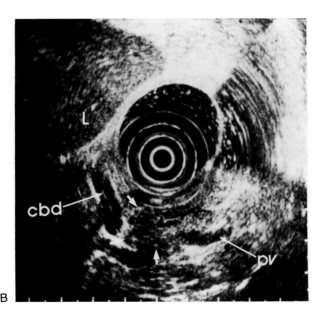

Fig. 8-165. Ampullary neoplasm. **(A)** Noninvasive, well-circumscribed adenoma (arrows) (frequency 7.5 MHz; range, 6 cm). **(B)** Invasive irregular neoplasm (arrows) (frequency, 7.5 MHz; range, 9 cm). (*cbd,* common bile duct; *pv,* portal vein; *L,* liver.) (From Nickl and Cotton,[213] with permission.)

nodes at a distance from the primary lesion will escape endosonographic detection.[222]

Recently a colonoscope combined with ultrasound has been developed for evaluation of the colon; it allows for visual examinations, biopsy, and endosonography throughout the colon.[222] The echoendoscope is the instrument of choice for visualization of the proximal colonic carcinomas, because the transducer can be maneuvered into the proximal colonic segments, allowing endoscopic location of target lesions.[215] Applications of colonoscopic ultrasound would include the evaluation of large sessile adenomas and the follow-up examinations of anastomoses after tumor resection[222] (Figs. 8-166 and 8-167). At present the precise role of colonoscopic ultrasound in diagnostic evaluation of colorectal disease has not been fully defined, and further comparative trials are needed.[222]

Lesions may not always be successfully visualized since the lumen of the colon is relatively narrow and passage of the colonoscope becomes difficult when cancer has resulted in stenosis.[223] Estimation of the cancer invasion is more often accurate when the lesion is less circumferential with less narrowing, is less advanced, and is protruded rather than depressed; the major factor impairing visualization of lesions is the degree of narrowing.[223]

Evaluation of colorectal disease by ultrasound coupled with a colonoscope has evolved. This technique has been shown to correctly estimate the depth of cancer invasion in 84.9 percent of cases in which the lesion was appropriately visualized.[224] By using this modality, paraintestinal lymph node metastases can be detected in 38.1 percent.[223] This technique is not as successful in the evaluation of polyps, since histologic types cannot be differentiated.[223]

SUMMARY

During the first 10 years of use, endoscopic ultrasound appears to have an acceptable success rate in obtaining accurate diagnostic images.[213] In the literature, there continues to be some controversy regarding the clinical application of endoscopic ultrasound.[213] Some suggest that this technique will "become standard in major hospitals in the not-too-distant future," while others suggest caution and continue to regard the technique as investigational.[213]

Several indications of endoscopic ultrasound have been established: (1) to distinguish benign from malignant processes; (2) to further clarify the nature of benign processes; and (3) to stage suspected or known neoplasm to establish operability, to plan the surgical approach, to monitor the response to therapy, and to search for recurrence.[213]

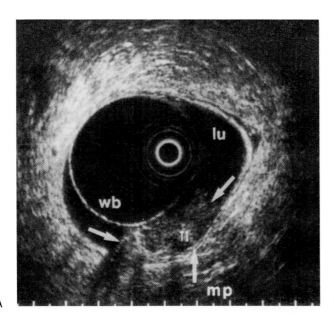
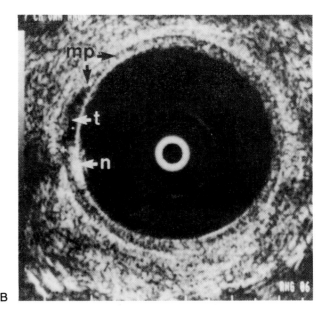

A   B

Fig. 8-166. Colon ultrasound. **(A)** Transcolorectal endosonography (TES) scan (Olympus EU-M2 echoduodenoscope) showing a polypoid hypoechoic tumor (arrows) located in the mucosa and submucosa *(T1)* without penetration into the muscularis propria *(mp)*. (*wb,* water-filled balloon; *lu,* water-filled rectal lumen.) **(B)** TES scan (5 MHz) showing a hypoechoic tumor *(t)* with penetration into the adjacent muscularis propria *(mp)* and an ulcer covered with some necrotic material *(n)*. Note the clear transection between the tumor and normal rectal wall architecture. (From Tio et al,[215] with permission.)

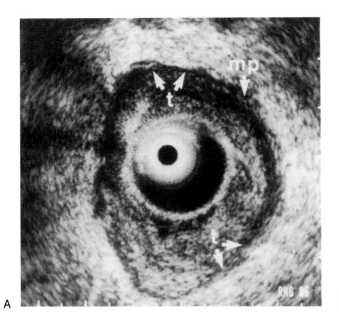
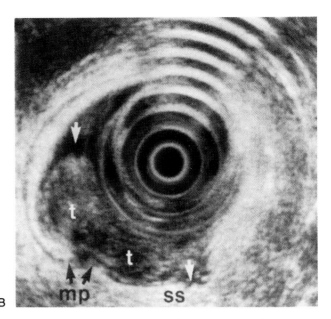

A   B

Fig. 8-167. Colon ultrasound. **(A)** TES scan (7.5-MHz nonoptic instrument) showing a circular hypoechoic tumor *(t)* with penetration into the muscularis propria *(mp)*. **(B)** TES scan (7.5-MHz echocolonoscope) revealing a polypoid tumor *(t)* protruding into the water-filled lumen (white arrows) and through the muscularis propria *(mp)* into the adjacent subsacral layer *(ss)* of the sigmoid, corresponding to a T3 carcinoma. (From Tio et al,[215] with permission.)

With regard to esophageal carcinoma, endoscopic ultrasound has demonstrated a 75 to 88 percent accuracy when compared with surgical resection.[213] Other authors have demonstrated an accuracy of 89 to 90 percent in evaluation of esophageal carcinoma and assessing the depth of tumor infiltration.[224,225] The limiting factor is stenosis.[225] Endoscopic ultrasound is the most reliable method of demonstrating small (<1 cm) intra- and extramural esophageal lesions, and it should be applied early in the work-up of patients with dysphagia.[226]

With gastric carcinoma, endoscopic ultrasound has an accuracy of 83 percent.[224,225] This technique can distinguish early carcinomas from advanced cancers and is accurate in diagnosing lymph node metastases.[224] It is valuable for studying many submucosal lesions of the upper GI tract.[227,228] An accuracy of over 95 percent has been reported in the accurate characterization of such tumors, including leiomyomas, leiomyosarcomas, lipomas, carcinoids, and extrinsically compressing tumors.[213]

Endoscopic ultrasound is a sensitive method (95 percent) for the detection of locally recurrent upper gastrointestinal tumors at the surgical anastomosis, with a specificity of 80 percent.[216] This technique appears to be important when selecting the patients likely to benefit from surgical treatment and planning the strategy of nonsurgical treatment such as laser photocoagulation, radiotherapy and/or chemotherapy.[229]

In the future, ultrasound probes may be developed as alternatives to the dedicated endoscopes.[230] These may be "blind" transducers, without an endoscope, inserted into the GI tract for visualization of the anatomy. Work is in progress to develop such transducers.

CONCLUSION

It is not suggested that ultrasound should replace the barium study and gastroscopy in the diagnosis of GI disease. Since ultrasound scanning is usually performed prior to these procedures, it is important to recognize features of GI lesions on ultrasound to streamline the patient's workup.[231] The pattern caused by concentric thickening of the infiltrated bowel wall holds true for lesions involving the wall of any portion of the alimentary tract.[13] Although inflammation and neoplastic infiltration of the wall are primary considerations when bowel wall thickening is demonstrated, other possible diagnoses include Crohn's disease, ileocecal tuberculosis, periappendiceal tumor, extensive ulcerative or hyperplastic coarse giant folds in Ménétrier's disease, and edema of the intestinal wall in thrombosis of the mesenteric veins.[232] Ultrasound is usually performed as the first diagnostic measure in cases of palpable abdominal masses and can usually show whether the mass originates from a parenchymal organ or the GI tract.[15] Ultrasound is not suitable for diagnosing the early stage of GI tumors confined to the mucosa and submucosa or for definitively excluding advanced tumors.[232]

REFERENCES

1. Gooding GAW, Laing FC: Rapid water infusion: a technique in the ultrasonic discrimination of the gas-free stomach from mass in the pancreatic tail. Gastrointest Radiol 1979;4:139

2. Kremer H, Grobner W: Sonography of polypoid gastric lesions by the fluid-filled stomach method. J Clin Ultrasound 1981;9:51

3. Weighall SL, Wolfman NT, Watson N: The fluid-filled stomach: a new sonic window. J Clin Ultrasound 1979;7:353

4. Worlicek H, Dunz, Engelhard K: Ultrasonic examination of the wall of the fluid-filled stomach. J Clin Ultrasound 1989;17:5

5. Cohen HL, Haller JO, Mestel AL et al: Neonatal duodenum: fluid aided US examination. Radiology 1987;1164:805

6. Abu-Yousef MM: Sonography of the right iliac fossa. Ultrasound Q 1990;8:73

7. Rubin C, Kurtz AB, Goldberg BB: Water enema: a new ultrasound technique in defining pelvic anatomy. J Clin Ultrasound 1978;6:28

8. Limberg B: Sonographic features of colonic Crohn's disease: comparison of in vivo and in vitro studies. J Clin Ultrasound 1990;18:161

9. Limberg B: Diagnosis of acute ulcerative colitis and colonic Crohn's disease by colonic sonography. J Clin Ultrasound 1989;17:25

10. Limberg B: Diagnosis of large bowel tumours by colonic sonography. Lancet 1990;335:144

11. Limberg B: Diagnosis of inflammatory and neoplastic large bowel diseases by conventional abdominal and colonic sonography. Ultrasound Q 1988;6:151

12. Hirooka N, Ohno T, Misonoo M et al: Sono-enterocolonography by oral water administration. J Clin Ultrasound 1989;17:585

13. Peterson LR, Cooperberg PL: Ultrasound demonstration of lesions of the gastrointestinal tract. Gastrointest Radiol 1978;3:303

14. Fleischer AC, Muhletaler CA, James AE Jr: Detection of bowel lesions during abdominal and pelvic sonography. JAMA 1980;244:2096

15. Fakhry JR, Berk RN: The "target" pattern: characteristic sonographic features of stomach and bowel abnormalities. AJR 1981;137:969

16. Fleischer AC, Muhletaler CA, James AE Jr: Sonographic patterns arising from normal and abnormal bowel. Radiol Clin North Am 1980;18:145

17. Fleischer AC, Muhletaler CA, Kurtz AB, James AE Jr: Real-time sonography of bowel. p. 117. In Winsberg F, Cooperberg PL (eds): Clinics in Diagnostic Ultrasound: Real-Time Ultrasonography. Vol. 10. Churchill Livingstone, New York, 1982

18. Torp-Pedersen S, Gronvall S, Holm HH: Ultrasonically guided fine-needle aspiration biopsy of gastrointestinal mass lesions. J Ultrasound Med 1984;3:65

19. Ennis MG, MacErlean DP: Biopsy of bowel wall pathology under ultrasound control. Gastrointest Radiol 1981;6:17

20. Bluth EI, Merritt CRB, Sullivan MA: Ultrasonic evaluation of the stomach, small bowel and colon. Radiology 1979;133:677

21. Fleischer AC, Muhletaler CA, James AE Jr: Sonographic assessment of the bowel wall. AJR 1981;136:887

22. Weinberg B, Rao PS, Shah KD et al: Ultrasound demonstration of an intramural leiomyoma of the gastric cardia with pathologic correlation. J Clin Ultrasound 1988;16:580

23. Miyamoto Y, Tsujimoto F, Tada S: Ultrasonographic diagnosis of submucosal tumors of the stomach: the "bridging layers" sign. J Clin Ultrasound 1988;16:251

24. Oliva L, Biggi E, Derchi LE, Cicio GR: Ultrasonic anatomy of the fluid-filled duodenum. J Clin Ultrasound 1981;9:245

25. Fleischer AC, Dowling AD, Weinstein ML, James AE, Jr: Sonographic patterns of distended, fluid filled bowel. Radiology 1979;133:681

26. Yeh H-C, Rabinowitz JG: Ultrasonography of gastrointestinal tract. Semin Ultrasound CT MR 1982;3:331

27. Wright LL, Baker KR, Meny RG: Ultrasound demonstration of gastroesophageal reflux. J Ultrasound Med 1988;7:471

28. Westra SJ, Wolf BHM, Staalman CR: Ultrasound diagnosis of gastroesophageal reflux and hiatal hernia in infants and young children. J Clin Ultrasound 1990;18:477

29. Gomes H, Menanteau B: Gastroesophageal reflux: comparative study between sonography and pH monitoring. Pediatr Radiol 1991;21:168

30. Komaiko MS: Gastric neoplasms: ultrasound and CT evaluation. Gastrointest Radiol 1979;4:131

31. Maglinte DDT, Lappas JC, Ng AC: Sonography of Bouveret's syndrome. J Ultrasound Med 1987;6:675

32. Teele RL, Henschke CI, Tapper D: The radiographic and ultrasonographic evaluation of enteric duplication cysts. Pediatr Radiol 1980;10:9

33. Moccia WA, Astacio JE, Kaude JV: Ultrasonographic demonstration of gastric duplication in infancy. Pediatr Radiol 1981;11:52

34. Kangarloo H, Sample WF, Hansen G et al: Ultrasonic evaluation of abdominal gastrointestinal tract duplication in children. Radiology 1979;131:191

35. Gorelik I, Goldman SM, Minkin SD et al: Gastric duplication originating from the tail of the pancreas ultrasonically demonstrated. J Clin Ultrasound 1976;4:429

36. Haller JO, Cohen HL: Hypertropic pyloric stenosis: diagnosis using US. Radiology 1986;161:335

37. Strauss S, Itzchak Y, Manor A et al: Sonography of hypertrophic pyloric stenosis. AJR 1981;136:1057

38. Robbins SL, Cotran RS: The gastrointestinal tract. p. 918. In Pathologic Basis of Disease. WB Saunders, Philadelphia, 1979

39. Sauerbrei EE, Paloschi GGB: The ultrasonic features of hypertrophic pyloric stenosis with emphasis on the postoperative appearance. Radiology 1983;147:503

40. Ball TI, Atkinson GO Jr, Gay BB Jr: Ultrasound diagnosis of hypertrophic pyloric stenosis: real-time application and the demonstration of a new sonographic sign. Radiology 1983;147:499

41. Blumhagen JD, Noble HGS: Muscle thickness in hypertrophic pyloric stenosis: sonographic determination. AJR 1983;140:221

42. Blumhagen JD, Coombs JB: Ultrasound in the diagnosis of hypertrophic pyloric stenosis. J Clin Ultrasound 1981;9:289

43. Finkelstein MS, Mandell GA, Tarbell KV: Hypertrophic pyloric stenosis: volumetric measurement of nasogastric aspirate to determine the imaging modality. Radiology 1990;177:759

44. Graif M, Itzchak Y, Avigad I et al: The pylorus in infancy: overall sonographic assessment. Pediatr Radiol 1984;14:14

45. Wilson DA, Vanhoutte JJ: The reliable sonographic diagnosis of hypertrophic pyloric stenosis. J Clin Ultrasound 1984;12:201

46. Teele RL: The pancreas, spleen, mesentery and gastrointestinal tract. p. 104. In Haller JO, Shkolnik A (eds): Clinics in Diagnostic Ultrasound: Diagnostic Ultrasound in Pediatrics. Vol. 8. Churchill Livingstone, New York, 1981

47. Teele RL, Smith EH: Ultrasound in the diagnosis of idiopathic hypertrophic pyloric stenosis. N Engl J Med 1977;296:1149

48. Stunden RJ, LeQuesne GW, Little KET: The improved ultrasound diagnosis of hypertrophic pyloric stenosis. Pediatr Radiol 1986;16:200

49. Blumhagen JD, Maclin L, Krauter D et al: Sonographic diagnosis of hypertrophic pyloric stenosis. AJR 1988;150:1367

50. Cohen HL, Schechter S, Mestel AL et al: Ultrasonic "double track" sign in hypertrophic pyloric stenosis. J Ultrasound Med 1987;6:139

51. O'Keeffe FN, Stransberry SD, Swischuk LE, Hayden CK Jr: Antropyloric muscle thickness at US in infants: what is normal? Radiology 1991;178:827

52. Westra SJ, DeGroot CJ, Smits NJ, Staalman CR: Hypertrophic pyloric stenosis: use of the pyloric volume measurement in early US diagnosis. Radiology 1989;172:615

53. Weiskittel DA, Leary DL, Blane CE: Ultrasound diagnosis of evolving pyloric stenosis. Gastrointest Radiol 1989;14:22

54. Jackson VP, Holden RW, Doering PR, Lappas LC: Sonographic diagnosis of adult hypertrophic pyloric stenosis. J Ultrasound Med 1985;4:505

55. Joharjy IA, Mustafa MA, Zaidi AJ: Fluid-aided sonography of the stomach and duodenum in the diagnosis of peptic ulcer disease in adult patients. J Ultrasound Med 1990;9:77

56. Tomooka Y, Onitsuka H, Goya T et al: Ultrasonography of benign gastric ulcers: characteristic features and sequential follow-ups. J Ultrasound Med 1989;8:513

57. Madrazo BL, Hricak H, Sandler MA, Eyler WR: Sonographic findings in complicated peptic ulcer disease. Radiology 1981;140:457

58. Chang-Chien CS, Lin HH, Yen CL et al: Sonographic demonstration of free air in perforated peptic ulcers: comparison of sonography with radiography. J Clin Ultrasound 1989;17:95

59. Hayden CK Jr, Swischuk LE, Rytting LE: Gastric ulcer disease in infants: US findings. Radiology 1987;164:131

60. Kopen PA, McAlister WH: Upper gastrointestinal and ultrasound examinations of gastric antral involvement in chronic granulomatous disease. Pediatr Radiol 1984;14:91

61. Bidula MM, Rifkin MD, McCoy RI: Ultrasonography of gastric phytobezoar. J Clin Ultrasound 1986;14:49

62. McCracken S, Jongeward R, Silver RM, Jafri SZH: Gastric trichobezoar: sonographic findings. Radiology 1986;161:123

63. Malpani A, Ramani SK, Wolverson MK: Role of sonography in trichobezoars. J Ultrasound Med 1988;7:661

64. Lambrecht L, Robberecht E, Deschynkel K, Afschrift M: Ultrasonic evaluation of gastric clearing in young infants. Pediatr Radiol 1988;18:314

65. Stringer DA, Daneman A, Brunelle F et al: Sonography of the normal and abnormal stomach (excluding hypertrophic pyloric stenosis) in children. J Ultrasound Med 1986;5:183

66. McAlister WH, Katz ME, Perlman JM, Tack ED: Sonography of focal foveolar hyperplasia causing gastric obstruction in an infant. Pediatr Radiol 1988;18:79

67. Gassner I, Strasser K, Gart G, Maurer H: Sonographic appearance of Ménétrier's disease in a child. J Ultrasound Med 1990;9:537

68. Shirahama M, Morita SI, Koga T et al: Gastrointestinal amyloidosis associated with multiple myeloma: sonographic features. J Clin Ultrasound 1991;19:493

69. Leekam RN, Matzinger MA, Gray RR: Gastric amyloidosis simulating antral malignancy on ultrasound. J Clin Ultrasound 1985;13:485

70. Morimoto K, Hashimoto T, Choi S et al: Ultrasonographic evaluation of intramural gastric and duodenal hematoma in hemophiliacs. J Clin Ultrasound 1988;16:108

71. Schabel SI, Rittenberg GM, Bubanj R, Warren E: Pedunculated gastric leiomyoma: a wandering abdominal mass demonstrated by ultrasound. J Clin Ultrasound 1979;7:211

72. Morgan CL, Trought WS, Oddson TA et al: Ultrasound

patterns of disorders affecting the gastrointestinal tract. Radiology 1980;135:129

73. Mascatello VJ, Carrera GF, Telle RL et al: The ultrasonic demonstration of gastric lesions. J Clin Ultrasound 1977;5:383

74. Yeh H-C, Rabinowitz JG: Ultrasonography and computed tomography of gastric wall lesions. Radiology 1981;141:147

75. Walls WJ: The evaluation of malignant gastric neoplasms by ultrasonic B-scanning. Radiology 1976;118:159

76. Cerri GG, Zeitune JMR, Hashimoto MS et al: The calcified target lesion: mucinous carcinoma of the stomach. J Clin Ultrasound 1985;13:431

77. Derchi LE, Biggi E, Rollandi GA et al: Sonographic staging of gastric cancer. AJR 1983;140:273

78. Derchi LE, Banderali A, Bossi MC et al: The sonographic appearance of gastric lymphoma. J Ultrasound Med 1984;3:251

79. Bolondi L, Casanova P, Caletti GC et al: Primary gastric lymphoma versus gastric carcinoma: endoscopic US evaluation. Radiology 1987;165:821

80. Salem S, Hiltz CW: Ultrasonographic appearance of gastric lymphosarcoma. J Clin Ultrasound 1978;6:429

81. Carroll BA, Ta HN: The ultrasonic appearance of extranodal abdominal lymphoma. Radiology 1980;136:419

82. Goerg C, Schwerk WB, Goerg K: Gastrointestinal lymphoma: sonographic findings in 54 patients. AJR 1990;155:795

83. Subramanyam BR, Balthazar EJ, Raghavendra BN, Madamba MR: Sonography of exophytic gastrointestinal leiomyosarcoma. Gastrointest Radiol 1982;7:47

84. Kaftori JK, Aharon M, Kleinhaus U: Sonography features of gastrointestinal leiomyosarcoma. J Clin Ultrasound 1981;9:11

85. Sandler MA, Ratanaprakarn S, Madrazo BL: Ultrasonic findings in intramural exogastric lesions. Radiology 1978;128:189

86. DeWilde V, Voet D, Dhont T et al: Ultrasound diagnosis of a solitary gastric metastasis. J Clin Ultrasound 1989;17:678

87. Scheible W, Goldberger LE: Diagnosis of small bowel obstruction: the contribution of diagnostic ultrasound. AJR 1979;133:685

88. Pozderac RV, Doust BD: Confusing appearance of a dilated jejunal loop. J Clin Ultrasound 1978;6:165

89. Pon MS, Scudamore C, Harrison RC, Cooperberg PL: Ultrasound demonstration of radiographically obscure small bowel obstruction. AJR 1979;133:145

90. Miller JH, Kemberling CR: Ultrasound scanning of the gastrointestinal tract in children: subject review. Radiology 1984;152:671

91. Bedi DG, Fagan CJ, Nocera RM: Sonographic diagnosis of bowel obstruction presenting with fluid-filled loops of bowel. J Clin Ultrasound 1985;13:23

92. Hayden CK Jr, Boulden TF, Swischuk LE, Lobe TE: Sonographic demonstration of duodenal obstruction with midgut volvulus. AJR 1984;143:9

93. Leonidas JC, Magid N, Soberman N, Glass TS: Midgut

volvulus in infants: diagnosis with US. Radiology 1991;179:491

94. Brambs HJ, Spamer C, Volk B, Holstege A: Diagnostic value of ultrasound in duodenal stenosis. Gastrointest Radiol 1986;11:135

95. Derchi LE, Ierace T, DePra L et al: The sonographic appearance of duodenal lesions. J Ultrasound Med 1986;5:269

96. Lee DH, Lim JH, Ko YT: Afferent loop syndrome: sonographic findings in seven cases. AJR 1991;157:41

97. Hopens T, Coggs GC, Goldstein HM, Smith BD: Sonographic diagnosis of afferent loop obstruction. AJR 1982;138:967

98. Hauser JB, Stanley RJ, Geisse G: The ultrasound findings in an obstructed afferent loop. J Clin Ultrasound 1974;2:287

99. Yeh H-C, Rose J, Rabinowitz JG: Sonography of an obstructive ileovesical anastomosis. J Clin Ultrasound 1980;8:160

100. Smithuis RHM, OpdenOrth J: Gastric fluid detected by sonography in fasting patients: relation to duodenal ulcer disease and gastric-outlet obstruction. AJR 1989;153:731

101. Tuncel E: Ultrasonic features of duodenal ulcer. Gastrointest Radiol 1990;15:207

102. Mostbeck G, Mallek R, Gebauer A, Tscholakoff D: Hepatic penetration by duodenal ulcer: sonographic diagnosis. J Clin Ultrasound 1990;18:726

103. Lee TG, Brickman FE, Avecilla LS: Ultrasound diagnosis of intramural intestinal hematoma. J Clin Ultrasound 1977;5:423

104. Chau WK, Na AT, Loh IW et al: Real-time ultrasound diagnosis of intramural intestinal hematoma. J Clin Ultrasound 1989;17:382

105. Orel SG, Nussbaum AR, Yale-Loehr A, Sanders RC: Duodenal hematoma in child abuse: sonographic detection. AJR 1988;151:147

106. Miyamoto Y, Fukuda Y, Urushibara K et al: Ultrasonographic findings in duodenum caused by Schönlein-Henoch purpura. J Clin Ultrasound 1989;17:299

107. Foley LC, Teele RL: Ultrasound of epigastric injuries after blunt trauma. AJR 1979;132:593

108. Hernanz-Schulman M, Genieser NB, Ambrosino M: Sonographic diagnosis of intramural duodenal hematoma. J Ultrasound Med 1989;8:273

109. Bar-Ziv J, Katz R, Nobel M, Antebi E: Duodenal duplication cyst with enteroliths: computed tomography and ultrasound diagnosis. Gastrointest Radiol 1989; 14:220

110. Fried AM, Pulmano CM, Mostowycz L: Duodenal duplication cyst: sonographic and angiographic features. AJR 1977;128:863

111. Burke LF, Clark E: Ileocolic intussusception. A case report. J Clin Ultrasound 1977;5:346

112. Weissberg DL, Scheible W, Leopold GR: Ultrasonographic appearance of adult intussusception. Radiology 1977;124:791

113. Swischuk LE, Hayden CK Jr, Boulden T: Intussusception: indications for ultrasonography and an explanation

of the doughnut and pseudokidney signs. Pediatr Radiol 1985;15:388

114. Bowerman RA, Silver TM, Jaffe MH: Real-time ultrasound diagnosis of intussusception in children. Radiology 1982;143:527

115. Skaane P, Skjennald A: Ultrasonic features of ileocecal intussusception. J Clin Ultrasound 1989;17:590

116. Morton ME, Blumenthal DH, Tan A, Li YP: The ultrasonic appearance of ileocolic intussusception. J Clin Ultrasound 1981;9:516

117. Alzen G, Funke G, Truong S: Pitfalls in the diagnosis of intussusception. J Clin Ultrasound 1989;17:481

118. Montali G, Croce F, De Pra L, Solbiati L: Intussusception of the bowel: a new sonographic pattern. Br J Radiol 1983;56:621

119. Holt S, Samuel E: Multiple concentric ring sign in the ultrasonographic diagnosis of intussusception. Gastrointest Radiol 1978;3:307

120. Sarti DA, Zablen MA: The ultrasonic findings in intussusception of the blind loop in a jejunoileal bypass for obesity. J Clin Ultrasound 1979;7:50

121. Kaude JV, McDowall JD, Neustein CL et al: Intussusception after jejunoileal bypass as diagnosed by ultrasound. Gastrointest Radiol 1981;6:135

122. Mulvihill DM: Ultrasound findings of chronic intussusception in a patient with cystic fibrosis. J Ultrasound Med 1988;7:353

123. Larson JM, Ellinger DM, Zbybel PJ, Peirce JC: Acute Meckel's diverticulitis: diagnosis by ultrasonography. J Clin Ultrasound 1989;17:682

124. Dorne HL, Jequier S: Sonography of intestinal lymphangiectasia. J Ultrasound Med 1986;5:13

125. Vijayaraghaven SB: Sonographic features of pneumatosis of the small bowel. J Clin Ultrasound 1990;18:579

126. Tennenhouse JE, Wilson SR: Sonographic detection of a small-bowel bezoar. J Ultrasound Med 1990;9:603

127. Peck RJ: Ultrasonography of intestinal ascaris. J Clin Ultrasound 1990;18:741

128. Avni EF, Gansbeke DV, Rodesch P et al: Sonographic demonstration of malabsorption in neonates. J Ultrasound Med 1986;5:85

129. DiCandio G, Mosca F, Campetelli A et al: Sonographic detection of postsurgical recurrence of Crohn disease. AJR 1986;146:523

130. Yeh H-C, Rabinowitz JC: Granulomatous enterocolitis: findings by ultrasonography and computed tomography. Radiology 1983;149:253

131. Gonzalez AC, Hanes JD: Retrorenal abscess secondary to a ruptured retrocecal appendix diagnosed by ultrasound B scan and 67 Ga radionuclide scan. J Clin Ultrasound 1977;5:114

132. Dunne M, Haney P, Sun C-CJ: Sonographic features of bowel perforation and calcific meconium peritonitis in utero. Pediatr Radiol 1983;13:231

133. Blumenthal DH, Rushovich AM, Williams RK, Rochester D: Prenatal sonographic findings of meconium peritonitis with pathologic correlations. J Clin Ultrasound 1982;10:350

134. Garb M, Risenborough J: Meconium peritonitis presenting as fetal ascites on ultrasound. Br J Radiol 1980;53:602

135. Bowen A, Mazer J, Zarabi M, Fujioka M: Cystic meconium peritonitis: ultrasonographic features. Pediatr Radiol 1984;14:18

136. Silverbach S: Antenatal real-time investigation of meconium cyst. J Clin Ultrasound 1983;11:455

137. Carroll BA, Moskowitz PS: Sonographic diagnosis of neonatal meconium cyst. AJR 1981;137:1262

138. Barki Y, Bar-Ziv J: Meconium ileus: ultrasonic diagnosis of intraluminal inspissated meconium. J Clin Ultrasound 1985;13:509

139. Wu CC: Sonographic findings of generalized meconium peritonitis presenting as neonatal ascites. J Clin Ultrasound 1988;16:48

140. Miller JH, Hindman BW, Lam AH: Ultrasound in the evaluation of small bowel lymphoma in children. Radiology 1980;135:409

141. Sener RN, Alper H, Demirci A, Diren HB: A different sonographic "pseudokidney" appearance detected with intestinal lymphoma: "hydronephrotic-pseudokidney." J Clin Ultrasound 1989;17:209

142. Morin ME, Panella J, Baker DA, Engle J: Ultrasound detection of a carcinoid tumor. Gastrointest Radiol 1979;4:359

143. Walecki JK, Hales ED, Chung EB, Laster HD: Ultrasound contribution to diagnosis of Peutz-Jeghers syndrome. Pediatr Radiol 1984;14:62

144. Derchi LE, Solbiati L, Rizzatto G, De Pra L: Normal anatomy and pathologic changes of the small bowel mesentery: US appearance. Radiology 1987;164:649

145. Perez-Fontan FJ, Soler R, Sanchez J et al: Retractile mesenteritis involving the colon: barium enema, sonographic, and CT findings. AJR 1986;147:937

146. Puylaert JBCM: Mesenteric adenitis and acute terminal ileitis: US evaluation using graded compression. Radiology 1986;161:691

147. Puylaert JBCM: Bacterial ileocaecitis. p. 63. In Ultrasound of Appendicitis and its Differential Diagnosis. Springer-Verlag, New York, 1990

148. Matsumoto T, Iida M, Sakai T et al: Yersinia terminal ileitis: sonographic findings in eight patients. AJR 1991;156:965

149. Puylaert JBCM, Lalisang RI, VanderWerf SDJ, Doornbos L: Campylobacter ileocolitis mimicking acute appendicitis: differentiation with graded-compression US. Radiology 1988;166:737

150. Puylaert JBCM, Kristjansdottir S, Golterman KL et al: Typhoid fever: diagnosis by using sonography. AJR 1989;153:745

151. Puylaert JBCM: Acute appendicitis: US evaluation using graded compression. Radiology 1986;158:355

152. Abu-Yousef MM, Bleicher JJ, Maher JW et al: High-resolution sonography of acute appendicitis. AJR 1987;149:53

153. Jeffrey RB Jr, Laing FC, Lewis FR: Acute appendicitis: high-resolution real-time US findings. Radiology 1987;163:11

154. Parulekar SG: Ultrasonographic findings in diseases of the appendix. J Ultrasound Med 1983;2:59

155. Deutsch A, Leopold GR: Ultrasonic demonstration of the inflamed appendix: case report. Radiology 1981;140:163

156. Jeffrey RB Jr, Laing FC, Townsend RR: Acute appendicitis: sonographic criteria based on 250 cases. Radiology 1988;167:327

157. Schwerk WB, Wichtrup B, Rothmund M, Ruschoff J: Ultrasonography in the diagnosis of acute appendicitis: a prospective study. Gastroenterology 1989;97:630

158. Gaensler EHL, Jeffrey RB Jr, Laing FC, Townsend RR: Sonography in patients with suspected acute appendicitis: value in establishing alternative diagnosis. AJR 1989;152:49

159. Worrell JA, Drolshagen LF, Kelly TC et al: Graded compression ultrasound in the diagnosis of appendicitis: a comparison of diagnostic criteria. J Ultrasound Med 1990;9:145

160. Poljak A, Jeffrey RB Jr, Kernberg ME: The gas-containing appendix: potential sonographic pitfall in the diagnosis of acute appendicitis. J Ultrasound Med 1991;10:625

161. Slovis TL, Haller JO, Cohen HL et al: Complicated appendiceal inflammatory disease in children: pylephlebitis and liver abscess. Radiology 1989;171:823

162. Vignault F, Filiatrault D, Brandt ML et al: Acute appendicitis in children: evaluation with US. Radiology 1990;176:501

163. Kao SCS, Smith WL, Abu-Yousef MM et al: Acute appendicitis in children: sonographic findings. AJR 1989;153:375

164. Ceres L, Lopez P, Parra G, Echeverry J: Ultrasound study of acute appendicitis in children with emphasis upon diagnosis of retrocecal appendicitis. Pediatr Radiol 1990;20:258

165. Puri P, O'Donnell B: Management of appendiceal mass in children. Pediatr Surg Int 1989;4:306

166. Borushok KF, Jeffrey RB Jr, Laing FC, Townsend RR: Sonographic diagnosis of perforation in patients with acute appendicitis. AJR 1990;154:275

167. Baker DE, Silver TM, Coran AG, McMillin KI: Postappendectomy fluid collections in children: incidence, nature, and evolution evaluated using US. Radiology 1986;161:341

168. Puylaert JBCM, Hoekstra F, DeVries B et al: Radiation appendicitis: demonstration with graded compression US. Radiology 1987;164:342

169. Sandler MA, Pearlberg JL, Madrazo BL: Ultrasonic and computed tomographic features of mucocele of the appendix. J Ultrasound Med 1984;3:97

170. Horgan JG, Chow PP, Richter JO et al: CT and sonography in the recognition of mucocele of the appendix. AJR 1984;143:959

171. Dachman AH, Lichtenstein LE, Friedman AC: Mucocele of the appendix and pseudomyxoma peritonei. AJR 1985;144:923

172. Athey PA, Hacken JB, Estrada R: Sonographic appearance of mucocele of the appendix. J Clin Ultrasound 1984;12:333

173. Bahia JO, Wilson MH: Mucocele of the appendix presenting as an adnexal mass. J Clin Ultrasound 1989;17:62

174. Skaane P, Ruud TE, Haffner J: Ultrasonographic features of mucocele of the appendix. J Clin Ultrasound 1988;16:584

175. Li YP, Morin ME, Tan A: Ultrasound findings in mucocele of the appendix. J Clin Ultrasound 1981;9:406

176. Tan A, Lau PH: Sonography of primary adenocarcinoma of the appendix with pathological correlation. Am J Gastroenterol 1983;78:488

177. Oppenheimer DA, Carroll BA, Shochat SJ: Sonography of imperforate anus. Radiology 1983;148:127

178. Schuster SR, Teele RL: An analysis of ultrasound scanning as a guide in determination of "high" or "low" imperforate anus. J Pediatr Surg 1979;14:798

179. Derchi LE, Musante F, Biggi E et al: Sonographic appearance of fecal masses. J Ultrasound Med 1985;4:573

180. Glass-Royal MC, Choyke PL, Gottenberg JE, Grant EG: Sonography in the diagnosis of neutropenic colitis. J Ultrasound Med 1987;6:671

181. Teefey SA, Montana MA, Goldfogel GA, Shuman WP: Sonographic diagnosis of neutropenic typhlitis. AJR 1987;149:731

182. Hussain S, Dinshaw H: Ultrasonography in amebic colitis. J Ultrasound Med 1990;9:385

183. Downey DB, Wilson SR: Pseudomembranous colitis: sonographic features. Radiology 1991;180:61

184. Bolondi L, Ferrentino M, Trevisani F et al: Sonographic appearance of pseudomembranous colitis. J Ultrasound Med 1985;4:489

185. Ball TI, Wyly JB: Enterocyst formation: a late complication of neonatal necrotizing enterocolitis. AJR 1986;147:806

186. Patel U, Leonidas JC, Furie D: Sonographic detection of necrotizing enterocolitis in infancy. J Ultrasound Med 1990;9:673

187. Brill PW, Olson SR, Winchester P: Neonatal necrotizing enterocolitis: air in Morison pouch. Radiology 1990;174:469

188. Avni EF, Rypens S, Cohen E, Pardou A: Pericholecystic hyperechogenicities in necrotizing enterocolitis: a specific sonographic sign? Pediatr Radiol 1991;21:179

189. Vernacchia FS, Jeffrey RB, Laing FC, Wing VW: Sonographic recognition of pneumatosis intestinalis. AJR 1985;145:51

190. Parulekar SG: Sonography of colonic diverticulitis. J Ultrasound Med 1985;4:659

191. Wilson SR, Toi A: The value of sonography in the diagnosis of acute diverticulitis of the colon. AJR 1990;154:1199

192. Wada M, Kikuchi Y, Doy M: Uncomplicated acute diverticulitis of the cecum and ascending colon: sonographic findings in 18 patients. AJR 1990;155:283

193. Veranck J, Lambrecht S, Rutgeerts L et al: Can sonography diagnose acute colonic diverticulitis in patients with acute intestinal inflammation? A prospective study. J Clin Ultrasound 1989;17:661

194. Chen SS, Chou YH, Tiu CM, Chang T: Sonographic

features of colovesical fistula. J Clin Ultrasound 1990;18:589

195. Townsend RR, Jeffrey RB Jr, Laing FC: Cecal diverticulitis differentiated from appendicitis using graded-compression sonography. AJR 1989;152:1229

196. Skaane P: Ultrasonic demonstration of a pedunculated colonic polyp. J Clin Ultrasound 1987;15:204

197. Kelvin FM, Maglinte DDT: Colorectal carcinoma: a radiologic and clinical review. Radiology 1987;164:1

198. Schabel SI, Rittenberg GM, Johnson EG III: Carcinoma of the colon demonstrated by ultrasound. J Clin Ultrasound 1978;6:436

199. Gooding GAW: Ultrasonography of the cecum. Gastrointest Radiol 1981;6:243

200. Kremer H, Lohmoeller G, Zollner N: Primary ultrasonic detection of a double carcinoma of the colon. Radiology 1977;124:481

201. Becking WB, Puylaert JBCM, Feldberg MAM, VanLeeuwen MS: Appendiceal involvement in cecal carcinoma: demonstration by ultrasound. Gastrointest Radiol 1989;14:170

202. Parker LA, Vincent LM, Ryan FP, Mittelstaedt CA: Primary lymphoma of the ascending colon: sonographic demonstration. J Clin Ultrasound 1986;14:221

203. Hildebrandt U, Feifel G, Dhom G: The evaluation of the rectum by transrectal ultrasonography. Ultrasound Q 1988;6:167

204. Rifkin MD, Ehrlich SM, Marks G: Staging of rectal carcinoma: prospective comparison of endorectal US and CT. Radiology 1989;170:319

205. Jochem RJ, Reading CC, Dozois RR et al: Endorectal ultrasonographic staging of rectal carcinoma. Mayo Clin Proc 1990;65:1571

206. St. Ville EW, Jafri SZH, Madrazo BL et al: Endorectal sonography in the evaluation of rectal and perirectal disease. AJR 1991;157:503

207. Rifkin MD, Marks GJ: Transrectal US as an adjunct in the diagnosis of rectal and extrarectal tumors. Radiology 1985;157:499

208. Orrom WJ, Wong WD, Rothenberger DA et al: Endorectal ultrasound in the preoperative staging of rectal tumors. Dis Colon Rectum 1990;33:654

209. Mascagni D, Corbellini L, Urciuoli P, DiMatteo G: Endoluminal ultrasound for early detection of local recurrence of rectal cancer. Br J Surg 1989;76:1176

210. Grant TH, Eisenstein MM, Brandt T, Leland J: Supralevator abscess: evaluation with transrectal sonography. Gastrointest Radiol 1989;14:354

211. Botet JF, Lightdale C: Endoscopic sonography of the upper gastrointestinal tract. AJR 1991;156:63

212. Botet JF, Lightdale CJ, Zauber AG et al: Preoperative staging of esophageal cancer: comparison of endoscopic US and dynamic CT. Radiology 1991;181:419

213. Nickl NJ, Cotton PB: Clinical application of endoscopic ultrasonography. Am J Gastroenterol 1990;85:675

214. Vilgrain V, Mompoint D, Palazzo L et al: Staging of esophageal carcinoma: comparison of results and endoscopic sonography and CT. AJR 1990;155:277

215. Tio TL, Coene PLLO, VanDelden OM, Tytgat GNJ:

216. Lightdale CJ, Botet JF, Kelsen DP et al: Diagnosis of recurrent upper gastrointestinal cancer at the surgical anastomosis by endoscopic ultrasound. Gastrointest Endosc 1989;35:407

217. Tio TL, Coene PPLO, den Hartog Jager FCA, Tytgat GNJ: Preoperative TNM classification of esophageal carcinoma by endosonography. Hepato-Gastroenterology 1990;37:376

218. Nakamura H, Endo M, Shimojuu K et al: Esophageal varices evaluated by endoscopic ultrasonography: observation of collateral circulation during non-shunting operations. Surg Endosc 1990;4:69

219. Nakazawa S, Yoshino J, Nakamura T et al: Endoscopic ultrasonography of gastric myogenic tumor: a comparative study between histology and ultrasonography. J Ultrasound Med 1989;8:353

220. Fujishima H, Misawa T, Chijiiwa Y et al: Scirrhous carcinoma of the stomach versus hypertrophic gastritis: findings at endoscopic US. Radiology 1991;181:197

221. Botet JF, Lightdale CJ, Zauber AG et al: Preoperative staging of gastric cancer: comparison of endoscopic US and dynamic CT. Radiology 1991;181:426

222. Rosch T, Lorenz R, Classen M: Endoscopic ultrasonography in the evaluation of colon and rectal disease. Gastrointest Endosc 1990;36:S33

223. Shimizu S, Tada M, Kawai K: Use of endoscopic ultrasonography for the diagnosis of colorectal tumors. Endoscopy 1990;22:31

224. Tio TL, Coene PPLO, Luiken GJHM, Tytgat GNJ: Endosonography in the clinical staging of esophagogastric carcinoma. Gastrointest Endosc 1990;36:52

225. Tio TL, Coene PPLO, Schouwink MH, Tytgat GNJ: Esophageal carcinoma: preoperative TNM classification with endosonography. Radiology 1989;173:411

226. Dancygier H, Classen M: Endoscopic ultrasonography in esophageal diseases. Gastrointest Endosc 1989;35:220

227. Yasuda K, Cho E, Nakajima M, Kawai K: Diagnosis of submucosal lesions of the upper gastrointestinal tract by endoscopic ultrasonography. Gastrointest Endosc 1990;36:S17

228. Caletti G, Zani L, Bolondi L et al: Endoscopic ultrasonography in the diagnosis of gastric submucosal tumor. Gastrointest Endosc 1989;35:413

229. Tio TL, Schouwink MH, Cikot RJLM, Tytgat GNJ: Preoperative TNM classification of gastric carcinoma by endosonography in comparison with the pathologic TNM system: a prospective study of 72 cases. Hepato-gastroenterology 1989;36:51

230. Kimmey MB, Martin RW, Silverstein FE: Endoscopic ultrasound probes. Gastrointest Endosc 1990;36:S40

231. Salem S, O'Malley BP, Hiltz CW: Ultrasonographic appearance of gastrointestinal masses. J Can Assoc Radiol 1980;31:163

232. Schwerk W, Braun B, Dombrowski H: Real-time ultrasound examination in the diagnosis of gastrointestinal tumors. J Clin Ultrasound 1979;7:425

9

Peritoneal Cavity and Abdominal Wall

Lawrence M. Vincent

Because the bulk of intra-abdominal, extraorgan pathology consists of fluid or fluid-containing structures or is associated with intraperitoneal fluid, ultrasound is often an ideal diagnostic modality. In those disease entities perhaps better studied by other modalities, findings detected by ultrasound screening may play a pivotal role in directing speedy and cost-effective management. Ultrasound may also have a wide application in the assessment of the abdominal wall and superficial soft tissues.

To realize the full diagnostic potential of ultrasound, the sonologist must combine a meticulous scanning technique with knowledge of anatomic relationships—not always a simple task in certain pathologic states. In this chapter, technique and pertinent sonographic anatomy are reviewed. Sonographic appearances of a variety of intraperitoneal collections are detailed, including ascites, pus or inflammatory fluid, blood, bile, and cerebrospinal fluid (CSF). Since a general overview of intra-abdominal fluid collections is a major part of my intention, discussion is not limited to the confines of the peritoneum. Thus, retroperitoneal collections of lymph and urine, as well as intraorgan and extraperitoneal cystic lesions and gynecologic pathology that may enter the differential diagnosis of intraperitoneal fluid collections are highlighted. Finally, noncystic lesions involving the peritoneum, omentum, and mesentery, as well as abnormalities of the abdominal wall, are considered.

TECHNIQUE

As with all ultrasound imaging, strict adherence to appropriate transducer selection, correct gain and tissue attenuation compensation, and proper positioning of the patient are imperative. A systematic real-time survey may be initially performed, followed by further specific evaluation of regions of interest as determined by clinical presentation and findings. While conventional real-time scanning is adequate for demonstration of peristalsis (to identify a mass as bowel, distinguish a mass from bowel, or document adhesions) and for identification of pertinent vascular structures, color Doppler and duplex ultrasound should be employed for anatomic and diagnostic clarification as necessary. Abnormal collections should be characterized according to size, pattern of distribution, internal echo characteristics, and relationship to anatomic structures.

Optimal visualization of the superficial abdomen requires the use of a higher frequency transducer than normally employed for routine intra-abdominal work (i.e., 5 or 7.5 MHz short or medium focus), as depth of penetration may be sacrificed for increased resolution. The major limitation of most sector scanheads in evaluating superficial structures is the restricted near field of view, a disadvantage readily overcome with current wide-head real-time scanheads (linear or curved phased array). Another important advantage of wide-head scanheads over sector scanheads relates to detection of specular reflectors (primarily membranes delimiting muscle groups or anatomic compartments), an ability dependent on the orientation of the ultrasound beam relative to the reflecting surface. Because conventional sector scanheads direct the sound beam from a single angle, and because specular reflectors are best seen when the beam is perpendicular to the surface, a slight change in ultrasound beam inclination to the planar surface of the reflector greatly reduces the intensity of the returning echo. This, in combination with the limited field of view, compromises the usefulness of sector scanheads in evaluation of the anterior peritoneum and the abdominal wall, as identification of tissue layers is required for localization of pathology.[1]

Although examination with ultrasound is the preferred means of characterizing fluid-containing lesions, the "classic" sonographic findings of absence of internal echoes, smooth posterior wall margins, and distal acoustic enhancement are not necessarily reliable (or even primary) criteria for the diagnosis of these lesions. More specific criteria relating to the fluid nature of a mass, if present, include the presence of refraction shadows (acoustic shadowing occurring because of refraction of the sound beam at the boundary of a fluid and solid structure), internal septations, fluid-fluid levels, and anterior reverberation artifact.[2-4] Not only may homogeneous solid masses simulate cystic structures, but cystic masses, particularly complicated ones, manifest echopatterns that mimic solid lesions. Thus, even with careful technique, echotexture may be misleading and technical pitfalls unavoidable, a limitation of which the sonologist must be ever mindful.

PERITONEAL CAVITY

ANATOMY AND LOCALIZATION OF ABNORMALITIES

Determination of Intraperitoneal Location

The clinical importance of distinguishing intraperitoneal processes from pleural, subcapsular, retroperitoneal, and other extraperitoneal processes is obvious. Accurate sonographic localization may confirm or narrow the differential diagnosis and aid in decision-making regarding possible ultrasound guidance for diagnostic or therapeutic drainage. Awareness of patterns of distribution and recognition of normally placed and displaced anatomic structures is crucial for localization, particularly with large collections in the right upper quadrant posteriorly and in the lower abdomen and pelvis.

Pleural versus Subdiaphragmatic

Because of the coronary ligament attachments, collections in the right posterior subphrenic space cannot extend between the bare area of the liver and the diaphragm (Figs. 9-1 and 9-2). Conversely, because the right pleural space extends medially to the attachment of the right superior coronary ligament, pleural collections may appear apposed to the bare area; in fact, unless loculated, pleural fluid will tend to distribute posteromedially (Fig. 9-3). Similarly, subcapsular collections need not be limited to the lateral aspect of the right upper quadrant. Transverse ultrasound images demonstrating perihepatic collections extending medially to the coronary ligamentous attachments must therefore represent either a pleural or subcapsular, rather than a subphrenic process.[5,6]

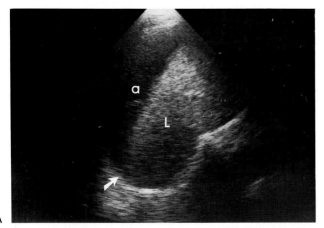
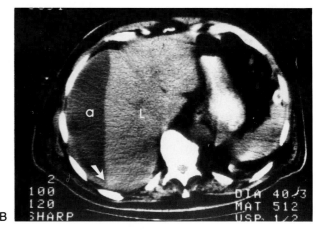

A   B

Fig. 9-1. Right subphrenic abscess. **(A)** Transverse ultrasound and **(B)** corresponding CT scan demonstrate clear demarcation of abscess *(a)* from adjacent liver *(L)*. Note that the collection does not extend medial to the attachment of the right superior coronary ligament, thus delineating the lateral margin of the bare area of the liver (arrow).

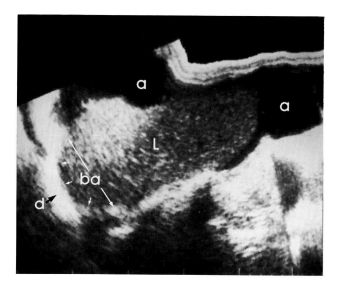

Fig. 9-2. Ascites. Longitudinal image 12 cm to right of midline demonstrates limitation of distribution of free intraperitoneal fluid *(a)* in the right upper quadrant by coronary ligamentous attachments. Note that the fluid does not extend between the bare area *(ba)* of the liver *(L)* and the diaphragm *(d)*.

Unfortunately, due to rib interference and obliquity of the sound beam to the dome of the liver, technically useful transverse scans of the high upper abdomen may be difficult to obtain. Differentiation of subpulmonic effusions from subphrenic fluid collections by ultrasound is usually made by longitudinal imaging. Recognition of the distinct curvilinear echoes that form the diaphragmatic echocomplex and identification of its

relationship to the fluid allow compartmentalization (Fig. 9-4). Although a pleural effusion may produce a diminution in the diaphragmatic echo, the dome of the liver remains sharply marginated, whereas the well-defined liver border is generally lost with subphrenic collections[7] (Fig. 9-1A).

Subcapsular versus Intraperitoneal

Subcapsular liver and spleen collections are readily identified when seen inferior to the diaphragmatic echocomplex unilaterally and conforming to the shape of the organ capsule (Fig. 9-5). Subcapsular liver collections will also be confined by the falciform ligament, and unlike intraperitoneal fluid, may extend medially to the attachment of the superior coronary ligament. With respiration, there is characteristically a lack of change in the subcapsular collection relative to the organ.

Retroperitoneal versus Intraperitoneal

Retroperitoneal location of a mass is confirmed when anterior renal displacement (or anterior displacement of visualized, dilated ureters) can be documented (Fig. 9-6). A mass interposed anteriorly and/or superiorly to the kidneys, however, can be located either intraperitoneally or retroperitoneally (i.e., in the perirenal or anterior pararenal spaces). Determination of the anatomic origin of large masses in the posterior right upper quadrant may be possible on the basis of retroperitoneal fat displace-

A
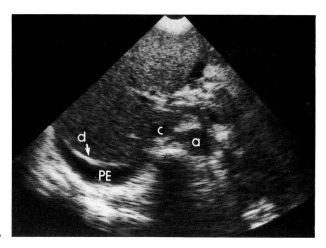

B
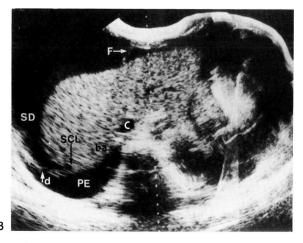

Fig. 9-3. Pleural effusion. **(A)** Transverse scan demonstrates a fluid collection *(PE)* posterior to the distinct curvilinear diaphragmatic echocomplex *(d)*, extending posteromedially. *(a,* aorta; *c,* inferior vena cava.) **(B)** Transverse scan in a different patient with ascites in addition to pleural effusion *(PE)* demonstrates fluid outlining both sides of the diaphragm *(d)*. The ascites cannot extend medial to the attachment of the superior coronary ligament *(SCL)*, in contrast to the pleural effusion, which extends into the medial costophrenic angle. *(ba,* bare area of the liver; *c,* inferior vena cava; *SD,* subphrenic space; *F,* falciform ligament.) (Fig. B from Rubenstein et al,[5] with permission.)

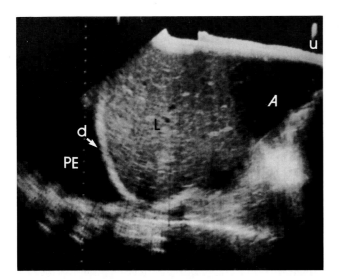

Fig. 9-4. Pleural effusion. Longitudinal scan demonstrates a fluid collection *(PE)* superior to the distinct curvilinear diaphragmatic echocomplex *(d)*. Free intraperitoneal fluid *(A)* is also present in the right subhepatic space. (*L*, liver; *u*, level of umbilicus.)

ment, vascular displacements, or dynamic motion of the mass against adjacent organs.

Fatty and collagenous connective tissues in the perirenal (or anterior pararenal space) produce echoes that are best demonstrated on longitudinal scans. Since retroperitoneal lesions displace the echo ventrally and often cranially, while hepatic and subhepatic lesions produce inferior and posterior displacement, the vector of displacement of this retroperitoneal fat may permit diagnosis of the origin of right upper quadrant masses. How-

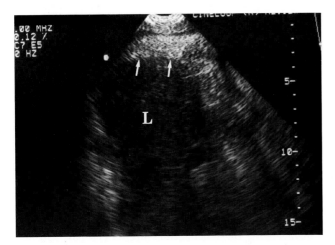

Fig. 9-5. Subcapsular liver hematoma. Oblique image of the right upper quadrant in a patient post liver biopsy demonstrates a band of hyperechogenicity (arrows) conforming to the anterolateral margin of the liver *(L)*.

ever, since this sign is dependent on adequate retroperitoneal fat, it is usually not present in children or in cachectic patients.[8]

Anterior displacement of the superior mesenteric vessels, splenic vein, renal vein, and inferior vena cava (except for the retrohepatic portion, which may be similarly displaced by posterior hepatic masses) excludes an intraperitoneal location. Large right-sided retroperitoneal masses distinctively rotate the intrahepatic portal veins to the left, such that the right portal vein is oriented in a posteroanterior direction instead of its normal left to right horizontal course. Similarly, the left portal vein may course horizontally from right to left, rather than the umbilical portion entering the liver in a posteroanterior direction. Right posterior hepatic masses of similar dimension produce only minor displacement of the intrahepatic portal vein.[9]

Observing dynamic motion of a mass against adjacent organs during respiration or extrinsic pressure may be used to diagnose its origin. Primary liver masses should move simultaneously with the liver and slide against the kidney, masses of renal origin should slide against the inferior liver surface, and adrenal or other retroperitoneal tumors should slide against both the liver and kidney. Application of this sign may be limited in obese patients, patients who are unable to cooperate with deep respirations, or in cases of tumor mass directly invading the adjacent organ.[10]

Extraperitoneal versus Intraperitoneal

Delineation of an undisrupted peritoneal line demarcates extraperitoneal from intraperitoneal locations. Although extraperitoneal fluid collections generally are lenticular with an acute superior angle (as commonly seen with fluid within the confines of the rectus sheath or in the prevesical space) (Fig. 9-7), collections caudal to the linea semicircularis may have a more variable configuration and be confused with abdominopelvic pathology. Demonstration of posterior or lateral bladder displacement suggests an extraperitoneal (i.e., prevesical space) or retroperitoneal location, respectively (see under Abdominal Wall).

Sonographic Identification of Intraperitoneal Compartments

Once the intraperitoneal location of a collection or mass is confirmed, further compartmentalization within the confines of the peritoneal cavity may suggest specific etiologies and influence the subsequent diagnostic workup. Accurate localization of abnormalities detected by ultrasound may depend on identification of liga-

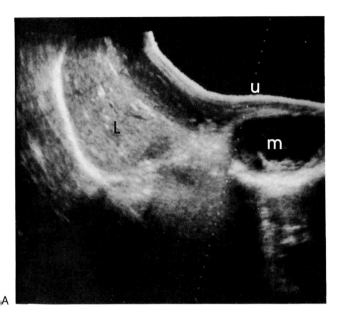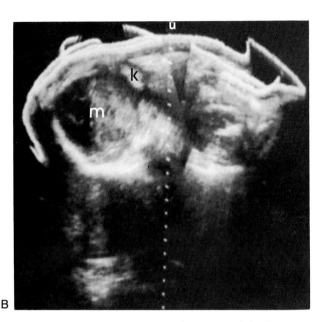

Fig. 9-6. Psoas hematoma. **(A)** Right longitudinal and **(B)** transverse scans demonstrate a large mass *(m)* of mixed echogenicity in the area of the psoas muscle. Retroperitoneal location is confirmed on the basis of anteromedial displacement of the right kidney *(k)*. (*u*, level of umbilicus; *L*, liver.)

ments and peritoneal attachments not normally visualized (Fig. 9-8). The sonographic appearance of intraperitoneal ligaments and reflections and the compartments they define are described in this section. The visualization of this normal anatomy by ultrasound is dependent on the pathologic presence of intraperitoneal fluid.

Perihepatic and Upper Abdominal Compartments

The ligaments on the right side of the liver form the subphrenic and subhepatic spaces. The falciform ligament, which courses over the anterior surface of the liver and attaches to the lower surface of the diaphragm and

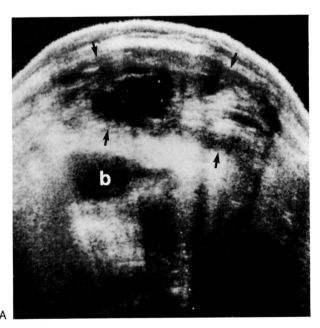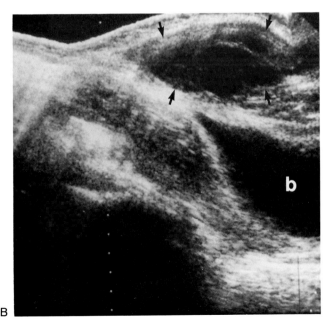

Fig. 9-7. Abdominal wall hematoma. **(A)** Transverse and **(B)** midline sagittal scans demonstrate a complex, largely anechoic collection (arrows) anterior to the bladder *(b)*. Note the lenticular configuration with an acute superior angle in the longitudinal image.

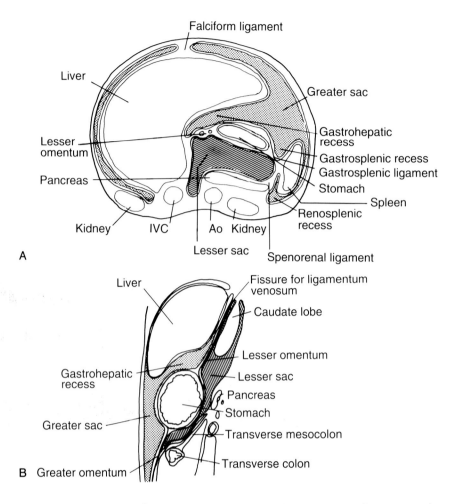

A

B

Fig. 9-8. Intraperitoneal compartments and their borders. **(A)** Transverse and **(B)** midline sagittal anatomic sections of the abdomen. Note that the lesser sac is separated from the more anterior gastrohepatic recess by the lesser omentum and stomach. The gastrosplenic ligament and splenorenal ligaments separate the gastrosplenic recess and the renosplenic recess from the lesser sac, respectively. Also note that the caudate lobe projects into the lesser sac, the latter extending upward to the inferior surface of the diaphragm and then around the caudate lobe to the fissure for the ligamentum venosum.

the ventral abdominal wall, divides the subphrenic space into right and left components (Fig. 9-9). The ligamentum teres hepatis, the remnant of the umbilical vein, ascends from the umbilicus to the umbilical notch of the liver within the free margin of the falciform ligament prior to coursing within the liver (Fig. 9-10). The bare area of the liver is delineated by the right superior and inferior coronary ligaments, which separate the posterior subphrenic space from the right superior subhepatic space (Morison's pouch). Lateral to the bare area and the

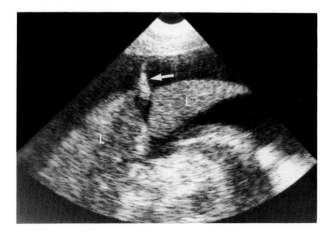

Fig. 9-9. Falciform ligament. Transverse image of a patient with ascites. The falciform ligament (arrow) courses over the anterior surface of the liver and attaches to the lower surface of the diaphragm and the ventral abdominal wall. It divides the anterior subphrenic space into right and left components. (*L*, liver.)

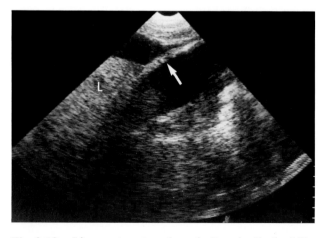

Fig. 9-10. Ligamentum teres hepatis. Longitudinal midline scan of a patient with ascites. The ligamentum teres hepatis (arrow) ascends from the umbilicus to the umbilical notch of the liver within the free margin of the falciform ligament (*L*, liver.)

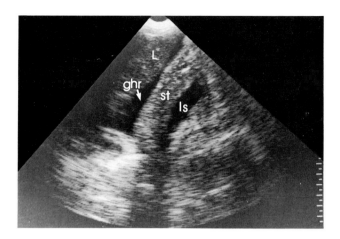

Fig. 9-11. Stomach. Identification of the stomach *(st)* and more posterior structures is dependent on the presence of surrounding fluid and the absence of a significant amount of gastric air. In this longitudinal image to the left of midline, the stomach can be seen delineating the posterior lesser sac fluid *(ls)* from the more anteriorly located fluid in the gastrohepatic recess *(ghr)*. (L, liver.)

right triangular ligament (formed by the fused right superior and inferior coronary ligaments), the posterior subphrenic and subhepatic spaces are continuous.

A single large and irregular perihepatic space surrounds the superior and lateral aspects of the left lobe of the liver, with the left coronary ligaments anatomically separating the subphrenic space into an anterior and a posterior compartment. The left subhepatic space is likewise divided into an anterior compartment (gas-

trohepatic recess) and a posterior compartment (lesser sac) by the lesser omentum and the stomach. Simplistically (and often misleadingly), the lesser sac lies anterior to the pancreas and posterior to the stomach. Definition of the stomach borders and more posterior structures by ultrasound is dependent on the presence of surrounding fluid and the absence of a significant amount of gastric gas. If stomach position is adequately localized, ultrasound can distinguish fluid collections involving the lesser and greater omental cavities (Fig. 9-11).

With fluid present in both the lesser and greater omental cavities, the lesser omentum may be identified as a linear, undulating echodensity extending from the stomach to the porta hepatis (Fig. 9-12). Similarly, the gastrosplenic ligament, a left lateral extension of the greater omentum that connects the gastric greater curvature to the superior splenic hilum and forms a portion of the left lateral border of the lesser sac (demarcating it from the gastrosplenic recess of the greater sac), may be identified on transverse ultrasound images (Fig. 9-13). Thus, identification of the lesser omentum, stomach, and/or gastrosplenic ligament allows for accurate compartmentalization of the lesser sac (posteriorly) from the greater omental bursa (anteriorly).

Other boundaries of the lesser sac occasionally may be visualized by ultrasound in the presence of fluid. The splenorenal ligament, formed by the posterior reflection of the peritoneum off the spleen and passing inferiorly to overlie the left kidney, forms the posterior portion of the left lateral border of the lesser sac and separates the lesser sac from the renosplenic recess (Fig. 9-14). The trans-

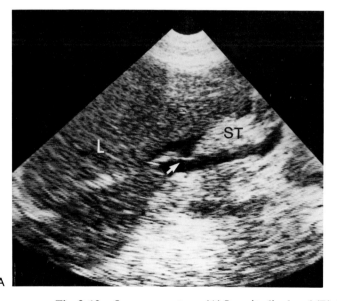

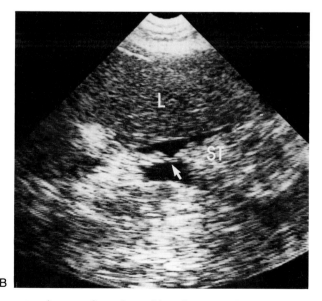

A   B

Fig. 9-12. Lesser omentum. **(A)** Longitudinal and **(B)** transverse images of a patient with ascites secondary to alcoholic liver disease demonstrate the lesser omentum (arrow) as a linear echodensity extending from the lesser curvature of the stomach *(ST)* to the porta hepatis. This landmark separates the fluid in the anterior gastrohepatic recess from that in the posterior lesser sac. (*L*, liver.)

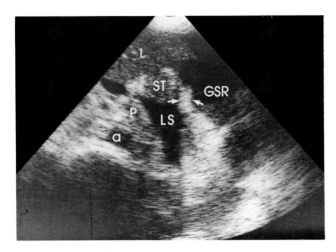

Fig. 9-13. Gastrosplenic ligament. Transverse oblique image of a patient with metastatic adenocarcinoma and ascites demonstrates the gastrosplenic ligament (arrows) forming a portion of the left lateral border of the lesser sac. (*ST*, stomach; *P*, pancreas; *GSR*, gastrosplenic recess; *LS*, lesser sac; *L*, liver; *a*, aorta.)

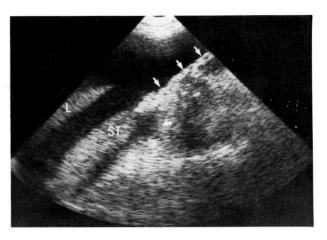

Fig. 9-15. Greater omentum. Left longitudinal image of a patient with intraperitoneal fluid in both the greater and lesser peritoneal cavities demonstrates the greater omentum (arrows) draping from the greater curvature of the stomach *(ST)* and folding back on itself to attach to the transverse colon and mesocolon. The greater omentum defines the inferoanterior extent of the lesser sac, while the transverse mesocolon (curved arrow) delimits the lesser sac inferiorly. (*L*, liver.)

verse mesocolon defines the inferoposterior extent of the lesser sac, and the greater omentum, which drapes from the greater curvature of the stomach and folds back on itself to attach to the transverse colon and mesocolon, forms the inferoanterior border (Fig. 9-15).

The Lesser Omental Bursa

The lesser sac itself is subdivided into a larger lateroinferior space and a smaller mediosuperior recess by the

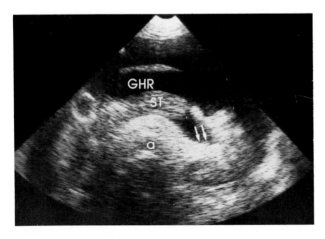

Fig. 9-14. Splenorenal ligament. Transverse scan in same patient as seen in Fig. 9-13 demonstrates the location of the splenorenal ligament (arrows), which forms the left posterolateral portion of the lesser sac, and separates the latter from the renosplenic recess. (*ST*, stomach; *GHR*, gastrohepatic recess; *a*, aorta).

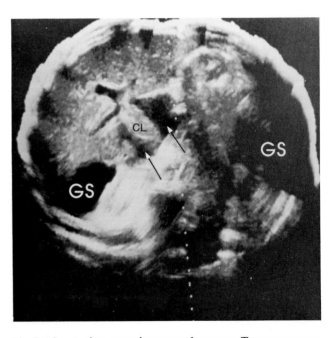

Fig. 9-16. Ascites, superior recess, lesser sac. Transverse scan of the upper abdomen in a peritoneal dialysis patient with both free and loculated upper abdominal fluid. In addition to the greater sac ascites *(GS)*, fluid surrounds the caudate lobe *(CL)* both anteriorly and posteriorly (arrows). This "floating" caudate implies fluid within the superior recess of the lesser sac, since fluid limited to the gastrohepatic recess will not occupy the posterior location. (From Vincent et al,[12] with permission.)

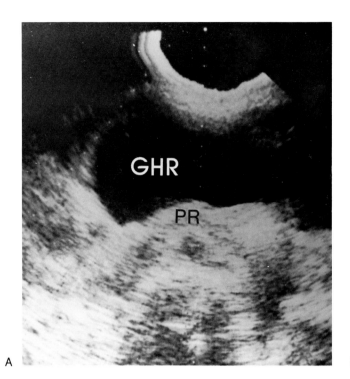

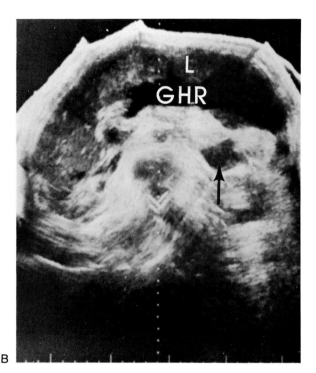

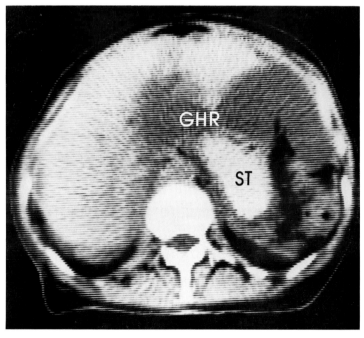

Fig. 9-17. Ascites, gastrohepatic recess. **(A)** Transverse scan of a patient with ovarian adenocarcinoma. A large fluid collection *(GHR)* is noted anterior to the pancreatic region *(PR)*. **(B)** Transverse scan at higher level than in Fig. A. The previously seen collection appears apposed to the left lobe of the liver *(L)*, thus occupying the gastrohepatic recess *(GHR)*. A smaller amount of lesser sac ascites can be appreciated (arrow). **(C)** CT scan of approximately the same level as in Fig. B documents a large fluid collection in the gastrohepatic recess *(GHR)* with posterior stomach *(ST)* displacement. A small lesser sac collection was also identified on additional CT images. (From Vincent et al,[12] with permission.)

gastropancreatic folds, which are produced by the left gastric and hepatic arteries. Superiorly and to both sides of midline, the lesser sac extends to the diaphragm. The superior recess of the bursa surrounds the anterior, medial, and posterior surfaces of the caudate lobe, making the caudate a lesser sac structure. Thus, the appearance of a caudate lobe that is "floating" in fluid confirms a lesser sac component, since fluid strictly confined to the gastrohepatic recess should not extend posterior to the caudate (Fig. 9-16).

Large upper abdominal fluid collections, particularly when loculated, may distort anatomic landmarks by displacing and compressing organs and vascular structures. If the stomach is satisfactorily identified, the location of the fluid may be inferred by the manner of gastric displacement. Large lesser sac collections displace the lesser curvature of the stomach laterally and the posterior portion of the stomach anteriorly, while collections in the gastrohepatic recess displace the anterior portion of the stomach posteriorly[11] (Figs. 9-17 and 9-18).

Because of the anatomic boundaries of the lesser sac, large lesser sac collections may appear more superiorly, anteriorly, or inferiorly than would be anticipated.[12] With lateral displacement of the stomach, lesser sac fluid

may appear directly apposed to the ventral abdominal wall in the midline (Fig. 9-19). Although the caudal extent of the lowermost portion of the lesser sac is at the level of the transverse mesocolon, a well-defined inferior recess may persist between the anterior and posterior reflections of the greater omentum. Thus, lesser sac collections may extend a considerable distance below the plane of the pancreas by inferiorly displacing the transverse mesocolon or extending into the inferior recess of the greater omentum.[13,14]

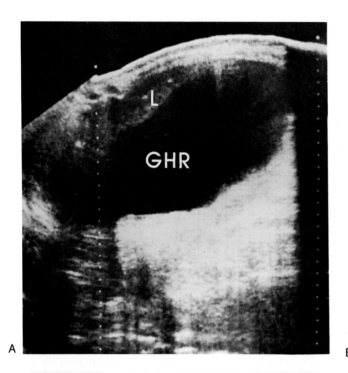

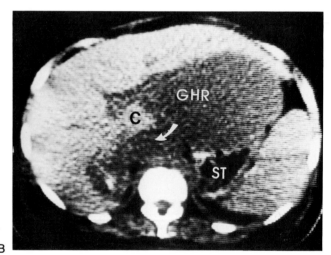

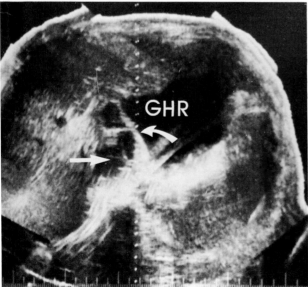

Fig. 9-18. Ascites, greater and lesser sacs. **(A)** Left longitudinal scan of a patient on chronic peritoneal dialysis demonstrates a large fluid collection *(GHR)* extending to the anterior abdominal wall. *(L,* liver.) **(B)** CT scan of the same patient documents a large collection in the gastrohepatic recess *(GHR)*, with posterior displacement and compression of the stomach *(ST)*. Note fluid (curved arrow) located posterior to the caudate lobe *(C)*. **(C)** Transverse ultrasound image at the level of the previous CT image demonstrates the large gastrohepatic collection *(GHR)*. In addition, fluid is seen in the superior recess of the lesser sac (straight arrow), posterior to the caudate lobe. The lesser omentum is seen as a linear echodensity separating these two collections (curved arrow). (From Vincent et al,[12] with permission.)

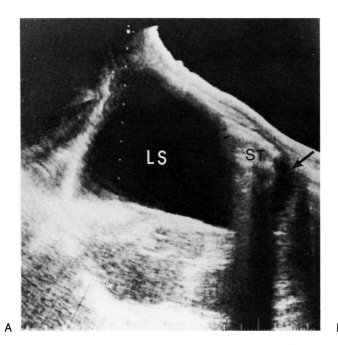
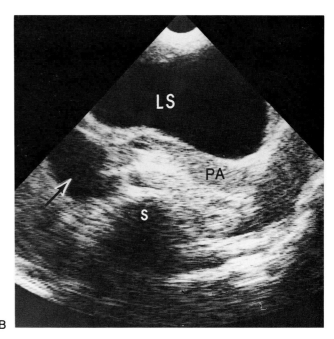

Fig. 9-19. Loculated lesser sac ascites. **(A)** Left longitudinal scan of a renal failure patient presenting with an epigastric mass. The large lesser sac fluid collection *(LS)* displaces the stomach *(ST)* anteriorly, laterally, and inferiorly. Greater sac fluid is noted inferiorly to the displaced stomach (arrow). Note similarity in appearance of this image to Fig. 9-18A. **(B)** Transverse ultrasound image of the same patient, demonstrating the apposition of the large fluid collection *(LS)* to the pancreas *(PA)*. Stomach cannot be identified in this plane because of its inferolateral displacement. A smaller subhepatic fluid collection is noted on the right (arrow). Note similarity in appearance to Fig. 9-17A. (*s*, spine.) (From Vincent et al,[12] with permission.)

Lower Abdominal and Pelvic Compartments

The supravesical space and medial and lateral inguinal fossae represent intraperitoneal paravesical spaces formed by indentation of the anterior parietal peritoneum by the bladder, obliterated umbilical arteries, and inferior epigastric vessels. A more posterior intraperitoneal recess — the rectovesical space — is divided by the uterus into an anterior vesicouterine recess and the posterior rectouterine sac, or pouch of Douglas. Free pelvic fluid is often identified only in the posterior cul-de-sac, but larger amounts may surround the uterus and broad ligaments, and even extend into the inguinal or femoral canals (Fig. 9-20). The peritoneal reflection over the dome of the bladder may have an inferior recess extending anterior to the bladder (the cavum peritonei or the anterior paravesical fossa), and fluid contained within this space may appear rounded or ovoid when imaged transversely.[15]

Intraperitoneal paravesical fluid collections are generally easy to differentiate from extraperitoneal paravesical fluid with ultrasound. Ascites displaces the distended urinary bladder inferiorly, but not posteriorly (although posterior displacement of the partially filled bladder may occur with ascites). Also, intraperitoneal fluid will compress the bladder from its lateral aspect only in cases of loculation.[16] Conversely, fluid collections in the extraperitoneal prevesical space have a "yoke over a bell" or a "molar tooth" configuration, displacing the bladder posteriorly and compressing it from the sides along its entire length.[17,18] With sagittal scanning, prevesical collections in the retropubic space (also known as the space of Retzius) are characterized by an acute superior angle.[18]

FLUID COLLECTIONS AND FLUID-CONTAINING MASSES

Ascites

Typical serous ascites appears as echofree fluid regions indented and shaped by the organs and viscera it surrounds or between which it is interposed. In early experimental cadaver work with A-mode ultrasound, as little as 100 ml of infused intraperitoneal fluid could be detected (in prone and right lateral decubitus positions).[19] Using volume estimates of the hepatorenal recess, 30 to 40 ml of fluid in this specific location could be detected.[20] In a subsequent study, 10 to 15 ml of fluid in

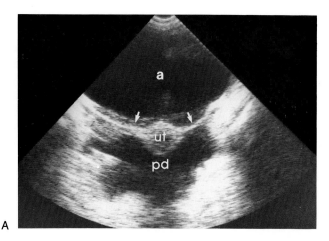

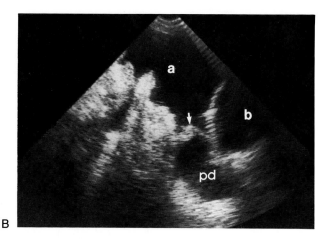

Fig. 9-20. Pelvic ascites. (**A**) Transverse pelvic scan in a patient with massive ascites demonstrates the uterus *(ut)* and broad ligaments (arrows) forming a dividing septum between the pelvic fluid in the anterior and posterior compartments. (*a*, ascites, anterior compartment; *pd*, ascites, pouch of Douglas.) (**B**) Right longitudinal image in the same patient again demonstrates the right broad ligament (arrow) separating anterior pelvic fluid *(a)* from fluid in the pouch of Douglas *(pd)*. (*b*, bladder.)

the pouch of Douglas (patient supine) and in the hepatorenal recess pouch (after Trendelenburg and right decubitus positioning) was reliably detected with transabdominal scanning.[21] The amount of intraperitoneal fluid necessary for recognition by ultrasound is dependent on location as well as volume. Presumably even smaller volumes might be detectable in the cul-de-sac with endovaginal scanning. Regardless, ultrasound is the primary imaging modality for the detection of intra-abdominal fluid.[22]

Factors other than fluid volume that affect the distribution of intraperitoneal fluid include peritoneal pressure, patient position, area from which the fluid originates, rapidity of fluid accumulation, presence or absence of adhesions, density of the fluid with respect to other abdominal organs, and degree of bladder fullness.[23,24] The dynamic pathways of flow of intraperitoneal fluid in vivo have been established by peritoneography; they are pertinent not only for anatomic explanation of preferential location of ascitic fluid, but also directly relate to the intraperitoneal spread of exudates and intraperitoneal seeding of malignant disease. Briefly summarized, fluid in the inframesocolic compartments preferentially seeks the pelvic cavity from the left infracolic space via the right side of the rectum and from the right infracolic space via the small bowel mesentery. After first filling the pouch of Douglas and then the lateral paravesical recesses, the fluid ascends both paracolic gutters. Since the left paracolic gutter is shallower than its counterpart, and since its cephalad extent is limited by the phrenicocolic ligament, the major flow from the pelvis is via the right paracolic gutter, which

serves as the main communication between the upper and lower abdominal compartments in both directions[25] (Fig. 9-21).

Ascites may also involve the chest, extending from the abdomen into the posterior mediastinum through the esophageal hiatus in patients with concomitant hiatal hernia. Stretching of the phrenoesophageal ligament with hiatal hernia permits rising of the esophagogastric junction, accompanied anteriorly and on the left side by the anterior layer of lesser omentum. Peritoneum posterior and to the right of the hiatus may extend into the chest with larger hernias[26] (Fig. 9-22).

The smallest volumes of fluid in the supine patient first appear around the inferior tip of the right lobe of the liver, in the superior portion of the right flank, and in the pelvic cul-de-sac, followed by collection in the paracolic gutters and lateral and anterior to the liver.[27] In a prospective study in men with varying degrees of ascites secondary to liver disease, ascites was around the liver in 92 percent, in the pelvis in 77 percent, in the paracolic gutters in 69 percent, and in Morison's pouch in 63 percent. Of those with moderate or modest ascites, fluid was seen in Morison's pouch in 57 percent and 24 percent of patients, respectively.[28]

Transudative ascites in Morison's pouch is less frequently encountered than might be expected, particularly since this recess is a preferential drainage site for contaminated collections. An explanation for this phenomenon is that the liver ordinarily sinks in ascitic fluid, which results in obliteration of this space in the supine position; with a large amount of ascites, the liver may become suspended under the distended abdominal wall

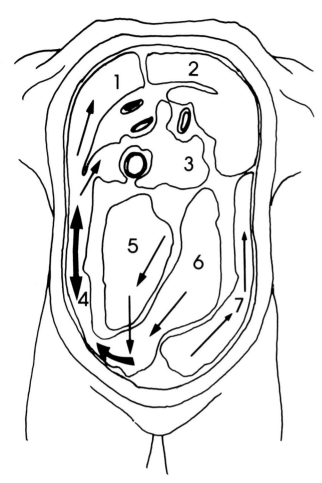

Fig. 9-21. Dynamic pathways of intraperitoneal fluid flow. Fluid from the inframesocolic compartments preferentially seeks the pelvic cavity. After filling the pouch of Douglas and the lateral paravesical recesses, fluid ascends both paracolic gutters. The right paracolic gutter, deeper than its left counterpart, serves as the main communication between the upper and lower abdominal compartments in both directions. (*1*, right subphrenic space; *2*, left subphrenic space; *3*, lesser sac; *4*, right paracolic gutter; *5*, right infracolic space; *6*, left infracolic space; *7*; left paracolic gutter.)

by the falciform ligament, and the pouch may open up to accommodate fluid.[29] Similarly, relatively smaller amounts of fluid in the lesser sac are present with benign, transudative ascites, which suggests that the foramen of Winslow is more a potential than a real communicating pathway in most adults.[30]

Small bowel loops will sink or float in surrounding ascitic fluid depending on relative gas content and amount of fat in the mesentery (Fig. 9-23). The middle portion of the transverse colon usually floats on top of the fluid because of its gas content, whereas the ascending portions of the colon, which are fixed retroperitone-

ally, remain in their normal location with or without gas[31] (Fig. 9-24). Floating loops of small bowel, anchored posteriorly by mesentery and with fluid between the mesenteric folds, have a characteristic anterior convex fan shape or arcuate appearance (Fig. 9-25). In severely emaciated patients with scant mesenteric fat, the entire small bowel mesentery complex may sink in ascitic fluid.[29] With "tense" ascites, bowel loops may be asymmetrically displaced and appear compressed (Fig. 9-26).

Although the pouch of Douglas is the most common site for intraperitoneal pelvic fluid accumulation, an overdistended bladder may mask small quantities of fluid. Partial bladder emptying may permit detection of subtle cul-de-sac collections not initially appreciated. Displaced cul-de-sac fluid from bladder overdistension, migrating to the peritoneal reflection adjacent to the anterior and superior aspect of the uterine fundus, may be visible as a well-defined triangular fluid "cap" on longitudinal sonograms[24] (Fig. 9-27).

Certain deviations from the usual sonographic patterns associated with ascites suggest an exudative (i.e., inflammatory or malignant) rather than a transudative collection. These include fine or coarse internal echoes, loculation or unusual distribution, matting or clumping of bowel loops, and thickening of interfaces between the fluid and neighboring structures[32] (Figs. 9-28 and 9-29). In one series, the overall accuracy of ultrasound in differentiating transudates from exudates was approximately 82 percent. Absence of these findings, however, does not exclude exudative fluid, since approximately one-fourth of exudates in the study just described demonstrated a transudative sonographic pattern.[27] Chylous ascites may also present with diffuse fine high-amplitude echoes.[33] Obviously the demonstration of sonographically visible liver metastases, abdominal masses, or adenopathy associated with intraperitoneal fluid suggests malignant ascites regardless of its appearance.

Because a disproportionate amount of fluid within the lesser sac is not typical for generalized peritoneal ascites, its presence should direct a search for pathology in adjacent organs (i.e., acute pancreatitis and its complications or penetrating posterior gastric ulcer) or consideration of a malignant etiology, such as carcinoma of the pancreas or ovary.[30] Exceptions to this pattern may be encountered in renal failure patients on long-term intraperitoneal dialysis with prior episodes of peritonitis[12] (Fig. 9-19). While fluid in the hepatorenal recess may be a manifestation of generalized ascites, its detection in the context of an acute abdomen may represent inflammatory fluid from acute cholecystitis, fluid due to pancreatic autolysis, or blood from a ruptured hepatic neoplasm or ectopic gestation.[20] Fluid isolated to the hepatorenal recess is particularly bothersome for exu-

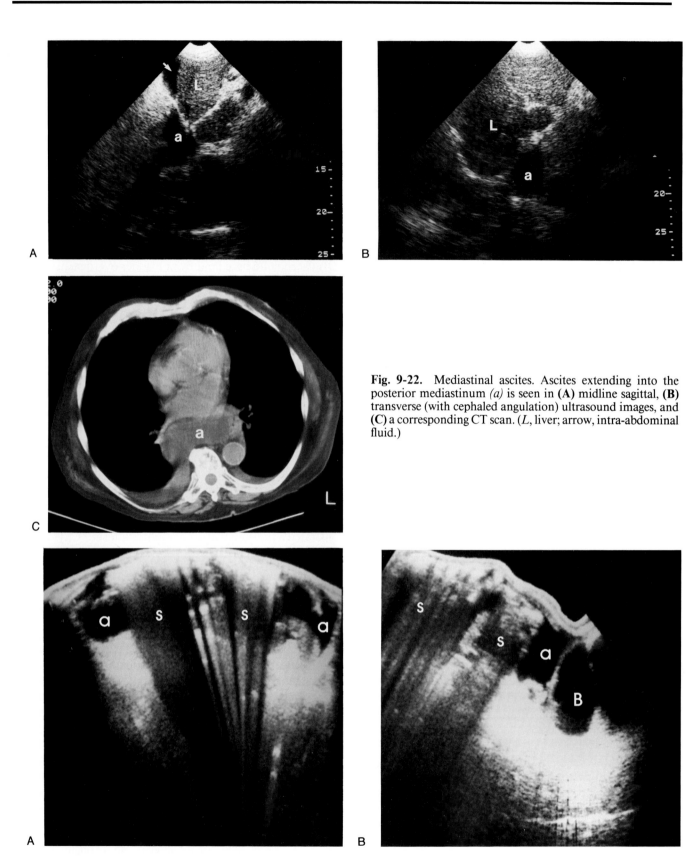

Fig. 9-22. Mediastinal ascites. Ascites extending into the posterior mediastinum *(a)* is seen in **(A)** midline sagittal, **(B)** transverse (with cephaled angulation) ultrasound images, and **(C)** a corresponding CT scan. (*L*, liver; arrow, intra-abdominal fluid.)

Fig. 9-23. Floating small bowel loops. **(A)** Transverse and **(B)** midline sagittal ultrasound images demonstrate acoustic shadowing *(s)* from gas-filled small bowel loops that are floating to the anterior abdominal surface in a patient with ascites. (*a*, ascites; *b*, bladder.)

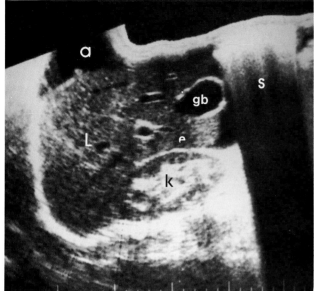

Fig. 9-24. Floating transverse colon. Longitudinal scan to the right of midline in a patient with ascites demonstrates bowel gas shadowing *(s)* from transverse colon floating on ascitic fluid. Ascending portions of the colon, fixed retroperitoneally, will remain in the normal location in the presence of ascites, with or without intraluminal gas. *(L,* liver; *k,* right kidney; *gb,* gallbladder; *a,* ascites.)

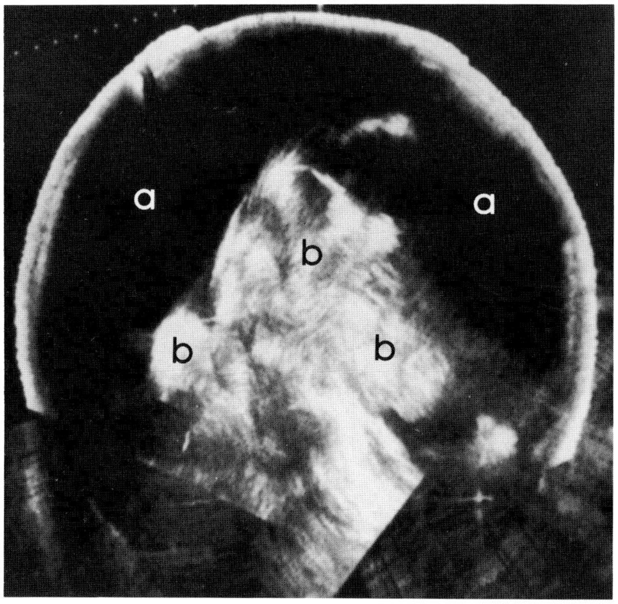

Fig. 9-26. Tense ascites. Transverse scan in a patient with pancreatic ascites demonstrates nonfloating bowel loops *(b)* completely surrounded and compressed by the ascitic fluid *(a).* The presence of floating bowel loops in ascites is dependent on relative gas content within the bowel, the amount of fat in the mesentery, and the degree of tenseness of the ascites.

date, as confinement to this location is not typical for simple ascites.

Localized intra-abdominal fluid collections are commonly encountered in patients who have undergone recent abdominal surgery. Fluid in the gallbladder fossa has been identified in 24 percent of 105 cholecystectomy patients 2 to 4 days postoperatively, with 92 percent

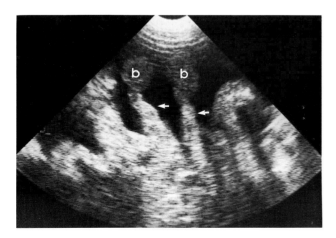

Fig. 9-25. Ascites in mesenteric folds. Longitudinal scan of the abdomen of a patient with ascites demonstrates floating small bowel *(b)* with fluid between the mesenteric folds (arrows), producing the characteristic fan-shaped appearance.

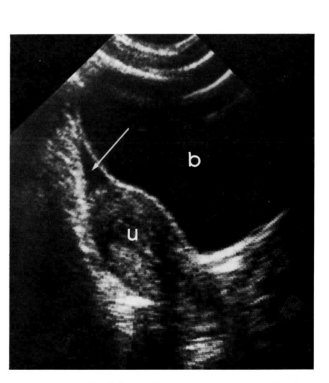

Fig. 9-27. Pelvic fluid, uterine fundal "cap." Longitudinal scan demonstrates a triangular fluid collection (arrow) at the interface of the uterine fundus *(u)* and the bladder *(b).* (From Nyberg et al,[24] with permission.)

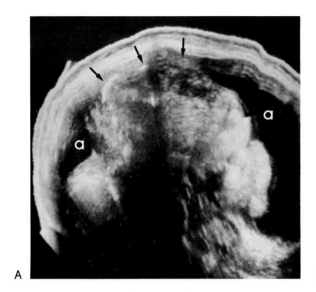
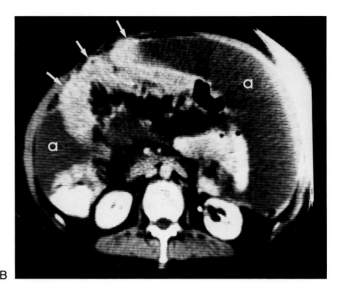

Fig. 9-28.   Malignant ascites. **(A)** Transverse scan and **(B)** CT scan at comparable level in a patient with malignant ascites demonstrate adherence and clumping of bowel loops to a portion of the anterior abdominal wall (arrows), a pattern suggesting exudative ascites. (*a*, ascites.)

being of no clinical significance.[34] Interestingly, patients closed without drains did not develop fluid, suggesting that the presence of drains may predispose to fluid accumulation, possibly by preventing apposition of tissue surfaces. In a study of 80 asymptomatic postoperative patients following a variety of abdominal surgical procedures, localized abdominal fluid collections were seen in 19 percent (15 patients) on postoperative day 4 and 6 percent (5 patients) on postoperative day 8. Collections identified in two patients 12 days after surgery were both abnormal (abscess and hematoma).[35] In a subsequent

similar study of 52 patients, 8 percent (4 patients) had detectable fluid collections on the seventh postoperative day; the two collections not in the gallbladder fossa proved abnormal.[36] Thus, as a general rule, abdominal fluid collections do not persist as a normal part of the healing process 1 week after abdominal surgery.

Transudative ascites, when exhibiting the typical sonographic characteristics as described, is not likely to be confused with other entities. Nonetheless, bilious, chylous, urinary, or CSF ascites may appear indistinguishable, and fresh hematomas or inflammatory collections

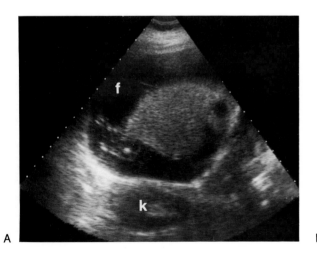
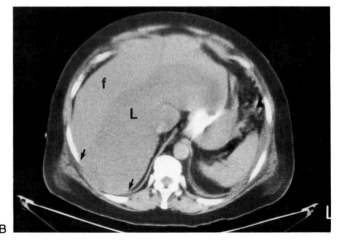

Fig. 9-29.   Infected ascites. **(A)** Fluid with internal echoes *(f)* is seen surrounding the inferior right hepatic lobe in a transverse scan, beam centered laterally on the right (*k*, right kidney). **(B)** CT scan at a higher level demonstrates the fluid collection *(f)*, which is characterized by relatively high attenuation values. Note demarcation of the bare area (arrows). (*L*, liver.)

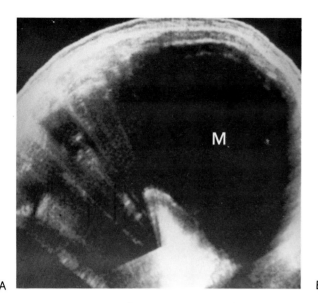
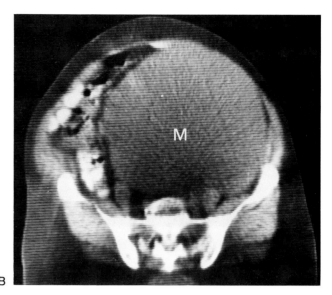

A   B

Fig. 9-30. Ovarian cystadenoma. **(A)** Transverse scan demonstrates an enormous anechoic abdominopelvic mass *(M)*, correlating with **(B)** CT scan findings. Large cystic neoplasms of this nature may occasionally mimic ascites, although bowel loop displacement by the tumor mass is distinct from the floating bowel loop pattern that is more commonly seen with transudative ascites. Evaluation may be even more difficult when loculated ascitic fluid collections are present, or when cystic neoplasms exist concurrently with free or loculated ascites.

may occasionally pose similar problems. Large cystic neoplasms, in particular cystadenocarcinoma of the ovary, may mimic ascites,[37] although bowel loop displacement by tumor mass is clearly distinct from the central "floating" bowel loop pattern commonly seen with transudative ascites (Fig. 9-30). Excess preperitoneal fat in the anterior abdominal wall may occasionally simulate a shallow collection of ascites, but its characteristic location (anterior to liver) and appearance (low-

amplitude echoes and the lack of positional variation or interface with bowel) should obviate any possible confusion.

Loculated or exudative collections of ascites may be more difficult to distinguish from other intraperitoneal cystic masses such as abscess, hematoma, lymphocele, pancreatic inflammatory fluid, or cystic neoplasm.[38,39] Loculated ascitic collections incorporating bowel loops may add to the confusing sonographic picture, as will the

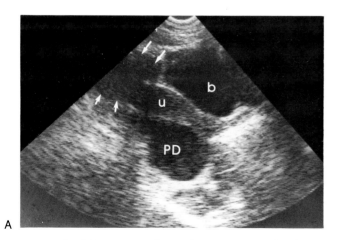
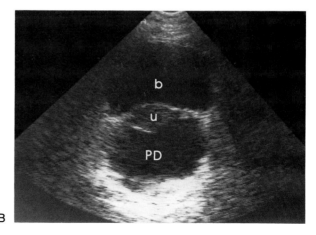

A   B

Fig. 9-31. Appendiceal abscess. **(A)** Longitudinal midline and **(B)** transverse scans of the pelvis in a septic 14-year-old girl demonstrate ovoid hypoechoic collections anterosuperior to the uterus (arrows) and within the pouch of Douglas *(PD)*. Low-amplitude echoes are seen within both collections, along with slightly increased posterior acoustic enhancement. (*u*, uterus; *b*, bladder.)

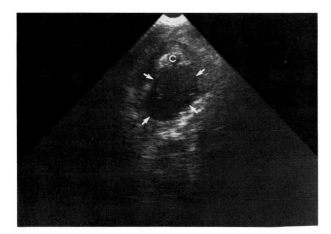

Fig. 9-32. Postappendectomy abscess. Longitudinal image of the right lower quadrant demonstrates a fairly well-delineated ovoid hypoechoic collection (arrows) adjacent to the cecum *(c)*, with mild posterior acoustic enhancement.

coexistence of ascites and a large cystic neoplasm. Compared with cystic masses, loculated ascites tends to be more irregular in outline, generally shows less mass effect, and may change shape slightly with positional variation.[27] This generalization need not hold true, however, since fluid confined within an anatomic compartment (such as the lesser sac) may appear regular in outline and produce significant displacement of stomach or bowel, mimicking a pancreatic pseudocyst or abscess. Extrapancreatic inflammatory fluid in atypical locations is especially prone to confusion with loculated ascites.

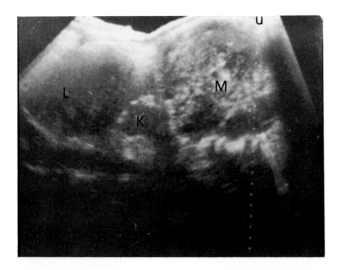

Fig. 9-33. Retroperitoneal abscess. Right longitudinal image demonstrates a large, solid-appearing hyperechoic complex mass *(M)*. A total of 13,000 ml of pus were ultimately removed from this large retroperitoneal abscess by needle aspiration and incisional drainage. (*L*, liver; *K*, kidney; *u*, level of umbilicus.)

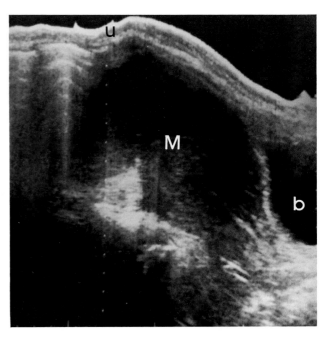

Fig. 9-34. Postpartum pelvic abscess. Longitudinal midline scan in a postpartum woman with fever demonstrates a large, complex but predominantly anechoic pelvis mass *(M)*, with internal echoes present dependently. (*b*, bladder; *u*, level of umbilicus.)

Abscesses

The gamut of sonographic appearances of abscess collections ranges from a cyst-like, fluid appearance to a solid pattern, the variability reflecting the physical characteristics of the collection at the time of

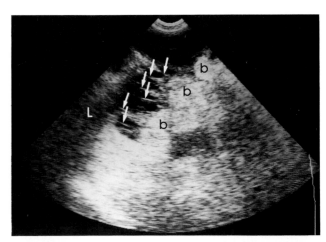

Fig. 9-35. Intra-abdominal abscess. Longitudinal scan demonstrates strandy echodensities (arrows) within an anechoic collection surrounding bowel loops in the right upper abdomen of a patient following cecal perforation. (*L*, liver; *b*, bowel loops.)

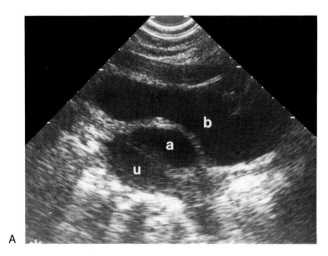 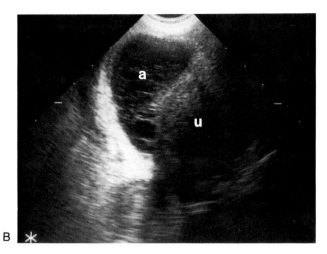

A

B

Fig. 9-36. Diverticular abscess. **(A)** Transabdominal midline sagittal scan demonstrates an oval hypoechoic collection *(a)* interposed between bladder *(b)* and uterus *(u)*. **(B)** Sagittal transvaginal image more clearly characterizes the strandy internal echoes within the abscess *(a)*. *(u,* uterus.)

examination[40-42] (Figs. 9-31 to 9-33). In a large percentage of cases, weak echoes are dispersed throughout the collection, although well-defined fluid-debris levels may be seen. Large amounts of strongly echoing debris may also be encountered, often dependently, as well as septa or band-like internal echoes corresponding to the walls of loculi (Figs. 9-34 to 9-36). Gas-containing abscesses reveal scattered air reflectors (Fig. 9-37); less commonly, they may appear as a region of acoustic shadowing or an echogenic mass with or without acoustic shadowing.[43] A horizontal echogenic line representing an air-fluid level in a large gas-containing abscess may be recognized

when the collection is viewed from a posterior position[44] (Fig. 9-38).

Although parenchymal abscesses are usually round or ellipsoidal, the configuration of intraperitoneal abscesses depends on the anatomic compartment involved (Figs. 9-39 and 9-40). Abscesses tend to hold their shape and displace or indent neighboring structures unless they meet with resistant boundaries such as the liver capsule or sacral promontory. Thus, a right-sided subphrenic abscess may have a curvilinear border and mimic ascites; however, if under enough pressure, the collection may have convex rather than curvilinear margins[45,46] (Fig.

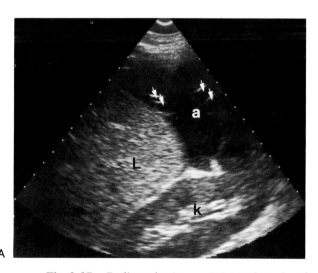 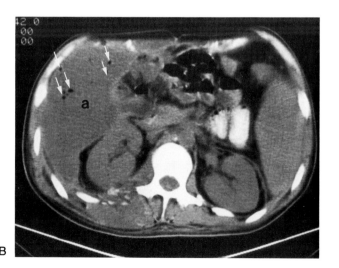

A

B

Fig. 9-37. Perihepatic abscess. **(A)** Multiple air reflectors (arrows) are apparent in this right sagittal scan of a large perihepatic abscess collection *(a)*. *(L,* liver; *k,* right kidney.) **(B)** Corresponding CT scan illustrates scattered small gas collections (arrows) within the abscess *(a)*.

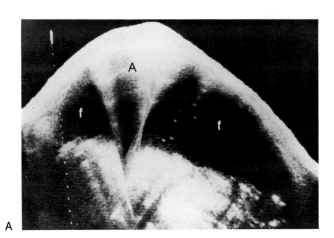

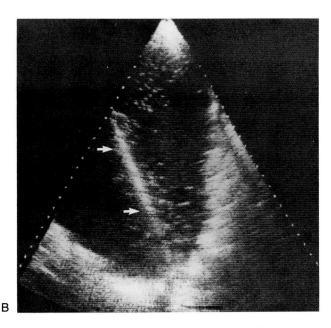

Fig. 9-38. Air-containing abscess. **(A)** Transverse scan of the upper abdomen demonstrates a large fluid collection *(f)*. Ring-down artifacts *(A)* seen anteriorly result from air in the nondependent portion of the cavity. **(B)** Real-time sector scan of the same patient, with the beam aimed anteromedially from a left posterolateral approach, demonstrates a linear echo (arrows) representing the air-fluid level. Since the position of the transducer corresponds to the top of the display, the entire image is rotated more than 90 degrees; thus, the echogenic line of the air-fluid level appears past the vertical rather than horizontal (From Golding et al,[44] with permission.)

9-41). Non-solid-appearing and non-gas-containing abscesses generally transmit sound well, although the degree of potentiation of deep echoes is less than that of simple fluid collections. The walls of abscesses are typically finely irregular, although gross wall irregularity has been reported in 25 percent of abscesses in one series.[42]

Retained surgical sponges may result in an aseptic fibrinous response or an exudative response with abscess formation. Sonography typically identifies a complex, predominantly hypoechoic mass containing highly echogenic foci; the latter is often associated with a strong posterior shadow[47-49] (Fig. 9-42). Distinction between the two types of foreign body reaction does not appear possible on the basis of ultrasound criteria.

Potential difficulties with abscess searches using ultrasound include lack of specificity, the presence of inci-

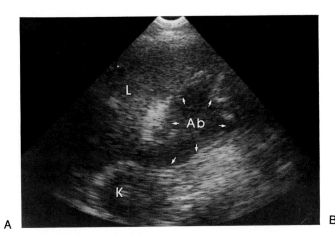

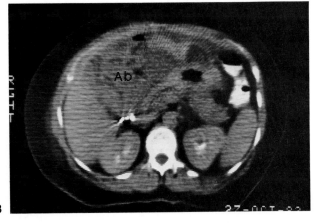

Fig. 9-39. Subhepatic abscess. **(A)** Transverse oblique scan of the right upper abdomen in a febrile patient following a gastrectomy demonstrates a homogeneous hypoechoic mass *(Ab)* occupying the right subhepatic space. *(L,* liver; *K,* kidney.) **(B)** CT scan confirms abnormal soft tissue density *(Ab)* in the subhepatic region. Subsequent surgical drainage confirmed a large right subhepatic abscess.

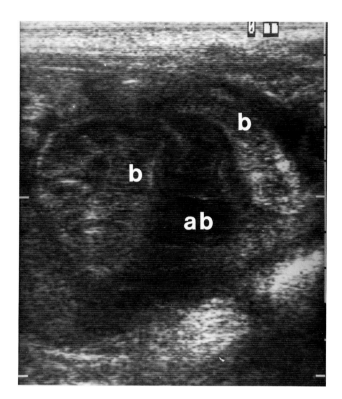

Fig. 9-40. Diverticular abscess. Sagittal image of the left lower quadrant in a febrile patient with known diverticular disease demonstrates an irregular fluid collection with fine strandy densities *(ab)* surrounding, and indented by, distal colonic bowel loops *(b)*.

sions, drains, or ostomies, and obscuration by bowel gas. However, with meticulous examination and manipulation of patient position, the presence of bowel gas need not always severely limit ultrasound evaluation. Because the liver serves as a nearly constant window into both the right and left subhepatic spaces, as well as into the right subdiaphragmatic space, and since the bladder similarly provides a window into the pouch of Douglas and the supravesical pelvis, the right upper quadrant and pelvis are the anatomic regions best suited for ultrasound evaluation. With the spleen present, the left upper quadrant and left subphrenic region can frequently be evaluated by scanning intercostally or coronally with the patient in the right lateral decubitus position. Thus, many abscesses tend to occur in regions where obscuration by bowel gas is technically not a major factor. In certain intra-abdominal locations, particularly the anterior pararenal space, intervening bowel gas will preclude visualization of an abscess unless the collection is extensive enough to displace interposed bowel loops. If the patient is examined in the decubitus position, gas-distended bowel will usually not interfere with visualization of paracolic gutter abscesses. Similarly, the posterior pararenal space, the perirenal space, and the lesser sac may be demonstrated sonographically with the patient in the prone or decubitus position.[50]

The overall accuracy of ultrasound in patients with a suspected abscess has been reported to be as high as 96.8 percent, with a sensitivity of 93 percent, and a specificity of 98.6 percent.[51] Other investigators have reported sen-

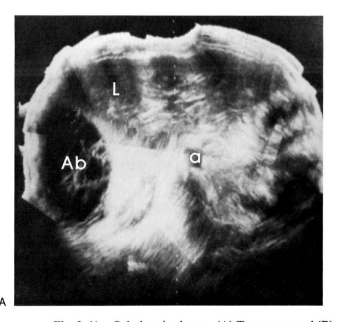

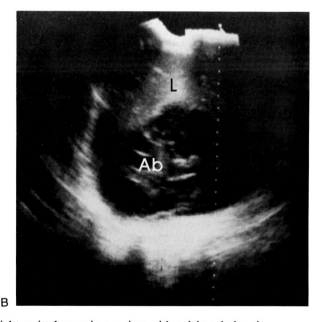

A

B

Fig. 9-41. Subphrenic abscess. **(A)** Transverse and **(B)** right sagittal scans in a patient with a right subphrenic abscess show a complex but largely anechoic mass *(Ab)* with a convex medial margin, with indentation of liver parenchyma *(L)*. *(a*, aorta.)

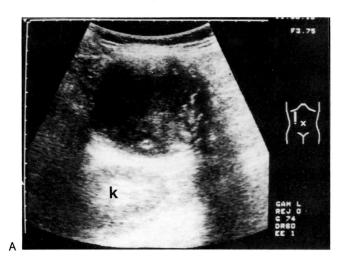

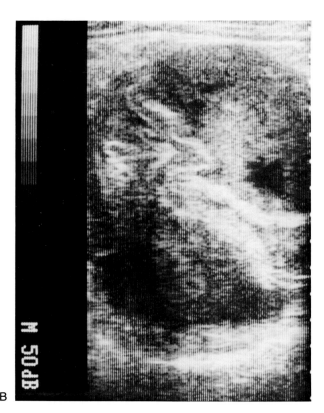

Fig. 9-42. Retained surgical sponge. Two examples of well-defined cystic-appearing masses with irregular internal echoes, identified intraperitoneally and retroperitoneally respectively, in patients imaged **(A)** 18 years after cholecystectomy and **(B)** 8 years after partial nephrectomy. (*k*, right kidney.) (From Kokubo et al,[49] with permission.)

sitivities of less than 93 percent, although greater than 80 percent.[50,52-55] Nonetheless, there have been occasional jarring discrepancies in the literature, with one report of a 44 percent sensitivity for abscess detection using ultrasound.[56] This variance emphasizes the dependence of ultrasound on the technique employed by the examiner, and perhaps to a lesser extent on the equipment utilized.

A multi-imaging approach to abscess detection is often superior to the use of any single modality. Computed tomography (CT) appears to have a well-documented advantage over ultrasound in the accuracy of abscess detection.[46,53-55] Ultrasound studies in the upper abdomen are generally more diagnostic than those in the lower abdomen, and the diagnostic rate is increased when there is a clinical direction to a specific location or quadrant.[55] Because ultrasound scanning is rapid and flexible, and because of its relatively low cost and lack of ionizing radiation, it is often preferred as the initial screening examination for evaluation of a suspected abscess, particularly when there are localizing signs or symptoms. However, in some critically ill patients or patients with localized findings, CT may be the prefera-

ble initial modality depending on patient habitus, the suspected location of abnormality, presence of ileus, or presence of wounds and dressings. Despite demonstration of an abnormal collection by ultrasound, CT evaluation may still be desirable to further depict the extent of the process and relate it to surrounding structures, or to define a safe access route for aspiration biopsy or therapeutic drainage.

Ultrasound-directed needle aspiration of fluid collections is generally preferable to CT-directed aspiration because of speed and cost advantages, although CT localization is advisable when precise anatomic detail is necessary with small or deep-seated lesions. Large superficial collections are ideal for ultrasound localization, but smaller collections may be aspirated successfully with the employment of transducer biopsy guides. With aspiration of fluid collections, transgression of bowel loops with the biopsy needle should be avoided, since an uninfected collection may become contaminated by the needle passage, and/or a false-positive diagnosis may be obtained with the culturing of inadvertent aspiration of bowel contents.[46]

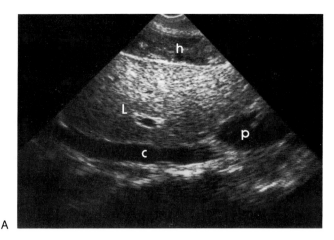

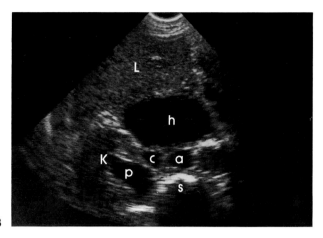

A

B

Fig. 9-43. Intra-abdominal hematoma. Hematomas *(h)* are identified **(A)** anterior to the liver on sagittal scan and **(B)** in the right subhepatic region on transverse scan. Note that diffuse echoes are seen within both hematomas, although they appear somewhat more coarse in the former. Also noted incidentally is right hydronephrosis. (*L*, liver; *K*, kidney; *p*, dilated renal pelvis; *c*, inferior vena cava; *a*, aorta; *s*, spine.)

Hematomas

The echo characteristics of hematomas are highly variable and dependent on age of the collection and transducer frequency. In the acute phase of hemorrhage, hematomas imaged with abdominal transducer frequencies (2.25 to 3.0 MHz) typically are echofree with increased through transmission. In vitro studies have shown, however, that fresh clots are highly echogenic when imaged with higher frequency transducers, while hemolyzed clots become anechoic after 96 hours regardless of transducer frequency.[57]

Subsequent organization of a laminated clot or fragmentation of a hemolyzed clot within a hematoma results in the generation of internal echoes, which most commonly disperse throughout the collection but may layer dependently (Figs. 9-43 and 9-44). Coarse clumps of highly echogenic material may be a striking feature of chronic hematomas (Fig. 9-45). Because of continued clot lysis, late hematomas contain significantly fewer echoes than those less than 30 days old, and may eventually become completely anechoic. Old hematomas, when anechoic, may contain either a thin serosanguinous fluid or a solid gelatinous material.[57,58]

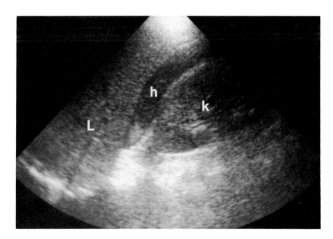

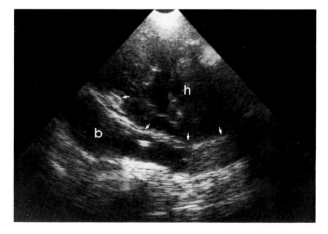

Fig. 9-44. Morison's pouch hematoma. Sagittal image of the right upper abdomen in a patient with ruptured corpus luteum cyst demonstrates clotting blood *(h)* in the hepatorenal recess, with internal echoes seen layering dependently. (*L*, liver; *k*, right kidney.)

Fig. 9-45. Pelvic hematoma. Sagittal midline pelvic scan in a young adult following a motor vehicle accident demonstrates bladder *(b)* compression by a large complex pelvic mass (*h*, arrows). The coarse clumps of echogenic material as seen in this case are characteristic of subacute hematomas.

The shape of hematomas appears determined primarily by location, with intraperitoneal collections generally ovoid or spherical and tending to displace rather than conform to adjacent structures.[45] A lenticular configuration, as well as conformity to surrounding organs, is more likely to be encountered in instances when hemorrhage dissects along well-defined tissue planes, as with hematomas in the anterior abdominal wall or in a subcapsular location[58] (Figs. 9-5 and 9-7). The presence of wall irregularity and septations is variable and of no real diagnostic aid, although thick, angular septae have been described as characteristic of incisional hematomas.[59] The walls of fresh or older hematomas may be sharply defined; however, in one series (including intraorgan as well as intra- and extraperitoneal hematomas), 88 percent demonstrated irregularity of the wall by ultrasound at some time in their course.[58] The incidence of septations within hematomas ranges from 10 to 44 percent among separate series of hematomas in all locations.[42,58]

Intramural intestinal hemorrhage in hemophilia has been demonstrated sonographically as a tubular anechoic mass (hemorrhage) containing a core of strong echoes (bowel lumen), an appearance not unlike that of neoplastic or inflammatory diseases of bowel or other causes of bowel wall thickening.[60] Mesenteric hematomas arising spontaneously as a complication of long-term anticoagulant therapy or following trauma have also been documented by ultrasound as primarily anechoic masses containing internal echoes and/or septa.[61,62]

The sonographic appearance of hematomas is not specific; in particular, there may be considerable overlap with that of abscesses. Cystic masses containing clotted blood may appear indistinguishable from simple hematomas.[63] Nonetheless, the presence of a highly echogenic fluid collection in the pouch of Douglas may be of significant value in diagnosing pelvic hemoperitoneum, since most other fluid collections in the pelvis are predominantly anechoic with low-level echoes.[64] Of course, clinical correlation (i.e., history of trauma, bleeding diathesis, and/or drop in hematocrit) will permit sonographic diagnosis with a high degree of confidence in many cases.

Since there is no reliable means of detecting the presence of infection in a hematoma by ultrasound, needle aspiration must be relied on in certain clinical situations. Skinny needle aspiration of a collection may be unsuccessful despite the "cystic" sonographic appearance if solid gelatinous material is contained within it. In one series, however, all attempted aspirations of hematomas yielded a bloody aspirate when the collections contained echoes.[58]

Bilomas

Extrahepatic loculated collections of bile may develop because of iatrogenic, traumatic, or spontaneous rupture of the biliary tree. While most arise secondary to postoperative bile leakage after gallbladder or liver surgery or nonoperative trauma, bilomas may also be a complication of percutaneous diagnostic transhepatic cholangiography (PTC), biliary drainage procedures, endoscopic retrograde cholangiopancreatography (ERCP), gallbladder neoplasm, liver transplantation, and sickle cell disease (in the latter two instances as a consequence of hepatic arterial occlusion/infarction).[65-71]

On ultrasound, these collections characteristically appear cystic, although they may contain weak internal echoes or a fluid-fluid level if clots or debris are present[65-67,69] (Fig. 9-46). Those containing purulent bile are associated with a more complex internal echopattern (Fig. 9-47). Bilomas typically have sharp margins; when extrahepatic, they are usually crescentic, both surrounding and compressing structures with which they come in contact. While most collections are located in the right or mid-upper abdomen in continuity with the liver or biliary structures, a surprisingly large percentage are localized in the left upper quadrant; 4 of 11 cases in one series, and 5 of 21 cases in another.[66,69]

As with other intraperitoneal cystic collections, the appearance of bilomas is nonspecific, but a correct diagnosis may be suggested from the sonographic findings

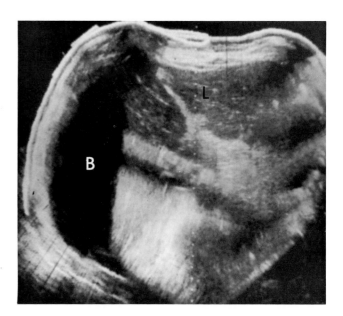

Fig. 9-46. Biloma. A large, anechoic lenticular collection *(B)* is seen lateral to the liver *(L)* in a postcholecystectomy patient. (Transverse scan, 14 cm above the umbilicus.)

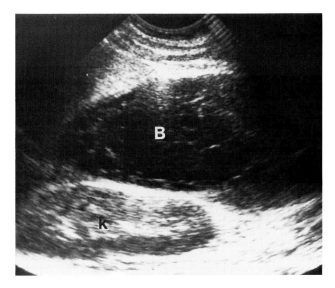

Fig. 9-47. Infected biloma. Right longitudinal scan of a patient with an infected biloma *(B)* demonstrates internal echoes and thin septations within an otherwise anechoic intraperitoneal mass. *(k,* right kidney.) (Courtesy of Harry A. Grant, MD, Eastside Radiology Associates, Bellevue, WA.)

when they are correlated with the clinical history of recent trauma or biliary surgery. Needle aspiration is essential in confirming the diagnosis, and ultrasound-directed guidance may be useful in this regard. The initial appearance of the aspirate may be deceiving in those cases presenting as frank abscesses, with the purulent material not taking on a more bilious appearance until 24 to 48 hours of subsequent drainage.[66]

Inflammatory Fluid of Pancreatic Origin

Inflammatory fluid collections of pancreatic origin, including frank pancreatic pseudocysts, are perhaps the most variable in appearance of all intra-abdominal fluid collections. They may be uni- or multilocular, ovoid or irregular in shape, and have smooth or ragged walls. They may be anechoic or contain a widely variable amount of debris, including multiple septations or nondependent internal echoes due to contained and adherent inflammatory masses (Figs. 9-48 and 9-49). When filled with organizing hematoma, they may mimic a solid mass. Posterior acoustic enhancement is not necessarily present and in some instances its absence may be due to peripheral calcification. Differentiation from abscess and hematoma may be impossible based on ultrasound criteria alone, although pseudocysts are often accompanied by diffuse or focal pancreatic swelling. Change in internal echo characteristics with serial scanning may suggest intervening infection, hemorrhage, or rupture. In addition, evolution over a time interval may help to differentiate a left renal or adrenal cyst from a pancreatic tail mass.[41,42,45,72]

Extrapancreatic fluid collections (i.e., fluid that has tracked beyond the bounds of the pancreas into the surrounding tissues) need not be "cyst-like" or fixed by a dense fibrous capsule, particularly in the acute phase, when most distend an already existing anatomic space or conform to the borders of surrounding viscera. Extrapancreatic fluid collections may involve the lesser sac, the anterior and posterior pararenal spaces, or the peri-

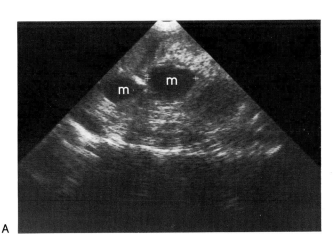

A

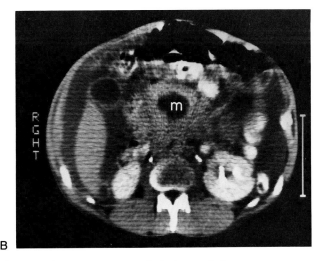

B

Fig. 9-48. Pancreatic pseudocysts. **(A)** Longitudinal midline scan demonstrates two relatively anechoic masses *(m)* with scattered low-amplitude echoes and increased through transmission. **(B)** CT scan through the lowermost lesion, revealing a somewhat irregular ovoid low-density area *(m)* within the body of the pancreas.

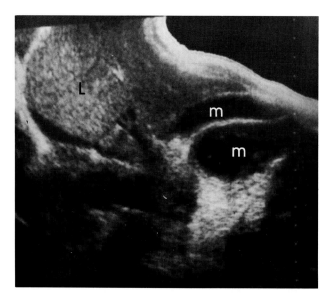

Fig. 9-49. Pancreatic pseudocysts. Longitudinal scan to the right of midline demonstrates adjacent, predominantly anechoic masses in the right upper quadrant *(m)*. (*L*, liver.)

hepatic and juxtasplenic regions, or may reside within the liver or splenic parenchyma or extend into the mediastinum.[73,74] This potential for a remote location does not simplify sonographic diagnosis.

When hemorrhagic, pancreatic fluid collections vary in sonographic appearance depending on the age of the hemorrhage. Acute hemorrhage may appear as well-defined masses with homogeneous echoes of medium intensity, with or without posterior enhancement. In the subacute phase (approximately 1 week after an event), cystic structures containing clumps of internal echoes or

septations may be seen, while remote hemorrhage may be visualized as a purely anechoic lesion.[75]

Cystic Lesions of the Mesentery, Omentum, and Peritoneum

Cystic lesions of the mesentery, omentum, and peritoneum are uncommon lesions not sharing a single etiologic mechanism in their development. Abdominal cysts in general have been categorized as (1) embryologic and developmental, (2) traumatic or acquired, (3) neoplastic, and (4) infective and degenerative.[76,77] The first category includes lesions of lymphatic (e.g., lymphangioma), enteric, and urogenital origin. The terms *mesenteric cyst* and *omental cyst* are often associated with chyle-containing lesions; however, both terms are descriptive only, referring to location and gross appearance. From an imaging perspective, this spectrum may include, in addition to lymphangiomas, nonpancreatic pseudocysts, enteric cysts, enteric duplication cysts, and mesothelial cysts.[78] Specific identification as to etiology of these cystic lesions, if possible, lies in the domain of the pathologist.

Mesenteric and omental cysts characteristically are uni- or multilocular cystic structures with smooth walls[78-82] (Fig. 9-50). Internal septations are typically thin; a single thick septation may correspond to a loop of small bowel trapped by mass.[78] When present, internal echoes correlate with fat globules, debris, superimposed hemorrhage, or infection. Diffuse low-amplitude drifting or swirling echos may be seen in chyle-containing cysts[83]; complicated collections may contain fluid-debris

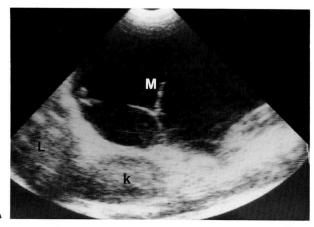
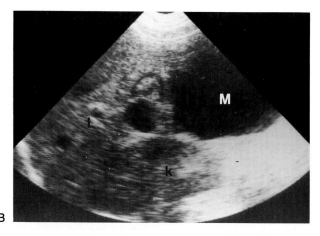

Fig. 9-50. Mesenteric cyst. **(A)** Right sagittal scan demonstrates a large, primarily anechoic intraperitoneal mass *(M)* with scattered septations and diffuse low-amplitude echoes. The mass could not be shown to originate from any specific organ. (*L*, liver; *k*, right kidney.) **(B)** In another patient, right longitudinal scan reveals a similar, apparently non-organ-related mass *(M)*, in this instance without internal echoes. This latter lesion was histologically shown to represent a gastric duplication. (*L*, liver; *k*, right kidney.)

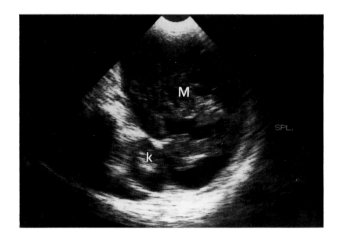

Fig. 9-51. Hemorrhagic mesenteric cyst. A complex left upper quadrant mass *(M)* with a "honey-comb" appearance is seen in a 7-year-old boy on a left transverse oblique scan. (*k*, kidney.) (From Geer et al,[86] with permission.)

or fat-fluid levels or grossly irregular and heterogeneous solid components[78,84-86] (Fig. 9-51).

Although mesenteric cysts may present as a discrete round mass, both mesenteric and particularly omental cysts may follow the contours of the underlying bowel and conform closely to the anterior abdominal wall rather than produce distension (Fig. 9-52). In these instances, the collection may change configuration with

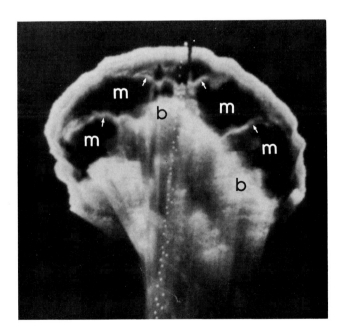

Fig. 9-52. Omental cyst. Omental cyst appears on transverse scan as an extensive septated fluid-filled mass *(m)* closely conforming to the anterior abdominal wall and displacing the bowel *(b)* posteriorly. (From Geer et al,[86] with permission.)

changes in patient position.[87,88] Careful attention to distribution (e.g., anterior location of fluid with none posterior or between bowel loops) can help exclude free intraperitoneal fluid, but not necessarily a loculated collection of ascites. To muddle the diagnostic picture even further, hemorrhage into omental or mesenteric cysts may cause rapid abdominal distension and clinically mimic the sudden onset of ascites.[89]

Benign cystic peritoneal mesothelioma is a rare multicystic lesion with a predilection for the peritoneal and omental surfaces of the pelvic viscera. More common in females, it is felt to represent an intermediate form between the benign adenomatoid tumor of the peritoneum and malignant peritoneal mesothelioma.[90-92] Sonographically, this lesion has a nonspecific thin-walled multicystic appearance[93,94] (Fig. 9-53). The relationship of this entity to so-called peritoneal inclusion cysts is currently unclear; the latter may result from trapping of fluid by peritoneal adhesions. Peritoneal inclusion cysts should be considered in the differential diagnosis when large adnexal cystic structures are identified in a young woman, particularly if there is a history of abdominal surgery or trauma[95-97] (Fig. 9-54).

Fungal infections uncommonly present as peritoneal cystic lesions. Blastomycosis involving the genitourinary tract may present as a cystic multiseptate mass, indistinguishable sonographically from an ovarian epithelial neoplasm or other intraperitoneal cystic lesions.[98] Encysted peritoneal hydatidosis has been reported as a cystic multiseptate mass extending from an intact liver cyst into the peritoneal cavity.[99] Peritoneal echinococcus confined to the peritoneal cavity has also been reported; the mass displayed a homogeneous internal echotexture

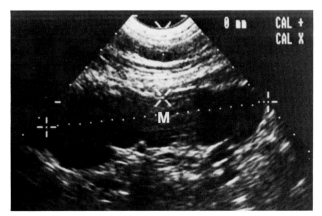

Fig. 9-53. Cystic mesothelioma. Longitudinal scan of lower abdomen and pelvis demonstrates a nonspecific thin-walled cystic mass *(M)* that contained septations (not shown here). (Courtesy of Pablo R. Ros, MD, University of Florida, Gainesville, FL.)

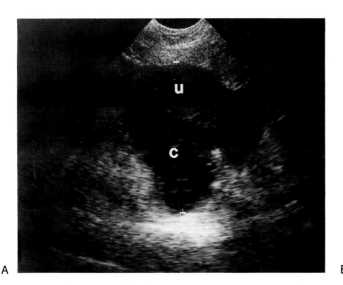
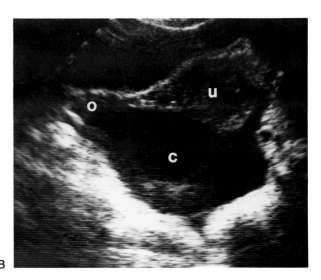

Fig. 9-54. Peritoneal inclusion cyst. **(A)** Transverse scan of the pelvis in a 20-year-old patient status-post colectomy and endorectal pullthrough reveals cysts of mixed echogenicity *(c)* posterior to the uterus *(u)*. No recognizable ovarian tissue was identified. **(B)** Transverse scan in a different patient with prior history of trauma, status-post splenectomy and partial pancreatectomy, demonstrates a large cystic mass *(c)* contiguous with the right ovary *(o)*, with leftward displacement of the uterus *(u)*. (From Hoffer et al,[97] with permission.)

but with a strong posterior wall echo/posterior enhancement. The "solid" cystic appearance in this case was the result of innumerable acoustic interfaces from a multitude of small daughter cysts.[100]

Pseudomyxoma Peritonei

Pseudomyxoma peritonei, which arises from mucinous tumors of the appendix and ovary, is characterized by diffuse involvement of the peritoneal surfaces and omentum with gelatinous mucinous implants, often with massive gelatinous ascites.[101] Ultrasound findings most frequently reported include mantle-like echogenic masses consisting of numerous tiny cysts, echogenic ascites (representing gelatinous ascites), or multiple complex cystic masses surrounding and displacing bowel[102-105] (Figs. 9-55 and 9-56). Other reported appearances include multiple floating or dependent 5 to 20 mm "mucin balls" within ascites[106] or multiple rounded echodense masses (amorphous calcification present in the latter instance).[107] Occasionally, findings

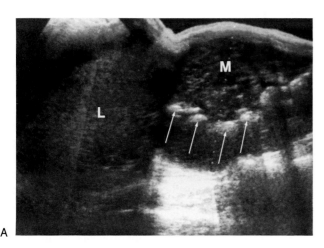
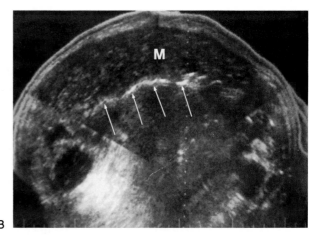

Fig. 9-55. Pseudomyxoma peritonei. **(A)** Right longitudinal and **(B)** transverse scans demonstrate an extensive mantle-like echogenic mass *(M)*, representing gelatinous ascites, with posterior displacement of bowel loops. (*L*, liver; arrows, intraluminal air.)

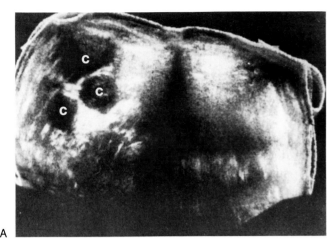

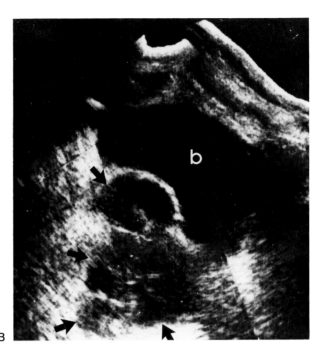

Fig. 9-56. Pseudomyxoma peritonei. **(A)** Transverse scan at the inferior margin of the liver demonstrates several thick wall cysts *(c)* with the appearance of intervening septa. On other scans, the inferior edge of the liver was indented by these cysts (peritoneal scalloping), although the liver itself appeared normal. **(B)** Longitudinal scan over bladder *(b)* in the same patient demonstrates numerous retrovesical cysts (arrows) with intervening septa. (From Hopper,[103] with permission.)

may suggest only an exudative ascites, with nonfloating posterior position of bowel loops.[108] If identified, infiltration along the umbilical vein remnant may provide a differentiating feature between pseudomyxoma peritonei and ascites.[101] Indentation of the liver edge by extrinsic pressure from implants, so-called scalloping, may be sonographically detectable, but this finding is more consistently demonstrated by CT.[103,104,108]

Cerebrospinal Fluid Ascites and Pseudocysts

Cerebrospinal fluid ascites, a rare complication of ventriculoperitoneal shunting, is a diffuse, nonloculated collection of CSF that occurs secondary to a primary failure of the peritoneal cavity to absorb spinal fluid.[109] Sonographically this will be indistinguishable from transudative ascites, but the presence of generalized intraperitoneal fluid in an infant with a ventriculoperitoneal shunt in place should suggest this rare entity.

Encystation of CSF fluid producing distal end obstruction of a ventriculoperitoneal shunt is a more common complication, with a reported incidence of 1.75 percent in one series.[110] The pathophysiology of the intraperitoneal pseudocyst apparently involves an inflam-

matory response to either the catheter or some component of the draining CSF fluid. The inflammatory reaction around the catheter tip is presumed secondary to a low-grade shunt infection and localized peritonitis. A small collection may form around the tip of the shunt tubing and preclude escape of the CSF fluid into the general peritoneal space, or a relatively large area of the peritoneal cavity may become isolated by dense adhesions that produce a multiloculated, poorly absorbing space. The pseudocyst wall may be a thick fibrous capsule (e.g., intestinal loops matted together by connective tissue) or it may be formed solely of inflamed serosal surfaces.[109,111,112]

Ultrasound demonstrates a typical intra-abdominal cystic mass in association with the distal end of the shunt tube[113–119] (Figs. 9-57 and 9-58). Shunt tubing is identified as a linear echogenic structure with acoustic shadowing. Internal echoes or septae may be seen with superimposed infection; abscess formation around the shunt tip may present as a well-circumscribed mass of mixed internal echodensities with an irregular inner border and a surrounding hypoechoic zone.[120]

A small amount of free intraperitoneal CSF fluid is a normal concomitant of satisfactory ventriculoperitoneal shunt function, although its absence does not indicate shunt malfunction. A localized collection of fluid in as-

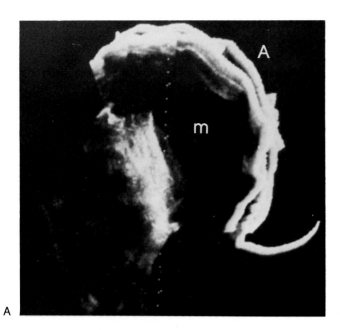 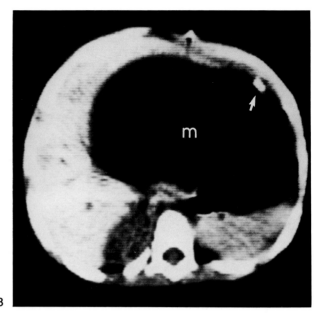

A   B

Fig. 9-57. CSF pseudocyst. **(A)** Transverse decubitus ultrasound and **(B)** corresponding abdominal CT scan demonstrate a large cystic intra-abdominal mass *(m)* in a 4-year-old with a ventriculoperitoneal shunt and abdominal distension. The distal end of the shunt tube (arrow) is identified on CT scan. (*A*, anterior.)

sociation with the abdominal end of a ventriculoperitoneal shunt, however, is pathologic and indicates a malfunction in the system.[121] Although CSF pseudocysts may also be diagnosed by CT, ultrasound is the initial modality of choice in the evaluation of shunt patients who present with abdominal symptoms or an abdominal mass, with or without associated neurologic findings.

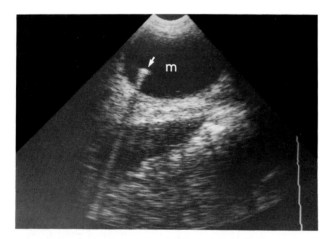

Fig. 9-58. CSF pseudocyst. Elderly patient following a ventriculoperitoneal shunt placement for normal pressure hydrocephalus, presenting with palpable abdominal mass. Longitudinal scan demonstrates an anechoic collection *(m)* associated with shunt tubing (arrow). This superficial collection is extraperitoneal.

DIFFERENTIAL DIAGNOSTIC CONSIDERATIONS

Lymphocele

Lymphocele, a lymph-filled space usually resulting from surgical disruption of lymphatic channels, is a well-recognized complication of radical gynecologic procedures, extensive pelvic urologic operations including staging lymphadenectomy for prostatic or bladder carcinoma, and renal transplantation.[122-125] Lymphoceles are most often unilocular and typically located retroperitoneally in the pelvis, although upper abdominal lymphoceles may occur secondary to aortofemoral bypass or para-aortic/renal hilar node dissections.[126,127]

Sonographically, lymphoceles are generally elliptical, with sharp margins or varying degrees of wall irregularity. They are characterized by increased through transmission and no internal echoes, although thin septations have been seen in as many as 50 percent of cases in one reported series.[42] Since an uncomplicated lymphocele should not contain debris or internal echoes (other than possibly thin septa), these findings suggest the presence of an abscess or hematoma, or a lymphocele complicated by infection. Pelvic lymphoceles may markedly compress and displace the bladder to one side, but in general they displace organs to a lesser extent than an abscess, and may themselves be indented by adjacent solid organs[29,45] (Figs. 9-59 and 9-60).

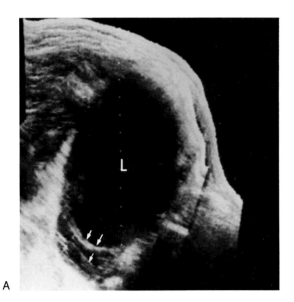
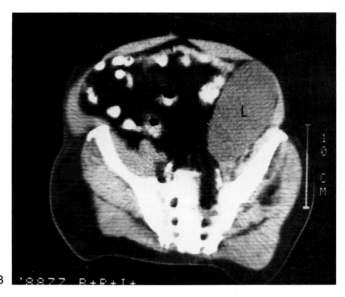

Fig. 9-59. Lymphocele. **(A)** Transverse scan of the left lower abdomen and **(B)** corresponding CT scan in a man following radical prostatectomy. Ultrasound demonstrates the characteristic elliptical shape of the lymphocele *(L),* with sharp margins and slight wall irregularity, and increased through transmission. Also noted are septations and internal echoes present posteriorly (arrows), a finding not appreciated on the CT scans.

Lymphoceles in the posterior pararenal compartment may be the result of cephalad spread from processes originating in the extraperitoneal pelvis, but the retroperitoneal location (and thus exclusion of loculated ascites) may be inferred by anterior kidney or ureter displacement. The retroperitoneal origin of the collection may be more difficult to ascertain sonographically if it is in an atypical location, such as a midlumbar lym-phocele that is anteroinferior rather than posterior to the kidney.[127] Urinomas and lymphoceles may be indistinguishable by ultrasound.[45] As with all fluid collections demonstrated by ultrasound, correlation with history, physical examination, and available radiographic studies may suggest the origin of the collection, but needle aspiration of the visualized fluid may be the only way to establish the diagnosis.

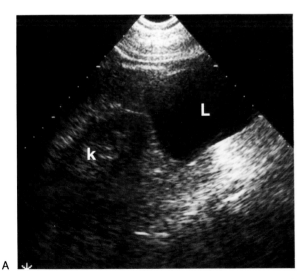
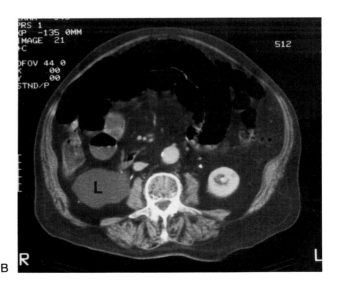

Fig. 9-60. Lymphocele. In another patient status-post radical prostatectomy, **(A)** right sagittal ultrasound and **(B)** corresponding CT image demonstrate a thin-walled, simple-appearing retroperitoneal fluid collection inferior to the right kidney. *(L,* lymphocele; *k,* right kidney.)

Lymphangioma and Mature Teratoma of the Retroperitoneum

Lymphangiomas are believed to represent developmental anomalies of dilated lymphatic vessels. When they involve the retroperitoneum, sonography characteristically demonstrates an elongated mass containing uncomplicated fluid, with or without septa. Internal debris, sometimes layering, is common; septations, when present, tend to be thick[128-130] (Fig. 9-61). Ultrasound findings overlap those of a mature teratoma of the retroperitoneum. The latter lesion contains uncomplicated fluid in roughly three-fourths of cases; on the basis of sonographic pattern alone, fat in retroperitoneal teratomas cannot be reliably differentiated from other types of soft tissue. Identifiable calcium is much more common in mature teratomas than in lymphangiomas, however[131] (Fig. 9-62).

Urinoma

An encapsulated collection of urine may result from closed renal injury or surgical intervention, or may arise spontaneously secondary to an obstructing lesion (e.g., posterior urethral valves, ureteropelvic junction obstruction in neonates; ureteral obstruction secondary to pelvic neoplasm or retroperitoneal adenopathy in adults). Extraperitoneal extravasation may be subcapsular or perirenal, the latter collections are sometimes termed *uriniferous pseudocysts*.[132,133]

Urine leakage tends to remain localized to the perinephric space, the obvious exceptions being in instances of renal trauma or after disruption of tissue boundaries by major surgery. However, collections under high enough pressure may potentially leak around the ureter, where the perinephric fascia is the weakest, or even into adjoining fascial planes and the peritoneal cavity. Par-

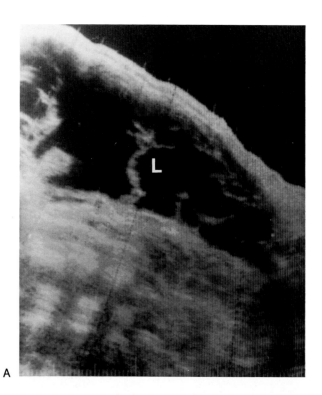

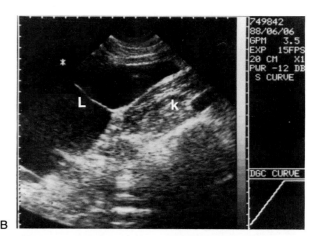

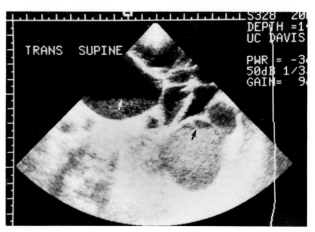

Fig. 9-61. Lymphangioma. **(A)** Longitudinal image of the pelvis in a newborn demonstrates a multiloculated lymphangioma *(L)* with thick septations but otherwise uncomplicated fluid. **(B)** Left parasagittal scan in another patient demonstrates a multiloculated lymphangioma *(L)* anterior to the left kidney *(k)*. **C** In a third patient, transverse sonogram demonstrates a mass consisting of multiple locules with echogenic debris and fluid-debris levels (arrows). At surgery, this lymphangioma was located in the anterior pararenal space, adherent to the pancreas, and evidenced recent and prior hemorrhage. (From Davidson and Hartman,[130] with permission.)

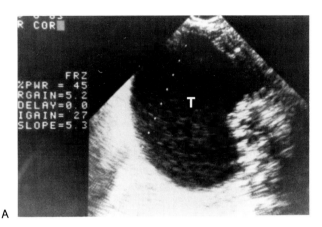
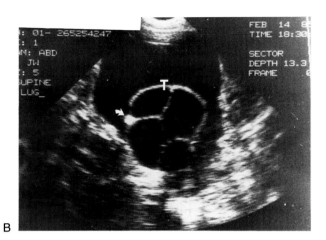
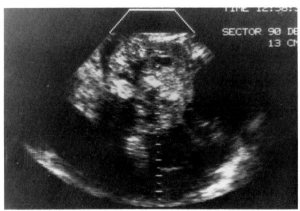

Fig. 9-62. Teratoma. **(A)** Sagittal scan of a 6-month-old girl demonstrates a fluid-filled teratoma *(T)* with echogenic debris layering dependently. **(B)** In a 1-year-old girl, a mature teratoma *(T)* is composed primarily of uncomplicated fluid, with an eccentrically located multiloculated component. Note echogenic focus consistent with calcification (arrow). **C** In a 2-month-old girl, this large mature teratoma (filling entire image) is heterogeneous and complex, with fluid and soft tissue components of the mass roughly equal. (From Davidson et al,[131] with permission.)

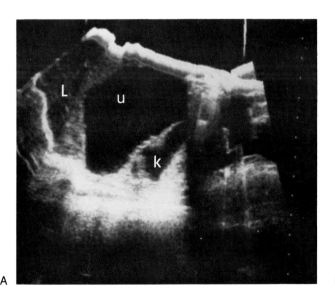
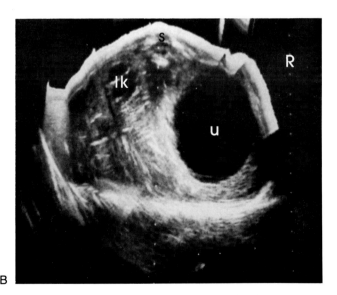

Fig. 9-63. Urinoma. **(A)** Right longitudinal supine and **(B)** transverse prone scans in a male newborn with posterior urethral valves demonstrate the encapsulated extravasated urine collection as a large anechoic retroperitoneal mass *(u)* interposed between the hydronephrotic right kidney *(k)* and liver *(L)*. Left hydronephrosis is also apparent *(lk)*. *(s,* spine; *R,* right.)

tially because of gravity, these cystic masses are most often oriented inferomedially with upward and lateral displacement of the lower pole of the kidney along with medial displacement of the ureter.[134] Circumferential perirenal urinomas may produce pseudonephromegaly on excretory urography; ultrasound can easily eliminate diagnostic confusion in these instances.[135]

Sonographically, urinomas may be anechoic or contain low-level internal echoes, and have good increased through transmission. They characteristically have sharp margins and tend to be elliptical in shape, although they may be indented by adjacent solid organs[41] (Figs. 9-63 and 9-64). In one small series, thin septa were present in 60 percent.[42] A more complex septated appearance has been described in neonates, presumably the result of blood and proteins extravasated into the perirenal space at the time of renal parenchymal rupture. Solid-appearing regions may also be attributable to blood products layering within such loculations.[136]

Urachal Cyst

The adult urachus, the remnant of the embryologic connection between the ventral cloaca and the umbilicus, is normally a functionally closed fibrous cord located extraperitoneally in the midline between the peritoneum and the transversalis fascia. Incomplete regression of the urachus during development may result in various anomalies, including patent urachus, urachal diverticulum, urachal sinus, or urachal cyst.[137] The latter entity, representing persistence of the urachal midpor-

tion with both cephalic and caudal ends closed, typically remains silent unless symptoms related to size or secondary infection supervene.[138]

The ultrasound appearance of urachal cysts ranges from a small cystic mass in the lower abdomen between the umbilicus and bladder[139,140] to a giant multiseptated cystic structure extending into the upper abdomen, with compression and elongation of the bladder[141] (Figs. 9-65 and 9-66). Mixed echogenicity may be encountered within the cyst when infection is present.[142] Examination should be performed with bladder distension to identify anatomic relationships. In the pediatric age group, change in configuration of the cystic mass postvoiding, with elongation and inferior extension of the caudal portion, suggests bladder communication (e.g., patent urachus instead of urachal cyst).[143]

A normal urachal remnant, appearing as a small elliptical hypoechoic structure overlying the anterosuperior surface of the bladder, appears to be a common finding in the pediatric population, reportedly depicted in 62 of 100 bladder sonograms. A small central echogenic component, presumably corresponding to the mucosal lining within such a remnant, was identified in 16 percent of cases in this series[144] (Fig. 9-67).

Organ-Associated Fluid and Cystic Masses

Renal, hepatic, splenic, pancreatic, and adrenal cysts in adults usually are easily localized to their respective organ with ultrasound, with certain exceptions (e.g., distinguishing a left adrenal cyst or renal cyst from a pan-

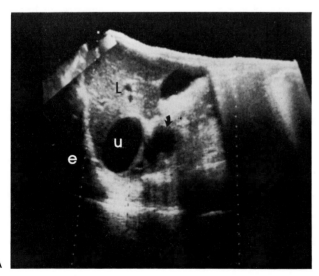

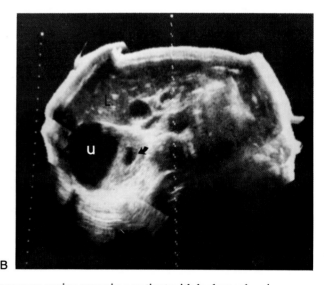

Fig. 9-64. Urinoma. **(A)** Right longitudinal and **(B)** transverse supine scans in a patient with hydronephrosis (arrow) and a right urinoma *(u)* secondary to obstructing lymph nodes from prostatic carcinoma. The anechoic mass is noted supralaterally to the kidney, producing compression on both the liver *(L)* and kidney. Incidentally noted on longitudinal images is a pleural effusion *(e)*.

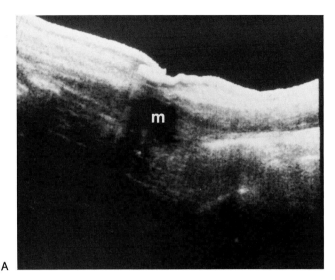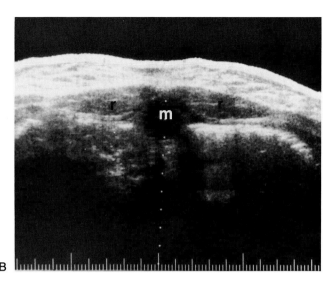

Fig. 9-65. Infected urachal cyst. **(A)** Midline sagittal and **(B)** transverse images of the lower abdomen demonstrate an irregularly marginated cystic mass *(m)* between the umbilicus and bladder (not shown). Although the relationship between the mass and the transversalis fascia and peritoneum cannot be distinctly imaged (i.e., the lesion separates them), focality and location nonetheless suggest an extraperitoneal location and the appropriate diagnosis. (*r*, rectus muscles.)

creatic tail lesion) (Fig. 9-68). Anatomic relationships may be less clearcut when cysts are associated with displaced or malpositioned organs. Similarly, ischemic bowel may mimic a complex cystic mass if continuity with more normal-appearing bowel is not recognized (Fig. 9-69). Massive hydro- or pyonephrosis may initially be disorienting, but the diagnosis is suggested when an ipsilateral kidney cannot be visualized (Figs. 9-70 and 9-71). Extensive polycystic kidney/liver disease and cystadenoma/adenocarcinoma of the biliary tree or pancreas may also disorient the unwary or inexperienced sonologist.

A variety of nongynecologic cystic masses may be encountered in the pelvis in relation to the bladder, including obstructed pelvic kidney, bladder diverticula, ureterocele and hydroureter, seminal vesicle cysts, prostatic cysts, urachal cysts, varices, and iliac artery aneurysms.[145,146]

Abnormalities that originate supradiaphragmatically, such as a large aneurysm involving the anteroinferior aspect of the left ventricle, may severely depress the diaphragm and mimic intraperitoneal pathology.[147] The differential diagnosis of a cystic midepigastric or lower abdominal mass includes aneurysm of a branch vessel or

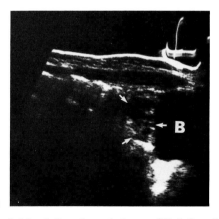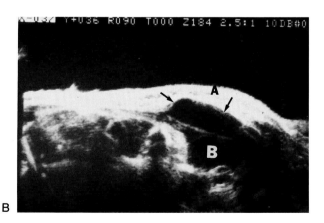

Fig. 9-66. Infected urachal cyst. **(A)** Infected urachal cyst is seen on a longitudinal scan as a mass of mixed echogenicity (arrows) adherent to and involving the dome of the bladder *(B)*. **(B)** Longitudinal scan in a different patient shows apposition of an infected, abscess-forming urachal cyst (arrows) to the anterior wall of the bladder *(B)*. (*A*, anterior abdominal wall.) (From Spataro et al,[142] with permission.)

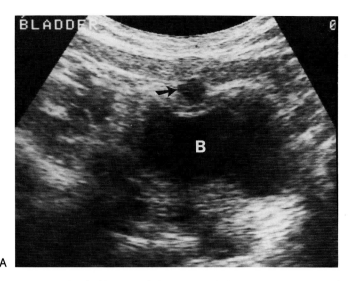
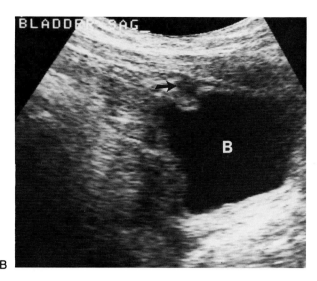

Fig. 9-67. Urachal remnant. **(A)** Transverse bladder image demonstrates a urachal remnant (arrow) in the midline. **(B)** Urachal remnant (arrow) is seen anterosuperior to bladder on sagittal scan. (*B*, bladder.) (From Cacciarelli et al,[144] with permission.)

the aorta itself; demonstration of flow with color Doppler and/or duplex ultrasound or continuity with vasculature structures is basic to diagnosis (Fig. 9-72).

In the neonate, organ-associated fluid collections such as ovarian cyst, choledochal cyst, hydrometrocolpos, and hydronephrosis secondary to ureteropelvic junction obstruction may sometimes be difficult to localize with complete confidence. Bowel-associated cystic abdominal masses in the neonate include duplication cysts, cystic meconium peritonitis/pseudocyst, segmental dilatation of bowel, and volvulus with pseudocyst formation.[148]

Cystic-Appearing Solid Lesions and Necrotic Lesions

Lymphomatous masses at times appear extremely hypoechoic, exhibiting many features of fluid-filled or cystic masses.[149] Other solid masses, including sarcomas, hypernephromas, and adenocarcinomas (such as metastatic breast lesions) may be diffusely hypoechoic or have localized areas of necrosis or fluid.[2,4,45,150] Uterine leiomyomas may also appear hypoechoic or contain large cystic components[4,45,151,152] (Fig. 9-73). Hemorrhagic/

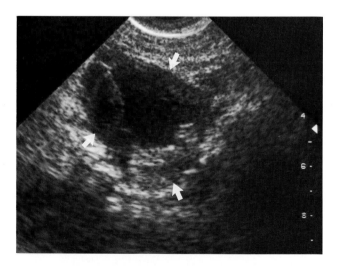

Fig. 9-68. Adrenal cyst. Prone right sagittal scan demonstrates an oval hypoechoic mass *(c)* with good increased through transmission anterior to the upper pole of the right kidney *(k)*. Similar lesions, when occurring on the left side, may be difficult to distinguish from processes involving the pancreatic tail.

Fig. 9-69. Ischemic bowel. Sagittal scan of the left lower quadrant in a patient status-post repair of ruptured aortic aneurysm illustrates a markedly thickened loop of ischemic distal colon, seen in cross-section (arrows). Continuity with bowel could be easily established when the scan plane traversed the long axis of the involved loop.

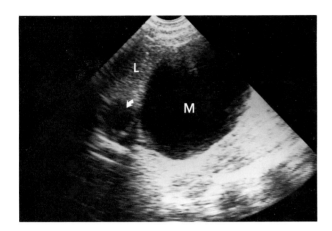

Fig. 9-70. Ureteropelvic junction obstruction. Transverse scan demonstrates a large cystic abdominal mass *(M)* adjacent to the right kidney. Right caliectasis is also seen (arrow). Left kidney was normal in appearance. (*L*, liver.)

necrotic tumors typically contain an irregular cystic center surrounded by an echogenic rim of tissue that is distinct from adjacent soft tissues.[42]

Gynecologic Pathology

Gynecologic abnormalities that may mimic or present sonographically as abdominopelvic fluid-containing masses include leiomyoma/leiomyosarcoma (Fig. 9-73), ovarian neoplasms (Figs. 9-30, 9-74 to 9-76), endometriomas (Fig. 9-77), pyometra, pelvic inflammatory disease (Fig. 9-78), ovarian/parovarian cysts (Fig. 9-79), peritoneal inclusion cysts (Fig. 9-54), and chronic ectopic pregnancy (Fig. 9-80).[96,97,151-162]

Pseudolesions

Distended, fluid-filled bowel may be confused with an abnormal fluid collection by ultrasound, although in most instances bowel can be identified by contour, echo characteristics, and detection of peristalsis with real-time sonography (Fig. 9-81). Differentiation may be considerably more difficult, however, if multiple loops of bowel are matted together in the shape of a mass by adhesions from prior surgery, or if wads of omentum are involved in an inflammatory process or fill in prior surgical defects.[163,164]

Gastric distension, particularly in the neonate, may be mistaken for a cystic abdominal mass (Fig. 9-82); similarly, gallbladder distension secondary to parenteral hyperalimentation may be erroneously perceived as a cystic mass[165] (Fig. 9-83).

Excessive fat in the supradiaphragmatic region, appearing as a homogeneous well-defined hypoechoic area beneath the anterior abdominal wall, may stimulate processes such as subdiaphragmatic abscess, subpulmonic effusion, ascites, or tumor[166] (Fig. 9-84).

Since liver parenchyma is less echogenic than that of spleen, the lateral extent of the normal left lobe of liver may mimic a left subphrenic abscess or subcapsular/perisplenic hematoma.[167,168] Typically, a relatively hypoechoic crescent-shaped structure is identified superior to the spleen with imaging in the coronal plane (Fig.

(Text continues on page 630)

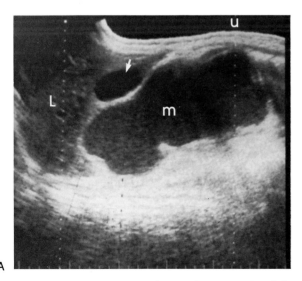

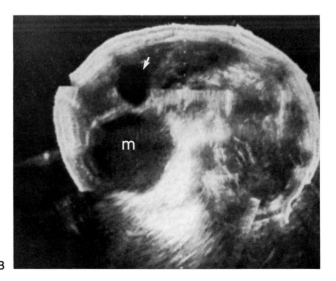

A B

Fig. 9-71. Pyonephrosis. Massive pyonephrosis in a pregnant woman with congenital right ureteropelvic junction obstruction is seen on **(A)** right longitudinal and **(B)** transverse scans as a large hypoechoic mass *(m)*. Diffuse low-amplitude echoes are seen within the mass, and are increased in amplitude in the more dependent portions of the dilated renal collecting system. (arrow, gallbladder; *L*, liver; *u*, level of umbilicus.)

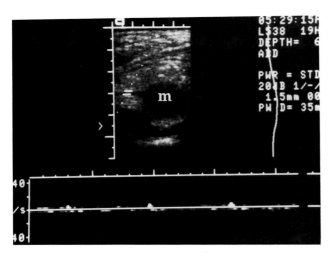

Fig. 9-72. Bacterial aneurysm. A man 2 weeks post-aortic valve replacement for subacute bacterial endocarditis presented with abdominal pain. Sagittal image below the level of the aortic bifurcation demonstrates a 2.5 cm oval anechoic mass *(m).* Color Doppler (not shown) demonstrated swirling flow; a feeding arterial branch was documented with color Doppler and duplex ultrasound *(sampled region and corresponding waveform).* At surgery, a bacterial aneurysm arising from an iliocolic artery branch was identified and resected.

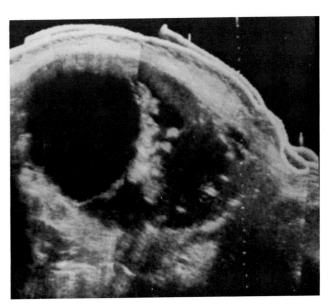

Fig. 9-74. Papillary serous cystadenocarcinoma of the ovary. Right longitudinal scan of the lower abdomen and pelvis demonstrates a large mass characterized by anechoic regions with intervening septations and mural nodules.

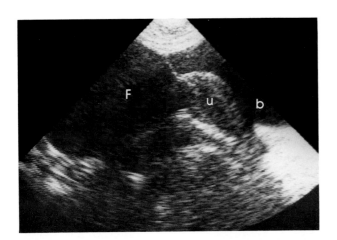

Fig. 9-73. Leiomyoma. Longitudinal scan of the lower abdomen and pelvis demonstrates a large hypoechoic fibroid *(F)* emanating superiorly from the uterine fundus. *(u,* uterus; *b,* bladder.)

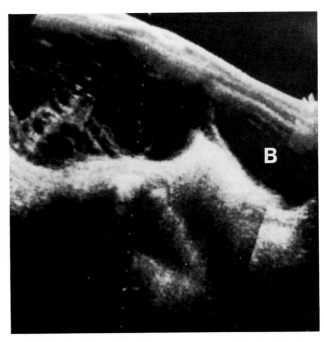

Fig. 9-75. Granulosa thecal cell tumor. Midline sagittal scan of the lower abdomen and pelvis in a child with precocious puberty demonstrates a large, predominantly anechoic mass with prominent septations. (B, bladder.)

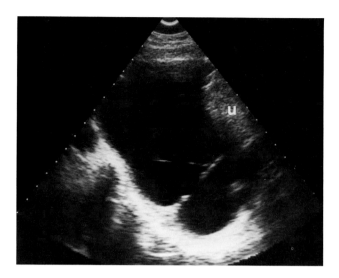

Fig. 9-76. Dermoid. Longitudinal scan to the right of midline demonstrates an anechoic abdominopelvic mass with minimal septations/solid components surrounding the uterus *(u)*.

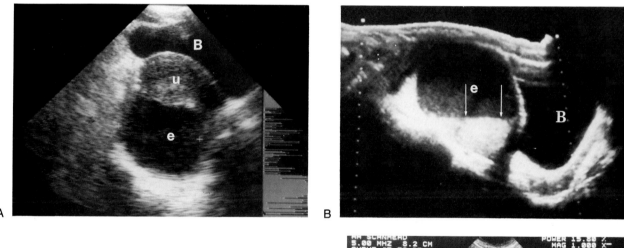

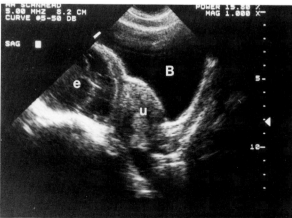

Fig. 9-77. Endometrioma. **(A)** In this sagittal scan of the pelvis, the endometrioma *(e)* appears as a fluid-containing mass posterior to the uterus *(u)* with diffuse low-amplitude internal echoes. **(B)** In a longitudinal midline scan of another patient, a large endometrioma *(e)* contains a discrete fluid-fluid level (arrows). **(C)** In a third patient, the endometrioma *(e)* appears as a more complex fluid-containing mass superior to the uterine fundus *(u)*. *(B,* bladder.)

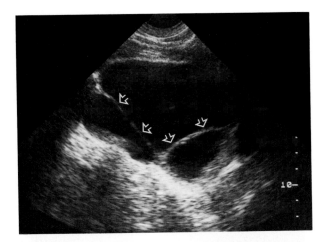

Fig. 9-78. Hydrosalpinx. A sagittal pelvic scan off-midline demonstrates a fluid-filled mass with the appearance of septations (open arrows). These linear echoes in fact represent folds of the distended, convoluted fallopian tube.

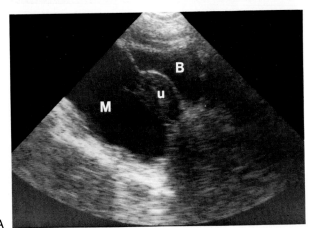

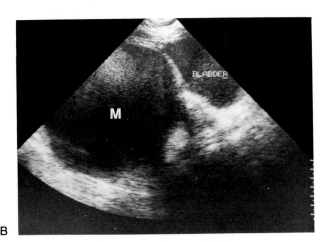

Fig. 9-79. Parovarian cysts. **(A & B)** Large simple-appearing cystic adnexal masses are seen off-midline in longitudinal scans of two different patients. Reverberation artifact is present anteriorly within the mass in Fig. B. (*M*, cystic mass; *u*, uterus; *B*, bladder.)

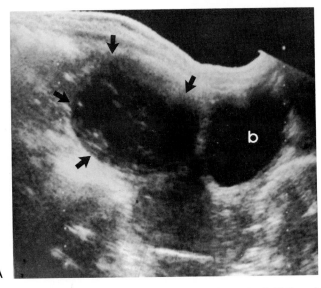

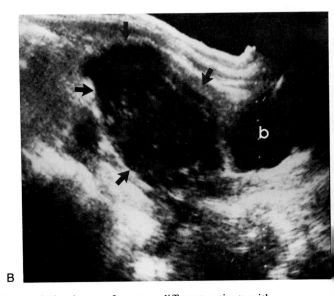

Fig. 9-80. Chronic ectopic gestations. **(A & B)** Longitudinal midline images from two different patients with chronic ectopic gestation demonstrate primarily anechoic complex pelvic masses (arrows) with increased through transmission. (*b*, bladder.)

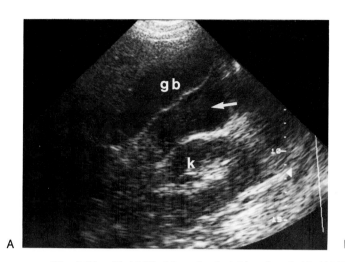
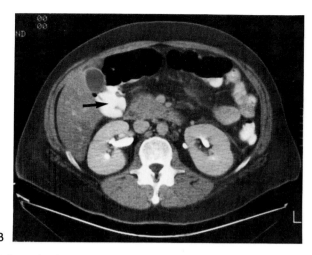

A   B

Fig. 9-81. Fluid-filled bowel mimicking free fluid. **(A)** Right sagittal scan. What was initially interpreted as extrapancreatic inflammatory fluid (arrow) contiguous with the gallbladder in a patient with acute pancreatitis was subsequently shown on **(B)** CT examination to represent a fluid-filled bowel loop (arrow). (*gb*, gallbladder; *k*, right kidney.)

Fig. 9-82. Distended stomach. Left lateral decubitus sagittal scan of a neonate demonstrates a large complex mass *(ST)* in the left upper abdomen, representing normal stomach distended with infant formula. (*s*, spleen tip.)

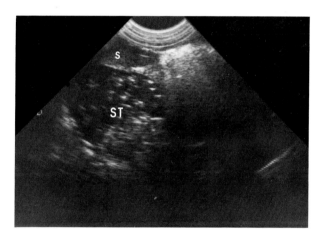

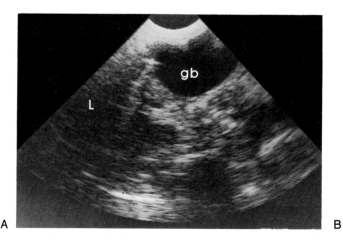
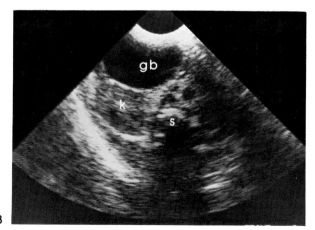

A   B

Fig. 9-83. Gallbladder pseudotumor. An abdominal mass was palpated in this 2-year-old premature infant. **(A)** Longitudinal and **(B)** transverse scans identify the "mass" as a distended gallbladder (*L*, liver; *k*, kidney; *gb*, gallbladder; *s*, spine.) (From Durrell et al,[254] with permission.)

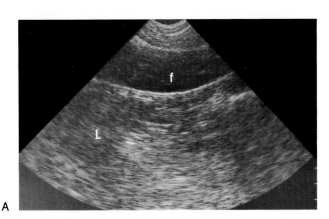

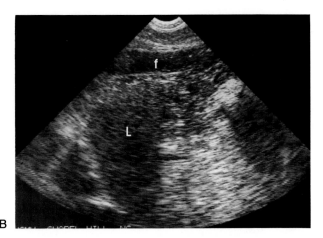

A   B

Fig. 9-84. Preperitoneal fat. **(A)** Transverse and **(B)** longitudinal scans in different obese patients demonstrate excess preperitoneal fat *(f)*, which appears relatively hypoechoic and which may occasionally mimic a shallow collection of ascites. (*L*, liver.)

9-85). Avoiding this pitfall depends on recognizing the solid acoustic properties of the pseudolesion (i.e., no increased through transmission or refraction artifact) and identifying continuity with the liver. Demonstration of a portal triad and "sliding" of the elongated left lobe over the spleen with respiration are additional confirmatory findings.[169]

NONCYSTIC INTRAPERITONEAL EXTRAORGAN LESIONS

Peritoneal Metastases

Peritoneal metastases usually develop from cellular implantation across the peritoneal cavity, although metastases may also be lymph or blood borne. The most common primary sites are the ovaries, stomach, and colon. Other potential primary sites include the pancreas, biliary tract, kidneys, testicles, and uterus; similarly, sarcomas, melanomas, teratomas, and embryonic tumors of childhood may secondarily involve the peritoneum.[170]

Sonographically, peritoneal metastases may exhibit a nodular, sheet-like, or irregular configuration, the last pattern resulting from irregular growth or consolidation of sheet-like masses (Figs. 9-86 and 9-87). Small nodules may appear attached to the peritoneal line, with the integrity of the line preserved, while larger masses will generally obliterate the line. Adhesion of bowel loops to the masses is not uncommon.[171]

In the presence of ascites, appendices epiploicae of the large bowel may be identified with ultrasound. These small pouches of fat-filled peritoneum may mimic primary or metastatic tumors of the peritoneum unless

their regularly spaced relationship to the outer surface of the large bowel is recognized.[172]

Leiomyomatosis peritonealis disseminata, a rare benign proliferation of submesothelial nodules involving peritoneal surfaces, will be suggestive of disseminated malignant neoplasm of the peritoneum. In the active stage of the disease, the nodules are microscopically indistinguishable from leiomyomas; differentiation from metastatic sarcoma may be particularly challenging for the pathologist when the process is spontaneously regressing. This entity occurs only in women during the reproductive years, and is often associated with pregnancy. Solid intra-abdominal masses and the absence of ascites in a pregnant woman, particularly with asso-

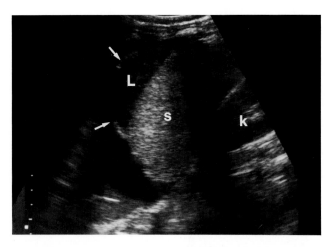

Fig. 9-85. Pseudosubcapsular hematoma. This leukemia patient with low platelets was evaluated for a drop in hematocrit. A left coronal oblique scan demonstrates the lateral extension of the left lobe of the liver *(L)* mimicking a subcapsular splenic hematoma. A large pleural effusion is also present. (arrows, diaphragm; *s*, spleen; *k*, left kidney.)

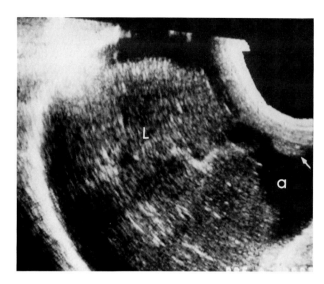

Fig. 9-86. Peritoneal metastasis. Longitudinal scan of right hypochondrium in patient with gastric antral carcinoma demonstrates a metastatic peritoneal implant (arrow) surrounded by ascitic fluid *(a)*. Metastatic liver disease is also present. (*L*, liver). (From Derchi et al,[255] with permission.)

ciated uterine myomas, should suggest the diagnosis.[173,174]

Lymphoma of Omentum and Mesentery

Lymphomatous cellular infiltration of the greater omentum may be seen as a uniformly thick, hypoechoic band-shaped structure that follows the convexity of the anterior and lateral abdominal wall, which has been termed the *omental band*.[175-177] Mesenteric lymphomatous involvement characteristically presents as a lobulated confluent hypoechoic mass surrounding a centrally positioned echogenic area. This appearance, the result of a mass infiltrating the mesenteric leaves and encasing the superior mesenteric artery and veins, has been termed the *sandwich sign*.[178] (Fig. 9-88).

Generally, mesenteric lymphomatous involvement is accompanied by para-aortic or retroperitoneal adenopathy, and isolated mesenteric involvement is more commonly accompanied by metastatic carcinoma. Nonetheless, isolated lymphomatous mesenteric masses occasionally may be encountered, particularly with nodular undifferentiated lymphocytic lymphoma.[178,179] Despite the characteristic relatively anechoic appearance of lymphoma, metastatic nodes may have a similar appearance.[149] Thus, the presence of the sandwich sign may be more helpful in distinguishing lymphoma from metastatic carcinoma than reliance on the presence of associated adenopathy or the internal echo characteristics of the mesenteric masses. Since mesenteric involvement is significantly less frequent in Hodgkin's lymphoma compared with non-Hodgkin's lymphoma, documentation of the sandwich sign with ultrasound is more suggestive of the latter.[180,181]

Primary Tumors of the Peritoneum, Omentum, and Mesentery

Secondary tumors and lymphoma are the neoplasms that most commonly involve the peritoneum and mes-

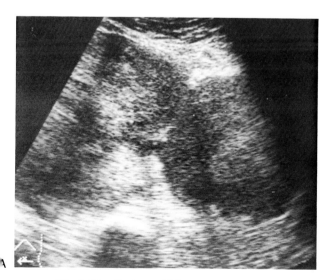

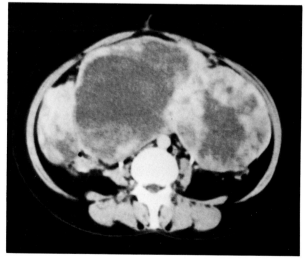

B

Fig. 9-87. Peritoneal leiomyosarcomatosis. **(A)** Transverse scan of the midabdomen reveals two large, heterogeneous and predominantly solid-appearing intra-abdominal masses. **(B)** CT scan shows well-defined, large masses containing extensive, irregular areas of low attenuation, indicating central necrosis. Posterior displacement of small bowel loops (not shown) confirmed intraperitoneal origin of the masses. Note absence of ascites or lymphadenopathy, characteristic of this uncommon presentation of metastatic leiomyosarcoma. (Case provided courtesy of Dr. Byung Ihn Choi, Department of Radiology, Seoul National University Hospital.)

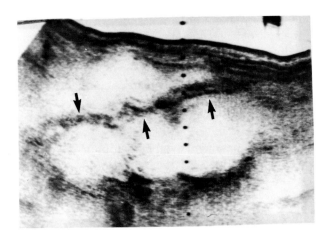

Fig. 9-88. Mesenteric lymphoma, the sandwich sign. Longitudinal scan demonstrates a homogeneous, hypoechoic mass surrounding a central area of linear echogenicity representing the mesentery (arrows). (From Mueller et al,[178] with permission.)

entery. Rarely, the peritoneum, mesentery, or omentum are the site for primary tumor involvement, including fibrous, lipomatous, smooth muscle, and vascular tumors.

Fibrous tumors appear to represent the most common primary solid neoplasm of the mesentery, while smooth muscle tumors, which are also relatively frequent in the mesentery, are the most common lesions found in the greater omentum. Interestingly, lipomatous tumors are not dominant in either location and are relatively more common in the retroperitoneum. Also, almost the only important vascular tumor type in the mesentery and omentum appears to be the uncommon hemangiopericytoma. Whether benign or malignant, most of the primary tumors of the mesentery tend to grow to a large size. Just as in the omentum, where tumors can also reach massive proportions, the mobility of the mesentery often permits large growth before symptoms other than a palpable mass are produced. Mesenteric masses are often freely movable, characteristically from side to side but not in the craniocaudad direction.[182–184]

Fibromatoses and Fibrosing Mesenteritis

A fibromatosis is defined as an infiltrating fibroblastic proliferation showing none of the features of an inflammatory response and no features of unequivocal neo-

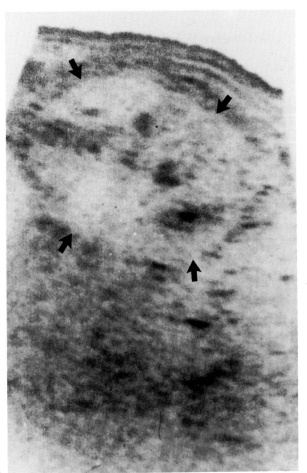

A

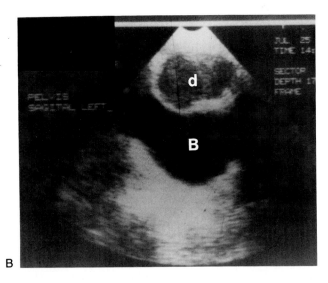

B

Fig. 9-89. Desmoid tumor. **(A)** Transverse scan of the midabdomen with the patient supine demonstrates a well-circumscribed solid mass (arrows) containing scattered high-amplitude echoes. (Courtesy of R.L. Baron, MD, and J.K.T. Lee, MD.) **(B)** In a different patient, sagittal sonogram demonstrates a predominantly homogeneous echogenic mass with a hyperechoic rim *(d)* anterior to the bladder *(B)*. (From Mantello et al,[191] with permission.)

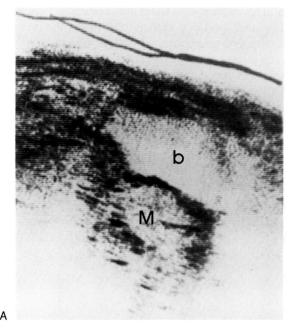

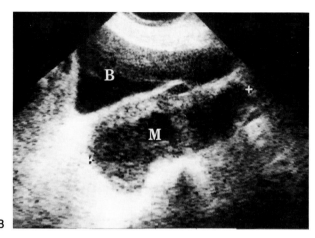

A   B

Fig. 9-90. Fibrosing/retractile mesenteritis. **(A)** Midline longitudinal scan demonstrates a retrovesical mass *(M)* containing multiple internal echoes. The patient had a prior hysterectomy. (*b*, bladder.) (From Bendon et al,[195] with permission.) **(B)** In a different patient, oblique pelvic sonogram shows a solid mass *(M)* with central hypoechoic areas in a similar location. This mass correlated with concentric stricture of the rectosigmoid colon on barium enema. (*B*, bladder.) (From Pérez-Fontán et al,[194] with permission.)

plasm.[185] Desmoids are a category of fibromatosis that arise from musculoaponeurotic structures in any area of the body, although they most frequently arise in the anterior abdominal wall. Fibroblastic masses that are localized intra-abdominally may constitute an isolated abnormality or may be associated with subcutaneous soft tissue tumors and Gardner syndrome. Fibromatoses involving the mesentery and omentum most commonly arise in the mesentery of the small intestine.[185-187]

Fibrous tissues generally have a homogeneously hypoechoic sonographic appearance, while typically appearing hyperdense relative to muscles and solid viscera on CT.[188] Reports of mesenteric desmoids with ultrasound correlation characterize these lesions as well circumscribed and predominantly hypoechoic, often containing scattered higher level echoes. The variable echogenicity depends on the degree of cellularity as well as incorporated fat and blood vessels[189-191] (Fig. 9-89). Areas of acoustic shadowing arising from within the mass and not originating from echogenic foci have also been noted and are believed secondary to focal fibrotic areas with increased collagen content.[190]

Fibroinflammatory thickening of the mesentery, referred to by terms such as *fibrosing mesenteritis, sclerosing mesenteritis, retractile mesenteritis,* and *mesenteric/ intra-abdominal panniculitis,* probably represents a reparative process initiated by damage of mesenteric adipose tissue.[187,192,193] Sonographic appearances vary from an irregularly shaped hypoechoic area to a hyperechoic mass with central hypoechoic areas[194,195] (Fig. 9-90). Fat necrosis of the mesentery secondary to pancreatitis may also simulate a primary mesenteric tumor, appearing as a well-demarcated solid mass with both solid and cystic elements[196,197] (Fig. 9-91).

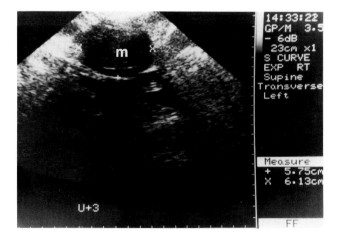

Fig. 9-91. Fat necrosis. Scan of an 8-cm moveable nontender left upper quadrant intra-abdominal mass in a man with a history of abdominal trauma 20 years earlier demonstrates a complex, hypoechoic, spherical mass *(m)*, its solid nature evidenced by significant attenuation of the sound beam. (From Kordan and Payne,[197] with permission.)

Smooth Muscle, Lipomatous, and Other Nonfibroblastic Neoplasms

As with all noncystic primary tumors involving the mesentery and omentum, sonographic descriptions in the literature are only infrequently encountered. This is particularly true of the nonfibroblastic lesions, which are rarer than other primary mesenteric neoplasms—

uncommon themselves. Those entities more typically found in other locations, such as the retroperitoneum or in association with abdominal hollow viscera, are discussed in greater detail elsewhere in this text.

Four sonographic patterns have been observed in extrahepatic mesenchymal sarcomas (including leiomyosarcoma, liposarcoma, fibrosarcoma, and rhabdomyosarcoma) involving mesentery, abdominal hollow

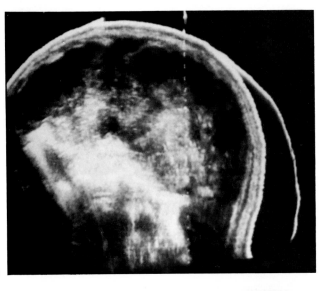

A

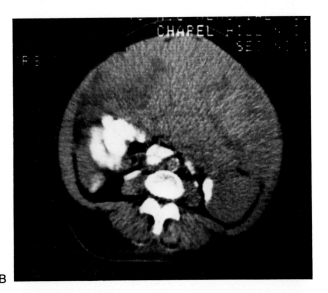

B

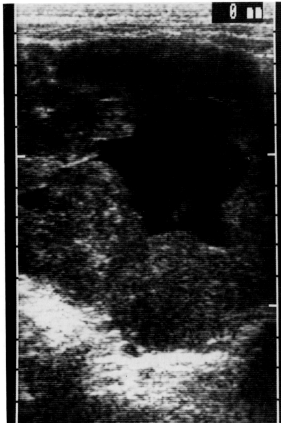

C

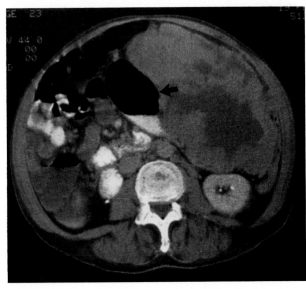

D

Fig. 9-92. Leiomyosarcoma. **(A)** Transverse sonogram and **(B)** corresponding CT scan demonstrate an extensive intra-abdominal mass of mixed echogenicity. The more anterior portions of the mass are noted to be relatively hypo- and anechoic. **(C)** Sonogram and **(D)** corresponding CT scan in another patient show a large mass with central hemorrhage/necrosis. CT reveals continuity with and medial displacement of stomach (arrow), consistent with a gastric origin.

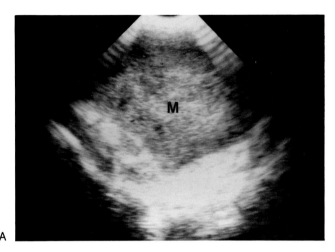 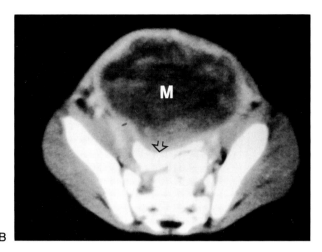

A   B

Fig. 9-93. Rhabdomyosarcoma. **(A)** Transverse sonogram and **(B)** corresponding CT scan of a child with rhabdomyosarcoma *(M)* of bladder origin demonstrate fairly homogeneous hyperechoic echo characteristics with ultrasound. Note continuity with and posterior displacement of bladder on CT (arrow).

viscera, and retroperitoneal areas: (1) hyperechoic masses intermixed with anechoic zones, (2) hyperechoic masses with central fluid-filled zones, (3) homogeneous hyperechoic masses, and (4) homogeneous hypoechoic masses[198] (Figs. 9-92 and 9-93). Because sarcomas have a tendency to develop central necrosis with cavitation and hemorrhage, the sonographic appearance of a large tumor mass with signs of necrosis should suggest the possibility of a sarcoma. However, in the series of 24 tumors just cited, 54 percent of the sarcomas were classified as homogeneous sonographically. When extensive necrosis is present, sarcomatous lesions may potentially mimic a benign fluid-filled mass such as a pancreatic pseudocyst.

Among the mesenchymal sarcomas in the series cited above, five liposarcomas demonstrated a spectrum of ultrasound appearances, including homogeneously hypoechoic, homogeneously hyperechoic, and hyperechoic with hypoechoic zones[198] (Fig. 9-94). Since subcutaneous lipomas and adipose tissue may be either relatively echofree or echogenic, depending on the ratio of lipid to aqueous constituents,[199] this variation in the echopattern of homogeneous lipomatous lesions is not surprising. It is also not surprising that ultrasound descriptions of mesenteric or omental lipomas are sparse in the literature, as most are small and discovered only incidentally. In addition, echogenic fat appears to be the most prevalent form in vitro, and with high-level internal echoes blending with the echopattern of bowel gas (or retroperitoneal fat), lipomatous abdominal masses may be easily overlooked.

Gastrointestinal teratomas, including those involving the mesentery and lesser omentum, vary in appearance from a predominantly cystic mass to a predominantly solid mass with multiple cysts. Septations may be of variable thickness, and solid areas are inhomogeneous with moderate intensity echoes. Focal bright reflectors with acoustic shadowing, representing calcification, may also be encountered.[200]

Castleman disease, an uncommon disorder of lymphoid tissue usually occurring in the mediastinum, has been reported in the greater omentum. This benign hy-

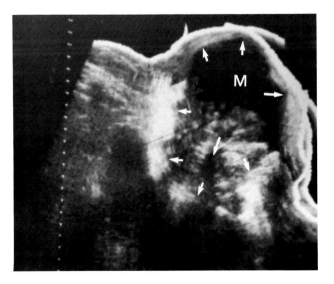

Fig. 9-94. Liposarcoma. Longitudinal scan of the lower abdomen demonstrates an extensive mass *(M,* arrows) with large anechoic components, presumably originating from the abdominal wall. The tumor was grossly necrotic and hemorrhagic at laparotomy.

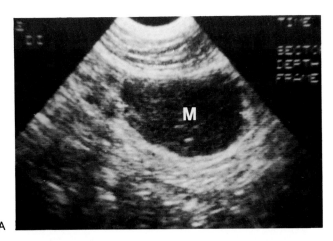

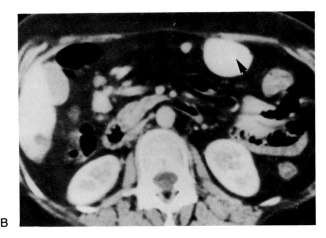

A   B

Fig. 9-95. Castleman disease of the greater omentum. **(A)** A homogeneous hypoechoic mass in the greater omentum *(M)*, discovered incidentally in a 56-year-old asympomatic woman, appears **(B)** on CT as a well-marginated, enhancing mass (arrow). (From Volta et al,[201] with permission.)

pervascular mass appeared as a homogeneously hypoechoic omental mass with ultrasound.[201] (Fig. 9-95).

Peritoneal and Omental Mesothelioma

Mesotheliomas involve the peritoneum as a primary lesion much less commonly than the pleura, but the intra-abdominal variety tends to follow a more virulent course. Regardless of the site of origin, mesotheliomas usually occur in middle-aged men; asbestos exposure is considered an etiologic factor. The most frequent initial

symptom is abdominal pain, accompanied by significant weight loss and ascites. On gross examination, peritoneal mesotheliomas may present as a large tumor mass with discrete smaller nodules scattered over larger areas of the visceral and parietal peritoneum, or as diffuse nodules and plaques that coat the abdominal cavity and envelop and matt together the abdominal viscera.[202,203]

Ultrasound typically demonstrates sheet-like or irregular masses of relatively low echogenicity contiguous with the anterior abdominal wall, which may or may not be accompanied by ascites[204] (Fig. 9-96). The inner surface of the mass is characteristically lobular, and may either encase small bowel loops or be separated from them by a hypoechoic line representing ascitic fluid or thickening of the bowel wall.[205,206] Mesenteric involvement is common, resulting in adhesions, bowel fixation, and an ultrasound pattern that has been described as pleated or fan-like; entrapped intra-abdominal and omental fat may appear as scattered bright reflectors within the mass[205] (Fig. 9-97). The tumor itself may mimic ascites, appearing as a homogeneous hypoechogenicity surrounding the liver[207] (Fig. 9-98).

A large nodular or globular mass, a pattern of presentation that may be encountered in carcinomatosis, is not likely to be seen with mesothelioma.[204] Other differential points from carcinomatosis include a disproportionately small amount of ascites and relatively more common mesenteric involvement with peritoneal mesothelioma.[205] Diffuse mesenteric amyloidosis, presenting as a large homogeneous intra-abdominal mass appearing to engulf mesenteric vessels and bowel, is a benign process that may potentially mimic both of these entities.[206]

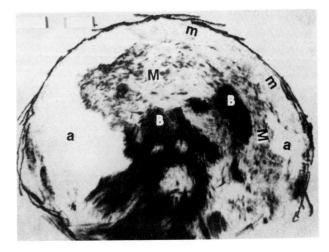

Fig. 9-96. Peritoneal mesothelioma. Transverse scan 6 cm above the umbilicus demonstrates an omental mass *(M)* fusing with a diffuse peritoneal mass *(m)*. Bowel loops *(B)* are displaced posteriorly. Ascites *(a)* is also present. (From Yeh and Chahinian,[204] with permission.)

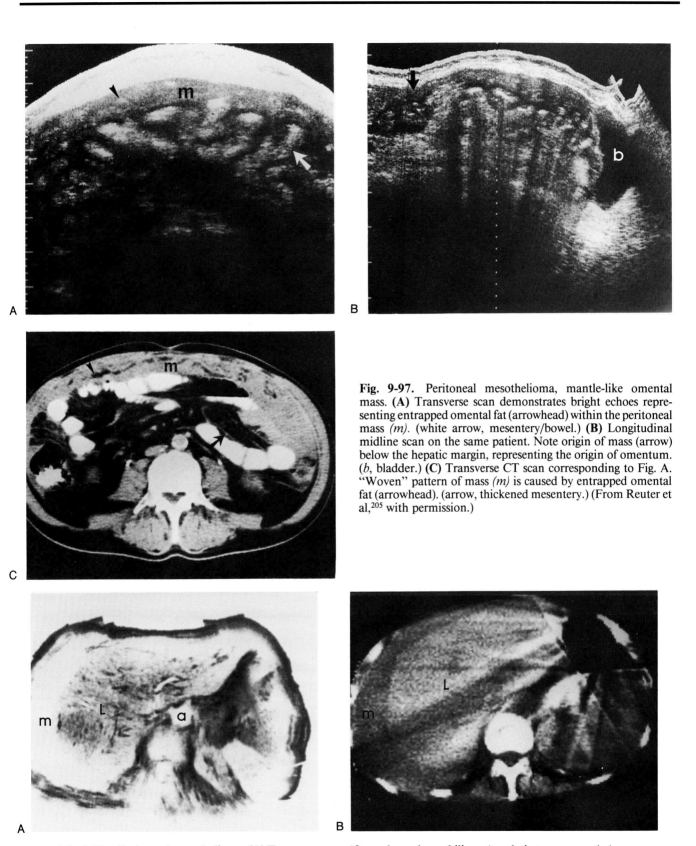

Fig. 9-97. Peritoneal mesothelioma, mantle-like omental mass. **(A)** Transverse scan demonstrates bright echoes representing entrapped omental fat (arrowhead) within the peritoneal mass *(m)*. (white arrow, mesentery/bowel.) **(B)** Longitudinal midline scan on the same patient. Note origin of mass (arrow) below the hepatic margin, representing the origin of omentum. (*b*, bladder.) **(C)** Transverse CT scan corresponding to Fig. A. "Woven" pattern of mass *(m)* is caused by entrapped omental fat (arrowhead). (arrow, thickened mesentery.) (From Reuter et al,[205] with permission.)

Fig. 9-98.   Peritoneal mesothelioma. **(A)** Transverse scan 12 cm above the umbilicus. Anechoic tumor mass *(m)* surrounding liver *(L)*, mimicking ascites. No acoustic enhancement is present. (*a*, aorta.) **(B)** Transverse CT scan 13 cm above umbilicus after ingestion of oral contrast. Low-density tumor mass *(m)* surrounds the liver *(L)*. (From Dach et al,[207] with permission.)

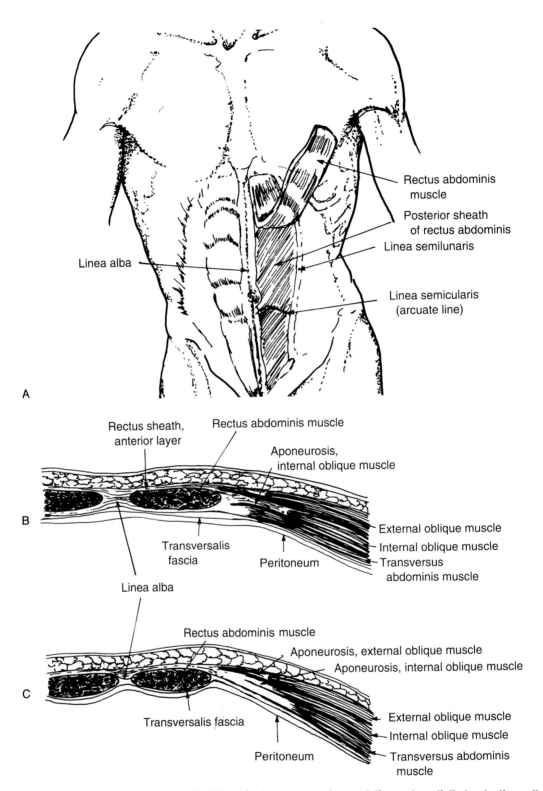

Fig. 9-99. Abdominal wall anatomy. **(A)** The paired rectus muscles are delineated medially by the linea alba, and laterally by the linea semilunaris. The linea semicircularis, or arcuate line of Douglas, demarcates the inferior margin of the posterior rectus sheath. **(B)** Cross-section schematic above the level of the arcuate line illustrates that the rectus muscle is enveloped by its sheath both anteriorly and posteriorly. **(C)** More caudally the muscle is separated from the anterior abdominal contents only by the transversalis fascia and the peritoneum.

ABDOMINAL WALL

Superficial abdominal lesions are readily evaluated with ultrasound. In addition to characterizing and localizing clinically palpable abnormalities, ultrasound may be useful in the patient who has undiagnosed abdominal complaints, suspected hernia, or postoperative incisional complaints.

NORMAL ANATOMY

The paired rectus abdominis muscles are delineated medially in the midline of the body by the linea alba, while laterally, the aponeuroses of the external oblique, internal oblique, and transversus abdominis muscles unite to form a band-like vertical fibrous groove called the linea semilunaris, or spigelian fascia. Through the upper two-thirds of the anterior abdominal wall, the aponeurotic sheath of the three anterolateral abdominal muscles invests the rectus both anteriorly and posteriorly. Approximately midway between the umbilicus and the symphysis pubis, at the linea semicircularis (or arcuate line of Douglas), the entire aponeurotic sheath passes anteriorly to the rectus only. Thus, while the posterior rectus sheath is composed of aponeuroses from both the internal oblique and transversus abdominis muscles above the arcuate line, below the line the rectus muscle is separated from the intra-abdominal contents only by the transversalis fascia and the peritoneum (Fig. 9-99).

With a high-frequency, short-focused transducer, the midline and anterolateral muscle groups can be identified beneath the superficial fascia and subcutaneous tissue; the distinctness of the individual muscle groups is largely dependent on the degree of patient muscular development (Fig. 9-100). On transverse images, the rectus muscles can be visualized as a biconvex muscle group delimited by the linea alba and the linea semilunaris. On both longitudinal and transverse images, the peritoneal line is seen as a discrete linear echogenicity in the deepest layer of the abdominal wall (Fig. 9-101). Although this line usually represents a combination of the peritoneum and the deep abdominal fascia, with abundant extraperitoneal fat the peritoneum and deep fascia may be appreciated as two separate linear echodensities.[209] On longitudinal images on either side of the midline linea alba, the region of the arcuate line can be identified at the zone of transition in which the peritoneal line becomes less distinct sonographically (Fig. 9-102).

PATHOLOGY

The basic categories of disease processes involving the abdominal wall include hematoma, inflammatory lesions, neoplasm, hernia, and postsurgical lesions. Other

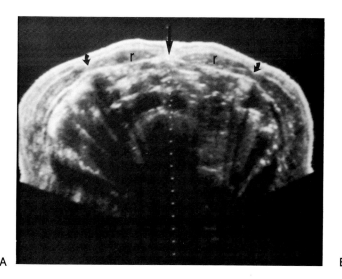

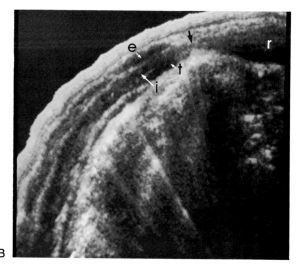

A   B

Fig. 9-100. Abdominal wall anatomy. **(A)** Transverse scan 1 cm above the umbilicus demonstrates the paired rectus abdominis muscles *(r)* delineated by the midline linea alba (straight arrow) and the linea semilunaris (curved arrows). **(B)** Magnified view again demonstrates the rectus muscle group *(r)*, the linea semilunaris (black arrow), and the anterolateral muscle groups. (*e*, external oblique; *i*, internal oblique; *t*, transversus abdominis.)

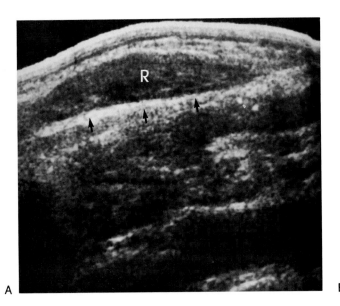

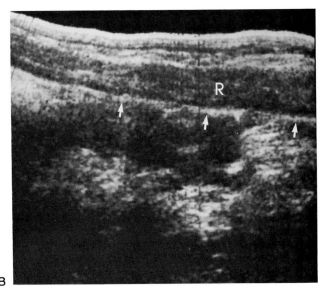

Fig. 9-101. Rectus abdominis muscle. **(A)** Right transverse and **(B)** right sagittal scans demonstrate a normal rectus abdominis muscle *(R)*. The peritoneal line can be seen in both transverse and longitudinal images as a discrete linear echogenicity in the deepest layer of the abdominal wall (arrows). Echogenic subcutaneous tissues are noted anteriorly to the muscle group.

abnormalities that may present in the anterior abdominal wall include endometriosis and venous collaterals. Regardless of the amount of fat or muscle present, the left and right sides of the abdominal wall should appear symmetrical, with asymmetry representing an important clue to superficial disease.

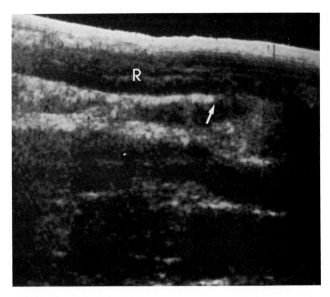

Fig. 9-102. Rectus abdominis muscle. Longitudinal scan to the right of midline, at a lower level than in Fig. 9-101B, again demonstrates a distinct peritoneal line, which becomes less distinct sonographically at the level of the arcuate line of Douglas (arrow). (*R*, rectus abdominis.)

Extraperitoneal Hematomas

Rectus sheath hematomas are acute or chronic collections of blood lying either within the rectus muscle or between the muscle and its sheath. Vascular disruption and hemorrhage may be the result of direct trauma, pregnancy, cardiovascular and degenerative muscle diseases, surgical injury, anticoagulation therapy, long-term steroid therapy, extremes of certain types of physical exercise, or sudden vigorous uncoordinated muscular contraction (e.g., an episode of coughing or sneezing). Onset is often acute, usually with a sharp, persistent nonradiating pain that may mimic intra-abdominal pathology, particularly if the hemorrhage is below the arcuate line, where peritoneal irritation is more likely. When occurring above the arcuate line, a mass may be palpable within the confines of the rectus sheath.[210-215]

With ultrasound, rectus sheath hematomas typically appear largely anechoic, with scattered internal echoes dependent on the stage of clot breakdown (Figs. 9-103 and 9-104). Above the arcuate line, the hematoma is limited laterally by the linea semilunaris and medially by the linea alba. Confined also by the rectus sheath anteriorly and posteriorly, these hematomas characteristically are biconvex in shape, appearing spindle-like on longitudinal images and ovoid when demonstrated transversely.[216,217] Below the linea semicircularis, where there is no posterior fascial sheath and the retrorectus space communicates with the prevesicular space of Retzius,

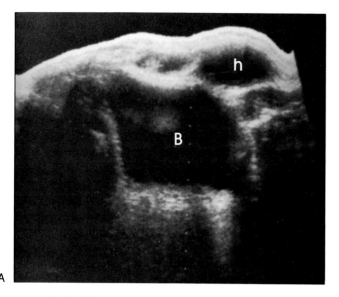

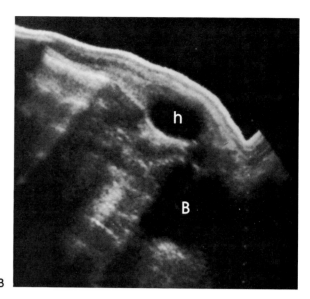

A   B

Fig. 9-103. Rectus sheath hematoma. **(A)** Lower abdominal transverse and **(B)** left longitudinal scans demonstrate an elliptical anechoic collection *(h)* involving the left rectus muscle inferiorly. The patient was a known hypertensive secondary to a pheochromocytoma. *(B,* bladder.)

hematomas can expand extensively into the extraperitoneal space passing inferiorly, laterally, and posteriorly to impinge on the bladder and potentially mimic primary pelvic pathology[218,219] (Fig. 9-105).

Intramuscular hemorrhages associated with muscle tears or separations, as might be encountered in sports-related abdominal wall injuries, show irregularly shaped hypoechoic or anechoic areas within the muscle.

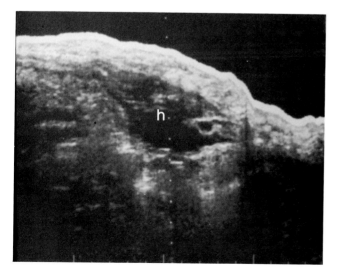

Fig. 9-104. Abdominal wall hematoma. Left longitudinal scan of the lower abdomen and pelvis in this woman receiving subcutaneous heparin demonstrates an anechoic abdominal wall collection *(h)* containing areas of increased echogenicity.

Chronic or recurrent muscular injuries demonstrate ill-defined echogenic areas and heterogeneous echotexture corresponding to fibrosis, inflammatory change, and occasionally small amounts of fluid[220] (Fig. 9-106).

Bladder-flap hematoma refers to a collection of blood between the bladder and lower-uterine segment, resulting from a lower-uterine transverse cesarean section and bleeding from uterine vessels.[221,222] This should be distinguished from blood in the prevesical space caused by disruption of the inferior epigastric vessels or their branches during cesarian delivery, the latter termed *subfascial hematoma.* Subfascial hematomas are located posterior to the rectus muscle, distinguishing them from superficial wound hematomas, the latter located anterior to the rectus muscle[223] (Fig. 9-107 and 9-108).

Inflammatory Lesions

Abdominal wall abscesses may appear anechoic or demonstrate variable internal echoes, depending on the extent of cellular debris, and usually exhibit good through transmission. Gas bubbles producing strong echoes and acoustic shadowing are highly suggestive of abscess, but, when present, the abnormality must be distinguished from a hernia on the basis of the presence or absence of peristalsis, abdominal wall defect, or accompanying swelling and/or pus. Although the margins are usually irregular due to the dissecting nature of the infectious process, an abscess is usually more well defined

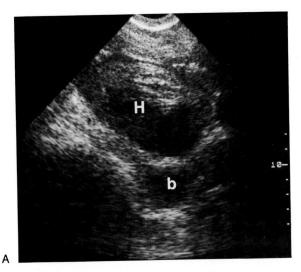
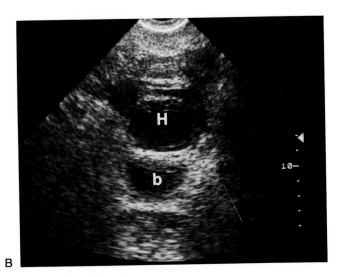

Fig. 9-105. Extraperitoneal hematoma. **(A)** Midline longitudinal and **(B)** transverse scans of the pelvis demonstrate a large, fairly well-demarcated complex mass *(H)* anterior to, and posteriorly displacing, the bladder *(b)*. Rectus hematomas arising inferior to the arcuate line may extend to both sides of midline and simulate pelvic pathology.

when compared with the more diffuse, ill-defined lateral margins of cellulitis or a phlegmon. With phlegmon involving different layers of the abdominal wall, the boundaries between the layers remain intact.[209]

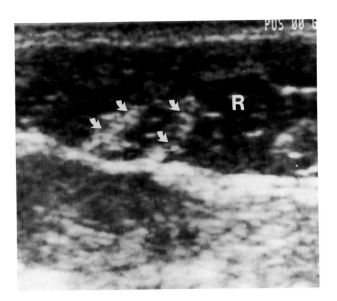

Fig. 9-106. Chronic rectus abdominis tear/fibrosis. This right-handed collegiate varsity tennis player sustained an acute muscle injury to his abdomen several months prior to this examination and continued to be limited by pain associated with serving and overhead slams. Transverse scan of the abdominal wall to the left of midline demonstrates irregular linear echogenic foci (arrows) within the left rectus abdominis *(R)*, corresponding to the location of persistent tightness and discomfort. Ill-defined echogenic areas are characteristic of the fibrosis associated with chronic or recurrent muscular injuries.

Abscesses are usually flat, spindle-shaped, or ovoid in shape, with configuration depending on size, location, and extension (Figs. 9-109 and 9-110). For example, they may appear flat or spindle-shaped when widely spread, ovoid when distended with pus, and bonnet-shaped when an intramuscular or subcutaneous collection has a wider extension into the extraperitoneal fat space.[209] When large, abscesses involving the extraperitoneal fat may appear intraperitoneal, but delineation of the peritoneal line will prevent misdiagnosis. In the pelvoabdominal region, where the peritoneal line may be harder to document, posterior displacement of the bladder suggests the extraperitoneal location.

Incision-Related Abnormalities

When evaluating for subincisional fluid collections, the greatest care possible must be taken to remove bandages and surgical appliances. When indicated, the ultrasound transducer can be sterilely draped and a sterile conducting medium utilized. Incisional abscesses typically present as a clearly defined fluid collection associated with the incisional line.[224,225] Although irregular margins or internal echoes might suggest infection, absence of these findings does not permit unequivocal differention from hematomas or wound seromas, the latter appearing characteristically anechoic with smooth margins, superficial and intimately related to the wound, and associated with a localized mass effect[217] (Fig. 9-111).

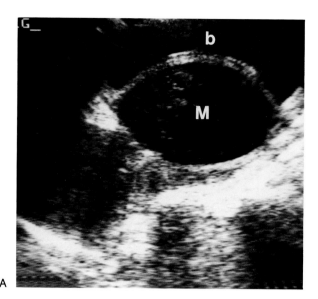
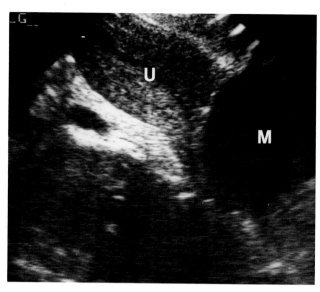

A   B

Fig. 9-107. Bladder flap hematoma. **(A)** Longitudinal pelvic sonogram over lower uterine segment and **(B)** higher longitudinal sonogram in a cesarean section patient demonstrate a large complex mass *(M)* interposed between bladder *(b)* and lower segment of the enlarged postpartum uterus *(U)*. (From Baker et al,[221] with permission.)

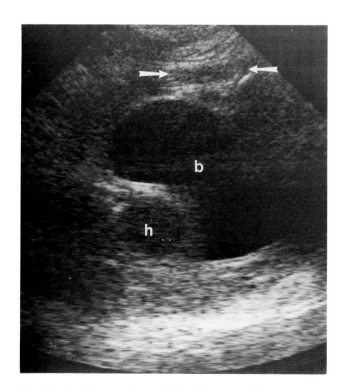

Fig. 9-108. Concomitant subfascial and bladder-flap hematomas. Longitudinal scan of a cesarean section patient shows a bladder-flap hematoma *(h)* posterior to the bladder, as well as a subfascial hematoma (arrows) anterior to the bladder *(b)*. (From Wiener et al,[223] with permission.)

Neoplasms

Neoplasms of the abdominal wall include lipomas, desmoid tumors, metastases (e.g., melanoma), and rarely, malignant tumors arising from muscle or fat. Omental tumors or peritoneal metastases may involve the anterior abdominal wall and appear sonographically inseparable from it, but the relative extent of involvement demonstrated by ultrasound may be helpful in determining the site of origin. Tumors of the abdominal wall as a rule are hypoechoic, even cystic in appearance; the exception being lipomas, which may be difficult to separate from adjacent subcutaneous tissues because of their echogenic nature[225-227] (Figs. 9-112 and 9-113).

One of the more likely primary tumors to be encountered in the anterior abdominal wall is the desmoid tumor, a benign fibrous neoplasm of aponeurotic structures, which most commonly arises in relation to the rectus abdominis and its sheath. In a series of 38 patients with abdominal wall desmoids, the overwhelming sex preponderance was female (76 percent), with roughly 16 percent directly related to pregnancy. One-fifth of cases involved the linea alba, and approximately 16 percent were associated with surgical scars.[228] The generally accepted etiologic factors are trauma (including injury during pregnancy) and hormonal disturbances, in addition to the known association with familial intestinal polyposis.[228]

Abdominal wall desmoid tumors appear anechoic or hypoechoic, typically with smooth and sharply defined

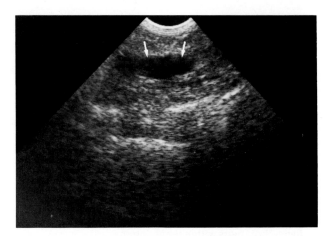 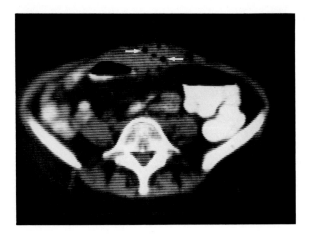

Fig. 9-109. Abdominal wall abscess. **(A)** Transverse midline scan in the lower abdomen of a patient with Crohn's disease demonstrates an elliptical anechoic collection within the abdominal wall (arrows). **(B)** CT scan in same patient through slightly different plane demonstrates abnormal soft tissue density within the anterior abdominal wall containing multiple air lucencies (arrows).

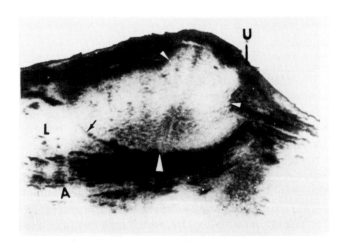

Fig. 9-110. Abdominal wall abscess. Midline longitudinal scan demonstrates a huge bonnet-shaped abscess causing marked protrusion of the abdomen in a patient with Crohn's disease. The abscess extends through a defect (small arrowheads) in the abdominal wall muscle into the extraperitoneal fat space, which is markedly distended with pus (large arrowhead). The huge abscess in the extraperitoneal fat space was shown to produce compression (arrow) on the liver *(L).* Numerous echoes within the abscess are due to necrotic tissue debris. (*A,* aorta; *U,* level of umbilicus.) (From Yeh and Rabinowitz,[209] with permission.)

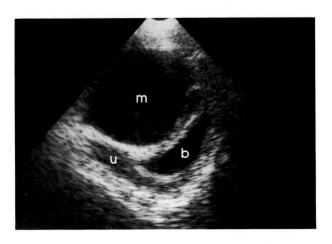

Fig. 9-111. Postsurgical infected abdominal wall hematoma. Longitudinal scan of the pelvis demonstrates a well-defined hypoechoic mass with diffuse low-amplitude echoes *(m).* Note posterior displacement of the bladder *(b),* indicating the extraperitoneal location of the collection. This scan was obtained after a right salpingo-oophorectomy for benign cystic teratoma, the patient subsequently presenting with fever and lower abdominal pain. (*u,* uterus.)

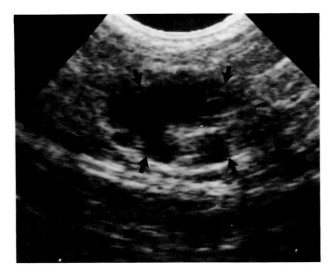

Fig. 9-112. Abdominal wall plasmacytoma. In a patient with known multiple myeloma and a palpable abdominal wall mass, a complex but primarily hypoechoic lesion (arrows) is identified in the subcutaneous tissues. Note the absence of increased through transmission.

margins, although lateral borders may appear somewhat ill defined or irregular. Posterior transmission of sound may be poor, although in many instances posterior acoustic enhancement is present[229-231] (Fig. 9-114).

Endometriosis

Endometriosis in the superficial soft tissues is an uncommon occurrence, usually developing within the umbilicus or in surgical incisions and scars. Possible

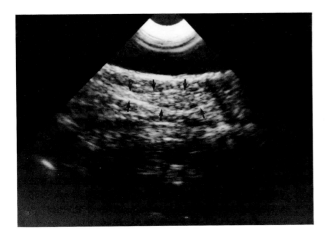

Fig. 9-113. Lipoma. Scan of the superficial abdomen using an intervening water bath demonstrates a focal lesion (arrows) that is nearly isoechoic to surrounding subcutaneous fat. Because of their echogenic nature, lipomas may frequently be difficult to delineate from adjacent tissues, as in this example.

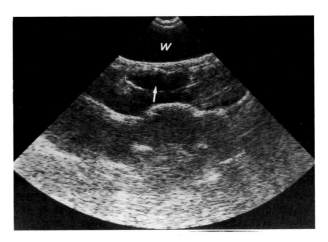

Fig. 9-114. Abdominal wall desmoid tumor. Transverse scan obtained through a water bath *(W)* demonstrates an ellipsoid hypoechoic mass within the abdominal wall (arrow). Posterior transmission of sound appears diminished.

mechanisms of development include proliferation of endometrial cells transported to an abnormal location, metaplasia of endometrial tissue at an ectopic site, or an interdependent mechanism in which endometrial cells, when transmitted by any means to a susceptible tissue, themselves stimulate imitative metaplasia.[232] In a review of 82 patients with cutaneous endometriosis in all loca-

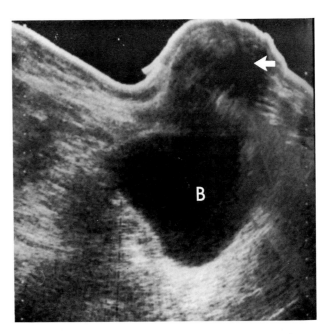

Fig. 9-115. Abdominal wall (subcutaneous) endometrioma. Longitudinal image of the pelvis demonstrates an anechoic mass (arrow) within the superficial tissues adjacent to the bladder *(B)*. Patient had undergone a cesarean section 8 years before the examination and first noticed the midline mass 4 years later. (From Vincent and Mittelstaedt,[236] with permission.)

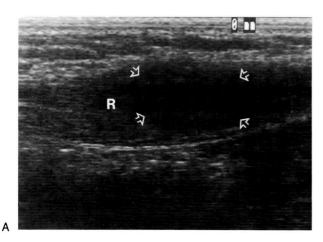

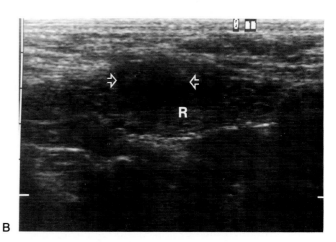

A   B

Fig. 9-116. Abdominal wall (intramuscular) endometrioma. **(A)** Longitudinal and **(B)** transverse scans of the right rectus abdominis muscle *(R)* reveal a subtle relatively hypoechoic region of differing echotexture (arrows) within the muscle. This abnormality corresponded to the patient's region of tenderness and was directly adjacent to a transverse cesarian section scar. The correct diagnosis was suggested preoperatively on the basis of these findings.

tions, 54 percent had pain or tenderness, 40 percent demonstrated exacerbation of symptoms during menstruation, and 12 percent manifested cyclical bleeding. Nearly one-third of cases arose in scars from cesarian section, and all but 5 cases arose either in surgical wounds or in the physiologic scar of the umbilicus.[232] Development of abdominal wall endometriosis has also been reported as a sequela of amniocentesis for hypertonic saline abortion.[233,234]

The sonographic appearance of superficial endometrioma is variable, with both mixed, primarily anechoic and solid-type echopatterns (echotexture similar to adjacent muscle) having been reported[235,236] (Figs. 9-115 and 9-116). The diagnosis of endometriosis should be seriously entertained with the identification of any subcutaneous or intramuscular mass associated with a surgical scar or the umbilicus, given the appropriate clinical setting, regardless of sonographic appearance.

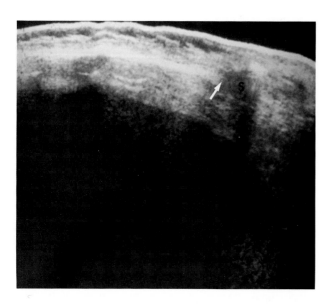

Fig. 9-117. Ventral hernia. Right longitudinal scan directly over a large palpable ventral hernia demonstrates disruption of the peritoneal line (arrow) and echodensity within the mass with distal air shadowing *(s)*. Peristalsis within bowel loops was identified during real-time examination.

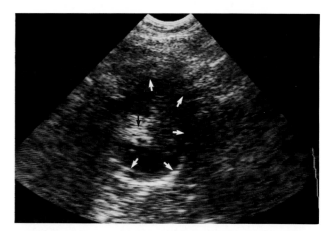

Fig. 9-118. Ventral hernia. Longitudinal real-time image in a patient with a tender right lower quadrant mass (white arrows). No peristalsis was identified within the abnormality, but the tubular mass contained a mixed echopattern and was associated with adjacent increased echoes (black arrow); the latter thought to represent mesenteric fat. The hernia was clinically reduced, and the patient returned later for elective hernia repair. Note that on these real-time sector images, delineation of the peritoneal line is difficult, as is definite compartmentalization of the mass.

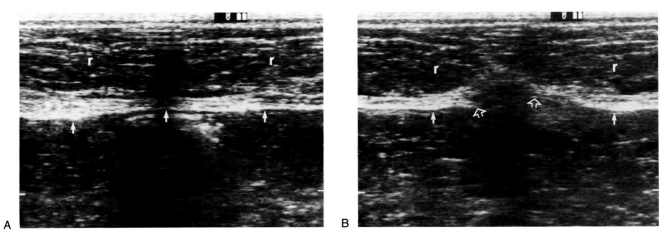

Fig. 9-119. Ventral hernia. **(A)** Transverse midline scan just cephalad to the hernia demonstrates an intact peritoneal line (arrows) and the paired rectus abdominis muscles *(r)*. **(B)** Scanning plane just inferior to that in Fig. A. demonstrates fascial disruption (open arrows) at the site of herniation. (*r*, rectus abdominis muscles.)

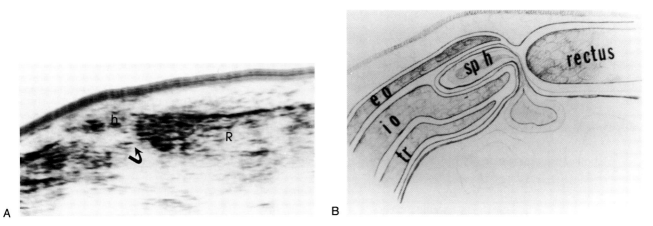

Fig. 9-120. Spigelian hernia. **(A)** Transverse scan of the right lateral abdomen and **(B)** corresponding schematic diagram demonstrate a defect in the anterior abdominal wall in the region of the spigelian fascia (arrow), with interposed bowel contents *(h)* penetrating the aponeuroses of the internal oblique *(io)* and transversus abdominis *(tr)* muscles but restricted by the external oblique *(eo)* aponeurosis. (*R*, rectus abdominis.) (From Engel and Deitch[240] with permission.)

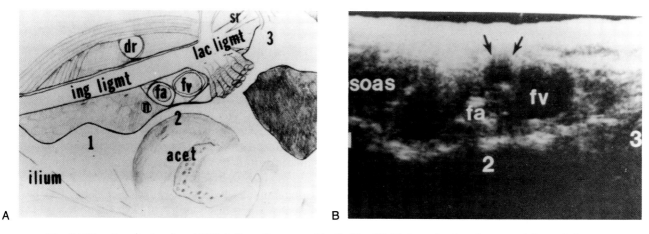

Fig. 9-121. Inguinal region. **(A)** Relation of sonographically identifiable bony landmarks to overlying soft tissue with oblique scanning of inguinal region. (*1*, anterior inferior iliac spine; *2*, iliopubic junction; *3*, pubic crest; *ing ligmt,* inguinal ligament; *lac ligmt,* lacunar ligament; *fa,* femoral artery; *fv,* femoral vein; *n,* femoral nerve; *dr,* deep inguinal ring; *sr,* superficial inguinal ring; *acet,* acetabulum.) **(B)** Corresponding scan, right groin. Femoral artery *(fa)* definitely identified at real-time sonography; femoral vein *(fv)* accentuated by Valsalva maneuver; deep inguinal ring (arrows). (From Engel and Deitch,[240] with permission.)

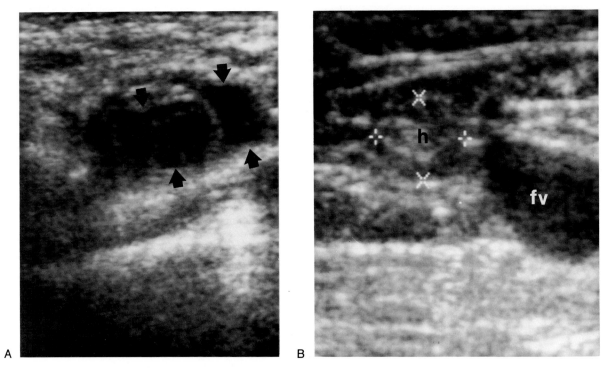

Fig. 9-122. Femoral hernia. **(A)** Incarcerated small bowel with surrounding fluid (arrows) is shown in this oblique scan of the right groin. Medial relationship to the femoral vein was established at real-time. **(B)** In another patient with herniation of fat only, a relatively echogenic mass *(h)* is identified medially to the left femoral vein *(fv)*.

Hernia

Ultrasound is of established value in hernia detection, especially in the patient in whom definitive clinical evidence is lacking or ambiguous.[237-242] Although real-time

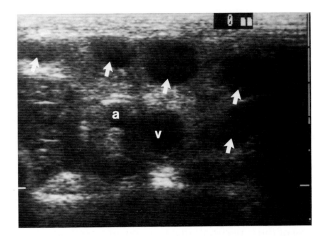

Fig. 9-123. Inguinal adenopathy. Multiple hypoechoic lymph nodes (arrows) are identified in this oblique scan of the right groin. Note femoral artery *(a)* and vein *(v)* in cross-section, seen overlying the bony reflection from the iliopubic junction.

identification of peristalsing bowel within a palpable mass presents no diagnostic dilemma, peristalsis may be absent with incarceration, and herniation may involve the omentum only. In addition, because the echopattern of bowel may suggest a solid, fluid-filled, and/or gas-containing structure, hernia may potentially mimic other superficial masses such as cysts, hematomas, abscesses, metastases, or desmoid tumors. Thus, care must be taken to sonographically document fascial disruption for definitive diagnosis (Figs. 9-117 to 9-119).

Herniation of deep tissues through a defect in the linea semilunaris, or spigelian hernia, is often difficult to appreciate clinically, as classic findings are frequently lacking. Most commonly originating near the junction of the linea semilunaris and the arcuate line, the spigelian hernia sac itself may dissect between the muscle layers or subcutaneous tissues to move elsewhere. The hernia usually penetrates both the transversus abdominis muscle and the internal oblique muscle, expanding laterally in the space between the two oblique muscles. The hernia may be quite small, with only a tag of omentum intermittently trapped within the peritoneal defect. Careful sonographic imaging, particularly using transverse images, may demonstrate the fascial disruption

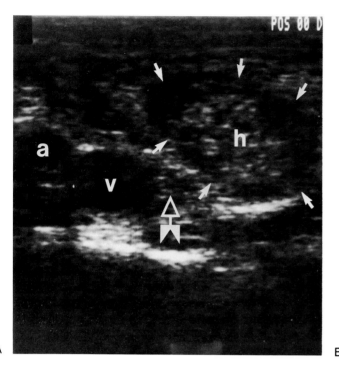
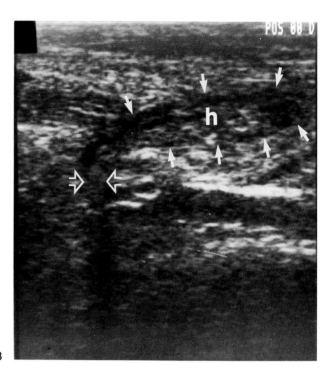

Fig. 9-124. Indirect inguinal hernia. **(A)** Oblique scan of the right groin demonstrates a well-defined complex mass (*h*, arrows) approaching the superficial inguinal ring (not seen). Note its relationship to the femoral artery *(a)* and vein *(v)*; in particular, the mass is anterior to the femoral canal (open arrow). No peristalsis could be seen at real-time examination. **(B)** With a change in scanning angle, the hernia sac (*h*, arrows) can be traced superiorly, where it is clearly shown penetrating the deep inguinal ring (open arrows).

and the hernial contents limited ventrally by the external oblique aponeurosis[217,237,240,243-247] (Fig. 9-120).

Evaluation of the inguinal and femoral regions is best performed by oblique scanning between the anterior su-

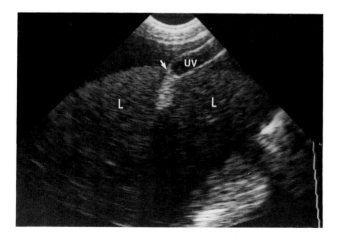

Fig. 9-125. Venous collateral. Transverse scan of the upper abdomen in a chronic alcoholic with portal hypertension demonstrates a tubular anechoic structure (*uv*, umbilical vein) anterior to the liver *(L)*. The structure could be followed along the anterior abdominal wall, and is seen to enter the liver in the region of the ligamentum teres (arrow). Ascites is also present.

perior iliac spine and the pubic crest, along the course of the inguinal ligament. Normal soft tissue structures are related to the anterior superior iliac spine, the iliopubic junction, and the pubic crest. The femoral artery and vein are identified just anterior to the iliopubic junction; the femoral vein is located more medially and will be shown to distend with the Valsalva maneuver. The psoas muscle and lymphatic channels occupy the space between the anterior superior iliac spine and the iliopubic junction[240] (Fig. 9-121).

Masses arising in relation to the femoral vessels and beneath the inguinal ligament include femoral hernias (located medial to the femoral vein), lipomas, soft tissue sarcomas, and lymph nodes (Figs. 9-122 and 9-123). Abnormalities arising superior to the femoral vessels and inguinal ligament (in the region of the deep inguinal ring) include direct and indirect inguinal hernias, ectopic testicles, and extension of femoral hernias. Extensions of inguinal hernias, ectopic testicles, varicoceles, and other cord masses can be identified sonographically in the region of the superficial ring or in the area extending from the deep ring medially and inferiorly toward the pubic crest[240,248] (Fig. 9-124).

Because the patient is examined in the supine position and a small nonpalpable hernia may not be identifiable

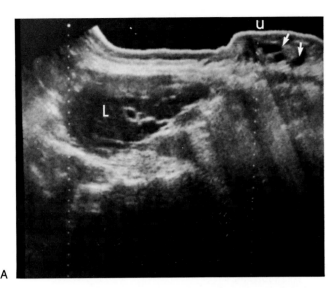
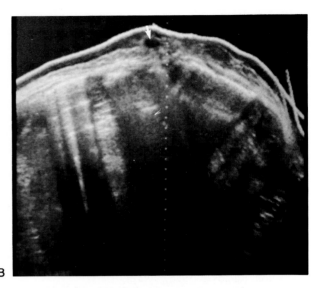

A   B

Fig. 9-126. Venous collaterals (superficial epigastrics). **(A)** Midline longitudinal and **(B)** transverse scans at the level of the umbilicus *(u)* demonstrate multiple tubular anechoic structures within the superficial soft tissues (arrows). No patent umbilical vein or connection with the left portal vein could be demonstrated. The patient was known to have a long-standing occlusion of the inferior vena cava secondary to deep venous thrombosis. (*L*, left lobe of liver.)

even with straining, sonography appears more reliable in the diagnosis of occult disease in the femoral than in the inguinal region.[249]

Venous Collaterals

In portal hypertension, recanalization of the umbilical vein may provide a collateral pathway between the left portal vein and the superficial epigastric veins. Sonographically, the vein appears as a tubular anechoic structure coursing beneath the anterior abdominal wall in the midline, extending from the region of the umbilicus to the expected location of the ligamentum teres[250,251] (Fig. 9-125). With periumbilical epigastric varices (caput medusae), the vessel may be seen entering a conglomerate of round and oval anechoicities distally.[252] The sonographic appearance of these portosystemic collaterals and their obvious connection with the liver, in the clinical setting of portal hypertension, should preclude confusion of these structures with the other abdominal wall abnormalities described earlier. The use of color Doppler or conventional duplex ultrasound to document flow has simplified diagnosis even more.

Superficial collateral vessels need not imply portal hypertension, as they may also be associated with obstruction of the inferior vena cava. When present under these circumstances, however, the pathways do not involve the umbilical vein in general, and the inferior and superficial epigastric veins drain into the internal mammary and thoracoabdominal veins, respectively[253] (Fig. 9-126).

REFERENCES

1. Slasky BS, Lenkey JL, Skolnick ML et al: Sonography of soft tissues of extremities and trunk. Semin Ultrasound 1982;3:288
2. Callen PW, Marks WM: Lymphomatous masses simulating cysts by ultrasonography. J Can Assoc Radiol 1979;30:244
3. Sommer FG, Filly RA, Minton MJ: Acoustic shadowing due to refractive and reflective effects. AJR 1979;132:973
4. Bree RL, Silver TM: Differential diagnosis of hypoechoic and anechoic masses with gray scale sonography: new observations. J Clin Ultrasound 1979;7:249
5. Rubenstein WA, Auh YH, Whalen JP, Kazam E: The perihepatic spaces: computed tomographic and ultrasound imaging. Radiology 1983;149:231
6. Griffin DJ, Gross BH, McCracken S, Glazer GM: Observations on CT differentiation of pleural and peritoneal fluid. J Comput Assist Tomogr 1984;8:24
7. Landay M, Harless W: Ultrasonic differentiation of right pleural effusion from subphrenic fluid on longitudinal scans of the right upper quadrant: importance of recognizing the diaphragm. Radiology 1977;123:155
8. Gore RM, Callen PW, Filly RA: Displaced retroperitoneal fat: sonographic guide to right upper quadrant mass localization. Radiology 1982;142:701
9. Engel IA, Auh YH, Rubenstein WA et al: Large posterior abdominal masses: computed tomographic localization. Radiology 1983;149:203

10. Lim JH, Ko YT, Lee DH: Sonographic sliding sign in localization of right upper quadrant mass. J Ultrasound Med 1990;9:455

11. Whalen JP: Radiology of the Abdomen: Anatomic Basis. Lea & Febiger, Philadelphia, 1976

12. Vincent LM, Mauro MA, Mittelstaedt CA: The lesser sac and gastrohepatic recess: sonographic appearance and differentiation. Radiology 1984;150:515

13. Jeffrey RB, Federle MP, Goodman PC: Computed tomography of the lesser peritoneal sac. Radiology 1981;141:117

14. Dodds WJ, Foley WD, Lawson TL et al: Anatomy and imaging of the lesser peritoneal sac. AJR 1985;144:567

15. Callen PW, Filly RA, Korobkin M: Ascitic fluid in the anterior paravesical fossa: misleading appearance on CT scans. AJR 1978;130:1176

16. Auh YH, Rubenstein WA, Markisz JA et al: Intraperitoneal paravesical spaces: CT delineation with US correlation. Radiology 1986;159:311

17. Auh YH, Rubenstein WA, Schneider M et al: Extraperitoneal paravesical spaces: CT delineation with US correlation. Radiology 1986;159:319

18. Spring DB, Deshon GE Jr, Babu S: The sonographic appearance of fluid in the prevesical space. Radiology 1983;147:205

19. Goldberg BB, Goodman GA, Clearfield HR: Evaluation of ascites by ultrasound. Radiology 1970;96:15

20. Weill F, LeMouel A, Bihr E et al: Ultrasonic diagnosis of intraperitoneal fluid in Morison's pouch (and in the splenoperitoneal recess): the moon crescent sign. J Radiol 1980;61:251

21. Forsby J, Henriksson L: Detectability of intraperitoneal fluid by ultrasonography. Acta Radiol Diagn 1984;25:375

22. Bundrick TJ, Cho S-R, Brewer WH, Beachley MC: Ascites: comparison of plain film radiographs with ultrasonograms. Radiology 1984;152:503

23. Proto AV, Lane EJ, Marangola JP: A new concept of ascitic fluid distribution. AJR 1976;126:974

24. Nyberg DA, Laing FC, Jeffrey RB: Sonographic detection of subtle pelvic fluid collections. AJR 1984;143:261

25. Meyers MA: Intraperitoneal spread of infections. p. 1. In Meyers MA (ed): Dynamic Radiology of the Abdomen. Springer-Verlag, New York, 1976

26. Godwin JD, MacGregor JM: Extension of ascites into the chest with hiatal hernia: visualization on CT. AJR 1987;148:31

27. Gefter WB, Arger PH, Edell SL: Sonographic patterns of ascites. Semin Ultrasound 1981;2:226

28. Gooding GAW, Cummings SR: Sonographic detection of ascites in liver disease. J Ultrasound Med 1984; 3:169

29. Yeh H-C, Wolf BS: Ultrasonography in ascites. Radiology 1977;124:783

30. Gore RM, Callen PW, Filly RA: Lesser sac fluid in predicting the etiology of ascites: CT findings. AJR 1982;139:71

31. Jolles H, Coulam CM: CT of ascites: differential diagnosis. AJR 1980;135:315

32. Edell SL, Gefter WB: Ultrasonic differentiation of types of ascitic fluid. AJR 1979;133:111

33. Franklin JT, Azose AA: Sonographic appearance of chylous ascites. J Clin Ultrasound 1984;12:239

34. Elboim CM, Goldman L, Hann L et al: Significance of post-cholecystectomy subhepatic fluid collections. Ann Surg 1983;198:137

35. Neff CC, Simeone JF, Ferrucci JT Jr et al: The occurrence of fluid collections following routine abdominal surgical procedures: sonographic survey in asymptomatic postoperative patients. Radiology 1983;146:463

36. Gold JP, Canizaro P, Kazam E et al: The reliability of the results of ultrasound detection of fluid collections in the early postceliotomy period. Surg Gynecol Obstet 1985;161:5

37. Grobe JL, Kozarek RA, Sanowski RA, Earnest DL: "Pseudo-ascites" associated with giant ovarian cysts and elevated cystic fluid amylase. Am J Gastroenterol 1983;78:421

38. Baer JW: Extraperitoneal mass effect by ascites under tension. Gastrointest Radiol 1990;15:3

39. Vincent LM, Parker LA, Mittelstaedt CA: Sequela of continuous ambulatory peritoneal dialysis (CAPD) mimicking primary gynecologic pathology. J Ultrasound Med 1987;6:483

40. Schwerk WB, Dürr HK: Ultrasound gray-scale pattern and guided aspiration puncture of abdominal abscesses. J Clin Ultrasound 1981;9:389

41. Doust BD, Quiroz F, Stewart JM: Ultrasonic distinction of abscesses from other intra-abdominal fluid collections. Radiology 1977;125:213

42. Hill M, Sanders RC: Gray scale B scan characteristics of intra-abdominal cystic masses. J Clin Ultrasound 1978;6:217

43. Kressel HY, Filly RA: Ultrasonographic appearance of gas-containing abscesses in the abdomen. AJR 1978;130:71

44. Golding RH, Li DKB, Cooperberg PL: Sonographic demonstration of air-fluid levels in abdominal abscesses. J Ultrasound Med 1982;1:151

45. Doust BD, Thompson R: Ultrasonography of abdominal fluid collections. Gastrointest Radiol 1978;3:273

46. Mueller PR, Simeone JF: Intraabdominal abscesses: diagnosis by sonography and computed tomography. p. 425. In Federle MP (ed): Symposium on CT and Ultrasonography in the Acutely Ill Patient. Vol. 21. WB Saunders, Philadelphia, 1983

47. Sekiba K, Akamatsu N, Niwa K: Ultrasound characteristics of abdominal abscesses involving foreign bodies (gauze). J Clin Ultrasound 1979;7:284

48. Choi BI, Kim SH, Yu ES et al: Retained surgical sponge: diagnosis with CT and sonography. AJR 1988;150:1047

49. Kokubo T, Itai Y, Ohtomo K et al: Retained surgical sponge: CT and US appearance. Radiology 1987;165:415

50. Filly RA: Annual oration: detection of abdominal abscesses: a combined approach employing ultrasonography, computed tomography and gallium-67 scanning. J Can Assoc Radiol 1979;30:202

51. Taylor KJW, Wasson JFM, deGraaff C et al: Accuracy of grey-scale ultrasound diagnosis of abdominal and pelvic abscesses in 220 patients. Lancet 1978;1:83

52. Gross BH, Chinn DH, Callen PW, Filly RA: Real-time vs. static scanning in the diagnosis of abdominal and pelvic abscesses. J Ultrasound Med 1983;2:223

53. Carroll B, Silverman PM, Goodwin DA, McDougall IR: Ultrasonography and indium 111 white blood cell scanning for the detection of intraabdominal abscesses. Radiology 1981;140:155

54. Knochel JQ, Koehler PR, Lee TG, Welch DM: Diagnosis of abdominal abscesses with computed tomography, ultrasound, and ¹¹¹In leukocyte scans. Radiology 1980;137:425

55. Moir C, Robins RE: Role of ultrasonography, gallium scanning, and computed tomography in the diagnosis of intraabdominal abscess. Am J Surg 1982;143:582

56. Lundstedt C, Hederström E, Holmin T et al: Radiological diagnosis in proven intraabdominal abscess formation: a comparison between plain films of the abdomen, ultrasonography and computerized tomography. Gastrointest Radiol 1983;8:261

57. Coelho JCU, Sigel B, Ryva JC et al: B-mode sonography of blood clots. J Clin Ultrasound 1982;10:323

58. Wicks JD, Silver TM, Bree RL: Gray scale features of hematomas: an ultrasonic spectrum. AJR 1978;131:977

59. Rankin RN, Hutton L, Grace DM: Postoperative abdominal wall hematomas have a distinctive appearance on ultrasonography. Can J Surg 1985;28:84

60. Lee TG, Brickman FE, Avecilla LS: Ultrasound diagnosis of intramural intestinal hematoma. J Clin Ultrasound 1977;5:423

61. Fon GT, Hunter TB, Haber K: Utility of ultrasound for diagnosis of mesenteric hematoma. AJR 1980;134:381

62. Raghavendra BN, Grieco AJ, Balthazar EJ et al: Diagnostic utility of sonography and computed tomography in spontaneous mesenteric hematoma. Am J Gastroenterol 1982;77:570

63. Frank B, Bolich P, Reichert J: Sonographic appearance of organized blood within a cyst: two case reports. J Clin Ultrasound 1975;3:233

64. Jeffrey RB, Laing FC: Echogenic clot: a useful sign of pelvic hemoperitoneum. Radiology 1982;145:139

65. Zegel HG, Kurtz AB, Perlmutter GS, Goldberg BB: Ultrasonic characteristics of bilomas. J Clin Ultrasound 1981;9:21

66. Mueller PR, Ferrucci JT Jr, Simeone JF et al: Detection and drainage of bilomas: special considerations. AJR 1983;140:715

67. Kuligowska E, Schlesinger A, Miller KB et al: Bilomas: a new approach to the diagnosis and treatment. Gastrointest Radiol 1983;8:237

68. Dupas J-L, Mancheron H, Sevenet F et al: Hepatic subcapsular biloma: an unusual complication of endoscopic retrograde cholangiopancreatography. Gastroenterology 1988;94:1225

69. Vazquez JL, Thorsen MK, Dodds WJ et al: Evaluation and treatment of intraabdominal bilomas. AJR 1985;144:933

70. Kaplan SB, Zajko AB, Koneru B: Hepatic bilomas due to hepatic artery thrombosis in liver transplant recipients: percutaneous drainage and clinical outcome. Radiology 1990;174:1031

71. Middleton JP, Wolper JC: Hepatic biloma complicating sickle cell disease: a case report and a review of the literature. Gastroenterology 1984;86:743

72. Laing FC, Gooding GAW, Brown T, Leopold GR: Atypical pseudocysts of the pancreas: an ultrasonographic evaluation. J Clin Ultrasound 1979;7:27

73. Siegelman SS, Copeland BE, Saba GP et al: CT of fluid collections associated with pancreatitis. AJR 1980;134:1121

74. Weill F, Brun PH, Rohmer P, Belloir A: Migrations of fluid of pancreatic origin: ultrasonic and CT study of 28 cases. Ultrasound Med Biol 1983;9:485

75. Hashimoto BE, Laing FC, Jeffrey RB Jr, Federle MP: Hemorrhagic pancreatic fluid collections examined by ultrasound. Radiology 1984;150:803

76. Beahrs OH, Judd ES Jr, Dockerty MB: Chylous cysts of the abdomen. Surg Clin North Am 1950;30:1081

77. Baker AH: Developmental mesenteric cysts. Br J Surg 1961;48:534

78. Ros PR, Olmstead WW, Moser RP Jr et al: Mesenteric and omental cysts: histologic classification with imaging correlation. Radiology 1987;164:327

79. Mittelstaedt C: Ultrasonic diagnosis of omental cysts. Radiology 1975;117:673

80. Nordshus T, Løtveit T: Multiple mesenteric cysts diagnosed by ultrasound. Ann Chir Gynaecol 1976;65:234

81. Takeuchi S, Yamaguchi M, Sakurai M et al: A case of mesenteric cyst diagnosed by ultrasound examination and a review of Japanese literatures. Jpn J Surg 1979;9:359

82. Rifkin MD, Kurtz AB, Pasto ME: Mesenteric chylous (lymph-containing) cyst. Gastrointest Radiol 1983;8:267

83. Longmaid HE III, Tymkiw J, Rider EA: Sonographic diagnosis of a chylous mesenteric cyst. J Clin Ultrasound 1986;14:458

84. Nicolet V, Grignon A, Filiatrault D, Boisvert J: Sonographic appearance of an abdominal cystic lymphangioma. J Ultrasound Med 1984;3:85

85. van Mil JBC, Laméris JS: Unusual appearance of a mesenteric cyst. Diagn Imaging 1983;52:28

86. Geer LL, Mittelstaedt CA, Staab EV, Gaisie G: Mesenteric cyst: sonographic appearance with CT correlation. Pediatr Radiol 1984;14:102

87. Haller JO, Schneider M, Kassner EG et al: Sonographic evaluation of mesenteric and omental masses in children. AJR 1978;130:269

88. Wicks JD, Silver TM, Bree RL: Giant abdominal masses in children and adolescents: ultrasonic differential diagnosis. AJR 1978;130:853

89. Gordon MJ, Sumner TE: Abdominal ultrasonography in a mesenteric cyst presenting as ascites. Gastroenterology 1975;69:761

90. Katsube Y, Mukai K, Silverberg SG: Cystic mesothelioma of the peritoneum: a report of five cases and review of the literature. Cancer 1982;50:1615

91. Schneider V, Partridge JR, Gutierrez F et al: Benign cystic mesothelioma involving the female genital tract: report of four cases. Am J Obstet Gynecol 1983;145:355

92. Nirodi NS, Lowry DS, Wallace RJ: Cystic mesothelioma of the pelvic peritoneum. Two case reports. Br J Obstet Gynaecol 1984;91:201

93. Schneider JA, Zelnick EJ: Benign cystic peritoneal mesothelioma. J Clin Ultrasound 1985;13:190

94. O'Neil JD, Ros PR, Storm BL et al: Cystic mesothelioma of the peritoneum. Radiology 1989;170:333

95. McFadden DE, Clement PB: Peritoneal inclusion cysts with mural mesothelial proliferation. a clinicopathological analysis of six cases. Am J Surg Pathol 1986;10:844

96. Cancelmo RP: Sonographic demonstration of multilocular peritoneal inclusion cyst. J Clin Ultrasound 1983;11:334

97. Hoffer FA, Kozakewich H, Colodny A, Goldstein DP: Peritoneal inclusion cysts: ovarian fluid in peritoneal adhesions. Radiology 1988;169:189

98. Bundy AL, Fleischer AC, Thieme GA, James AE: Blastomycosis presenting as a peritoneal inflammatory cyst. J Clin Ultrasound 1985;13:205

99. Niron EA, Özer H, Dolunay H: Encysted peritoneal hydatidosis, unusual ultrasonographic and clinical presentation of liver echinococcosis. Br J Radiol 1981;54:339

100. Davies RP, Kennedy G, Chatterton BE: Noncystic appearance of intraperitoneal echinococcus on ultrasound examination. J Clin Ultrasound 1986;14:55

101. Dachman AH, Lichtenstein JE, Friedman AC: Mucocele of the appendix and pseudomyxoma peritonei. AJR 1985;144:923

102. Yeh H-C, Shafir MK, Slater G et al: Ultrasonography and computed tomography in pseudomyxoma peritonei. Radiology 1984;153:507

103. Hopper KD: Ultrasonic findings in pseudomyxoma peritonei. South Med J 1983;76:1051

104. Hann L, Love S, Goldberg RP: Pseudomyxoma peritonei: preoperative diagnosis by ultrasound and computed tomography. Cancer 1983;52:642

105. Merritt CB, Williams SM: Ultrasound findings in a patient with pseudomyxoma peritonei. J Clin Ultrasound 1978;6:417

106. Hayashi N, Tamaki N, Yamamoto K et al: Sonography of pseudomyxoma peritonei. J Ultrasound Med 1986;5:401

107. Seale WB: Sonographic findings in a patient with pseudomyxoma peritonei. J Clin Ultrasound 1982;10:441

108. Seshul MB, Coulam CM: Pseudomyxoma peritonei: computed tomography and sonography. AJR 1981;136:803

109. Davidson RI: Peritoneal bypass in the treatment of hydrocephalus: historical review and abdominal complications. J Neurol Neurosurg Psychiatry 1976;39:640

110. Agha FP, Amendola MA, Shirazi KK et al: Abdominal complications of ventriculoperitoneal shunts with emphasis on the role of imaging methods. Surg Gynecol Obstet 1983;156:473

111. Fischer EG, Shillito J Jr: Large abdominal cysts: a complication of peritoneal shunts. Report of three cases. J Neurosurg 1969;31:441

112. Parry SW, Schuhmacher JF, Llewellyn RC: Abdominal pseudocysts and ascites formation after ventriculoperitoneal shunt procedures. Report of four cases. J Neurosurg 1975;43:476

113. Cunningham JJ: Evaluation of malfunctioning ventriculoperitoneal shunts with gray scale echography. J Clin Ultrasound 1976;4:369

114. Nakagaki H, Matsunaga M, Maeyama R, Mizoguchi R: Intraperitoneal pseudocyst after ventriculoperitoneal shunt. Surg Neurol 1979;11:447

115. Goldfine SL, Turetz F, Beck AR, Eiger M: Cerebrospinal fluid intraperitoneal cyst: an unusual abdominal mass. AJR 1978;130:568

116. Raghavendra BN, Epstein FJ, Subramanyam BP, Becker MH: Ultrasonographic evaluation of intraperitoneal CSF pseudocyst. Report of three cases. Childs Brain 1981;8:39

117. Briggs JR, Hendry GMA, Minns RA: Abdominal ultrasound in the diagnosis of cerebrospinal fluid pseudocysts complicating ventriculoperitoneal shunts. Arch Dis Child 1984;59:661

118. Lee TG, Parsons PM: Ultrasound diagnosis of cerebrospinal fluid abdominal cyst. Radiology 1978;127:220

119. Brenbridge ANAG, Buschi AJ, Lees RF, Sims T: Sonography of CSF pseudocyst. Am J Dis Child 1979;133:646

120. Grunebaum M, Ziv N, Kornreich L et al: The sonographic signs of peritoneal pseudocyst obstructing the ventriculo-peritoneal shunt in children. Neuroradiology 1988;30:433

121. Fried AM, Adams WE Jr, Ellis GT et al: Ventriculoperitoneal shunt function: evaluation by sonography. AJR 1980;134:967

122. Dodd GD, Rutledge F, Wallace S: Postoperative pelvic lymphocysts. AJR 1970;108:312

123. Basinger GT, Gittes RF: Lymphocyst: ultrasound diagnosis and urologic management. J Urol 1975;114:740

124. Morin ME, Baker DA: Lymphocele: a complication of surgical staging of carcinoma of the prostate. AJR 1977;129:333

125. Starzl TE, Groth CG, Putnam CW et al: Urological complications in 216 human recipients of renal transplants. Ann Surg 1970;172:1

126. Fitzer PM, Sallade RL, Graham WH: Computed tomography and the diagnosis of giant abdominal lymphocele. Va Med 1980;107:448

127. Fried AM, Williams CB, Litvak AS: High retroperitoneal lymphocele: unusual clinical presentation and diagnosis by ultrasonography. J Urol 1980;123:583

128. Rossi L, Mandrioli R, Rossi A, Ugolotti U: Retroperitoneal cystic lymphangioma. Br J Radiol 1982;55:676

129. Radin R, Weiner S, Koenigsberg M et al: Retroperitoneal cystic lymphangioma. AJR 1983;140:733

130. Davidson AJ, Hartman DS: Lymphangioma of the retroperitoneum: CT and sonographic characteristics. Radiology 1990;175:507

131. Davidson AJ, Hartman DS, Goldman SM: Mature tera-

toma of the retroperitoneum: radiologic, pathologic, and clinical correlation. Radiology 1989;172:421

132. Macpherson RI, Gordon L, Bradford BF: Neonatal urinomas: imaging considerations. Pediatr Radiol 1984;14:396

133. Healy ME, Teng SS, Moss AA: Uriniferous pseudocyst: computed tomographic findings. Radiology 1984;153:757

134. McInerney D, Jones A, Roylance J: Urinoma. Clin Radiol 1977;28:345

135. Tien R, Shirkoda A, David R: Circumferential perirenal urinoma mimicking nephromegaly on urography. Urol Radiol 1989;11:92

136. Feinstein KA, Fernbach SK: Septated urinomas in the neonate. AJR 1987;149:997

137. Blichert-Toft M, Nielsen OV: Congenital patent urachus and acquired variants. Acta Chir Scand 1971;137:807

138. Bauer SB, Retik AB: Urachal anomalies and related umbilical disorders. p. 195. In Jeffs RD (ed): Symposium on Congenital Anomalies of the Lower Genitourinary Tract. WB Saunders, Philadelphia, 1978

139. Morin ME, Tan A, Baker DA, Sue HK: Urachal cyst in the adult: ultrasound diagnosis. AJR 1979;132:831

140. Bouvier J-F, Pascaud E, Mailhes F et al: Urachal cyst in the adult: ultrasound diagnosis. J Clin Ultrasound 1984;12:48

141. Williams BD, Fisk JD: Sonographic diagnosis of giant urachal cyst in the adult. AJR 1981;136:417

142. Spataro RF, Davis RS, McLachlan MSF et al: Urachal abnormalities in the adult. Radiology 1983;149:659

143. Anderson ML, Miller JH, Reid BS, Gilsanz V: 'How's urachus.' Proceedings from American Institute of Ultrasound in Medicine, (Abstract 723), p. 221, 1983

144. Cacciarelli AA, Kass EJ, Yang SS: Urachal remnants: sonographic demonstration in children. Radiology 1990;174:473

145. Rifkin MD, Needleman L, Kurtz AB et al: Sonography of nongynecologic cystic masses of the pelvis. AJR 1984;142:1169

146. Friedman AP, Haller JO, Schulze G, Schaffer R: Sonography of vesical and perivesical abnormalities in children. J Ultrasound Med 1983;2:385

147. Hansen GR, Laing FC: Sonographic evaluation of a left ventricular aneurysm presenting as an upper abdominal mass. J Clin Ultrasound 1980;8:151

148. Effman EL, Griscom NT, Colodny AH, Vawter GF: Neonatal gastrointestinal masses arising late in gestation. AJR 1980;135:681

149. Hillman BJ, Haber K: Echographic characteristics of malignant lymph nodes. J Clin Ultrasound 1980;8:213

150. Yeh H-C, Wolf BS: Ultrasonography and computed tomography in the diagnosis of homogeneous masses. Radiology 1977;123:425

151. Lev-Toaff AS, Coleman BG, Arger PH et al: Leiomyomas in pregnancy: sonographic study. Radiology 1987;164:375

152. Nocera RM, Fagan CJ, Hernandez JC: Cystic parametrial fibroids mimicking ovarian cystadenoma. J Ultrasound Med 1984;3:183

153. Ouimette MV, Bree RL: Sonography of pelvoabdominal cystic masses in children and adolescents. J Ultrasound Med 1984;3:149

154. Athey PA, Malone RS: Sonography of ovarian fibromas/thecomas. J Ultrasound Med 1987;6:431

155. Sheth S, Fishman EK, Buck JL et al: The variable sonographic appearances of ovarian teratomas: correlation with CT. AJR 1988;151:331

156. Quinn SF, Erickson S, Black WC: Cystic ovarian teratomas: the sonographic appearance of the dermoid plug. Radiology 1985;155:477

157. Walsh JW, Taylor KJW, Rosenfield AT: Gray scale ultrasonography in the diagnosis of endometriosis and adenomyosis. AJR 1979;132:87

158. Swayne LC, Love MB, Karasick SR: Pelvic inflammatory disease: sonographic-pathologic correlation. Radiology 1984;151:751

159. Baltarowich OH, Kurtz AB, Pasto ME et al: The spectrum of sonographic findings in hemorrhagic ovarian cysts. AJR 1987;148:901

160. Alpern MB, Sandler MA, Madrazo BL: Sonographic features of parovarian cysts and their complications. AJR 1984;143:157

161. Athey PA, Cooper NB: Sonographic features of parovarian cysts. AJR 1985;144:83

162. Bedi DG, Fagan CJ, Nocera RM: Chronic ectopic pregnancy. J Ultrasound Med 1984;3:347

163. Cunningham JJ: False-positive gray-scale ultrasonography for intra-abdominal abscesses. Arch Surg 1976;111:810

164. Engel JM, Deitch EA: Omentum mimicking cystic masses in the pelvis. J Clin Ultrasound 1980;8:31

165. Barth RA, Brasch RC, Filly RA: Abdominal pseudotumor in childhood: distended gallbladder with parenteral hyperalimentation. AJR 1981;136:341

166. Rao KG, Woodlief RM: Excessive right subdiaphragmatic fat: a potential diagnostic pitfall. Radiology 1981;138:15

167. Arenson AM, McKee JD: Left upper quadrant pseudolesion secondary to normal variants in liver and spleen. J Clin Ultrasound 1986;14:558

168. Crivello MS, Peterson IM, Austin RM: Left lobe of the liver mimicking perisplenic collections. J Clin Ultrasound 1986;14:697

169. Middleton WD: Pseudosubcapsular splenic hematoma due to elongation of left hepatic lobe (case 3, sonography case of the day). AJR 1989;152:1325

170. Daniel O: The differential diagnosis of malignant disease of the peritoneum. Br J Surg 1951;39:147

171. Yeh H-C: Ultrasonography of peritoneal tumors. Radiology 1979;133:419

172. Derchi LE, Reggiani L, Rebaudi F, Bruschetta M: Appendices epiploicae of the large bowel: sonographic appearance and differentiation from peritoneal seeding. J Ultrasound Med 1988;7:11

173. Williams LJ, Pavlick FJ: Leiomyomatosis peritonealis disseminata: two case reports and review of the medical literature. Cancer 1980;47:1726

174. Renigers SA, Michael AS, Bardawil WA et al: Sono-

graphic findings in leiomyomatosis peritonealis disseminata: a case report and literature review. J Ultrasound Med 1985;4:497

175. Stein MA: Omental band: new sign of metastasis. J Clin Ultrasound 1977;5:410

176. D'amico RJ: The omental band sign in reticulum cell sarcoma. J Med Soc NJ 1979;76:441

177. Yaghoobian J, Demeter E, Colucci J: Ultrasonic demonstration of lymphomatous infiltration of the greater omentum. Med Ultrasound 1984;8:65

178. Mueller PR, Ferrucci JT Jr, Harbin WP et al: Appearance of lymphomatous involvement of the mesentery by ultrasonography and body computed tomography: the 'sandwich sign.' Radiology 1980;134:467

179. Bernardino ME, Jing BS, Wallace S: Computed tomography diagnosis of mesenteric masses. AJR 1979;132:33

180. Kadin ME, Glatstein E, Dorfman RF: Clinicopathologic studies of 117 untreated patients subjected to laparotomy for the staging of Hodgkin's disease. Cancer 1971;27:1277

181. Goffinet DR, Castellino RA, Kim H et al: Staging laparotomies in unselected previously untreated patients with non-Hodgkin's lymphomas. Cancer 1973;32:672

182. Yannopoulos K, Stout AP: Primary solid tumors of the mesentery. Cancer 1963;16:914

183. Stout AP, Hendry J, Purdie FJ: Primary solid tumors of the great omentum. Cancer 1963;16:231

184. Weinberger HA, Ahmed MS: Mesenchymal solid tumors of the omentum and mesentery: report of four cases. Surgery 1977;82:754

185. MacKenzie DH: The fibromatoses: a clinicopathological concept. Br Med J 1972;4:277

186. DasGupta TK, Brasfield RD, O'Hara J: Extra-abdominal desmoids: a clinicopathological study. Ann Surg 1969;170:109

187. Sacks B, Joffe N, Harris N: Isolated mesenteric desmoids (mesenteric fibromatosis). Clin Radiol 1978;29:95

188. Rubenstein WA, Gray G, Auh YH et al: CT of fibrous tissues and tumors with sonographic correlation. AJR 1986;147:1067

189. Baron RL, Lee JKT: Mesenteric desmoid tumors. Radiology 1981;140:777

190. Sampliner JE, Paruleker S, Jain B et al: Intra-abdominal mesenteric desmoid tumors. Am Surg 1982;48:316

191. Mantello MT, Haller JO, Marquis JR: Sonography of abdominal desmoid tumors in adolescents. J Ultrasound Med 1989;8:467

192. Reske M, Namiki H: Sclerosing mesenteritis. Report of two cases. Am J Clin Pathol 1975;64:661

193. Katz ME, Heiken JP, Glazer HS, Lee JKT: Intraabdominal panniculitis: clinical, radiographic, and CT features. AJR 1985;145:293

194. Pérez-Fontán FJ, Soler R, Sanches J et al: Retractile mesenteritis involving the colon: barium enema, sonographic, and CT findings. AJR 1986;147:937

195. Bendon JA, Poleynard GD, Bordin GM: Fibrosing mesenteritis simulating pelvic carcinomatosis. Gastrointest Radiol 1979;4:195

196. Haynes JW, Brewer WH, Walsh JW: Focal fat necrosis

presenting as a palpable abdominal mass: CT evaluation. J Comput Assist Tomogr 1985;9:568

197. Kordan B, Payne SD: Fat necrosis simulating a primary tumor of the mesentery: sonographic diagnosis. J Ultrasound Med 1988;7:345

198. Bree RL, Green B: The gray scale sonographic appearance of intraabdominal mesenchymal sarcomas. Radiology 1978;128:193

199. Behan M, Kazam E: The echographic characteristics of fatty tissues and tumors. Radiology 1978;129:143

200. Bowen B, Ros PR, McCarthy MJ et al: Gastrointestinal teratomas: CT and US appearance with pathologic correlation. Radiology 1987;162:431

201. Volta S, Carella I, Gaeta M et al: Castleman disease of the greater omentum (letter to the editor). AJR 1990;154:652

202. Moertel CG: Peritoneal mesothelioma. Gastroenterology 1972;63:346

203. Banner MP, Gohel VK: Peritoneal mesothelioma. Radiology 1978;129:637

204. Yeh H-C, Chahinian AP: Ultrasonography and computed tomography of peritoneal mesothelioma. Radiology 1980;135:705

205. Reuter K, Raptopoulos V, Reale F et al: Diagnosis of peritoneal mesothelioma: computed tomography, sonography, and fine-needle aspiration biopsy. AJR 1983;140:1189

206. Shah JM, King DL: Gray scale sonographic presentation of a mesothelioma of the greater omentum. J Clin Ultrasound 1979;7:147

207. Dach J, Patel N, Patel S, Petasnick J: Peritoneal mesothelioma: CT, sonography, and gallium-67 scan. AJR 1980;135:614

208. Allen HA III, Vick CW, Messmer JM, Parker GA: Diffuse mesenteric amyloidosis: CT, sonographic and pathologic findings. J Comput Assist Tomogr 1985;9:196

209. Yeh H-C, Rabinowitz JG: Ultrasonography and computed tomography of inflammatory abdominal wall lesions. Radiology 1982;144:859

210. Lee PWR, Bark M, Macfie J, Pratt D: The ultrasound diagnosis of rectus sheath haematoma. Br J Surg 1977;64:633

211. Manier JW: Rectus sheath hematoma. Six case reports and a literature review. Am J Gastroenterol 1972;54:443

212. Hopper KD, Smazal SF Jr, Ghaed N: CT and ultrasonic evaluation of rectus sheath hematoma: a complication of anticoagulant therapy. Milit Med 1983;148:447

213. Trias A, Boctor M, Echave V: Ultrasonography in the diagnosis of rectus abdominis hematoma. Can J Surg 1981;24:524

214. Tromans A, Campbell N, Sykes P: Rectus sheath haematoma: Diagnosis by ultrasound. Br J Surg 1981;68:518

215. Spitz HB, Wyatt GM: Rectus sheath hematoma. J Clin Ultrasound 1977;5:413

216. Kaftori JK, Rosenberger A, Pollack S, Fish JH: Rectus sheath hematoma: ultrasonographic diagnosis. AJR 1977;128:283

217. Fried AM, Meeker WR: Incarcerated spigelian hernia: ultrasonic differential diagnosis. AJR 1979;133:107

218. Wyatt GM, Spitz HB: Ultrasound in the diagnosis of rectus sheath hematoma. JAMA 1979;241:1499

219. Benson M: Rectus sheath haematomas simulating pelvic pathology: the ultrasound appearances. Clin Radiol 1982;33:651

220. Fornage BD, Touche DH, Segal P, Rifkin MD: Ultrasonography in the evaluation of muscular trauma. J Ultrasound Med 1983;2:549

221. Baker ME, Bowie JD, Killam AP: Sonography of post-cesarean-section bladder-flap hematoma. AJR 1985;144:757

222. Winsett MZ, Fagan CJ, Bedi DG: Sonographic demonstration of bladder-flap hematoma. J Ultrasound Med 1986;5:483

223. Wiener MD, Bowie JD, Baker ME, Kay HH: Sonography of subfascial hematoma after cesarean delivery. AJR 1987;148:907

224. Cunningham J, Thomas JL, Detection and localization of subincisional abscesses with gray scale echography. Am Surg 1979;45:388

225. Goldberg BB: Ultrasonic evaluation of superficial masses. J Clin Ultrasound 1975;3:91

226. Miller EI, Rogers A: Sonography of the anterior abdominal wall. Semin Ultrasound 1982;3:278

227. O'Malley BP, Qizilbash AH: Mesenchymal chondrosarcoma of the rectus sheath. Case report with ultrasonic findings. J Clin Ultrasound 1977;5:348

228. Brasfield RD, DasGupta TK: Desmoid tumors of the anterior abdominal wall. Surgery 1969;65:241

229. Hanson RD, Hunter TB, Haber K: Ultrasonographic appearance of anterior abdominal wall desmoid tumors. J Ultrasound Med 1983;2:141

230. Wallace JHK: Ultrasonic diagnosis of abdominal wall desmoid tumor. J Can Assoc Radiol 1980;31:120

231. Yeh H-C, Rabinowitz JG, Rosenblum M: Complementary role of CT and ultrasonography in the diagnosis of desmoid tumor of abdominal wall. Comput Radiol 1982;6:275

232. Steck WD, Helwig EB: Cutaneous endometriosis. Clin Obstet Gynecol 1966;9:373

233. Ferrari BT, Shollenbarger DR: Abdominal wall endometriosis following hypertonic saline abortion. JAMA 1977;238:56

234. Kaunitz A, Di Sant' Agnese PA: Needle tract endometriosis: an unusual complication of amniocentesis. Obstet Gynecol 1979;54:753

235. Miller WB Jr, Melson GL: Abdominal wall endometrioma. AJR 1979;132:467

236. Vincent LM, Mittelstaedt CA: Sonographic demonstration of endometrioma arising in cesarean scar. J Ultrasound Med 1985;4:437

237. Spangen L: Ultrasound as a diagnostic aid in ventral abdominal hernia. J Clin Ultrasound 1975;3:211

238. Thomas JL, Cunningham JJ: Ultrasonic evaluation of ventral hernias disguised as intraabdominal neoplasms. Arch Surg 1978;113:589

239. Deitch EA, Engel JM: Ultrasonic diagnosis of surgical diseases of the anterior abdominal wall. Surg Gynecol Obstet 1980;151:484

240. Engel JM, Deitch EE: Sonography of the anterior abdominal wall. AJR 1981;137:73

241. Lineaweaver W, Vlasak M, Muyshondt E: Ultrasonic examination of abdominal wall and groin masses. South Med J 1983;76:590

242. Yeh H-C, Lehr-Janus C, Cohen BA, Rabinowitz JG: Ultrasonography and CT of abdominal and inguinal hernias. J Clin Ultrasound 1984;12:479

243. Sutphen JH, Hitchcock DA, King DC: Ultrasonic demonstration of spigelian hernia. AJR 1980;134:174

244. Deitch EA, Engel JM: Spigelian hernia: an ultrasonic diagnosis. Arch Surg 1980;115:93

245. Nelson RL, Renigers SA, Nyhus LM et al: Ultrasonography of the abdominal wall in the diagnosis of spigelian hernia. Am Surg 1980;46:373

246. Balthazar EJ, Subramanyam BR, Megibow A: Spigelian hernia: CT and ultrasonography diagnosis. Gastrointest Radiol 1984;9:81

247. Spangen L: Spigelian hernia. Surg Clin North Am 1984;64:351

248. Deitch EA, Soncrant MC: The value of ultrasound in the diagnosis of nonpalpable femoral hernias. Arch Surg 1981;116:185

249. Deitch EA, Soncrant MC: Ultrasonic diagnosis of surgical disease in the inguinal-femoral region. Surg Gynecol Obstet 1981;152:319

250. Glazer GM, Laing FC, Brown TW, Gooding GAW: Sonographic demonstration of portal hypertension: the patent umbilical vein. Radiology 1980;136:161

251. Subramanyam BR, Balthazar EJ, Madamba MR et al: Sonography of portosystemic venous collateral in portal hypertension. Radiology 1983;146:161

252. Jüttner H-U, Jenney JM, Ralls PW et al: Ultrasound demonstration of portosystemic collaterals in cirrhosis and portal hypertension. Radiology 1982;142:459

253. Ferris EJ, Vittimberga FJ, Byrne JJ et al: The inferior vena cava after ligation and plication. Radiology 1967;89:1

254. Durrell CA, Vincent LM, Mittelstaedt CA: Gallbladder ultrasonography in clinical context. Semin Ultrasound CT MR 1984;5:315

255. Derchi LE, Biggi E, Rollandi GA et al: Sonographic staging of gastric carcinoma. AJR 1983;140:273

10

Spleen

Carol A. Mittelstaedt

On abdominal sonograms, the liver, spleen, gallbladder, pancreas, aorta, kidneys, and other abdominal structures are easily identified, and many abnormalities are diagnosed. As a rule, the only remark concerning the spleen is splenomegaly, otherwise, no statement is made.

In the past, the spleen was often ignored on conventional ultrasound because it was difficult to visualize. In the supine position, a normal-sized spleen lies high under the rib cage and posterior to the stomach and splenic flexure of the colon, which are strongly reflective structures. Using real-time ultrasound, this is no longer a problem.[1] In addition, ultrasound is a relative newcomer to the diagnostic armamentarium for evaluation of the spleen. Its potential, restrictions, and diagnostic capabilities have still not been fully ascertained. Some investigators have described the variability of ultrasonic patterns,[2-4] and have analyzed amplitude histograms of splenic texture or consistency.[5] Still, ultrasound can often be useful in evaluating disease processes of the spleen. Most abnormalities involving the spleen produce enlargement, which permits excellent sonographic visualization.

TECHNIQUE

Preparation

There is no special patient preparation prior to an ultrasound of the spleen.

Ultrasound Technique

The spleen can be scanned with the patient in various positions. If the spleen is quite large, it can be adequately evaluated with the patient supine by employing both longitudinal and transverse planes (Fig. 10-1). Although the normal-sized spleen can be visualized in the supine position, the minimally enlarged to normal-sized spleen may also be examined with the patient in the right-lateral decubitus or prone position[3] (Figs. 10-2 and 10-3). However, the spleen is easily visualized using a left posterolateral, lower intercostal approach in the supine position.[1] Both longitudinal and transverse scans are obtained during held inspiration. The right-lateral decubitus position (coronal view) is my preferred position for evaluating the spleen because in this position the spleen is closest to the near field of the transducer and the best detail of the splenic architecture is obtained (Fig. 10-2). Careful attention should be paid to the time-gain-compensation (TGC) and transducer characteristics because incorrect use of either can produce misleading artifacts.[6] The normal splenic echopattern should be homogeneous, with the internal echoes slightly less[6] or equal to the liver.[3,4]

Studies can be adequately done with real-time ultrasound. If the spleen is quite large and a comparison is necessary between the spleen and liver echopattern, then comparison views of the right and left upper quadrant (liver and spleen) may be obtained using the same transducer and machine setting.

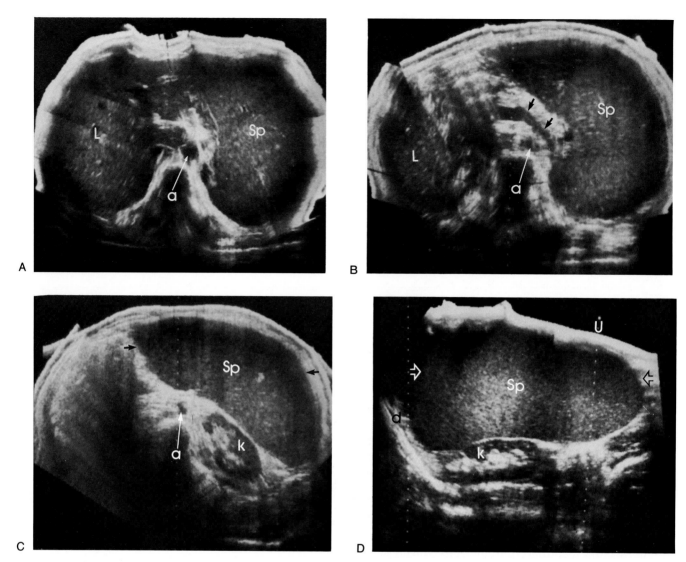

Fig. 10-1. Enlarged spleen, static scans. Supine transverse views at **(A)** 18 cm, **(B)** 10 cm, and **(C)** 2 cm above the umbilicus as well as **(D)** a longitudinal scan at 8 cm to the left of midline demonstrate a markedly enlarged spleen (*Sp*), with an isoechoic (same density as liver [*L*] parenchyma) echopattern in this patient with non-Hodgkin's lymphoma. To determine the splenic volumetric index (SI), the splenic width (black arrows) can be measured on Fig. C, with the anteroposterior dimension measured on Fig. A or Fig. B. The length (open arrows) can be measured on Fig. D. The values obtained are multiplied and the product is divided by 27. In this case, the SI is 156 with normal being 8 to 34. (*a*, aorta; solid black arrows, splenic vein; *k*, left kidney; *d*, diaphragm; *U*, level of the umbilicus.)

NORMAL ANATOMY

The spleen, the largest unit of the reticuloendothelial system, plays an important role in the defense mechanism of the body and is involved in pigment and lipid metabolism. With its architecture consisting of the white pulp (lymphoid tissue) and the intervening red pulp (red blood cells and reticulum cells), the spleen is normally

devoid of hematopoietic activity.[7] Rarely the primary site of disease, it is often affected by systemic disease processes.

The spleen, an intraperitoneal structure lying between the left hemidiaphragm and stomach, is related to the eighth through eleventh ribs. Its superior surface is in contact with the left hemidiaphragm; its medial surface is related to the stomach, tail of pancreas, left kidney,

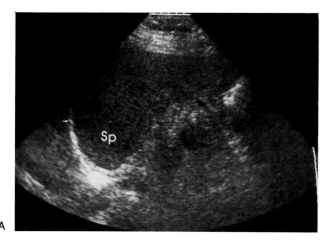
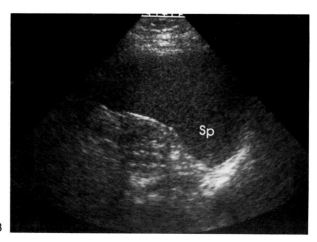

A

B

Fig. 10-2. Normal spleen. (**A**) Coronal sagittal and (**B**) transverse scans of a normal spleen (*Sp*). It has a uniform echopattern that cannot be compared with liver on the same scan, since with real-time both are not uniformly visualized. To compare the echodensity, separate scans of the liver and spleen must be performed using the same technique. (arrow, diaphragm.)

and splenic flexure of the colon (Fig. 10-4). The left hemidiaphragm is seen as a bright curvilinear echogenic structure that is close to the proximal superolateral surface of the spleen (Figs. 10-1D and 10-2A). The spleen is covered with peritoneum except for its hilum. It is held in position by the lienorenal, gastrosplenic, and phrenicocolic ligaments,[6] which are derived from layers of the peritoneum that form the greater and lesser sac. The spleen's close proximity to the left kidney, pancreas, and

gastrointestinal tract facilitates the extension of inflammatory processes.[6]

Splenic Size

Various studies have evaluated splenic size. One investigation has determined a splenic volumetric index (SVI)[8]; the breadth, thickness, and height are obtained

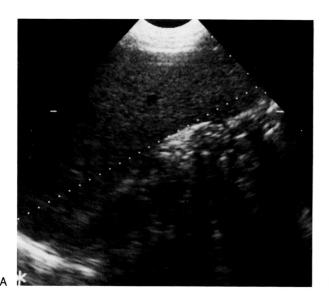
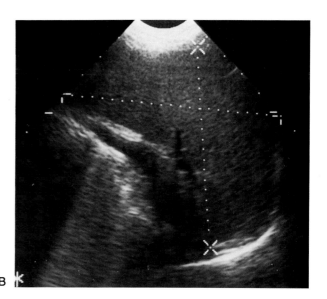

A

B

Fig. 10-3. Minimally enlarged spleen. (**A**) Sagittal and (**B**) transverse scans of a spleen that is in the upper limits of normal for size (length, 11.5 cm; transverse, 8.7 cm; and anteroposterior, 7.7 cm) with the patient in the supine position. The spleen appears uniform in echotexture. While the echopattern of the spleen cannot be compared with the liver on this image (since the liver is not visualized), it can be compared by viewing images of the liver taken without changing the machine settings.

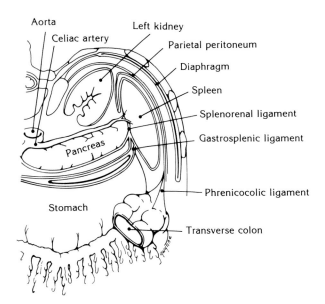

Fig. 10-4. Normal spleen. The spleen is related to the left hemidiaphragm superiorly, and to the stomach, pancreatic tail, and splenic flexure of the colon medially. It is covered with peritoneum except for its hilum and is held in position by the splenorenal, gastrosplenic, and phrenicocolic ligaments.

on a compound scan with each measurement taken at the largest point (Figs. 10-1 and 10-3). The breadth (width) and thickness (anteroposterior [AP]) may be measured on a transverse, supine scan at the level of the xyphoid in a normal to minimally enlarged spleen or at the widest portion in an enlarged spleen. On a longitudinal scan in the mid-axillary line in the normal to minimally enlarged spleen, the height (length) is measured (Fig. 10-3A). In the enlarged spleen, the longest length is obtained on a supine scan (Fig. 10-1D). The values obtained are multiplied by each other and the product is divided by 27 (the cube of the three values). The SVI was found to be 8 to 34 in 95 percent of normal cases.[8] There were no statistically significant differences related to age, sex, or morphology. From this study, it was believed that a distinction could be made between a normal and abnormal spleen on the basis of the SVI.

Another study has evaluated splenic size by using the following formula: $SI = a \times b$, where SI is splenic index, a is the transverse diameter in centimeters, and b is the vertical diameter in centimeters of the maximum cross-sectional image of the spleen.[9] The SI is graded as follows: grade 0, 0 to 30 cm²; grade I, 31 to 60 cm²; grade II, 61 to 90 cm²; grade III, 91 to 120 cm²; and grade IV, more than 120 cm².[9] The following weights correspond to the grades: grade 0, 0 to 120 g; grade I, 121 to 190 g;

grade II, 191 to 260 g; grade III, 261 to 330 g; and grade IV, greater than 330 g.[9] Grades 0 and I are not palpable, grade II may or may not be palpable, and grades III and IV are palpable. There is good correlation between spleen weights and SIs.[9]

Splenic size can also be estimated as a sectional area using the following formula: $S = 0.9 \times a \times b$, where S is sectional area in square centimeters, a is the maximum length (in centimeters) of the spleen across the splenic hilum, and b is the short length (in centimeters) from the hilus, perpendicular to a.[9]

Other authors have evaluated splenic size by taking two measurements with the patient in the right-lateral decubitus position.[10] The maximum length *(L)* is measured as a line joining the two organ poles and the spleen thickness *(D)* as the shortest distance between the apex of the spleen convexity and the hilus. A length up to 11 cm and a thickness of up to 5 cm are considered the upper limits of normal.[10] This group of investigators divided splenic size into three categories: (1) normal, up to 11 by 5 cm; (2) moderate splenomegaly, 11 cm by 5 cm to 20 cm by 8 cm; and (3) severe splenomegaly, over 20 cm by 8 cm.[10]

Normal splenic size in infants and children has also been evaluated[11] and is measured by obtaining a coronal view that includes the hilum, while the patient is breathing quietly. The length is obtained with the patient in a supine or slightly right-lateral decubitus position. Correlating with age, height, and weight, the greatest longitudinal distance between the dome of the spleen and the tip (splenic length) is measured. The following guidelines are proposed for the upper limit of normal splenic length based on one measurement: 3 months, 6 cm; 6 months, 6.5 cm; 12 months, 7 cm; 2 years, 8 cm; 4 years, 9 cm; 6 years, 9.5 cm; 8 years, 10 cm; 10 years, 11 cm; 12 years, 11.5 cm; 15 years or older, 12 cm for girls and 13 cm for boys.[11] These measurements can serve as a guide for selecting patients who require more quantitative estimations of splenic size.

Splenomegaly can be found in various disorders. The spleen can enlarge with reactive proliferation of lymphocytes or reticuloendothelial cells, with infiltration by lymphoma cells or other neoplastic cells or by lipid-laden macrophages, with extramedullary hematopoiesis, and with proliferation of phagocytic cells or vascular congestion. In one study, splenomegaly was found in 71.9 percent of patients with hepatitis and cirrhosis, in 79.2 percent of those with leukemia, in 73.1 percent of those with collagen disease, and in 68.8 percent of those with autoimmune diseases.[9] More than 50 percent of patients with chronic myelogenous leukemia have grade IV spleens.[9] Ultrasound can be most useful in estimating splenic size in cases of nonpalpable spleens.

Splenic Echopattern

Depending on patient position and machine control settings, the normal splenic echopattern can vary considerably. It may be weakly echogenic (hypoechoic), homogeneous, and transonic or strongly echogenic (hyperechoic), similar in echodensity to the liver. The gain and TGC controls are usually set to obtain adequate echoes within the liver when the patient is supine. The normal spleen appears to have the same relative echodensity as the liver in the supine position (Fig. 10-1).

To establish a standard technique for the spleen and other organs, a gray-scale phantom is needed. Without such a phantom the next best way, at this time, for establishing a standard technique is internal control within each patient. Amplitude histograms of splenic texture or consistency have been analyzed by some investigators[12] and the variability of gray-scale ultrasonic patterns has been reported.[2] It has been my experience in determining the echodensity of the spleen that the liver echodensity in the supine position serves as an adequate standard provided the liver is normal (i.e., no hepatocellular or metastatic disease). The splenic pattern is described as isoechoic if the spleen and liver have the same relative echodensity (Figs. 10-1 to 10-3), and hypoechoic if the echopattern within the spleen is relatively less echogenic than the liver. Focal lesions within the spleen are described as hypoechoic or hyperechoic depending on their relationship to the rest of the splenic echodensity. Perisplenic lesions are also described as hypoechoic or hyperechoic depending on their comparative echodensity to the spleen.

Normal Variant

One group of investigators has reported a "pseudo perisplenic" lesion, which was secondary to normal liver and spleen echogenic texture.[1] It is particularly noted in thin young women and children and represents a potential pitfall that can simulate a fluid collection superior and lateral to the spleen. This appearance actually represents an elongated left lobe of the liver that extends to the left side of the abdomen and presents posteriorly in the left subphrenic space as an echopoor crescent around the superior and lateral aspect of the spleen (Fig. 10-5).[1] The key to the identification is that the "perisplenic abnormality" is seen to slide over the spleen during shallow respiration.[1] It occurs predominantly in thin individuals, in whom visualization of the upper abdominal anatomy is not easy. In these thin patients, the liver stretches across the upper abdomen to the left upper quadrant since there is not enough anteroposterior depth to ac-

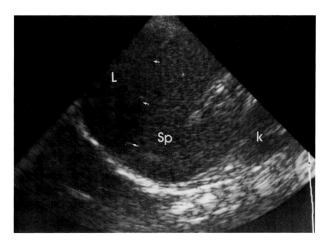

Fig. 10-5. Pseudo perisplenic lesion. Sagittal view through the left upper quadrant in a child that demonstrates a hypoechoic crescent area (representing left lobe of the liver [*L*]) anterosuperior to spleen (*Sp*). The liver was seen to move as a separate structure (arrows) from spleen during real-time examination. (*k*, left kidney.)

commodate its bulk entirely on the right side.[1] Even though the liver has been described as either isoechoic or more echogenic than the spleen, in this phenomenon the liver is less echogenic than the spleen.[1] Also, with this phenomenon, although the liver and spleen are imaged simultaneously at the same depth within the same field of view using the same gain and TGC curve, the difference in the echopattern cannot be explained.[1]

FOCAL DISEASE

Focal defects in the spleen may be single or multiple, and may be found in normal-sized or enlarged spleens. The major nontraumatic causes for focal splenic defects include tumors (benign and malignant), infarction, abscesses, and cysts. Detection may be incidental (e.g., unsuspected splenic defect demonstrated as part of a technetium sulfur colloid [TcSC] study of the liver), or may be encountered in the evaluation of clinically suspected splenic disease (e.g., splenic infarct or abscess).[13]

Ultrasound not only allows differentiation between solid and cystic lesions but also permits evaluation of adjacent abdominal structures. However, ultrasound examination of the spleen may be hampered by rib artifact or excessive bowel gas in the left upper quadrant. In addition, ultrasound is less sensitive for detection of focal abnormalities in patients without splenomegaly and, therefore, is usually not the primary screening procedure for possible focal splenic lesions.

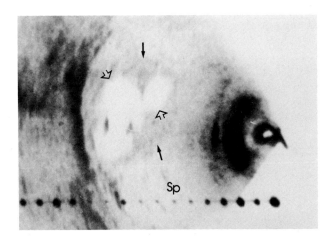

Fig. 10-6. Splenic hamartoma. Transverse scan, right-lateral decubitus position. A mass (arrows) is seen within the spleen that is more dense than the spleen (*Sp*). Note the cystic component (open arrows) within the mass. (From Brinkley and Lee,[14] with permission.)

Tumors of the Spleen

Benign Primary Neoplasms

Hamartomas, cavernous hemangiomas, and cystic lymphangiomas are the most common benign neoplasms involving the spleen.

Hamartomas. Typically, splenic hamartomas have both solid and cystic components, with the solid portion appearing hyperechoic on ultrasound[14] (Fig. 10-6). These lesions are usually discovered as incidental findings at autopsy because patients are usually asymptomatic. The importance in recognizing these benign neoplasms rests in differentiating them from other lesions. Splenic hamartomas, which may be solitary or multiple and are well defined but not encapsulated,[14] are composed either of lymphoid tissue or a combination of sinuses and structures that are equivalent to the pulp cords of normal splenic tissue.

Hemangiomas. Hemangiomas are the most common primary neoplasm of the spleen.[15] The overall incidence is 1 in 600 cases or 0.3 to 14 percent based on autopsy series occurring in adults 30 to 50 years of age.[15,16] Pathologically, this lesion is defined by a proliferation of vascular channels of variable size, capillary to cavernous, lined by a single layer of endothelium and filled with erythrocytes.[15] There may be calcification in either a central (mottled) or peripheral (curvilinear) pattern.[15]

Most splenic hemangiomas are small and usually the patients are asymptomatic,[16] which may be attributable to the very slow growth of the lesion.[15] Splenic hemangiomas, however, can become large. When patients are symptomatic, the symptoms are related to the size of the spleen, which has compressed neighboring organs, ane-

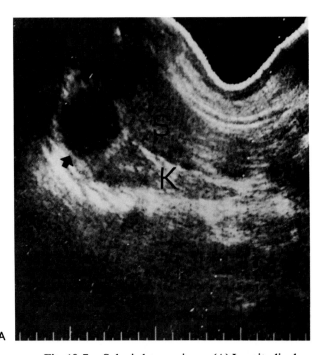
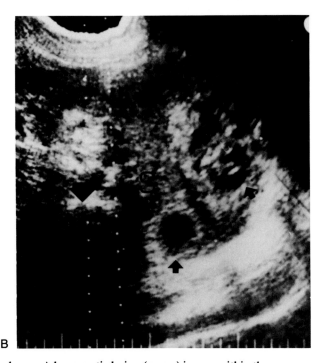

Fig. 10-7. Splenic hemangioma. **(A)** Longitudinal coronal scan. A large cystic lesion (arrow) is seen within the spleen (*S*) with acoustic enhancement. (*K*, kidney.) **(B)** Transverse scan demonstrating a mixed lesion in the spleen (*S*). Hypoechoic areas are seen (arrows). (Large arrow, spine.) *(Figure continues.)*

mia, or low-grade infection with fever and malaise.[16] Splenic rupture with peritoneal symptoms can occur in up to 25 percent of cavernous hemangiomas. When these lesions are multiple, they may be part of a generalized angiomatosis that involves multiple organs, especially the liver and the skeleton.[15]

A splenic hemangioma has been typically described as a large inhomogeneously echogenic mass on ultrasound with multiple small hypoechoic areas[17] (Figs. 10-7 to 10-10). Two distinctive sonographic patterns have been described: (1) a predominantly echogenic mass and (2) a complex mass.[15] Solid hemangiomas correspond to the echogenic mass (Figs. 10-7C, 10-8, and 10-9A). Tumors that contain well-defined cystic chambers filled with fluid (ranging from hemorrhagic to serous) and debris correspond to the complex pattern, which demonstrates multiple cystic areas (some anechoic and others containing echoic debris) within a splenic mass[15] (Figs. 10-7B, 10-9B, and 10-10). A mixed ultrasound appearance can be accounted for by infarction with coagulated blood or fibrin in the cavities.

A characteristic pattern on color Doppler has been reported in hemangiomas with and without compres-

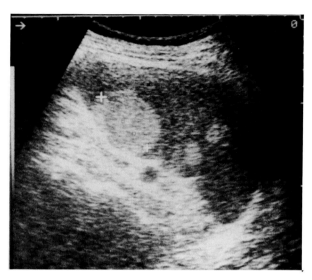

Fig. 10-8. Splenic hemangioma. Sonogram in an asymptomatic patient shows multiple, sharply marginated, hyperechoic lesions. Contrast-enhanced CT confirmed splenic hemangioma. (From Goerg et al,[32] with permission.)

sion.[18] Color echoes demonstrated within the lesion disappeared during compression and reappeared immediately after. This phenomenon suggests that the tumor is vascular and soft. Using this technique, it may be possible to differentiate splenic vascular tumors from infarction and to distinguish these hemangiomas from other splenic masses.[18]

The ultrasound features described above are not specific, and therefore, lesions such as hydatid cyst, abscess, dermoid, or metastasis cannot be excluded.[16] Since the sonographic pattern associated with splenic hemangiomas may vary, the differential diagnosis for these lesions must include both solid and cystic splenic masses.[15] The solid lesions include hamartoma, metastasis, infarct, lymphoma, angiosarcoma, and rare malignant mesodermal neoplasms (fibrosarcoma, carcinosarcoma, and malignant fibrous histiocytoma).[15] The cystic lesions include abscess, cyst, lymphangioma, lymphoma, metastasis, and hematoma. As a rule, surgery is not indicated unless rupture is likely, the hemangioma is very large, or in cases associated with coagulopathy.[15]

Lymphangioma. Cystic lymphangiomatosis, a benign malformation of the lymphatics composed of endothelium-lined cystic spaces, appears as a mass with extensive cystic replacement of the splenic parenchyma[3,4,19-21] (Fig. 10-11). Now considered a type of congenital anomaly,[21] lymphangiomatosis affects predominately the somatic soft tissue and is found in the neck, axilla, mediastinum, retroperitoneum, and soft

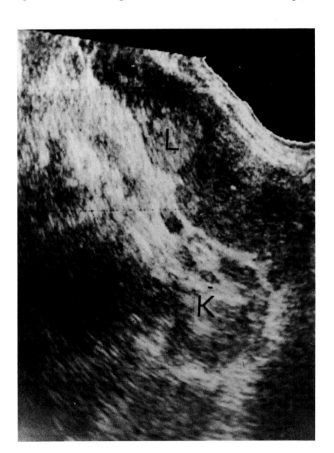

Fig. 10-7 (Continued). **(C)** Transverse scan of the spleen (S) with a well-circumscribed echodense lesion (L). (K, kidney.) (From Manor et al,[16] with permission.)

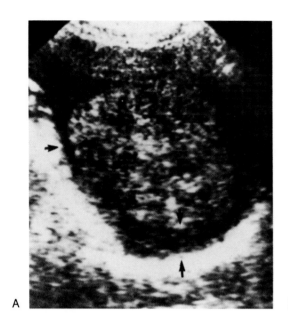
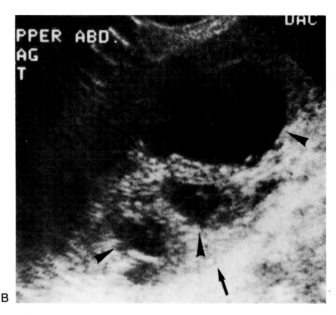

A   B

Fig. 10-9.   Splenic hemangioma. **(A)** Large solid mass. Sonogram reveals a large, solid, echogenic mass occupying most of the spleen at this location. There is a surrounding rim of hypoechogenic splenic tissue (arrows). **(B)** Complex mass (with both cystic and solid components). Longitudinal sonogram in another patient shows a complex mass within the spleen. Multiple, predominantly anechoic, cystic areas (arrowheads) are noted, surrounded by echodense solid hemangioma (arrows). (From Ros et al,[15] with permission.)

tissues of the extremities.[19] The process may diffusely involve multiple organ systems or may be confined to a solitary organ such as liver, spleen, kidney, or colon. Splenic involvement is rare.[19]

Histologically, lymphangiomatosis is characterized by a lesion that consists of a honeycomb of large and small thin-walled cysts containing a clear fluid resembling lymph and separated by bands of fibrous tissue. The multicystic appearance on ultrasound is fairly characteristic with multiseptate cystic spaces present within the spleen (Fig. 10-11). Color Doppler can provide additional information about intratumoral vascularization

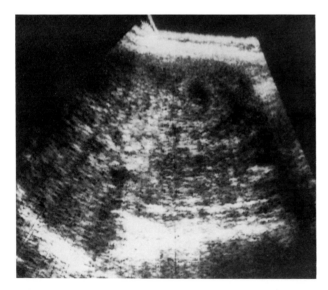

Fig. 10-10.   Splenic hemangioma. Coronal scan of a cavernous hemangioma. The enlarged spleen contains areas of increased echoes and a few small hypoechoic areas. (From Solbiati et al,[17] with permission.)

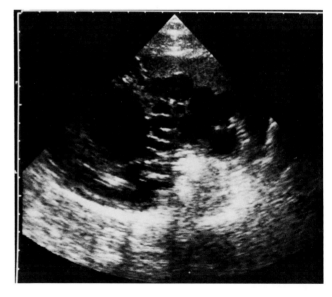

Fig. 10-11.   Splenic lymphangioma. Sonography of the spleen shows a group of multiple cysts with thin septa (left intercostal scan). (From Tsurui et al,[21] with permission.)

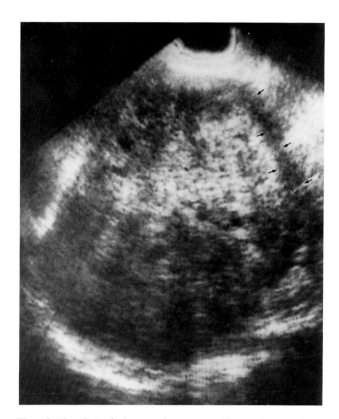

Fig. 10-12. Splenic hemangiosarcoma. Coronal scan with a large, inhomogeneous, mainly echogenic spleen with a pattern similar to Figure 10-10. A rim of normal splenic tissue (arrows) is seen in the lower pole. (From Solbiati et al,[17] with permission.)

and can clearly define many fine vessels, indicative of the intrasplenic arteries and veins running along the septa.[21]

Malignant Primary Neoplasm

Hemangiosarcoma, a rare malignant neoplasm arising from the vascular endothelium of the spleen, predominately affects patients between the ages of 50 and 59 years.[22] Chemicals such as polyvinyl chloride, thorium, and arsenic are known to induce angiosarcoma of the liver but they have not been linked with similar tumors of the spleen.[22] Patients with these lesions may have nonspecific signs and symptoms; about 70 percent of patients may demonstrate anemia, possibly hemolytic in nature, secondary to damaging of red blood cells as they traverse irregular vascular channels in the spleen.[22] Pathologically, these lesions arise from sinus epithelium and may represent either degeneration of hemangiomas or de novo tumors.[22] Approximately 90 percent of primary splenic angiosarcomas metastasize.[22] There is a poor survival rate associated with these lesions; a 20 percent 6-month survival has been reported.[22] Patients who undergo a splenectomy prior to rupture appear to have a prolonged survival.[22]

Findings with ultrasound have been scantily reported.[17,22] These lesions may, however, look similar to cavernous hemangiomas on ultrasound with a mixed to cystic pattern (Figs. 10-12 and 10-13). In one reported case[17] the lesion appeared as a large mass with a nonhomogeneous, mainly hyperechoic pattern; it was similar to that observed with hemangiomas, except for the lack of hypoechoic areas.

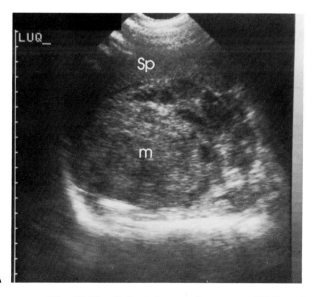

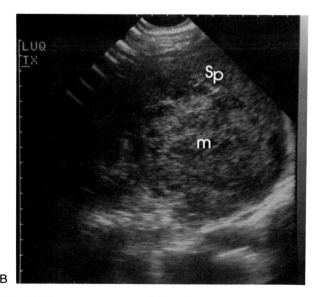

A   B

Fig. 10-13. Splenic hemangiosarcoma. **(A)** Longitudinal and **(B)** transverse scans of the spleen (*Sp*) demonstrating a poorly defined hyperechoic mass (*m*). The mass is inhomogeneously echogenic. (Courtesy of Jerome J. Cunningham, M.D., Department of Radiology, Ohio State University, Columbus, OH.)

Lymphoma

The spleen is commonly involved in lymphoma; in 32 percent of patients with non-Hodgkin's lymphoma[23] and in 39 percent of patients with Hodgkin's disease,[24] the spleen was involved at initial presentation. In one series, 4 of 12 patients with Hodgkin's disease and 9 of 12 patients with histiocytic lymphoma had discrete masses in the spleen, while such focal "tumorous" involvement was not found in any of 24 other cases of non-Hodgkin's lymphoma.[25] One recent group of investigators evaluated patients with splenic involvement and malignant lymphoma in which 75 percent exhibited splenomegaly while 23 percent did not.[10] Hodgkin's lymphoma is associated with both focal and diffuse splenic disease. All non-Hodgkin's lymphoma cases with high-grade malignancy demonstrate focal lesions that were larger than 3 cm in diameter. In non-Hodgkin's lymphoma cases with low-grade malignancy, both focal and diffuse disease was detected and the lesions were less than 3 cm.[10]

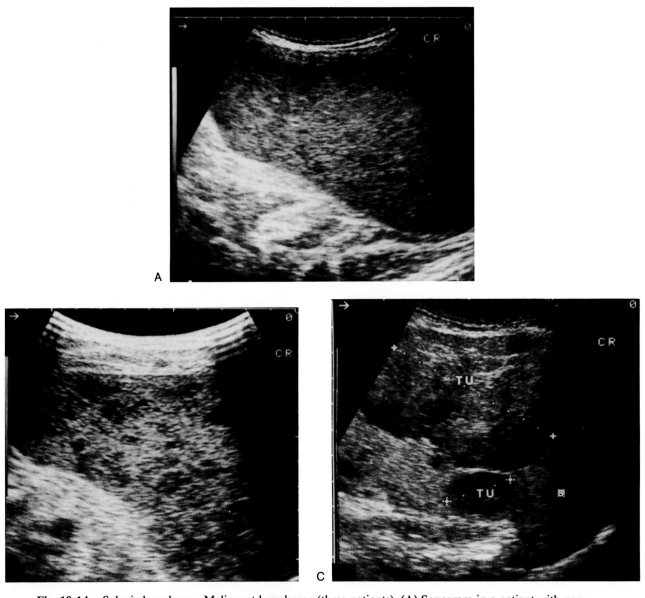

Fig. 10-14. Splenic lymphoma. Malignant lymphoma (three patients). **(A)** Sonogram in a patient with non-Hodgkin's lymphoma of low-grade malignancy shows diffuse inhomogeneity of spleen with hypoechoic lesions smaller than 1 cm in diameter. **(B)** Sonogram in a patient with Hodgkin's disease shows small, focal, nodular, hypoechoic lesions larger than 1 cm in diameter. **(C)** Sonogram in a patient with non-Hodgkin's lymphoma of high-grade malignancy shows large, focal, nodular, hypoechoic lesions (*TU*). (*S*, spleen.) (From Goerg et al,[32] with permission.)

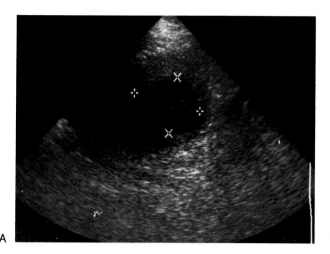
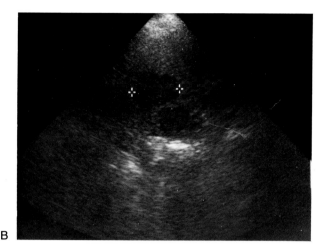

Fig. 10-15. Non-Hodgkin's lymphoma. **(A)** Sagittal and **(B)** transverse scans of the spleen demonstrate multiple focal hypoechoic lesions (calipers) greater than 3 cm in size.

Unfortunately, detection of splenic lymphoma is quite difficult. A sensitivity of 22 percent has been reported for detection of lymphomatous involvement of the spleen with either TcSC or contrast-enhanced computed tomography (CT).[26] Previous studies utilizing TcSC scanning were also discouraging, with only 10 percent sensitivity.[27] Similarly disappointing was gallium citrate imaging with only 41 percent of splenic sites of lymphoma detected in one large series of patients with both Hodgkin's disease and non-Hodgkin's lymphoma,[28] and 26 percent sensitivity for detection of splenic sites in a series of patients with non-Hodgkin's lymphoma.[29] Nonenhanced CT studies detected lymphomatous involvement of the spleen in only 5 of 11 proven cases (45 percent).[30] There has been a recent report of similar sensitivity results for contrast-enhanced CT examinations: 45 percent for non-Hodgkin's lymphoma and 61 percent for Hodgkin's disease of the spleen.[31]

Although focal splenic lesions in lymphoma are typically hypoechoic at ultrasound[3,4,20] (Figs. 10-14 to 10-16), focal echogenic areas have also been described[17] (Fig. 10-17). Recent reports described all lesions associated with lymphatic malignant tumors to be hypoechoic; therefore the hyperechoic pattern unlikely.[10,32] Several splenic patterns associated with lymphoma are described: (1) diffuse infiltration (multiple small nodules covering the entire spleen) characteristic of Hodgkin's lymphoma and non-Hodgkin's lymphoma of low-grade malignancy; (2) small nodular foci of medium size (less than 3 cm) characteristic of low-grade malignant lymphomas; (3) larger foci of more than 3 cm characteristic of lymphomas of high-grade malignancy; (4) non-Hodgkin's lymphoma of high-grade malignancy with sharply

defined focal lesions; (5) Hodgkin's lymphoma associated with diffuse and focal lesions; and (6) all patients with Hodgkin's lymphoma and non-Hodgkin's lymphoma with splenic lesions by ultrasound have abdominal lymphoma involvement. In 33 percent of patients with malignant lymphoma in one series, diffuse splenic involvement with hypoechogenic lesions smaller than 1 cm in diameter was found.[32]

One investigator claimed a 78 percent sensitivity for ultrasound in the detection of splenic lymphoma;

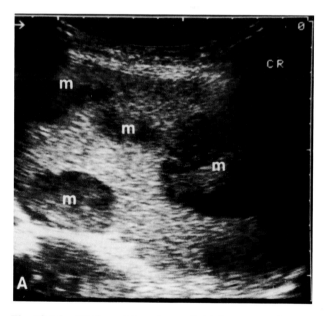

Fig. 10-16. Malignant lymphoma. Initial sonogram in a patient with high-grade non-Hodgkin's lymphoma shows large, rounded, hypoechoic lesions (*m*). (From Goerg et al,[32] with permission.)

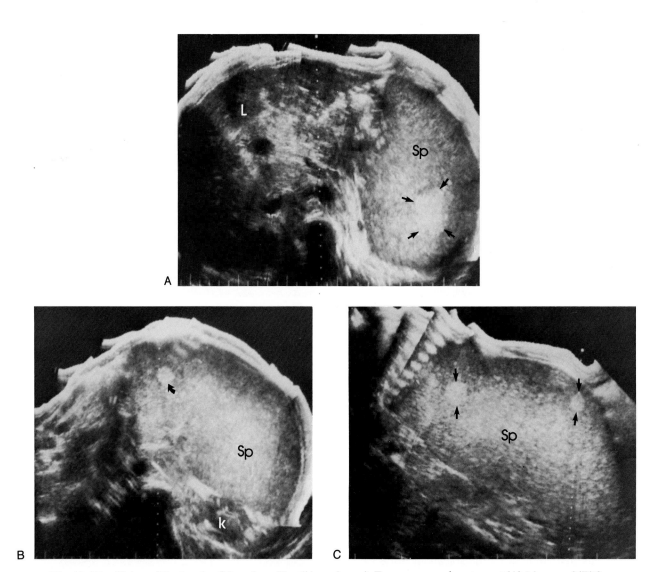

Fig. 10-17. Hairy cell leukemia of the spleen (B-cell lymphoma). Transverse supine scans at **(A)** 14 cm and **(B)** 2 cm above the umbilicus and **(C)** a longitudinal scan in the left midaxillary line demonstrate multiple focal echogenic areas (arrows) within an enlarged and echodense spleen (*Sp*). (*L*, liver; *k*, left kidney.)

splenomegaly and low-level echoes were the criteria employed, not focal abnormality.[33] Since there is a low incidence of focal splenic lesions, hypoechoic splenic lesions in a patient with lymphoma may be regarded as neoplastic with a high degree of certainty.[10] This group of investigators did not find splenic size a reliable criterion for evidence of disease.[10]

Metastases

Splenic metastases are generally the result of hematogenous spread.[34,35] In a postmortem study, the spleen was the 10th most common site of metastatic disease, with the most common sites of origin being breast (21 percent), lung (18 percent), ovary (8 percent), stomach (7

percent), melanoma (6 percent), and prostate (6 percent). Frequency of splenic involvement, expressed as the percentage of each primary tumor that had splenic metastases, was melanoma (34 percent), breast (12 percent), ovary (12 percent), lung (9 percent), prostate (6 percent), and stomach (4 percent).[34]

In most instances, splenic metastases are associated with metastatic involvement of other organs,[35] and are usually associated with widely disseminated malignancy.[36] In an autopsy series, up to 10 percent of patients with cancer may be found to have splenic metastases.[36] Metastases confined to the spleen are extremely rare. Despite the presumed rarity of isolated splenic metastases, one group found liver metastases to be absent in 70 percent of cases of splenic metastases.[37] Frequently these

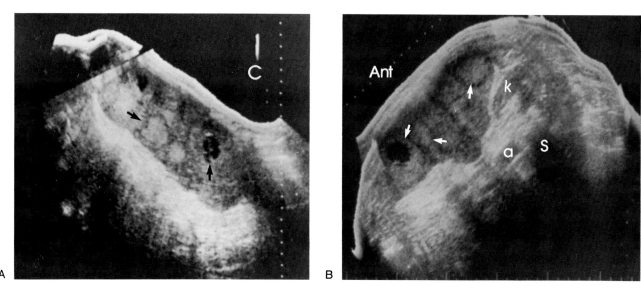

Fig. 10-18. Splenic metastases. Carcinoma of the lung. **(A)** Longitudinal and **(B)** transverse scans in the right-lateral decubitus position demonstrate multiple hyperechoic lesions (arrows) within the spleen. Some have a bull's-eye pattern and some have necrotic (hypoechoic) centers. (*C*, level of the iliac crest; *a*, aorta; *S*, spine; *k*, kidney; *Ant,* anterior.) (From Mittelstaedt,[3] with permission.)

metastatic deposits are only microscopically evident (32 percent of cases in one series).[34] As a result, splenic metastases are only rarely symptomatic, though splenic infarction with associated perisplenitis has been attributed to tumor emboli.[38]

Ultrasound may delineate focal metastases as either hypoechoic, mixed, hyperechoic, or target lesions[3,4,20,36,39-41] (Figs. 10-18 and 10-19). One series[32] reported that splenic metastases were predominantly hypoechoic. The ultrasound pattern associated with

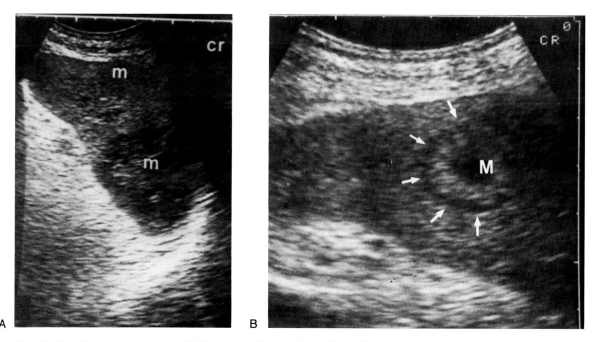

Fig. 10-19. Splenic metastases. **(A)** Sonogram in a patient with malignant melanoma shows multiple hypoechoic metastases (*m*) of the spleen, confirmed at autopsy. **(B)** Sonogram in a patient with colonic carcinoma with diffuse liver metastasis shows splenic lesions (*M*) with a hypoechoic rim (arrows) and central liquefied area. Autopsy revealed splenic metastasis. (From Goerg et al,[32] with permission.)

these lesions is variable; individual tumors do not give rise to a particular type of pattern.[36] Melanoma deposits appear as hypoechoic lesions, but of higher echo amplitude than lymphoma; some are echodense.[17] There has been one case report of splenic plasmacytoma in which the lesion appeared hyperechoic.[41] Metastatic splenic lesions may be solitary (31.5 percent) or multiple (60 percent) nodular lesions, or diffuse infiltrating lesions (8.5 percent).[36] While focal or diffuse splenic lesions may not be specific for a tumor type, they may be presumed to be metastatic in a patient with a known primary tumor.[36] Fine needle biopsy of the splenic lesion may be performed if further evaluation is needed. Splenic metastases seen at ultrasound tend to indicate a poor prognosis and suggest disseminated malignancy, which will probably be beyond treatment.[36]

Correlative Imaging

All the standard noninvasive imaging modalities (TcSC, ultrasound, and CT) have been shown to be effective in the detection of focal splenic lesions.[13] TcSC, though quite sensitive in the detection of focal defects, is nonspecific and only evaluates the spleen and liver. Because CT requires intravenous contrast injection for optimal detection of focal disease, the utility of this modality may be limited in patients with contrast allergy.

Systematic comparisons of the relative effectiveness of imaging modalities (TcSC, ultrasound, and CT) for the detection of focal splenic lesions are lacking. However, comparative imaging studies evaluating suspected liver metastases may serve as a basis for modality selection for splenic imaging.[42-45] Most studies have shown TcSC and CT to have similar sensitivities for the detection of hepatic lesions but with CT having a greater specificity.[42-45] In the one series including ultrasound as well as TcSC and CT, ultrasound had the lowest sensitivity.[44]

Infarction

Infarction of the spleen occurs owing to septic emboli and local thromboses in patients with pancreatitis, subacute bacterial endocarditis, leukemia, lymphomatous disorders, myeloproliferative disorders, sickle cell anemia, hemolytic anemia, sarcoidosis, or polyarteritis nodosa.[17,46,47] Clinical symptoms may include the sudden onset of pain in the upper left abdomen, which is occasionally associated with a painful restriction of the respiratory excursion, local pain on palpation, or diffuse abdominal pain, the infarction may be asymptomatic.

The sonographic appearances of infarcts vary widely according to the time since onset.[17,47] The age of the infarct, however, does not necessarily correlate with the ultrasound pattern.[47] The following patterns have been

seen with infarcts: predominantly wedge-shaped or round, irregularly delineated or smooth, hypoechoic, and anechoic[47,48] (Figs. 10-20 and 10-21). A fresh hemorrhagic infarct appears hypoechoic (Figs. 10-20A & C and 10-21), while a healed infarction, because of scar tissue formation, appears as echogenic wedge-shaped lesions with their base toward the subcapsular surface on the spleen[17] (Fig. 10-20B). A wedge-shaped hypoechoic or hyperechoic lesion with its apex toward the splenic hilum and its base located in the periphery is more immediately recognizable as an infarct.[32,48] In the earlier stages, a presumptive diagnosis is possible since the detection of changes (in echogenicity and/or in size) over a period of time strongly suggests an infarct.[48]

These various patterns appear to be related to edema, bleeding, necrosis, and inflammation.[47] Edema, inflammation, and necrosis can account for the poor or absent echogenicity of early infarcts in the acute stage.[48] Fibrosis and shrinkage, which occur later, give rise to the gradually increasing echogenicity and reduction in size of the infarcted area, eventually progressing to the dense hyperechoic appearance of the old healed infarct.[48]

Ultrasound, which has been used to evaluate the spleen for infarcts following splenic embolization,[49] is able to detect wedge-shaped defects with well-demarcated borders. While both abscesses and infarcts are hypoechoic, these lesions could be distinguished. Abscesses as a rule were poorly defined, irregular with variable shape, and sometimes had thick and/or shaggy walls. Infarcts were seen as wedge-shaped hypoechoic lesions with well-demarcated borders. With follow-up, these investigators found that the infarcts became smaller and increasingly echogenic but retained their triangular shape[49] (Fig. 10-20B).

When examining patients 24 hours after therapeutic embolization of the splenic artery for treatment of portal hypertension, splenic infarcts appear as wedge-shaped, hypoechoic, and well-defined lesions on ultrasound.[47] Without complications, this is the typical ultrasound pattern for acute infarction. Months later, scar states of infarction may be seen as inhomogeneity of splenic texture.

No correlation has been found for predicting complications between the size of the spleen, and the number, the configuration, or the extent of the infarct.[47] The following are predictors for patients requiring surgical intervention: increasing subcapsular hemorrhage, extravasation of blood into the peritoneal cavity, and flow phenomena in the area of infarction as seen with pulsed Doppler.[47] Histologic examination reveals superinfection of the infarct when arterial signals are demonstrated within the infarction area with Doppler. Splenectomy should be reserved for those patients in whom there are clear ultrasound signs of life-threatening splenic rupture.[47] Even though splenic infarctions tend to self-heal,

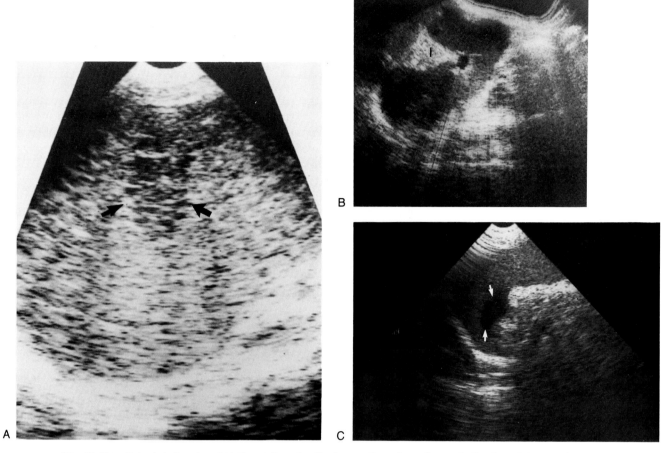

Fig. 10-20. Splenic infarction. **(A)** Case 1. Longitudinal scan of a patient after embolization of the splenic artery. A wedge-shaped hypoechoic area (arrows) is seen. (From Weingarten et al,[49] with permission.) **(B)** Case 2. Longitudinal scan with a triangular, highly echogenic area (*I*) due to a scar seen. (From Solbiati et al,[17] with permission.) **(C)** Case 3. Longitudinal supine view demonstrating a hypoechoic area (arrows), which appears round on transverse scan and somewhat triangular on longitudinal view.

short-term follow-up with ultrasound is recommended for early recognition of these possible complications.[47]

Acute Splenic Sequestration Crisis

Acute splenic sequestration crisis (ASSC), a rare complication in adults with sickle cell disease, is diagnosed by evidence of sudden splenic enlargement, a rapid fall in hematocrit, and evidence of marrow activity such as a reticulocyte count greater than or equal to steady-state values.[50] This complication accounts for almost 50 percent of deaths in children under 2 years of age with sickle cell disease.[50] Past the age of 8 years, ASSC is rare owing to progressive splenic fibrosis. In adults, the rarity of ASSC may be due to a relatively low susceptibility or to underdiagnosis, particularly of minor episodes.[50] Investigators report that ultrasound shows patency of the splenic vein and multiple hypoechoic lesions on the periphery of an enlarged spleen that is of low attenuation

on CT[50] (similar to Fig. 10-22). These findings may be secondary to subacute hemorrhage.

Initially, the treatment of ASSC is transfusion; the spleen responds rapidly, returning to baseline size. Splenectomy is not performed in adults unless there are recurrent episodes or red blood cell alloantibodies that might hamper transfusion.[50]

Partial Splenic Embolization

A relatively new technique, partial splenic embolization with antibiotic prophylaxis is increasingly utilized as a method of treatment for hypersplenism.[51] Following surgical splenectomy, there is an increased incidence of severe sepsis in patients undergoing splenectomy because of trauma (i.e., 1 to 2 percent, 50 times higher than the general population). The incidence is even higher in those undergoing a splenectomy for idiopathic thrombocytopenic purpura, Hodgkin's disease, acquired he-

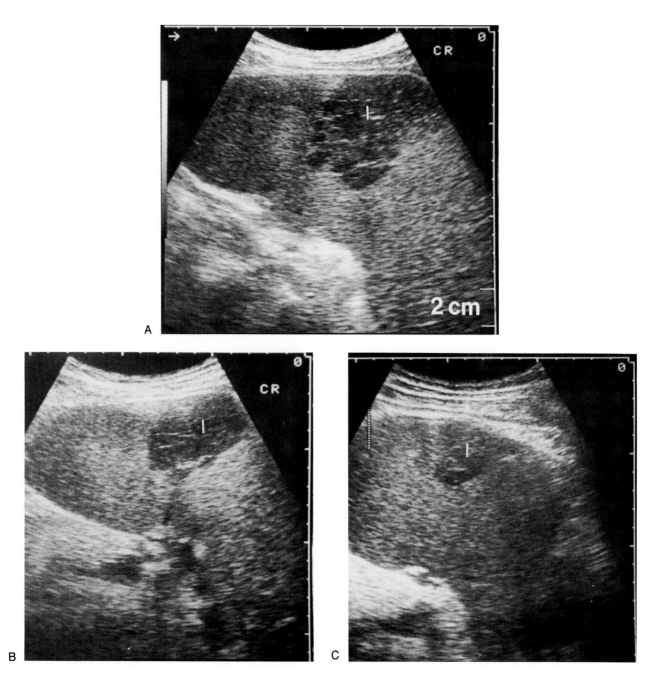

Fig. 10-21. Splenic infarction. Longitudinal scans of a patient with chronic myeloid leukemia, splenomegaly, and follow-up observation of acute splenic infarct (*I*). **(A)** Sonogram at diagnosis. **(B)** Follow-up sonogram 3 weeks later. **(C)** Third examination 7 weeks after primary diagnosis. The hypoechoic infarct became smaller but retained the triangular shape. (From Goerg and Schwerk,[47] with permission.)

molytic anemia, or other hematologic disorders. The highest incidence is in children undergoing splenectomy for blood dyscrasias.

Ultrasound and CT can be used after embolization for identification of viable and infarcted splenic tissue after partial splenic embolization. Ultrasound may demonstrate hypoechoic areas characteristic of infarcted areas and tiny, linear echoes scattered throughout the spleen

that are typical of postinfarction intravascular gas[51] (Fig. 10-23). The intravascular gas may be seen within infarcted tissue even without infection. The linear echoes disappear within a few months when the spleen typically becomes smaller and more homogeneously echogenic.

It is still to be proven whether the normal immune function of the spleen can be preserved by partial splenic embolization.[51] It is believed that postsplenectomy, 30

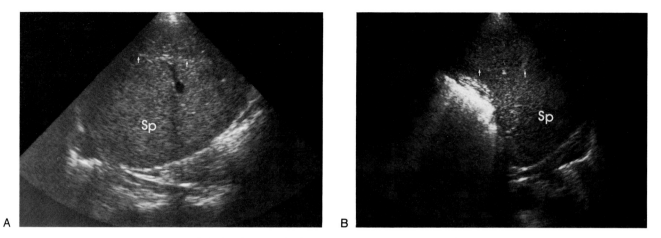

Fig. 10-22. Peripheral splenic infarction. **(A)** Sagittal and **(B)** transverse scans of the spleen (*Sp*) demonstrate a subtle relative hypoechoic area anteriorly (arrows) containing fine echogenic foci. The area on CT scan was lucent and represented a large splenic infarction.

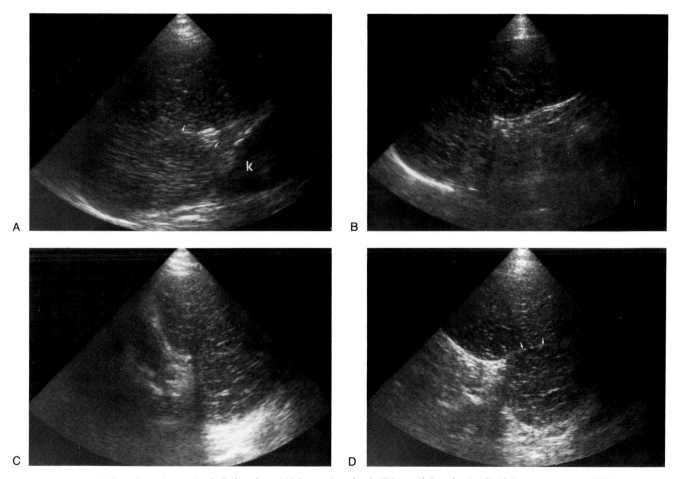

Fig. 10-23. Complete splenic infarction. **(A)** Lateral sagittal, **(B)** medial sagittal, **(C)** high transverse, and **(D)** lower transverse scans demonstrate a relatively hypoechoic spleen with multiple fine linear echogenic areas. At splenectomy, the spleen was found to be totally necrotic with the fine dense areas representing fibrous trabeculation. The spleen was enlarged (18 cm in length) with a lobular configuration more laterally in Fig. A and inferiorly in Fig. D in the region of the splenic hilum (arrows). (*k*, kidney.)

to 50 percent of the normal functioning splenic parenchyma must remain functioning to prevent the high incidence of sepsis seen in all age groups, particularly in children under the age of 5 years. Longer follow-up of larger numbers of patients undergoing partial splenic embolization will be needed before it is known whether this procedure does lower or prevent the occurrence of this disastrous syndrome, postsplenectomy sepsis.[51]

Abscess

Bacterial

Splenic abscesses are relatively uncommon; an incidence of only 0.14 to 0.22 percent was reported in a large autopsy series.[6,52,53] The infrequency of splenic abscess is probably related to the phagocytic activity of its efficient reticuloendothelial system and leukocytes. This effective defense system may be breached in several ways, such as overwhelming hematogenous seeding from bacterial endocarditis, septicemia, depressed immunologic states, or intravenous drug abuse.[52-55] In 75 percent of cases there is hematogenous spread from distant foci.[6] Infective endocarditis is the most common single source of splenic abscesses and is seen in up to 40 percent of cases.[56] *Streptococcus* is the most common etiologic organism, followed by *Staphylococcus, Salmonella,* and *Escherichia coli.*[6,53] Nidus formation from underlying splenic damage (traumatic hematoma or infarction in sickle cell disease, leukemia, other hemaglobinopathies, or other conditions) may also cause abscess.[52-56] In 15 percent of cases, there is an association with a history of trauma.[6] Invasion by an extrinsic process (perinephric or subphrenic abscess, perforated gastric or colonic lesions, or pancreatic abscess) may occur.[52-56] Direct extension of inflammatory processes from adjacent organs occurs in 10 percent of cases.[6]

The high mortality associated with delay in diagnosis of splenic abscess emphasizes the need for prompt detection and therapy.[6,55-58] Despite antibiotic therapy, the mortality is high.[56] The overall mortality for splenic abscess is 41 percent.[6] TcSC will show a splenic abscess as a nonspecific focal defect. Gallium scanning may add specificity by showing a rim of increased activity around the splenic lesion, but this approach may delay diagnosis by 48 hours.[57,59]

Patients with splenic abscesses may present with various symptoms, making diagnosis difficult, and clinical findings may be subtle. In one series, 95 percent of the patients had fever while 42 percent had left upper quadrant tenderness.[56] One-third of the patients had an elevated left hemidiaphragm or pleural effusion.[56] Fever and tachycardia (90 percent), abdominal pain (60 percent), left chest pain, and left shoulder and flank pain are

the most common symptoms.[6,53] Splenomegaly (40 percent), a vague mass, and/or left upper quadrant tenderness may also be found.[6,53]

Ultrasound has proven quite effective in the detection of splenic abscess. These lesions generally exhibit mixed echopatterns that are predominately hypoechoic but often contain hyperechoic foci that represent debris or gas[6,53,55,58,60] (Figs. 10-24 and 10-25). Some authors report a pattern varying from an anechoic, mainly fluid pattern with a few nonreverberatory echoes, to a complex solid pattern.[32] Some investigators describe anechoic lesions.[53,56] The definition of these lesions is usually poor and they may have thick and/or shaggy walls.[49,53,58] As a rule, there is no increased through transmission associated with these lesions,[58] although some investigators describe a variable amount of associated acoustic enhancement.[6] Gas within an abscess appears as scattered hyperechoic areas with acoustic shadowing or reverberation artifact[6,56] (Fig. 10-25). In contrast to the echofree acoustic shadow caused by foci of calcium, the shadow caused by gas contains ill-defined low-level echoes and has poorly defined margins.[6]

The ultrasound appearance of abscess is not entirely characteristic and as such, the lesion cannot be totally differentiated from infarct, neoplasm, or hematoma on the basis of the ultrasound pattern alone.[6,56] Ultrasound also has the advantage of delineating abnormalities in the adjacent left subphrenic and perinephric spaces, and has been reported to have an accuracy of 96 percent in detecting abscesses and to be 99 percent accurate in correctly excluding abscesses.[6] The accuracy of CT varies from 75 to 100 percent, while that of gallium scanning varies from 60 to 82 percent with a higher false-positive rate.[6] Ultrasound is the method of choice for the early diagnosis of patients with suspected splenic abscess and represents a good screen for patients with fever and nonspecific abdominal symptoms.[6] To establish the diagnosis, an ultrasound-guided percutaneous fine needle aspiration is recommended by some authors.[32]

Computed tomography shows splenic abscesses as focal areas of decreased attenuation, best demonstrated when intravenous contrast is used to enhance the normal splenic parenchyma.[60-62] An abscess may appear loculated or may contain fluid layers with different attenuation.[61,62] Owing to its sensitivity for detection of air, CT provides a more specific diagnosis in cases of air-containing abscesses.[60,62]

Fungal

Fungal splenic abscesses, including candidal ones, consist of pus, necrotic tissue, and fungus surrounded by layers of histiocytes, chronic inflammatory cells, and fibrosis.[63] They occur almost exclusively in immunosup-

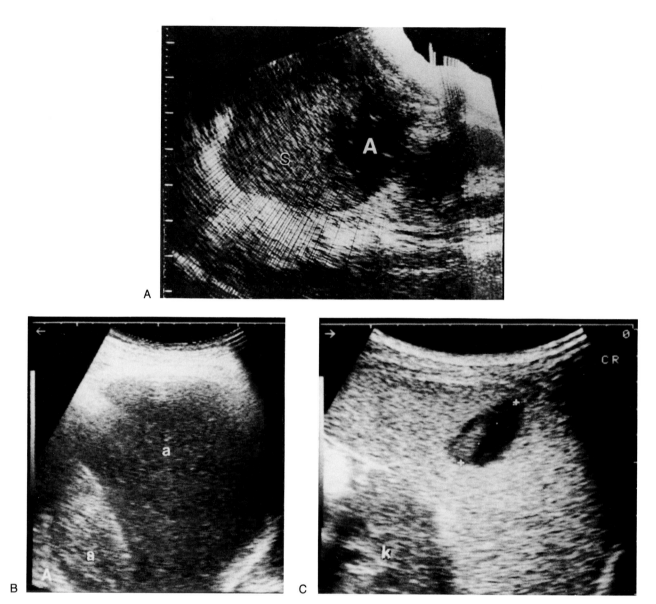

Fig. 10-24. Splenic abscess. **(A)** Coronal scan with a large anechoic mass (*A*) in the inferior aspect of the spleen (*S*). The mass contains scattered echoes due to debris. (From Pawar et al,[60] with permission.) **(B)** Sonogram in a patient with severe septic disease of unknown origin shows a large hypoechoic splenic lesion. Sonographically guided percutaneous puncture confirmed the presence of an abscess (*a*). (*S*, spleen.) **(C)** Sonogram in a patient with fever shows a small, rounded, hypoechoic lesion. Pus was aspirated by fine needle puncture. (*k*, kidney.) (Figs. B & C from Goerg et al,[32] with permission.)

pressed patients receiving multidrug chemotherapy. The signs and symptoms are nonspecific and include persistent fevers, malaise, and weight loss. The pathogens most frequently involved include *Candida, Aspergillus,* and *Cryptococcus.*

Various ultrasound patterns associated with candidiasis have been described: a "wheel-within-a-wheel" appearance with a peripheral hypoechoic zone (fibrosis), an enclosed hyperechoic zone (inflammatory cells), and a hyperechoic center (pus, necrotic debris, and fungal elements); hypoechoic lesions with a hyperechoic center (fibrosis surrounding inflammatory cells without central necrosis); and healing lesions that become uniformly hyperechoic (fibrosis without central inflammatory mass) and eventually small and hyperechoic (scan, often calcified)[63] (Fig. 10-26). Splenomegaly is common and the lesions are usually smaller than 2 cm.[63] Splenectomy is the usual treatment.

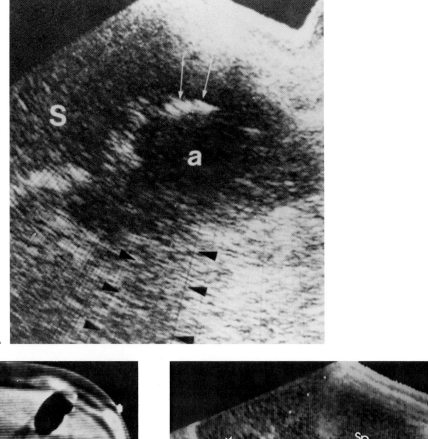

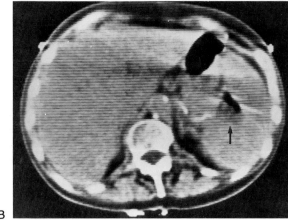

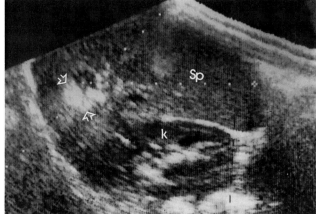

Fig. 10-25. Splenic abscess. **(A)** Case 1. Coronal scan of the spleen (*S*) with a large relatively anechoic abscess (*a*) with scattered internal echoes. Increased echogenicity (arrows) and acoustic shadowing (arrowheads) are due to the gas within the abscess. **(B)** This was confirmed on CT as an area of diminished attenuation (arrow) with a collection of gas in its anterior aspect. (From Pawar et al,[60] with permission.) **(C)** Case 2. Longitudinal scan with an abscess with increased echogenicity of the walls (arrows). (*k*, left kidney; *Sp* spleen.) (From Kay et al,[6] with permission.)

Other

Other less common pathogens involved in splenic abscesses include tuberculous[64] and amebic[65] pathogens. In the report of a tuberculous splenic abscess, the lesion was described as irregular and hypoechoic that contained scattered internal echoes and calcium deposition. Except for tuberculous splenic abscesses, calcification is rarely seen in splenic abscesses. Both gas-containing pyogenic abscesses and cholesterol-containing congenital splenic cysts may also show echogenic internal echoes.[64] A sonographic-guided aspiration might yield the diagnosis and the lesion may be cured by medical treatment in some cases.[64] Although amebic liver abscesses have been reported in endemic areas, there have been few reports with regard to splenic involvement.[65] In

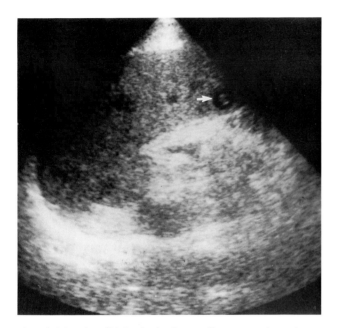

Fig. 10-26. Candidal splenic abscess. Sonogram shows hypoechoic splenic lesions, one with a "wheel-within-a-wheel" appearance (arrow). (From Chew et al,[63] with permission.)

the case reported, the lesions in the liver showed multiple, anechoic space-occupying lesions with posterior enhancement. In the same case, a splenic lesion was detected as an echogenic lesion with posterior enhancement and an irregular wall. Ultrasound-guided needle aspiration yielded the diagnosis.[65]

Acquired Immunodeficiency Syndrome

There have been recent reports dealing with visceral calcification in patients with acquired immunodeficiency syndrome (AIDS).[66,67] Since extrapulmonary *Pneumocystis carinii* infection is common in patients with AIDS, it is not usually considered in the differential diagnosis or diffuse sonographic parenchymal abnormalities in the thyroid, liver, spleen, or kidneys in the imaging literature.[66] The use of aerosol pentamidine in patients with disseminated *P. carinii* infection may be important. Affecting nearly 80 percent of AIDS patients, *P. carinii* pneumonia is a major cause of morbidity and mortality in this group of patients.[66] Although *P. carinii* pneumonia may be prevented by the prophylactic use of aerosol pentamidine, subclinical pulmonary infections with occult systemic seeding might occur.[66] Thus, aerosol pentamidine may put users at risk for disseminated *P. carinii* pneumonia. It might be advantageous to sonographically examine AIDS patients for disseminated *P. carinii,* if they are receiving aerosol pentamidine.[66]

An unusual sonographic pattern has been reported — that of innumerable tiny, bright, and highly reflective nonshadowing foci scattered diffusely throughout the liver, kidneys, pancreas, and spleen[66] (Fig. 10-27). On biopsy of liver and thyroid involvement, no calcium was seen to account for the tiny reflective echoes; as such these echoes may not be due to the presence of calcium initially.[66] On CT, the diffuse parenchymal abnormality demonstrated on ultrasound was not visualized. There-

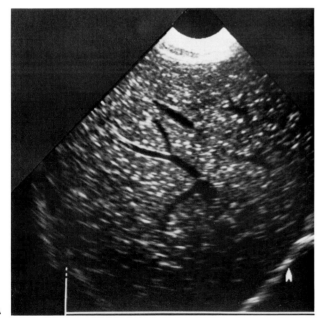

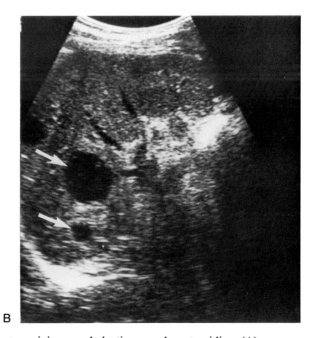

A   B

Fig. 10-27. *Pneumocystis carinii* infection in AIDS patient receiving prophylactic aerosol pentamidine. **(A)** Sagittal sonogram shows innumerable echogenic foci in liver. **(B)** Coronal sonogram of spleen shows multiple bright parenchymal echoes and focal hypoechoic masses (arrows). (From Spouge et al,[66] with permission.)

fore, ultrasound appears to be more sensitive than CT in detecting extrapulmonary *P. carinii* in the early stages. The ultrasound findings may represent a manifestation of relatively early disease.[66,67] Additionally, ultrasound can be employed to followup a patient who has been on systemic therapy.

Other authors have reported a similar echopattern in the liver, spleen, kidneys, lungs, and small intestine in an AIDS patient with widespread cytomegalovirus (CMV) infection.[67] Biopsy of the liver and kidneys demonstrated changes due to CMV infection. Since the patient had had an episode of *P. carinii* pneumonia earlier, which had been treated with intravenous pentamidine, it is possible the echopattern demonstrated could be secondary to an early infection with *P. carinii* rather than due to the CMV infection.[67] A second patient in this series had widespread small echogenic foci in the liver. Biopsy showed small granulomas associated with *Mycobacterium avium-intracellulare* infection. Therefore, organisms other than *P. carinii,* mainly CMV and *M. avium-intracellulare,* may cause discrete visceral calcifications in patients with AIDS.[67]

Cysts

Splenic cysts, which are relatively rare, have been classified as parasitic or nonparasitic in origin.[68]

Hydatid Cysts

Echinococcus is the only parasite that forms splenic cysts. While hydatid cysts are the most common cause of splenic cysts worldwide, they are uncommon in the United States.[69,70] Hydatid disease, caused by the larval form of the genus *Echinococcus,* of which *Echinococcus granulosus* is the most common, involves the spleen in less than 2 percent of all human infestations by *Echinococcus;* it more frequently involves the liver and lungs.[71] The signs and symptoms may be nonspecific and include abdominal pain, enlarged spleen, and fever; however, secondary infection, cyst rupture, and anaphylactic shock may develop. The most reliable laboratory finding in human hydatidosis is the presence of the arc 5 of Capron on immunoelectrophoresis. The appearance of splenic involvement varies and is affected by the location and age of the cyst and associated complications, such as secondary infection and rupture.

Parasitic cysts appear as anechoic lesions with possible daughter cysts and calcifications or as solid masses with fine internal echoes and poor distal enhancement.[17] The ultrasound findings with splenic involvement are not specific, even if the typical findings of solitary, anechoic lesions are demonstrated[71] (Fig. 10-28A). Most often, an anechoic pattern is observed, although a mixture of infolded membranes, scoleces, and hydatid sand may produce a highly echogenic (solid) pattern because of the large acoustic impedance difference between the intracystic components[71] (Fig. 10-28B). It is often difficult to differentiate splenic hydatidosis from other splenic cystic lesions. It should be particularly suspected in patients in endemic areas. The diagnosis is favored if daughter cysts are present within a large cystic lesion or if cystic lesions are observed in other organs such as the liver.[71]

Nonparasitic Cysts

Nonparasitic splenic cysts have been categorized as either (1) true or "primary" cysts (epidermoid cysts), which contain an epithelial lining and considered to be of congenital origin; or (2) false or "secondary" cysts, which lack a cellular lining, probably develop as a result of prior trauma to the spleen, and account for approximately 80 percent of nonparasitic splenic cysts.[70] A false cyst might also be secondary to either infarction or splenic infection.[72]

Epidermoid (epithelial-lined) cysts are lined by cells thought to arise from mesothelial cells that migrate during embryogenesis from the primitive coelomic cavity into the splenic analge.[73] Epidermoid cysts may be due to squamous metaplasia within preexisting mesothelial cysts. These may arise from invagination of the surface mesothelium during spleen formation or trapping of peritoneal mesothelium after rupture of the splenic capsule, collection of peritoneal mesothelial cells trapped in splenic sulci, or they may originate from normal lymph spaces.[72,74] Epithelial cysts are uncommon, comprising approximately 10 percent of the benign nonparasitic cysts.[74,75] These cysts are usually solitary, unilocular, and rarely contain calcification. The internal surface of the cyst may be smooth or trabeculated. The fluid within the cyst may be clear or turbid and may contain protein, iron, bilirubin, fat, and cholesterol crystals.[73]

Epidermoid cysts occur more commonly in females, with 50 percent occurring in patients younger than 15 years old.[73] The mean age of those diagnosed with epidermoid cysts is 20 years with a range of 6 months to 62 years.[74] While one series reported no strong sexual predominance,[74] others have reported a female predominance.[75] Epidermoid cysts, which have been found in siblings of patients with such cysts, might, in these cases, be an autosomal recessive, organ-specific defect of mesothelial migration.[74] However, a natural history of sporadic or familial occurrence has not yet been provided.[74] Since ultrasound is a noninvasive procedure, it might be warranted to screen siblings of persons with epidermoid cysts so that appropriate precautions and prophylaxis can be initiated if necessary.[74] If the diagnosis is in ques-

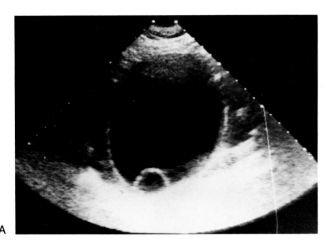

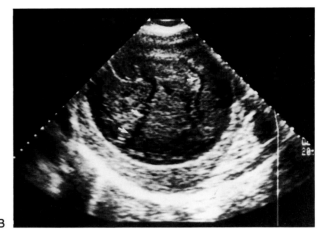

A   B

Fig. 10-28. Splenic hydatid disease. **(A)** A 48-year-old woman with splenic hydatidosis. Oblique sonogram of left upper quadrant shows spherical anechoic mass containing small cystic lesion. **(B)** Splenic hydatid cyst in 45-year-old woman with abdominal pain. Oblique sonogram shows echogenic (solid) mass corresponding to hydatid cyst. Cyst is filled by echogenic material composed of hydatid sand, infolded membranes (arrows), and debris. (From Franquet et al,[71] with permission.)

tion, an ultrasound-guided aspiration might be performed to verify it.[76] Treatment options depend on presentation and the life-style of the patient and include observation, partial or complete splenectomy, marsupialization, and percutaneous aspiration.[72,74]

Although most patients present with an asymptomatic left upper quadrant mass, symptoms, when present, include mild left-sided abdominal discomfort or pain and postprandial fullness. Seventy percent of patients are asymptomatic.[75] Although an infrequent complication, rupture requires immediate surgery.[75] On ultrasound, rupture is diagnosed if a cystic splenic mass is observed to have discontinuous cyst margins in association with free peritoneal fluid.[75]

Ultrasound findings are distinctive: hypoechoic or anechoic foci with well-defined walls and increased through transmission (Figs. 10-29 to 10-32). The sonographic appearance of epidermoid cysts may include increased internal echoes at higher gain settings, although even at these settings post-traumatic cysts tend to remain echofree[73,77] (Fig. 10-32). Their complex pattern with irregularities and thickness of the posterior wall may be due to epithelial trabeculations and internal echoes from blood clots[17] (Figs. 10-31 and 10-32). One case of a splenic cyst that was homogeneously echogenic has been reported[73] (Fig. 10-30). There may be layering of two fluids within the cyst when hemorrhage occurs, with the dependent layer being relatively echogenic[72,78] (Fig. 10-31). In up to one-fourth of false cysts, curvilinear or plaquelike calcification is present; it is less common in true cysts.[72] Ultrasound has the advantage of identifying the splenic origin of the mass.

In the differential diagnosis, a false cyst is favored if the patient is older than the fourth decade, if there is hematoma elsewhere in the spleen, or if the cyst wall is calcified.[72] Also consistent with the diagnosis of a splenic cyst is a predominantly cystic mass containing low-level echoes. However, the differential diagnosis should include echinococcal cyst, a large solitary abscess or hematoma, the rare intrasplenic pancreatic pseudocyst, and cystic neoplasm of the spleen.[72]

Biopsy

In many cases, an imaging technique may only lead to a differential, not a specific diagnosis. For a definitive diagnosis and as a possible alternate to laparotomy, a fine needle biopsy may be performed with a high degree of safety.[17,79,80] One investigator has performed more than 1,000 splenic punctures without complication.[79,80] Others have performed needle biopsies in 45 cases of diffuse and focal splenic disease without immediate or subsequent adverse reactions.[17] No intrasplenic hematomas or lesions along the needle path were seen in the 23 patients who underwent splenectomy soon after fine needle aspirations. Real-time ultrasound guidance was used in eight cases of splenic masses in which the final diagnoses, without surgery, were made in five cases. Two of these were cysts that were drained percutaneously and were not seen to recur on follow-up examination. Fine needle aspiration should be considered as a major diagnostic tool in evaluation of focal splenic lesions of unknown etiology.

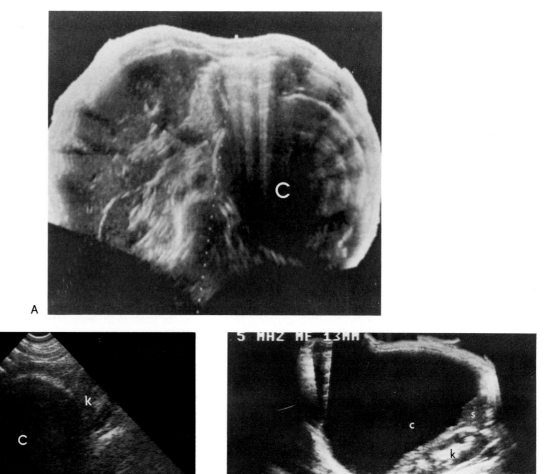

Fig. 10-29. Splenic cyst. Simple. **(A)** Case 1. Supine transverse scan at 12 cm above the umbilicus and **(B)** prone longitudinal scan demonstrating an anechoic mass (*C*) with dense borders in the area of the spleen. The wall of the cyst was calcified. (*k*, left kidney.) (Fig. A from Mittelstaedt et al,[13] with permission.) **(C)** Case 2. Longitudinal scan showing a large rounded echofree cyst (*c*) with surrounding margin of normal splenic tissue (*s*) inferiorly and posteriorly. The left kidney (*k*) is pushed inferiorly and the upper pole is squashed anteroposteriorly. (Fig. C from Daneman and Martin,[73] with permission.)

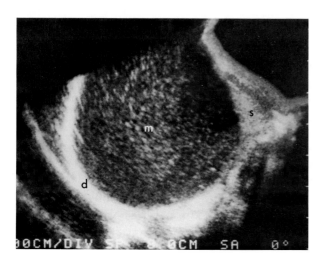

Fig. 10-30. Splenic cyst. Echogenic. Longitudinal scan demonstrating a large rounded echogenic mass (*m*) surrounded by normal splenic tissue (*s*) inferiorly. (*d*, diaphragm.) Echoes within the cyst were due to the high content of fat droplets within the cyst fluid. (From Daneman and Martin DJ,[73] with permission.)

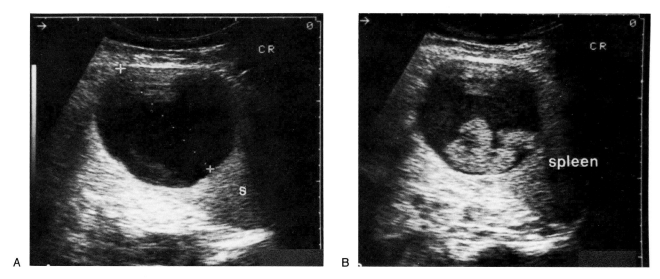

Fig. 10-31.   Splenic cyst. **(A)** Initial sonogram shows a large echofree cyst with echo enhancement in distal area. (*S*, spleen.) **(B)** Sonogram 3 years later shows echoes at bottom of cyst, probably caused by hemorrhage. (From Goerg et al,[32] with permission.)

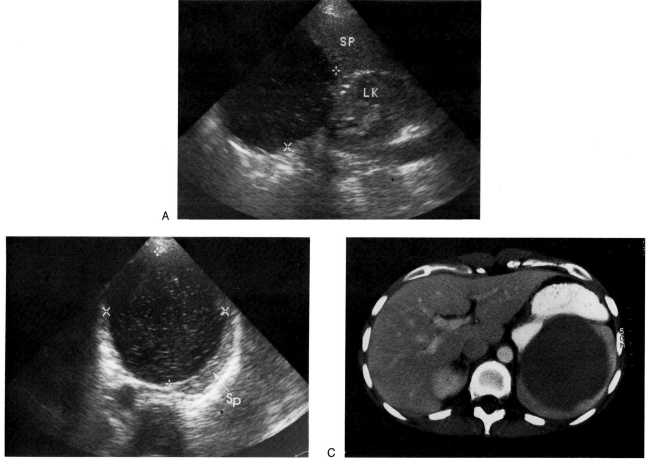

Fig. 10-32.   Splenic cyst **(A)** Sagittal and **(B)** transverse sonograms in the right-lateral decubitus position demonstrate a cystic mass (76 × 72 × 79 mm) containing fine internal echoes secondary to trabeculation. (*Sp*, spleen; *LK*, left kidney.) **(C)** Enhanced CT scan of the splenic cyst.

One group of investigators report their experience with interventional procedures in the spleen.[81] These included biopsies, diagnostic and therapeutic fluid aspiration, and catheter drainage of abscesses, hematomas, intrasplenic pancreatic pseudocysts, and necrotic tumor.[81] No complications occurred with biopsies performed using 22- or 20-gauge needles only. These procedures resulted in diagnoses of primary and secondary malignancies and an infectious process. As shown, interventional radiologic procedures in the spleen are feasible and there are methods to promote their safe application.

DIFFUSE DISEASE

Hematopoietic Abnormalities

Hematopoietic abnormalities include those disease processes affecting erythropoiesis, granulocytopoiesis, and lymphopoiesis.[82] The myeloproliferative disorders are classified as abnormalities of both erythropoiesis and granulocytopoiesis.[82]

Erythropoietic Abnormalities

The erythropoietic abnormalities include sickle cell disease, hereditary spherocytosis, hemolytic and chronic anemias, polycythemia vera, thalassemia, and the myeloproliferative disorders. Congestion of the red pulp and reticuloendothelial cell hypertrophy are often seen pathologically.[7,82]

Erythropoietic abnormalities generally produce an isoechoic splenic pattern on ultrasound (same density as the liver)[3,4] (similar to Fig. 10-33). One author has described an isoechoic splenic pattern in a case of hereditary spherocytosis.[83]

Granulocytopoietic Abnormalities

Cases of reactive hyperplasia due to acute and chronic infection, as well as splenitis associated with chronic granulomatous disease (e.g., sarcoid, tuberculosis, etc.) are included in this category. Pathologically, these spleens demonstrate lymphoid hyperplasia of the white pulp, and lymphocytes, neutrophils, and/or phagocytic cells in the red pulp.[7,82]

Other than splenomegaly, no definite abnormalities are usually demonstrated on TcSC or CT scans. By contrast, ultrasound has been shown to exhibit a specific pattern—a spleen that is diffusely hypoechoic (less dense than liver).[3,4]

Myeloproliferative Disorders

The diseases in this category include acute and chronic myelogenous (granulocytic or myelocytic) leukemias, polycythemia vera, myelofibrosis, megakaryocytic leukemia, and erythroleukemia. All of these appear to have a common myeloproliferative stimulus.[82] Extramedullary hematopoiesis may replace the normal splenic architecture. In the myelogenous leukemias, the spleen is infiltrated by leukemic cells of the granulocytic series.[7]

In acute and chronic myelogenous leukemia, the spleen exhibits an isoechoic ultrasound pattern similar to that seen with the erythropoietic abnormalities[3,4] (Fig. 10-33). A case has been described in which the red pulp was dominant, with infiltration by the hematopoietic elements pathologically.[84] Although other authors describe cases of chronic myelogenous leukemia and myelofibrosis as having an increased splenic echopattern, their examples appear to demonstrate a hypoechoic pattern when splenic echogenicity is compared with that of the liver.[83] Still others have illustrated a case of chronic myelogenous leukemia that appeared to have an isoechoic splenic pattern.[85]

Lymphopoietic Abnormalities

Pathologically, spleens involved by lymphopoietic abnormalities demonstrate infiltration of the normal splenic architecture by cells of lymphopoietic origin.[7] This category includes the lymphocytic leukemias, lymphoma, and Hodgkin's disease.

On ultrasound, most spleens affected with lymphocytic leukemia, lymphoma, or Hodgkin's disease demonstrate a diffusely hypoechoic splenic pattern.[3,4,12,33,83,85,86] Focal hypoechoic lesions may also be present in both Hodgkin's and non-Hodgkin's lymphoma[3,4] (Figs. 10-14 to 10-16). Non-Hodgkin's lymphoma and "lymphoid malignancy" have also been reported to have an isoechoic echopattern.

Reticuloendothelial Disorders

Diseases having reticuloendothelial hyperactivity and varying degrees of lipid storage in phagocytes are included in this category.[82] Examples include Wilson's disease, Felty syndrome, Still's disease, and reticulum cell sarcoma. On ultrasound scan, the splenic pattern appears isoechoic[3,4] (similar to Fig. 10-33).

Gaucher's Disease

A familial disorder of lipid metabolism, Gaucher's disease results in accumulation of glucocerebrosides in

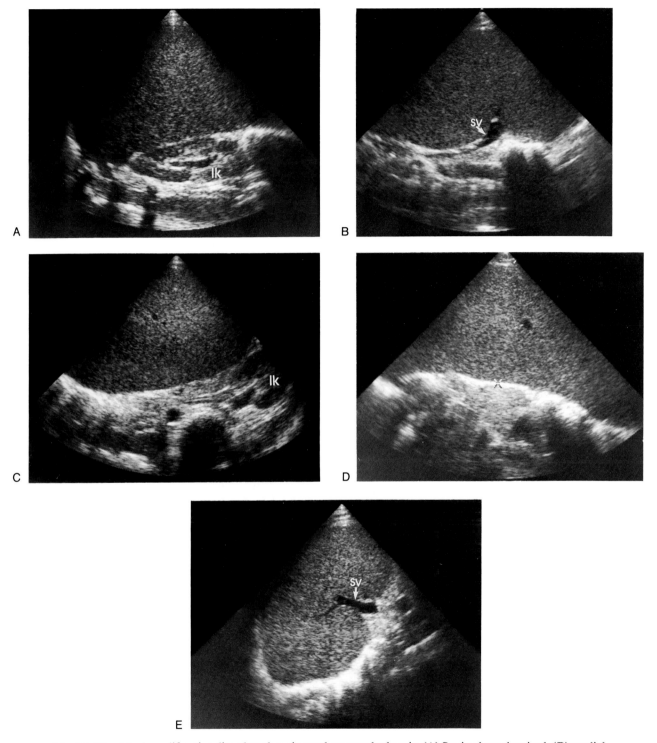

Fig. 10-33. Myeloproliferative disorder: chronic myelogenous leukemia. **(A)** Supine lateral sagittal, **(B)** medial sagittal, and **(C)** transverse scans as well as **(D)** right-lateral decubitus sagittal and **(E)** transverse scans demonstrate a massively enlarged homogeneous spleen. It was similar in echopattern to the liver. (*sv*, splenic vein; *lk*, left kidney.)

the reticuloendothelial cells. This is caused by a deficiency of glucocerebrosidase. Three variants have been reported: type I (adult or chronic nonneuronopathic)—patients present at any age with hepatosplenomegaly, bone infarctions, and hemorrhagic diathesis; type II (infantile or acute neuronopathic)—patients have rapid progression of central nervous system involvement that results in death, usually within the first years of life; type III (juvenile or subacute neuronopathic)—patients have central nervous system involvement but typically live until adolescence.[87] Hepatosplenomegaly is present in all forms.[87,88]

There have been reports in the literature of the ultrasound findings in the spleen associated with Gaucher's disease.[87,88] The most common ultrasound pattern described was that of focal hypoechoic areas throughout a markedly enlarged spleen[87,88] (Fig. 10-34); these lesions did not exhibit acoustic enhancement. The oldest patients had hyperechoic lesions.[87] Pathologically, the splenic lesions were composed of circumscribed areas of fibrosis with entrapped Gaucher cells or focal homogeneous clusters of Gaucher cells.[87,88] Most spleens in cases of Gaucher's disease have a normal appearance aside from being enlarged.[88] Abdominal sonograms in patients with Gaucher's disease should always include the spleen since a significant number of patients have demonstrated a variety of Gaucher pathology in the spleen with ultrasound.[87] This should be kept in mind when evaluating such a patient who has left upper quadrant pain.

Congestion

There is thickening of the trabeculae, fibrosis of the red pulp, and atrophy of lymphoid tissue with chronic

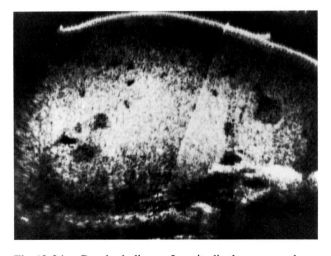

Fig. 10-34. Gaucher's disease. Longitudinal sonogram shows multiple hypoechoic masses in a markedly enlarged spleen. (From Hill et al,[87] with permission.)

passive congestion.[82] In most cases, the congestion is secondary to hepatocellular disease.

In most cases of congestive splenomegaly due to cirrhosis, there is increased uptake of the radionuclide in the spleen relative to the liver, and increased uptake in the bone marrow.[89] Some patients may have normal splenic uptake with increased marrow uptake.[89]

On ultrasound scan, the spleen may either demonstrate an isoechoic or hypoechoic pattern.[3,4] Because the liver is abnormal in these cases, it cannot be used as an internal standard for comparison.

TRAUMA

The spleen is the intra-abdominal organ most commonly injured as a result of blunt abdominal trauma.[90] Automobile accidents are responsible for most of these injuries. Splenic trauma is often associated with injuries of other structures including (in decreasing order of incidence) chest wall (rib fractures), left kidney, spinal cord, liver, lung, craniocerebral structures, small and large intestines, pancreas, and stomach.[91]

Trauma to the spleen may result in linear or stellate lacerations, capsular tears secondary to traction from adhesions or suspensary ligaments, puncture wounds from foreign bodies or rib fractures, subcapsular hematomas, avulsion of the vascular pedicle, and laceration of the short gastric vessels. Free intraperitoneal blood is most often seen acutely (i.e., immediately after injury). However, delayed rupture, occurring days to weeks following the traumatic event, occurs in 10 to 15 percent of patients with free intraperitoneal blood. Delayed ruptures are probably related to a slowly enlarging subcapsular hematoma with subsequent rupture, or a small splenic laceration that was temporarily tamponaded. *Occult splenic rupture* is a term applied to a post-traumatic pseudocyst, which is generally secondary to an organized intrasplenic or parasplenic hematoma.[91] Splenic trauma may result in autotransplantation of splenic tissue on to peritoneal surfaces, a condition termed *splenosis.* Patients with splenosis may subsequently develop adhesions leading to intestinal obstruction.[92]

Clinically, 10 to 20 percent of splenic lacerations are not obvious.[93] The main presenting symptoms include left upper quadrant pain (100 percent), left shoulder pain (50 percent), left flank pain (36 percent), and postural dizziness (21 percent).[94] The most frequent clinical signs are left upper quadrant tenderness (100 percent), hypotension (36 percent), and decreased hemoglobin level (43 percent).[94] Peritoneal lavage is a sensitive technique for the detection of intraperitoneal bleeding but is invasive, may be falsely positive, and will not detect either

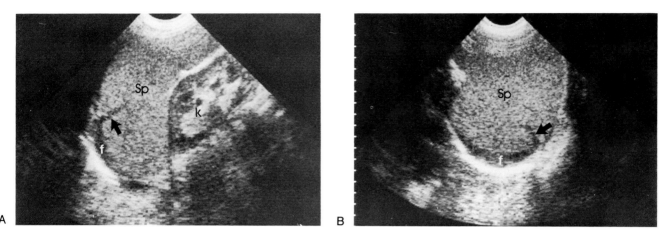

Fig. 10-35. Splenic laceration. **(A)** Coronal scan 4 days after injury demonstrating a small peripheral splenic laceration (arrow) in continuity with a perisplenic fluid collection (*f*). (*Sp*, spleen; *k*, kidney.) **(B)** Transverse scan showing the laceration (arrow) and the perisplenic fluid collection (*f*). (*Sp*, spleen.) (From Lupien and Sauerbrei,[94] with permission.)

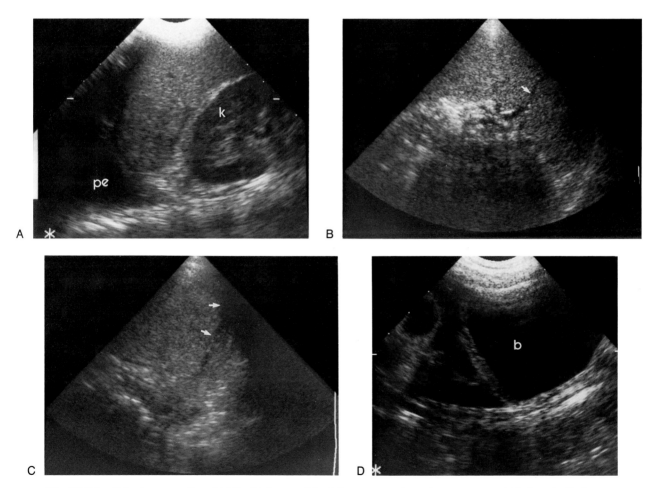

Fig. 10-36. Splenic transection. **(A)** Sagittal scan of the left upper quadrant demonstrates a left pleural effusion (*pe*) in this child with splenic trauma. (*k*, left kidney.) **(B & C)** Coronal transverse scans at higher and lower levels, respectively, in the right-lateral decubitus position with visualization of an extensive splenic fracture line (arrows). **(D)** Sagittal view of the pelvis reveals peritoneal fluid (blood). (*b*, urinary bladder.)

retroperitoneal hemorrhage or a subcapsular splenic hematoma without free intraperitoneal blood. Although splenectomy is the most common treatment for splenic trauma, simple observation, splenorrhaphy (suture repair of laceration), partial splenectomy, and percutaneous aspiration are now being performed for some cases of subcapsular hematoma and for small lacerations.[95-97] Splenectomy may predispose patients to subsequent septicemia and therefore should not be performed unnecessarily. It is clear, therefore, that splenic trauma must be detected as well as characterized in an attempt to define those patients who can benefit from conservative management.

Because plain films are most often normal or equivocal in cases of subcapsular hematoma, imaging modalities may assume great importance in the evaluation of splenic trauma. Selection of the proper examinations will help in achieving an accurate appraisal of the spleen and other intra-abdominal structures and thus expedite the patient's diagnostic workup.

Ultrasound

Ultrasound has not been shown to be as reliable as either TcSC or CT in the evaluation of splenic trauma. Technically inadequate examinations occur in as many as 20 percent of cases secondary to accompanying rib fractures and contusions of chest tubes.[98] With the advent of the newer high-resolution sector real-time systems, ultrasound has become a rapid, accurate examination in many cases. Ultrasonic signs of splenic trauma include splenomegaly or progressive splenic enlargement, an irregular splenic border, intrasplenic fluid (hematoma), splenic inhomogeneity (contusion), subcapsular and pericapsular fluid collections (subcapsular hematoma), free intraperitoneal blood, and left pleural effusion[94,96,99] (Figs. 10-35 to 10-39). A small peripheral laceration appears as a linear echopoor defect (Fig. 10-35A). With transection, a more extensive plane of fluid may be seen transversing the entire thickness of the splenic pulp, or the spleen may have an inhomogeneous

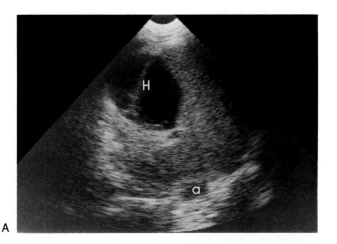

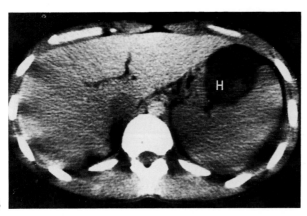

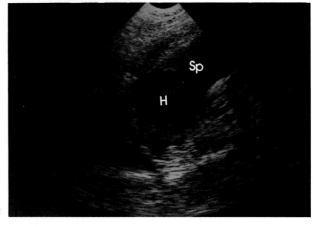

Fig. 10-37. Intrasplenic hematoma. **(A)** Case 1. Transverse, supine real-time scan. There is a hypoechoic mass (*H*) in the region of the splenic hilum. (*a*, aorta.) **(B)** CT scan, enhanced, demonstrating the hematoma (*H*) in the area of the splenic hilum. (From Mittelstaedt et al,[13] with permission.) **(C)** Case 2. Longitudinal right-lateral decubitus scan. A poorly defined hypoechoic area (*H*) is seen within the spleen (*Sp*).

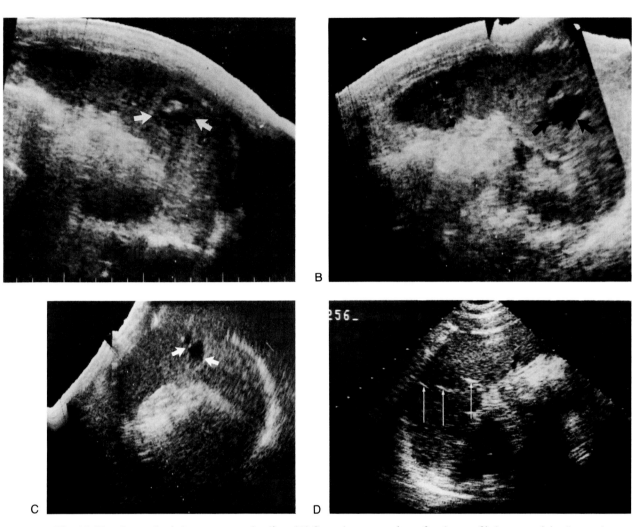

Fig. 10-38. Intrasplenic hematoma — healing. **(A)** Scan demonstrating a focal area of inhomogenicity (arrows) 3 days after initial injury. **(B)** Ten days later the lesion has become echofree (arrows). **(C)** Two weeks after Fig. B was taken, Fig. C shows a decrease in the size of the intrasplenic fluid collection (arrows). **(D)** Sixteen months after the initial trauma, only small echogenic lines (arrows) are seen in the area of the previous splenic lesion. These are likely fibrous scars. (From Lupien and Sauerbrei,[94] with permission.)

echopattern (Fig. 10-36). Focal hematomas are represented by intrasplenic fluid collections (Figs. 10-37 and 10-38). With a subcapsular hematoma, perisplenic fluid is seen (Fig. 10-39).

On ultrasound, sonographic patterns of splenic trauma can change considerably in a short period of time. Blood exhibits varying echopatterns depending on the age of the trauma. In less than 24 hours, intraparenchymal hemorrhage may appear hyperechoic.[94] Therefore, a fresh hematoma may be indistinguishable from normal splenic tissue, giving only the appearance of splenomegaly or a double contour to the spleen.[96] As the protein and cells resorb and the hematoma becomes organized, the fluid collection becomes hyperechoic. Focal areas of inhomogeneity probably represent tiny splenic

lacerations that give rise to small collections of blood interspersed with disrupted splenic pulp (contusion). With time, the hematoma will appear more fluid or lucent (Fig. 10-38). Echofree intraperitoneal fluid probably represents blood, perhaps intermixed with peritoneal transudate due to the presence of blood within the cavity[94] (Fig. 10-36D).

The pattern of splenic healing and the time it takes depend on the nature and size of the initial lesion[94] (Fig. 10-38). Larger lesions persist for longer periods of time, while small peripheral lacerations tend to disappear several weeks after the injury. Free fluid collections disappear more quickly because fluid is transported across pleural and peritoneal membranes rapidly; pleural effusion and intraperitoneal fluid disappears quickly (2 and

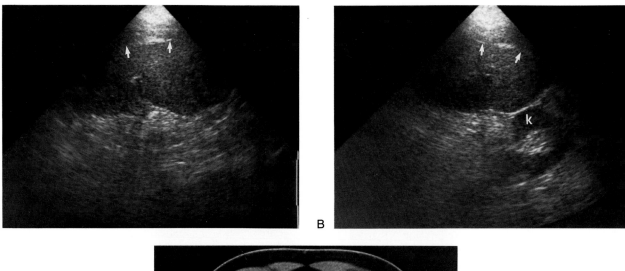

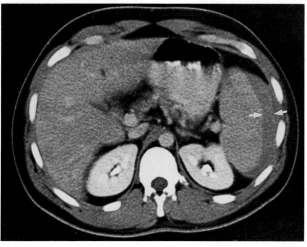

Fig. 10-39. Subcapsular hematoma. **(A)** Right-lateral decubitus sagittal and **(B)** transverse scans of the spleen demonstrate a double outline (arrows) along the periphery of the spleen secondary to the subcapsular hematoma. (*k*, left kidney.) **(C)** Enhanced CT scan similarly demonstrating the subcapsular hematoma (arrows).

4 weeks, respectively). Intrasplenic hematoma and contusion usually resorb over a period of months (7 to 66 weeks). The longer time is probably because the fluid, protein, and necrotic debris must be resorbed from within a solid organ in which the blood supply has already been focally disrupted.[94] When followed to complete resolution, the spleen may become normal, or small irregular foci may be present that are echogenic and probably represent scar[94] (Fig. 10-38). As a rapid, noninvasive diagnostic technique, ultrasound can be used for multiple follow-up examinations if warranted.

Computed Tomography

In a series evaluating the spleen following blunt abdominal trauma using CT, the spleen was noted to increase in volume on serial studies.[100] This increase in volume (defined as an increase over 10 percent), which was seen in 57 percent of the patients, did not correlate with clinical deterioration or the need for splenectomy. It is postulated to be due to a marked adrenergic stimulation after injury and to changing fluid volumes.[100] Initially there is a decrease in splenic size and eventual return to normal size owing to the systemic effect of trauma rather than to the local abdominal injury. The peak in size occurs 6 days after trauma.[100]

There have been several CT studies dealing with grading systems to classify splenic trauma and predict prognosis and treatment.[101-103] The goal is to preserve splenic tissue whenever possible since there is the occurrence of overwhelming postsplenectomy infection.[101] Postsplenectomy sepsis has a frequency of 4.25 percent, a mortality rate of 2.25 percent, and may occur up to 15 years after splenectomy.[101] One group of authors[101] believed that the post-traumatic outcome of the injured spleen is not predictable with use of the various grading methods. The ultimate decision for laparotomy should be based on clinical status and not on radiographic findings.[101] Another study[102] demonstrated that while CT remains an accurate method of identifying and quantifying initial splenic injury, as well as documenting progression or healing of critical injury, it cannot reliably predict the outcome of blunt splenic injury in adults. Treatment choices should be based on the hemodynamic status of the patient and results of serial laboratory and bedside assessments.[102]

Still other authors believe that a CT grading system is reproducible and useful in quantitating splenic injury.[103] The following grades were developed: grade I, splenic laceration or linear parenchymal defect, equals 1 point; grade II, splenic fracture or thick irregular defects, equals 2 points; grade III, shattered spleen, equals 3 points.[103] Fluid around the spleen, around the liver, and in the pelvis scored 1 point each. Questionable observations were assigned a half point. Patients with scores of 2.5 or less could be treated conservatively; patients with scores over 2.5 are more likely to require surgery.

Because of the reduction in immunologic competence and the increased risk of sepsis in patients who have undergone splenectomy, clinicians now adopt a nonsurgical approach in the treatment of patients with an injured spleen.[94] The nonoperative management requires careful clinical observation, bed rest, and serial hematocrit.[104] Patients are selected for nonoperative management on the basis of a stable clinical status and laboratory evidence of cessation of bleeding.[104] An initial ultrasound might be valuable to serve as a baseline for those with repeated trauma and/or new symptoms.[94] The decision to operate should be based on a combination of clinical and ultrasound/or CT findings.[94]

Percutaneous Aspiration

In recent years nonoperative management of splenic rupture has been recommended and used increasingly because postsplenectomy patients have been shown to have an increased susceptibility to overwhelming infection.[97] With ultrasound guidance, fine needle aspiration of the perisplenic or subcapsular fluid can confirm the diagnosis and often be therapeutic.[96] One author reports three patients with infectious mononucleosis and splenic rupture diagnosed and followed as outpatients by ultrasound; laparotomy was avoided in these cases. One of the hematomas was aspirated percutaneously with ultrasound guidance, and did not recur on the follow-up examination.

OTHER

Variant Orientation and Contour

The normal spleen is highly variable in both contour and orientation. These variations are generally without clinical significance and are commonly noted as incidental findings during imaging procedures. Nonetheless, unusual splenic configurations and positions may mimic pathologic entities and may complicate, or even precipitate, diagnostic workups. Appropriate image procedures and a knowledge of these variations may easily obviate this confusion and eliminate the necessity for further unwarranted or invasive procedures.

Three major splenic configurations have been described: orange-segment (44 percent), tetrahedral (42 percent), and triangular (14 percent) (Fig. 10-40). Additionally, splenic configuration has been categorized into two major types: (1) a compact spleen, with a narrow hilus and even borders; and (2) a distributed spleen, with a widespread hilus, a notched anterior border, a thumblike lobe at the inferior pole, and an expanded portion or "tubercle" at the upper medial pole[105] (Figs. 10-23 and 10-41). In most individuals there is good splenic contact with the diaphragm and the lateral abdominal wall; poor contact can often be accounted for by enlargement of the left lobe of the liver, ascites, deformity of the left hemidiaphragm, or a small, horizontally positioned spleen.[106]

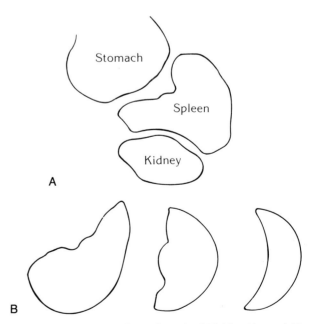

Fig. 10-40. Splenic configurations. **(A & B)** Note the variable splenic contours on cross-section at the splenic hilum, where a prominent ridge or lobulation may be seen. (Modified from Piekarski et al,[37] with permission.)

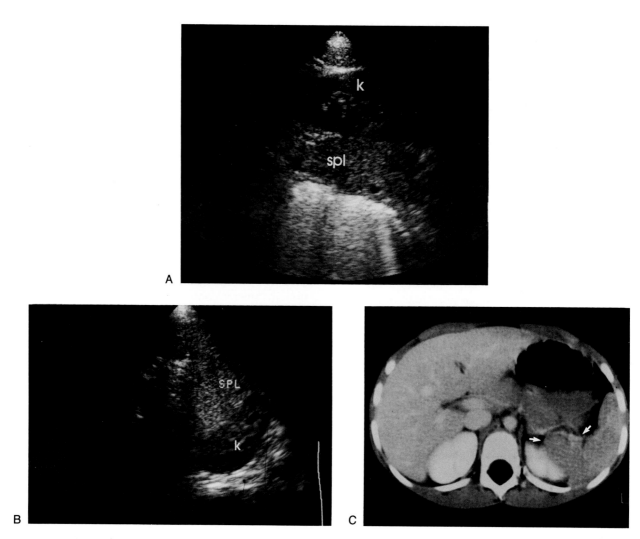

Fig. 10-41.   Normal splenic variant. **(A)** Right-lateral decubitus sagittal and **(B)** transverse views (coronal) of the left kidney (*k*) demonstrate the spleen (*spl*) projecting as a "mass" anterior to the kidney. **(C)** The mass represents a medial projection (arrows) from the spleen as seen on the CT scan.

Left upper quadrant masses, or even gastric dilatation, may displace the spleen inferiorly, producing "pseudo-splenomegaly."[107] Caudad displacement may also be secondary to subdiaphragmatic abscesses, splenic cysts or abscesses, left pleural effusion, or marked cardiomegaly; cephalad displacement may be caused by left lung volume loss, left pneumonectomy, paralysis of the left hemidiaphragm, or a large intra-abdominal mass.[108] In patients whose status is postrepair of congenital ventral hernia, the spleen and the liver may have an abnormal shape and be ventrally located.[109]

The so-called upside down spleen is most likely due to developmental rotation of the spleen on its longitudinal-anteroposterior axis, causing the hilus to be directed cephalad or laterally[110] (Fig. 10-42). The typical scintigraphic pattern (a concave superior and convex inferior margin) of a spleen with its hilus oriented superiorly should not be confused with splenic trauma or infarction. On abdominal radiographs or ultrasound, the upside down spleen can mimic a left suprarenal mass.[111]

Other splenic variations may simulate renal or suprarenal masses on routine radiographic studies. Although downward and/or medial displacement of the entire left kidney by an enlarged spleen is common and easily recognized, localized flattening of the upper pole of the left kidney can be the result of a "distributed" spleen with a "lumpy" contour, a transverse spleen, a rotated and ptotic spleen, or an accessory spleen [112] (Fig. 10-1). Similarly, variant splenic configurations may suggest a retrogastric mass or a fundal lesion on barium study.[113,114] A normal-sized spleen with a medial lobulation projecting between the pancreatic tail and the left kidney may be

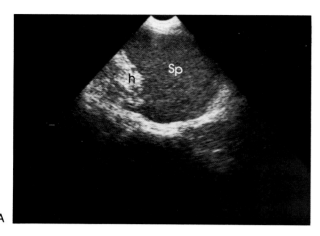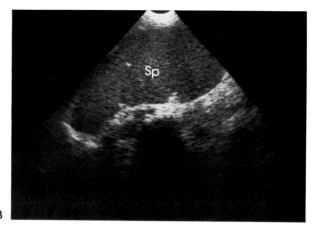

A   B

Fig. 10-42. "Upside-down" spleen. **(A)** Longitudinal and **(B)** transverse scans of the spleen (*Sp*). Note that the splenic hilum (*h*) is directed superiorly on the longitudinal scan (Fig. A). (Fig. A from Mittelstaedt et al,[13] with permission.)

confused with a cystic mass in the tail of the pancreas on prone ultrasound examination[115] (Fig. 10-41).

Documentation that splenic variation is to blame for suspected left upper quadrant mass can often be provided by ultrasound or TcSC (Figs. 10-1, 10-41, and 10-42). Satisfactory ultrasound evaluation, however, can be difficult in an obese or gaseous patient. In addition, upper quadrant examination in the prone position is not without pitfalls. Although TcSC will delineate splenic variation, relationships between splenic tissue and adjacent structures are not always clear-cut, and anomalous bulges of splenic tissue are not necessarily seen to best advantage in standard views. In many instances, CT scanning with oral contrast administration is the most successful imaging modality in clarifying splenic configuration and orientation as it relates to adjacent organs (i.e., as the cause of a retrogastric or suprarenal mass effect).

Wandering Spleen/Splenic Torsion

Wandering spleen, (also known as *ectopic spleen, aberrant spleen, floating spleen, splenic ptosis*) refers to migration of the spleen from its normal location in the left upper quadrant. This relatively rare variant is most probably the result of embryologic anomaly of the supporting ligaments of the spleen, although splenomegaly and abdominal laxity (the latter sometimes associated with multiparity and hormonal effects of pregnancy) have been considered predisposing factors.[116,117] Based on several large series of splenectomies, the incidence of wandering spleen is less than 0.5 percent.[118] As proliferating surface peritoneal cells on the left side of the greater omentum (dorsal mesogastrium), the splenic anlage em-

bryologically is first present in the fifth week of fetal development.[118] The cells break free and invade the underlying mesenchyma where they undergo splenic differentiation. There is a close proximity of the left urogenital fold to the developing spleen. The spleen may remain on a long pedicle and lie in an ectopic intra-abdominal location if there is incomplete fusion of the dorsal mesogastrium.[118]

Clinical presentations include an asymptomatic abdominal or pelvic mass, mild discomfort (from splenic congestion and perhaps ligamentous/visceral pressure), intermittent abdominal pain (attributed to spontaneous torsion and detorsion of the splenic pedicle), and abdominal catastrophe (resulting from splenic volvulus).[119] Bleeding gastric varices have been reported as presenting findings, and are presumed to be secondary to splenic vein occlusion associated with chronic torsion of the vascular pedicle.[120]

Splenomegaly is an important cause in the development of an acquired wandering spleen.[118] The spleen may initially occupy its normal position and subsequently migrate caudally when marked splenomegaly develops.[118] Other predisposing factors to the development of a wandering spleen include abdominal musculature laxity (e.g., prune belly syndrome) and pregnancy (hormonal influences).[118]

While splenic torsion associated with a wandering spleen has been reported, there have been few reports of splenic torsion in the left upper quadrant.[121] The identification of a normal-sized spleen below and lateral to the lower pole of the left kidney on ultrasound would suggest the possibility of change in the axis of the spleen. Evidence of infarction (hypoechoic areas) may also be demonstrated along with subcapsular fluid seen with hematoma.[121]

Ultrasound is often the preliminary study for evaluation of abdominal pain or mass, and sonographic imaging should strongly suggest the diagnosis of wandering spleen when a solid "mass" is demonstrated and splenic echoes are absent from their normal location[122] (Figs. 10-42 and 10-43). Demonstration of a "feeding vessel" associated with the mass should heighten suspicion further.[123]

In the case of uncomplicated splenic displacement, TcSC or ultrasound will confirm the abnormal spleen location.[124] However, as the spleen moves into and out of normal position, sequential TcSC or ultrasound scanning may be required for documentation. Obviously, in the case of a "transient" abdominal mass, scans must be wisely timed to coincide with the mass being palpable.[125] If torsion has occurred, the spleen may not be visualized by scintigraphy, or splenic uptake may be relatively diminished, dependent on the degree of vascular supply

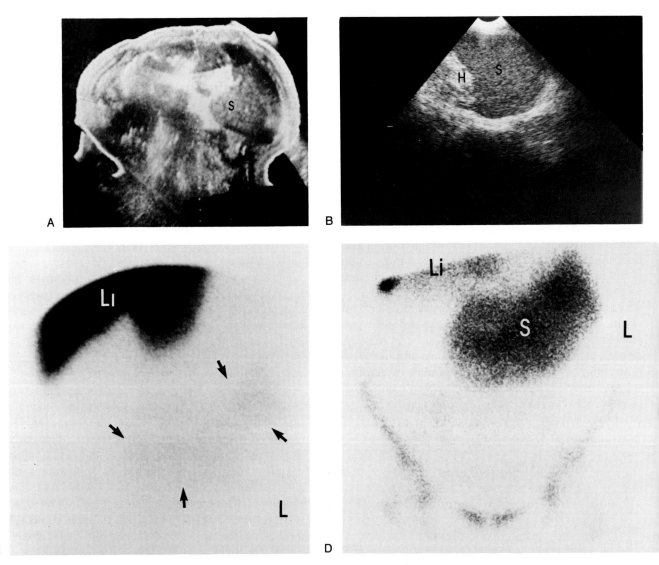

Fig. 10-43. Wandering spleen with torsion. Patient with pain and an abdominal mass. **(A)** Supine, transverse scan at the level of the umbilicus. The spleen (*S*) is seen at this level instead of in the left upper quadrant. **(B)** Supine, longitudinal real-time image of the spleen. The image appears to be reversed because the splenic hilum (*H*) is superior to the spleen (*S*). The patient was referred for technetium 99m-sulfur colloid radionuclide splenic scintigraphy (TcSC) to confirm the diagnosis and evaluate splenic vascularity. **(C)** Anterior view of TcSC scan with the camera centered over the spleen located at the level of the umbilicus. Uptake in the spleen (arrows) is barely visible when scans are taken for a predetermined count. (*L*, left; *Li*, liver.) **(D)** Anterior view of a TcSC scan centered over the spleen with the scan taken for a predetermined time instead of for counts. The liver (*Li*) is shielded. The spleen (*S*) appears reversed from its normal orientation. The decreased activity in the spleen is compatible with vascular compromise. (*L*, left.) *(Figure continues.)*

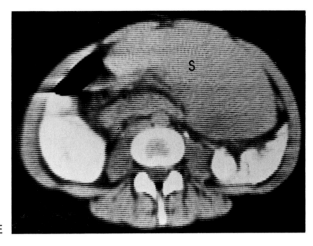 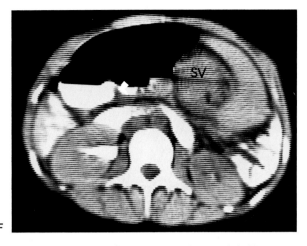

Fig. 10-43 *(Continued).* **(E)** CT scan confirms the presence of a rotated spleen (*S*) in the lower abdomen. **(F)** CT scan at a higher level in the abdomen than the CT scan in Fig. E. The dilated splenic vessels (*SV*) are noted in the splenic hilum. Angiography demonstrated a 720 degree torsion. (From Mittelstaedt et al,[13] with permission.)

compromise.[126] Absence of splenic visualization with TcSC is not entirely specific because nonvisualization may be secondary to acquired functional asplenia.[127] Nonetheless, in the absence of preexisting disease (most commonly, sickle cell anemia), splenic nonvisualization in the face of an abdominal mass or an acute abdomen should provide a key clue to the diagnosis of splenic volvulus.

Accessory Spleens/Splenosis

Accessory spleens, resulting from failure of fusion of the separate splenic masses forming on the dorsal mesogastrium, are most commonly located in the splenic hilum or along splenic vessels or associated ligaments. Their occurrence has also been reported from the diaphragm to the scrotum.[128] They are solitary in 88 percent of cases, double in 9 percent, and greater than two in 3 percent.[129] Despite a reported autopsy incidence of 10 to 31 percent, accessory spleens are detected incidentally in only about 0.05 percent of routine TcSC scans.[130] This discrepancy may be explained by the difficulty in visualizing accessory splenic tissue owing to obscuration by surrounding splenic radionuclide accumulation or relatively low tracer accumulation in the accessory tissue. Additionally, the field of view in routine TcSC scanning will not include less characteristic locations.[131]

Customarily, accessory spleens remain small and do not present as clinical problems. Rarely, torsion and infarction of an accessory spleen may present as an acute abdomen.[132,133] Accessory spleens may also simulate pancreatic, suprarenal, and retroperitoneal tumors,[134,135] and may even be mistaken as such at arte-

riography[136] or mimic an intragastric neoplasm on upper gastrointestinal examination.[137] An accessory spleen that has undergone compensatory hypertrophy after splenectomy may present as an abdominal mass. Although the appearance of a well-defined, almost spherical or uniform soft tissue density in the region of the splenectomy bed should be suggestive of accessory spleen on CT, this appearance is not specific, and could be produced by primary or secondary retroperitoneal neoplasms.[138] Similarly, accessory splenic tissue may resemble recurrent renal tumor after nephrectomy.[139]

Ultrasound has enabled the identification and documentation of accessory spleens based on their appearance, location, and most importantly blood supply.[129] They are round or oval solid structures with echogenicity similar to that of the main spleen[129] (Figs. 10-44 to 10-46), and are surrounded by high-amplitude interfaces that separate them from adjacent parenchymal organs. In one series, most were found in the splenic hilum, with a smaller number in the splenocolic ligament and anterior to the tail of the pancreas. In 90 percent, the blood supply of the accessory spleen can be identified with ultrasound[129] (Figs. 10-44 and 10-45). In 34 percent, the arterial supply from the splenic artery can be seen as a single tortuous arterial branch originating from the splenic artery near the splenic hilum[129] (Fig. 10-46). In 66 percent, a single straight vein is seen originating from the accessory spleen and draining into the splenic vein[129] (Fig. 10-45).

Scintigraphy is the most sensitive modality for the detection and localization of functional accessory splenic tissue. Aside from its utility in instances of simulated mass lesions, detection of residual splenic tissue may have important clinical implications in postsple-

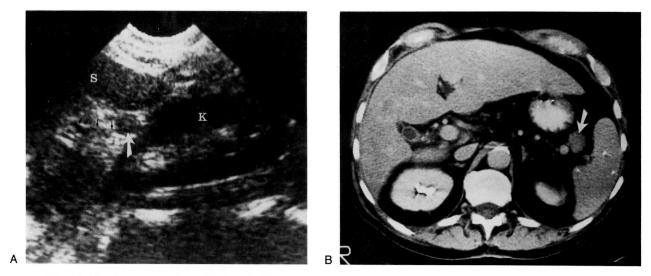

Fig. 10-44.   Accessory spleen. **(A)** Longitudinal scan with accessory spleen (white arrow) separated from main spleen (*S*) and left kidney (*K*) by high-amplitude interface. The blood supply (black arrows) is from the splenic artery. **(B)** Enhanced CT scan, with accessory spleen (arrow) isodense to main spleen. (From Subramanyam et al,[129] with permission.)

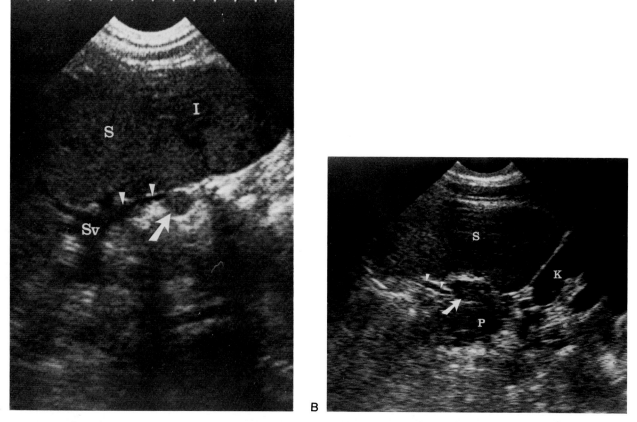

Fig. 10-45.   Accessory spleen. **(A)** Longitudinal scan in a patient with splenomegaly (*S*) and an area of infarct (*I*). The accessory spleen (arrow) is drained by a branch (arrowheads) of the splenic vein (*Sv*). **(B)** Oblique scan demonstrating an oval accessory spleen (arrow) with venous drainage (arrowheads). Note its relationship to spleen (*S*), tail of pancreas (*P*), and left kidney (*K*). (From Subramanyam et al,[129] with permission.)

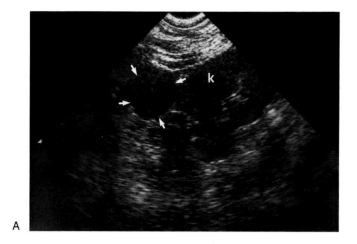

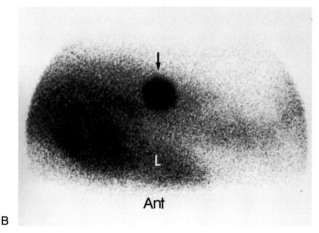

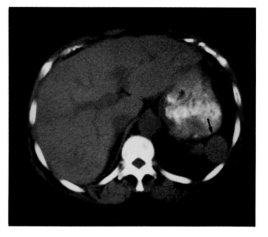

Fig. 10-46. Accessory spleen. Patient with idiopathic thrombocytopenic purpura and prior splenectomy. (A) On longitudinal right-lateral decubitus scan, a round echodense mass (arrows) is seen in the area of the splenic bed. The left kidney (*k*) is separate from the mass. (B) Left lateral view of a scan with ^{99m}Tc heat-damaged red blood cells demonstrates a round area (arrow) of increased activity in the area of the spleen. (*L,* liver; *Ant,* anterior.) (C) Unenhanced CT scan demonstrating the accessory spleen (arrow).

nectomy patients with autoimmune hemolytic anemias, idiopathic thrombocytopenic purpura, or hereditary spherocytosis. A possible cause of relapsing disease after splenectomy in these patients is recurrent splenic function, be it from hypertrophy of a previous small accessory spleen or the growth of new tissue from seeded spleen tissue.[140,141] Scanning may initially be performed with a radiocolloid, but because hepatic uptake may obscure small amounts of splenic tissue, repeat scanning may be performed with a spleen-specific agent, such as chemical or heat denatured technetium 99m (^{99m}Tc) labeled red blood cells[142] (Fig. 10-46B).

Splenosis, or post-traumatic autotransplantation of splenic tissue in the pleural or peritoneal cavities, may also be diagnosed by TcSC.[143,144] Unlike accessory spleens, the functioning tissue in splenosis does not follow the pattern of splenic embryologic development and

is often more numerous and widespread. Recent evidence suggests that splenosis is a frequent occurrence after splenectomy for trauma.[145] Although the diagnosis is usually made incidentally at surgery for obstruction or abdominal pain, the history of prior trauma, with or without splenectomy, may provide the clue for appropriate imaging and a correct preoperative diagnosis.[146] Multiple splenic foci may not be visualized routinely on liver-spleen scanning without modification of the technique, in particular, the use of a higher intensity setting on the gamma camera.[147]

Usually subsequent to traumatic rupture of the spleen, splenosis is the autotransplantation of splenic tissue.[148] The peritoneal cavity is the most commonly involved site when there is disruption of the spleen, resulting in seeding of splenic tissue throughout the body. The diagnosis of splenosis may be made by the absence of How-

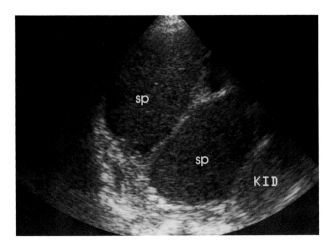

Fig. 10-47. Polysplenia. Sagittal scan of the right abdomen in this patient with multiple congenital anomalies (including situs inversus) demonstrates two splenic structures (*sp*). The patient also had interruption of the inferior vena cava with azygos continuation. (*KID,* left kidney.)

ell-Jolly bodies, siderocytes, and other postsplenectomy abnormalities on peripheral blood smear.[148] Ultrasound may be able to identify splenosis nodules as round hypoechoic masses.[149] A more specific diagnosis may be made on radionuclide scans. Splenosis and accessory spleens may be characterized by (1) association with medical history of spleen trauma with splenectomy (absent in accessory spleens), (2) numerous round masses of variable size shape (much fewer in accessory spleens), and (3) round masses distributed throughout the peritoneum and the retroperitoneum (in accessory spleen the masses are near the left side of the dorsal mesogastrium).[149]

The Spleen and Congenital Heart Disease

The infrequent asplenia/polysplenia syndromes occur in association with a variable constellation of complex cardiac malformations, bronchopulmonary abnormalities, and visceral heterotaxia (anomalous placement of organs or major blood vessels). The latter includes a horizontal liver, malrotation of the gut, and interruption of the inferior vena cava with azygous continuation[150] (Fig. 10-47). Although CT has recently been employed to demonstrate various components of polysplenia in a relatively older patient,[151] nuclear medicine techniques offer the most assistance in evaluation of these syndromes. Ultrasound, as a rule, is not used for evaluation in these instances.

There are several congenital cardiosplenic syndromes that may occur that consist of complex malformations, splenic anomalies, and intermediate situs.[152] Predominant in females, the asplenia type has bilateral right-sided features of a horizontal midline liver, Howell-Jolly bodies in the peripheral blood resulting from asplenia, and bilateral right lung morphology. Occurring mainly in males, the polysplenic type has bilateral left-sided features consisting of absence of a gallbladder and bilateral left lung morphology.[152] Both of these may be associated with situs ambiguous of the gastrointestinal tract.

TcSC may be the initial imaging agent utilized; however this agent may be unable to definitely establish the presence or absence of splenic tissue, owing to superimposition of a midline liver or inadequate resolution. In these instances, selective imaging of the spleen with heat-natured red blood cells labeled with ^{99m}Tc appears to be a complementary and superior technique.[153] Comparison of TcSC scans with scans employing hepatobili-

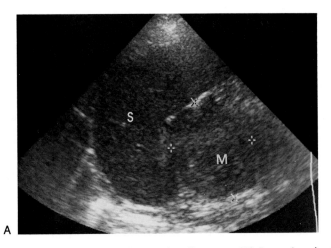

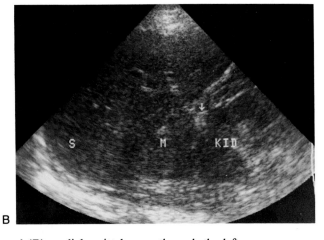

Fig. 10-48. Pancreatic tail tumor. **(A)** Lateral sagittal and **(B)** medial sagittal scans through the left upper quadrant demonstrate a solid mass (*M*, 52 × 44 mm) that is noted to be separate from spleen (*S*) and left kidney (*KID*). On CT scan, the mass could not be separated from spleen.

ary agents may be of use in suspected asplenia. A discrepancy in organ morphology between the two studies indicates the presence of the spleen, whereas similarity of the image suggests asplenia.[154]

Following injection of radionuclide agents into the foot veins, it is possible to image the inferior vena cava, and thus demonstrate inferior vena cava anomalies, including absence of the renal-to-hepatic portion with azygous extension, left-sided inferior vena cava, and double inferior vena cava.[155] Because the location of the inferior vena cava has great significance in establishing situs or abdominal heterotaxia, such radionuclide venography in conjunction with TcSC studies may obviate the need for arteriography in some instances. Similarly, this technique may be of considerable aid in the selection of the appropriate approach for cardiac catheterization in those patients who will undergo palliative or corrective surgery.

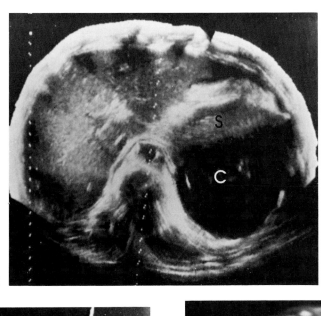

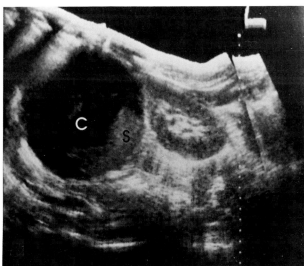

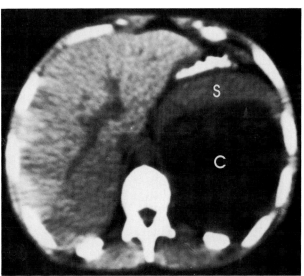

Fig. 10-49. Pancreatic pseudocyst involving spleen. **(A)** Supine, transverse scan at 16 cm above the umbilicus. A cystic mass (*C*) is seen in the left upper quadrant posterior to the spleen (*S*). **(B)** Prone, longitudinal scan demonstrating the relationship of the pseudocyst (*C*) to the spleen (*S*) and the left kidney. On ultrasound alone, this pseudocyst could not be differentiated from a splenic hematoma. (Fig. B from Mittelstaedt,[3] with permission.) **(C)** Enhanced CT scan. A large low-density area (pseudocyst, *C*) is seen posterior to the spleen (*S*). As with ultrasound, the relationship to pancreas could not be established and a splenic hematoma could not be excluded. (Figs. A & C from Mittelstaedt et al,[13] with permission.)

PERISPLENIC ABNORMALITIES

Lesions of the pancreas, left kidney, left adrenal gland, and left lobe of the liver may impinge on the spleen and mimic primary splenic disease.[156] Ultrasound is a valuable technique in differentiating primary splenic disease from perisplenic abnormalities.

Pancreatic Disease

Lesions of the body and tail of the pancreas can mimic a primary splenic process when extension of the inflammatory or neoplastic lesion occurs by direct extension or by extension along the splenorenal ligament (Figs. 10-48 and 10-49). This ligament attaches the tail of the pancreas to the visceral parietal covering of the spleen. Exudation of pancreatic fluid in the anterior pararenal space from acute pancreatitis may track along this ligament to produce a perisplenic or intrasplenic fluid accumulation that may mimic a splenic cyst or perisplenic abscess or hematoma[157,158] (Fig. 10-49).

TcSC scanning typically demonstrates an extrinsic impression on the spleen in the case of perisplenic abnormalities, whereas an intrasplenic lesion often shows a rim of functioning tissue around the photon-deficient area. However, the TcSC scan is frequently unable to differentiate primary splenic lesions from perisplenic abnormalities such as pancreatic disease, although it does provide a sensitive method for initial detection of such abnormalities.

Ultrasound examination may show a relatively anechoic fluid collection located posterior and lateral to the spleen, which is often anteromedially displaced (Fig. 10-49). Differentiation between an intrasplenic cyst, splenic hematoma, and an anechoic intrasplenic pancreatic pseudocyst may be extremely difficult unless the radiologist is aware of this uncommon entity and the clinical situation is appropriate. If the pseudocyst contains debris that produced internal echoes, it may be difficult to exclude necrotic tumor or abscess on the basis of the ultrasound appearance alone.

Computed tomography may help differentiate an intrasplenic pseudocyst from a primary splenic cyst by showing secondary signs of pancreatitis, thereby suggesting a pancreatic etiology. Secondary signs detected by CT include loss of the fat planes separating the pancreas from adjacent organs and thickening of Gerota's fascia lateral to the left kidney in the left paracolic gutter.[157]

The optimal radiographic assessment of a splenic defect or perisplenic fluid collection seen on TcSC or ultrasound includes confirmation of associated secondary findings of pancreatitis by CT scan. Needle aspiration of the perisplenic fluid collection using ultrasound or CT guidance may confirm an inflammatory pancreatic etiology by showing an elevated amylase. The aspirate may also be positive for carcinoma by cytology or demonstrate an unsuspected perisplenic abscess or hematoma.

Renal Disease

The upper pole of the left kidney impinges on the splenic hilum and the medial surface of the spleen is cupped around the lateral border of the left kidney. The

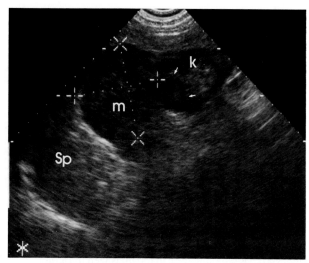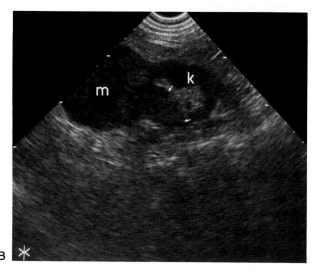

Fig. 10-50. Renal neoplasm. The left upper quadrant mass in this patient was demonstrated to be a mass (*m*) separate from spleen (*Sp*) on **(A)** sagittal supine and **(B)** right-lateral decubitus scans. It is seen to extend from the left kidney (*k*, arrows).

splenorenal ligament provides the attachment between the left kidney's perirenal space and the visceral parietal coat of the spleen.

A peripheral renal cyst that is situated in the lateral or superior left kidney may indent the splenic parenchyma and produce an impression on TcSC scan or ultrasound that is difficult to differentiate from a splenic cyst. If an extrinsic impression in the spleen is detected by TcSC scan, ultrasound of the spleen may demonstrate both the cyst and a "beak" of renal parenchyma surrounding it. This beak sign, as with excretory urography, is helpful in both CT and ultrasound demonstration of cysts. Used in conjunction, the ultrasound examination may confirm the cystic nature of the lesion and the CT scan with contrast enhancement may demonstrate the beak sign of renal parenchyma surrounding the cyst. CT alone is not entirely reliable in detection of benign cystic renal disease versus solid low-density neoplasm.

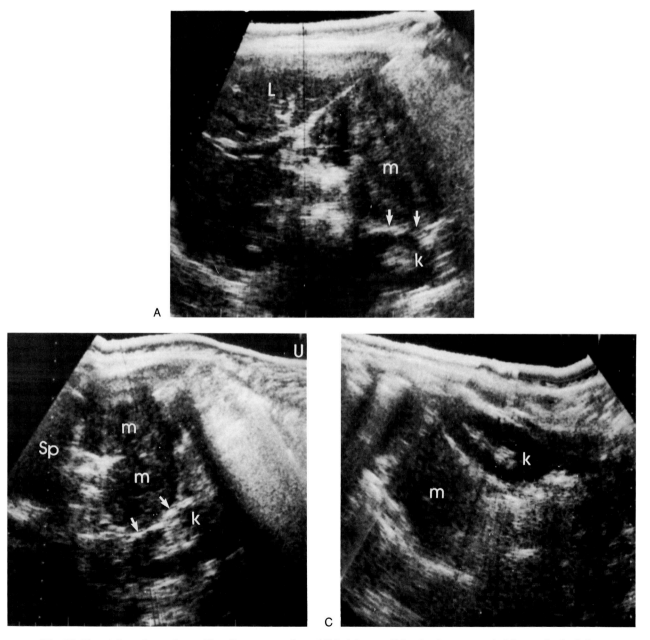

Fig. 10-51. Adrenal neoplasm. Ganglioneuroma in a child. A large solid, echodense mass (*m*) is seen in the left upper quadrant on (**A**) a transverse scan at 3 cm below the xyphoid and on (**B**) a longitudinal scan 4 cm to the left of midline. It cannot be entirely separated from spleen (*Sp*), although it seems to be separate (arrows) from the left kidney (*k*). (*L*, liver; *U*, level of the umbilicus.) (**C**) On a prone longitudinal scan at 4 cm to the left, the mass (*m*) appears separate from the left kidney (*k*). Spleen as such is not identified on this scan.

Neoplastic or inflammatory involvement of the kidney may extend retroperitoneally along the splenorenal ligament or directly into the spleen's medial surface (Fig. 10-50). Again, in confusing cases, needle aspiration may reveal the primary site of a neoplastic lesion or lead to percutaneous catheter drainage of a perisplenic or renal abscess.

Adrenal Lesions

The left adrenal gland may be the source of tumors or cysts that extrinsically compress the spleen (Fig. 10-51). Hemorrhage of the adrenal gland or adrenal cysts is usually confined to the perirenal space. If a cyst, tumor, or hematoma is not large enough to impinge on the spleen's medial border and be detected on TcSC scan, CT or ultrasound may suggest the adrenal etiology of this finding.

With the advent of high resolution CT scanning using 1.5-mm, 2-mm, or 4-mm slice thickness, the adrenals can be reliably imaged in nearly all patients. However, if an adrenal neoplasm is large enough to impress on the spleen, there may be some difficulty differentiating adrenal from renal primary, especially with tumor invasion of the left kidney on CT or ultrasound.

CONCLUSION

In general, screening for lesions suspected in the spleen can be done with TcSC techniques and/or ultrasound. Lesions in the left upper quadrant, whether they are within the spleen and adjacent organs or structures such as the kidney or diaphragm, can be effectively investigated with ultrasound. When localization is less certain, evaluation of the patient should probably be initiated with CT.

REFERENCES

1. Li DKB, Cooperberg PL, Graham MF, Callen P: Pseudo perisplenic "fluid collections": a clue to normal liver and spleen echogenic texture. J Ultrasound Med 1986;5:397
2. Taylor KJW: Atlas of Gray Scale Ultrasonography. Churchill Livingstone, New York, 1978
3. Mittelstaedt CA: Ultrasound of the spleen. p. 233. In Raymond HW, Zwiebel WJ (eds): Seminars in Ultrasound. Vol. 2. Grune & Stratton, Orlando, FL, 1981
4. Mittelstaedt CA, Partain CL: Ultrasonic-pathologic classification of splenic abnormalities: gray-scale patterns. Radiology 1980;134:697
5. Taylor KJW, Milan J: Differential diagnosis of chronic

splenomegaly by gray-scale ultrasonography: clinical observations and digital A-scan analysis. Br J Radiol 1976;49:519
5. Kay CJ, Pawar S, Rosenfield AT: Sonography of splenic abscesses. p. 91. In Raymond HW, Zwiebel WJ (eds): Seminars in Ultrasound: Abscesses. Vol. 4. Grune and Stratton, Orlando, FL, 1983
7. Robbins S, Cotran RS (eds): Spleen. p. 803. In Pathologic Basis of Disease. WB Saunders, Philadelphia, 1979
8. Pietri H, Boscaini M: Determination of a splenic volumetric index by ultrasonic scanning. J Ultrasound Med 1984;3:19
9. Ishibashi H, Higuchi N, Shimamura R et al: Sonographic assessment of grading of spleen size. J Clin Ultrasound 1991;19:21
10. Goerg C, Schwerk B, Goerg K, Havemann K: Sonographic patterns of the affected spleen in malignant lymphoma. J Clin Ultrasound 1990;18:569
11. Rosenberg HK, Markowitz RI, Kolberg H et al: Normal splenic size in infants and children: sonographic measurements. AJR 1991;157:119
12. Vicary FR, Souhami RL: Case reports: ultrasound and Hodgkin's disease of the spleen. Br J Radiol 1977;50:521
13. Mittelstaedt CA, McCartney WH, Mauro MA et al: Spleen. p. 235. In Simeone J (ed): Clinics in Diagnostic Ultrasound: Coordinated Diagnostic Imaging. Churchill Livingstone, New York, 1984
14. Brinkley AA, Lee JKT: Cystic hamartoma of the spleen: CT and sonographic findings. J Clin Ultrasound 1981;9:136
15. Ros PR, Moser RP Jr, Dachman AH et al: Hemangioma of the spleen: radiologic-pathologic correlation in ten cases. Radiology 1987;162:73
16. Manor A, Starinsky R, Garfinkel D et al: Ultrasound features of a symptomatic splenic hemangioma. J Clin Ultrasound 1984;12:95
17. Solbiati L, Bossi MC, Bellotti E et al: Focal lesions in the spleen: sonographic patterns and guided biopsy. AJR 1983;140:59
18. Niizawa M, Ishida H, Morikawa P et al: Color Doppler sonography in a case of splenic hemangioma: value of compressing the tumor. AJR 1991;157:965
19. Rao BK, AuBuchon J, Lieberman LM et al: Cystic lymphangiomatosis of the spleen: a radiologic-pathologic correlation. Radiology 1981;141:781
20. Shirkhoda A, McCartney WH, Staab EV et al: Imaging of the spleen: a proposed algorithm. AJR 1980;135:195
21. Tsurui N, Ishida H, Morikawa P et al: Splenic lymphangioma: report of two cases. J Clin Ultrasound 1991;19:244
22. Nahman B, Cuningham JJ: Sonography of splenic angiosarcoma. J Clin Ultrasound 1985;13:354
23. Stein RS: Saturday conference: non-Hodgkin's lymphoma. South Med J 1978;71:1261
24. Kaplan HS: Hodgkin's Disease. Harvard University Press, Cambridge, 1980
25. Ahmann DL, Kiely JM, Harrison EG, Payne WS: Malignant lymphoma of the spleen. Cancer 1966;19:461
26. Zornoza J, Ginaldi S: Computed tomography in hepatic lymphoma. Radiology 1981;138:405

27. Silverman S, DeNardo GL, Glatstein E, Lipton MJ: Evaluation of the liver and spleen in Hodgkin's disease. Am J Med 1972;52:362

28. McCaffrey JA, Rudders RA, Kahn PC et al: Clinical usefulness of Gallium-67 scanning in the malignant lymphomas. Am J Med 1976;60:523

29. Longo DL, Schilsky RL, Blei L et al: Gallium-67 scanning: limited usefulness in staging patients with non-Hodgkin's lymphoma. Am J Med 1980;68:695

30. Breiman RS, Castellino RA, Harell GS et al: CT-pathologic correlations in Hodgkin's disease and non-Hodgkin's lymphoma. Radiology 1978;126:159

31. Castellino RA: Noninvasive evaluation of lymphoma. Radiologic techniques. Presented at the 68th Annual Meeting of the Radiological Society of North America, Chicago, 1982

32. Goerg C, Schwerk WB, Goerg K: Sonography of focal lesions of the spleen. AJR 1991;156:949

33. Glees JP, Taylor KJW, Gazet JC et al: Accuracy of grayscale ultrasonography of liver and spleen in Hodgkin's disease and other lymphomas compared with isotope scans. Clin Radiol 1977;28:233

34. Berge T: Splenic metastases: frequencies and patterns. Acta Pathol Microbiol Scand 1974;82:499

35. Marymont JH, Gross S: Patterns of metastatic cancer in the spleen. Am J Clin Pathol 1963;40:58

36. Siniluoto T, Paivansalo M, Lahde S: Ultrasonography of splenic metastases. Acta Radiol 1989;30:463

37. Piekarski J, Federle MP, Moss AA, London SS: Computed tomography of the spleen. Radiology 1980;135:683

38. Verheyden CN, Van Heerden JA, Carney JA: Symptomatic metastatic melanoma of the spleen. Minn Med 1974;57:693

39. Murphy JF, Bernardino ME: The sonographic findings of splenic metastases. J Clin Ultrasound 1979;7:195

40. Paling MR, Shawker TH, Love IL: The sonographic appearance of metastatic malignant melanoma. J Ultrasound Med 1982;1:75

41. Adler DD, Silver TM, Abrams GD: The sonographic appearance of splenic plasmacytoma. J Ultrasound Med 1982;1:323

42. MacCarty RL, Wanner HW, Stephens DH et al: Retrospective comparison of radionuclide scans and computed tomography of the liver and pancreas. AJR 1977;129:23

43. Biello DR, Levitt RG, Siegel BA et al: Computed tomography and radionuclide imaging of the liver: a comparative evaluation. Radiology 1978;127:159

44. Snow JH, Goldstein HM, Wallace S: Comparison of scintigraphy, sonography, and computed tomography in the evaluation of hepatic neoplasm. AJR 1979;132:915

45. Knopf DR, Torres WE, Fajman WJ, Sones PF: Liver lesions: comparative accuracy of scintigraphy and computed tomography. AJR 1982;138:623

46. Kim EE: Focal splenic defect. Semin Nucl Med 1979;9:320

47. Goerg C, Schwerk WB: Splenic infarction: sonographic patterns, diagnosis, follow-up, and complications. Radiology 1990;174:803

48. Maresca G, Mirk P, De Gaetano AM et al: Sonographic patterns in splenic infarct. J Clin Ultrasound 1986;14:23

49. Weingarten MJ, Fakhry J, McCarthy J et al: Sonography after splenic embolization: the wedge-shaped acute infarct. AJR 1984;141:957

50. Roshkow JE, Sanders LM: Acute splenic sequestration crisis in two adults with sickle cell disease: US, CT, and MR imaging findings. Radiology 1990;177:723

51. Kumpe DA, Rumack CM, Pretorius DH et al: Partial splenic embolization in children with hypersplenism. Radiology 1985;155:357

52. Lawhorne TW, Zuidema GD: Splenic abscess. Surgery 1976;79:686

53. Hertzanu Y, Mendelsohn DB, Goudie E, Butterworth A: Splenic abscess: a review with the value of ultrasound. Clin Radiol 1983;34:661

54. Gadacz T, Way LW, Dunphy JE: Changing clinical spectrum of splenic abscess. Am J Surg 1974;128:182

55. Ralls PW, Quinn MF, Colletti P et al: Sonography of pyogenic splenic abscess. AJR 1982;138:523

56. Rudick MG, Wood BP, Lerner RM: Splenic abscess diagnosed by ultrasound in the pediatric patient: report of three cases. Pediatr Radiol 1983;13:269

57. Chulay JD, Landerani MR: Splenic abscess: report of ten cases and review of the literature. Am J Med 1976;61:513

58. Laurin S, Kaude JV: Diagnosis of liver-spleen abscesses in children with emphasis on ultrasound for the initial and followup examinations. Pediatr Radiol 1984;14:198

59. Brown JJ, Sumner TE, Crowe JE, Staffner LD: Preoperative diagnosis of splenic abscess by ultrasonography and radionuclide scanning. South Med J 1979;72:575

60. Pawar S, Kay CJ, Gonzalez R et al: Sonography of splenic abscess. AJR 1982;138:259

61. Grant E, Mertens MA, Mascatello VJ: Splenic abscess: comparison of four imaging methods. AJR 1979;132:465

62. Moss ML, Kirschner LP, Peereboom G, Fereis RA: CT demonstration of a splenic abscess not evident at surgery. AJR 1980;135:159

63. Chew FS, Smith PL, Barboriak D: Candidal splenic abscesses. AJR 1991;156:474

64. Wu CC, Chow KS, Lu TN et al: Tuberculous splenic abscess: sonographic detection and follow-up. J Clin Ultrasound 1990;18:205

65. Gupta RK, Pant CS, Ganguly SK: Ultrasound demonstration of amebic splenic abscess. J Clin Ultrasound 1987;15:555

66. Spouge AR, Wilson SR, Gopinath N et al: Extrapulmonary pneumocystis carinii in a patient with AIDS: sonographic findings. AJR 1990;155:76

67. Towers MJ, Withers CE, Hamilton PA et al: Visceral calcification in patients with AIDS may not always be due to pneumocystis carinii. AJR 1991;156:745

68. Fowler RH: Non-parasitic benign cystic tumors of the spleen. Int Abstr Surg 1953;96:209

69. Volpe JA, DeNardo GL: The preoperative diagnosis of spleen cysts by scintiscanning. AJR 1965;94:839

70. Shanser JD, Moss AA, Clark RE, Palubinskas AJ: Angiographic evaluation of cystic lesions of the spleen. AJR 1973;119:166

71. Franquet T, Montes M, Lecumberri FJ et al: Hydatid

disease of the spleen: imaging findings in nine patients. AJR 1990;154:525

72. Dachnan AH, Ros PR, Murari PJ et al: Nonparasitic splenic cysts: a report of 52 cases with radiologic-pathologic correlation. AJR 1986;147:537

73. Daneman A, Martin DJ: Congenital epithelial splenic cysts in children. Emphasis on sonographic appearances and some unusual features. Pediatr Radiol 1982;12:119

74. Ragozzino MW, Singletary H, Patrick R: Familial splenic epidermoid cyst. AJR 1990;155:1233

75. Rathaus V, Zissin R, Goldberg E: Spontaneous rupture of an epidermoid cyst of spleen: preoperative ultrasonographic diagnosis. J Clin Ultrasound 1991;19:235

76. Goldfinger M, Cohen MM, Steinhardt MI et al: Sonography and percutaneous aspiration of splenic epidermoid cyst. J Clin Ultrasound 1986;14:147

77. Moran C, Geisse G: Epidermoid cysts of the spleen. J Can Assoc Radiol 1977;28:150

78. Propper RA, Weinstein BJ, Skolnick ML, Kisloff B: Ultrasonography of hemorrhagic splenic cysts. J Clin Ultrasound 1979;7:18

79. Soderstrom N: How to use cytodiagnostic spleen puncture. Acta Med Scand 1976;199:1

80. Soderstrom N: Cytology of the spleen. p. 229. In Zajicek J (ed): Aspiration Biopsy Cytology, Part 2 Cytology of Infradiaphragmatic Organs. S Karger AG, Basle, Switzerland, 1979

81. Quinn SF, VanSonenberg E, Casola G et al: Interventional radiology in the spleen. Radiology 1986;161:289

82. Anderson WAD: Pathology. CV Mosby, St. Louis, 1971

83. Siler J, Hunter TB, Weiss J, Haber K: Increased echogenicity of the spleen in benign and malignant disease. AJR 1980;134:1011

84. Hunter TB, Haber K: Unusual sonographic appearance of the spleen in a case of myelofibrosis. AJR 1977;128:138

85. Cooperberg P: Ultrasonography of the spleen. p. 244. In Sarti DA, Sample WF (eds): Diagnostic Ultrasound: Text and Cases. GK Hall, Boston, 1980

86. Cunningham JJ: Ultrasonic findings in isolated lymphoma of the spleen simulating splenic abscess. J Clin Ultrasound 1978;6:412

87. Hill SC, Reinig JW, Barranger JA et al: Gaucher disease: sonographic appearance of the spleen. Radiology 1986;160:631

88. Stevens PG, Kumari-Subaiya SS, Kahn LB: Splenic involvement in Gaucher's disease: sonographic findings. J Clin Ultrasound 1987;15:397

89. Beckerman C, Gottschalk A: Diagnostic significance of the relative uptake of liver compared with spleen in 99m Tc sulfur colloid scintiphotography. J Nucl Med 1971;12:237

90. Stivelman RL, Glaubitz JP, Crampton RS: Laceration of the spleen due to nonpenetrating trauma: one hundred cases. Am J Surg 1963;106:888

91. Schwartz SI: Spleen. p. 1285. In Schwartz SI, Hume DM, Lillenei RC et al (eds): Principles of Surgery. McGraw-Hill, New York, 1974

92. Gentry LR, Brown JM, Lindren RD: Splenosis: CT demonstration of heterotopic autotransplantation of splenic tissue. J Comput Assist Tomogr 1982;6:1184

93. Villarreal-Rios A, Mays ET: Efficacy of clinical evaluation and selective splenic arteriography in splenic trauma. Am J Surg 1974;127:310

94. Lupien C, Sauerbrei EE: Healing in the traumatized spleen: sonographic investigation. Radiology 1984;151:181

95. Goodman PC, Federle MP: Splenorrgraphy: CT appearance. J Comput Assist Tomogr 1980;4:251

96. Johnson MA, Cooperberg PL, Boisvert J et al: Spontaneous splenic rupture in infectious mononucleosis: sonographic diagnosis and followup. AJR 1981;136:111

97. Ein SH, Shandling B, Simpson JS, Stephens CA: Nonoperative management of traumatic spleen in children: how and why. J Pediatr Surg 1978;113:117

98. Froelich JW, Simeone JF, McKusick DA et al: Radionuclide imaging and ultrasound in liver/spleen trauma: a prospective comparison. Radiology 1982;145:457

99. Asher WM, Parvin S, Virgillio RW, Haber K: Echographic evaluation of splenic injury after blunt trauma. Radiology 1976;118:411

100. Goodman LR, Aprahamian C: Changes in splenic size after abdominal trauma. Radiology 1990;176:629

101. Umlas SL, Cronan JJ: Splenic trauma: can CT grading systems enable prediction of successful nonsurgical treatment? Radiology 1991;178:481

102. Mirvis SE, Whitley NO, Gens DR: Blunt splenic trauma in adults: CT-based classification and correlation with prognosis and treatment. Radiology 1989;171:33

103. Scatamacchia SA, Raptopoulos V, Fink MP, Silva WE: Splenic trauma in adults: impact of CT grading on management. Radiology 1989;171:725

104. Morgenstern L, Uyeda RY: Nonoperative management of injuries of the spleen in adults. Surgery 1983;157:513

105. Michels NA: The variational anatomy of the spleen and splenic artery. Am J Anat 1942;70:21

106. Kreel L, Mindel S: The radiographic position of the spleen. Br J Radiol 1969;42:830

107. Landgarten S, Spencer RP: Splenic displacement due to gastric dilatation. J Nucl Med 1971;13:223

108. Go RT, Tonami N, Schapiro RL, Christie JH: The manifestations of diaphragmatic and juxta-diaphragmatic diseases in the liver-spleen scintigraph. Radiology 1975;115:119

109. Viamonte M, Sheldon JJ: Computed tomography. p. 320. In Margulis AR, Burhenne HJ (eds): Alimentary Tract Radiology (Abdominal Imaging). Vol. III. CV Mosby, St. Louis, 1979

110. Westcott JL, Krufky EL: The upside-down spleen. Radiology 1972;105:517

111. D'Altorio RA, Cano JY: Upside-down spleen as cause of suprarenal mass. Urology 1978;11:422

112. Madayag M, Bosniak MA, Beranbaum E, Becker J: Renal and suprarenal pseudotumors caused by variations of the spleen. Radiology 1972;105:43

113. Brown RB, Dobbie RP: Splenic indentation of the gastric fundus resembling gastric neoplasm. AJR 1959;81:599

114. Font RG, Sparks RD, Herbert GA: Ectopic spleen mim-

icking an intrinsic fundal lesion of the stomach. Am J Digest Dis 1970;15:49

115. Gooding GAW: The ultrasonic and computed tomographic appearance of splenic lobulations: a consideration in the ultrasonic differential of masses adjacent to the left kidney. Radiology 1978;126:719

116. Abell I: Wandering spleen with torsion of the pedicle. Ann Surg 1933;98:722

117. Woodward DAK: Torsion of the spleen. Am J Surg 1967;114:953

118. Kinori I, Rifkin MD: A truly wandering spleen. J Ultrasound Med 1988;7:101

119. Gordon DH, Burrell MI, Levin DC et al: Wandering spleen: the radiological and clinical spectrum. Radiology 1977;125:39

120. Sorgen RA, Robbins DI: Bleeding gastric varices secondary to wandering spleen. Gastrointest Radiol 1980;5:25

121. Kinare AS, Ambardekar ST, Pande SA: Sonographic diagnosis of splenic torsion in a spleen situated in the left upper quadrant. J Clin Ultrasound 1990;18:586

122. Hunter TB, Haber KK: Sonographic diagnosis of a wandering spleen. Am J Roentgenol 1977;129:925

123. Setiawan H, Harrell RS, Perret RS: Ectopic spleen. A sonographic diagnosis. Pediatr Radiol 1982;12:152

124. Isikoff MB, White DW, Diaconis JN: Torsion of the wandering spleen, seen as a migratory abdominal mass. Radiology 1977;123:36

125. Barnett SM, Poole JR, Briggs RC: Sequential liver-spleen scanning for documentation of wandering spleen. Clin Nucl Med 1981;6:528

126. Broker FHL, Khettry J, Filler RM, Treves S: Splenic torsion and accessory spleen: a scintigraphic demonstration. J Pediatr Surg 1975;10:913

127. Spencer RP, Dhawan V, Suresh K et al: Causes and temporal sequence of onset of functional asplenia in adults. Clin Nucl Med 1978;3:17

128. Curtis GM, Movitz D: The surgical significance of the accessory spleen. Ann Surg 1946;123:276

129. Subramanyam BR, Balthazar EJ, Horii SC: Sonography of the accessory spleen. AJR 1984;143:47

130. Spencer RP, Wasserman I, Dhawan V, Suresh K: Incidence of functional splenic tissue after surgical splenectomy. Clin Nucl Med 1977;2:63

131. Wahner-Roedler DL, Hoagland HC, Wahner HW: Idiopathic thrombocytopenic purpura: detection of accessory splenic tissue. Clin Nucl Med 1981;6:141

132. Babcock TL, Coker DD, Haynes JL, Conklin HB: Infarction of an accessory spleen causing an acute abdomen. Am J Surg 1974;127:336

133. Bass RT, Yao ST, Freeark RJ: Torsion of an accessory spleen of the cecum presenting as acute appendicitis. N Eng J Med 1967;277:1190

134. Stiris MG: Accessory spleen versus left adrenal tumor: computed tomographic and abdominal angiographic evaluation. J Comput Assist Tomogr 1980;4:543

135. Rosenkranz W, Kamhi B, Horowitz M: Retroperitoneal accessory spleen simulating a suprarenal mass. Br J Radiol 1969;42:939

136. Clark RE, Korobkin M, Palubinskas AJ: Angiography of accessory spleens. Radiology 1972;102:41

137. DasGupta TK, Busch RC: Accessory splenic tissue producing indentation of the gastric fundus resembling gastric neoplasm. N Engl J Med 1960;263:1360

138. Beahrs JR, Stephens DH: Enlarged accessory spleens: CT appearance in post-splenectomy patients. AJR 1980;135:483

139. Alter AJ, Uehling DT, Zwiebel WJ: Computed tomography of the retroperitoneum following nephrectomy. Radiology 1979;133:663

140. Spencer RP: Accessory splenic tissue and recurrence of idiopathic thrombocytopenic purpura or other hematologic disorders. Clin Nucl Med 1976;1:62

141. Verheyden CN, Beart RW, Clifton MD, Phyliky RL: Accessory splenectomy in management of recurrent idiopathic thrombocytopenic purpura. Mayo Clin Proc 1978;53:442

142. Atkins HL, Goldman AG, Fairchild RG et al: Splenic sequestration of 99m-Tc labeled, heat treated red blood cells. Radiology 1980;136:501

143. Moinuddin M: Splenosis: first scintigraphic demonstration of extension splenic implants. Clin Nucl Med 1982;7:67

144. Jacobson SJ, DeNardo GL: Splenosis demonstrated by splenic scan. J Nucl Med 1971;12:570

145. Pearson HA, Johnston D, Smith KA, Touloukian RJ: The born-again spleen: return of splenic function after splenectomy for trauma. N Engl J Med 1978;298:1389

146. Fitzer PM: Preoperative diagnosis of splenosis by 99m-Tc sulfur colloid scanning. Clin Nucl Med 1977;2:348

147. Andrus MS, Johnston GS: Visualization of residual splenic tissue: a high intensity technique. Clin Nucl Med 1981;6:577

148. Delamarre J, Capron JP, Drouard F et al: Splenosis: ultrasound and CT findings in a case complicated by an intraperitoneal implant traumatic hematoma. Gastrointest Radiol 1988;13:275

149. Maillard JC, Menu Y, Scherrer A et al: Intraperitoneal splenosis: diagnosis by ultrasound and computed tomography. Gastrointest Radiol 1989;14:179

150. Randall PA, Moller JH, Amplatz K: The spleen and congenital heart disease. AJR 1973;119:551

151. DeMaeyer P, Wilms G, Baert AL: Polysplenia. J Comput Assist Tomogr 1981;5:104

152. Dodds WJ, Taylor AJ, Erickson SJ et al: Radiologic imaging of splenic anomalies. AJR 1990;155:805

153. Ehrlich CP, Papanicolaou N, Treves S et al: Splenic scintigraphy using Tc-99m labeled heat-denatured red blood cells in pediatric patients: concise communication. J Nucl Med 1982;23:209

154. Rao BK, Shore RM, Lieberman LM, Polcyn RE: Dual radiopharmaceutical imaging in congenital asplenia syndrome. Radiology 1982;145:805

155. Freedom RM, Treves S: Splenic scintigraphy and radionuclide venography in the heterotaxy syndrome. Radiology 1973;107:381

156. Raymond HW, Zwiebel WJ: Gaumut: fluid filled left upper quadrant masses. p. 151. In Raymond HW, Zwiebel WJ (eds): Seminars in Ultrasound. Vol. 1. Grune & Stratton, Orlando, FL, 1980

157. Vick CW, Simeone JF, Ferrucci JT et al: Pancreatitis associated fluid collections involving the spleen: sonographic and computed tomographic appearance. Gastrointest Radiol 1981;6:247

158. Okuda K, Taguchit T, Tshinara K, Kono A: Intrasplenic pseudocyst of the pancreas. Clin Gastroenterol 1981;3:37

11

Vascular Evaluation

Gretchen A. W. Gooding

TECHNIQUE

Sonography of the blood vessels of the abdomen is usually performed to answer the following questions: Is there flow, and, if so, what are its characteristics? Do the veins have normal respiratory rhythmicity? Are the arteries triphasic or of low resistance on spectral analysis? Is there tortuosity, dissection, stenosis, occlusion, aneurysm, or arteriovenous communication?

Preparation

No particular preparation is necessary to visualize the great vessels of the abdomen. If visualization is obscured by bowel gas when the patient is supine and scanned in standard parasagittal and transverse planes, a coronal approach may be helpful, scanning in the plane of the midaxillary line. Alternatively, the patient can be turned to a lateral decubitus position and scanned coronally; this position places the aorta posterior to the inferior vena cava (IVC). This is a particularly effective way to see the renal artery origins and the iliac bifurcation (Fig. 11-1).[1,2] With splenomegaly, a right lateral decubitus scanning plane can be effective for seeing the great vessels.

Fasting for 8 to 12 hours may be beneficial for left renal artery visualization since both the stomach and colon can obscure that vessel.

Instrumentation

Vascular sonography requires not only real-time capability, but also flow characterization capacity provided by either duplex ultrasound or color Doppler. Spectral analysis of the flow is essential to distinguish artery from vein, to determine stenoses and low-flow states, and to verify occlusion, arteriovenous fistulae, or dissection.

Abdominal vessels such as the aorta and the IVC can be examined with a variety of transducers: linear, sector, phased, mechanical, or annular array. The thinner the patient, the higher the transducer frequency that can be effective; this allows for better resolution. Greater depth of penetration requires a lower-frequency transducer. The typical imaging frequencies used for these great vessels is 3.5 to 5 MHz. Doppler frequencies vary with the manufacturer and may be the same as or less than the imaging frequency. To sample for velocity, duplex sonography requires an ability to place a cursor in a particular area of the vessel, and this range gate can then be opened wide or narrow to fit the needs of the examination. Estimated flow volume determinations require the range gate to be opened fully to encompass the whole vessel on longitudinal scan. The timed average velocity generated can be multiplied by the area times 60 to yield an estimated volume in milliliters per minute. When stenosis is the abnormality to be evaluated, a narrow range gate may detect just where the greatest narrowing exists in the vessel. Angle correction enables the examiner to verify the angle of insonation, so that it can be

705

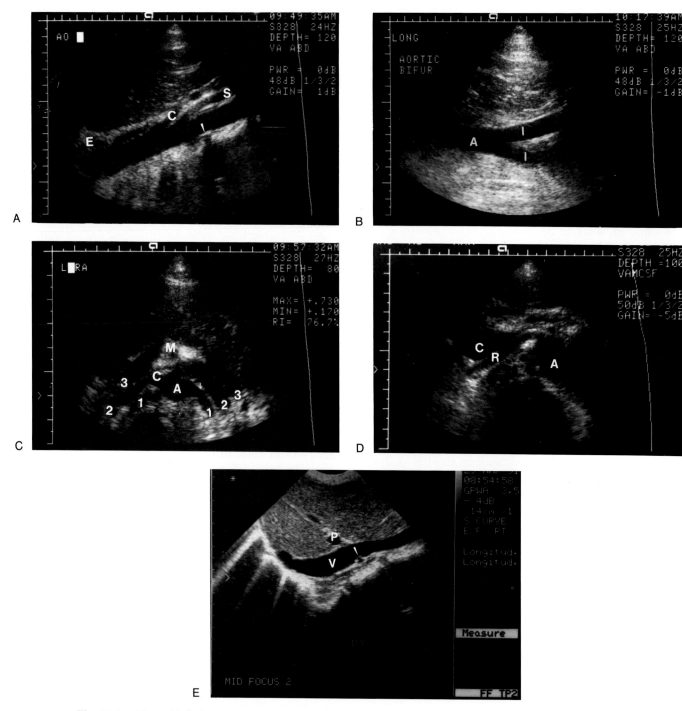

Fig. 11-1. Normal inferior vena cava and aorta. **(A)** Longitudinal sonogram of the abdominal aorta showing the normal celiac *(C)* and superior mesenteric *(S)* arteries and the cardioesophageal junction *(E)*. There is a calcified plaque on the posterior aorta wall, which casts an acoustic shadow (arrowhead). **(B)** Coronal image of the abdominal aorta *(A)* showing the iliac bifurcation *(I)*. **(C)** Transverse sonogram showing a normal aorta *(A)*, inferior vena cava *(C)*, the renal arteries *(1)*, the renal veins *(2)*, the splenoportal confluence *(3)*, and the superior mesenteric artery *(M)*. **(D)** Transverse scan of the abdominal aorta *(A)* demonstrating the right renal artery *(R)* behind the inferior vena cava *(C)*. **(E)** A longitudinal sonogram showing the inferior vena cava *(V)* and portal vein *(P)* surrounded by the liver and right renal artery (arrowhead).

adjusted to less than 60 degrees for a more accurate determination of velocity. An angle correction larger than reality will result in greater velocities than actually exist. This has more relevance in the carotid artery when diagnoses are made on the basis of abnormalities of velocity.

An audible Doppler signal helps to direct the interrogation of the vessel to the correct area as well.

Color Doppler is designed to recognize flow direction, the usual distinctions based on red and blue colors indicating opposite directions of flow in relation to the transducer. A lighter color indicates higher velocity. Turbulence produces disorganized color patterns in all directions, which can cause color to extend beyond the vessel lumen to the adjacent soft tissues.[3]

Color Doppler requires some change in the technique of scanning, since an oblique approach rather than the classic perpendicular gives greater color information and a better Doppler profile. The Doppler equation is such that the cosine of a 90-degree scanning angle is zero and so, theoretically, no Doppler information is generated.

Certain artifacts are inherent in the present systems. With color Doppler, mirror image artifacts can cause discrete focal flow reversals.[4] Tiny vessels of a few millimeters can be misregistered[5] or not detected. With increased gain settings, artificial color can occur in nonvascular anechoic areas.[6] High-pass filters set too high can eliminate low-level diastolic flow and cut off the initial systolic window at the baseline.

Ultrasonic contrast agents, one of which is human albumin microspheres,[7] offer potential to enhance arterial Doppler signals. Theoretically, this could be of value when areas of focal infarction are suspected and nonenhanced flow is minimal.

Scan Technique

The great vessels of the abdomen, the IVC and the aorta, are scanned by ultrasound in parasagittal and transverse planes from the diaphragm to the bifurcation at the umbilicus (Fig. 11-1). For the aorta, images are obtained in the proximal aorta, the midportion, and the distal area with a specific transverse view of the iliac bifurcation. In examining the IVC, normally only the portion subtended by the liver is apparent consistently. If the entire extent of the IVC is visible, this usually means that the patient has congestion.

NORMAL ANATOMY

Aorta

The abdominal aorta is an anechoic tapering tube just to the left of the midline that emanates from a diaphragmatic hiatus and divides at the level of the umbilicus into the common iliac arteries (Figs. 11-1 and 11-2). The aorta is mapped longitudinally and transversely by sonography throughout its length from the posterior diaphragm to a more anterior position at the umbilicus. By duplex sonography, the normal aorta has a triphasic waveform of high resistance on spectral analysis (Fig. 11-3). In plug flow (the type of flow found in the normal aorta), the column of blood travels at nearly the same velocity from the center of this large vessel to the walls. Peripheral flow in smaller vessels is parabolic, with the greatest velocity of flow in the center and the slowest flow along the walls. With color Doppler, slower arterial flow is red; high-velocity or stenotic flow is white. In the normal aorta, the entire vessel tends to be uniformly red, while the IVC is characteristically blue. Peak systolic velocities normally diminish proximally to distally both in native vessels and in peripheral grafts[8,9]; the peak systolic velocity in the aorta is greater than in the popliteal artery. Blood pressure, on the other hand, is higher in the ankles than in the upper extremities.

The bright double line at the interface of the aortic lumen noted by sonography has been reported as artifact[10] rather than intima, media, and adventitia.

In contrast to the IVC, the aorta is not readily compressible and maintains its shape when surrounded by extraneous masses such as adenopathy or horseshoe kidney (Fig. 11-4).

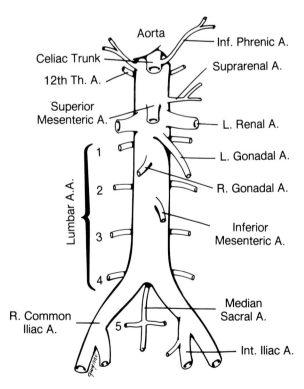

Fig. 11-2. Abdominal aorta and its branches.

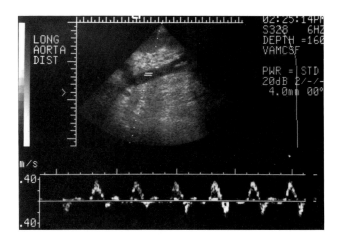

Fig. 11-3. Normal aorta. Longitudinal coronal scan of the aorta and the bifurcation of the iliac arteries showing a typical triphasic waveform on spectral analysis.

If color Doppler is available, the entire study may be videotaped in color and a few pertinent images photographed for the patient record. Alternatively, the study may be done in standard gray-scale and a few color images taken of the most important findings.

After images are obtained and recorded, spectral data are gathered from the duplex or color-coded images. The angle of insonation is adjusted to less than 60 degrees to document an accurate flow velocity and waveform. Flow velocity has more relevance for the arteries than the veins. In the IVC and the feeding branches, flow velocity is low and the actual velocity is of little importance. The main features of venous flow that should be determined by spectral analysis are the character and direction of the flow, its response to respiratory and augmentation maneuvers, and, in the iliac and more peripheral veins, the compressibility of the veins to external transducer pressure.

The atherosclerotic aorta is often tortuous and may twist and turn to either side of midline. To ensure accurate measurements in the transverse plane, the transducer is rotated at 90 degrees from the parasagittal plane of the aorta rather than rotating the transducer to a true transverse of the abdomen. Tortuosity will be recognized on color Doppler by the red and blue colors of disorganized flow. Increased velocity will be represented in white by most machines. However, the particular assignment of other colors varies with the manufacturer.

Aortic expansion should be measured in three planes: (1) sagittal; (2) transverse, at the greatest dilatation; and

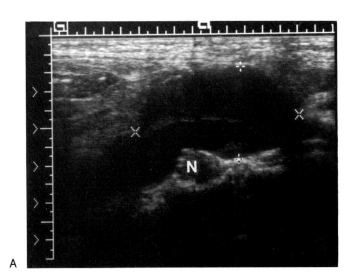

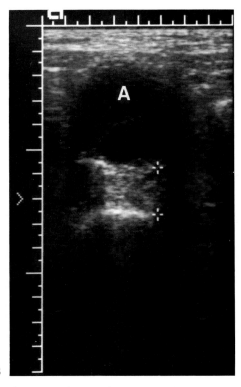

Fig. 11-4. Abdominal aortic aneurysm. **(A)** Longitudinal sonogram of an abdominal aortic aneurysm (calipers) showing a small node *(N)* posterior to the aorta. **(B)** The same aortic aneurysm *(A)* seen on transverse scan with the posterior lymph node (calipers).

(3) longitudinal, although the length is often an estimation if the aneurysm is longer than the field of view (Fig. 11-4). Outer wall to outer wall measurements are the norm, although consistency in where the measurements are taken is the most important factor, since these patients tend to be monitored over several years.

Aortic Branches

Renal Arteries

Most aortic aneurysms are well below the renal arteries, but an attempt should be made to verify the position of the renal arteries in relation to an aortic aneurysm. The approximate level of the renal arteries can be found by locating the longitudinal IVC, the transverse portal vein, and common hepatic duct in the same image, with the patient in a left lateral decubitus position (Fig. 11-1C–E). In this position, the right renal artery is posterior to the IVC just obliquely inferior to the common duct. In the same position, visualization of the longitudinal aorta in coronal section may reveal the bilateral origin of the renal arteries from the aorta.

The renal arteries are lateral branches of the inferior abdominal aorta and can be multiple (Fig. 11-1C). The typical renal arterial signal on duplex sonography is that of low resistance with a prominent forward diastolic component.

The renal arteries are not always identified by sonography, particularly on the left because they may be obscured by overlying air-filled stomach and bowel.

On transverse scan, the renal arteries are usually at the same level as the renal veins (Fig. 11-1C). The left renal vein crosses the midline between the superior mesenteric artery (SMA) and the aorta to empty into the IVC, while the left renal artery emanates directly lateral from the aorta to the left kidney. The right renal artery crosses posteriorly behind the IVC from the lateral aorta (Figs. 11-1C–E and 11-5), while the right renal vein empties directly into the IVC anterior to the renal artery.

MRI, CT, and angiography may be used to visualize renal artery involvement in abdominal aortic aneurysms when ultrasound fails.[11] The right renal artery can often be partially visualized when the patient is in a left lateral decubitus position. The renal origin is noted transversely on a longitudinal scan behind the IVC just obliquely opposite the portal vein and common hepatic duct (Fig. 11-1).

Mesenteric Branches

The celiac artery is the first anterior proximal branch of the abdominal aorta to be seen sonographically (Figs. 11-1A, 11-2, 11-6, and 11-7). On transverse images, the hepatic artery and splenic artery branches are consistently seen, while the left gastric is less consistently noted (Fig. 11-6B).

The SMA exits anteriorly from the aorta immediately inferior to the celiac artery (Figs. 11-1A & C, 11-2, and 11-7). On transverse scan, it is one of the markers of the position of the pancreas, the body of which is anterior, separated by the splenic/portal venous confluence (Fig. 11-1C). The left renal vein interposes between the SMA and the aorta.

The inferior mesenteric artery is not apparent routinely, but becomes enlarged and visible as a collateral pathway with obstruction of the celiac and superior mesenteric arteries.

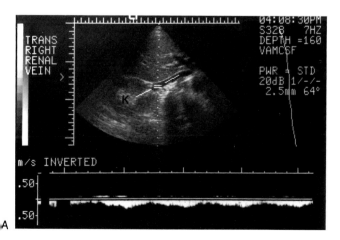

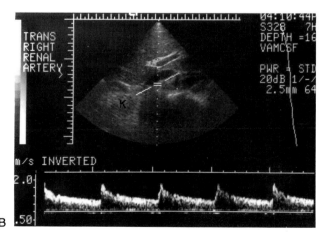

Fig. 11-5. Right renal vein and artery. **(A)** Transverse scan showing the length of the right renal vein. The spectral analysis documents a normal venous signal. (*K*, kidney.) **(B)** Transverse scan demonstrating a renal arterial signal, which has a characteristic low-impedance waveform, with prominent diastolic flow. (*K*, kidney.)

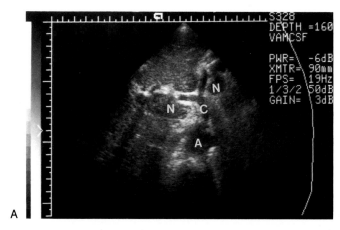
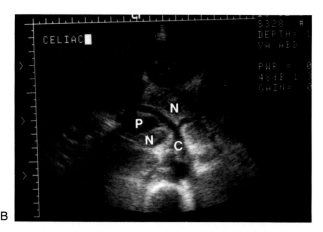

Fig. 11-6. Celiac artery. **(A)** Transverse sonogram of the aorta *(A)* showing the origin of the celiac axis *(C)* with nodes *(N)* adjacent in a patient with acquired immunodeficiency syndrome (AIDS). **(B)** Transverse scan demonstrating the celiac axis *(C)*, with the hepatic artery branch on the right of the patient and the splenic artery branch on the left. A node *(N)* is in the crotch of this bifurcation, and another is posterior to the portal vein *(P)*. This patient has AIDS.

The celiac artery and SMA are the first and second branches, respectively, of the abdominal aorta (Figs. 11-6 and 11-7). These are midline and anterior vessels. The celiac artery feeding the liver, spleen, and stomach has a low-impedance signal on spectral analysis.[12] The SMA is more highly resistant in the fasting state, but converts to a low-resistance waveform after eating[13]; this is accompanied by elevated velocities of increased flow.[13-15] In malrotation, the sonographic image of the SMA on transverse scan is reversed to the right of the midline rather than to the left.[16]

The SMA occasionally gives off an accessory or replaced hepatic artery, which, on transverse scan, is noted as a little tube emanating from the SMA on the right that travels to the lines posterior to the portal vein, rather than the typical anterior pathway.

Iliac Arteries

The iliac artery and vein lie in the posterior pelvis and can be obscured by overlying bowel gas (Figs. 11-1B, 11-2, 11-3, and 11-8).[17]

Coronal scans of the distal aorta may identify the proximal origin of the common iliac arteries (Figs. 11-1B and 11-3). The scanning plane most successfully used to visualize the iliac arteries is an oblique one from the

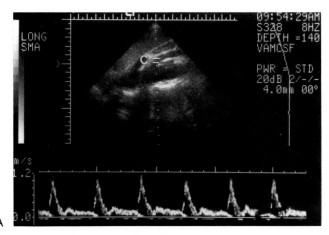
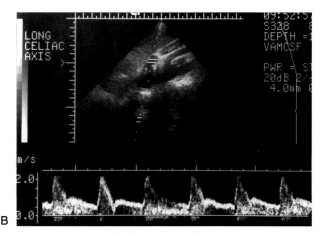

Fig. 11-7. Celiac and superior mesenteric arteries. **(A)** Longitudinal scan of the aorta showing the proximal origin of the celiac artery *(C)* followed by the origin of the superior mesenteric artery (caliper). The superior mesenteric artery has high-resistance flow and is triphasic. **(B)** Longitudinal sonogram of the abdominal aorta showing a caliper in the celiac artery and a waveform that has more diastolic flow than the superior mesenteric artery.

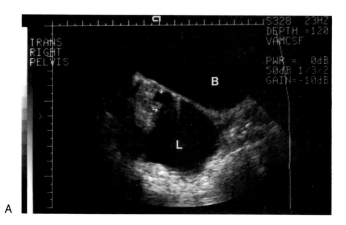

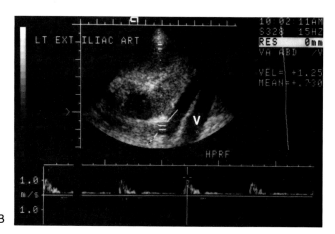

A   B

Fig. 11-8. Iliac artery and vein. **(A)** Transverse oblique sonogram of the pelvis showing the bladder anteriorly *(B)*, a lymphocele *(L)* posteriorly, immediately adjacent to the iliac artery (top arrow) and the iliac vein (bottom arrow). **(B)** Oblique sonogram in the pelvis defining the normal external iliac artery (caliper, origin of the renal artery to a renal transplant) and the external iliac vein posterior to it *(V)*.

umbilicus to the femoral artery at the inguinal ligament. A full bladder is an aid to sighting.

The internal iliac artery and veins are not reliably identified by sonography, but the external iliac artery and vein are; they both track from deep in the pelvis to a superficial position at the inguinal ligament.

The iliac artery has a well-defined triphasic waveform on spectral analysis, and the vein has a typical venous Doppler signal hovering near baseline and responsive to respiratory maneuvers and augmentation. An augmented venous signal is produced by a peripheral squeeze of the soft tissues of the thigh, which, when no obstruction intervenes, renders a bolus of venous flow of increased velocity into the iliac vessels.

Inferior Vena Cava

The IVC, formed from the junction of the common iliac veins, is an expandable channel to the right of midline, parallel to the adjacent aorta and, typically, homogeneously blue on color coding (Figs. 11-1C–E and 11-9 to 11-11). Curving upward proximally, the IVC empties into the right atrium while the adjacent aorta is more posterior at this diaphragmatic level.

Ordinarily, the IVC is well seen proximally as it enters and traverses the liver. More distally it is not typically seen in its entirety unless expanded by congestive failure, tricuspid regurgitation,[18] constrictive pericardial disease,[19] or right atrial tumor. Cardiac tamponade from pericardial effusion[20] causes the IVC to become enlarged and unresponsive to respiratory maneuvers, as does an aortocaval fistula.

The normal IVC is readily affected by changes in respiration, but the effects are difficult to monitor in progress by real-time sonography since the IVC tends to move out of the field of view of the transducer. During a Valsalva maneuver, increased abdominal pressure compresses the IVC, as does inspiration. Nephrologists[21] have used the diameter of the IVC and its normal ability

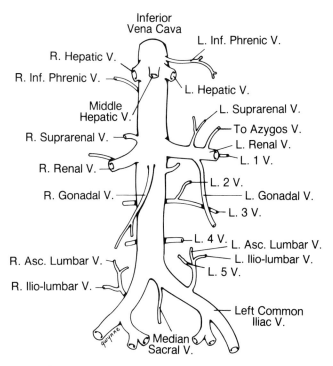

Fig. 11-9. Inferior vena cava and its tributaries.

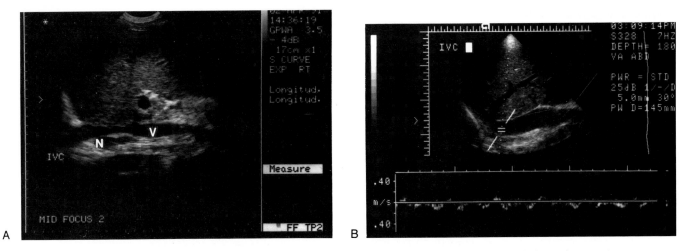

Fig. 11-10. Normal inferior vena cava. **(A)** Longitudinal sonogram of the inferior vena cava *(V)* showing a node *(N)* posterior to it in a patient with AIDS. **(B)** Longitudinal sonogram of the inferior vena cava showing a less than perfect waveform on spectral analysis, because the angle has not been corrected to the inferior vena cava flow, but is still adjusted for the hepatic vein.

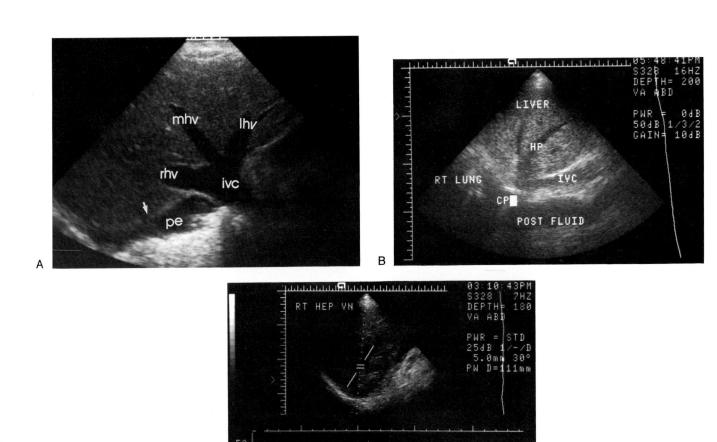

Fig. 11-11. Hepatic veins. **(A)** Transverse scan through the junction of the hepatic veins with the inferior vena cava *(ivc)* in a patient with congestive failure that is producing dilatation of the hepatic veins. *(rhv,* right hepatic vein; *mhv,* middle hepatic vein; *lhv,* left hepatic vein; *pe,* pleural effusion; arrow, diaphragm.) **(B)** Longitudinal sonogram of the inferior vena cava *(IVC)* and the hepatic veins *(HP)* showing fluid in the costophrenic sulcus *(CP)* and a large retroperitoneal fluid collection *(POST FLUID)* posterior to the inferior vena cava following surgery. **(C)** Longitudinal sonogram of the right hepatic vein showing the typical waveform on spectral analysis, that of transmitted atrial contractions. The angle of insonation is correct, and excellent flow is noted.

to decrease in size on deep inspiration as an indicator of fluid equilibration in patients on hemodialysis.

Patients receiving intermittent positive-pressure ventilation respond physiologically to increased intrathoracic pressure by developing an increased IVC diameter during both inspiration and expiration[22]; these changes are related to venous stasis and diminished venous return to the heart.

Cardiologists use the expiratory/inspiratory IVC diameters near the junction with the right atrium to develop a caval index of the percent collapse as a function of right atrial pressure.[23] A caval index of 50 percent or greater indicates a right atrial pressure less than 10 mmHg,[23] and indices less than that indicate elevation greater than 10 mmHg.

The typical waveform of the IVC on spectral analysis is one that reflects both respiratory variation and transmitted atrial contractions. This is damped by partial thrombosis or compression, whether from external pressure or from internal neoplastic or fibrotic involvement. With damping, the IVC waveform converts to a continuous low-velocity signal reminiscent of the normal portal vein signal.[24] IVC flow can actually be monitored by Doppler in utero.[25]

When extremely congested, the IVC may exhibit low level echoes posteriorly, a layering effect of slowly moving red blood cells, which resolves with improved circulation following treatment. This phenomenon of layering is probably related to abnormally low shear rates of flow.[26]

Inferior Vena Cava Branches

Hepatic Veins

The first branches to the IVC are the hepatic veins (right, middle, and left), which are identified on both longitudinal and transverse scans of the liver and can be followed to their convergence into the right atrium (Figs. 11-9 and 11-11). The spectral waveform of the hepatic veins is identical to that of the IVC, and the changes that affect the IVC, such as damping of the signal by partial thrombosis, are translated to the hepatic veins (Figs. 11-10B and 11-11B & C). Right-heart failure and tricuspid insufficiency accentuate the signal formed on the basis of transmitted atrial contractions and respiratory motion.

Renal Veins and Gonadal Veins

The next major set of veins draining into the IVC are the renal veins, which are anterior to the renal arteries (Figs. 11-1C, 11-5A, and 11-9). The renal veins are best seen on transverse scan at the level of the pancreas (Figs.

11-1C, and 11-5A). On transverse scan, dilatation of the left renal vein is typically noted as a normal finding on the left, before it narrows to traverse between the aorta and the SMA (Fig. 11-1C).[27] Abnormal dilatation of the left renal vein may result from collateral flow in portal hypertension or in arteriovenous fistula. Thrombosis or tumor can also expand the vein unilaterally. Bilateral renal vein enlargement occurs in congestive heart failure or proximal IVC obstruction.

Occasionally, the gonadal veins are recognized sonographically, the right emptying into the IVC and the left emptying into the left renal vein (Fig. 11-9).

Ascending Lumbar Vein

The right ascending lumbar vein may be noted sonographically as a 2-mm tiny tube dorsal to the IVC and the aorta on transverse scan, behind the right renal artery (Fig. 11-12).[28] With congenital absence of the IVC or obstruction to flow in the IVC, the lumbar veins enlarge to become major collateral flow channels to the azygous and hemiazygous systems (Fig. 11-13).

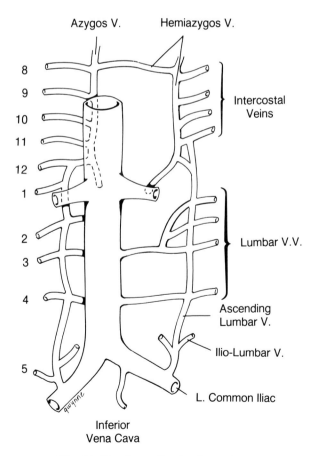

Fig. 11-12. Ascending lumbar vein.

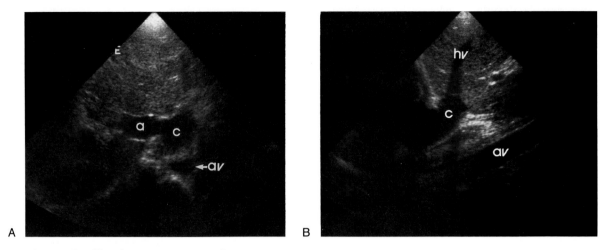

Fig. 11-13. Situs inversus and congenital absence of the inferior vena cava. **(A)** High transverse scan demonstrating the aorta *(a)* on the right, the hepatic vein confluence *(c)*, and the dilated azygos vein *(av)*. **(B)** Sagittal view of the left upper quadrant with visualization of the hepatic vein confluence *(c)*, hepatic vein *(hv)*, and dilated azygos vein *(av)*.

Iliac Veins

The iliac veins converge to form the IVC and have all the characteristics of normal venous flow (i.e., respiratory rhythmicity, response to augmentation) and of the external branches, which are more superficial in position and more amenable to transducer pressure than the deeper common iliac veins (Figs. 11-8 and 11-9). As abdominal vessels, the iliac veins diminish in size with a Valsalva maneuver because of increased abdominal pressure.

AORTIC ABNORMALITIES

Fetal Aorta

Normal fetal aortic flow can be monitored during gestation.[29] By measuring fetal mean aortic velocities, investigators have predicted fetal anemia in isoimmunized fetuses[30]; there is a positive correlation between increased aortic velocity and decreased hemoglobin levels. Normal fetal aortic flow is continuous and positive throughout the cardiac cycle.[31] Fetal aortic blood flow

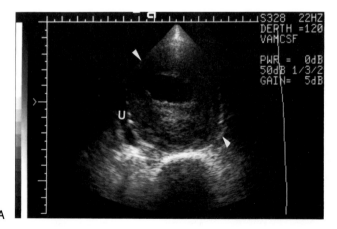
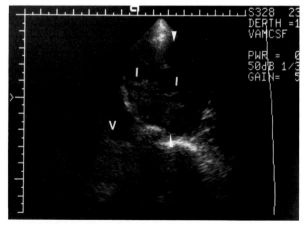

Fig. 11-14. Abdominal aortic aneurysm. **(A)** Transverse scan of the abdominal aorta demonstrating a large aortic aneurysm (arrowheads) with circumferential thrombus. A lucency to the right of the aorta *(U)* raised the possibility of free fluid, but this proved to be the ureter on CT. **(B)** More distal transverse sonogram showing the common iliac limbs *(I)* surrounded by the circumferential thrombus (arrowheads) extending from the aorta. *(V,* inferior vena cava.)

with an absent end diastole on spectral analysis indicates high resistance to flow[32] and is related to fetal distress and growth retardation.[31] Reverse diastolic flow in the descending aorta of the fetus appears to be an indicator of severe fetal asphyxia suggestive of impending fetal demise.[33]

Prenatal echocardiographic studies of coarctation of the fetal aorta[34] show reduced aortic blood flow, a large right ventricle, and a large pulmonary artery, but these findings are not specific. In children, color Doppler has been used in the diagnosis of coarctation of the aorta, with marked turbulence noted at the site of stenosis.[35]

Atherosclerosis

With development of atherosclerosis, the aortic wall becomes irregular from plaque formation. Calcifications along the wall are common and cast a typical acoustic shadow (Fig. 11-1A).

Abdominal Aortic Aneurysm

Abdominal aortic aneurysms (AAAs) are rarely congenital.[36] Most occur in elderly men with a genetic predisposition, are atherosclerotic in origin, and are distal to the renal arteries (97 percent) (Figs. 11-4, 11-14, and 11-15).[37] The sonographic criterion is focal dilatation of the aorta of 3 cm in AP diameter or greater. The sonographic diagnosis of AAA is highly accurate (98 percent). Since AAAs tend to be monitored at routine intervals by sonography, accurate measurements of their height, width, and length are important. These aneurysms, whether saccular (Fig. 11-16) or fusiform (Fig. 11-17), tend to be slowly progressive, averaging an increase in diameter of 0.4 to 0.5 cm/yr in one study[38] and only 0.21 cm/yr in another study.[39] Dramatic increases in size even without symptoms occur unpredictably.[40] In an early experience with color Doppler, abdominal aneurysms tended to have either (1) laminar flow that was red, with large amounts of thrombus restricting the

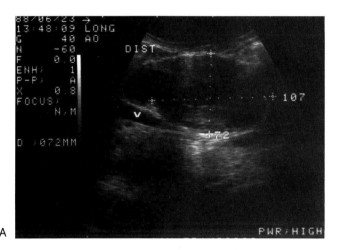

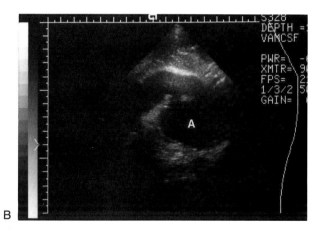

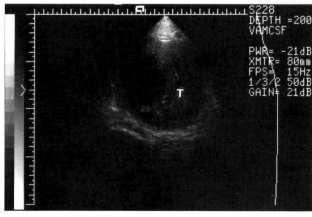

Fig. 11-15. Abdominal aortic aneurysm. **(A)** Longitudinal sonogram showing a large abdominal aortic aneurysm, 7 cm in diameter (calipers), that compresses the inferior vena cava *(V)*. **(B)** Longitudinal sonogram showing a remarkably tortuous aorta and an aortic aneurysm *(A)*. **(C)** Transverse scan of an abdominal aortic aneurysm showing eccentric thrombus *(T)*.

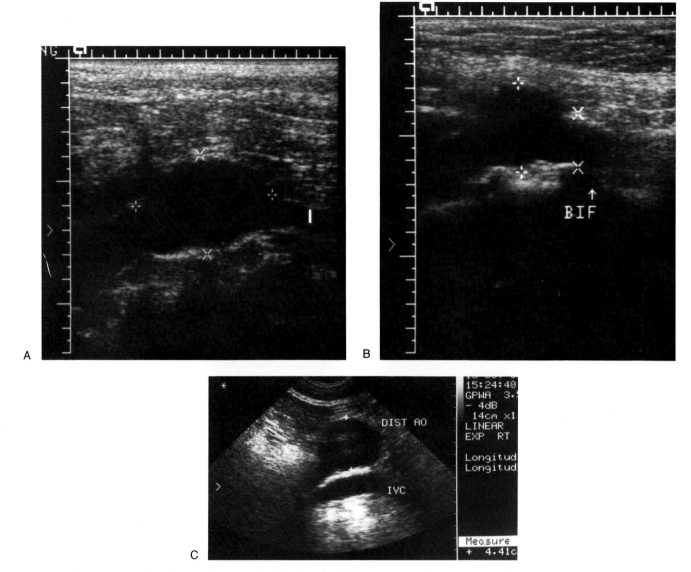

Fig. 11-16. Saccular aortic aneurysm. **(A)** Longitudinal sonogram of the aorta showing a saccular focal distal abdominal aortic aneurysm (calipers) and a normal iliac artery *(I)*. **(B)** Longitudinal sonogram of the aorta showing a small saccular aneurysm (calipers) that extends into the iliac artery *(X)*. **(C)** Longitudinal sonogram of the aorta showing a saccular aneurysm and demonstrating with tortuosity how the aorta *(DIST AO)* may be anterior to the inferior vena cava *(IVC)*.

lumen size, or (2) in large aneurysms without much thrombus, turbulent chaotic flow with pixels of different colors.[41] Calcifications are common in the aneurysmal wall, along the inner lumen, and within the thrombus itself.

Large AAAs (6 cm or larger) have a natural tendency to expand (Fig. 11-15A). Over 5 years, 25 percent of AAAs 5 cm or more may rupture.[39] AAAs smaller than 5 cm have a low risk of rupture.[39] No rupture occurred in one study of 130 patients with an AAA less than 5 cm.[39]

Occasionally, infrarenal AAAs extend above or are adjacent to the renal artery origins and are misinterpreted by ultrasound or CT as actually involving the renal arteries.[42] Since renal artery involvement has a much more serious prognosis, this misinterpretation may be avoided by proceeding to angiography for a definitive diagnosis. Occasionally, the entire aorta and iliac arteries are markedly dilated throughout their course. This has been related to an abnormality of the media.

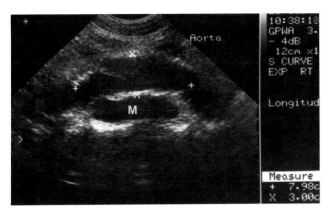

Fig. 11-17. Fusiform aneurysm. Longitudinal sonogram of the aorta showing a fusiform aortic aneurysm (calipers). The aneurysm is elevated by a lymphomatous mass posteriorly *(M)*.

Dissection

Abdominal aortic dissection is as a rule an extension of a thoracic aortic disease process that arises distal to the subclavian artery (type B) and occurs predominantly in hypertensive males (Figs. 11-18 and 11-19). Of these hypertensive men, 16 percent are likely to have renovascular hypertension from renal artery stenosis.[43] Marfan syndrome and bicuspid aortic valve, coarctation, and trauma are other etiologies. Thoracic dissecting aneurysms can be detected by transesophageal color Doppler, but experience is limited.[44,45] Acute aortic dissection confined to the abdomen is rare, although isolated instances occur.[46] Sonography of the classic abdominal aortic dissection shows a highly mobile pulsating, sharp zigzag interface of the intima media separated from the media-adventitia (Fig. 11-20).[47-49] Reentry is usually in the iliac artery. In the carotid artery, Kotval et al[50] have demonstrated reversed systolic flow in one compartment of the dissection and forward flow in the other.

During interventional procedures a focal area of intimal flap may be raised; this is usually more rigid in sonographic appearance than the classic aortic dissection.

Anechoic thrombus dorsal to hyperechoic thrombus in an aortic aneurysm[51] can be mistaken for chronic thrombosed dissection. CT may clarify the issue. Chronic dissections (Fig. 11-18)[52] have a lower mortality than (1) acute dissections, (2) those associated with pain, (3) those involving the visceral vessels, and (4) those that rupture. Angiography is the definitive diagnostic test. In the acute case, focal aortic replacement with a graft is the appropriate therapy.

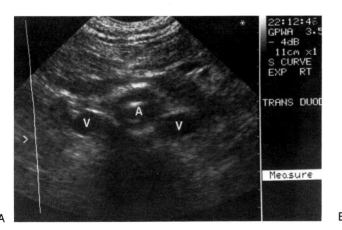

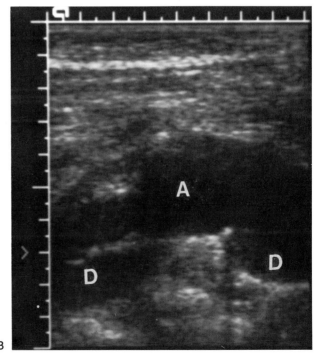

Fig. 11-18. Aorta dissection. **(A)** Transverse sonogram of the midline aorta *(A)* showing evidence of a chronic dissection. On either side of the aorta is a duplicated inferior vena cava *(V)*. **(B)** Longitudinal sonogram of a distal aortic aneurysm *(A)* also demonstrating a chronic dissection *(D)*, proven by CT.

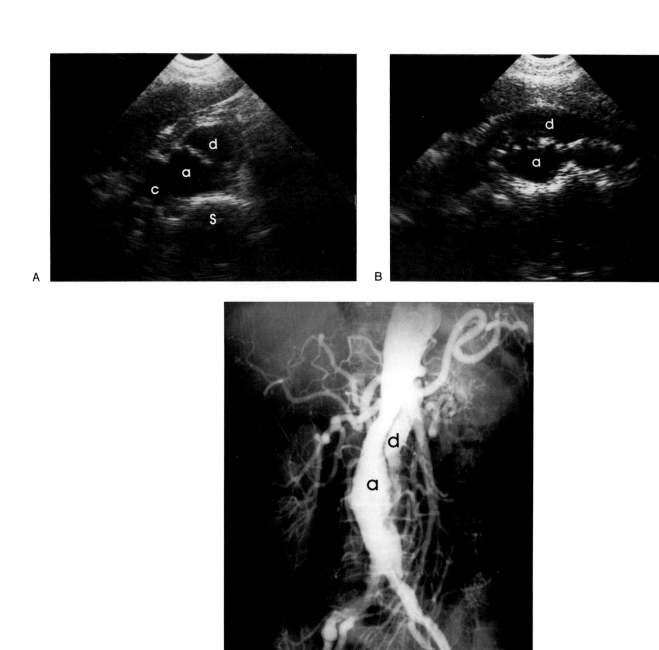

Fig. 11-19. Dissecting aortic aneurysm. False lumen. **(A)** Transverse scan. The aorta *(a)* is displaced to the right by the false lumen *(d)* anterolaterally. The inferior vena cava *(c)* is compressed on this scan (S, spine.) **(B)** Longitudinal scan of a dissecting aortic aneurysm. Two lumens, true *(a)* and false *(d),* are seen. **(C)** Angiogram demonstrating the true *(a)* and false *(d)* lumens.

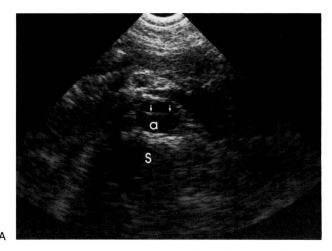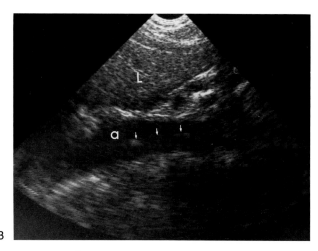

Fig. 11-20. Aortic dissection: intimal flap. **(A)** Transverse and **(B)** sagittal scans of aortic dissection. A small linear echodensity (arrows) is seen within the aortic *(a)* lumen. This represented an intimal flap that moved in real-time. (S, spine; *L,* liver.)

Ruptured Aortic Aneurysm

Patients with ruptured AAA have a high mortality (70 to 90 percent),[53] and those suspected of rupture require emergent surgery. Although sonography is used to show large aneurysms, again usually below the renal artery, one study demonstrated that it was not particularly sensitive (4 percent)[54] in detecting large fluid collections related to hemorrhage, which are often in the area of the retroperitoneal psoas muscle (commonly on the left side) (Fig. 11-21).[55] After repair of aortic rupture, these large collections take months to resolve.

Death from aortic rupture is largely preventable. Elective resection of an aortic aneurysm based on physiologic rather than actual age has a low mortality (<5 percent).[56] Because the rate of clinical detection of AAA by palpation, is not great (positive predictive value of only 14.7 percent[57-59]), sonographic screening of those at risk is recommended, particularly in men over 65 years old with peripheral vascular disease, especially those who smoke, have hypertension, and chronic obstructive pulmonary diseases.[58-62] Because of a genetic predisposition, their siblings over 55 should also be monitored since about 25 percent of brothers and 7 percent of sisters are at risk[63] for AAA in middle age.

Aortocaval Fistulae

About 5 percent of patients with AAA, regardless of its size, present with distal embolization as the first indication of disease,[64] and these patients have an associated high morbidity. Aortocaval fistulae rarely are (1 percent of patients) a complication of AAA (Fig. 11-22).[65,66]

They produce highly turbulent, high-volume, continuous low-resistance flow on duplex ultrasound and color Doppler. The IVC is enlarged. Aortocaval fistulae also occur from blunt trauma[67] and in 4 percent of ruptured aortic aneurysms.[65]

Six cases of traumatic aorta left renal vein fistulae have been reported[68,69]; one occurred spontaneously as a result of rupture of an AAA.

High-volume flow is a reliable characteristic of arteriovenous communication. The veins enlarge, and the arteries are prominent. Estimated flow can be calculated by determining a peak velocity and an average velocity over time from a longitudinal image. Then, an area of the vessel in cross-section is obtained. The average velocity over time multiplied by the area times 60 equals the estimated volume of flow in milliliters per minute. This calculation is subject to a number of errors but may help confirm that increased flow actually exists.

Aortic Coarctation

Aortic coarctation can develop in the abdominal aorta as a congenital or acquired lesion, located above the renal arteries, interrenal or infrarenal in position. Sonography reveals a focal aortic narrowing. This sometimes occurs in Takayasu's arteritis.

Aortic Thrombosis

Aortic thrombosis is not an entity detectable by B-mode ultrasound since the sonographic appearance is identical to that of the normal aorta, an anechoic taper-

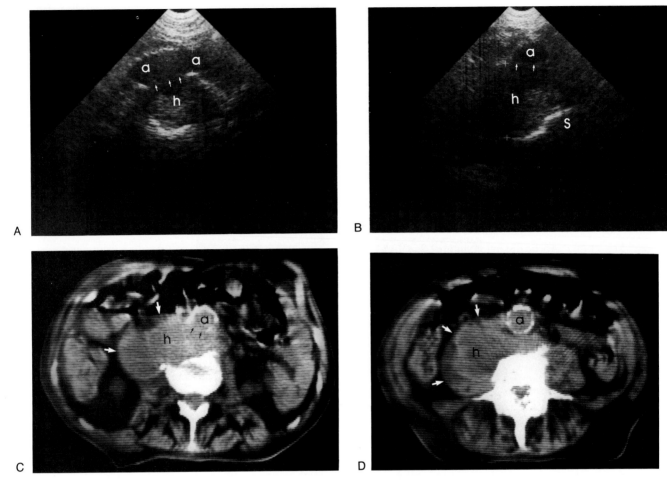

Fig. 11-21.   Ruptured aortic aneurysm. **(A)** Longitudinal scan of a ruptured aortic aneurysm with what appears to be discontinuity in the posterior wall (arrows) of the aorta *(a)*. There is an echogenic mass representing a hematoma *(h)* posterior in that area and to the right of midline. **(B)** Transverse scan of the same ruptured aortic aneurysm. *(S,* spine.) **(C & D)** CT scans displaying the ruptured aortic wall *(a,* black arrows) with a hematoma *(h,* white arrows) seen as a soft tissue density mass in the right retroperitoneum.

ing midline tube (Fig. 11-23).[70] With duplex ultrasound or color Doppler, no signal is evident. In neonates, aortic thrombosis is a complication of umbilical artery catheterization,[71] and long-term follow-up of these infants indicates related complications, including renovascular hypertension and leg growth abnormalities, even though flow documented by Doppler had been restored[72] to normal.

Other Complications

About 4 percent of AAA are associated with perianeurysmal fibrosis, which is especially prominent anteriorly and laterally.[73] These so-called inflammatory aneurysms[74] are more likely to cause back and abdominal pain, are less likely to rupture, and tend to be accompa-

nied both by an elevated sedimentation rate[75] and elevated creatinine levels; the latter are related to fibrosis around the ureters, causing hydronephrosis.[76] The cause is not known.

Curiously, cholelithiasis is present in about 50 percent of those with AAA.[77]

In one series following AAA repair, hydronephrosis developed transiently in 12 percent but creatinine only resolved spontaneously by the end of the first year.[78]

Large AAAs can compress the ureter to produce unilateral hydronephrosis or narrow the renal artery, which results in hypertension and renal ischemia (Fig. 11-14A).[79] Renal artery involvement is more accurately evaluated by angiography, MRI, or CT.[80]

Suprarenal aortic aneurysms are more likely to be mycotic,[81] syphilitic, or traumatic or to be extensions of thoracic aneurysms.[82] Digital subtraction angiography

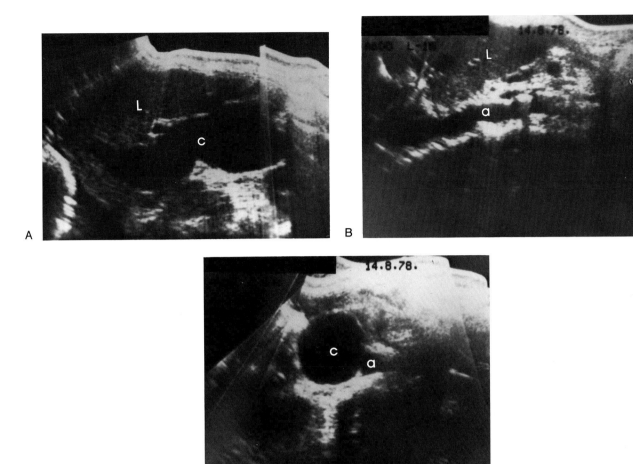

Fig. 11-22. Aortocaval fistula. **(A)** Longitudinal scan of an aortocaval fistula 7 cm to the right of midline. The inferior vena cava *(c)* is markedly dilated. *(L*, liver.) **(B)** Longitudinal scan of an aortocaval fistula 1 cm to the left of midline. The abdominal aorta *(a)* does not exhibit aneurysmal dilatation. (L, liver.) **(C)** Transverse scan of an aortocaval fistula 8 cm below the xyphoid. The markedly distended inferior vena cava *(c)* and normal aorta *(a)* are seen. At angiography the patient was found to have a right common iliac artery aneurysm with fistulous communication with the lower end of the inferior vena cava and a large left-to-right shunt through the fistula. (From Khoo,[197] with permission.)

may be more sensitive in detecting aneurysms in this location than is either CT or ultrasound.[83] Adjacent fluid without a Doppler signal can suggest abscess or hematoma.

The sonographic detection of thoracic aortic aneurysms and dissections was not possible until the recent advent[84,85] of transesophageal echocardiography, studies of which suggest that it may be a reliable diagnostic tool. Although patient sedation is required, it is operator dependent and the distal ascending aorta is poorly seen.[86]

The aorta is not compressed by periaortic masses. Common ones are hematoma (Fig. 11-24), adenopathy (Figs. 11-4A and 11-17), retroperitoneal fibrosis, and retroperitoneal neoplasm including primary tumors, metastases, and lymphoma. Horseshoe kidney typically produces a narrow band of soft tissue mass on sonography anterior to the distal aorta that can be initially mistaken for adenopathy.

Aortic Grafts

In aortic aneurysm repair, a focal tube graft may be placed, surrounded by the incised walls of the aneurysm, which is wrapped around the graft. Fluid between the aneurysmal wall and the graft is a common finding early after the surgical repair. A less common repair is division of the aorta with proximal and distal closure of the distal aneurysm followed by an end-to-end vessel bypass.[87]

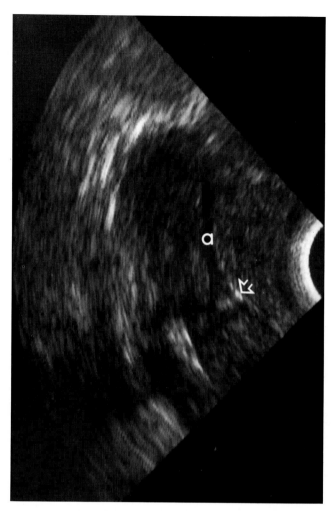

Fig. 11-23. Aortic thrombosis: umbilical catheter complications. No femoral pulses were palpable in this patient. At longitudinal real-time scan through the left flank, a nonpulsatile aorta *(a)* was seen. There was a dense echogenic (arrow) plaque in the left common iliac artery.

The aneurysm, which is left in place but isolated to flow, occludes.

Other procedures that may be performed when iliac disease is also present are (1) the aortoiliac graft, done for aneurysmal extension involving the iliac arteries, and (2) the aortofemoral graft, placed for arterial obstructive disease. These grafts can be end to end at the proximal anastomosis or end to side, with the graft anterior to the native aorta (Fig. 11-25).[88,89] Grafts of knitted Dacron at the distal aortic bifurcation tend to dilate over long-term follow-up.[90] The distal anastomosis may also be end to end (usually the case in aortoiliac grafts) or end to side (Fig. 11-26). Since the native vessels are diseased, they may not be well seen by sonography, but if they are not occluded, they also have a detectable signal on duplex

ultrasound. The grafts normally have a triphasic waveform of a peripheral vessel. Distal stenosis at the anastomosis causes elevated focal peak systolic velocity.

Although anastomotic aneurysms are uncommon (<2 percent), they are most likely to occur at the distal anastomosis of an aortofemoral graft or at the femoral anastomosis of a femoral-femoral graft (Fig. 11-27). This may be related to poor surgical technique or increased stress at a site of frequent motion. Whatever the cause, the false aneurysm tends to expand over time and can rupture. Sonography reveals an expansile mass, with or without thrombus, that has a holosystolic waveform on duplex sonography, which translates to a mosaic of color on color Doppler, reflecting the turbulent flow. Thrombosed pseudoaneurysms have no Doppler signal and can be confused with fluid collections.[91] Fluid collections around these grafts present as anechoic masses without an intrinsic Doppler signal, although those immediately adjacent to the graft can have a transmitted signal.[91,92]

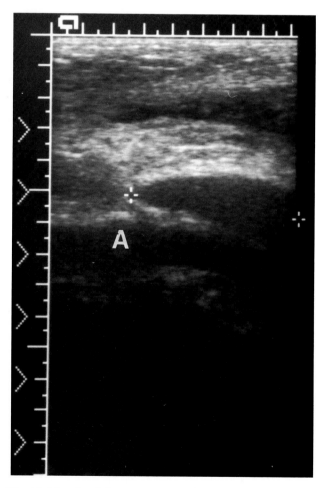

Fig. 11-24. Aortic hematoma. Longitudinal sonogram of the aorta *(A)* showing an oval hypoechoic mass anteriorly (calipers), which proved to be a hematoma following aortic surgery.

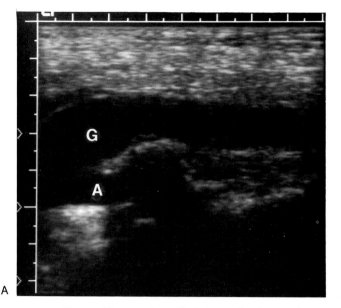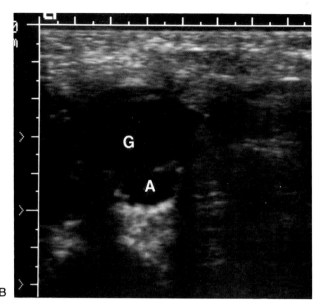

Fig. 11-25. Aortic graft. **(A)** Longitudinal oblique scan showing a proximal end-to-side aortofemoral bypass graft *(G)*. The distal native aorta *(A)* is posterior. **(B)** Transverse sonogram of the same aortofemoral graft at the proximal anastomosis demonstrating that the proximal graft *(G)* is mildly dilated. *(A,* aorta.)

These fluid collections all have a similar appearance and can be seromas, hematomas, lymphoceles, or abscesses. Aspiration, when feasible, leads to the correct diagnosis, but noninfected retroperitoneal collections in the abdomen can become infected if the bowel is traversed during the procedure. Hematomas, abscesses, and lymphoceles can also present with varying echogenicities (Fig. 11-28).

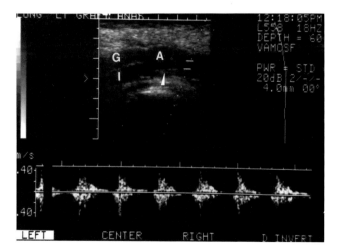

Fig. 11-26. Aortic graft. Longitudinal sonogram of the groin showing the common femoral artery *(A)*, an aortofemoral graft anastomosis *(G)*, the native external iliac artery *(I)*, a holosystolic waveform indicating turbulence, and a small plaque in the posterior wall of the common femoral artery (arrowhead). (From Gooding,[200] with permission.)

Anastomotic aneurysms or pseudoaneurysms occur at aortoiliac surgical anastomoses of grafts, but are far more common in aortofemoral grafts or femoral-femoral graft anastomoses at the femoral implantation site (Fig. 11-27).[91,93] These aneurysms typically have holosystolic turbulent flow which on color imaging has a multicolored mosaic appearance. Thrombosed aneurysms have no Doppler signal.

Abscesses usually require graft excision although percutaneous drainage may suffice.[94]

AORTIC BRANCH ABNORMALITIES

Renal Artery

Renal Artery Stenosis

Stenosis of the renal arteries is typically due to progressive atherosclerosis, but fibrodysplasia, trauma, extension of aortic aneurysm, dissection, arteritis, entrapment by the diaphragmatic crus (rarely), and emboli are other reasons for the narrowing or occlusive disease. Other vascular abnormalities of the renal arteries are isolated aneurysm and arteriovenous malformation.

In the evaluation of renal artery stenosis, it is much easier to define the renal arteries in renal transplants than in the normal flank position of the kidneys, because the vessels are more superficial. Color Doppler examinations also improve visualization and are used to detect

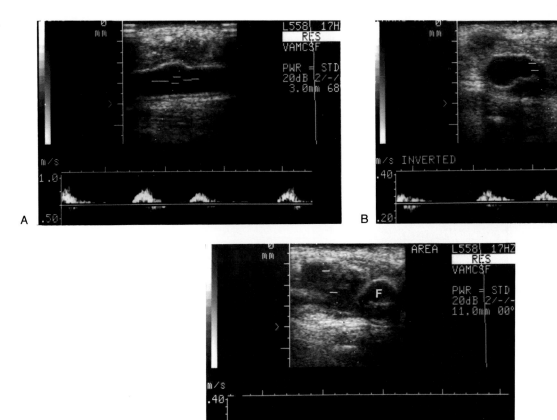

Fig. 11-27. Femoral-femoral graft. **(A)** Longitudinal sonogram of a femoral-femoral graft showing an unusual mild central dilatation. Spectral analysis shows the graft to be patent. **(B)** Transverse scan of a femoral-femoral anastomosis showing minimal dilatation of 1.5 cm in diameter. The normal femoral artery is about 1 cm in diameter. The spectral waveform documents patency. **(C)** Longitudinal sonogram of the area near a femoral-femoral graft showing a soft tissue mass on which a caliper is placed with the gate opened to the fullest extent to detect flow, which was absent. (*F*, femoral artery.) Clinically, this mass was thought to be a false aneurysm but is consistent with resolving hematoma.

the vascular complications of renal allografts, including renal artery stenosis, arteriovenous (AV) fistula, renal vein thrombosis, and infarction.[95] When pseudoaneurysms or arteriovenous fistula develop in renal transplants as complications of renal biopsy, duplex sonography[96] and color Doppler are the screening tools for diagnosis[97] and are used again in the intraoperative treatment, especially when percutaneous embolization is used.

A sonographic search for renal artery stenosis takes about 2 hours following a 12-hour fast, since the entire course of all renal arteries has to be followed and sampled by duplex ultrasound.[98] Successful visualization occurs in about 90 percent of cases in the most experienced hands.[98] Stenoses typically cause jets of flow with focal steep elevations of peak systolic velocity above 125 cm/s. With near-occlusive critical disease, the peak systolic velocity is markedly dampened and diastole disap-

pears. Another clue to renal artery stenosis is the determination of the renal artery/distal aorta ratio of peak systolic velocity. A ratio greater than 3.5 is indicative of renal artery stenosis.[99] This technique can be 93 percent accurate in skilled hands[100] and is also used to monitor the results of renal artery angioplasty or aortorenal bypass graft.

Renal Artery Aneurysm

Renal artery aneurysms are congenital or acquired; the latter are two-thirds more common than the former (Fig. 11-29).[101] With the advent of color Doppler, the distinction between the avascular renal cyst and the vascular aneurysm is immediate. The renal aneurysm, whether true or false, is remarkable for a turbulent mosaic of color within its boundaries and holosystolic flow

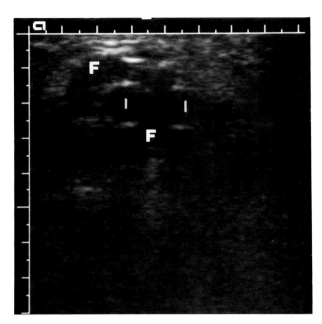

Fig. 11-28. Aortic graft. Transverse scan of the iliac limbs *(I)* at the bifurcation showing surrounding fluid *(F)* following aortic surgery.

on spectral analysis. Intraparenchymatous renal artery aneurysms usually have iatrogenic causes from biopsy or are related to polyarteritis or infection.

Arteriovenous Fistula

Both pseudoaneurysms and AV fistulas, produce turbulent flow, but AV fistulas, whether congenital or acquired, characteristically produce continuous flow with a prominent diastolic component as opposed to the ho-

losystolic flow in pseudoaneurysms. Both can cause perivascular color artifacts, but AV fistulas alone can cause arterialization of the feeding veins which are enlarged (Figs. 11-30 and 11-31).

Other

The resistive index of the renal arteries (i.e., the peak systole minus end diastole divided by peak systole) tends to fall with elevated heart rate[102] and rise with external renal compression, in hydronephrosis, and in acute vascular rejection.

Mesenteric Artery

Stenosis

Color Doppler is a potential way to examine the celiac artery and SMA for origin stenosis when patients present with abdominal angina (i.e., abdominal pain after eating) and weight loss. With stenosis of both the celiac artery and SMA, the inferior mesenteric vein becomes an enlarged collateral visible on ultrasound. To date, angiography has been the only effective way to examine these vessels. Celiac stenosis also results from ligamentous compression of the celiac axis by the median arcuate ligament of the diaphragm.[103]

Aneurysm

Splanchnic aneurysms occur in about 10 percent of patients with chronic pancreatitis[104] and affects the splenic artery most commonly, but also the hepatic and

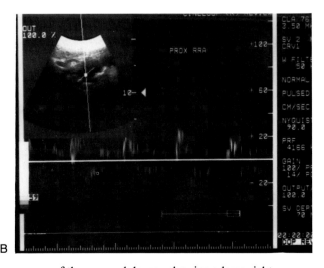

Fig. 11-29. Renal artery aneurysm. **(A)** Longitudinal sonogram of the upper abdomen showing a large right renal artery aneurysm *(RRA)*, filled with thrombus, which abuts into and compresses the inferior vena cava *(IVC)*. **(B)** Longitudinal sonogram demonstrating a caliper at the origin of the right renal artery, which has some flow.

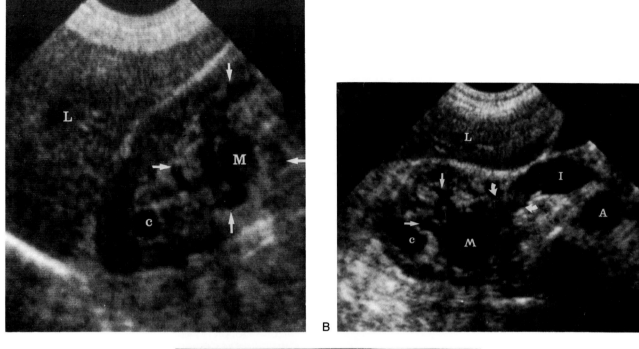

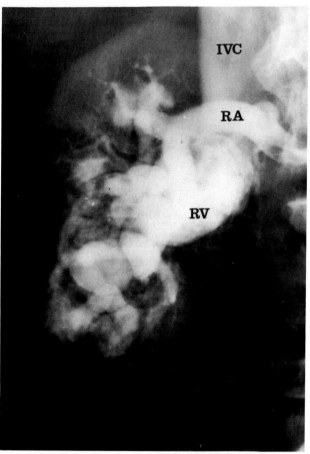

Fig. 11-30. Renal arteriovenous fistula. Crisoid type. **(A)** Longitudinal real-time scan through the liver *(L)* and right kidney revealing multiple anechoic tubular structures (arrows) ending in an anechoic mass *(M)* constituting a cirsoid arteriovenous malformation. (*c*, dilated upper-pole calyx.) **(B)** Transverse real-time scan at the renal hilum. The arteriovenous malformation *(M)* is supplied by multiple vessels (straight arrows) and drained by a dilated renal vein containing thrombus (curved arrows). (*c*, dilated calyx; *L*, liver; *I*, inferior vena cava; *A*, aorta.) **(C)** Selective renal angiogram revealing a hypertrophied renal artery *(RA)* supplying the malformation with arteriovenous shunting and early opacification of the renal vein *(RV)* and inferior vena cava *(IVC)*. (From Subramanyam et al,[96] with permission.)

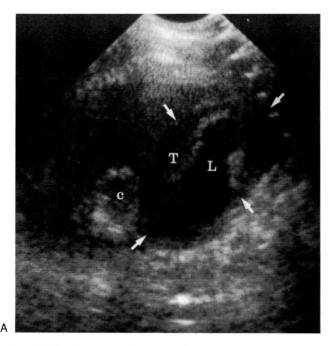

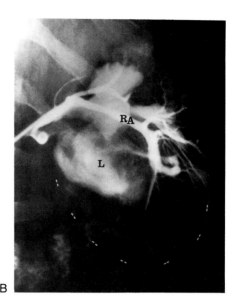

A

B

Fig. 11-31. Renal arteriovenous fistula. Aneurysmal type. **(A)** Longitudinal real-time scan revealing a large mass (arrows) involving the lower half of the kidney. Note the solid periphery representing thrombus *(T)* and a central hypoechoic tubular lumen *(L). (c,* calyx.) **(B)** Left renal angiogram revealing an enlarged segmental renal artery *(RA),* filling the lumen *(L)* of the aneurysm. (dotted lines, thrombosed segment of the aneurysm.) (From Subramanyam et al,[96] with permission.)

celiac arteries, the SMA,[104,105] and the gastroduodenal artery (Figs. 11-32 and 11-33). Other causes of these aneurysms are traumatic, congenital, and mycotic. Since many are asymptomatic, the danger lies in the significant risk of rupture. Rapid recognition of such aneurysms is possible with color Doppler; distinction from the avascular pseudocyst of the pancreas is simple. By contrast, small fluid collections in the pancreas were probably overcalled as pseudocysts prior to color Doppler capability; it becomes apparent that some of these cases represent pancreatic varices, with obvious venous characteristics on color coding.

Other

Hepatic portal venous gas has been found sonographically in mesenteric artery occlusion[106] and after liver transplantation[107] as fleeting, hyperechoic, nonshadowing echoes traveling in the veins.

Since the SMA lies directly posterior to the pancreas, its root may become thickened in cancer of the pancreas, which by sonography is a sign of neoplastic vascular involvement.[108] The sign has limited specificity since this thickening can also occur in obesity, pancreatitis, and other gastrointestinal cancers.

Iliac Artery

Iliac Artery Aneurysm

The iliac arteries are subject to aneurysm formation, but much less so than the aorta. These aneurysms are usually extensions from aortic aneurysmal disease and are atherosclerotic in origin but can form from trauma, infection, and congenital disease (Figs. 11-34 to 11-36). On ultrasound, these aneurysms can be obscured by overlying bowel gas,[109] at which point CT or MRI should be considered.

Isolated iliac aneurysms are typically silent clinically. They tend to expand inexorably and eventually are subject to rupture, often into the colon and occasionally into the ureter. Expansion can produce unilateral hydronephrosis, since the iliac artery and the ureter are in close association, the ureter crossing anteriorly (Fig. 11-34B). Large iliac aneurysms can bulge into the lateral walls of the bladder; on sonography, the impressions are similar to those of large lymphoceles (Fig. 11-36). Again, color Doppler can be used to show the vascular character of these lesions. Patients who have had aortic aneurysm resection should also be monitored for the development of iliac aneurysmal disease, which may proceed asymptomatically.[11]

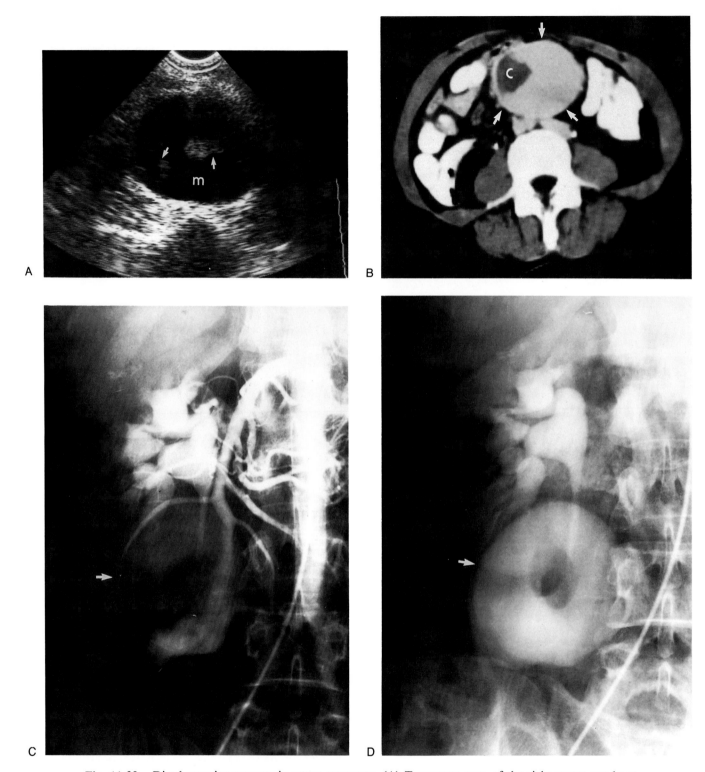

Fig. 11-32. Distal superior mesenteric artery aneurysm. **(A)** Transverse scan of the right upper quadrant revealing a 6.5-cm mass *(m)* which exhibited flow on Doppler. An internal clot (arrows) is seen. **(B)** Enhanced CT scan showing the enhancing aneurysm (arrows) with some internal clot *(c)*. **(C & D)** Arteriograms demonstrating the superior mesenteric aneurysm (arrows).

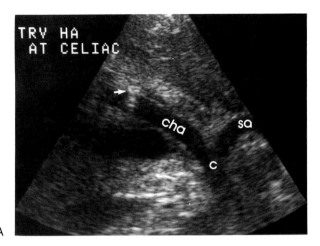
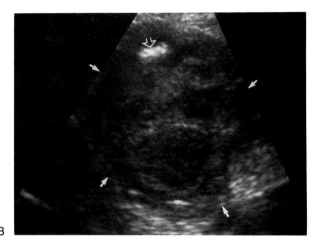

A   B

Fig. 11-33. Gastroduodenal artery aneurysm: postembolization. **(A)** Transverse view of the celiac artery *(c)* branches with coil (arrow) at the takeoff of the gastroduodenal artery. *(cha,* common hepatic artery; *sa,* splenic artery.) **(B)** Transverse scan of a previously pulsatile mass (arrows, 57 × 77 mm) in the region of the pancreatic head. The coil (open arrow) is seen in the anterior aspect of the aneurysm. Doppler demonstrated no flow within the aneurysm, indicating adequate embolization.

Aortoiliac Stenosis

Aortoiliac stenosis is best identified sonographically by duplex ultrasound or color Doppler. With mild stenosis,[110] initially the triphasic waveform on spectral analysis develops some spectral broadening (1 to 19 percent stenosis). More severe (20 to 49 percent) stenosis results in maintenance of reverse flow but an elevation in peak systolic velocity of 30 to 100 percent from the segment immediately preceding it.[110] With increased involvement (50 to 99 percent stenosis), the reversed diastole component disappears and peak systole rises,[111] only to eventually fall in preocclusive states.

A focal elevation of peak systolic velocity of 100 to 200 percent compared with that of both proximal and distal[112] iliac segments was associated with an accuracy of

88 percent in one study of iliac stenosis.[112] Velocity changes of 150 percent in another study were 92 percent sensitive in detecting a greater than 50 percent stenosis.[113] In that particular study,[113] greater end-diastolic velocities were associated with more severe stenosis (75 to 99 percent stenosis) than with moderate disease. Real-time assessment alone is not sensitive to such flow abnormalities. Detection of aortoiliac occlusion by lack of signal on duplex ultrasound or color Doppler is highly sensitive.[113]

Percutaneous Procedure Complications

Since most percutaneous catheterizations are done at the common femoral artery, this area is subject to traumatic complications (in approximately 0.2 to 9 percent)

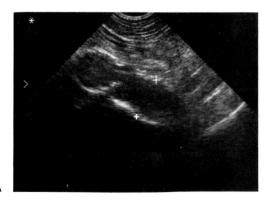
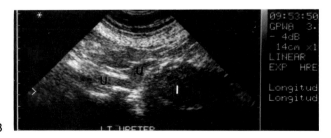

A   B

Fig. 11-34. Iliac aneurysm. **(A)** Oblique sonogram in the pelvis showing a large lobular iliac aneurysm (calipers). **(B)** The ureter *(U)* is dilated, takes a sharp turn up to the iliac aneurysm *(I),* and then tapers as it is compressed by the iliac aneurysm. This has caused hydronephrosis.

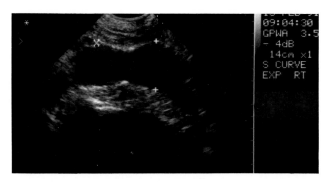

Fig. 11-35. Iliac aneurysm. Transverse sonogram showing the distal aorta dividing into bilateral iliac aneurysms (calipers).

of pseudoaneurysm, AV fistula, and hematoma.[114] Kotval et al have shown in three patients that pseudoaneurysms can spontaneously thrombose over time.[115] Of interest is that under color Doppler surveillance, these pseudoaneurysms tend to thrombose spontaneously with persistent manual compression[116] if treated initially after diagnosis.

Arteriovenous Malformation

Arteriovenous malformations can also occur in the area; these are either congenital, primary,[117] neoplastic, or traumatic.[118] They are especially well seen with color Doppler, which depicts the random, turbulent, low-resistance, high-volume flow.[119]

These AV fistulas and those surgically created for hemodialysis manifest turbulence in a distinct way. With color Doppler, a distinct bleeding of random color in the soft tissues occurs beyond the actual involved vessels,[1] a phenomenon caused by the highly turbulent flow.[120]

Other

Lymphoceles are typical fluid collections in the area around the iliac vessels, particularly in those patients who have had a lymph node dissection, a common postoperative finding in staging of cancer of the prostate (Figs. 11-8A and 11-37).

INFERIOR VENA CAVA ABNORMALITIES

Congenital

Absence of the IVC is very rare[121] and is associated with multiple superficial and deep venous collaterals.

The major anomalies of the IVC[122] relate to embryologic development at 6 to 10 weeks' gestation. Devia-

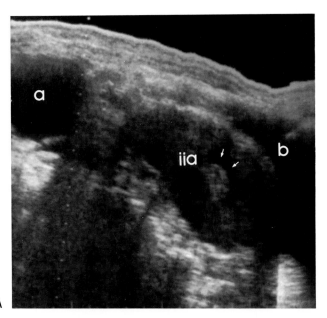

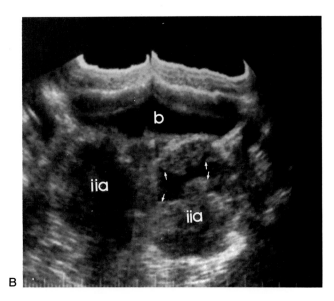

Fig. 11-36. Internal iliac aneurysms. **(A)** Longitudinal scan at 3 cm to the left of midline. The dilated distal aorta *(a)* at the level of the umbilicus is seen, as well as a mass *(iia)* posterior to the bladder *(b)*. (arrows, lumen.) **(B)** Transverse scan through the bladder *(b)*. Bilateral internal iliac aneurysms *(iia)* are noted. The one on the right was clotted off and was not pulsatile on real-time ultrasound. The lucency in the left one represents lumen (small arrows).

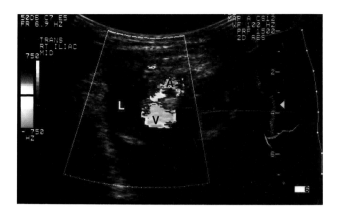

Fig. 11-37. Lymphocele. Transverse sonogram of the pelvis showing a lymphocele *(L)* lateral to the iliac artery *(A)* and vein *(V)* (done in color, photographed in black and white). The common femoral vein compressed and augmented normally, but did not respond to a Valsalva maneuver, although it had done so before pelvic surgery. Such a response is indicative of either deep venous thrombosis in the iliac veins or external compression of them, as in this case.

tions from normal embryogenesis result in four major anomalies (Fig. 11-38)[122]:

1. Duplication of the IVC (Fig. 11-18)[123]
2. Transposition of the IVC to the left side of the aorta[124]
3. Retroaortic renal vein[125] (2 to 3 percent)
4. Circumaortic left renal vein (1.5 to 8.7 percent)

Sonography lends itself best to the diagnosis of the first three, while CT can define them all. The major importance of the recognition of these anomalies is to avoid complications related to their presence during aortic or caval surgery.

When both the IVC and aorta are on the same side, asplenia or polysplenia is suggested.[126,127]

The scimitar syndrome is an anomaly of the pulmonary venous drainage. Part of or all of the right lung venous return empties into the IVC,[128] which can be stenotic. This has been diagnosed by echocardiogram and occurs in conjunction with other vascular anomalies

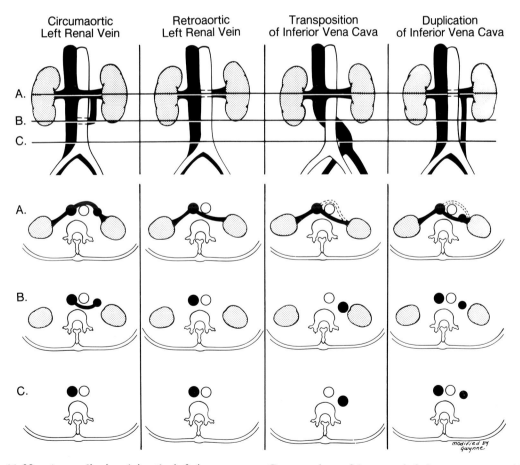

Fig. 11-38. Anomalies involving the inferior vena cava. Cross-sections of the aorta, inferior vena cava, and left renal vein showing anomalies of the inferior vena cava and left renal vein. In transposition and duplication, a venous structure may pass either anterior or posterior (dashed line) to the aorta at the level of the renal vein. (Modified from Royal and Callen,[198] with permission.)

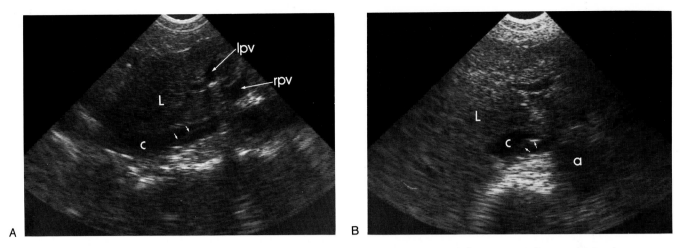

Fig. 11-39. Inferior vena cava web. **(A)** Longitudinal and **(B)** transverse real-time scans. A linear echodensity (arrows) is seen within the inferior vena cava *(c).* This moved at real-time in the dilated inferior vena cava. (*lpv,* left portal vein; *rpv,* right portal vein; *L,* liver; *a,* aorta.)

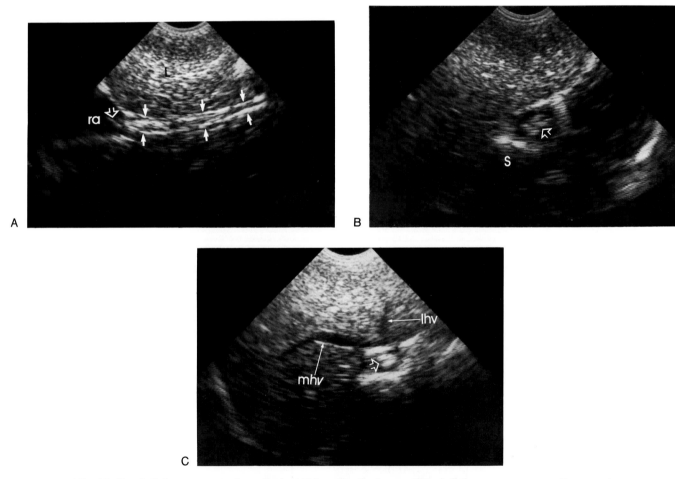

Fig. 11-40. Inferior vena cava thrombosis. **(A)** Longitudinal scan of the inferior vena cava revealing an echogenic "cast" (arrows) filling the lumen of the inferior vena cava. A portion of the thrombus (open arrow) projects into the right atrium *(ra).* (*L,* liver.) **(B)** High transverse scan. The thrombus (open arrow) is surrounded by the anechoic lumen of the inferior vena cava. (*S,* spine.) **(C)** Transverse scan at the level of the hepatic veins. Only the left *(lhv)* and middle *(mhv)* veins are demonstrated; the right hepatic vein was never seen. On this scan, as well as on the lower scans, no inferior vena cava lumen was demonstrated. An echogenic thrombus (open arrow) is seen.

including sequestration, dextrocardia, and pulmonary hypoplasia.

Coarctation of the IVC, while rare,[129] is a congenital cause of Budd-Chiari syndrome that can be suggested by sonography. Early surgical repair can prevent irreversible liver disease. One approach to treatment of this condition is the use of a mesocaval shunt, which has been traditionally assessed by angiography. Early limited data[130] suggest that both MRI and duplex sonography may be used to assess shunt patency, stenosis, or occlusion.

Duplication of the IVC[123] can be confused with adenopathy on a transverse sonogram (Fig. 11-18A). Also, the duplicated portion of the IVC can be a source of pulmonary emboli. Color Doppler imaging has potential to improve the detection of this anomaly by ultrasound.

Congenital absence of the infrahepatic segment of the IVC with azygos and hemiazygous continuation is another anomaly of the abdominal cava (Fig. 11-13).[131] This anomaly has a well-known association with polysplenism, and an associated unique infrarenal IVC aneurysm has been described.[132]

Retrocaval ureter can sometimes be suggested sonographically from hydronephrosis and a dilated ureter, which courses, usually on the right, behind the IVC. Another name for this congenital anomaly of the IVC is circumcaval ureter.[133]

When unsuspected, circumaortic and retroaortic renal veins can complicate vascular surgery in the area and should be considered sonographically as possibilities when aortic or caval surgery is contemplated. These are well recognized with CT.

Budd-Chiari Syndrome

Budd-Chiari syndrome produces abnormal hepatic vein thrombosis, collateralization of the hepatic veins, and venous flow reversals.[134,135] Extension of the process leads to secondary thrombosis of the IVC.[136] Another rare cause of Budd-Chiari syndrome is membranous obstruction of the IVC, which causes hepatosplenomegaly, ascites, and multiple venous collaterals. This has been reported both in isolated instances and in a series of children in Namibia.[137]

Thrombosis

General

Inferior vena cava obstruction occurs from membranes or webs, thrombosis, intrinsic tumor, or local invasion (Fig. 11-39).[138]

Thrombosis of the IVC may be partial or complete. The occluded IVC can be anechoic or filled with visible echoes. No Doppler signal is present, and no respiratory rhythmicity is apparent. Complete occlusion may elimi-

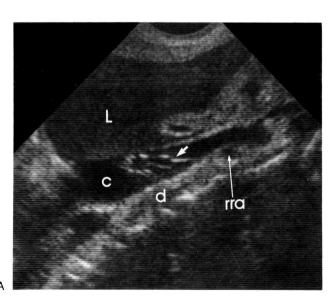

A

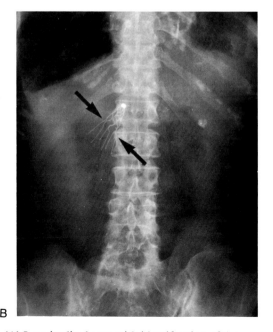

B

Fig. 11-41. Inferior vena cava filter. Kimray-Greenfield filter. **(A)** Longitudinal scan with identification of the filter (arrow) in the inferior vena cava *(c)* superior to the right renal artery *(rra)*. (*L*, liver; *d*, right crus of the diaphragm). **(B)** Radiograph of the filter device showing the metallic prongs (arrows) by which it attaches itself to the caval wall. (From Hill and Sanders,[28] with permission.)

nate any trace of the vessel as distinguished from the soft tissue. Partial thrombosis results in a damped spectral signal without phasicity.

Long-standing IVC thrombus can calcify[139]; on sonography this produces bright echoes that cast acoustic shadows (Fig. 11-40). IVC thrombus is occasionally associated with hydrops fetalis.[140]

IVC thrombosis can also develop as a complication of right heart catheterization,[141] but fortunately the thrombus may lyse spontaneously in some situations.[142]

Bladder distension in the neonate is an unusual cause of IVC obstruction that is amenable[143] to sonographic detection.

Infection

Septic thrombosis of the IVC by a variety of pathogens including *Candida*[144] results in no Doppler signal and no color depiction on color Doppler imaging. IVC thrombosis, noted by ultrasound, has also been reported as a complication of amebic liver abscess.[145] Another study[146] reports that real-time sonography has detected transient, bright hyperechoic signals in the IVC as a result of air produced by an adjacent renal abscess. Still another study reports dissemination of pulmonary hydatid cyst rupture into the IVC.[147]

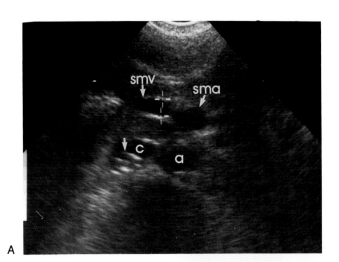

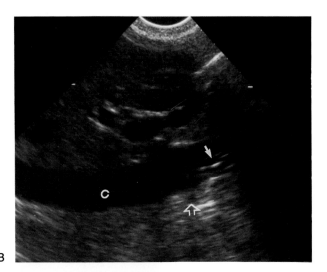

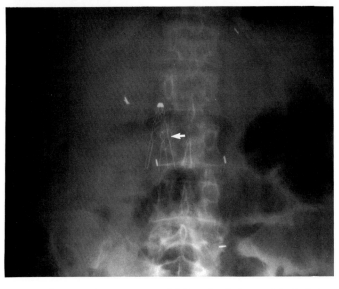

Fig. 11-42. Inferior vena cava filter. **(A)** Transverse and **(B)** sagittal views of the inferior vena cava *(c)* demonstrating a filter (arrow) just below the level of the right renal artery (open arrow). (*smv,* superior mesenteric vein; *sma,* superior mesenteric artery; *a,* aorta.) **(C)** Radiograph of the filter (arrow) showing the metallic prongs.

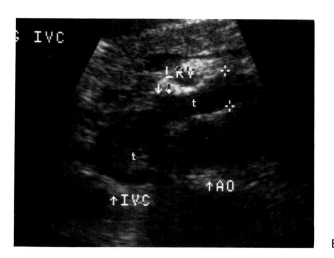

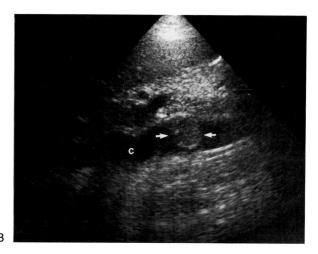

A

B

Fig. 11-43. Inferior vena cava tumor: renal cell carcinoma. **(A)** Transverse view in a patient with a large left renal cell carcinoma with tumor *(t)* extending into the left renal vein *(LRV)* and inferior vena cava *(IVC)*. *(AO, aorta.)* **(B)** Sagittal view of the inferior vena cava *(c)* containing tumor (arrows) seen at the level of the left renal vein.

Treatment

Filter. To prevent pulmonary emboli, IVC filters provide a physical blockade to thrombus while maintaining IVC patency. These filters are seen on sonography as bright, hyperechoic interfaces in the proximal vessel (Figs. 11-41 and 11-42).[148] They can perforate or migrate, can have associated extravascular hematoma, or can be malpositioned.[149] A case can be made for performing echocardiography before inserting such a filter, to exclude right atrial embolus.[150]

The venotomy site of insertion of the filter is subject to thrombosis (14 to 19 percent)[151,152] as determined by duplex sonography or color Doppler.

Graft. To treat unilateral occlusion of the iliac vein, some patients have a femoral-femoral venous crossover graft placed in the superficial soft tissues of the pubis, a location easily amenable to duplex sonographic interrogation. A normal graft is compressible and has a venous signal responsive to respiration and augmentation.[153] With occlusion, no signal can be detected.

Surgical Ligation. After surgical ligation of the IVC, the peripheral venous flow is only mildly affected[154] because of adequate collateral flow. Doppler ultrasound shows that in this situation the IVC is not a source of peripheral venous reflux, as might be expected; such reflex tends to develop as a result of peripheral deep venous thrombosis.

Tumor

Primary

Primary tumor of the IVC is rare but is most likely to be leiomyosarcoma. On sonography, this tumor presents as a large, expansible, intraluminal, fusiform heterogeneous soft tissue mass of medium echo intensity.[155–157] One complication of this neoplasm is the development of an acute Budd-Chiari syndrome[158] with concomitant leg swelling, ascites, and renal failure.[159]

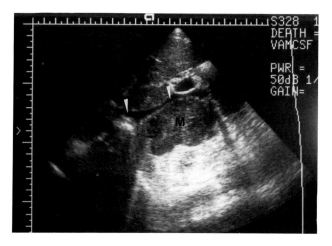

Fig. 11-44. Inferior vena cava compression. A large adrenal metastasis *(M)* impresses on the posterior inferior vena cava (arrowheads) on this longitudinal sonogram.

Secondary

A hepatic vein tumor can extend into the IVC[159] and vice versa.

Renal neoplasms are particularly prone to IVC extension; they include renal cell carcinoma (Fig. 11-43),[160–162] with a sensitivity of detection by sonography of 100 percent,[162] Wilms' tumor, and angiomyolipoma.[163]

Other metastases can extend into the IVC[164] from the adrenal glands (including, rarely, pheochromocytoma),[165,166] the retroperitoneum, the uterus,[165,167] and the liver.[168] In these situations, the intraluminal mass is echo producing and expands the IVC, but cannot be distinguished from nonneoplastic thrombus.

Aggressive neoplasms may proceed to the right atrium,[165,168] where they can be recognized by echocardiography.[169] Right atrial myxoma can actually obstruct the IVC. Review of the experience with Wilms' tumor extension shows that the level of IVC involvement has no effect on survival; surgical resection of the tumor, even when involving the IVC and right atrium, is recommended when possible.[168]

Compression

Medial indentation of the IVC on transverse scans has been reported as a sonographic sign of fluid in the superior recess of the lesser sac.[170] Another typical finding of fluid distribution in the upper recess of the lesser sac is fluid encirclement of the medial border of the caudate lobe of the liver.

Adenopathy, adjacent liver lesion, aortic aneurysms (Figs. 11-11B and 11-44), and primary or secondary retroperitoneal masses tend to compress the IVC as they enlarge (Fig. 11-10A). Examples are hepatoma of the medial right or caudate lobes of the liver, adrenal metastases (Fig. 11-44), renal tumors, neurogenic neoplasms, sarcoma of the retroperitoneum, and even osteophytes

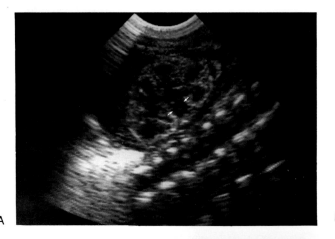

A

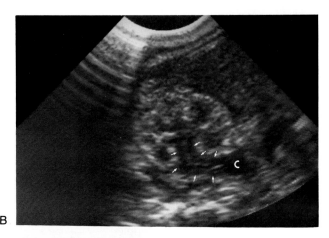

B

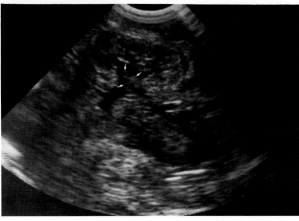

C

Fig. 11-45. Renal vein thrombosis. Newborn with anuria. **(A)** Longitudinal and **(B)** transverse scans of the right kidney demonstrating a distorted renal echopattern. Thrombus (arrows) is seen within the renal veins. The right renal vein was distended and full of echoes at real-time (Figs. A & B), while **(C)** a mobile thrombus was seen with the left renal vein. (*c*, inferior vena cava.)

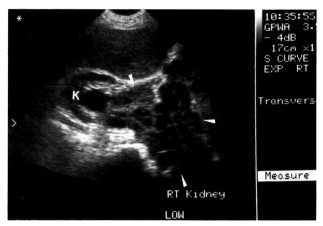

Fig. 11-46. Renal vein compression. Transverse sonogram of the right kidney *(K)* demonstrating hydronephrosis and multiple lymph nodes obscuring the renal artery and vein (arrowheads).

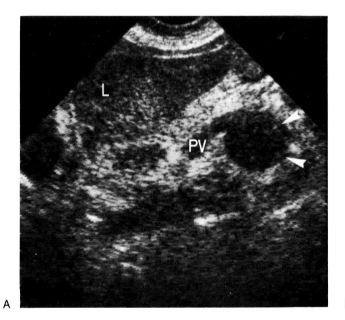

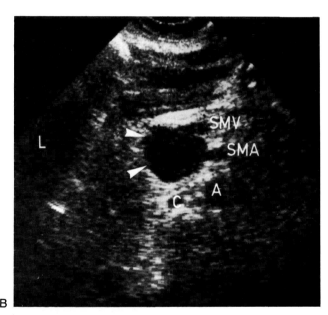

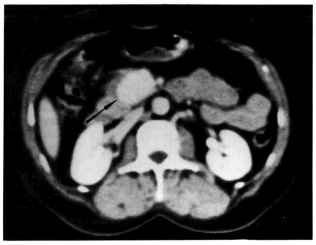

Fig. 11-47. Superior mesenteric vein aneurysm. **(A)** Longitudinal and **(B)** transverse scans of a cystic, compressible tumor (arrowheads) in the vicinity of the superior mesenteric vein *(SMV)*. (*L*, liver; *PV*, portal vein; *C*, inferior vena cava; *A*, aorta; *SMA*, superior mesenteric artery.) **(C)** CT scan with enhancement (arrow) during venous phase. (From Schild et al,[199] with permission.)

of the anterior lumbar spine. Fluid collections, hematoma, and adjacent splanchnic, aortic, or renal aneurysms can also impress the IVC (Figs. 11-10A, 11-15B, and 11-29). Marked narrowing of the IVC from external compression can lead to diminished venous return with peripheral edema and a propensity to develop deep venous thrombosis distally.

INFERIOR VENA CAVA BRANCH ABNORMALITIES

Renal Vein

Thrombosis

Child. In infants or fetuses in utero, renal vein thrombosis produces echogenic linear markings in the interlobular veins, which can extend to the IVC (Fig. 11-45).[171] Duplex ultrasound interrogation detects no venous signal, and the renal arterial flow shows increased impedance,[172] (i.e., diminished diastolic flow).

Thrombosis appears related to diminished renal blood flow and dehydration. Although initially the kidney is enlarged, venous infarction can lead to atrophy of the affected kidney.[173] The thrombosis can occur in a variant left retroaortic renal vein.[174] Sonography also is used to monitor the response to treatment.

Adult. In adults, renal vein thrombosis is likely to be related to renal disease, often in association with the nephrotic syndrome, but hypercoagulable states and extension of IVC thrombosis or tumor are other causes (Fig. 11-43). External compression of the renal vein is another cause of renal vein thrombosis.

Other. Renal vein thrombosis occurs in 1 to 4 percent of renal transplants.[175] Calcifications of the renal vein and IVC have been reported sonographically from prior thrombosis,[176] prenatally,[177] and in neonates.

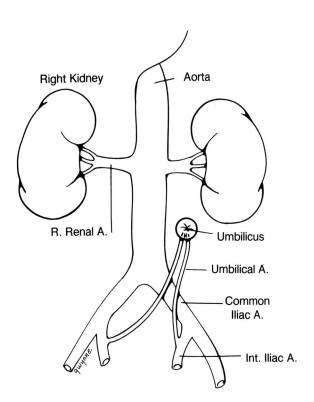

Fig. 11-48. Pathway of umbilical arterial catheter. The arterial catheter passes through either of the paired umbilical arteries traveling inferiorly toward the ipsilateral internal iliac artery. After entering the internal iliac artery, the catheter turns cephalad to pass up the common iliac artery and aorta.

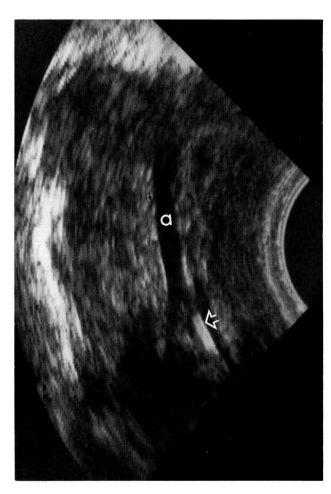

Fig. 11-49. Umbilical arterial catheter. Longitudinal (coronal) scan through the right flank. The abdominal aorta *(a)* is easily seen, as are the renal arteries (arrows) and iliac vessels. The catheter tip (open arrow) can be seen within the right iliac artery.

Entrapment

Left renal vein entrapment[178] has been touted as a cause of left renal vein compression and postcompression dilatation as the vein proceeds between the SMA and the aorta. It is associated with isomorphic red blood cells, hematuria, left flank pain, normal venography, and a typical sonographic appearance.[178]

Tumor

Because renal neoplasia commonly extends to the renal vein, the sonographer should look carefully for that extension and include the IVC and the right atrium in the examination when aggressive neoplastic expansion is suspected (Fig. 11-45). One ultrasound report documents renal neoplastic extension into the contralateral renal vein.[179] Another documents primary leiomyosarcoma of the renal vein[180] as a homogeneous hyperechoic mass. Renal neoplasms commonly invade the renal veins, but adrenal cancer and left gonadal cancers also can extend to the renal veins.

Other

Portal hypertension may result in collateralization via the left renal veins with retrograde flow. The renal veins can be compressed by adjacent masses, including lymphoma, aneurysms, and retroperitoneal hemorrhage (Fig. 11-46).

Iliac Vein

Even when the external or common iliac vein cannot be seen, abnormalities can be suspected from an examination of the common femoral vein. The common femoral vein normally has respiratory phasicity, expands readily by at least 50 percent in response to a Valsalva maneuver, completely compresses to transducer pressure, and augments on spectral analysis when the more distal leg is squeezed and a bolus of venous flow is forced forward.

When the iliac venous system is occluded by thrombosis or compressed by adjacent fluid, such as lymphocele or hematoma, or by neoplasia, the common femoral vein loses its respiratory rhythmicity (Fig. 11-37). The femoral vein normally compresses to transducer pressure, but the response to a Valsalva maneuver is lost or damped. Other abnormalities such as ascites or congestive heart failure can also affect respiratory phasicity and the response to a Valsalva maneuver.

Other

Sonography is well documented to be accurate in the diagnosis of portal vein thrombosis (see Ch. 5). Superior mesenteric vein obstruction[181-183] can also be demon-

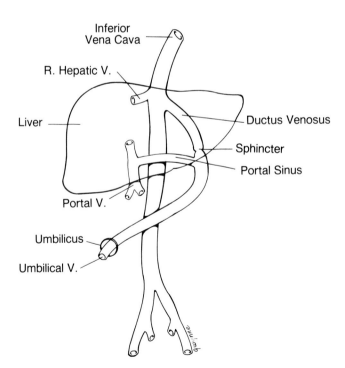

Fig. 11-50. Pathway of umbilical venous catheter. The umbilical venous catheter passes superiorly in the midline through the umbilical vein as it courses through the falciform ligament and enters the liver where the umbilical vein joins the left portal vein. Then the catheter ascends through the ductus venosus to enter an hepatic vein close to their confluence in the inferior vena cava.

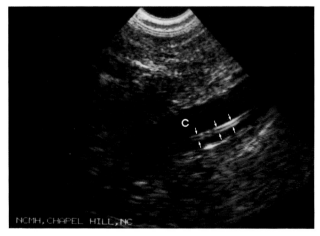

Fig. 11-51. Femoral catheter, adult. An inferior vena cava *(c)* catheter (arrows) inserted through the femoral vein in an adult can be seen in this longitudinal scan as a double echogenic line.

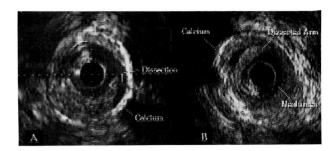

Fig. 11-52. Intravascular ultrasound: dissection. Transverse intravascular image of the iliac vessels demonstrating a dissection on these transverse images. (Courtesy of PJ Fitzgerald, Department of Medicine and Cardiology, University of California, San Francisco.)

strated sonographically and is a cause of mesenteric ischemia.

Rarely, a spontaneous mesenteric vein–systemic shunt is documented by ultrasound[184]; a specific report details an inferior mesenteric vein-to-internal iliac vein communication. Splanchnic vein aneurysm occasionally develops (Fig. 11-47).

INTERVENTIONAL

Umbilical Catheters

Arterial and venous umbilical catheter localization by ultrasound is another real contribution to noninvasive diagnosis. The arterial umbilical catheter is ideally placed in the distal aorta below the renal arteries (Fig. 11-48). The catheter enters the internal iliac artery di-

rectly from the umbilical artery and is advanced to the distal aorta (Fig. 11-49).

The venous umbilical catheterization allows the catheter tip to advance to the most proximal position of the IVC via the portal vein and the ductus venosus to a hepatic vein near the confluence (Fig. 11-50).

Miscellaneous Catheters

Catheters can be identified intraluminally in both arteries and veins as bright, hyperechoic, linear structures (Fig. 11-51).[185] Moving the catheter under real-time visualization exaggerates its location by sonography.

During interventional procedures, catheters may break and fragment within the vessel. Ultrasound has been used to find these migrating foreign bodies.[186]

Inappropriate position of the catheter, as well as thrombosis, dissection, and perforation are complications to be alert for.[187]

Intraoperative Vascular Ultrasound

Palpation to detect vessel wall abnormality is not precise or particularly accurate. Surgeons use intraoperative sonography of the ascending aorta to try to reduce the risk of embolization of the atherosclerotic plaque that can potentially break away from the aorta to cause a stroke following vessel cannulation or clamping maneuvers of the aorta during cardiac surgery.[188] Others have used intraoperative sonography to evaluate the repair of aortic dissection,[189] to identify the integrity of graft anastomosis, and to evaluate stenosis and the presence of an intimal flap.

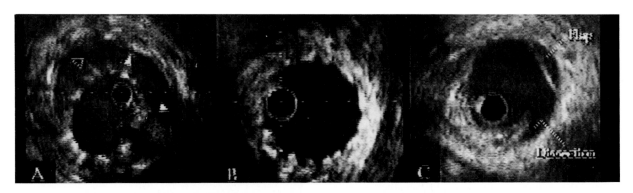

Fig. 11-53. Intravascular ultrasound: positioning. Transverse intravascular image of the iliac vessels shows **(A)** poor apposition of the probe within the vessel, **(B)** improved apposition of the probe to the vessel, and **(C)** a focal dissection and at the 2 o'clock position a linear flap. (Courtesy of PJ Fitzgerald, Department of Medicine and Cardiology, University of California, San Francisco.)

43. Rackson ME, Lossef SV, Sos TA: Renal artery stenosis in patients with aortic dissection: increased prevalence. Radiology 1990;177:555

44. Takamoto S, Omoto R: Visualization of thoracic dissecting aortic aneurysm by transesophageal Doppler color flow mapping. Herz 1987;12:187

45. Erbel R, Borner N, Steller D et al: Detection of aortic dissection by transoesophageal echocardiography. Br Heart J 1987;58:45

46. De Bock L, Van Schil PE, Vanmaele RG et al: Acute aortic dissection confined to the infrarenal segment. J Cardiovasc Surg 1989;30:867

47. Giyanani VL, Krebs CA, Nall LA et al: Diagnosis of abdominal aortic dissection by image-directed Doppler sonography. J Clin Ultrasound 1989;17:445

48. Chow WH, Tai YT, Cheung KL et al: Spontaneous dynamic echoes in aortic dissection. J Clin Ultrasound 1990;18:442

49. Rosen SA: Painless aortic dissection presenting as spinal cord ischemia. Ann Emerg Med 1988;17:840

50. Kotval PS, Babu SC, Fakhry J et al: Role of the intimal flap in arterial dissection: sonographic demonstration. AJR 1988;150:1181

51. King PS, Cooperberg PL, Madigan SM: The anechoic crescent in abdominal aortic aneurysms: not a sign of dissection. AJR 1986;146:345

52. Graham D, Alexander JJ, Franceschi D et al: The management of localized abdominal aortic dissections. J Vasc Surg 1988;8:582

53. Johansen K, Kohler TR, Nicholls SC et al: Ruptured abdominal aortic aneurysm: the Harborview experience. J Vasc Surg 1991;13:240

54. Shuman WP, Hastrup W Jr, Kohler TR et al: Suspected leaking abdominal aortic aneurysm: use of sonography in the emergency room. Radiology 1988;168:117

55. Gooding GAW: Ruptured abdominal aorta: postoperative ultrasound appearance. Radiology 1982;145:781

56. Campbell WB, Collin J, Morris PJ: The morality of abdominal aortic aneurysm. Ann R Coll Surg Engl 1986;68:275

57. Beede SD, Ballard DJ, James EM et al: Positive predictive value of clinical suspicion of abdominal aortic aneurysm. Implications for efficient use of abdominal ultrasonography. Arch Intern Med 1990;150:549

58. Lederle FA, Walker JM, Reinke DB: Selective screening for abdominal aortic aneurysms with physical examination and ultrasound. Arch Intern Med 1988;148:1753

59. Shapira OM, Pasik S, Wassermann JP et al: Ultrasound screening for abdominal aortic aneurysms in patients with atherosclerotic peripheral vascular disease. J Cardiovasc Surg 1990;31:170

60. Russell JG: Is screening for abdominal aortic aneurysm worthwhile? Clin Radiol 1990;41:182

61. Bengtsson H, Ekberg O, Aspelin P et al: Ultrasound screening of the abdominal aorta in patients with intermittent claudication. Eur J Vasc Surg 1989;3:497

62. Crawford ES: Ruptured abdominal aortic aneurysm: an editorial. J Vasc Surg 1991;18:348

63. Webster MW, Ferrell RE, St Jean PL et al: Ultrasound screening of first-degree relatives of patients with an abdominal aortic aneurysm. J Vasc Surg 1991;13:9

64. Baxter BT, McGee GS, Flinn WR et al: Distal embolization as a presenting symptom of aortic aneurysms. Am J Surg 1990;160:197

65. Ivert T, Lie M, Lunde P: Noninvasive diagnosis of fistula abdominal aortic aneurysm to the inferior vena cava. Case report. Acta Chir Scand 1988;154:669

66. Cook AM, Dyet JF, Mann SL: Ultrasonic and comparative angiographic appearances of a spontaneous aorto-caval fistula. Clin Radiol 1990;41:286

67. Daxini BV, Desai AG, Sharma S: Echo-Doppler diagnosis of aortocaval fistula following blunt trauma to abdomen. Am Heart J 1989;118:843

68. Batt M, Hassen-Khodja R, Bayada JM et al: Traumatic fistula between the aorta and the left renal vein: case report and review of the literature. J Vasc Surg 1989;9:812

69. Mansour MA, Russ PD, Subber SW et al: Aorto-left renal vein fistula: diagnosis by duplex sonography. AJR 1989;152:1107

70. Gooding GAW, Effeney DJ: Static and real-time B-mode sonography of arterial occlusions. AJR 1982;133:869

71. Seibert JJ, Taylor BJ, Williamson SL et al: Sonographic detection of neonatal umbilical-artery thrombosis: clinical correlation. AJR 1987;148:965

72. Seibert JJ, Northington FJ, Miers JF et al: Aortic thrombosis after umbilical artery catheterization in neonates: prevalence of complications on long-term follow-up. AJR 1991;156:567

73. Liu CI, Cho SR, Brewer WH et al: Inflammatory aneurysm of the abdominal aorta: diagnosis by computerized tomography and ultrasonography. South Med J 1987;80:1352

74. Fitzgerald EJ, Blackett RL: 'Inflammatory' abdominal aortic aneurysms. Clin Radiol 1988;39:247

75. Lindblad B, Almgren B, Bergqvist D et al: Abdominal aortic aneurysm with perianeurysmal fibrosis: experience from 11 Swedish vascular centers. J Vasc Surg 1991;13:231

76. Savarese RP, Rosenfeld JC, DeLaurentis DA: Inflammatory abdominal aortic aneurysm. Surg Gynecol Obstet 1986;162:405

77. Schuster JJ, Raptopoulos V, Baker SP: Increased prevalence of cholelithiasis in patients with abdominal aortic aneurysm: sonographic evaluation. AJR 1989;152:509

78. Goldenberg SL, Gordon PB, Cooperberg PL et al: Early hydronephrosis following aortic bifurcation graft surgery: a prospective study. J Urol 1988;140:1367

79. Lepke RA, Pagani JJ: Renal artery compression by an aortic aneurysm: an unusual cause of hypertension. AJR 1982;139:812

80. Pavone P, Di Cesare E, Di Renzi P et al: Abdominal aortic aneurysm evaluation: comparison of US, CT, MRI, and angiography. Magn Reson Imaging 1990;8:199

81. Wilde CC, Tan L, Cheong FW: Computed tomography and ultrasound diagnosis of mycotic aneurysm of the

abdominal aorta due to salmonella. Clin Radiol 1987;38:325

82. LaRoy LL, Cormier PJ, Matalon TAS et al: Imaging of abdominal aortic aneurysms. AJR 1989;152:785

83. Vowden P, Wilkinson D, Ausobsky JR et al: A comparison of three imaging techniques in the assessment of an abdominal aortic aneurysm. J Cardiovasc Surg 1989;30:891

84. De Simone R, Haberbosch W, Iarussi D et al: Transesophageal echocardiography for the diagnosis of thoracic aortic aneurysms and dissections. Cardiologia 1990;35:387

85. Adachi H, Kyo S, Takamoto S et al: Early diagnosis and surgical intervention of acute aortic dissection by transesophageal color flow mapping. Circulation 1990;82:19

86. Shively BK: Transesophageal echocardiography in the assessment of aortic pathology. J Thorac Imaging 1990;5:40

87. Shah DM, Chang BB, Paty PSK et al: Treatment of abdominal aortic aneurysm by exclusion and bypass: an analysis of outcome. J Vasc Surg 1991;13:15

88. Gooding GAW, Herzog KA, Hedgcock MW et al: B-mode ultrasonography of prosthetic vascular grafts. Radiology 1978;127:763

89. Gooding GAW, Effeney DJ, Goldstone J: The aortofemoral graft: detection and identification of healing complications by ultrasonography. Surgery 1981;89:94

90. Nunn DB, Carter MM, Donohue MT et al: Postoperative dilation of knitted Dacron aortic bifurcation graft. J Vasc Surg 1990;12:291

91. Polak JF, Donaldson MC, Whittemore AD et al: Pulsatile masses surrounding vascular prostheses: real-time US color flow imaging. Radiology 1989;170:363

92. Paes E, Paulat K, Hamann H et al: Early detection and differentiation of periprosthetic fluid accumulation after vascular reconstructive surgery. Surg Endosc 1988;2:256

93. Coughlin BF, Paushter DM: Peripheral pseudoaneurysms: evaluation with duplex US. Radiology 1988; 168:339

94. Tobin KD: Aortobifemoral perigraft abscess: treatment by percutaneous catheter drainage. J Vasc Surg 1988;8:339

95. Grenier N, Douws C, Morel D et al: Detection of vascular complications in renal allografts with color Doppler flow imaging. Radiology 1991;178:217

96. Subramanyam BR, Lefleur RS, Bosniak MA: Renal arteriovenous fistulas and aneurysms: sonographic findings. Radiology 1983;149:261

97. Middleton WD, Kellman GM, Melson GL et al: Postbiopsy renal transplant arteriovenous fistulas: color Doppler US characteristics. Radiology 1989;171:253

98. Strandness DE Jr: The renal arteries. p. 146. In Duplex Scanning in Vascular Disorders, Raven Press, New York, 1990

99. Taylor DC, Kettler MC, Moneta GL et al: Duplex ultrasound in the diagnosis of renal artery stenosis: a prospective evaluation. J Vasc Surg 1988;7:363

100. Taylor DC, Moneta GL, Strandness DE Jr: Follow-up of renal artery stenosis by duplex ultrasound. J Vasc Surg 1989;9:410

101. Hantman SS, Barie JJ, Glendening TB et al: Giant renal artery aneurysm mimicking a single cyst on ultrasound. J Clin Ultrasound 1982;10:136

102. Mostbeck GH, Gossinger HD, Mallek R et al: Effect of heart rate on Doppler measurements of resistive index in renal arteries. Radiology 1990;175:511

103. Patten RM, Coldwell DM, Ben-Menachem Y: Ligamentous compression of the celiac axis: CT findings in five patients. AJR 1991;156:1101

104. Gooding GAW: Ultrasound of a superior mesenteric artery aneurysm secondary to pancreatitis: a plea for real-time ultrasound of sonolucent masses in pancreatitis. J Clin Ultrasound 1981;9:255

105. Ugolotti U, Miselli A, Mandrioli R et al: Ultrasound diagnosis of superior mesenteric artery aneurysm: two case reports. J Clin Ultrasound 1984;12:581

106. Bloom RA, Cracium E, Jurim O et al: Sonographic demonstration of hepatic venous gas in mesenteric arterial thrombosis. J Clin Gatroenterol 1988;10:226

107. Chezmar JL, Nelson RC, Bernardino ME: Portal venous gas after hepatic transplantation: sonographic detection and clinical significance. AJR 1989;153:1203

108. Kosuge T, Makuuchi M, Takayama T et al: Thickening at the root of the superior mesenteric artery on sonography: evidence of vascular involvement in patients with cancer of the pancreas. AJR 1991;156:69

109. Gomes MN, Choyke PL: Pre-operative evaluation of abdominal aortic aneurysms: ultrasound or computed tomography? J Cardiovasc Surg 1987;28:159

110. Strandness DE Jr: Duplex scanning for diagnosis of peripheral arterial disease. Herz 1988;13:372

111. Langsfeld M, Nepute J, Hershey FB et al: The use of deep duplex scanning to predict hemodynamically significant aortoiliac stenoses. J Vasc Surg 1988;7:395

112. de Smet AA, Kitslaar PJ: A duplex criterion for aorto-iliac stenosis. Eur J Vasc Surg 1990;4:275

113. Legemate DA, Teeuwen C, Hoeneveld H: The potential of duplex scanning to replace aorto-iliac and femoropopliteal angiography. Eur J Vasc Surg 1989;3:49

114. Kresowik TF, Khoury MD, Miller BV et al: A prospective study of the incidence and natural history of femoral vascular complications after percutaneous transluminal coronary angioplasty. J Vasc Surg 1991;13:328

115. Kotval PS, Khoury A, Shah PM et al: Doppler sonographic demonstration of the progressive spontaneous thrombosis of pseudoaneurysms. J Ultrasound Med 1990;9:185

116. Fellmeth BD, Roberts AC, Bookstein JJ et al: Postangiographic femoral artery injuries: nonsurgical repair with US-guided compression. Radiology 1991;178:671

117. Walstra BR, Janevski BK, Jörning PJ: Primary arteriovenous fistula between common iliac vessels: ultrasound, computer tomographic, and angiographic findings—a case report. Angiology 1989;40:222

118. Helvie MA, Rubin J: Evaluation of traumatic groin arteriovenous fistulas with duplex Doppler sonography. J Ultrasound Med 1989;8:21

119. Liu JB, Merton DA, Mitchell DG et al: Color Doppler imaging of the iliofemoral region. RadioGraphics 1990;10:403

120. Igidbashian VN, Mitchell DG, Middleton WD et al: Iatrogenic femoral arteriovenous fistula: diagnosis with color Doppler imaging. Radiology 1989;170:749

121. Knudtzon J, Gudmundsen TE, Svane S: Congenital absence of the entire inferior vena cava. The diagnostic significance of varicose veins of the abdominal wall. Acta Chir Scand 1986;152:541

122. Giordano JM, Trout HH: Anomalies of the inferior vena cava. J Vasc Surg 1986;3:924

123. Senecail B, Lefevre C, Person H et al: Radiologic anatomy of duplication of the inferior vena cava: a trap in abdominal imaging. A report of 8 cases. Surg Radiol Anat 1987;9:151

124. Gollub MJ, Friedwald JP, Sceusa D: Sonographic diagnosis of transposition of the inferior vena cava. J Clin Ultrasound 1990;18:502

125. Kinard RE, Orrison WW: Ultrasound demonstration of the retroaortic left renal vein. J Clin Ultrasound 1986;14:151

126. Hernanz-Schulman M, Ambrosino MM, Genieser NB et al: Current evaluation of the patient with abnormal visceroatrial situs. AJR 1990;153:797

127. Tonkin ILD, Tonkin AK: Visceroatrial situs abnormalities: sonographic and computed tomographic appearance. AJR 1982;138:509

128. Jimenez M, Hery E, van Doesburg NH et al: Inferior vena cava stenosis in scimitar syndrome: a case report. J Am Soc Echocardiol 1988;1:152

129. Jayanthi V, Victor S, Dhala B et al: Pre-operative and post-operative ultrasound evaluation of Budd-Chiari syndrome due to coarctation of the inferior vena cava. Clin Radiol 1988;39:154

130. Chezmar JL, Bernardino ME: Mesoatrial shunt for the treatment of Budd-Chiari syndrome: radiologic evaluation in eight patients. AJR 1987;149:707

131. Roguin N, Lam M, Frenkel A et al: Radionuclide angiography of azygos continuation of inferior vena cava in left atrial isomerism (polysplenia syndrome). Clin Nucl Med 1987;12:708

132. Stiris MG, Finnanger AM: Postrenal segment aneurysm and infrahepatic interruption of the inferior vena cava. A case report. Acta Radiol 1987;28:545

133. Schaffer RM, Sunshine AG, Becker JA et al: Retrocaval ureter: sonographic appearance. J Ultrasound Med 1985;4:199

134. Ohnishi K, Terabayashi H, Tsunoda T et al: Budd-Chiari syndrome: diagnosis with duplex sonography. Am J Gastroenterol 1990;85:165

135. Brown BP, Abu-Yousef M, Farner R et al: Doppler sonography: a noninvasive method for evaluation of hepatic venocclusive disease. Am J Roentgenol 1990;154:721

136. Gentil-Kocher S, Bernard O, Brunelle F et al: Budd-Chiari syndrome in children: report of 22 cases. J Pediatr 1988;113:30

137. Hoffman HD, Stockland B, von der Heyden U: Membranous obstruction of the inferior vena cava with Budd-Chiari syndrome in children: a report of nine cases. J Pediatr Gastroenterol Nutr 1987;6:878

138. Park JH, Lee JB, Han MC et al: Sonographic evaluation of inferior vena caval obstruction: correlative study with vena cavography. AJR 1985;145:757

139. Uglietta JP, Woodruff WW, Effmann EL et al: Duplex Doppler ultrasound evaluation of calcified inferior vena cava thrombosis. Pediatr Radiol 1989;19:250

140. van der Vange N, Bruinse HW: Hydrops fetalis associated with inferior vena cava thrombosis. Eur J Obstet Gynecol Reprod Biol 1986;21:113

141. Bouwels LH, Cheriex EC, de Zwaan C et al: Diagnosis and follow-up of a large inferior caval vein thrombus following right heart catheterization. Eur Heart J 1987;8:198

142. Puylaert JB, Ulrich C: Spontaneous thrombolysis of a large caval thrombus after insertion of an inferior vena cava filter: diagnosis and follow-up by ultrasound. Diagn Imaging Clin Med 1986;55:121

143. Gallaher KJ, Gross G: Bladder distention as a cause of inferior vena caval obstruction in the newborn: demonstration with ultrasonography. Am J Perinatol 1989;6:424

144. Ashkenazi S, Pickering LK, Robinson LH: Diagnosis and management of septic thrombosis of the inferior vena cava caused by Candida tropicalis. Pediatr Infect Dis J 1990;9:446

145. Hodkinson J, Couper-Smith J, Kew MC: Inferior vena caval and right atrial thrombosis complicating an amebic hepatic abscess. Am J Gastroenterol 1988;83:786

146. James PN, Chalmers AG, Fowler RC: Ultrasound demonstration of gas in hepatic veins. Clin Radiol 1989;40:429

147. Segura JM, Conthe P, Martin R: Pulmonary hydatid seeding mimicking hematogenous metastases: sonographic diagnosis of hydatid rupture into the inferior vena cava. J Clin Ultrasound 1989;17:112

148. Liu GC, Angtuaco TL, Ferris EJ et al: Inferior vena caval filters: noninvasive evaluation. Radiology 1986;160:521

149. Guglielmo FF, Kurtz AB, Wechsler RJ: Prospective comparison of computed tomography and duplex sonography in the evaluation of recently inserted Kimray-Greenfield filters into the inferior vena cava. Clin Imaging 1990;14:216

150. Alberts WM, Tonner JA, Goldman AL: Echocardiography in planned interruption of the inferior vena cava. South Med J 1989;82:772

151. Dorfman GS, Cronan JJ, Paolella LP et al: Iatrogenic changes at the venotomy site after percutaneous placement of the Greenfield filter. Radiology 1989;173:159

152. Mewissen MW, Erickson SJ, Foley WD et al: Thrombosis at venous insertion sites after inferior vena caval filter placement. Radiology 1989;173:155

153. Harris JP, Kidd J, Burnett A et al: Patency of femorofemoral venous crossover grafts assessed by duplex scanning and phlebography. J Vasc Surg 1988;8:679

154. Perhoniemi V, Salmenkivi K, Vorne M: Venous haemo-

dynamics in the legs after ligation of the inferior vena cava. Acta Chir Scand 1986;152:23

155. Fong KW, Zalev AH: Sonographic diagnosis of leiomyosarcoma of the inferior vena cava: correlation with computed tomography and angiography. Can Assoc Rad J 1987;38:229

156. Cederlund CG, Edin R: Asymptomatic leiomyosarcoma of the inferior vena cava. Incidental finding at ultrasonography. Acta Radiol 1987;28:181

157. Bousquet JC, Goze A, Hassan M et al: Leiomyosarcoma of the inferior vena cava. Ultrasonographic appearance. J Ultrasound Med 1987;6:7

158. Kracht M, Becquemin JP, Anglade MC et al: Acute Budd-Chiari syndrome secondary to leiomyosarcoma of the inferior vena cava. Ann Vasc Surg 1989;3:268

159. Dunlap HJ, Udjus K: Atypical leiomyoma arising in an hepatic vein with extension into the inferior vena cava and right atrium. Report of a case in a child. Pediatr Radiol 1990;20:202

160. Hietala SO, Ekelund L, Ljungberg B: Venous invasion in renal cell carcinoma: a correlative clinical and radiologic study. Urol Radiol 1988;9:210

161. Webb JA, Murray A, Bary PR et al: The accuracy and limitations of ultrasound in the assessment of venous extension in renal carcinoma. Br J Urol 1987;60:14

162. Giuliani L, Giberti C, Martorana G et al: Value of computerized tomography and ultrasonography in the preoperative diagnosis of renal cell carcinoma extending into the inferior vena cava. Eur Urol 1987;13:26

163. Arenson AM, Graham RT, Shaw P et al: Angiomyolipoma of the kidney extending into the inferior vena cava: sonographic and CT findings. AJR 1988;151:1159

164. Didier D, Racle A, Etievent JP et al: Tumor thrombus of the inferior vena cava secondary to malignant abdominal neoplasms: US and CT evaluation. Radiology 1987;162:83

165. Godine LB, Berdon WE, Brasch RC et al: Adrenocortical carcinoma with extension into inferior vena cava and right atrium: report of 3 cases in children. Pediatr Radiol 1990;20:166

166. Dicke TE, Henry ML, Minton JP: Intracaval extension of pheochromocytoma simulating pulmonary embolism. J Surg Oncol 1987;34:160

167. Vargas-Barron J, Keirns C, Barragan-Garcia R et al: Intracardiac extension of malignant uterine tumors. Echocardiographic detection and successful surgical resection. J Thorac Cardiovasc Surg 1990;99:1099

168. Ritchey ML, Kelalis PP, Breslow N et al: Intracaval and atrial involvement with nephroblastoma: review of National Wilms Tumor Study-3. J Urol 1988;140:1113

169. Patel CC, Rees A, Bertolone SJ: Intracardiac extension of Wilms tumor. Am J Pediatr Hematol-Oncol 1989;11:46

170. Shapiro RS, Silvers AR, Halton KP et al: Medial indentation of the inferior vena cava. J Ultrasound Med 1991;10:227

171. Lalmand B, Avni EF, Nasr A et al: Perinatal renal vein thrombosis. Sonographic demonstration. J Ultrasound Med 1990;9:437

172. Reuther G, Wanjura D, Bauer H: Acute renal vein thrombosis in renal allografts: detection with duplex Doppler US. Radiology 1989;170:557

173. Wiggelinkkhuizen J, Oleszczuk-Raszke K, Nagel FO: Renal venous thrombosis in infancy. S Afr Med J 1989;75:413

174. Washecka R, Hulnick DH, Catanese A et al: Postpartum renal vein thrombosis with left retroaortic renal vein. Urology 1987;29:548

175. Delbeke D, Sacks GA, Sandler MP: Diagnosis of allograft renal vein thrombosis. Clin Nucl Med 1989;14:415

176. Jayogapal S, Cohen HL, Brill PW et al: Calcified neonatal renal vein thrombosis demonstration by CT and US. Pediatr Radiol 1990;20:160

177. Sanders LD, Jequier S: Ultrasound demonstration of prenatal renal vein thrombosis. Pediatr Radiol 1989;19:133

178. Wolfish NM, McLaine PN, Martin D: Renal vein entrapment syndrome: frequency and diagnosis. A lesson in conservatism. Clin Nephrol 1986;26:96

179. Carvalho P: Sonographic demonstration of renal tumour extension into the contralateral renal vein. Br J Radiol 1989;62:1093

180. Martin J, Garcia M, Duran A et al: Renal vein leiomyosarcoma: a case report and literature review. Urol Radiol 1989;11:25

181. Freling NJ, Schuur KH, Haagsma EB et al: Ultrasound as first imaging modality in superior mesenteric and portal vein thrombosis. J Clin Ultrasound 1986;14:554

182. Ida M, Arai K, Yoshikawa J et al: Therapeutic hepatic vein angioplasty for Budd-Chiari syndrome. Cardiovasc Interventional Radiol 1986;9:187

183. Kidambi H, Herbert R, Kidambi AV: Ultrasonic demonstration of superior mesenteric and splenoportal venous thrombosis. J Clin Ultrasound 1986;14:199

184. Horiguchi Y, Kitano T, Takagawa H: A large inferior mesenteric-caval shunt via the internal iliac vein. Gatrointest Jpn 1988;23:684

185. Gooding GAW, Bank WO: Ultrasound visualization of 5-F catheter. Radiology 1982;144:647

186. Woo VL, Gerber AM, Scheible W et al: Real-time ultrasound guidance for percutaneous transluminal retrieval of nonopaque intravascular catheter fragment. AJR 1979;133:760

187. Oppenheimer DA, Carroll BA, Garth KE: Ultrasonic detection of complications following umbilical arterial catheterization in the neonate. Radiology 1982;145:667

188. Marshall WG Jr, Barzilai B, Kouchoukos NT et al: Intraoperative ultrasonic imaging of the ascending aorta. Ann Thorac Surg 1989;48:339

189. Kyo S, Takamoto S, Adachi H: Intraoperative evaluation of repair of aortic dissection: surgical decision making. Int J Cardiac Imaging 1989;4:49

190. Nishimura RA, Welch TJ, Stanson AW et al: Intravascular US of the distal aorta and iliac vessels: initial feasibility studies. Radiology 1990;176:523

191. Isner JM, Rosenfield K, Losordo DW et al: Percutaneous intravascular US as adjunct to catheter-based interventions: preliminary experience in patients with peripheral vascular disease. Radiology 1990;175:61

192. Pandian NG, Kreis A, Weintraub A et al: Real-time intravascular ultrasound imaging in humans. Am J Cardiol 1990;65:1392

193. Harrison JK, Sheikh KH, Davidson CJ et al: Balloon angioplasty of coarctation of the aorta evaluated with intravascular ultrasound imaging. J Am Coll Cardiol 1990;15:906

194. Davidson CJ, Sheikh KH, Harrison JK et al: Intravascular ultrasonography vesus digital subtraction angiography: a human in vivo comparison of vessel size and morphology. J Am Coll Cardiol 1990;16:633

195. Gussenhoven WJ, Essed CE, Frietman P et al: Intravascular echographic assessment of vessel wall characteristics: a correlation with histology. Int J Cardiac Imaging 1989;4:105

196. Schmitz-Rode T, Günther RW, Müller-Leisse C: US-assisted aspiration thrombectomy: in vitro investigations. Radiology 1991;178:677

197. Khoo HT: The large inferior vena cava—a sign in arteriovenous fistula between the right common iliac artery and the inferior vena cava. J Clin Ultrasound 1982;10:291

198. Royal SA, Callen PW: CT evaluation of anomalies of the inferior vena cava and left renal vein. AJR 1979;132:759

199. Schild H, Schweder F, Braun B, Lang H: Aneurysms of the superior mesenteric vein. Radiology 1982;145:641

200. Gooding GAW: Peripheral vascular (arterial and venous). In Goldberg B (ed): Diagnostic Ultrasound. Williams & Wilkins, Baltimore (in press)

12

Retroperitoneum

Carol A. Mittelstaedt

For years, the retroperitoneum has been a difficult region to image radiographically. Additionally, signs and symptoms of retroperitoneal diseases are frequently vague and poorly localized. With the advent of ultrasound and computed tomography (CT), retroperitoneal disorders are readily identified and their spread through the various retroperitoneal compartments assessed.[1]

TECHNIQUE

Preparation

There is no specific preparation for an ultrasound examination of the retroperitoneal structure. Because the study is sometimes limited by bowel gas, an overnight fast is desirable to diminish this problem.

Adrenal

The overall success of visualization of the normal adrenal by ultrasound depends on the size of the patient, the amount of perirenal fat, and the effect of bowel gas.[2] It also depends in part on the persistence of the examiner since various projections must be tried before abandoning the examination. The development of new equipment with sophisticated beam-focusing capabilities has permitted better visualization of the adult adrenal gland.

One approach to examination of the adrenal is a specific alignment between the kidney and the ipsilateral paravertebral vessel (inferior vena cava [IVC] or aorta);

this is best accomplished in the decubitus position.[3,4] The scan is performed in a line connecting the center of the kidney and the paravertebral vessel by scanning from the anterolateral aspect of the patient[5,6] (Fig. 12-1). This approach visualizes the adrenal in its coronal section, which is in line with the central axis of the kidney.[7] To visualize the adrenal, as well as to separate it from the crus of the diaphragm, one must sector through the appropriate intercostal space (9th to 10th) between the junction of the anterior midaxillary line during suspended respiration.[8,9] A deep inspiration is essential to scan subcostally either in the midclavicular line or through the flank.[8] Small changes in the receiver sensitivity and/or transducer output are often required to distinguish the adrenal from surrounding retroperitoneal fibrofatty tissue.[4] The time-gain-compensation (TGC) and gain are adjusted by using the renal parenchyma as a reference; normally there are fine echoes within the parenchyma.

One of the most successful techniques for visualization of the adrenal is the coronal approach (Figs. 12-1 to 12-3). This scan may be performed in the supine, decubitus, or upright position with the transducer in the mid- to posterior axillary line. These coronal views may be performed with the patient in a 45 to 90 degree posterior oblique or opposite decubitus position — right lateral decubitus for left-sided structures and left lateral decubitus for right-sided structures.[10] Most often, coronal sections are performed with the patient in the left lateral decubitus position scanning from the right side in the subcostal or intercostal spaces. For the cephalic extent of these structures, the right hepatic lobe functions as an

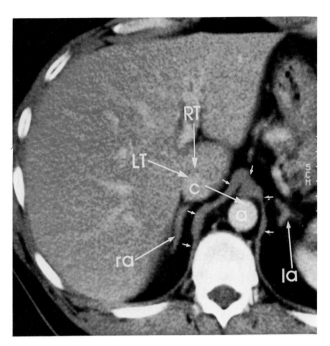

Fig. 12-1. Adrenal glands: CT scan. The relationship of the right *(ra)* and left *(la)* adrenal glands to the aorta *(a)* and inferior vena cava *(c)* can be seen. The right adrenal can be visualized with ultrasound by scanning directly anterior through the inferior vena cava with the patient supine *(RT)* or in the anterior axillary line with the patient in the left lateral decubitus position. The left adrenal may be best visualized by scanning sagittally in the midclavicular line (or anterior axillary line, *LT*) with the patient in the left lateral decubitus position, using the aorta and inferior vena cava as "acoustic windows." In this position, the left adrenal is seen posterior to the aorta on ultrasound. (arrows, diaphragmatic crura.)

acoustic window. When scanning from the left in the right lateral decubitus position, the window achieved does not produce images as reliably as does the window through the hepatic lobe.[10] One should slowly sector from lateral to posterolateral toward the inferior vena cava or aorta, which are used as references in the longitudinal and transverse planes.[11]

Sagittal scans angled slightly off the true coronal axis can be used to most favorably demonstrate the desired anatomy. On a sagittal scan along the axillary line, the IVC and aorta are first visualized; then the transducer is angled posteriorly toward the adrenal region. On a sagittal scan with the transducer angled anteriorly and the patient supine, the IVC is first seen; then the scan plane is slightly angled in a mediolateral direction. The right gland can be seen anterior to the right crus and posterior to the IVC at the level of the right portal branch.[12]

The left adrenal gland can be very difficult to visualize because it is often obscured by gastric or bowel gas. The left adrenal may be best visualized by scanning in the posterior axillary line with the patient in the right decubitus position.[6,8,9] It is seen medial to the spleen, lateral to the aorta and crus of the diaphragm, superomedial to the left kidney, and posterior to the stomach and pancreatic tail.[5,6] The aorta and crus of the diaphragm are visualized by using the spleen and the left kidney as "acoustic windows."[6] Ten percent of left adrenals have been reported to extend down to the area of the renal hilum.[5]

An additional technique for improved visualization of the left adrenal gland has been reported.[13] With this technique, the left adrenal gland is examined both in the conventional right posterior oblique (RPO) position and by using the new cava-suprarenal line (CSL) position[13] (Figs. 12-1 and 12-3). The patient is placed in the 45 degree left posterior oblique position, and transverse scans are made from the right side to localize the left adrenal gland.[13] By using the aorta and IVC as double windows, sagittal views can be obtained after localization (Fig. 12-3). Additionally, measurements of length and depth of the gland can be obtained.[13]

Others have evaluated the adrenal glands by using linear-array real-time equipment instead of a sector transducer.[12] With a 3.5-MHz electronically focused transducer and the patient supine or with the left flank slightly elevated, sagittal or oblique scans are performed along the axillary line[12] (Fig. 12-4). With the spleen as an acoustic window, the transducer is placed in the intercostal space with the scan plane angled toward the adrenal region.[12] On the left, the adrenal gland is delineated from the spleen, the left diaphragmatic crus, the aorta, and the upper pole of the kidney.[12] On the right, the adrenal gland is delineated from the liver, the right diaphragmatic crus, the IVC, and the upper pole of the kidney (Fig. 12-4). The right and left adrenal glands are visualized in 98.5 and 90 percent of patients, respectively, by using this technique.[12]

The normal adrenal glands are not visualized as often in the prone position as in other positions. Masses as large as 3 cm can be detected with this approach.

How often is the adrenal gland visualized on ultrasound? Previous reports have stated that the normal adrenal is visualized in 85 percent of cases and the normal adrenal area in 12 percent.[3] The normal gland on the right has been reported to be visualized in 78 to 90 percent, with the left visualized in 44 to 80 percent.[2,14] With real-time sonography, the right adrenal can be identified in 82 percent of sagittal scans and 78.5 percent of transverse scans at the midaxillary line in the 9th to 10th intercostal space.[8] When scanning in the anterior axillary line through the flank, the right adrenal gland can be visualized in 53.5 percent of scans; when scanning subcostally oblique in the midclavicular line parallel to the rib cage, it can be visualized in 39.2 percent of scans.[8]

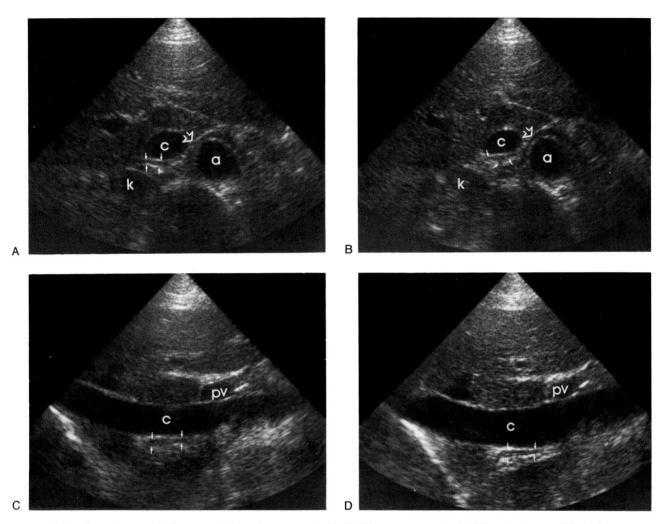

Fig. 12-2. Normal right adrenal. Anterior approach. **(A & B)** Transverse and **(C & D)** sagittal scans. The right adrenal (arrows) is seen as a lucent structure surrounded by echogenic fat posterior to the inferior vena cava *(c)* and lateral to the diaphragmatic crus (open arrow). Note that in Fig. A a different "limb" of the adrenal is visualized than from that in Fig. B. The same is true in Figs. C & D. (*a*, aorta; *k*, right kidney; *pv*, portal vein.)

The left adrenal can be seen in 41 percent of sagittal scans and 21.4 percent of transverse scans when scanning intercostally.[8] It is seen in 12.5 percent of sagittal scans when scanning in the flank in the posterior axillary line.[8] The least favorable approach for adrenal scanning is the posterior approach, in which the adrenal is seen only 1.7 to 3.5 percent of the time.[8]

With the development of new equipment with sophisticated beam-focusing capabilities, the adult adrenal gland can be better visualized. Ninety-nine percent of adrenals can be successfully visualized when imaged with the patient supine. The right lateral decubitus and upright positions are helpful when the adrenal region is obscured by interfering intestinal gas.[15] With a mean examination time of less than 1 minute, the right adrenal gland can be detected in 92 percent of patients.[15] The

mean examination time for the left adrenal is 2.5 minutes, with visualization in 71 percent.[15] Because of the complex shape of the adrenal gland, complete visualization necessitates multiple contiguous scan planes.

Use of the CSL position permits identification of the left adrenal gland in 90 percent of patients, in contrast to 60 percent when the RPO position is used. Additionally, the left adrenal examination takes half the time required for the examination of patients in the RPO position.[13] The most marked improvement with this technique is in obese and pediatric patients; there is improved ability to demonstrate the gland and reduction in time required for the examination.[13]

The reasons for poor adrenal visibility are the small size of the gland, poor lateral resolution of ultrasound, and small differences in impedance between adrenals

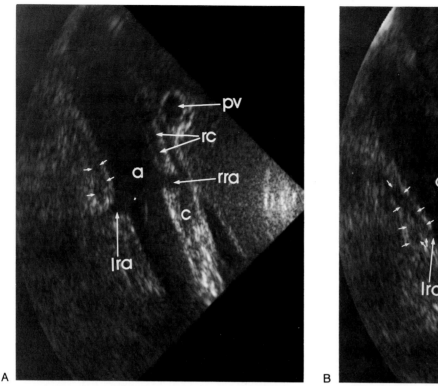
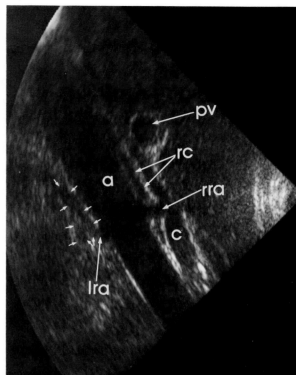

Fig. 12-3. Normal left adrenal. (**A & B**) With the patient in the left lateral decubitus position and the transducer in the midclavicular line angled to the left, the adrenal (small arrows) is seen posterior to the aorta *(a)*. Figs. A & B are at slightly different levels. Two limbs are seen to the adrenal in Fig. B. (*pv*, portal vein; *rc*, right crus; *c*, inferior vena cava; *lra*, left renal artery; *rra*, right renal artery.)

and surrounding fatty tissue.[8] Lesions as small as 12 to 20 mm have been identified by real-time ultrasound.[8] When the adrenal area is scanned, a tumor may be ruled out if no round or oval lesion is seen, even if the normal gland is not visualized. The sensitivity of this sort of scan is 97 percent, with a 96.5 percent specificity.[2]

Diaphragmatic Crura

With the recent improvements in resolution of the ultrasound equipment, extremely small anatomic structures are now being recognized with increasing frequency. The proper identification of these normal structures is important because they often serve as useful anatomic landmarks or may be misinterpreted as abnormalities.

The longitudinal coronal approach improves the visualization of the crura. These views may be obtained with the patient in a 45 to 90 degree posterior oblique or opposite decubitus position — right lateral decubitus for left-sided structures and left lateral decubitus for right-

sided structures.[10] Most often, coronal sections are performed with the patient in the left lateral decubitus position, scanning from the right side in the subcostal or intercostal spaces. When scanning from the left in the right lateral decubitus position, the window achieved does not produce images as reliably as does the window through the hepatic lobe.[10] For the cephalic extent of these structures, the right hepatic lobe functions as an acoustic window. Sagittal scans angled slightly off the true coronal axis can be used to most favorably demonstrate the desired anatomy. At times, coronal scans may be performed while the patient is supine.

The right crus is seen in a plane that passes through the right lobe of the liver, the kidney, and the adrenal gland (Figs. 12-1, 12-2, 12-5, and 12-6). When scanning transversely, the right diaphragmatic crus can be visualized on a view of the upper abdomen; its sagittal course between the IVC and aorta makes it particularly well visualized by coronal scanning.[10] The left is seen by using the spleen and left kidney as windows; the sound is perpendicular to the left crus, so it is to the left of the aorta[16] (Fig. 12-7).

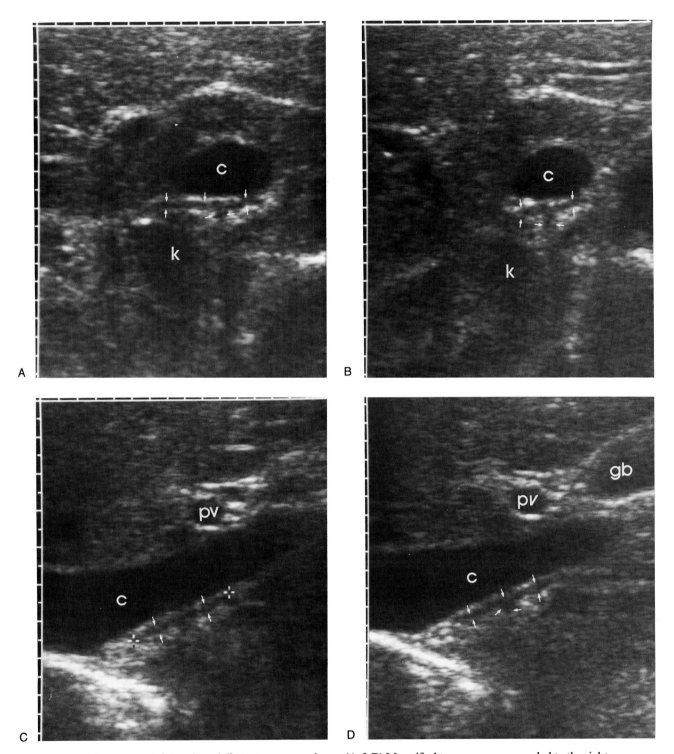

Fig. 12-4. Normal right adrenal, linear array transducer. **(A & B)** Magnified transverse scans angled to the right and left with the limbs (arrows) of the right adrenal seen. (*c*, inferior vena cava; *k*, right kidney.) **(C & D)** Magnified sagittal views through the inferior vena cava *(c)* demonstrate the right adrenal with a length of 3 cm. In Fig. D two limbs of the adrenal are seen. (*pv*, portal vein; *gb*, gallbladder.)

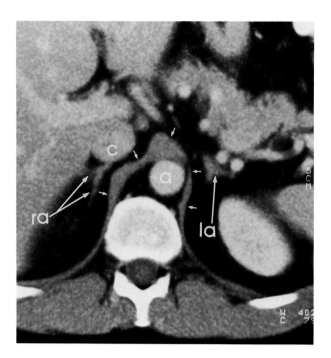

Fig. 12-5. Crura scanning approach. CT scan. The diaphragmatic crura (small arrows) can be seen as a linear soft tissue density between the adrenals and the aorta *(a).* On the right, it is seen in a plane that passes through the right lobe of the liver, inferior vena cava *(c),* and right adrenal *(ra).* It is also seen between the inferior vena cava and aorta *(a),* as well as anterior to the aorta. (*la,* left adrenal.)

Nodes

The para-aortic nodes are not visualized on ultrasound unless they are enlarged. They may be enlarged secondary to metastatic disease, lymphoma, or inflammation. As such, one must be able to identify their presence. To search for lymphadenopathy, it is necessary to identify the aorta and IVC and follow their course, looking for masses[17] (Figs. 12-8 and 12-9). In addition, the courses of the major branches of these vessels must be followed. Sometimes enlarged nodes are even seen posterior to the aorta (Fig. 12-10). Enlarged nodes may also be found in the porta hepatis, renal hila, and splenic hilum (Fig. 12-11). Sometimes these areas, as well as the para-aortic area, are difficult to visualize as a result of bowel gas. The study may be facilitated somewhat by the oral administration of water to help transmit the sound beam and displace the gas.

For better visualization, the patient may be scanned in various positions such as supine, lateral decubitus, and upright. When scanning through the anterior abdominal wall, the abdominal great vessels and the para-aortic and paracaval regions can often be obscured by overlying bowel gas and/or fat.[18] Most often, coronal sections are performed with the patient in the left lateral decubitus position scanning from the right side in the subcostal or intercostal spaces. With a coronal scan, the right lobe of the liver and the right kidney act as good acoustic transmitters and move anteriad and inferiad into the pathway

of the sound beam.[18] With the left kidney as an acoustic window, coronal scans may be obtained in the right posterior oblique position, although the left is usually less satisfactory because of the absence of the liver.[10,18] At times, coronal scans can be performed while the patient is supine. Sagittal scans angled slightly off the true coronal axis can most favorably demonstrate the desired anatomy. There is improved visibility of the para-aortic and paracaval nodes in the oblique view.[19] Generally, the prone position is not useful in evaluation of para-aortic and other abdominal nodes.

General Retroperitoneum

In some instances, the entire retroperitoneum must be scanned, for example, when looking for a hematoma, an abscess, retroperitoneal fibrosis, lymphoceles, or a tumor. With a real-time system, the entire area (the diaphragm to the iliac crest) can be scanned with the patient supine and then the upper abdomen can be scanned in the lateral decubitus or supine position by using a coronal approach (see above). To be complete, all scans of the retroperitoneum must include the kidneys, from which many processes originate; the kidneys can be used as landmarks. One should note whether the kidneys move with respiration, because in a perinephric inflammatory process they will not move. The retroperitoneum muscles should be identified.

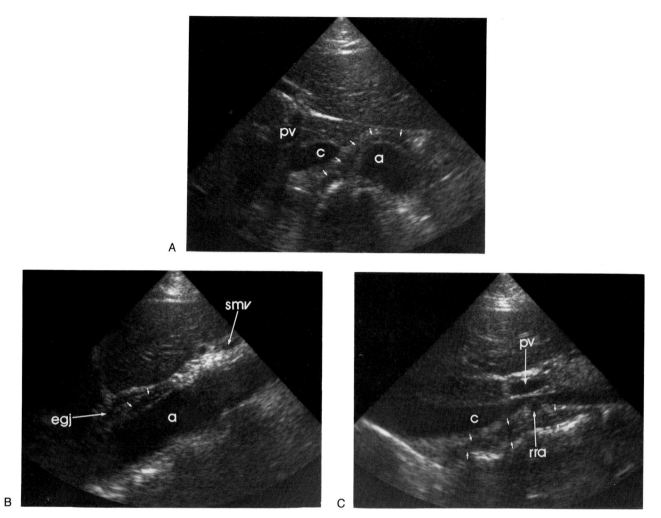

A

B

C

Fig. 12-6. Right crus. **(A)** Transverse scan from a directly anterior approach demonstrating the right crus (arrows) as a hypoechoic linear structure posterior to the inferior vena cava *(c)*; it runs between the inferior vena cava and aorta *(a),* as well as anterior to the aorta. (*pv,* portal vein.) **(B)** Directly anterior sagittal scan demonstrating the crus (arrows) as a hypoechoic structure anterior to the aorta *(a).* This represents the anterior decussation of the crus. It ends cephalically near the esophagogastric junction *(egj).* (*smv,* superior mesenteric vein.) **(C)** Sagittal scan from the anterior axillary line demonstrating the right crus (small arrows) as a hypoechoic structure posterior and parallel to the inferior vena cava *(c).* (*pv,* portal vein; *rra,* right renal artery.)

Fig. 12-7. Left crus. Transverse scan from a directly anterior approach demonstrating the left crus (arrows) as a hypoechoic structure running anterior and lateral to the aorta *(a).* The esophagogastric junction *(egj)* can be seen anteriorly. (*S,* spine; *c,* inferior vena cava; *L,* liver.)

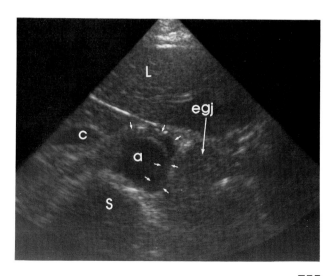

755

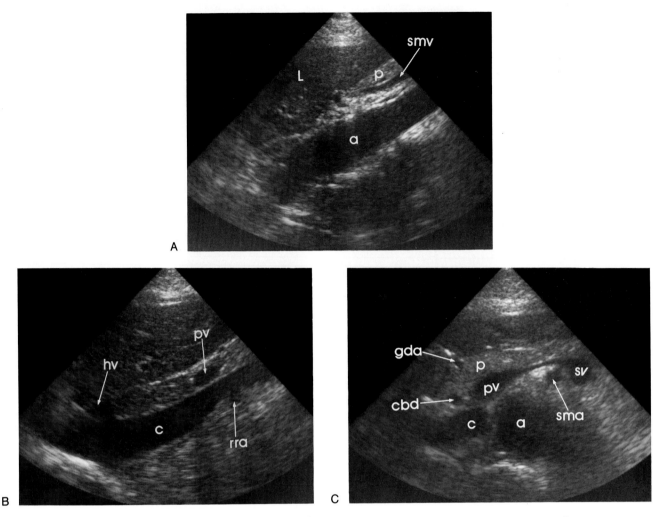

Fig. 12-8. Normal inferior vena cava and aorta. **(A)** Sagittal (long axis) view of the normal aorta *(a),* which runs posteriorly as it goes superiorly. (*L,* liver; *p,* pancreas; *smv,* superior mesenteric vein.) **(B)** Sagittal supine view demonstrating the inferior vena cava *(c)* as a tubular anechoic structure projecting anterior as it runs cephalad. (*hv,* hepatic vein; *pv,* portal vein; *rra,* right renal artery.) **(C)** Transverse supine view of the inferior vena cava *(c)* and aorta *(a).* No nodes are normally seen anterior to the inferior vena cava or aorta. (*p,* pancreas; *sv,* splenic vein; *gda,* gastroduodenal artery; *cbd,* distal common bile duct; *sma,* superior mesenteric artery; *pv,* portal vein.)

NORMAL ANATOMY

The retroperitoneum is delineated anteriorly by the posterior peritoneum, posteriorly by the transversalis fascia, and laterally by the lateral borders of the quadratus lumborum muscle and peritoneal leaves of the mesentery (Fig. 12-12). In its superior to inferior axes, the retroperitoneum extends from the diaphragm to the pelvic brim[1] (Fig. 12-13). Superior to the pelvic brim, the retroperitoneum can be partitioned into the lumbar and iliac fossae. The pararenal and perirenal spaces are included in the lumbar fossa.

To understand the patterns of spread and contain-ment of retroperitoneal pathologic processes, knowledge of the fascial layers of the retroperitoneum is essential. Although these layers are rarely directly visualized by ultrasound, their presence is suggested by the demonstration of pathologic processes or collections corresponding to known fascial compartments. Portions of the retroperitoneal connective tissue continue below the transversalis fascia of the abdominal wall. As such, pathologic processes can stretch from the anterior abdominal wall to the subdiaphragmatic space, mediastinum, and subcutaneous tissues of the back and flank. The retrofascial space, which includes the psoas, quadratus lumborum, and iliacus muscles (muscles posterior to the

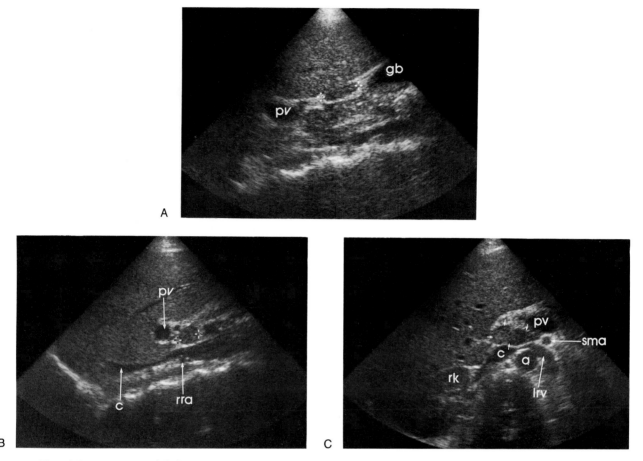

Fig. 12-9. Porta hepatis inflammatory nodes in a patient with AIDS. **(A & B)** Sagittal and **(C)** transverse scans in the porta hepatis region. An oblong node (calipers) is identified with a normal echopattern in Fig. A. A second node (calipers) is seen in Fig. B with the two (arrows) seen in Fig. C in cross-section. This appearance is seen with inflammatory reaction. (*pv*, portal vein; *gb*, gallbladder; *c*, inferior vena cava; *rra*, right renal artery; *a*, aorta; *rk*, right kidney; *sma*, superior mesenteric artery; *lrv*, left renal vein.)

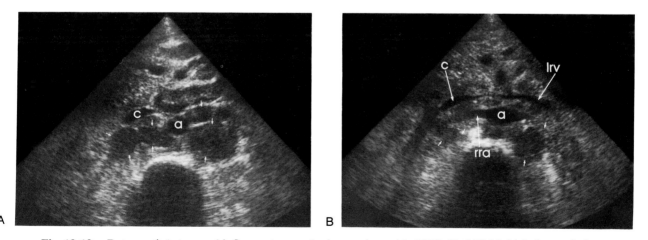

Fig. 12-10. Retroaortic/retrocaval inflammatory nodes in a patient with AIDS. **(A & B)** Multiple hypoechoic nodes are seen, with many (arrows) posterior to the aorta *(a)* and inferior vena cava *(c)* on these transverse views. (*lrv*, left renal vein; *rra*, right renal artery.)

757

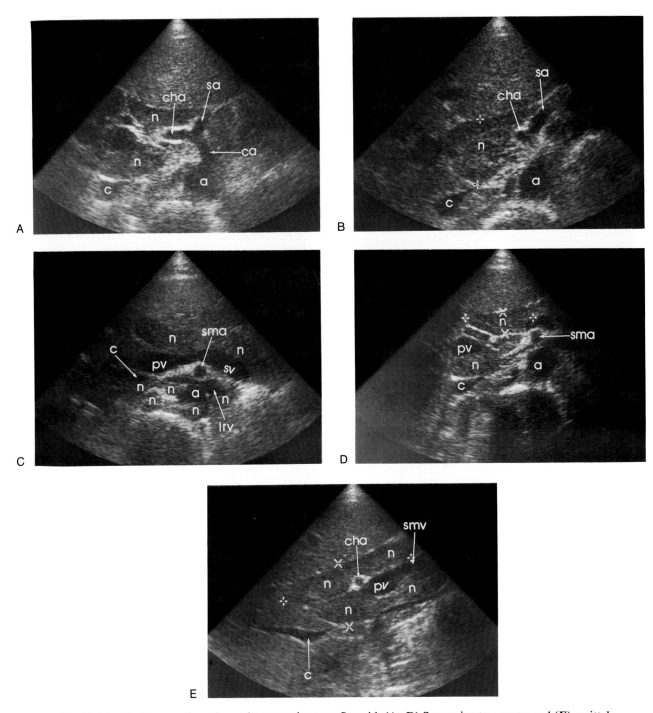

Fig. 12-11. Peripancreatic nodes and pancreatic mass. Sarcoid. **(A–D)** Successive transverse and **(E)** sagittal views demonstrating multiple masses *(n)* surrounding vessels and extending into the porta hepatis. In Fig. B, which is slightly lower than Fig. A, there is a mass (calipers, *n*) in the region of the pancreatic head. In Fig. E, the superior mesenteric vein *(smv)* and inferior vena cava *(c)* are compressed by the multiple nodes *(n)*. *(a,* aorta; *pv,* portal vein; *sma,* superior mesenteric artery; *sv,* splenic vein; *cha,* common hepatic artery; *sa,* splenic artery; *ca,* celiac artery; *lrv,* left renal vein.)

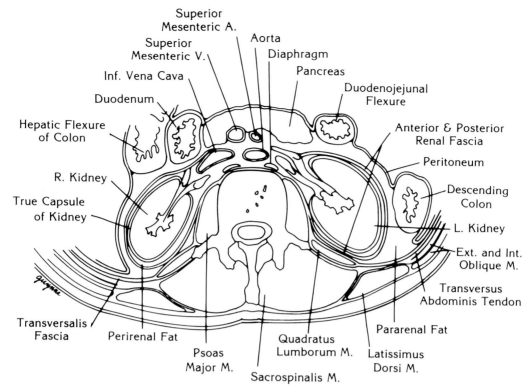

Fig. 12-12. Normal retroperitoneum. Cross-section of the lumbar fossa. The anterior pararenal space is bounded by the posterior peritoneum and anterior renal fascia and is continuous across the midline. The pancreas, common bile duct, duodenum, superior mesenteric vessels, and ascending and descending colon are included in this compartment. The perirenal spaces are separated by connective tissue sheaths surrounding the inferior vena cava and aorta. The lateral fusion of the anterior and posterior renal fascia forms the lateroconal fascia. Behind the posterior pararenal space is the transversalis fascia, which forms the anterior border of the retrofascial spaces (including the quadratus lumborum and psoas muscles).

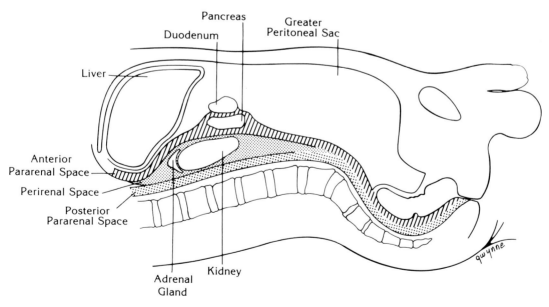

Fig. 12-13. Normal retroperitoneum. Right longitudinal section through the abdomen and pelvis. The anterior pararenal space is bounded anteriorly by the posterior peritoneum and posteriorly by the anterior renal fascia. The perirenal space is located between the anterior and posterior renal fascia. The posterior pararenal space is located between the posterior renal fascia and the transversalis fascia. The lumbar fossa extends from the diaphragm to the ilium. It is open inferiorly and merges as it enters the iliac fossa.

759

transversalis fascia), is often the site of extension of retroperitoneal pathologic processes.[1]

There have been several proposals to explain some of the retroperitoneal fluid collections observed: (1) the kidneys and renal fasciae develop within the domain of the primary retroperitoneum, whereas all alimentary structures develop in the intermesenteric domain; (2) these two domains communicate only at the mesenteric root; (3) the anterior renal fascia and lateroconal fascia cannot demarcate a retroperitoneal space that contains alimentary tract structures; (4) the secondary, or anterior, retroperitoneum is a laminated space, bounded by folded, fused leaves of mesentery, that contains distinct pancreaticoduodenal and colonic subcompartments; and (5) the anterior and posterior pararenal spaces do not normally communicate caudally in the iliac fossa.[20] These hypotheses may help to resolve the apparent conflict between certain findings on abdominal CT and current notions about retroperitoneal compartmental anatomy.[20]

Anterior Pararenal Space

Bounded anteriorly by the posterior parietal peritoneum and posteriorly by the anterior renal fascia, the anterior pararenal space is delineated laterally by the lateroconal fascia formed by the fusion of the anterior and posterior leaves of the renal fascia[5] (Figs. 12-12 and 12-13). The single lateroconal fascia is formed by the fusion of the anterior and posterior renal fascia, extending behind the ascending or descending colon; it extends to the flank and blends with the peritoneal reflection.[5] This space merges with the bare area of the liver by the coronary ligament. The pancreas, duodenal sweep, and ascending and transverse colon are the organs included in the anterior pararenal space (Fig. 12-12).

The ultrasound delineation of the normal anterior pararenal space is limited to identification of the pancreas and adjacent vasculature (Fig. 12-14). The pancreas extends in nearly a transverse plane from the region of the splenic hilum, posterior, inferior, and to the right. The splenic vein is posterior to the superior border of the pancreas (see Ch. 7).

The retroperitoneal portions of the intestinal tract lie within this space. The fluid-filled ascending and descending portions of the colon can sometimes be identified as tubular lucent structures. The duodenum can often be seen as a tubular or triangular fluid-filled space along the right lateral margin of the pancreatic head[1] (Fig. 12-14C). When there are pathologic processes involving the wall of this bowel, there is the production of the "bull's-eye" pattern caused by eccentric thickening. Most infections involving the anterior pararenal space

arise from the gastrointestinal tract (such as colon, retroperitoneal appendix, pancreas, and duodenum).[5] This retroperitoneal space is the most common site of infection (52.5 percent)[5] (see Ch. 8).

There have been reports of apparent extension of a pancreatic phlegmon or effusion from the anterior pararenal space into the posterior pararenal space. Investigators have shown that these posterior collections actually represent extension of pancreatitis from the anterior pararenal space to a potential space between the laminae of the posterior or renal fascia.[21] True involvement of the posterior pararenal space is very uncommon, as is extension into the perirenal space. The fibers of Gerota's fascia, as well as those connecting the lateroconal and anterior renal fasciae, serve as a relative barrier between the anterior pararenal space and the potential space created by the multilaminar nature of the posterior renal fascia.[21] The pathway of the commonly seen retrorenal extension of these effusions is confined by the retroperitoneal fasciae, which act as barriers of inflammation by intensely reacting to the offensive process rather than simply restricting it.[21]

Perirenal Space

The perirenal space is surrounded by the anterior and posterior layers of the renal fascia (Gerota's fascia) (Figs. 12-12, 12-13, and 12-15). These layers join and attach to the diaphragm superiorly, but they are united only loosely inferiorly at the level of the iliac crest, or superior border of the "false" pelvis. Collections in the perinephric space can communicate within the iliac fossa of the retroperitoneum. The lateroconal fascia, the lateral fusion of the renal fascia, proceeds anterior as the posterior peritoneum. The posterior renal fascia fuses medially with the psoas or quadratus lumborum fascia; the anterior renal fascia fuses medially with connective tissue surrounding the great vessels. This space contains the adrenal, kidney, and ureter; the great vessels, which also lie within this space, are largely isolated within their connective tissue sheaths[1] (Fig. 12-15).

The perirenal space contains the adrenal and kidney, which are enclosed in a variable amount of echogenic perinephric fat, the thickest portion being posterior and lateral to the lower pole of the kidney (Fig. 12-15). The kidney is located anterolateral to the psoas muscle, anterior to the quadratus lumborum muscle, and posteromedial to the ascending and descending colon. The second portion of the duodenum is anterior to the kidney hilum on the right. On the left, the kidney is bounded by the stomach anterosuperiorly, the pancreas anteriorly, and the spleen anterolaterally[1] (see Ch. 13).

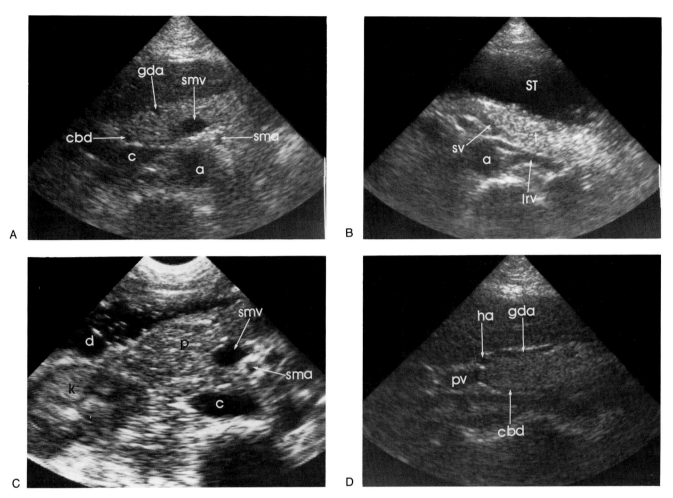

Fig. 12-14. Anterior pararenal space. **(A–C)** Transverse and **(D)** sagittal scans of the upper abdomen, demonstrating the pancreas. In Fig. B (slightly oblique and angled to the left) the stomach *(ST)* is distended for better visualization of the pancreatic tail *(t)*. In Fig. C (transverse right lateral decubitus) the duodenum *(d)* is distended for improved visualization of the pancreatic head. The relationship of the pancreas to the gastroduodenal artery *(gda),* and common bile duct *(cbd)* is seen in Figs. A & D. The ultrasound delineation of the normal anterior pararenal space is usually limited to the identification of the pancreas *(p)* and adjacent vasculature. (*sma,* superior mesenteric artery; *smv,* superior mesenteric vein; *a,* aorta; *c,* inferior vena cava; *k,* right kidney; *sv,* splenic vein; *pv,* portal vein; *lrv,* left renal vein; *ha,* hepatic artery.)

Adrenal

Adult. *Location.* The adrenal glands are generally anterior, medial, and superior to the kidneys (Fig. 12-1). The right adrenal is more superior to the kidney while the left is more medial (Figs. 12-1 and 12-2). The medial portion of the right gland is located immediately posterior to the IVC (to which the anteromedial ridge of the gland usually attaches), at or slightly above the level of the portal vein and lateral to the crus[22] (Figs. 12-1, 12-2, and 12-4). The lateral portion of the gland is posterior and medial to the right lobe of the liver and posterior to the duodenum.

The left adrenal is lateral or slightly posterolateral to the aorta and lateral to the crus[22] (Figs. 12-1 and 12-3). The superior portion is posterior to the lesser omental space, which is posterior to the stomach; the inferior portion is posterior to the pancreas. The splenic vein and artery pass between the pancreas and the left adrenal gland.[2] The left gland appears as a single-line structure that probably represents the lateral wing between the diaphragmatic crus and the medial aspect of the upper pole of the kidney, extending cranially to the kidney itself.[12]

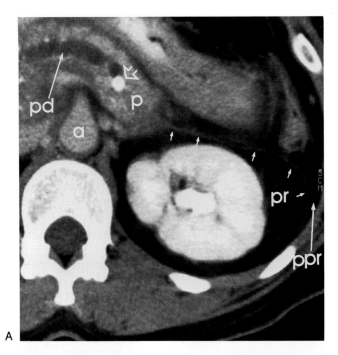

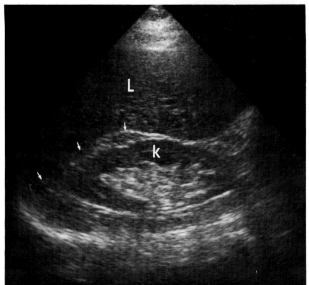

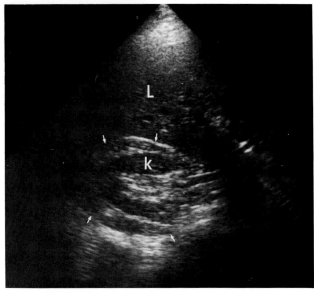

Fig. 12-15. Perirenal space. **(A)** Enhanced CT scan. The left kidney is seen within the perirenal space *(pr)* surrounded by perirenal fat. The anterior pararenal space is located anteriorly and contains the descending colon, duodenojejunal flexure, and pancreas *(p)*. In this patient with chronic pancreatitis, calcification (open arrow) and a dilated pancreatic duct *(pd)* are seen. The posterior pararenal space *(ppr)* is seen posterior to the perirenal space. *(a,* aorta.) On **(B)** sagittal and **(C)** transverse ultrasound scans of the right kidney *(k),* the perirenal space (arrows) can be identified by the abundant echodense perirenal fat. *(L,* liver.)

Shape and Configuration. The adrenal glands vary in size, shape, and configuration. The normal adrenal has been reported to be linear, curvilinear, triangular, trapezoidlike, fingerlike, or like an inverted V or Y on a coronal or sagittal oblique scan[5,7,8,15,23] (Figs. 12-2 and 12-

4). The right adrenal gland appears similar to an inverted Y or V when both its wings are within the scan plane, to a straight or curved line when only one wing is seen, and to a triangle when the lateral wings are not well developed on a transverse scan[12] (Figs. 12-2 and 12-4). Others describe the right gland as triangular.[5,7,22] A triangular shape is most frequently described, with the tail extending from the anteromedial aspect of the kidney.

The appearance of the left adrenal is rather Y-shaped or Z-shaped when both limbs are scanned simultaneously (Fig. 12-3). As such, when both wings of the gland are imaged simultaneously, the entire organ is not represented; the anteromedial bridge is not included in the scan plane. Additionally, there may be the false impression of enlargement of a wing.[15] The left may be seen as semilunar.[5,7,22]

Echopattern. Normally the adrenal appears as a distinct hypoechoic structure; at other times, only the highly echogenic fat is seen[8,12] (Figs. 12-2 to 12-4). The internal texture has intermediate consistency, and the cortex and medulla are usually not distinguished. At times, a few higher-level echoes can be seen arranged along a thin line within the center of the gland, suggesting a three-layered pattern.[12] The adrenal medulla may be seen as a highly echogenic linear structure in the gland. Differentiation of cortex and medulla has been identified in 13 percent of studies.[15]

Size. The adrenal is infrequently greater than 3 cm, with the normal adrenal being 3 to 6 cm long, 3 to 6 mm thick, and 2 to 4 cm wide.[2,4,5,6,9,22-24] The length (craniocaudal) and width (lateral) measurements of the adrenals vary widely depending on the portion of the gland within the scan plane.[12] Some report the maximum length as 4.2 cm and the maximum width as 3.5 cm.[12] The right may measure up to 6 cm when both wings of the gland are imaged simultaneously.[15] With the CSL view, the adult left adrenal appears as an elongated structure measuring 2 to 4 cm in length and 0.9 to 1.4 cm in anteroposterior thickness, with the left gland being slightly larger than the right.[13] The left adrenal measures 2 cm or less in length in the pediatric patient.[13] The distance from the skin to the adrenal is generally 4 to 8 cm when scanning in the decubitus position. The best ultrasound criterion for adrenal abnormality is a triangular shape ranging from a single convex margin to a perfectly round gland.[3,14]

Neonatal. In the neonate, the adrenal is characterized by a thin echogenic core surrounded by a thick transonic zone (Fig. 12-16). The thick rim of transonicity represents the hypertrophied adrenal cortex, while the echogenic core is the adrenal medulla. The cortex is composed of two layers: a thick fetal zone occupying 80 percent of the gland and a thin peripheral region that becomes the adult cortex.[25] The fetal cortex synthesizes a considerable amount of the precursors of maternal estrogens and is one of the main consumers of placental progesterone.[25] The decreased cortical echogenicity is probably a result of several factors. There are dilated blood-filled cortical sinusoids in the cortex as a result of vascular congestion. In addition, there is orderly parallel orientation of the cuboidal cells lining the cortical columns. After birth, the fetal zone of the adrenal cortex undergoes inevitable involution. The relative echogenicity of the adrenal medulla is probably secondary to the random orientation of its cell population. This structural disorder produces multiple reflective interfaces, resulting in an area of increased echogenicity. Increased amounts of collagen surrounding the central vessels may also add to the medullary echogenicity.[25]

The hyperechogenic area may be too large to be the medulla alone.[26] By correlating the appearance with postmortem macroscopic and histologic adrenal sections, investigators have found that the hyperechogenic central area represents not only the central vein and the medulla (which is very small in neonates) but also the congested sinusoids of the inner part of the fetal cortex.[26] The surrounding hypoechoic area appears to represent the less congested part of the fetal cortex, which is enclosed by the thin hyperechogenic definitive cortex and capsule.

There are marked involutional changes of the fetal zone of the neonatal adrenal gland (forming 80 percent of the adrenal cortex at term) during the early weeks and months of extrauterine life.[26] Accompanying this involution of the fetal zone are proliferation and development of the definitive zone.[26] During the first 3 months of life, the adrenal weight decreases; it then increases once more with further growth of the definitive zone.[26] The following adrenal sizes have been reported: a mean adrenal length of 17.3 ± 1.8 mm on day 1, decreasing to 7.7 ± 0.9 mm by day 42.[26] There is a rapid decrease in adrenal size in the first 10 days followed by a slower decrease over the next few weeks, consistent with the atrophy of the fetal zone of the adrenal.[26]

With increasing age, the cortex becomes smaller and the medulla becomes larger.[6] Until age 5 to 6 months, the cortex remains hypoechoic and the medulla hyperechoic. There is poor to absent ultrasound differentiation between the cortex and medulla by the time the gland becomes hyperechoic and smaller.[6] The gland appears similar to the adult gland, with straight or concave borders and a hypoechoic character, after 1 year of age.[6]

There is increased visualization of the neonatal adrenal as a result of several factors. The infant adrenal is proportionally larger than the adult adrenal. At birth, the adrenal is one-third the size of the kidney, whereas in the adult it is one-thirteenth the size of the kidney. In the neonate, there is a paucity of perirenal fat, which allows for easier resolution of the adrenal. In addition, the neonatal adrenal is closer to the skin surface, which allows

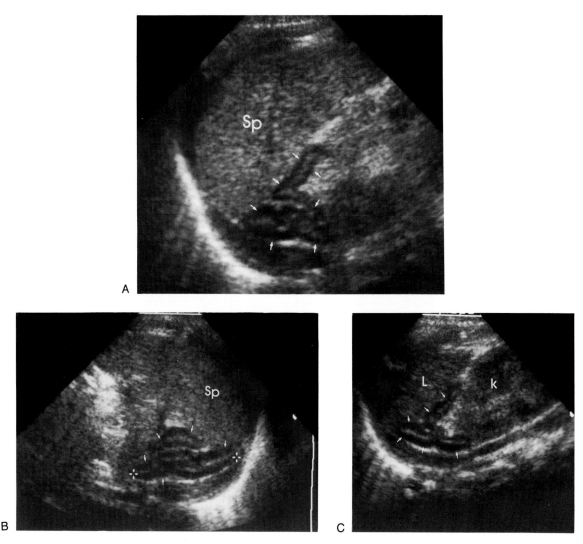

Fig. 12-16. Normal neonatal adrenal. Magnified **(A)** sagittal and **(B)** transverse views of the left adrenal. The normal adrenal (small arrows) is seen as a structure with an echogenic core and a hypoechoic rim. (*Sp*, spleen.) **(C)** Sagittal view of the right adrenal (same neonate), which appears similar to the left. (*k*, right kidney; *L*, liver.)

for the use of higher-frequency transducers, which in turn increases the resolution of small structures.[25] The right adrenal can be seen in 97 percent of cases, with the left seen in 83 percent.[5,25] The length of the neonatal adrenal varies from 0.9 to 3.6 cm (mean, 1.5 cm), and the width varies from 0.2 to 0.5 cm (mean, 0.3 cm).[25]

Investigators have evaluated adrenal gland size during the first year of life.[27] An adrenal size index (ASI) has been defined as part of the standardized adrenal sections. The following diameters are used to calculate the ASI: craniocaudal diameter *(c)* and the lengths of two lines running from the caudal end point of the craniocaudal diameter at an angle of 45 degrees to the ventrolateral and the dorsomedial borderline of the cross-section (S_1 and S_2). ASI = $(0.3536c)$ $(S_1 + S_2)$. The ASI is high in

newborns and decreases during the first year of life.[27] Degeneration begins in the central portion of the fetal zone between the first and fourth weeks of life; there is almost complete degeneration beyond the third month of life.[27] Accounting for 65 to 85 percent of the total adrenal tissue, the fetal zone consists of an abundantly capillarized homogeneous cell population without intracellular deposits of lipophilic material.[27] The adrenal size is maximal before the 15th day of life and decreases rapidly thereafter, with the most remarkable decrease occurring in the first 3 months of life.

It is especially important to recognize the characteristic appearance of the neonatal adrenal in renal agenesis, as the adrenal glands may simulate the appearance of the normal kidneys.[25,28] The adrenal preserves its characteristic echogenic medulla and anechoic cortex but enlarges when the normal renal tissue is not present; it loses its characteristic V or Y shape and appears more elliptical on ultrasound.[29] In these cases of renal agenesis, on the average the right and left adrenals are 3.4 and 2.9 cm long, respectively, and their thickness is increased to an average of 5 mm.[29] The elongation and thickening of the adrenal may be secondary to the lack of pressure exerted by the kidney against the developing adrenal gland.[29] This enlargement may also be seen in cases of renal ectopia.[29] When scanning, one should not mistaken the enlarged adrenal for the kidney.

Diaphragmatic Crura

The diaphragmatic crura begin as tendinous fibers from the lumbar vertebral bodies, disks, and transverse processes of L3 on the right and L1 on the left (Fig. 12-17). As it proceeds cephalad from its origin, the right crus, which is longer, larger, and frequently more lobular than the left, is closely associated with the anterior aspect of the lumbar vertebral bodies as it blends with the anterior longitudinal vertebral ligament (Figs. 12-5 to 12-7 and 12-17). The right renal artery crosses anterior to the crus and posterior to the IVC at the level of the right kidney. The right crus is bounded by the IVC anterolaterally and the right adrenal and right lobe of the liver posterolaterally in the upper abdomen (Figs. 12-5, 12-6, and 12-17). The fibers of the right crus diverge as it ascends superiorly. Laterally, most fibers insert in the central tendon of the diaphragm while the medial fibers ascend on the left side of the esophageal hiatus (Figs. 12-7 and 12-17). The medial tendinous margin of the

right crus extends anterior and decussates with the left anterior to the aorta.[16]

On a longitudinal scan, the entire right crus can be seen as a solid, longitudinally oriented structure immediately posterior to the IVC (Fig. 12-6). It should not be confused with the right renal artery.[30] The right crus is identified as a solid structure paralleling the aorta and IVC when scanning from the patient's right side with the patient in the left lateral decubitus position.[10] To the left of midline, the right crus is also visualized as a solid, longitudinal form anterior to the aorta[16] (Fig. 12-6). The right crus can be visualized in 50 percent of patients on longitudinal scans and in 90 percent on transverse scans.

The left crus courses superiorly along the anterior lumbar vertebral bodies and inserts into the central tendon of the diaphragm (Figs. 12-5, 12-7, and 12-17). During its ascent, it is closely associated with the celiac ganglion, left adrenal gland, splenic vasculature, and esophagogastric junction. Occasionally the medial fibers pass over the aorta and stretch obliquely to the fibers of the right, toward the IVC.[16] The left crus, which also parallels the aorta along the left, is shorter and smaller than the right crus.[10] It is particularly difficult to visualize on coronal or sagittal views.[10] It is never seen longitudinally, but can be seen on 50 percent of transverse scans[16] (Fig. 12-7).

Aorta

The aorta as a unit is in the perirenal space, although its dense perivascular connective tissue serves as a barrier to extension of perinephric processes. The aorta enters the abdomen posterior to the diaphragm at L1 and passes posterior to the left lobe of the liver (Fig. 12-8). It has a relatively straight course to L4, where it bifurcates. It has a slight anterior curve because of the lumbar lordosis. In a thin patient with exaggerated lumbar lordosis, the aorta may lie within 3 to 4 cm of the anterior abdominal wall and may be mistaken for an aneurysm on physical examination. It generally lies close to the anterior spine, which can be identified as an intense linear echo with distal shadow on longitudinal view and as an anterior concave echo on transverse scan (Fig. 12-8). If there is separation between the aorta and the spine, adenopathy, as well as fibrosis or hematoma, should be considered[1] (see Ch. 11).

Using the coronal approach and scanning from the right side places the aorta farther from the transducer.[10] Both the renal arteries and renal veins can often be visualized by this approach[10] (Fig. 12-3). Although this approach does not give optimal visualization of the superior mesenteric and celiac arteries, it is particularly well suited to visualization of the common iliac arteries.[10]

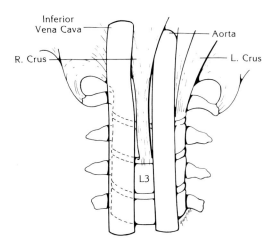

Fig. 12-17. Diaphragmatic crura. The relationship of the diaphragmatic crura, aorta, and inferior vena cava are illustrated. (Modified from Callen et al,[16] with permission.)

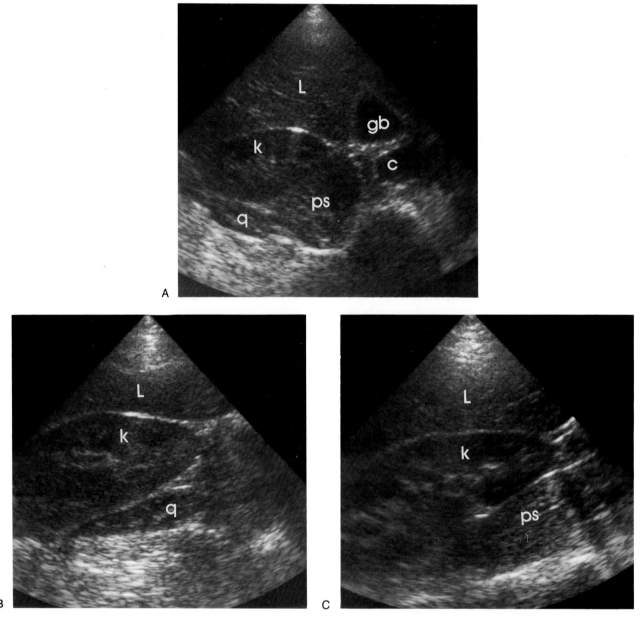

Fig. 12-18. Posterior pararenal space. **(A)** Transverse and **(B & C)** sagittal scans. The structures on the anterior and posterior boundaries of this space can be seen by ultrasound. Anteriorly in the perirenal space, the right kidney *(k)* can be seen with its perirenal fat. Posteriorly are components of the retrofascial space, the psoas *(ps)* and quadratus lumborum *(q)* muscles at this level. The quadratus lumborum muscle is a cephalically tapering elliptical hypoechoic structure, with the psoas muscle seen medial to the quadratus. (*c*, inferior vena cava; *gb*, gallbladder; *L*, liver.)

With the coronal approach, the renal arteries were visualized in 73 percent of patients without aneurysms in one series; the common iliac arteries were demonstrated in 82 percent[18] (Fig. 12-3). With an aortic aneurysm present, the frequency of visualization of the aortic bifurcation was 82 percent, with visualization of renal arteries in 45 percent.[18] In addition, the coronal view added the ability to see the aortic tortuosity as it appeared on aortogram.[18]

Inferior Vena Cava

The IVC has a longer intra-abdominal course than the aorta. It is seen as a tubular structure that is closest to the transducer during scanning from the coronal approach.[10] By altering the orientation slightly, the renal veins may be identified. The IVC extends from the junction of the two common iliac veins to the right of L5 and travels cephalad (Fig. 12-8); it then curves anteriorly toward its termination in the right atrium[1] (see Ch. 11).

Nodes

At ultrasound, normal lymph nodes appear as somewhat flattened hypoechoic structures.[31] The medullary portion of the lymph nodes contains lymphoid tissue, while the cortical portion contains lymph nodules or follicles.[31] A structure may be identified as a node when an echogenic central spot is visualized in a hypoechogenic nodule.[31]

Most nodes have a variable degree of lipomatosis, which is seen as an eccentric highly reflective defect.[31]

With chronic inflammation, obesity, and degenerative changes, there is benign fatty replacement of lymphoid tissue, which is responsible for the variations seen with high-resolution ultrasound. Beginning in the center of the lymph node and progressing toward the periphery, these fatty deposits are easily recognized as highly reflective defects in the hypoechogenic lymphoid tissue.[31] It is not unusual in obese people, in elderly patients (even without obesity), and after chronic infection to have a considerable part of the substance of the lymph nodes replaced by well-developed adipose tissue with preservation of only a peripheral and often incomplete zone of lymphoid tissue.[31] With extensive fatty infiltration, it can be hard to differentiate the nodes from the surrounding tissues.

Retroperitoneal nodes are known to surround the aorta and IVC and are sometimes located anterior to the spine (Figs. 12-10 and 12-11). When normal (≤ 1 cm) they are not seen on ultrasound scans. With the coronal oblique view, ultrasound can be 90 percent as effective as CT in detecting para-aortic, paracaval, and interaorticocaval lymph node enlargement.[18] This view helps differentiate enlarged lymph nodes from gonadal vessels or anomalies of the IVC.[18]

The common sites for nodes include para-aortic, paracaval, peripancreatic, renal hilar, and mesenteric (Figs. 12-9 to 12-11). Descriptions of ultrasound patterns associated with nodes include (1) rounded, focal echopoor lesions 1 to 3 cm in size; (2) larger, confluent echopoor masses often displacing the kidney laterally; (3) "mantle" of nodes in a paraspinal location; (4) "floating" or anteriorly displaced aorta; and (5) mesenteric "sandwich" sign representing anterior and posterior node masses surrounding mesenteric vessels.[1]

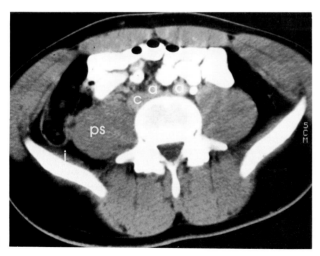

A

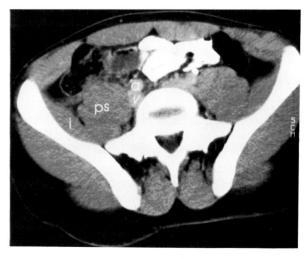

B

Fig. 12-19. Iliac fossa. **(A & B)** CT scans. The iliac fossa is the space between the peritoneum and transversalis fascia, which invests the iliacus *(i)* and psoas *(ps)* muscles. (*c*, inferior vena cava; *a*, iliac artery; *v*, iliac vein.)

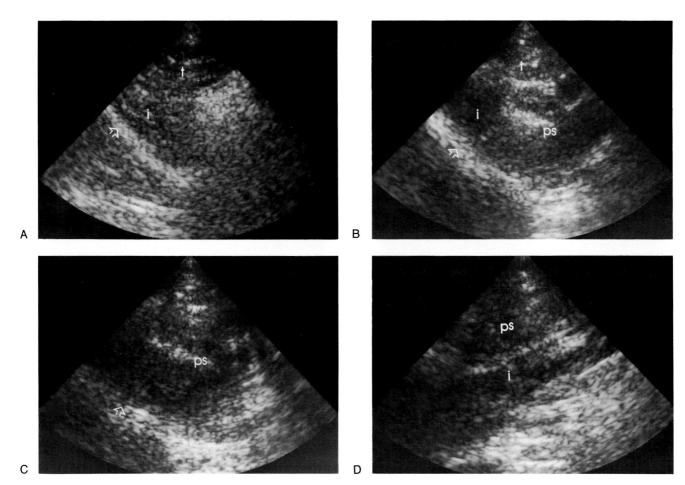

Fig. 12-20.   Iliac fossa. Iliacus and psoas muscles. The iliac fossa, the portion of the retroperitoneum between the posterior peritoneum and the transversalis fascia, is located between the internal surface of the iliac wing (open arrow) from the crest to iliopectal line. **(A–C)** Right successive transverse (Fig. C inferior and more medial) and **(D & E)** sagittal (Fig. D, sector transducer; Fig. E, linear transducer) scans display the structures visualized on ultrasound within this fossa, which include the psoas *(ps)* and iliacus *(i)* muscles. The transversus abdominis muscle *(t)* is seen anteriorly in Figs. A & B. The iliacus appears as a hypoechoic structure medial to the iliac wing. The psoas is seen posterior and medial to the iliacus. The anterior margins of the muscles are not sharply defined at this level. The psoas is not seen on the more superior scan (Fig. A) because of overlying bowel gas. The anatomy is not as well defined as on CT scan. *(Figure continues.)*

Posterior Pararenal Space and Iliac Fossa

The posterior pararenal space is located between the posterior renal fascia and the transversalis fascia (Figs. 12-12, 12-13, and 12-18). It extends laterally to the flank region and continues with the properitoneal (or extraperitoneal) fat space of the lateral abdominal wall.[5] It communicates with the properitoneal fat visualized on a radiograph as the "flank stripe," lateral to the lateroconal fascia. No organs are included within this space. Potentially, the two spaces are in communication through the properitoneal fat of the anterior abdominal wall.[5] Continuing from the diaphragm to the iliac crest,

this posterior space merges inferiorly with the anterior pararenal space and the retroperitoneal tissues of the iliac fossa. The psoas muscle, whose fascia merges with the posterior transversalis fascia, makes up the medial border of this posterior space. This space is open laterally and inferiorly.[1] Blood vessels and lymph nodes embedded in fat are found in the posterior pararenal space.

The iliac fossa is that region extending between the internal surface of the iliac wings from the crest to the iliopectineal line (Figs. 12-19 and 12-20). This space is also known as the "false" pelvis and contains the ureter and major branches of the distal great vessels and their accompanying lymphatics.[1] The transversalis fascia ex-

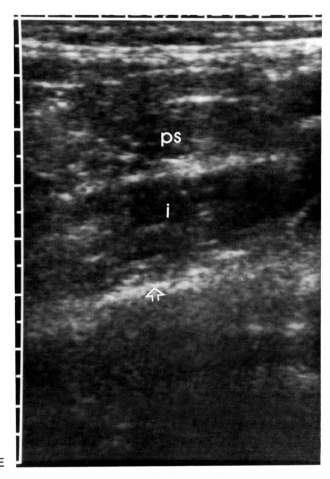

E

Fig. 12-20 *(Continued).*

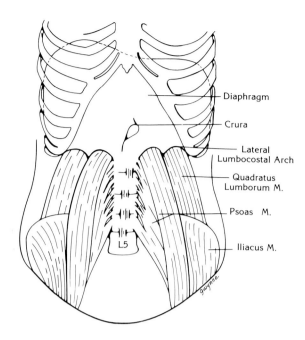

Fig. 12-21. Retrofascial space. The posterior abdominal wall components, muscles, nerves, lymphatics, and areolar tissue behind the transversalis fascia constitute this space. (Modified from Koenigsberg et al,[1] with permission.)

tends into the iliac fossa as the iliac fascia. The renal fascia terminates at the level of the superior margin of the iliac fossa and mixes loosely with the iliac fascia.

The usual fluid collections or hematoma in this space are due to spontaneous hemorrhage (hemorrhagic diathesis, anticoagulation, etc), ruptured abdominal aortic aneurysm, trauma, retroperitoneal lymphatic extravasation, or abscess.[5] In the retroperitoneal muscles, the most common site of abscess is the psoas muscle. This can be secondary to Crohn's disease, tuberculosis, pyelonephritis, diverticulitis, or appendicitis or can appear after surgical repair of abdominal aortic aneurysm.[5]

Retrofascial Space

The posterior abdominal wall components, muscles, nerves, lymphatics, and areolar tissue behind the transversalis fascia make up the retrofascial space (Fig. 12-21). It can be divided into three compartments, lumbar (quadratus lumborum), psoas, and iliac, by the leaves of the transversalis fascia, which invests each muscle and provides a barrier to the spread of infection.[1]

The quadratus lumborum originates from the iliolumbar ligament, the adjacent iliac crest, and the superior borders of the transverse process of the last three or four lumbar vertebrae and inserts into the inferior margin of the 12th rib (Fig. 12-21). It is adjoining and posterior to the colon, kidney, and psoas, depending on the level. On ultrasound, this muscle appears on transverse scan as a solid ovoid structure with low-amplitude internal echoes (Fig. 12-18). Sagittally, it is seen as a cephalically tapering elliptical structure (Fig. 12-18). Occasionally a linear echo is seen within the muscle substance, probably representing a cleft between muscle bundles.[32]

The psoas muscle spans from the mediastinum to the thigh (Figs. 12-18 to 12-22). With its fascia attaching to the pelvic brim, it extends to the thigh, joining with the inguinal ligament, iliacus fascia, and femoral sheath. It is seen as a tubular hypoechoic structure medial and posterior to the kidney on sagittal scan (Fig. 12-18). The psoas muscle may be easily visualized by using a coronal approach.[10] In this orientation, it appears as triangular tissue masses with the apices oriented cephalad. It passes obliquely from the abdomen into the pelvis. Its medial margins are the brightly reflective vertebral bodies, and its lateral margins are bordered by the kidneys or retroperitoneal fat.[10] On transverse scan, it is a rounded or

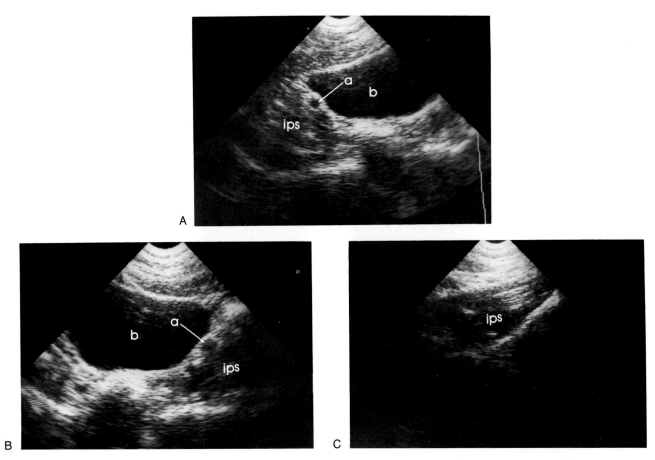

Fig. 12-22. Iliacus and iliopsoas muscles, pelvis. **(A)** Right and **(B)** left transverse and **(C)** right sagittal scans lower than that in Fig. 12-20. The iliacus and psoas muscles have joined to form the iliopsoas *(ips)* muscle. (*b*, bladder; *a*, external iliac artery.)

oval hypoechoic structure lateral to the spine[1] (Fig. 12-18).

The iliacus muscle, which makes up the iliac space, extends the length of the iliac fossa (Figs. 12-19 to 12-21). The psoas passes through the iliac fossa medial to the iliacus muscle and posterior to the iliac fascia. The two muscles merge as they extend into the true pelvis (Fig. 12-22). Proximal to their merger, the iliacus appears as a hypoechoic soft tissue layer medial to the iliac wings (Fig. 12-20). The iliopsoas muscle takes on a progressively more anterior location caudally to lie along the lateral pelvic sidewall (Figs. 12-22 and 12-23).

Pelvic Retroperitoneum

The pelvic portion of the retroperitoneum lies between the sacrum and pubis from back to front, pelvic peritoneal reflection above and pelvic diaphragm (coccygeus and levator ani muscles) below, and between the

fascial investment of the lateral pelvic wall musculature (obturator internus and piriformis)[1] (Fig. 12-23). There are four subdivisions of this pelvic space: prevesical, rectovesical, presacral, and bilateral pararectal (and paravesical) spaces.[1]

The extraperitoneal paravesical spaces have been evaluated by CT delineation and ultrasound correlation.[33] There is a large prevesical space, analogous to the anterior pararenal space, lying anterior and lateral to the umbilicovesical fascia. The umbilicovesical fascia divides the anterior extraperitoneal fat into a perivesical space (containing the bladder, umbilical arteries, and urachus) and a prevesical space (lying predominantly anterior and lateral to the umbilicovesical fascia).[33] The space of Retzius (retropubic space) is another name for the prevesical space. It spans from the pubis to the anterior margin of the bladder and is bordered laterally by the obturator fascia (Figs. 12-24 and 12-25). The prevesical space is noted to continue laterally with the extraperitoneal fat of the anterior abdominal wall, which is con-

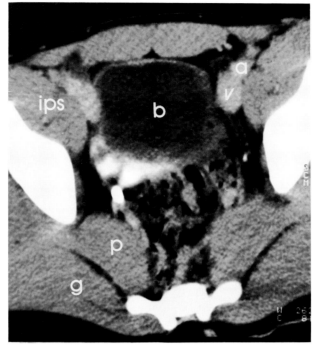

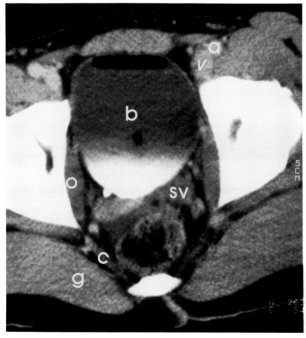

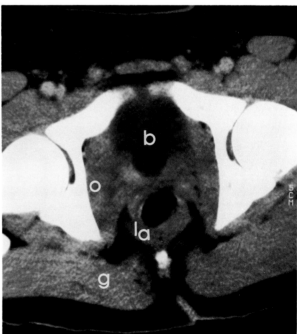

Fig. 12-23. Pelvic retroperitoneum. **(A–C)** Successive CT scans with Fig. C more inferior. The pelvic portion of the retroperitoneum lies between the sacrum and pubis, the pelvic peritoneal reflection and pelvic diaphragm, and the fascial investment of the lateral pelvic wall musculature. (*ips,* iliopsoas muscle; *p,* piriformis muscle; *b,* bladder; *sv,* seminal vesicles; *o,* obturator internus muscle; *v,* external iliac vein; *a,* external iliac artery; *g,* gluteus maximus muscle; *c,* coccygeus muscle; *la,* levator ani muscle.)

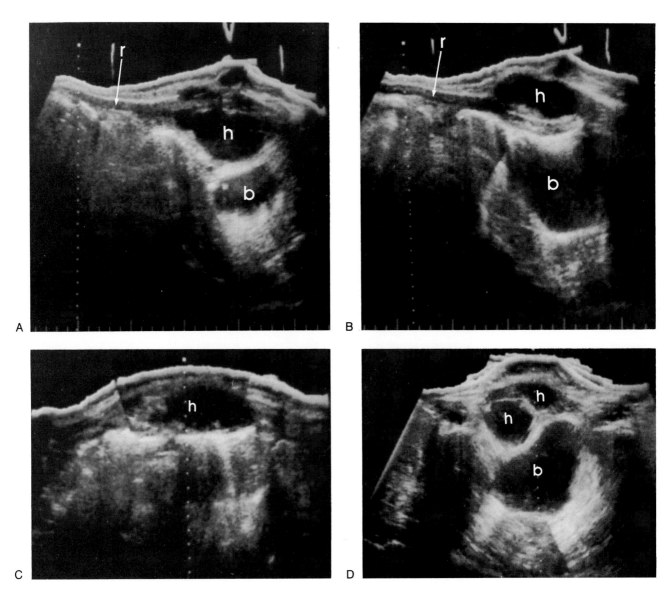

Fig. 12-24. Prevesical space. Postoperative hematoma. Sagittal scans (**A**) 2 cm to the right and (**B**) 2 cm to the left of midline and transverse scans (**C**) 6 cm and (**D**) 13 cm below the umbilicus demonstrating a hypoechoic septated mass *(h)* anterior to the bladder *(b)*. It appears to be continuous with the rectus abdominis *(r)* muscle, making it extraperitoneal.

tiguous with the properitoneal and retroperitoneal fat.[33] Connective tissue covering the bladder, seminal vesicles, and prostate is continuous with the fascial lamina within this space. The prevesical space extends up to the umbilicus and communicates with the properitoneal space in the anterolateral abdominal wall and flanks.[33]

Fluid in this prevesical space is most likely to collect anteriorly in front of the umbilicovesical fascia; a small amount may extend posteriorly in front of the peritoneum and behind the umbilicovesical fascia.[33] Effusions within the prevesical space may extend laterally around

the parietal peritoneum to come into contact with the iliopsoas muscles and external iliac vessels and then extend superiorly from the infrarenal retroperitoneal space into the pararenal compartments, especially the posterior pararenal and perinephric spaces (Fig. 12-26). Prevesical collections, which are more significant than those in the perivesical space, may result from a wide variety of disease processes and interventional procedures, including coagulation defects, pelvic or inguinal surgery, abscesses of the pelvic organs, and parametrial hematomas.[33]

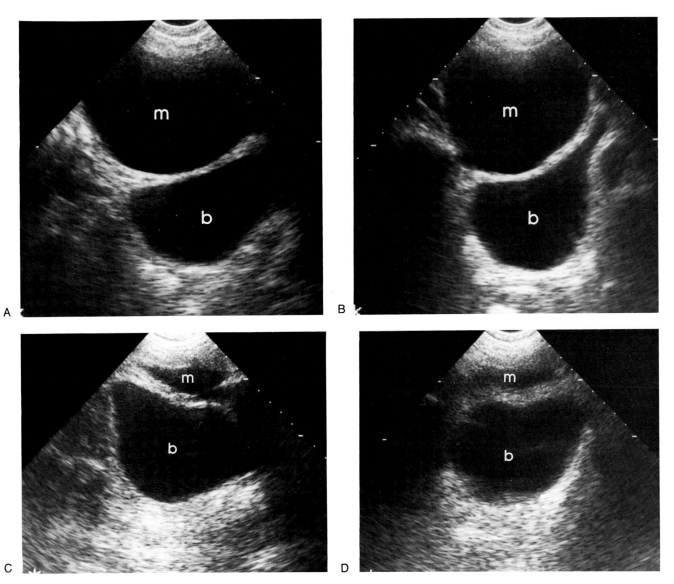

Fig. 12-25. Prevesical space. **(A)** Sagittal and **(B)** transverse scans in a patient after a radical prostatectomy. A large cystic mass *(m)* is seen in the prevesical space anterior to the urinary bladder *(b)*. The mass, which was a lymphocele, was drained percutaneously. Follow-up **(C)** sagittal and **(D)** transverse scans showing a significantly smaller fluid collection *(m)* anterior to the urinary bladder *(b)*.

The extraperitoneal space around the urinary bladder is lamellate, just like the retroperitoneal space around the kidneys. The anteroinferior boundary of both the prevesical and perivesical spaces is formed by the pubovesical ligament (or puboprostatic ligament in the male).[33] Lying within the perivesical space are the bladder, the urachus, and the obliterated umbilical arteries; these are surrounded by umbilicovesical fascia, analogous to the perinephric space within the renal fasciae.[33] The lower uterine segment or seminal vesicles, posterior to the urinary bladder, lie within the perivesical space, rather than in a separate compartment corresponding to the posterior pararenal space. Separating the posterior perivesical space from the rectum are the cul-de-sac and the inferolateral extension of its peritoneal layers as the rectovaginal or rectovesical septum.[33]

This space is an extension of the retroperitoneal space of the anterior abdominal wall deep to the rectus sheath, which is continuous with the transversalis fascia. The space between the bladder and rectum is the rectovesical

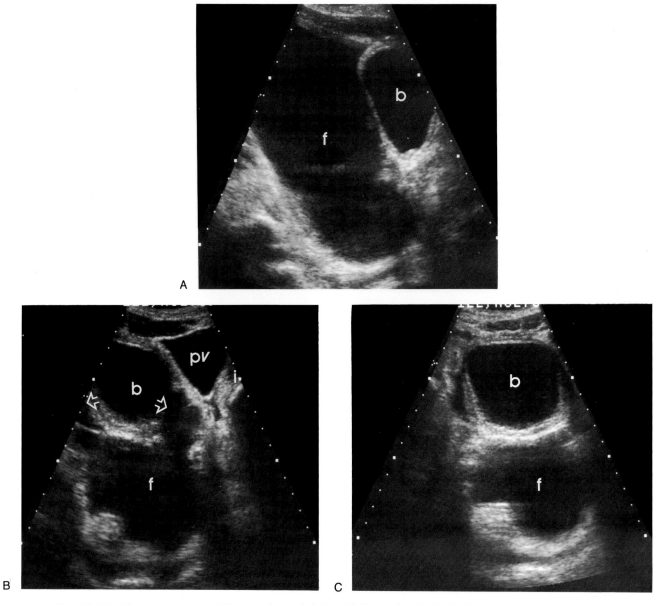

Fig. 12-26. Extraperitoneal and intraperitoneal fluid. **(A)** Sagittal and **(B & C)** transverse views showing peritoneal fluid *(f)* posterior to the urinary bladder *(b)*. The fluid does not extend anterior to the bladder. It does extend slightly lateral (open arrows) to the bladder in Fig. B. There is a noncommunicating fluid collection *(pv)* lateral to the bladder in Fig. B. This fluid was in the extraperitoneal perivesical space anterior to the iliacus *(i)* muscle.

space (Fig. 12-27). The presacral space is between the rectum and the fascia covering the sacrum and posterior pelvic floor musculature.[1] The bilateral pararectal space is bounded laterally by the piriformis and levator ani fascia and medially by the rectum. The paravesical space extends anteriorly from the bladder, medially to the obturator internus, and laterally to the external iliac vessels. The paravesical and pararectal spaces are traversed by the ureters.[1]

Many times, the most important differential diagnostic point is identification of a fluid collection within the extraperitoneal or intraperitoneal paravesical collections.[33] Both the extraperitoneal and intraperitoneal paravesical spaces are large, potential compartments that are separated by only a thin layer of anterior parietal peritoneum or, more medially, by only peritoneum and umbilicovesical fascia.[34] Fluid collections within the prevesical space have a "molar tooth" configuration

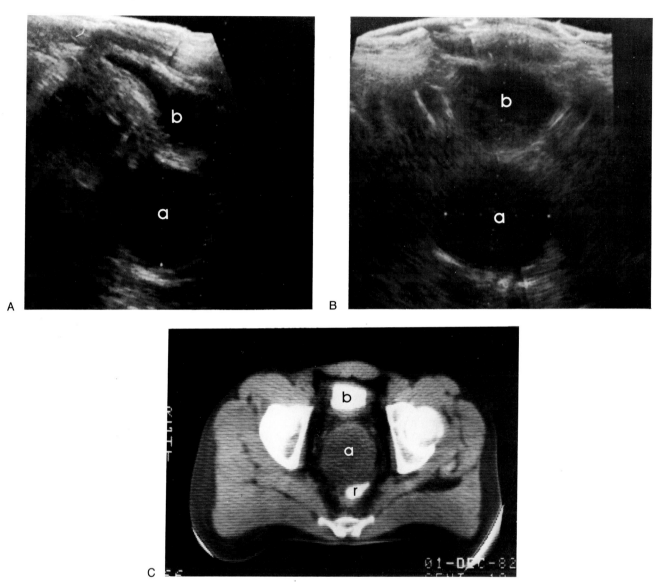

Fig. 12-27. Retrovesical space. Postoperative appendectomy abscess. **(A)** Sagittal and **(B)** transverse scans in a febrile male patient demonstrating a hypoechoic mass *(a)* posterior to the bladder *(b)*. **(C)** Similar to Fig. B, a low-density mass *(a)* is seen posterior to the bladder *(b)* and anterior to the rectum *(r)* on CT scan. This abscess was drained via a transrectal catheter.

around the urinary bladder, displacing the bladder posteriorly and compressing it from the sides along its entire length[34] (Figs. 12-25 and 12-26). Ascites displaces the distended urinary bladder inferiorly but not posteriorly and compresses it from the sides only if there is a focal loculation of fluid (Fig. 12-26).

When there are extraperitoneal perivesical collections, there is usually no associated prevesical fluid[34] (Fig. 12-26). Perivesical fluid can be distinguished from ascites by the lack of extension into the adjacent inguinal fossae (Fig. 12-26). At times, perivesical collections may

be loculated inferiorly around the bladder base or lower uterine segment, mimicking fluid in the cul-de-sac.[34]

The supravesical space and the medial and lateral inguinal fossae are intraperitoneal paravesical fossae formed by the indention of the anterior parietal peritoneum by the urinary bladder, obliterated umbilical arteries, and inferior epigastric vessels located within the extraperitoneal space of the anterior abdominal wall.[34] The supravesical space, the medial and lateral inguinal fossae, and the rectovesical or vesicouterine space are the intraperitoneal paravesical compartments.[34] Intraperi-

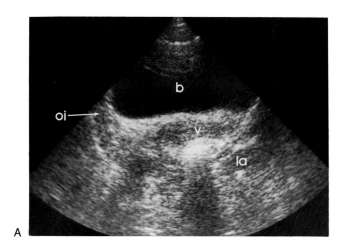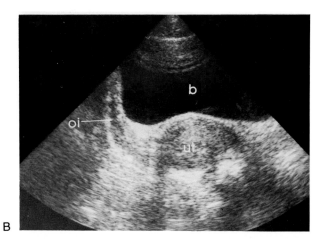

A   B

Fig. 12-28. Pelvic retroperitoneum. **(A & B)** Transverse scans through the pelvis from inferior (Fig. A) to superior (Fig. B) demonstrating the normal pelvic musculature that is frequently visualized on ultrasound. Ultrasound is limited by bowel gas within the pelvis. The pelvic musculature is better visualized by CT. The distended bladder *(b)* is seen in the midline. (*oi*, obturator internus muscle; *la*, levator ani muscle; *v*, vagina; *ut*, uterus.)

toneal fluid collections can be differentiated because they are inferior, but not posterior or lateral, by displacement of the distended urinary bladder, and by visualization of the umbilical folds and preservation of the properitoneal fat.[34]

The pelvic wall muscles, iliac vessels, ureter, bladder, prostate, seminal vesicles, and cervix are the retroperitoneal structures within the true pelvis (Figs. 12-23 and 12-28). Many of the posterior pelvic muscles are difficult to visualize by ultrasound because of overlying bowel gas. The obturator internus muscle lines the lateral aspect of the pelvis and is seen as a hypoechoic soft tissue structure with a concave medial border along the lateral aspect of the bladder (Figs. 12-23 and 12-28). Posteriorly, the piriformis muscle, a similar-appearing structure, is seen extending anterolaterally from the region of the sacrum (Fig. 12-23). Located medial to the obturator internus muscle is the internal iliac vein.[1]

Retroperitoneal Signs

Retroperitoneal Fat

At times it is difficult to determine the anatomic origin of a right upper quadrant mass. The reflection produced by right upper quadrant retroperitoneal fat (Fig. 12-15) is displaced in a characteristic manner by masses originating from this area. This pattern of displacement helps to localize the origin of the mass. Retroperitoneal lesions cause ventral and often cranial displacement of the echo. In addition, the lesion can be still further differentiated.

Fibrofatty echoes wedged in a triangular shape by masses in the upper pole of the kidney prove to be adrenal in origin. Lesions in the liver or in Morison's pouch displace the echoes posterior and inferior. Therefore, hepatic and subhepatic masses cause posterior displacement of this echo while renal and adrenal lesions cause anterior displacement of it.[35,36] Extrahepatic masses also shift the IVC anteromedially, resulting in anterior displacement of the right kidney.[36] This sign is absent or unreliable in a child or cachectic patient with a paucity of retroperitoneal fat. The displacement and/or visualization of the retroperitoneal fat is best seen on longitudinal scans and is inconsistent and poorly seen on transverse scans.[35,36] By knowing the vector of displacement of retroperitoneal fat, one can reliably diagnose the anatomic origin of the mass in the right upper quadrant.

Sliding Sign

Localization of a large tumor in the right upper quadrant of the abdomen is often very difficult.[37] A new sign to help identify the location of a mass has been identified. The sliding sign is the observation of dynamic motion of a mass against adjacent organs during respiratory movement or extrinsic pressure.[37] This sign is a very reliable criterion for the localization of the origin of the mass. If a mass moves with the liver and slides against the kidney, it should be hepatic; a mass moving with the kidney and sliding against the inferior surface of the liver is a renal tumor; and a mass sliding against both the liver and the kidney is an adrenal or other retroperitoneal tumor.[37]

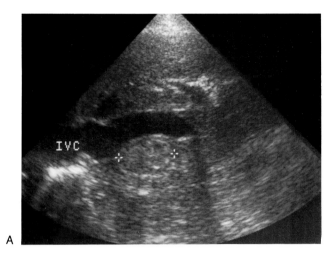

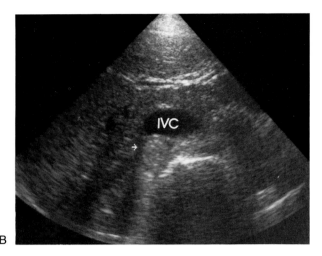

Fig. 12-29. Adrenal metastasis. **(A)** Sagittal and **(B)** transverse scans showing a mass (calipers, arrow, 18 × 18 × 32 mm) within the right adrenal gland posterior to the inferior vena cava *(IVC)*. The mass appears uniformly echogenic and represents an adrenal metastasis.

ABNORMALITIES

Adrenal

Ultrasound has been reported to have an overall accuracy of 95 percent in the evaluation of adrenal abnormalities.[3] The best criterion for diagnosing adrenal ab-

normalities is a change in the triangular shape ranging from a single convex margin to a perfectly round gland[3] (Fig. 12-29). To differentiate an adrenal mass from a renal mass, one must define an echo interface separating the mass from the upper pole of the kidney[24] (Fig. 12-30). At times, it may be difficult to differentiate a renal from an adrenal mass. By scanning carefully from mul-

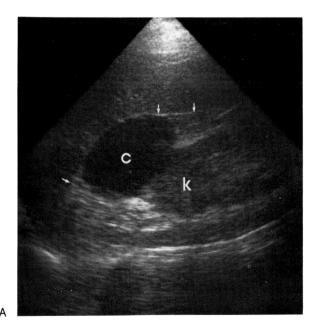

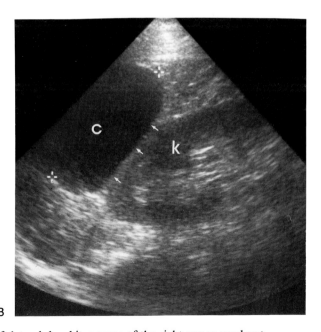

Fig. 12-30. Adrenal cyst. Sagittal **(A)** supine and **(B)** left lateral decubitus scans of the right upper quadrant demonstrating a cystic mass (*c*; 7.8 cm long) superior to the right kidney (*k*). A cleavage plane (arrows in Fig. B) is seen between the kidney and the mass. In Fig. A the cyst is noted to be within the perirenal space by its relationship to the perirenal fat (arrows).

tiple approaches, a demarcation between the mass and the kidney may be obtained.[5]

The upper pole of the kidney is displaced laterally when larger adrenal masses are present, since they are located anteromedial to the upper pole of the kidney.[5] The kidney may be displaced inferiorly with its upper pole compressed and flattened by the mass.[24] When the tumor grows inferiorly along the anterior surface of the kidney, there may be little downward displacement of the kidney.[7,38] Instead, there is a pressure deformity of the upper pole and the anterior surface of the kidney is compressed (Fig. 12-31). This may simulate tumor invasion on ultrasound.[7,38] There should be no distortion or splaying of the collecting system.

If downward extension anterior to the kidney occurs on the right, the mass may become posterior to the head of the pancreas, compress and displace the pancreas forward, and simulate a pancreatic mass on ultrasound.[38] However, with a pancreatic tumor the splenic vein will be displaced anteriorly instead of posteriorly.[38] A large right adrenal mass may displace the IVC forward. Compression of the posterior wall and/or anterior displacement of the IVC is seen in two-thirds of right adrenal tumors[22] (Fig. 12-31). A large left adrenal mass may extend forward and medial to partially surround the aorta.[38]

A tumor may involve the adrenal in a focal or diffuse fashion.[9] The usual solid adrenal mass is relatively hypo-echoic, because of the rather homogeneous cellular structure, with uniformly distributed echoes.[2,7,22,38] Usually round or oval, a focal tumor may be located in any part of the gland and ranges from 0.6 to 20 cm in diameter.[9] Small adrenal masses are easier to visualize than normal glands (incidence of visualization, 97 percent) since they are hypoechoic to surrounding fat and larger than the thickness of the normal adrenal gland.[5,9] When masses are small, they are usually round or oval. Masses 1 cm or smaller may be visualized by ultrasound.[5] It is often difficult to visualize adrenal masses less than 3 cm.[9]

It is much easier to delineate a moderate-sized (diameter, 3.5 to 5 cm) adrenal mass than a small one; it may be seen on anterior, lateral, or posterior scanning. In a large adrenal mass, focal areas of necrosis or hemorrhage are more likely to occur. As the mass grows, focal necrosis may develop, proceeding to liquefaction and becoming anechoic. A cavity surrounded by necrotic tissue may show an irregular and shaggy wall. As a general rule, large adrenal masses are more often malignant than smaller ones.[5]

The adrenal gland may be involved with multiple masses either unilaterally or bilaterally.[9] They may be seen with (1) metastatic disease (especially bronchogenic carcinoma, renal cell carcinoma, and melanoma), (2) pheochromocytoma, (3) lymphoma primarily in the adrenal or widespread, and (4) bilateral adrenal hyperplasia

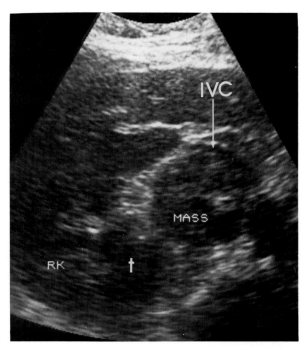

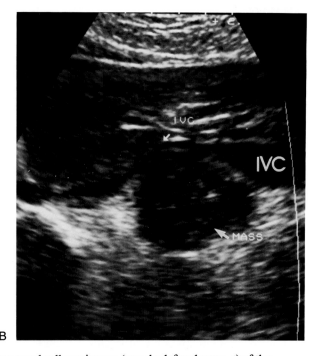

A   B

Fig. 12-31. Adrenal metastasis. In this patient with a large renal cell carcinoma (poorly defined mass, *t*) of the right kidney *(RK)*, there is an adrenal metastasis *(MASS)* causing compression and anterior displacement of the inferior vena cava *(IVC)* on **(A)** transverse and **(B)** sagittal views.

with multiple nodules usually less than 1 cm in diameter.[9]

A number of diseases are associated with diffuse enlargement; these include (1) diffuse bilateral hyperplasia; (2) neoplastic disease, most commonly lymphoma but sometimes bronchogenic or renal cell carcinoma; and (3) inflammatory disease, such as tuberculosis or histoplasmosis.[9]

Hemorrhage

Immediately after birth, the bulk of the primitive adrenal cortex undergoes atrophy. Already dilated vascular channels in the primitive cortex become more engorged and more vulnerable to hemorrhage.[5,7] The neonatal adrenals are susceptible to trauma and hemorrhage because of their relatively large size and vascularity; the bleeding is usually confined to the subcapsular space.[39] The exact cause of adrenal hemorrhage is unknown, but many factors are implicated, including (1) stress and trauma at birth, (2) anoxia, and (3) systemic disease (thrombocytopenia purpura, hemorrhagic disease of the newborn, septicemia, and congenital syphilis).[39,40]

Adrenal hemorrhage has been thought to be associated with fetal hypoxia. In one report, 32 percent of cases of neonatal asphyxia were associated with adrenal hemorrhage, usually occurring within the first few days of life.[41] The relationship of adrenal hemorrhage to hypoxia is not clearly understood. There may be redistribution of the blood flow to the brain, heart, and adrenal glands at the expense of the kidneys, spleen, and lungs. There is increased pressure within the capillary network as a result of congestion in the favored organs. Hemorrhage is more likely to occur in these organs; hypoxia also damages endothelial cells.[41]

Most frequently, these neonates present within 2 to 7 days of life with hyperbilirubinemia and an abdominal mass that is usually located on the right side.[40,42] Seventy percent are on the right side, with 5 to 10 percent bilateral.[40] The greater incidence of adrenal hemorrhage on the right side may be because the venous drainage of the right adrenal drains directly into the IVC.[42] These hemorrhages may be asymptomatic.[42]

Adrenal hemorrhage can be diagnosed by a combination of ultrasound and excretory urography without resorting to surgical exploration or invasive diagnostic procedures. On urography, there is downward displacement of the kidney on the affected side and a radiolucent suprarenal mass on body nephrogram phase. There is an anechoic suprarenal mass on ultrasound scans[2,39,40,43] (Fig. 12-32). There can be an echogenic component to the mass depending on the age of the hemorrhage; the echopattern is related to the state of liquefaction[2,7,39,40,43]

(Figs. 12-33 and 12-34). On follow-up examination, 2 to 4 weeks after the hemorrhage, typical suprarenal curvilinear calcifications can be seen radiographically, with a decrease in size of the mass seen on ultrasound scans[40] (Figs. 12-34 and 12-35).

When ultrasound shows enlarged adrenal glands of normal morphology in the proper clinical setting, impending hemorrhage should be included in the differential diagnosis. The pathologic stage of adrenal gland swelling that occurs prior to hemorrhage can be recognized by ultrasound.[41] When an enlargement of the adrenal is identified in a newborn, both hemorrhage and congenital hyperplasia should be considered.

Focal adrenal hemorrhages in the neonate have been reported.[44] The hemorrhage is focal with the uninvolved portion of the gland visualized adjacent to the hemorrhage (Fig. 12-36). The hemorrhage may be localized to the medulla primarily. The findings in this study conform to the gross patterns previously described: (1) bilateral central hematoma formation (involvement of the entire gland with loss of normal configuration and presence of medullary hematomas); (2) bilateral hemorrhagic necrosis without central hematoma (enlarged swollen glands with preservation of normal shape but loss of corticomedullary differentiation); (3) unilateral hemorrhagic necrosis; and (4) segmental lesions that are unilateral with a normal contralateral gland, unilateral with complete hemorrhagic necrosis of the contralateral gland, or bilateral.[44] As such, adrenal hemorrhage should also be considered when a focal adrenal mass is visualized in the appropriate clinical setting.

Besides being found as a complication of the neonatal period, adrenal hemorrhage may be spontaneous, traumatic, or related to anticoagulation[5,45] (Fig. 12-37). Spontaneous adrenal hemorrhage may occur in patients

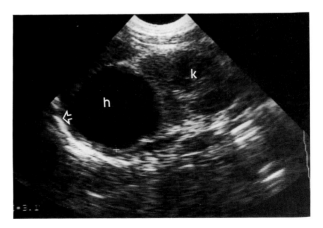

Fig. 12-32. Adrenal hemorrhage. Sagittal coronal scan on the right. A round, anechoic, suprarenal mass *(h)* is seen. (*k*, right kidney; open arrow, diaphragm.)

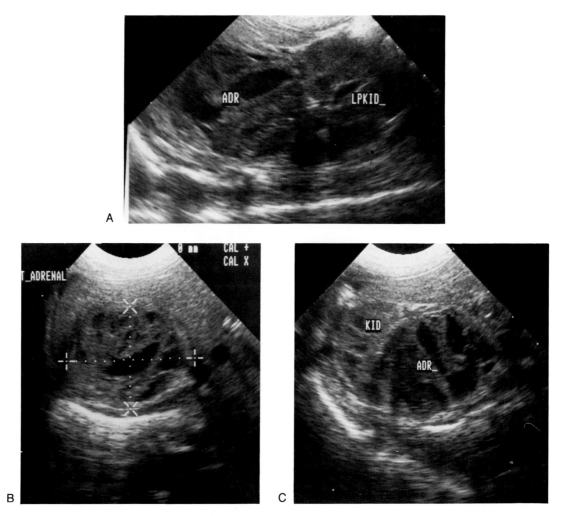

Fig. 12-33. Adrenal hemorrhage. **(A)** Sagittal and **(B & C)** transverse scans showing a large adrenal (37 × 38 mm) mass *(ADR,* calipers) with a mixed echopattern superiomedial to the right kidney *(KID, LPKID).*

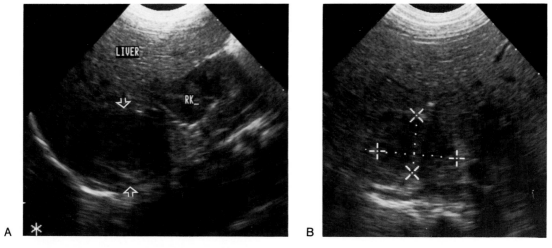

Fig. 12-34. Adrenal hemorrhage, follow-up. Follow-up **(A)** sagittal and **(B)** transverse scans 1 month later than Fig. 12-33 showing the mass (arrows, calipers), which has decreased in size and has become more hypoechoic. *(RK,* right kidney.)

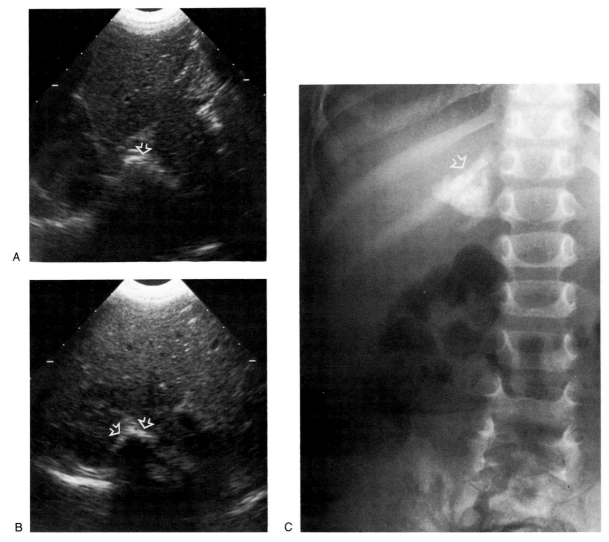

Fig. 12-35. Adrenal hemorrhage, old. **(A)** Sagittal and **(B)** transverse scans of the right upper quadrant in a baby showing a brightly echogenic focus (open arrows) with associated shadowing in the region of the right adrenal gland. **(C)** Radiograph demonstrating the characteristic calcification (open arrow) associated with an old adrenal hemorrhage.

with septicemia, hypertension, renal vein thrombosis, or adrenal disease such as tumor. In the older child or adult, it is often due to trauma or associated systemic illness or anticoagulation.[45] With Waterhouse-Friderichsen syndrome, there is fulminant bacterial sepsis, disseminated intravascular coagulation (DIC), shock, and necropsy evidence of bilateral adrenal hemorrhage.[46] With overwhelming bacterial septicemia, acute adrenocortical insufficiency may occur.[46] There appears to be a high association between decreased cortisol secretion and autopsy findings of massive bilateral adrenal hemorrhage.[46] In adults, adrenal hemorrhage may occur in a hypertrophic adrenal gland as a result of adrenocorticotropic hor-

mone (ACTH) therapy or severe stress.[5] The associated adrenocortical insufficiency associated with the fulminant meningococcemia is potentially reversible and warrants replacement corticosteroid therapy. As such, the identification of adrenal abnormalities antemortem has important prognostic and therapeutic implications. The greater occurrence on the right side may be due to an acute rise in venous pressure, which is more directly transmitted to the right adrenal gland because the right adrenal vein enters the IVC directly. All appear echofree, mixed, or echogenic at ultrasound, depending on the amount of clot versus serum or nonclotted blood present[46] (Fig. 12-37).

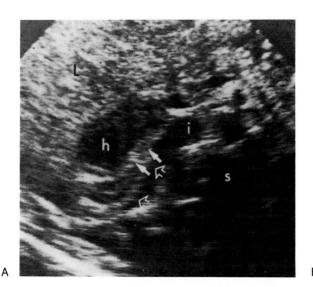
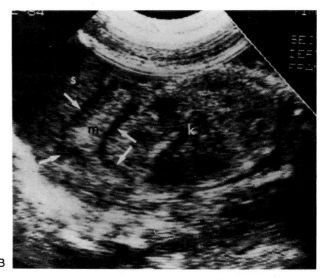

Fig. 12-36. Focal adrenal hemorrhage. **(A)** Transverse abdominal scan showing hemorrhage *(h)* in the lateral and anterior portions of the right adrenal gland. The medial limb of the adrenal gland (solid arrows) is not involved. (open arrows, right diaphragmatic crus; *s*, spine; *L*, liver; *i*, inferior vena cava.) **(B)** Left parasagittal scan showing normal hypoechoic adrenal cortex (arrows). However, the echogenic center *(m)* is markedly thickened. The spleen *(s)* and left kidney *(k)* are seen. (From Cohen et al,[44] with permission.)

In up to 25 percent of severely traumatized patients, adrenal hemorrhage may occur; 20 percent of cases are bilateral,[45,47] even though the adrenal is in the perirenal space surrounded by fat and enclosed by Gerota's fascia. There have been two proposed mechanisms of traumatic hemorrhage in the right adrenal: (1) direct compression of the gland between the spine and the liver; and (2) an acute rise in intra-adrenal venous pressure as a result of compression of the IVC, in which case hemorrhage is a secondary reaction, or the hemorrhage may be secondary to deceleration forces, which cause shearing of small vessels that perforate the adrenal capsule.[47] On ultrasound, the hemorrhagic adrenal appears as an enlarged, hyperechoic mass with a bright central echo that becomes cystic on follow-up examinations[47] (Fig. 12-37). The central echogenic area may reflect the acute nature of the hematoma, since blood tends to become less echogenic with time.

Hyperplasia

Neonates with congenital adrenal hyperplasia have been evaluated.[41,48,49] This abnormality results from an inborn enzyme deficiency in the biosynthetic pathway of adrenal steroid metabolism. As a result, there is ineffective production of adrenal steroids; overproduction and accumulation of cortisol precursors, some of which produce androgenic effects; and hyperplasia of the adrenal cortex. Growth of the adrenal cortex in the fetus is ACTH-dependent, and adrenal size is invariably increased in infants with the salt-wasting variety of congenital adrenal hyperplasia.[27]

Excessive accumulation of androgenic precursors results when there is adrenogenital syndrome (congenital hyperplasia) caused by deficiency of an enzyme (usually C-21 hydroxylase) necessary for adrenal production of cortisol.[49] There is inhibition of differentiation of the embryonic genital tract along female lines, resulting in masculinization in females with the overproduction of androgens.[48] In female infants, virilization of the genitalia is produced; this condition produces most cases of female pseudohermaphroditism. Its incidence is between 1 : 7,000 and 1 : 10,000.[49] An immediate diagnosis is important since early treatment with cortisol turns off the excessive androgen production and allows normal sexual development.[49]

Mineralocorticoid production is impaired in approximately 30 percent of cases, resulting in hyponatremia, hyperkalemia, hypoglycemia, and hypotension.[48] There is often a stormy neonatal period with shock, hyperkalemia, and hyponatremia. In any infant with salt-losing crisis, this diagnosis should be considered. In over 90 percent of cases, the most common enzymatic abnormality is C-21 hydroxylase deficiency.[48]

Ultrasound can be useful not only in evaluating adrenal size but also in identifying a uterus, which establishes the sexual identity of the infant. The diagnosis of congenital adrenal hyperplasia is highly likely when enlarged adrenals are seen, because none of the infants with ambiguous genitalia from other causes have enlarged

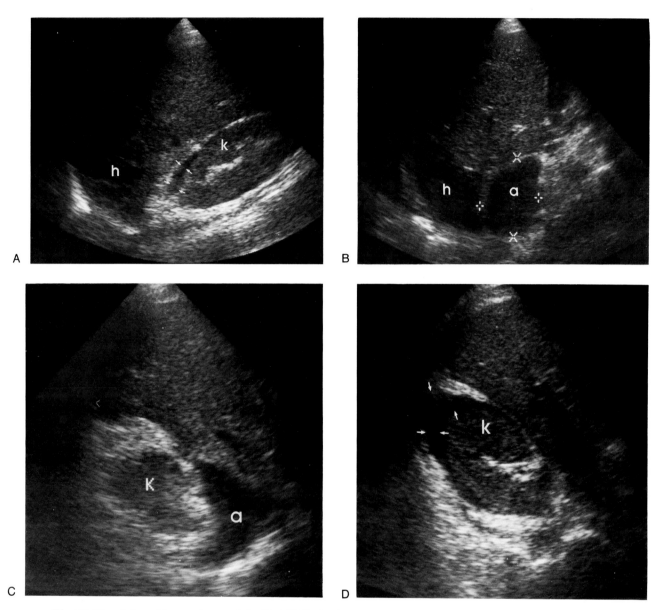

Fig. 12-37. Adrenal hemorrhage, adult. **(A & B)** Sagittal and **(C & D)** transverse scans through the right upper quadrant demonstrating several fluid collections in this traumatized adult. A hepatic hematoma *(h)* is seen as a lucent fluid collection within the liver in Figs. A & B. An adrenal hematoma *(a)* is seen in a suprarenal location as a lucent fluid collection in Figs. B & C. Fluid is seen in a perirenal location (arrows) (Figs. A & D) as well. (*k*, right kidney.)

adrenals.[49] On ultrasound, the adrenals may be enlarged, at the upper limits of normal or within normal limits. There is bilateral enlargement of the adrenal glands (normal length, 0.9 to 3.6 cm; normal width, 0.2 to 0.5 cm; normal ratio of adrenal width/adrenal pelvis, 0.38 : 0.70).[41] The mean adrenal length is 23.7 mm with a width of 5.3 mm; the asymptomatic infants studied demonstrate a length of 14.4 mm with a width of 1.9 mm.[48] The maximum cephalocaudal dimension is

defined as the length with the maximum dimension perpendicular to the length of the posterior wing, the width (Figs. 12-38 and 12-39). The ASI is markedly elevated in patients with the salt-wasting variety of C-21 hydroxylase deficiency, whereas in patients without severe salt loss, the ASI is in the upper normal range.[27] There may be loss of the normal corticomedullary differentiation. The cortex is affected more by the enlargement than is the medulla; this may be due to vascular congestion.[41]

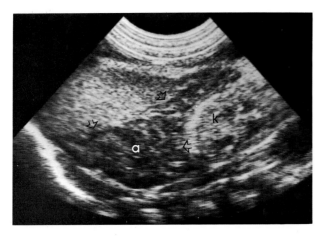

Fig. 12-38. Adrenal hyperplasia. Sagittal scan of the right adrenal in an infant demonstrating marked enlargement (*a*, arrows). The triangular shape of the adrenal is maintained. (*k*, kidney.) This patient with bilateral adrenal enlargement had a sibling with adrenal hyperplasia and showed biochemical changes consistent with this disease process.

Ultrasound can be an effective, noninvasive tool in the diagnosis of adrenal enlargement due to congenital adrenal hyperplasia. When normal-sized glands are seen, the diagnosis cannot be entirely excluded. The ultrasound finding of enlarged adrenal glands in addition to elevated 17-OH concentrations may alert the pediatri-

cian to anticipate impending salt loss, since unequivocal signs of salt wasting are not always present in the first days of life.[27]

Adrenal gland hyperplasia may also be found in adults.[50] Primary hyperaldosteronism is a disorder characterized by hypertension associated with an elevated plasma aldosterone concentration on at least one occasion and with a concurrent plasma renin concentration below the mean value.[50] Associated symptoms of hypokalemia such as muscle weakness, polyuria, nocturia, polydipsia, and, less commonly, paresthesia, tetany, and muscle paralysis are found. Also common is headache. This condition may be due to bilateral nodular hyperplasia of the adrenal glands (idiopathic primary hyperaldosteronism) or a single aldosterone-producing adenoma (Conn syndrome).[45,50]

Cushing syndrome may result from excess glucocorticoids from either exogenous (steroid treatment) or endogenous (overproduction of cortisol by the cortex) sources.[45] In 70 percent of patients with endogenous Cushing syndrome, the cause is bilateral adrenal hyperplasia.[45] Cushing syndrome is easier to detect since the gland is larger with bilateral adrenal enlargement of the entire adrenal gland without a focal mass. With Cushing's disease, there is overproduction of ACTH by a pituitary adenoma with bilateral adrenal hyperplasia. However, the associated ACTH may be produced by some tumors such as oat cell carcinoma; bronchial carcinoid adenomas; and tumors of the ovary, pancreas, thymus, and thyroid, as well as pheochromocytomas.[45]

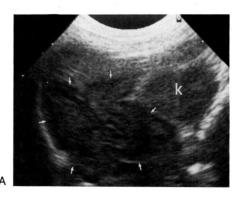
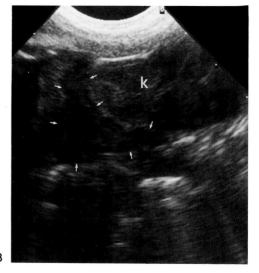

A   B

Fig. 12-39. Adrenal hyperplasia. Sagittal scans of the **(A)** right (2 cm AP) and **(B)** left (2.3 cm AP) adrenals demonstrating enlarged glands (arrows) that have lost the normal differentiation between the medulla and cortex. The infant was born with ambiguous genitalia and was a genotypic female. (*k*, kidney.)

In children, a rare cause of Cushing syndrome is primary pigmented nodular adrenocortical disease.

Infection

Abscess. In the neonate, adrenal abscess is a rare complication of adrenal hemorrhage.[51] Its diagnosis depends on correlation of perinatal history, clinical signs, and radiographic examination. There are two proposed theories for the development of adrenal abscess: (1) hematogenous bacterial seeding of a normal adrenal gland, with abscess formation; and (2) seeding of the neonatal adrenal hemorrhage, with abscess formation.[51]

In some cases of adrenal hemorrhage there may be organization and encapsulation of the hematoma with pseudocyst formation rather than resorption.[51] Neonatal septicemia and maternal infection may lead to seeding of the hematoma or pseudocyst, with formation of the adrenal abscess. To ensure appropriate clinical management, which may be lifesaving, early and accurate diagnosis of an adrenal abscess is very important.[51] In a case report, an adrenal abscess was seen to be a large, complex mass between the spleen and the inferiorly displaced kidney (Fig. 12-40). It contained diffuse low-level echoes and exhibited through transmission with enhancement at its posterior margin.[51]

Histoplasmosis. Chronic disseminated histoplasmosis usually affects older people who have a reduced immune response, and there may be a history of cancer, miliary tuberculosis, or systemic steroid therapy.[52] Weight loss, malaise, anorexia, and low-grade fever, which are nonspecific, are the most common clinical findings. Chronic disseminated histoplasmosis can be associated with bilateral adrenal gland enlargement similar in degree from side to side.[52] An important clue to the diagnosis of chronic disseminated histoplasmosis is bilateral adrenal gland enlargement, especially in patients with adrenal insufficiency in an area in which histoplasmosis is endemic.[52]

The most frequent ultrasound finding is bilateral and approximately symmetric adrenal gland enlargement.[52] The enlarged glands display an echodensity equal to or greater than that of the adjacent renal cortex (Fig. 12-41). Most characteristic is the finding of a triangular right adrenal and a cylindrical left adrenal.[52] Ultrasound may provide the first clue to this diagnosis.

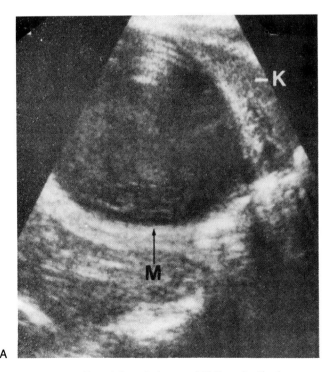
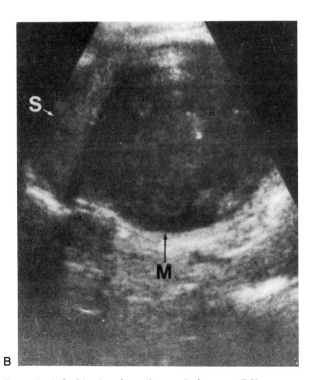

A

B

Fig. 12-40. Adrenal abscess. **(A)** Longitudinal sonogram from the left side showing a hypoechoic mass *(M)* containing diffuse, low-level echoes with displacement of the upper pole of the left kidney *(K)* inferiorly and laterally. **(B)** Longitudinal sonogram at a higher level showing the mass *(M)* inferior to the spleen *(S)*. (From Atkinson et al,[51] with permission.)

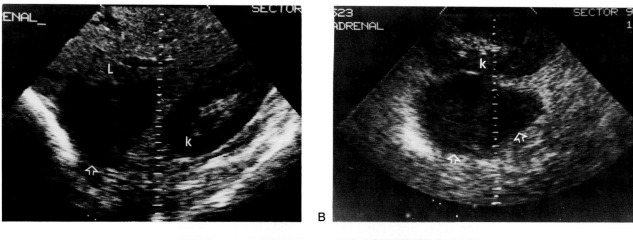

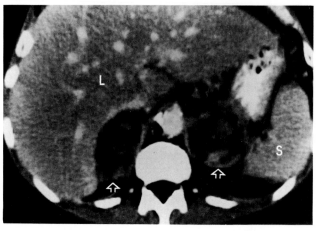

Fig. 12-41. Adrenal: chronic disseminated histoplasmosis. **(A)** Longitudinal sonogram through the right upper abdomen showing the enlarged, triangular right adrenal gland (arrow). A percutaneous biopsy of this gland with ultrasound guidance showed adrenal histoplasmosis. (*L*, liver; *k*, kidney.) **(B)** Longitudinal sonogram through the back with the patient prone showing the large left adrenal gland (arrows). (*k*, kidney.) **(C)** CT scan after infusion of contrast medium showing massively enlarged adrenal glands (arrows). (*L*, liver; *S*, spleen.) (From Wilson et al,[52] with permission.)

Insufficiency

After at least 90 percent of the adrenal cortex has been destroyed, primary adrenal insufficiency (Addison's disease) occurs.[45] The most common cause in the United States is idiopathic adrenal atrophy, and it is most probably an autoimmune disorder. Other causes include granulomatous disease (usually tuberculosis), infarction, amyloidosis, hemorrhage, or destruction by histoplasmosis, blastomyocosis, disseminated fungal infection, lymphoma, or metastatic tumor.[45] With this entity, it would be difficult to identify the adrenal glands by CT, let alone by ultrasound.

Cyst

Adrenal cysts are relatively infrequent lesions that seldom are manifested clinically. Most cysts are asymptomatic because of their small size. As uncommon lesions occurring at any age (usually presenting in the third to fifth decade), adrenal cysts involve the right and left glands equally but have a 3 : 1 female predilection.[45] The cysts may (very rarely) be bilateral.[53] They can be unilocular or multilocular and can vary immensely in size.

The most common type of adrenal cyst is the endothelial cyst, representing 44 to 45 percent of reported adrenal cysts.[5,45,53,54] These can be further subdivided

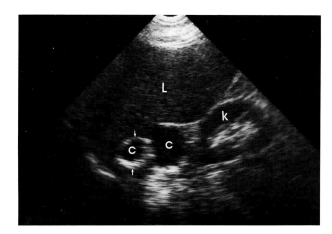

Fig. 12-42. Adrenal cyst. Sagittal scan showing multiple hypoechoic masses *(c)* in the adrenal area. One (arrows) has a very dense wall that is thought to represent calcification. Fluid obtained from an aspiration (the patient had a known primary tumor) was consistent with adrenal cyst fluid. (*k*, right kidney; *L*, liver.)

into lymphangiomatous (41 percent) and angiomatous (3 percent) cysts.[5,54] Pseudocyst (39 to 40 percent) is the next most frequent category and is the most likely to present clinically, as these cysts may be of considerable size.[45,53,54] Pseudocysts may be secondary to hemorrhage either into the normal adrenal or within an adrenal tumor such as an adenoma—this is the usual cause. The

remainder are sequelae of hemorrhage, epithelial glandular cysts, or echinococcal (7 percent) cysts.[5,37,53] Finally, the epithelial cyst (7 to 9 percent) represents cystic degeneration of adenomas and parasitic cysts and constitutes 6 percent of adrenal cysts.[37,45,54]

Adrenal cysts may range from small to very large. The cyst wall is thin and smooth. On ultrasound, the cyst is smooth, round, and echofree with thin walls and acoustic enhancement and is located suprarenally[2,7,45] (Figs. 12-30, 12-42, and 12-43). In 15 percent of cases, calcification may occur and can cause a thick, highly echogenic wall (peripheral and curvilinear) that casts an acoustic shadow[5,7,54] (Fig. 12-42). Because cysts are rarely symptomatic and thus are frequently encountered incidentally, a conservative approach to therapy is recommended. If the lesion is purely cystic, an ultrasound-guided aspiration may be performed to alleviate symptoms of pressure.[54] Cystic neuroblastoma (in the appropriate age group) should be considered in the differential diagnosis along with cystic degeneration of a metastasis or primary adrenal tumor when a cystic adrenal mass is encountered.[53]

Neoplasm

Adenoma. Abdominal CT scans encounter benign, nonhyperfunctioning adrenal adenomas commonly.[45] The incidence of these is higher among older patients and those with diabetes or hypertension. In 2 percent of

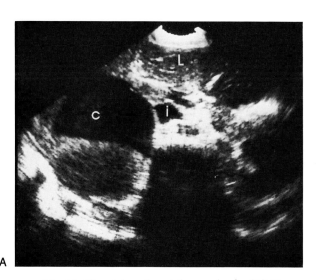

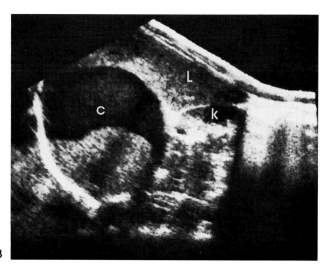

A   B

Fig. 12-43. Adrenal cyst, hemorrhagic. **(A)** Transverse supine scan at the level of the kidney showing a large retroperitoneal cystic mass *(c)* on the right. Note the straight fluid-fluid level and the echoes of different intensities within the mass. The liver *(L)* and inferior vena cava *(i)* are pushed anteriorly. **(B)** Parasagittal longitudinal scan through the right kidney *(k)* in the left lateral decubitus position. Note the undulation of the fluid-fluid level in the suprarenal cystic mass *(c)*. (From Barki et al,[53] with permission.)

adult autopsies, adrenal adenomas are noted; most are non-steroid-producing adenomas, but they may be part of an endocrine neoplastic syndrome. They are usually 1 to 5 cm in diameter and poorly encapsulated.[55] In 20 percent of cases of endogenous Cushing syndrome, a benign autonomous adrenal cortical adenoma is found, with primary adrenal cortical carcinoma in 10 percent of cases. In 80 percent of cases of primary aldosteronism there is a benign but unregulated aldosterone-secreting adenoma, which is the most common cause of primary aldosteronism.[45] The adenomas in Conn syndrome are the hardest to detect because they tend to be the smallest, averaging less than 2 cm in diameter.[45] On CT a nonhyperfunctioning adenoma is a well-defined rounded homogeneous mass.[45]

Hemangioma. As rare nonfunctioning tumors, hemangiomas are small and incidentally discovered at autopsy.[56] On ultrasound, this lesion has been shown to be a large mass with a heterogeneous nonspecific structural pattern — cystic, solid, and heterogeneous[56] (Fig. 12-44). On unenhanced CT, the lesion has a hypodense center with thick, irregular, higher-density peripheries.[56]

Myelolipoma. Adrenal myelolipoma is a rare cortical tumor (0.08 to 0.2 percent incidence at autopsy) composed of various proportions of fat and bone marrow elements.[2,7,55,57,58] The etiology of this lesion is unknown

but is suggested to be metaplasia of the mesenchymal stem cells, which are precursors of both adrenal and myeloid tissue. There has been no correlation between extramedullary hematopoiesis and adrenal myelolipomas. Hemorrhage and/or calcification may be present.[59] Chronic infection and trauma have been proposed as additional causative factors.[58] There is no malignant potential and the lesions are nonfunctioning.[59]

Most cases occur in the fourth to sixth decades, with equal frequency among men and women.[59] The lesion may vary from microscopic to 30 cm in diameter.[59] The patient may be asymptomatic or may complain of pain from hemorrhage, necrosis, or pressure on surrounding structures.[59]

The key factor for both identification and preoperative diagnosis by imaging methods is the presence of fat within these tumors.[57] Those with only small quantities of fat may be difficult to differentiate from other adrenal masses; these lesions may contain different proportions of fat and myeloid tissue. When a suprarenal fatty mass is demonstrated, the differential diagnosis includes myelolipoma, renal angiomyolipoma extending from the upper pole, and retroperitoneal lipoma and liposarcoma.[57]

The ultrasound appearance of an adrenal myelolipoma depends on its variable tissue components.[59] The right and left glands are affected with equal frequency. It is usually a well-defined discrete mass that may have a

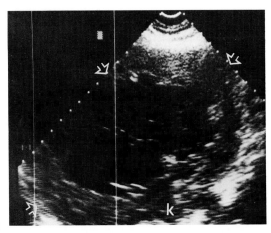
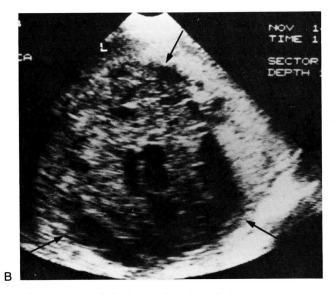

A   B

Fig. 12-44. Adrenal hemangioma. **(A)** Sagittal ultrasound scan of the left flank showing a large heterogeneous adrenal hemangioma (arrows) with a solid periphery and hypoechoic center. The left kidney *(k)* is compressed by the mass. **(B)** Sagittal ultrasound image of the right hypochondrium. The adrenal hemangioma (arrows) is seen as a large mass with complex structural pattern. Normal liver *(L)* is seen superior to the mass. (From Derchi et al,[56] with permission.)

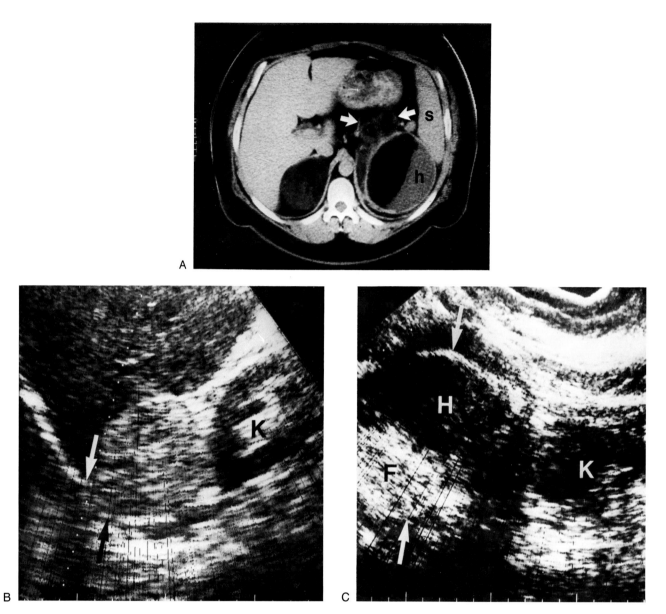

Fig. 12-45. Bilateral adrenal myelolipomas. **(A)** CT scan showing that the areas of lowest density within the right-sided myelolipoma are slightly higher density than normal fat, and that subtle areas of inhomogenicity are also evident. The left-sided myelolipoma contains areas of density equivalent to normal fat, and hemorrhage *(h)* has produced a blood-fat interface. Also on the left, there is extension of the tumor (arrows) beyond an apparent pseudocapsule and anterior displacement of the spleen *(S)*. **(B)** Right longitudinal ultrasound scan showing that the homogeneously fat myelolipoma has a relatively even pattern of high-amplitude echoes. A propagation speed artifact results in apparent discontinuity and posterior displacement of the diaphragm (arrows) deep to the mass. These ultrasound appearances are highly suggestive of a fatty mass. *(K,* right kidney.) **(C)** Coronal scan of the left myelolipoma (arrows) showing two distinct components: low-level echoes laterally corresponding to hemorrhage *(H)* and high-amplitude echoes medially caused by fat *(F).* The fatty component was recognized only in retrospect after review of the CT scan (Fig. A). *(K,* left kidney.) (From Vick et al,[59] with permission.)

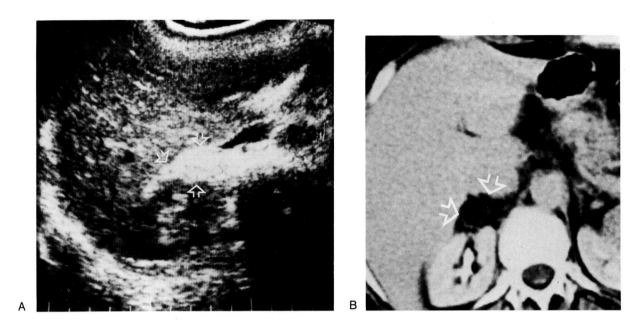

Fig. 12-46. Adrenal myelolipoma. **(A)** Axial sonogram of the right adrenal region showing a small, hyperechoic, homogeneous myelolipoma (arrows); no propagation speed artifact is seen posterior to mass. **(B)** Contrast-enhanced CT appearance of the same lesion. The tumor (arrows) has a slightly heterogeneous pattern owing to a few thin lines of increased density. (From Musante et al,[57] with permission.)

pseudocapsule and occasional involvement of extracapsular cortical tissue. It has been described as markedly echogenic on ultrasound[58,59] (Figs. 12-45 to 12-48). An additional finding that suggests a fat content is the apparent discontinuity and posterior displacement of an acoustic interface (e.g. diaphragm) distal to the fatty lesion, particularly when the tumor is larger than 4 cm[59] (Figs. 12-45 to 12-48). Owing to the slow propagation of ultrasound through fatty masses, this artifact is a valuable clue to the diagnosis.[57] It is easier to diagnose the

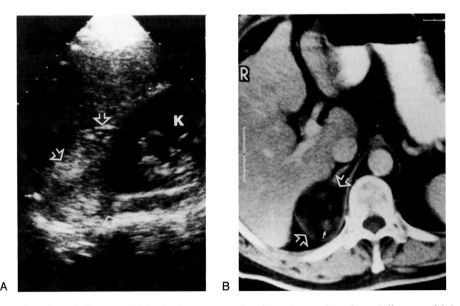

Fig. 12-47. Adrenal myelolipoma. **(A)** Sagittal sonogram showing a 6-cm adrenal myelolipoma with heterogeneous echopattern (open arrows). A propagation speed artifact causes apparent disruption of the right hemidiaphragm (small arrow). (*K*, kidney.) **(B)** The tumor is heterogeneous on contrast-enhanced CT image also. Enhancement of a small area of tumor (arrow) is noted. (From Musante et al,[57] with permission.)

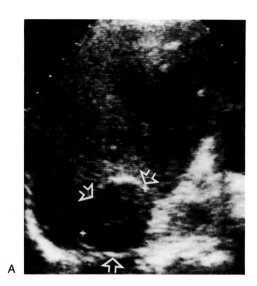 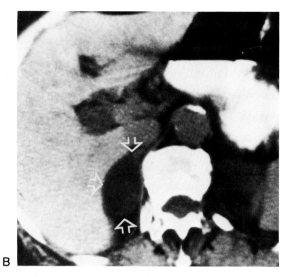

Fig. 12-48. Adrenal myelolipoma. **(A)** Axial sonogram of a 4-cm, homogeneous, hypoechoic myelolipoma (arrows); no propagation speed artifact is seen. **(B)** Before injection of contrast material, the tumor (arrows) has density values within range of fat. (From Musante et al,[57] with permission.)

larger lesions by ultrasound than the smaller ones.[57] Adjacent echogenic retroperitoneal fat may mask a small fatty myelolipoma. CT is recommended to confirm the fatty nature of the lesion (Figs. 12-45 to 12-48). The differential diagnosis includes lipoma, lymphangioma, myelolipoma, renal angiomyolipoma from upper pole, increased abdominal fat deposition, retroperitoneal teratoma, and liposarcoma.[59]

Pheochromocytoma. Pheochromocytomas are uncommon tumors, occurring in 0.5 to 1.0 percent of patients with hypertension. Ninety percent occur between the diaphragm and pelvic floor. These lesions arise from chromaffian cells, and most (90 percent) occur in the adrenal medulla; the remainder (7 to 10 percent) originate in the autonomic tissue, particularly the organs of Zuckerkandl and the parasympathetic ganglia.[60,61] Pheochromocytomas are malignant 5 to 10 percent of the time and are multiple 3 to 5 percent of the time. Paragangliomas or extra-adrenal pheochromocytomas, are found most commonly along the sympathetic chain in the retroperitoneum.[45]

Pheochromocytomas may be associated with multiple endocrine neoplasia (MEN) syndrome. The multiple lesions are frequently associated with heredofamilial syndromes. Type IIa includes medullary carcinoma of the thyroid, parathyroid hyperplasia, and pheochromocytoma. Type IIb comprises pheochromocytoma, medullary carcinoma of the thyroid, and mucocutaneous manifestations including mucosal neuromas, intestinal ganglioneuromatosis, and a marfanoid habitus.[45] The

sporadic pheochromocystomas are located outside the adrenal gland in up to 25 percent of cases, whereas those associated with the MEN II syndrome are always intra-adrenal.[45]

Clinically, patients present with hypertension (50 percent paroxysmal) in the fourth and fifth decades. The diagnosis can be confirmed by biochemical assay for catecholamines and metabolites in the urine.[61]

On ultrasound, pheochromocytomas may appear as purely solid masses of homogeneous or heterogeneous echoes. Hypoechoic areas indicate necrosis, and hyperechoic regions indicate hemorrhage. These lesions are usually quite large and sharply marginated and have a significant solid component with or without central necrosis or hemorrhage.[60]

Carcinoma. Primary adrenal cortical carcinoma is an uncommon cancer, occurring with an incidence of 1 to 2 per million per year.[45,62] Functional tumors are more common in females; otherwise the incidence is equal between men and women. Adrenal carcinomas usually produce steroids (90 percent) and are associated with one of the hyperadrenal syndromes. With functioning adrenocortical neoplasms, there may be Cushing syndrome, adrenogenital syndrome (virilization or feminization), precocious puberty, or, rarely, the clinical syndrome of hypertension with hypokalemic alkalosis (hyperaldosteronism).[62]

Tumor size varies from 3 to 22 cm[62] (Figs. 12-49 and 12-50). The smaller lesions (3 to 6 cm) appear hormonally active, and so the patients present earlier. There is a

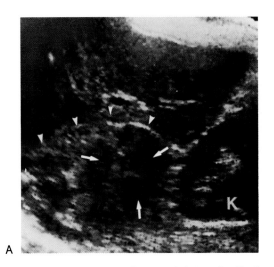
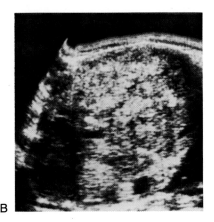

Fig. 12-49. Adrenocortical carcinoma. **(A)** Longitudinal sonogram of right adrenal gland showing a fairly well-defined heterogeneous adrenocortical carcinoma. Hypoechoic zones (arrows) correspond to necrotic tumor on pathologic examination. (*K*, right kidney; arrowheads, thick echogenic capsulelike rim.) **(B)** Longitudinal sonogram of left adrenal gland showing adrenocortical carcinoma with heterogeneous, predominantly echogenic pattern, corresponding to necrotic and hemorrhagic tumor on pathologic examination. (From Hamper et al,[62] with permission.)

greater probability of malignancy when the lesion is 3 to 4 cm, but adenomata can exceed 5 cm in diameter. Calcification may be associated with both benign and malignant disease. There is a strong tendency for these lesions to invade the adrenal vein, IVC, and lymph glands. Metastases to regional and periaortic nodes are common, with distant hematogeneous spread to the lungs and viscera.[55]

Adrenal carcinomas are more common on the left than the right, and up to 10 percent are bilateral.[45] These patients may present with abdominal pain or a palpable mass. Although extremely uncommon, childhood adrenocortical carcinoma is still the most common tumor occurring in the adrenal cortex.

Ultrasound allows rapid noninvasive confirmation when an adrenal tumor is suspected on clinical grounds. It can localize the lesion, serve as a guide for percutaneous needle aspiration biopsy, and assess metastatic spread preoperatively. However, no echopattern is specific enough to allow differentiation of adrenal adenoma from a small carcinoma.[62] A large adrenal carcinoma is usually described as a mass of complex echopatterns due to areas of hemorrhage, necrosis, or calcification (Fig. 12-49). In patients with the larger tumors, a complex predominantly echogenic pattern is demonstrated; some contain radiating linear echoes, the "scar sign." Although this finding is not specific, when it is present in a large adrenal mass the diagnosis of a cortical carcinoma should be suggested.[63] The smaller lesions exhibit a homogeneous echopattern similar to that of renal parenchyma; hypoechoic or hyperechoic lesions are seen with smaller lesions. Differentiation from neuroblastoma, adrenal cortical carcinoma, and adrenal adenoma by ultrasound may not be possible.

Neuroblastoma. Neuroblastoma is one of the most common tumors of childhood, with 80 percent occurring in patients less than 5 years of age and 35 percent in those less than 2 years. Seventy-five percent of patients are less than 4 years of age with 50 percent of patients less than 2 years of age; fewer than 10 percent are older than age 10 years. It is the most common extracranial solid malignant tumor in children and is the third most common cancer of childhood, surpassed in incidence only by acute leukemia and primary brain tumors.[64] There is a striking correlation between age and prognosis. After the age of 1 year, the tumor is usually malignant; before 1 year there is a remarkable tendency to spontaneous regression. The prognosis of this tumor remains extremely poor and has not been significantly affected by either irradiation or chemotherapy; the notable exception is in children less than 1 year of age.[64]

The main determinants of prognosis include the age of the patient, the site of the tumor, and the stage of the disease at initial diagnosis.[64] For all stages of neuroblastoma, the overall survival is 72 percent if the patient is less than 1 year of age, 28 percent at 1 to 2 years of age, and 12 percent at older than 2 years of age.[64] The highest mortality is associated with tumors arising within the abdomen and pelvis.[64] Compared with the 20 percent

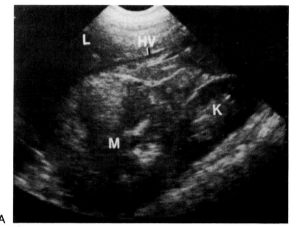

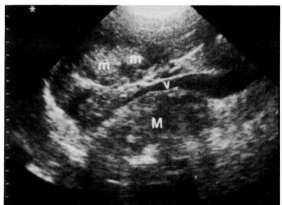

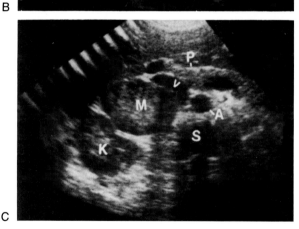

Fig. 12-50. Large adrenal carcinoma with liver metastases. **(A)** Longitudinal scan of right upper abdomen showing a large adrenal mass *(M)* superior to the right kidney *(K)*. The mass markedly indents the liver *(L)*. *(HV,* hepatic vein.*)* **(B)** Longitudinal scan more medially showing the medial portion of the mass *(M)* displacing the inferior vena cava *(v)* anteriorly. Two metastatic masses *(m)* are seen within the liver. **(C)** Transverse scan of epigastrium showing the inferior portion of the mass *(M)* indenting the right kidney *(K)* and compressing the inferior vena cava *(v)* from behind. The head of the pancreas *(P)* and the inferior vena cava are displaced anteriorly. (From Yeh,[9] with permission.)

survival for abdominal tumors, thoracic neuroblastomas have an overall 61 percent survival rate.[64]

There appears to be a benign course associated with neonatal neuroblastoma, with 50 percent of the patients classified with stage IV-S disease.[65] In younger children, less aggressive management may be warranted in the absence of stage IV disease, unlike that for neuroblastoma in older children, which is usually advanced at the time of clinical presentation. It is less crucial for extensive diagnostic investigation to identify all possible sites of neoplastic involvement since the treatment does not differ on the basis of the presence or absence of metastatic disease, especially in the liver.[65] The diagnosis of neonatal neuroblastoma is very likely when there is prenatal ultrasound detection of a solid suprarenal mass or the identification of liver lesions.[65] The diagnosis of neuroblastoma is confirmed without exception when liver involvement is detected. On prenatal ultrasound the findings may be nonspecific—hydramnios and hydrops fetalis—or consistent with a suprarenal mass. Postnatal ultrasound may confirm the adrenal location of the mass and evaluate the liver for metastatic disease.[65]

There are no clinical symptoms until the tumor invades or compresses adjacent structures, metastasizes, or produces paraneoplastic syndromes.[64] The clinical presentation is related to its rapid growth and secretory products. The symptoms include energy and weight loss, pallor, abdominal protrusion, irregular fever, and generalized malaise. Signs and symptoms including fever, weight loss, irritability, and anemia are nonspecific. In three-fourths of cases, the patients present with the metastases before the diagnosis of the primary lesion is made.[66] More than 90 percent of lesions produce catecholamines.

Most (50 to 80 percent) of these lesions occur in the adrenal glands, with 65 percent in the abdomen and with the posterior mediastinum being the second most common site.[64,66] The remainder of the abdominal/pelvic tumors originate in the paravertebral sympathetic chain or the presacral area, with an occasional abdominal tumor arising in the celiac axis or organ of Zuckerkandl. At times, a neuroblastoma may appear to be intrarenal.[66] Intrarenal neuroblastomas originate from adrenal rests found within renal tissue. Alternatively, an adrenal tumor may invade the kidney and appear within the renal tissue. The tumor metastasizes rapidly and widely through local infiltration and node metastases and is spread in the blood to the liver, lungs, and the bones.

This lesion arises from the primitive sympathetic neuroblasts of the embryonic neural crest.[64] Composed of entirely undifferentiated sympathoblasts, the neuroblastoma is a highly malignant tumor that is usually well demarcated and may contain gross or microscopic calcification, but lacks any capsular structures. Neuroblastoma may regress in the following ways: (1) it may disappear by cytolysis; (2) it may undergo hemorrhage and then necrosis, leading to fibrocalcific residuals; and/or (3) cytodifferentiation into ganglioneuroma and ganglioneuroblastoma may occur.[66] The degree of cellular maturation differentiates the three neural crest tumors —neuroblastoma, ganglioneuroblastoma, and ganglioneuroma. Various levels of differentiation are found.

A ganglioneuroma is composed of a fibrous background and is completely differentiated. It is an uncommon neurogenic neoplasm, and 60 percent occur in patients less than 20 years of age, with a slight female predominance.[67] It is a benign tumor containing mature ganglion cells, is well circumscribed, is encapsulated, and usually contains gross flecks of calcium.[64] It is found most frequently in the thorax, with 43 percent in the mediastinum, 32 percent in the abdomen, and 8 percent in the neck.[64,67] The intra-abdominal lesions are usually extra-adrenal.

A ganglioneuroblastoma is intermediate in differentiation. As a malignant tumor, it contains undifferentiated neuroblasts and mature ganglion cells; this tumor may be partially or totally encapsulated and frequently contains granular calcification.

Ultrasound is helpful in the detection of these tumors, as 70 percent arise in the abdomen. However, ultrasound is limited when the lesion arises in or extends into the chest and/or paraspinal area with extradural extension.[68] These lesions generally are heterogeneously echogenic with poorly defined margins[2,68] (Figs. 12-51 to 12-54). They are inhomogeneous in echogenicity because of the increased cellularity without collagenous stroma, hemorrhage, necrosis, or dystrophic calcification.[64] Tumor margins of neuroblastoma are poorly defined, and a capsule or pseudocapsule (rim of hyperechogenicity) is not seen.[65] Anechoic "cystic" areas and calcification frequently are present[65,68] (Figs. 12-52 and 12-54). Twenty percent of neuroblastomas demonstrate internal calcification on CT.[67] The areas of hyperechogencity may be related to calcification, hemorrhage, and necrosis. Seventy percent in one series were highly echogenic.[69]

An additional characteristic that seems to be specific for neuroblastoma is the ultrasound lobule.[70] The lobule is an area of increased echogenicity in a part of the larger tumor mass; this ultrasound appearance is secondary to the growth pattern of the tumor and is not cell specific. It consists of an oval or round "lobule" of homogeneously increased echogenicity that is round or ovoid with smooth margins and is easily demarcated from the surrounding tumor.[70]

Neuroblastomas and ganglioneuroblastomas frequently contain focal areas of necrosis, hemorrhage, and calcification.[67] As a result of this heterogeneous makeup, these masses contain more echoproducing interfaces than ganglioneuromas do. Other distinguishing factors between neuroblastomas and ganglioneuromas include the tendency of neuroblastomas to cross the midline and to have ill-defined edges[67] (Figs. 12-55 and 12-56). A careful examination should be performed to delineate the relationship of the mass to important vascular structures such as the IVC and aorta.[71] Although the mass

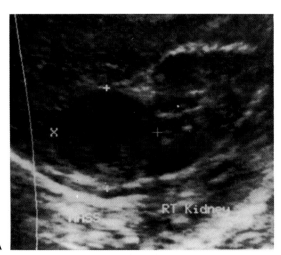

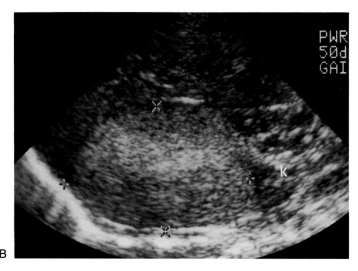

A   B

Fig. 12-51. Congenital neuroblastoma. **(A)** Longitudinal ultrasound scan of the right flank showing a right suprarenal cyst (mass). This scan was obtained when the patient was 4 weeks of age. The cyst was detected in utero and remained unchanged. (*RT,* right.) **(B)** Longitudinal ultrasound scan showing a solid right adrenal mass (calipers) depressing the right kidney *(k).* The adjacent liver is questionably inhomogeneous. (From Forman et al,[65] with permission.)

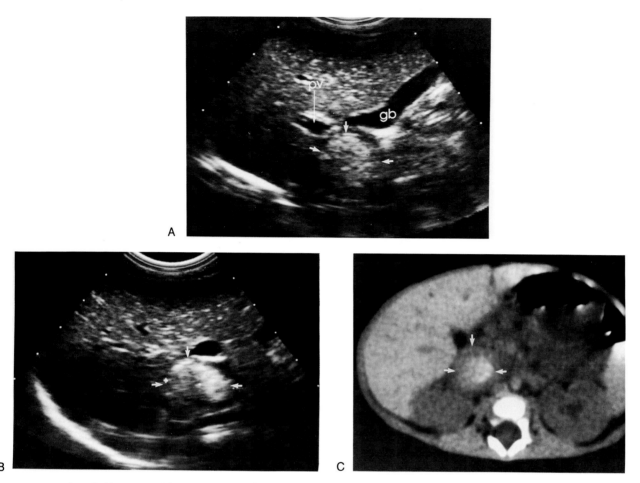

Fig. 12-52. Neuroblastoma, small with calcification. **(A)** Sagittal and **(B)** transverse scans demonstrating a highly echogenic mass (arrows) in the area of the right adrenal in this child. The highly echogenic pattern was thought to be secondary to internal calcifications as seen on **(C)** an unenhanced CT scan. (*pv*, portal vein; *gb*, gallbladder.)

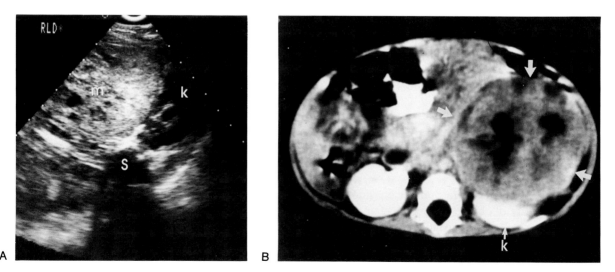

Fig. 12-53. Neuroblastoma, large and heterogeneous. **(A)** Transverse scan in the right lateral decubitus position demonstrating a large heterogeneous mass *(m)* anterior to the left kidney *(k)*. (*S*, spine.) **(B)** Similarly, the mass (arrows) is seen on an enhanced CT scan; it contains multiple low-density areas. (*k*, kidney.)

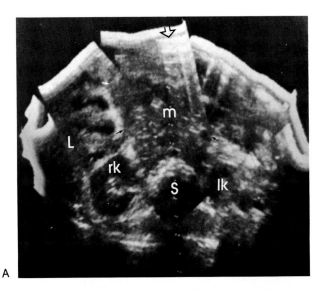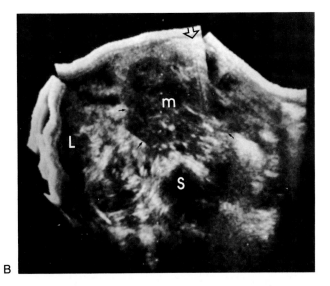

A   B

Fig. 12-54. Neuroblastoma. Transverse static scans at **(A)** 4 cm and **(B)** 3 cm above the umbilicus. A solid mass *(m)* is seen in the midline. It is difficult to define its borders (small arrows) especially on the left but it does extend to the left and right. Bowel gas anterior to the mass causes a reflective pattern (open arrow). (*L*, liver; *rk*, right kidney; *lk*, left kidney; *S*, spine). *(Figure continues.)*

may have well-defined margins, it also may adhere to adjacent structures, leading to involvement of those structures.[67]

The differential diagnosis of such a retroperitoneal mass in a child includes benign and malignant mesenchymal tumors; tumors of neurogenic origin such as schwannoma, neuroblastoma, and pheochromocytoma; Wilms' tumor; lymphoma; and metastases from testicular neoplasm.[67] When a large, solid, upper abdominal mass is identified within an infant or young child, the differential diagnosis should include neuroblastoma, Wilms' tumor, and hepatoblastoma.[72] Visualization of an intracaval mass makes Wilms' tumor or a primary liver tumor much more likely than neuroblastoma.[72] With Wilms' tumor, there is a relatively uniform echopattern, except where there are areas of hemorrhage, caliceal dilatation, or enlarged vascular spaces. Ultrasound is limited in the delineation of the extent of tumor and in monitoring the response to therapy. It has limited value in detecting metastatic disease to retroperitoneal and retrocrural lymph nodes. Additionally, it cannot detect extradural extension of tumor into the vertebral canal.

Despite its limitations, ultrasound is considered the screening modality of choice for neonatal or pediatric abdominal masses.[64] It can usually distinguish cystic from solid masses and determine whether a lesion is intra- or extrarenal. However, CT is the method of choice for evaluation of known neuroblastoma since it is able to detect calcification within the tumor as well as demonstrate local extension, lymph node involvement, and nonskeletal metastases.[64] It is essential for the con-

firmation, localization, and staging of neuroblastoma whether the tumor is abdominal, pelvic, thoracic, cervical, or intracranial.[64] Since total resolution of abdominal disease cannot always be accurately diagnosed by ultrasound, CT is recommended to further evaluate children in whom abdominal disease is thought to have resolved, since heavily calcified, residual neuroblastoma may be mistaken for bowel gas on ultrasound.[69]

Metastatic Tumor. Delineation of small adrenal masses in the normal adrenal gland presents a great challenge to the sonologist. Small and moderately sized (4 to 5 cm) masses characteristically are anteromedial to the upper pole of the kidney (Figs. 12-29, 12-31, and 12-57). They may indent the posterior wall of the IVC[2,73] (Fig. 12-31). The kidneys are displaced inferiorly by larger adrenal masses. Adrenal tumors are usually round or oval; the large ones are usually irregular. The tumors are usually somewhat hypoechoic[74-76] (Fig. 12-57). There may be strong areas of echoes with necrosis and hemorrhage.[2]

The adrenal glands are the fourth most common site in the body for metastases, after the lungs, the liver, and the bones.[75] Most commonly metastases to the adrenal are from squamous cell carcinoma of the lung (33 percent), with 30 percent from breast carcinoma and the remainder from melanoma, gastric carcinoma, and tumors of the colon, pancreas, kidney, and thyroid.[77] Up to 33 percent of patients with bronchogenic carcinoma of the lung have adrenal metastases.[76]

It is very rare for adrenal involvement to be the only manifestation of lymphoma.[45,78] Lymphomatous in-

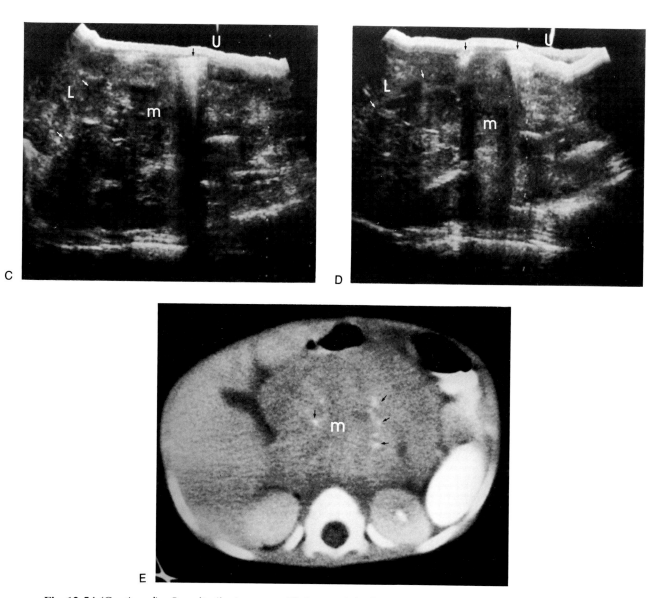

Fig. 12-54 *(Continued).* Longitudinal scans at **(C)** 1 cm to left of midline and **(D)** midline also demonstrate a solid mass *(m)* with poorly defined margins (white arrows). Bowel gas anterior to the mass causes a reflective pattern (black arrows). (*U*, level of the umbilicus; *L*, liver.) **(E)** Enhanced CT scan demonstrates the large mass *(m)* that extends to either side of midline. It does have internal calcification (arrows). The prevertebral vessels cannot be identified.

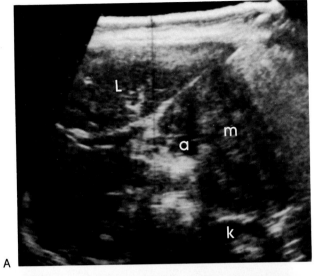

A

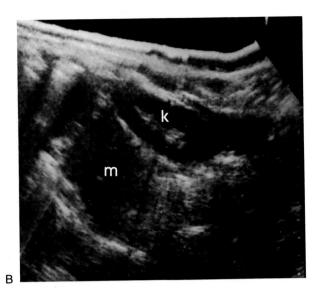

B

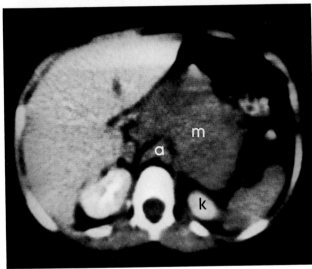

C

Fig. 12-55. Adrenal ganglioneuroma. **(A)** Transverse supine scan 13 cm above the umbilicus. A solid mass *(m)* is seen anterior, lateral, and posterior to the aorta *(a)*. It is separate from the posteriorly displaced left kidney *(k)*. (*L,* liver.) **(B)** Prone sagittal scan clearly demonstrating the solid mass *(m)* anterior to and separate from the left kidney *(k)*. **(C)** CT scan, enhanced. A soft tissue-density mass *(m)* is seen anterior to the left kidney *(k)* with a very similar appearance to Fig. A. (*a,* aorta.)

volvement of the adrenal is more common with non-Hodgkin's lymphoma than with Hodgkin's disease.[45] Although involvement at autopsy occurs 24 to 25 percent of the time, the adrenal glands are only diagnosed to be involved approximately 4 percent of the time in diffuse, non-Hodgkin's lymphoma.[75,78] As a rule, at the time of presentation there is evidence of disease elsewhere or at a site of tumor recurrence following therapy. Involvement of the adrenal is often bilateral (> 50 percent).[45,78] As such, lymphoma should be a major consideration when a hypoechoic solid mass is identified in the adrenal gland[74] (Fig. 12-58). Adrenal involvement with lymphoma may appear to have a very large cystic component containing several septations. The differential diagnosis for such a lesion would have to include adrenal carcinoma, necrotic metastasis, abscess, hemorrhage, and pheochromocytoma.[78]

Correlative Imaging

How do CT and ultrasound compare in imaging of the adrenal gland? Most institutions use CT when the primary question is whether there is an adrenal mass. CT can detect normal adrenal glands in most patients. In addition, it can detect slight or subtle enlargement. It is reported to have a sensitivity of 82 to 84 percent, a specificity of 95 to 98 percent, and an accuracy of 90 to 91 percent in the evaluation of the adrenal.[14,79,80] By contrast, with ultrasound it is much more difficult to identify the normal gland on a consistent basis. In the same studies, ultrasound had a sensitivity of 79 to 90 percent, a specificity of 61 to 97 percent, and an accuracy of 70 to 95 percent.[79]

Ultrasound does have a use in adrenal imaging. It is the modality of choice for evaluation of the neonatal

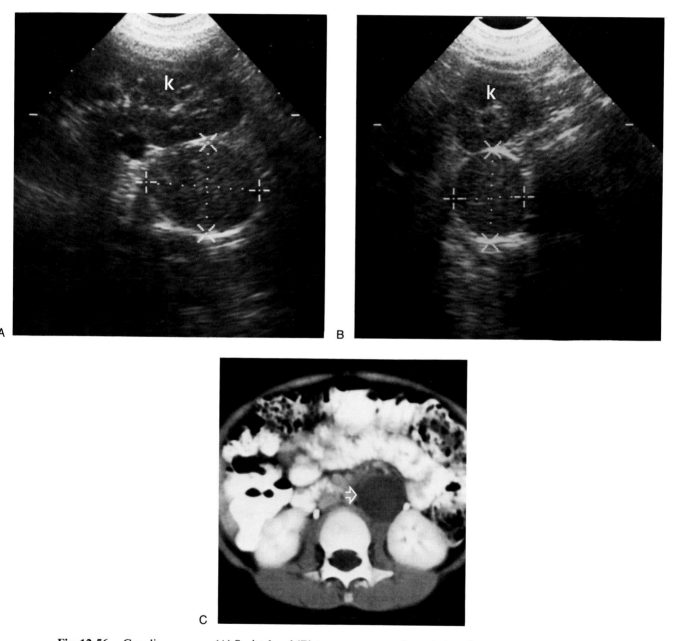

Fig. 12-56. Ganglioneuroma. **(A)** Sagittal and **(B)** transverse scans through the left kidney *(k)* demonstrating a homogeneous echogenic well-defined extrarenal mass (calipers, 25 × 32 × 39 mm). **(C)** CT scan demonstrating a low-density mass (arrow).

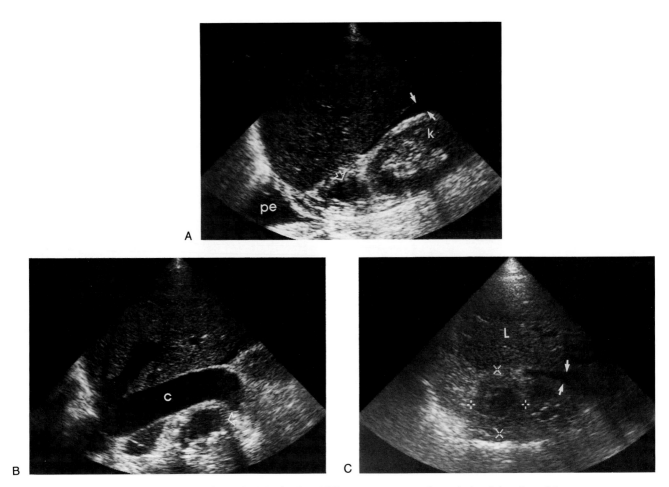

Fig. 12-57. Adrenal metastasis. **(A & B)** Sagittal and **(C)** transverse scans through the right adrenal demonstrating a relatively hypoechoic mass (open arrow, Figs. A & B; calipers, Fig. C; 40 × 35 mm) representing a metastatic lesion. (*pe*, pleural effusion; *k*, right kidney; arrows, ascitic fluid; *c*, inferior vena cava; *L*, liver.)

adrenal as well as that of the cachectic patient. At times it is difficult to define the adrenal as the origin of a mass on CT. By using sagittal scans, various body positions, and the retroperitoneal fat sign, ultrasound can often definitely identify the adrenal as the source of the mass.

General Retroperitoneum

Abscess

Abscesses remain a problem in clinical practice despite advances in antibiotic therapy and surgical technique. They present with increasing frequency in our enlarging population of patients who are immunocompromised by steroids or chemotherapy, in renal transplant patients, in leukemia patients, and in alcoholics.[81] Conventional radiography has inherent limitations in the delineation of retroperitoneal abscesses, which can

explain the increased morbidity and mortality (100 percent if untreated) associated with these lesions as compared with the morbidity and mortality associated with intraperitoneal abscesses.[82] Early diagnosis is crucial because surgical treatment prior to development of septicemia offers the greatest benefit.[82]

Retroperitoneal abscesses are usually secondary to infection (appendicitis, pyelonephritis, perinephric abscesses, bacterial spondylitis), trauma, bowel perforation, surgery, or cancer in adjacent retroperitoneal or intraperitoneal structures.[83,84] The most common abscesses in the anterior pararenal space are enteric in origin and result from pancreatitis, diverticulitis, or ulcer perforation. The abscesses in the perirenal space often occur postoperatively.[85] Perirenal abscesses have more irregular walls, are lobular in contour, and contain internal echoes. They often extend along the fascial plane to assume an elongated shape. They are commonly found

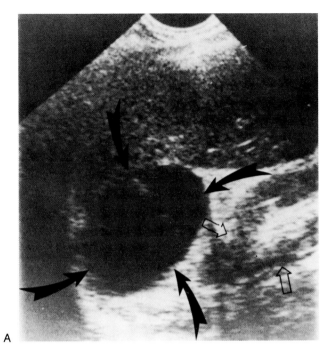
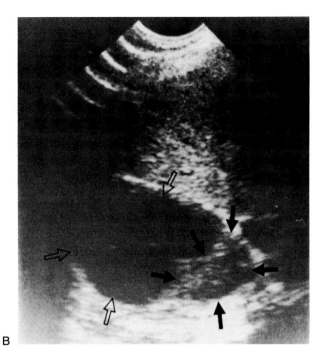

Fig. 12-58. Primary adrenal lymphoma. **(A)** Longitudinal ultrasonic scan of the right upper quadrant showing a large (8 × 10 cm) cystic adrenal mass (curved black arrows) with septations and solid components that was clearly demarcated from the liver and right kidney (open arrows). **(B)** Transverse ultrasonic scan again showing a large cystic component (open arrows) with a solid component (straight black arrows) in the medial aspect of the right adrenal mass. (From Vicks et al,[78] with permission.)

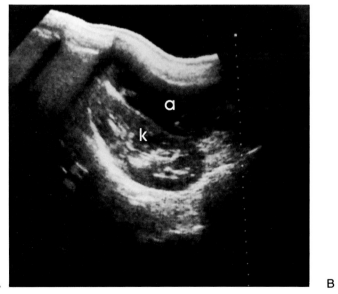
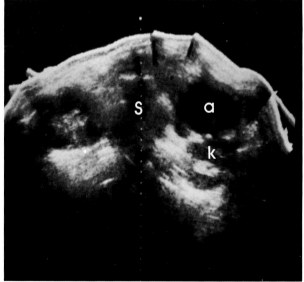

Fig. 12-59. Retroperitoneal abscess. **(A)** Prone sagittal scan. A poorly defined hypoechoic mass *(a)* is seen posterior to the right kidney *(k)*. **(B)** Prone transverse scan. The hypoechoic mass (*a*, abscess) is seen posterior to the right kidney *(k)*, displacing it anteriorly. The patient had a history of urinary tract infection, and the abscess was in the posterior pararenal space. (*S*, spine.)

in the psoas, as the abscess extends along the belly of the muscle.[85]

Iliopsoas abscesses have changed over the years relative to the pathogen. In most young patients, an iliopsoas abscess is primary, with the most frequently cultured organism being *Staphylococcus aureus*.[86] The majority in adults are secondary to inflammatory disease in the adjacent structures including the vertebrae, pancreas, kidney, and intestine; there is a lower incidence of primary abscess in adults. The most common presenting symptoms include pain in the flank, pelvis, or thigh; fever; and a limp or flexion deformity of the involved hip.[82,86] All patients present with fever, and 50 percent have a palpable flank mass or swelling.[82]

Retroperitoneal inflammatory disease is often elusive to detection by clinical and radiographic methods.[84] In one study, 90 percent of patients had radiographic signs of abnormality but the diagnosis was not made until postmortem in 25 to 30 percent of cases.[82] Almost half (40 to 50 percent) of patients with a retroperitoneal abscess die of the disease.[84] Ultrasound provides direct visualization of the abnormal retroperitoneal fluid collection. Although this modality cannot differentiate the different retroperitoneal fluid collections by echopattern alone, it can localize the lesion for percutaneous aspiration, which will lead to a definitive diagnosis.[82] Ultrasound can define the limits of the mass, identify displacement of adjacent organs, and demonstrate acoustic enhancement, confirming that the mass is indeed fluid-filled.[84] The fluid content of the space-occupying abscess allows it to assume a volumetrically economical shape, usually spherical or ellipsoid.[81] Its shape depends on its location. The fluid collection varies from uniformly echofree to mildly echogenic to highly echogenic[81] (Figs.

12-59 to 12-63). The mass may even have septation. The walls are usually convex and well defined but irregular.

The indications for percutaneous drainage of a retroperitoneal abscess include the identification of an abscess on ultrasound or CT and confirmation of the diagnosis by percutaneous aspiration. The contraindications are few; they include anticoagulant therapy and hematologic disorders that cause bleeding diatheses.[85] The catheter drainage may be accomplished by the modified Seldinger technique, which is similar to angiography. The patient's fever usually subsides within 24 to 48 hours following drainage, with the white blood cell count returning to normal within a week. If the patient's condition does not improve within 48 to 72 hours after drainage is begun and with appropriate antibiotics, a scan should be obtained to ascertain the location of the catheter and to evaluate the presence of undrained fluid. The catheter is usually removed 1 to 2 days after drainage stops (usually 10 to 14 days following the drainage procedure). If *S. aureus* is the organism of origin, the process is assumed to be primary and the purulent drainage will cease after 2 to 3 days with proper antibiotics.[86] Often a minimum of only 7 days of catheter drainage is sufficient; shorter drainage times may be used in the future. Before the catheter is withdrawn, the area is scanned to ensure that resolution is complete.[85]

Hemorrhage

In the child, a retroperitoneal hematoma is usually secondary to trauma or hemophilia. Of the bleeding episodes in hemophiliac patients, 80 percent occur within the musculoskeletal system. Hemorrhage into the hip

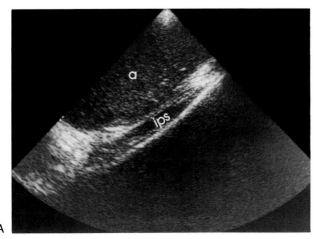

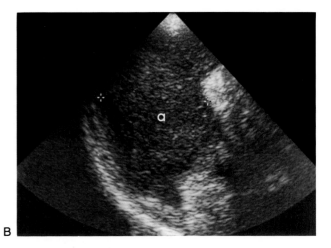

A   B

Fig. 12-60. Retroperitoneal abscess. **(A)** Sagittal and **(B)** transverse views of the right lower quadrant showing a large (25 × 38 mm) echogenic mass *(a)* anterior to the iliopsoas muscle *(ips)*. This patient had had an inguinal hernia repair in the distant past.

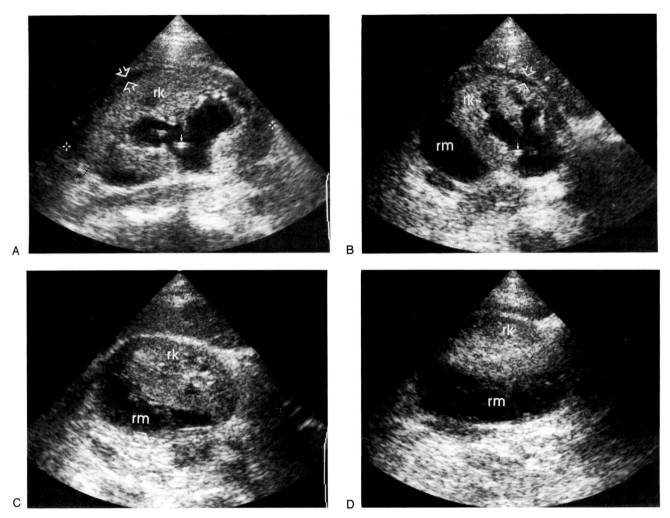

Fig. 12-61. Hematoma and/or abscess. Patient with bilateral percutaneous nephrostomies, decreased hematocrit, and fever. (**A**) Sagittal and (**B–D**) successive transverse views of the right kidney *(rk)* demonstrating hydronephrosis with a catheter (arrow) within the dilated collecting system. Perirenal fluid (open arrows) is seen, as well as a loculated fluid collection *(rm)* posterior to the kidney. By ultrasound alone, all these fluid collections could represent blood and/or infection.

joint, the rectus femoral muscle, the iliopsoas muscle, or even the anterior abdominal wall is considered in the differential diagnosis when a patient presents with hip flexion contracture (secondary to muscle spasm) and a positive iliopsoas sign.[87] The patient may present with flank pain and/or stiffness referred to the leg, hip, or groin. Although such bleeding may be clinically apparent, the exact location sometimes is difficult to establish, particularly when there is involvement of the retroperitoneal space, pelvic structures, muscle bundles, bowel loops, or mesentery.[88] Important in the management of these patients is the localization of the hemorrhage. Prolonged systemic treatment is not required in hemarthrosis in which the hemorrhage is self-limiting.

Early diagnosis of a psoas hematoma is extremely important in hemophilia because prompt therapy with plasma concentrate and appropriate plasma factor is highly effective in preventing femoral nerve entrapment and resulting nerve deficit.[83,89] Ultrasound can provide valuable information regarding the site of the hematoma in the hemophiliac patient. The examination of such patients should include evaluation of the iliopsoas muscle, retroperitoneal space, iliac fossa, anterior abdominal wall, hip joint, and thigh musculature and osseous components.[87] A small hematoma in a large muscle generally is resorbed without complication. A similar hematoma in a tight fascial compartment may cause significant ischemic myopathy and neuropathy.[88]

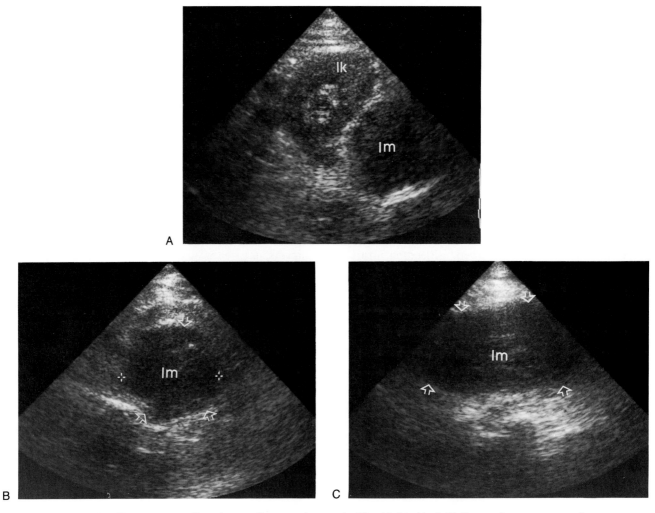

Fig. 12-62. Hematoma and/or abscess. Same patient as in Fig. 12-61. **(A & B)** Successive transverse views through the flank and left kidney *(lk)* with Fig. A higher than Fig. B. A lucent mass *(lm)* is seen in the area of the psoas muscle. **(C)** Sagittal view of the psoas mass *(lm)* demonstrating enlargement of the muscle with a decrease in the normal echopattern. By ultrasound alone, these findings involving the psoas could represent hematoma, but infection could not be excluded.

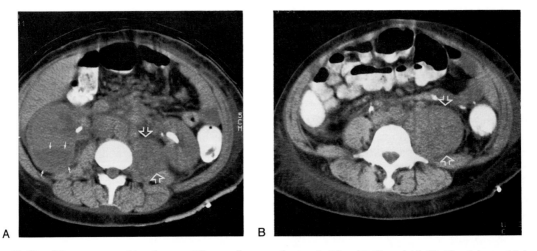

Fig. 12-63. Hematoma and/or abscess, CT scan. Same patient as in Figs. 12-61 and 12-62. Fig. A is at a higher level than Fig. B. The perirenal fluid (single arrow) is seen in Fig. A on the right along with the loculated fluid (small arrows) posterior to the kidney. The left psoas mass is seen on both scans as an enlarged psoas muscle (open arrows).

804

Ultrasound can be used to evaluate patients with hematomas.[87] Both the anatomic location of the hemorrhage and the ultrasound examination provide information about the nature of the hematoma.[87] When a focal anechoic or hypoechoic area with relative posterior acoustic enhancement is seen, an intramuscular hematoma should be considered[87] (Figs. 12-62 and 12-64). Other signs of loculations include displacement of muscular fibers and fascial planes. If a muscle is increased in thickness with a differing echopattern from the contralateral muscle, the hemorrhage is described as diffuse (interstitial); the internal striations representing muscle fibers and fasciculi are preserved.[87] Bleeding into the psoas causes it to enlarge and become more rounded.[83,89] The hematoma within the muscle is inseparable from the muscle (Figs. 12-62 and 12-64). It is important to differentiate between the two types of intramuscular hemorrhage since a loculated hematoma may be aspirated to relieve severe pain caused by compression of adjacent tissues and nerves.[87] Acutely after development, the hemorrhage may appear anechoic.[83,89] A hematoma cannot be distinguished from an abscess by ultrasound alone.

In the adult, a retroperitoneal hematoma may be secondary to trauma, bleeding diastheses, or a leaking aortic aneurysm (Figs. 12-62 to 12-64). A neoplasm may also rupture and bleed. The hematoma may be well localized or poorly defined as an infiltrative process. If the hemorrhage is recent in onset, it is typically anechoic. As clotting occurs, the pattern may change to complex with cystic and solid components; the degree of complexity varies with the ratio of clot to liquid blood within the hematoma.[11]

Fibrosis

Retroperitoneal fibrosis represents dense fibrous tissue proliferation in the form of a plaquelike or bulky mass 2 to 6 cm thick and generally confined to the central and paravertebral regions.[90] It usually extends from the perirenal space between the hila of the kidneys to the dome of the bladder. It has a potential to envelop rather than displace hollow structures such as ureters and blood and lymphatic vessels. It is an uncommon but progressive and serious illness that is usually clinically silent until it causes ureteral or vascular obstruction.[90] Its progressive course often results in significant obstructive uropathy.

The etiology of this disease process is obscure. In 70 percent of cases, it is idiopathic. There is evidence that there may be a hypersensitivity reaction (in 12 percent) to methysergide, which may be a cause; regression of the disease is variable after removal of the drug from the patient's therapy.[5,91] Patients with primary or metastatic retroperitoneal neoplasm exhibit retroperitoneal fibrosis. The cancer, irrespective of its type and/or source, apparently stimulates a fibrotic type of reaction indistinguishable from that of idiopathic fibrosis.[91]

Clinically, these patients present with back, flank, or abdominal pain often accompanied by nonspecific complaints of weight loss, nausea and vomiting, and

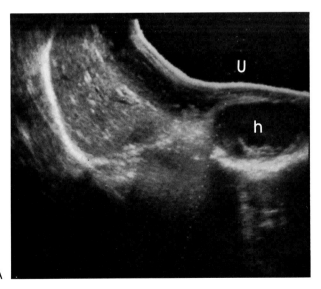

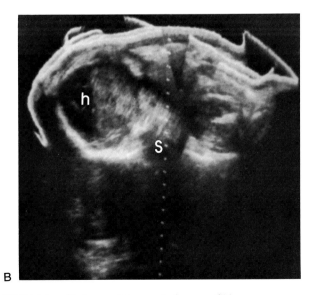

A   B

Fig. 12-64. Retroperitoneal hematoma in a hemophiliac. **(A)** Right sagittal scan. A hypoechoic mass *(h)* is seen in the area of the psoas/iliopsoas muscles. (*U*, level of the umbilicus.) **(B)** Transverse supine scan at 4 cm below the umbilicus. A hypoechoic mass *(h)* is seen in the area of the iliopsoas muscle. (*S*, spine.)

malaise.[90,91] There is a palpable abdominal or rectal mass in 30 percent of patients.[91] Hypertension and anuria are relatively common.[91] It has a peak incidence in the fifth to sixth decades with a male/female ratio of 2:1.[90,91] Clinical and radiographic features of retroperitoneal fibrosis are often varied and nonspecific.[91]

Excretory urography and retrograde studies are commonly used for the diagnosis. Bilateral or unilateral hydroureter associated with abdominal narrowing of the ureter or an encased appearance represents the diagnostic findings.[91] The combination of proximal hydroureter and medial deviation of the middle third of the ureter is thought to be almost pathognomonic.[91]

On ultrasound, this lesion is seen as either a large, bulky mass with ill-defined irregular margins or a flat, large mass with smooth margins located centrally and in the paravertebral region extending to the level of the sacral promontory and to the renal vessels.[90-93] A hypoechoic mass may be seen to surround the aorta and IVC; this may appear similar to lymphoma or metastatic disease.[5] It may be anechoic to hypoechoic[90-95] (Fig. 12-

65). The anterior margin appears to respect the peritoneal boundary and is clearly delineated, whereas the posterior margin is poorly defined and is not easily separated.[91,95] In one series, 87 percent of patients had associated hydronephrosis; this is often found to be the case.[90,93] It has a tendency to envelop but not displace structures such as the aorta, the IVC, and the ureters.[91,93,95] Its appearance is similar to that of retroperitoneal sarcoma, nodal metastases, lymphoma, and retroperitoneal hematoma.[91,93,95]

Lymphocele

Lymphoceles, which are lymph-filled spaces without a distinct epithelial lining, usually occur secondary to surgery. Their most common source is the pelvic lymphatics, although they may come from the para-aortic or renal hilar lymphatics.[96] There has been a report of a 3 percent incidence following pelvic lymphadenectomy for staging prostatic carcinoma.[97] They also occur fol-

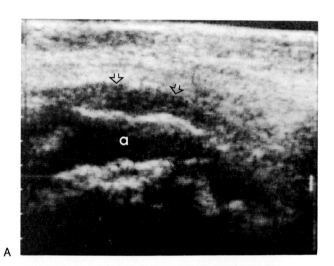

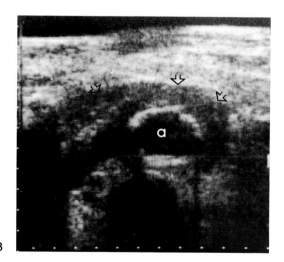

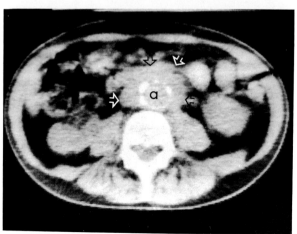

Fig. 12-65. Retroperitoneal fibrosis. **(A)** Transverse scan demonstrating a hypoechoic mass (arrows) encompassing the aorta *(a)* and the inferior vena cava. **(B)** Midline longitudinal scan. A hypoechoic mass (arrows) is seen anterior to the aorta *(a)*. **(C)** CT scan. The same mass (arrows) is seen surrounding the aorta *(a)*. (From Center et al,[93] with permission.)

lowing radical gynecologic procedures, extensive urologic operations, and renal transplants. A pelvic lymphocele represents an imbalance between inflow of lymph from the channels of the lower extremities, pelvic organs, and abdominal wall and outflow from the surgical bed into the central lymphatic structure.[97]

The characteristic pelvic location for this lesion is lateral to the bladder[97] (Figs. 12-25, 12-66, and 12-67). Although commonly located extraperitoneally in the pelvis, upper abdominal lymphoceles have been reported secondary to aortofemoral bypass, simple nephrolithotomies, and para-aortic/renal hilar node dissections. The anterior surface of the lymphocele may be within 3 cm of the anterior abdominal wall. The most common clinical presentation is a constellation of fullness and flank pain with or without pain extending into the pelvis and leg.[96]

Small (cross-sectional area less than 30 cm²) anechoic lymphoceles most probably undergo long-term spontaneous resolution. Those that are larger or more complex result in complications requiring surgical intervention. These lesions usually are ellipsoid with well-defined walls and never contain debris; they may be multilocular but are most often unilocular.[98] They are characterized by increased through transmission and no internal echoes, although thin septation has been seen (Figs. 12-66 and 12-67). Although ultrasound alone cannot differentiate lymphocele from hematoma, seroma, or abscess, a percutaneous aspiration may give a definitive diagnosis.[97] The fluid in lymphoceles is clear.

Lymphadenopathy

Lymph nodes are an important component of the widely dispersed lymphoreticuloendothelial system and are distributed throughout the body. These discrete structures are ovoid and measure 1 mm to between 1 and 2 cm in length. They are surrounded by a connective tissue capsule. They are rarely the site of primary disease but are secondarily involved in virtually all systemic infections and in many neoplastic disorders.[99]

Ultrasound evaluation of the nodes can help to differentiate between malignant and benign disease; specifically, evaluation of abdominal lymph nodes, echogenicity, shape, age of the patient, and a periaortic localization aid in differentiation between benign and malignant involvement. As for the architecture of the node, nodes associated with malignant disease are more hypoechoic than in benign disease.[100] Echogenicity is not an objective criterion because it depends not only on the tissue characteristics of the node itself, but also on the overlying structures, the transducer frequency, and the gain settings of the ultrasound equipment.[100] A sign of benignancy is the hilar fat sign, which represents a real anatomic structure. Lymph nodes associated with malignant diseases are in general larger and more numerous than in benign diseases.[100] Most involved with malignant disease tend to develop an ovoid or round shape, whereas in benign disease they tend to retain their original spindle shape[100] (Fig. 12-9).

Investigators have evaluated abnormal lymph nodes

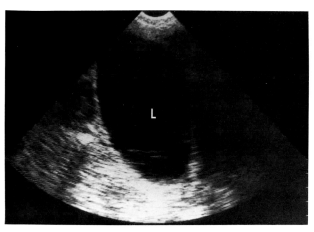

A

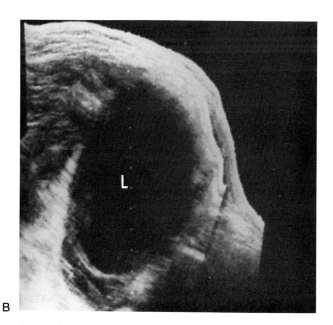

B

Fig. 12-66. Lymphocele. Postoperative prostatectomy patient with pelvic node dissection. An anechoic mass *(L)* is seen in the right pelvis on these **(A)** transverse and **(B)** transverse oblique scans.

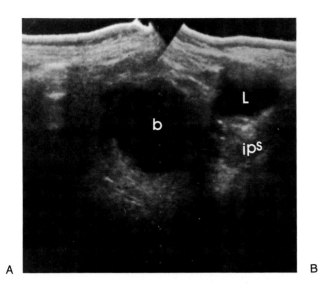
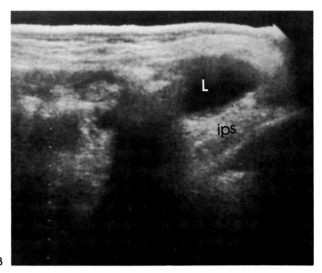

A   B

Fig. 12-67. Lymphocele. Postoperative ovarian carcinoma patient with node dissection. **(A)** Transverse supine scan at 8 cm above the symphysis. An anechoic mass *(L)* is seen to the left of the bladder *(b)* and anterior to the iliopsoas *(ips)* muscle. **(B)** Sagittal scan 6 cm to the left of midline. The anechoic lymphocele *(L)* is seen anterior to the iliopsoas *(ips)* muscle.

in vitro by ultrasound.[101] A central echogenic line has been found to be a valid diagnostic marker in 90 percent of cases; it is not found in any neoplastic lymph node.[101] The central echogenic line detected and previously described as the hilum is produced by numerous interfaces present in the internal part of the medulla, where the lymphatic sinuses converge at the hilum.[101] Small echogenic foci caused by calcium or amyloid deposits may be found in lymph nodes involved by metastases from medullary thyroid carcinoma, but the echogenic internal structure does not resemble the normal hilum.[101] Hypoechoic (liquefaction necrosis) or hyperechoic (fibrosis, coagulation necrosis) zones may be seen within both inflammatory and neoplastic lymph nodes (Figs. 12-9 to 12-11). In lymphoma, there is a characteristic micronodular configuration that corresponds perfectly to that seen on the cut surface. As such, the absence of the central echogenic line within nodes may be due to factors other than neoplastic disease, such as fatty replacement.[101] Therefore, roundness and absence of an echogenic hilum are considered signs of malignancy.

Others have investigated abdominal lymph nodes by ultrasound, evaluating nodes with regard to number, localization, dimensions, shape, and architecture.[100] Involvement with malignant metastatic disease often starts in the nearest group of lymph nodes adjacent to the involved organs. Surprisingly, a large number and variety of benign diseases are associated with detectable lymph nodes.[100] Many nodes are located in the epigastric and liver hilum in both malignant and benign diseases, whereas the periaortic and other retroperitoneal areas

are much more often involved in malignant disease[100] (Figs. 12-9 to 12-11 and 12-68).

A number of diseases are associated with lymphadenopathy; these include tuberculosis, sarcoidosis (Fig. 12-11), Crohn's disease, and inflammatory conditions (Figs. 12-9 and 12-10). Reactive hyperplasia of lymph nodes is also described with chronic liver disease and immune-mediated diseases such as celiac disease, mastocytosis, rheumatologic diseases, and acquired immunodeficiency syndrome (AIDS), and as an increased immunoresponse in intravenous drug abusers[100] (Figs. 12-9 and 12-10). As such, evaluation of enlarged retroperitoneal lymph nodes is important in the workup or follow-up of malignant neoplasm, lymphoma, metastatic disease, and certain inflammatory conditions.[5] The most important are the aortic and common iliac nodes (Fig. 12-68). Others detected by ultrasound include celiac, external and internal iliac, peripancreatic, perirenal, and pancreaticocaval nodes[5] (Figs. 12-10, 12-11, and 12-68).

If the appropriate technique is employed and the examination is performed thoroughly, the accuracy of the examination can be quite high.[5] With a decubitus coronal scan, a lymph node as small as 0.3 to 0.5 cm can be delineated[5] (Fig. 12-9). One series reported an accuracy as high as 90 percent in detecting para-aortic nodes compared with CT.[5]

Within the pelvis, iliac nodes are best visualized on a transverse scan with the patient supine.[5] The iliac artery is located anterior to the vein; both vessels are located medial or anteriomedial to the psoas muscle.[5] Iliac nodes

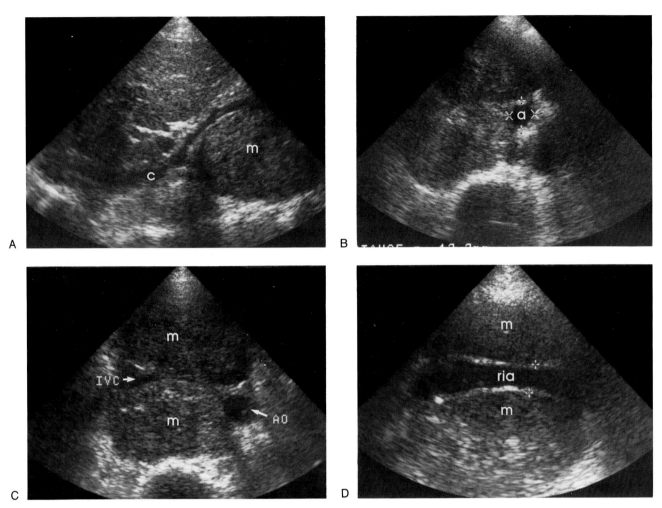

Fig. 12-68. Metastatic lymphadenopathy. **(A)** Sagittal and **(B & C)** transverse scans through the upper abdomen showing a large nodal mass *(m)* which displaces the inferior vena cava *(c)* anteriorly. There is a large mass of nodes *(m,* calipers) encasing the aorta *(a, AO)* and inferior vena cava *(IVC)* in Figs. B & C. The inferior vena caval lumen cannot be seen in Fig. B. **(D)** Sagittal view of the right iliac artery *(ria)* showing nodes *(m)* surrounding the vessel.

are usually located anteromedial or medial to the iliac vessels (Fig. 12-68). Large ones may indent a distended bladder, and those posterior to the iliac vessels may displace the latter anteriorly.[5]

Lymphoma. Lymphoma is the most common primary retroperitoneal tumor excluding those arising from the kidney, adrenals, and pancreas. It most commonly arises from the para-aortic and/or iliac nodes.[5] Malignant lymphomas are classified as Hodgkin's or non-Hodgkin's. Forty percent of newly diagnosed lymphomas are Hodgkin's disease, with the remainder being non-Hodgkin's lymphoma (nodular or diffuse). Effective therapeutic management with both radiation and chemotherapy in these patients requires not only accurate histologic classification but also reliable definition of the anatomic regions involved.[102-104]

Classically, the modality of lymphangiography has been proven to be accurate in the diagnosis of para-aortic and paracaval adenopathy, but fails to detect disease in other sites such as mesenteric, perisplenic, and perihepatic, as well as those in extranodal sites such as the liver and spleen. Ultrasound can detect retroperitoneal disease and provide additional information about the extent of abdominal involvement.[103,104] It is reported to be 80 to 90 percent accurate in detecting retroperitoneal nodal lymphoma.[102]

To evaluate for abdominal lymphoma or to determine the presence or absence of lymphadenopathy, the abdomen and pelvis must be scanned carefully.[105] Both the hepatic and splenic hila should be checked, and the liver, spleen, and kidneys should be scrutinized for changes in echopattern. There should be a search for nodes in the abdomen, at the origin of the celiac and the superior

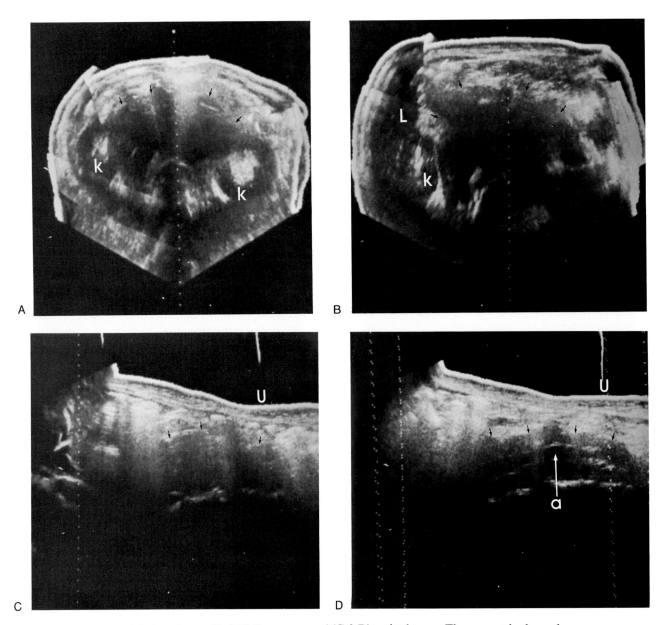

Fig. 12-69. Hodgkin's lymphoma. **(A & B)** Transverse and **(C & D)** sagittal scans. The prevertebral vessels are not well seen, and a mass effect (arrows) is seen. The aorta *(a)* lumen is encompassed by a mass (arrows) in Fig. D. (*k*, kidney; *L*, liver; *U*, level of the umbilicus.) *(Figure continues).*

mesenteric arteries, and in the para-aortic and renal hilar areas. The pelvis should be scanned with careful attention to the iliac areas.

Para-aortic Lymphadenopathy. There is involvement of the para-aortic nodes in 25 percent of Hodgkin's patients and 40 percent of non-Hodgkin's patients. More than 12 percent of patients with Hodgkin's disease demonstrate normal lymphangiograms with celiac, perisplenic, or mesenteric nodes. More than 40 percent of

patients with non-Hodgkin's lymphoma with normal lymphangiograms have mesenteric disease. The accuracy of ultrasound in the detection of retroperitoneal nodes has been reported to be 80 to 90 percent.[103,104,106] The detected nodal size is correct in 98.2 percent of cases, with nodes larger than 2 cm detected.[106] Bowel gas can obscure retroperitoneal structures, and mesenteric and retroperitoneal fat can degrade the ultrasound resolution, but there is a relatively high degree of accuracy in detection of nodes and extranodal disease, which sug-

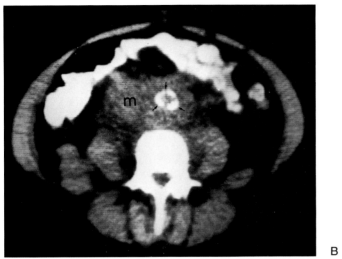

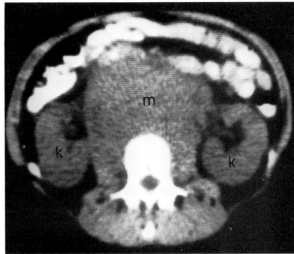

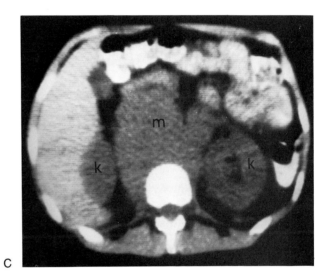

Fig. 12-69 *(Continued).* **(E–G)** CT scans. The aorta and inferior vena cava are not seen in Figs. F & G. In Fig. E, the aorta can be identified by the calcification (arrows) within the mass *(m)* surrounding it. The mass is much better defined on CT. (*k*, kidney.)

gests that ultrasound has a useful role in the initial staging process.[103,104]

The ultrasound appearance of lymphomatous nodes varies from hypoechoic to anechoic with very good sound transmission[103,104,107–109] (Figs. 12-69 and 12-70). Lymphomatous masses may be relatively echofree because of their homogeneous structure, which does not have sufficient interfaces to produce echoes.[107] At times the crus may be confused with nodes. Adenopathy secondary to nonlymphomatous disease or inflammatory process such as retroperitoneal fibrosis is indistinguishable (Fig. 12-9, 12-10, and 12-65). There is no correlation between the ultrasound appearance of the nodes and the histologic classification of the lymphoma. However, the largest para-aortic nodes usually result from non-Hodgkin's lymphoma[103,104] (Figs. 12-69 and 12-70).

Various ultrasound patterns of malignant lymphoma have been described, including (1) a mantlelike plaque of tumor seated on the vertebral body, especially in the para-aortic and paravertebral region (Fig. 12-69); (2) a conglomerated mass of tumor from mesenteric nodes surrounded by gastrointestinal gas; (3) organ compression or displacement by a mass of abdominal nodes; (4) compression or obscuration of the outlines of the aorta or IVC (Fig. 12-69 and 12-70); and (5) hypoechoic to anechoic images on ultrasound scans[107–111] (Figs. 12-69 and 12-70). Care should be taken to differentiate lymphadenopathy from collateral channels produced by portal and systemic venous systems, as both may have a lucent appearance.[112] Real-time or Doppler systems might help if pulsation is present. When portal hypertension and retroperitoneal masses are present, the possibility of varices should be considered.

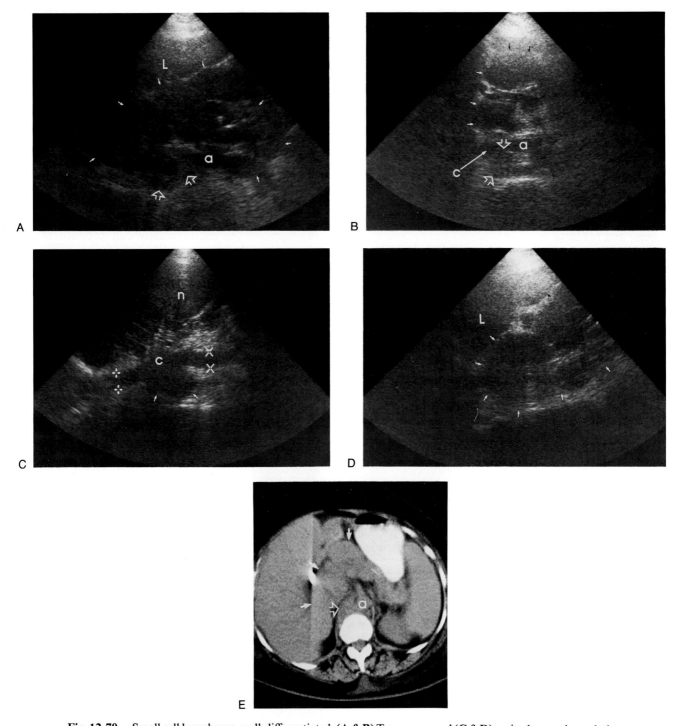

Fig. 12-70. Small cell lymphoma, well-differentiated. **(A & B)** Transverse and **(C & D)** sagittal scans through the upper abdomen in a large patient. A large, poorly defined mass (arrows) is seen anterior to the aorta *(a)*. Additionally, there is a mass (open arrows) posterior to the inferior vena cava *(c)* seen in Figs. A & B as well as in the sagittal view (Fig. C, arrows). In Figs. C & D the nodal mass *(n)* could not be separated well from the liver *(L)*. **(E)** CT scan showing the large mass of nodes (arrows) anterior to the aorta *(a)*. The retrocrural nodes (open arrow) are also seen. The crus was not identified on ultrasound (Figs. A & B).

Peripancreatic Lymphadenopathy. Enlarged nodes may appear as well-defined hypoechoic ovoid or rounded masses in the retropancreatic location or may surround and silhouette the region of the pancreatic head and body[113] (Figs. 12-69 and 12-70). It may be difficult to differentiate peripancreatic nodes from pancreatic masses.[5] Peripancreatic nodes represent paraduodenal, anterior paracaval, and superior mesenteric vessel nodes. These nodes, located within Gerota's fascia, may invade the kidney.[5] These nodes are infrequently opacified on contrast lymphangiogram scans.

Two major ultrasound patterns of peripancreatic lymphadenopathy have been described: (1) well-defined rounded or ovoid masses lateral and posterior to the pancreas but anterior to the level of the IVC, left renal vein, and aorta and easily distinguished from the pancreas; and (2) large confluent masses inseparable from and engulfing the pancreatic head[113] (Figs. 12-69 and 12-70). These lesions lie posterior to the splenic vein and the confluence of the splenic and portal veins.

Mesenteric Lymphadenopathy. The demonstration of mesenteric nodal involvement merits considerable attention because of the revision in therapy and prognosis

that follows. There is mesenteric adenopathy in more than 50 percent of patients with non-Hodgkin's lymphoma and in less than 4 percent of those with Hodgkin's lymphoma. The pattern of the adenopathy resembles retroperitoneal nodes; however, there is usually no "silhouette" sign involving the aorta and IVC.[103] Instead, the characteristic appearance is the presence of a lobulated confluent mass infiltrating the mesenteric leaves and encasing the superior mesenteric artery and vein, producing a "sandwich" appearance.[114]

Burkitt's Lymphoma. Burkitt's lymphoma is a clinically and histologically distinct tumor first described in African children.[115] It arises from the B lymphocytes and has a rapid doubling time but responds dramatically to combination chemotherapy.[115] Although it is potentially curable, the chemotherapy can produce rapid tumor lysis with subsequent life-threatening metabolic abnormalities, especially in a patient with a large tumor or compromised renal function.

The incidence of abdominal involvement in Burkitt's lymphoma is 69 percent. The abdominal masses tend to be large, solitary, and acoustically homogeneous. Most are found in the pelvis and upper abdomen as well as in

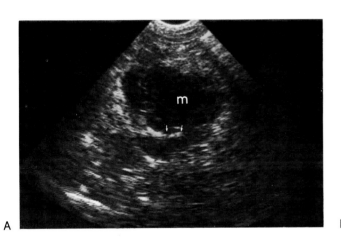

A

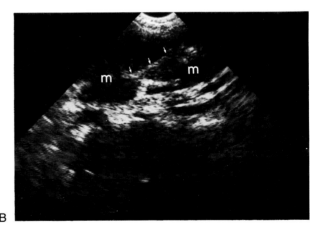

B

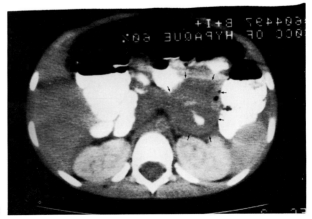

C

Fig. 12-71. Burkitt's lymphoma. **(A)** Transverse real-time scan. A large hypoechoic mass *(m)* is seen with a target pattern on the left. The echodense area (arrows) represents involved bowel lumen. **(B)** Sagittal scan through the hypoechoic mass *(m).* The bowel lumen (arrows) is within the mass. **(C)** CT scan demonstrating a soft-tissue mass (arrows) on the left involving bowel.

the retroperitoneum.[116] There is a high incidence of ileocecal, mesenteric, or ovarian involvement.[116] The terminal ileum is the most common site of gastrointestinal involvement.[115] These patients usually do not have the typical mantle of enlarged nodes seen in other types of lymphoma. The absence of lymph node disease and the presence of a bulky homogeneous extranodal tumor are characteristic ultrasound findings.[116]

The tumor bulk is the major prognostic factor in identifying patients likely to have metabolic complications resulting from chemotherapy. Because of the poor prognosis associated with large abdominal masses, surgical debulking is usually performed prior to chemotherapy. Ultrasound can be used to demonstrate the size and location of the tumor and the relationship between the tumor and normal organs. The tumor pattern varies from lucent to hyperechoic[107,115] (Fig. 12-71). In 76 percent of cases, the tumor is well defined, sharply marginated, and homogeneous. In 13 percent, there is ascites.[116]

Once Burkitt's lymphoma is suspected on the basis of the ultrasound scan, the kidneys should be assessed, as

there is a 5 percent incidence of direct renal involvement with this disease.[115,116] If there is abnormal renal function, an increased risk of metabolic complications with chemotherapy exists. Hydronephrosis is a recognized complication of nodal masses. There also may be tumor infiltration, poorly defined anechoic masses, or enlarged kidneys as a result of diffuse infiltration. If there is decreased renal function and a normal ultrasound appearance, uric acid nephropathy may be considered.[116]

Metastatic Lymphadenopathy. Metastatic disease can occur by lymphatic or hematogenous spread. It may be secondary to carcinoma of the breast, lung, or testis. There is often primary recurrence from previously resected urologic or gynecologic tumors.[11] Although the echopattern of these nodes, which are enlarged secondary to metastatic disease, may be varied, they are less commonly hypoechoic with metastatic disease than with lymphoma (Figs. 12-68 and 12-72 to 12-75). In one study it was found that 83 percent of lymphomatous nodes and only 53 percent of those secondary to soft

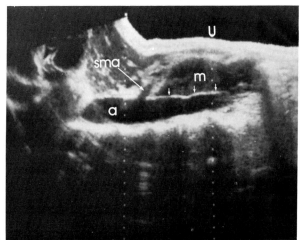

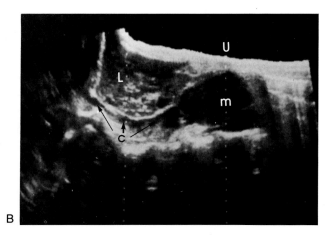

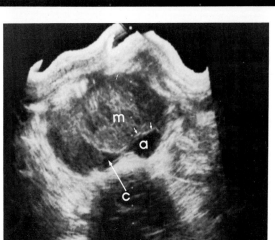

Fig. 12-72. Metastatic disease. Patient with known prostatic carcinoma and a pulsatile mass. Sagittal scans **(A)** in the midline and **(B)** 1 cm to the right of midline, as well as **(C)** a transverse scan 8 cm below the xyphoid, demonstrate an extra-aortic mass *(m)*. The outer wall (arrows) of the aorta *(a)* is the densest outline, and the mass is external to this wall, making it extra- or para-aortic. In addition, compression of the inferior vena cava *(c)* is seen in Figs. B & C. Percutaneous biopsy proved this to be prostatic carcinoma. (*L*, left lobe of the liver; *U*, level of the umbilicus; *sma,* superior mesenteric artery.)

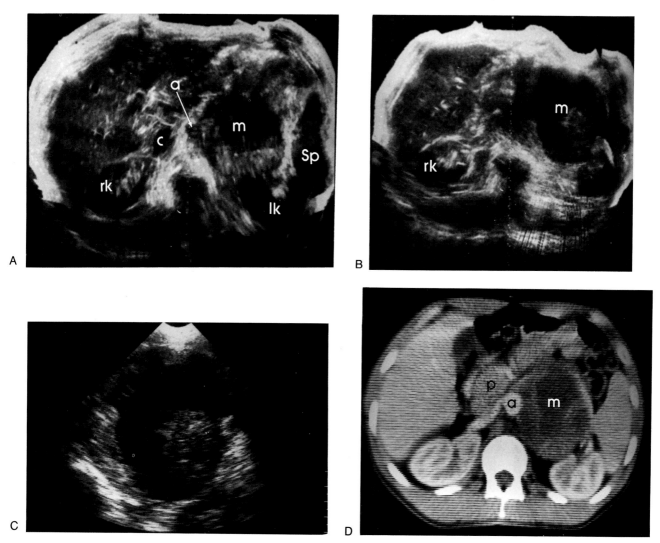

Fig. 12-73. Metastatic disease. Embryonal cell carcinoma. Transverse static scans at **(A)** 13 cm and **(B)** 10 cm above the umbilicus. A large mass *(m)* of mixed echodensity is seen. The left kidney *(lk)* appears displaced posteriorly and to the right. (*rk*, right kidney; *Sp*, spleen; *c*, inferior vena cava; *a*, aorta.) **(C)** Transverse scan of the mass. The mass appears to have a dense center and a hypoechoic periphery. **(D)** Enhanced CT scan. The mass *(m)* with a mixed density is seen lateral to the aorta *(a)*. It appears separate from the pancreas *(p)*.

tissue tumors were anechoic.[117] If ascites is found, invasion of the peritoneal surface is indicated.

Acquired Immunodeficiency Syndrome. Patients with abdominal lymphoma related to AIDS have been evaluated.[118] Both non-Hodgkin's lymphoma and Hodgkin's lymphoma have been reported associated with AIDS. These diseases manifest aggressive and atypical features in patients with AIDS, who frequently have advanced (stage 3 or 4) disease with extranodal involvement at the time of clinical presentation.[118] There is commonly extensive abdominal (retroperitoneal and mesenteric) adenopathy and parenchymal organ involvement.[118]

There is a dramatically greater frequency of non-Hodgkin's lymphoma in patients with AIDS than in the general population.[118] The incidence of the development of this disorder is 1,000 times higher than expected in human immunodeficiency virus (HIV)-positive males with persistent adenopathy.[118] In these patients, both non-Hodgkin's lymphoma and Hodgkin's lymphoma exhibit aggressive features. The lymphomas associated with AIDS have a higher histologic grade and are widespread. There is commonly involvement of the nervous system, bone marrow, and abdominal disease.[118]

Focal masses may be detected with ultrasound in 87 percent of these patients.[118] The liver is the most fre-

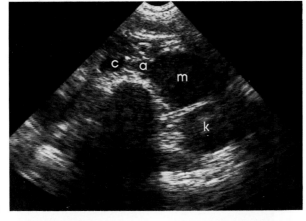

A

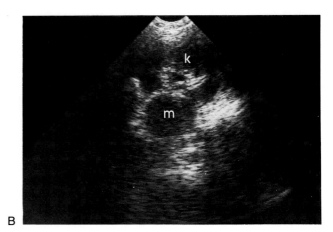

B

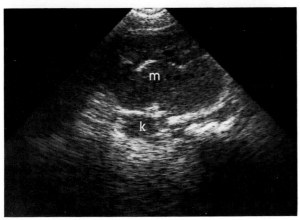

C

Fig. 12-74. Metastatic disease. Embryonal cell carcinoma. Twelve-year-old boy with weight loss, fever, and hematuria. **(A)** Transverse supine, **(B)** right lateral decubitus transverse coronal, and **(C)** sagittal scans demonstrating an echogenic mass *(m)* to the left of the aorta *(a)* and anterior to the left kidney *(k)*. The mass appears separate from the kidney. This mass was the metastatic tumor. (*c*, inferior vena cava.)

quently (45 percent) involved of the visceral organs. In patients without AIDS, the frequency of liver involvement with lymphoma is much lower (4.5 to 9.7 percent).[118] These lesions within the liver are hypoechoic; some are nearly anechoic. Focal lesions within the spleen are less commonly noted at ultrasound. A hypoechoic abdominal mass detected at ultrasound is suggestive of lymphoma when seen in patients with AIDS or at risk for AIDS.[118] The associated adenopathy may be due to reactive hyperplasia, but a specific abnormality (lymphoma, metastatic Kaposi sarcoma, or mycobacterial infection) is less likely with nodes greater than 1.5 cm in diameter.[118]

In one series, lymphadenopathy was present in 37 percent of patients in both risk groups (patients with AIDS, intravenous drug abusers)[119] (Figs. 12-9 and 12-10). Periportal and peripancreatic region nodes 1 to 2 cm in diameter are seen.[119] For more definitive evaluation, an ultrasound-guided percutaneous fine-needle aspiration biopsy can be helpful in establishing the diagnosis of abdominal lymphoma and for distinguishing it from other diagnostic considerations.[118] The most reliable finding that points to immune impairment in the appro-

priate clinical setting is adenopathy, which seems to be the least subjective ultrasound abnormality.[119]

The spleen and lymph nodes are the most common sites of involvement of extrapulmonary infection by *Pneumocystis carinii.*[120] Parenchymal calcifications can be found in the spleen, liver, kidneys, abdominal lymph nodes, adrenal glands, and mediastinal lymph nodes. Ultrasound may show diffuse tiny echogenic foci without shadowing in the liver, spleen, and kidneys (see Fig. 10-27). When calcifications or focal lesions are detected at one or more extrapulmonary sites in an immunodeficient patient, even if there is not history or evidence of *P. carinii* pneumonia, it should be suspected. The diagnosis can be confirmed by percutaneous fine-needle aspiration.[120]

Sarcoidosis. As a disease of unknown etiology, sarcoidosis is a multisystem granulomatous disorder primarily affecting the mediastinal and hilar lymph nodes, lungs, skin, and eyes.[121,122] The liver, spleen, peripheral lymph nodes, salivary glands, bones, heart, and nervous system are involved less often. Typical hilar adenopathy is usually present when there is involvement of intra-

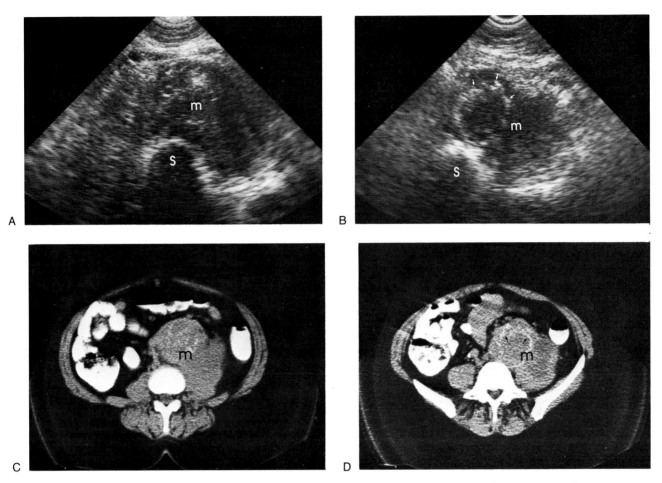

Fig. 12-75. Metastatic disease. Carcinoma of the cervix. **(A & B)** Transverse scans in the para-aortic area demonstrating a large solid mass *(m)*. The echodensities (arrows) in Fig. B represent calcifications. The aorta and inferior vena cava cannot be identified. *(S, spine.)* **(C & D)** CT scans demonstrating a similar finding to the ultrasound findings, with a para-aortic mass *(m)* that contains some calcification (arrows).

abdominal or retroperitoneal lymph nodes, which occurs rarely.[121] This disease usually affects young adults.

The abdominal manifestations of sarcoidosis include hepatomegaly (25 percent) and splenomegaly (25 percent).[122] With hepatic sarcoidosis, noncaseating granulomas are usually located in the portal spaces in patients without evidence of liver dysfunction.[122] In 24 percent, biopsy-proven hepatic granulomas compatible with hepatic sarcoidosis have been found.[122] Jaundice, chronic intrahepatic cholestasis, liver failure, and hepatic encephalopathy may be seen as other hepatic manifestations.[122] Lymphoma and metastatic disease are primarily considered when abdominal adenopathy is discovered[122] (Fig. 12-11). In the appropriate clinical setting, sarcoidosis should be considered in the differential diagnosis.

Biopsy. Nodal biopsy is performed for confirmation of the lymphangiographic findings and for histologic diagnosis in lieu of surgery.[123] In patients with lymphoma, 54 to 85 percent of biopsy specimens provide adequate cytologic information for a correct diagnosis.[123,124] As far as carcinoma to nodes is concerned, a fine-needle biopsy is diagnostically correct 72 percent of the time.[124]

Correlative Imaging. At most institutions, CT is the preferred modality for identification, staging, and follow-up of lymphoma. CT can detect smaller nodal enlargements than ultrasound can and is less likely to be nondiagnostic. In one study, 50 percent of the ultrasound scans ordered for staging the abdomen and pelvis were not sufficiently visualized for diagnostic conclusion.[125] On ultrasound scans, the presence or extent of the disease in nodal sites caudal to the pancreas was underestimated more commonly than in other areas.[125] Others report ultrasound to have an accuracy of 80 to 90 percent, a specificity of greater than 90 percent, and a sensitivity of 60 to 70 percent in the staging of lymphoma.[105]

Cysts

As rare pathologic conditions, primary retroperitoneal cysts lie in the retroperitoneal fatty tissues and have no apparent connection with any adult structure save areolar tissue.[126] The following classification has been devised: (1) wolffian cysts, (2) lymphatic cysts, (3) dermoids, (4) mesocolic cysts, and (5) parasitic lesions.[126] These lesions are commonly asymptomatic and are discovered on routine physical examination.

In the reported series, ultrasound was able to characterize the lesions as primary retroperitoneal cysts in all cases by showing them as separate from surrounding organs, containing clear fluid, and located within the retroperitoneum[126] (Fig. 12-76). The absence of internal debris and septations helps to differentiate them from abscesses, hematomas, and other cysts with complex structural patterns, such as dermoids and hydatids. The various types of retroperitoneal cysts cannot be differentiated by imaging methods.

These lesions may be seen as fluid-filled masses with anechoic content and regular margins; all exhibited increased through transmission[126] (Fig. 12-76). Ultrasound analysis of the different relationships of the kidney and the cysts during respiratory movements or the anterior displacement of surrounding structures allows the preoperative localization of the cyst within the retroperitoneum.

Primary Retroperitoneal Tumors

Most of the primary retroperitoneal tumors arise from the kidney and adrenal gland, with primary tumors other than lymphoma derived from mesenchymal and neurogenic tissue. Most are malignant.[11,127] Components may include fibrous tissue, muscle, fat, nerves, blood, and lymph vessels, as well as embryonic rests from the genitourinary or gastrointestinal system.[11] These primary retroperitoneal tumors may be classified as follows: (1) mesenchymal tumors — liposarcoma, leiomyosarcoma (leiomyoma), rhabdomyosarcoma (rhabdomyoma), fibrosarcoma, lymphangiosarcoma (lymphangioma); (2) vascular tumors — hemangiopericytoma, angiosarcoma (hemangioma), lymphangiosarcoma (lymphangioma); (3) neurogenic tumors — malignant schwannoma (neurilemoma, neurofibroma); (4) tumors of sympathetic nerve origin — neuroblastoma, ganglioneuroblastoma (ganglioneuroma), malignant paraganglioma (paraganglioma or extra-adrenal pheochromocytoma); and (5) germ cell tumors — malignant teratoma (benign teratoma), embryonal carcinoma, seminoma (occasionally arises from retroperitoneal space as a primary tumor).[5] Generally, retroperitoneal tumors are rapidly growing; the larger tumors are more likely to show evidence of necrosis and hemorrhage. The concurrence of

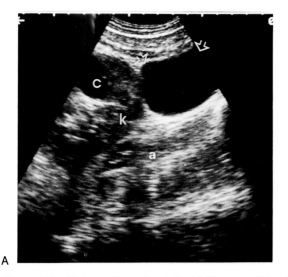 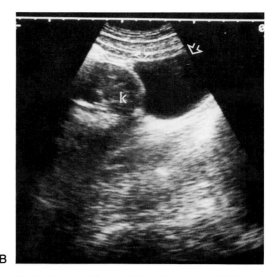

Fig. 12-76. Retroperitoneal cyst. Sagittal images of the right flank obtained during (**A**) expiration and (**B**) deep inspiration. The kidney moves inferiorly during inspiration, thus indenting the superior wall of the nonmovable retroperitoneal cyst (arrows). A small renal cyst *(c)* is associated. (*k*, right kidney; *a*, quadratus lumborum muscle.) (From Derchi et al,[126] with permission.)

the mass and ascites indicates invasion of the peritoneal surface.[1]

A number of signs are visualized on ultrasound that may suggest a retroperitoneal origin for a mass.[5] When there is anterior displacement of the pancreas or kidneys and anterior or lateral displacement of the aorta, IVC, and iliac arteries or veins, a retroperitoneal origin should be considered.[5] Retroperitoneal lesions frequently cause encasement of retroperitoneal structures, such as the aorta, IVC, renal arteries, kidney, and pancreas.[5] Additionally a retroperitoneal lesion may compress the iliopsoas or quadratus lumborum muscle.[5] When the lesion is very large, the assignment of the origin may be more difficult. A retroperitoneal origin should be questioned when a large abdominal lesion is visualized anterior to the aorta and/or IVC or iliopsoas or quadratus muscle without intervening bowel loops.[5] The location of the mass may help in suggesting the originating space of the mass. Masses in a paravertebral location may be neurogenic, whereas those of sympathetic nerve origin may be adrenal or para-aortic.[5] Paragangliomas or extra-adrenal pheochromocytomas may arise from the organ of Zuck-

erkandl, which is at the origin of the inferior mesenteric artery or slightly below the renal hilum.[5] The size of retroperitoneal masses is variable; many are large. Certain lesions tend to occur in children, including rhabdomyosarcoma, neuroblastoma, ganglioneuroblastoma, and teratoma.[5]

A variety of echopatterns are associated with these tumors. In malignant schwannoma, malignant fibrous histiocytoma, some rhabdomyosarcomas, and some lymphomas, a homogeneous tumor without necrosis or hemorrhage may be poorly echogenic or anechoic and simulate a cyst.[5] The ultrasound pattern of lipomas may vary from highly echogenic to poorly echogenic depending not on the fat content but on the number of fibrous stromas between fat globules.[5]

Mesenchymal Tumors. *Liposarcoma.* The most frequently described primary retroperitoneal tumor is the liposarcoma, which is often quite echoreflective, depending on its fat content[1,5,11] (Fig. 12-77). It is an uncommon tumor, but the third most common malignant tumor of soft tissue and the second most frequent retro-

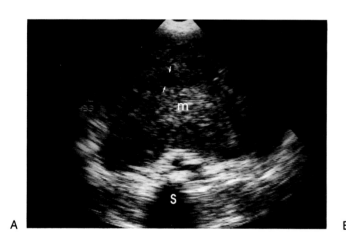

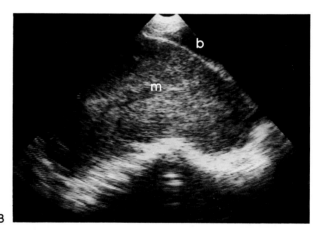

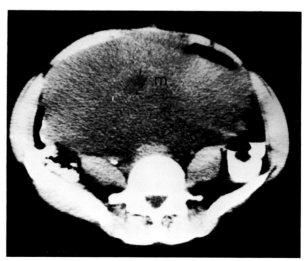

Fig. 12-77. Liposarcoma. **(A)** Transverse scan at the level of the umbilicus. An echodense mass *(m)* is seen anterior to the spine *(S)*. The aorta is not seen. There is a small anechoic area (arrows) within the mass. **(B)** Sagittal scan. The echodense mass *(m)* extends from the pelvis upward. The bladder *(b)* is seen anteriorly. **(C)** CT scan similar to Fig. A. The mass *(m)* is lower in density than soft tissue and contains a low-density area (arrows).

peritoneal malignant tumor. Thirteen percent of liposarcomas occur in the retroperitoneum, with more than one-third of these originating from the perirenal fat.[127] The diagnosis is rarely made preoperatively. On ultrasound, a mass with a complex echopattern and an irregularly thickened wall is seen[127] (Fig. 12-77). On the basis of ultrasound, liposarcoma cannot be differentiated from leiomyosarcoma and other retroperitoneal sarcomas.

Leiomyosarcoma and Other Sarcomas. Leiomyosarcomas are the second most common primary retroperitoneal tumors.[5] Leiomyosarcomas tend to undergo necrosis and cystic degeneration. Sarcomas other than liposarcoma present as complex or centrally necrotic soft tissue masses or as homogeneous soft tissue masses; on ultrasound, there are increased or decreased internal echoes or an echodense central area with a hypoechoic

periphery.[1,128] Fibrosarcomas and rhabdomyosarcomas (Fig. 12-78) are quite invasive and infiltrate widely into muscle and adjoining soft tissue.[11] Neurogenic tumors are common in the paravertebral region, where they arise from nerve roots or sympathetic chain ganglia (Fig. 12-79).

Some musculoskeletal tumors frequently have a soft tissue component in association with the bony abnormality. These include sacrococcygeal teratoma, giant cell tumor, and Ewing sarcoma.[129] In Ewing sarcoma, there is an extraosseous component in 90 percent of cases.[129] Ultrasound can be useful in evaluation of such pelvic and abdominal soft tissue masses (Figs. 12-80 and 12-81). This helps in assessment of the extent of disease, radiation planning, and follow-up.[129]

Malignant Fibrous Histiosarcoma. Malignant fibrous histiosarcoma is an uncommon neoplasm, making up

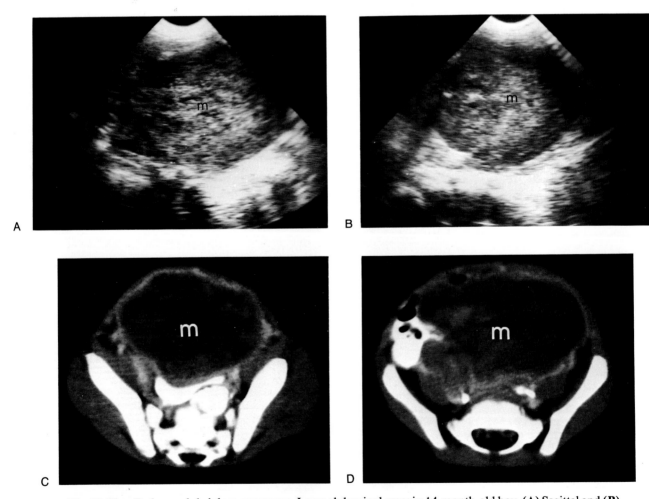

A B C D

Fig. 12-78. Embryonal rhabdomyosarcoma. Large abdominal mass in 14-month-old boy. **(A)** Sagittal and **(B)** transverse scans of the abdomen showing a solid, echodense mass *(m)* filling the entire lower abdomen. No anatomic structures are identified. **(C & D)** CT scans. The mass *(m)* appears to be low in density on CT and fills the entire lower abdomen.

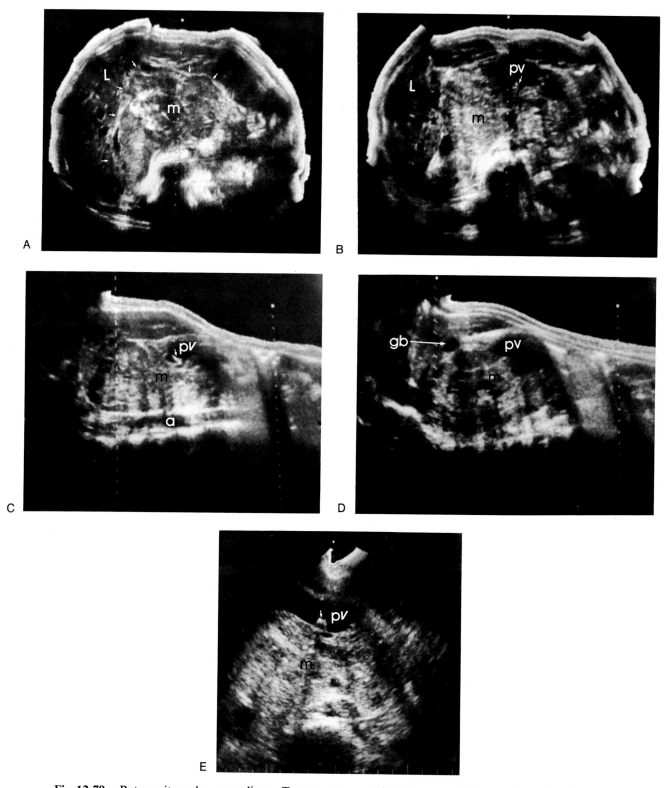

Fig. 12-79. Retroperitoneal paraganglioma. Transverse scans at **(A)** 16 cm and **(B)** 10 cm above the umbilicus and sagittal scans **(C)** in the midline and **(D)** 2 cm to the right of midline demonstrating a large, echodense prevertebral mass *(m)*. *(gb,* gallbladder; *a,* aorta; *L,* liver; *pv,* portal vein.) **(E)** Cone-down transverse view. The portal vein *(pv)* appears dilated and is located anterior to the mass *(m)*. It contains an echodense tumor nodule (arrows, Figs. B, C, & E) that moved on real-time scan but was attached to the wall of the portal vein. This patient had metastases to the liver, lung, and portal vein.

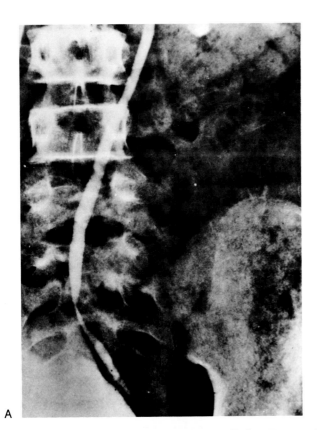

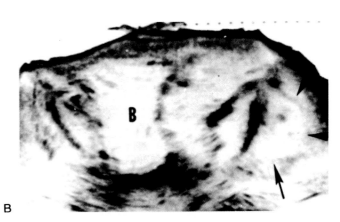

Fig. 12-80. Musculoskeletal tumor. Ewing sarcoma of the iliac crest. **(A)** Intravenous pyelogram demonstrating a permeative destructive process of the left iliac bone with considerable mass effect on the left ureter and urinary bladder. **(B)** Transverse scan showing a huge intrapelvic mass displacing the bladder *(B)*. Note the smaller extrapelvic component (arrows). (From deSantos and Goldstein,[129] with permission.)

about 10 percent of soft tissue sarcomas, and is thought to originate from undifferentiated mesenchymal cells.[130] It is composed of fibroblastlike and histiocytelike cell lines. The male/female ratio is slightly less than 2:1, with more than 70 percent of these tumors occurring in the fifth to seventh decades with a strong white predominance.[130] In one series, only 12 percent were found in the retroperitoneum with most found in the extremity (upper, 22 percent; lower, 48 percent) and 15 percent in the abdomen, with the thigh being the single most common site (34 percent).[130]

On ultrasound, a malignant histiocytic sarcoma is usually a well-defined mass with a variable echopattern secondary to the heterogeneity of the tumor[130] (Fig. 12-82). Frequently present are hypoechoic or anechoic areas, which may represent necrosis; marked inflammatory or myxoid cellularity may also cause the lower echogenicity.[130]

Lymphangiomyomatosis. Lymphangiomyomatosis is a rare tumorlike condition characterized by smooth muscle proliferation involving the major lymphatic trunks in the mediastinum and retroperitoneum, lymph nodes in these areas, and lymphatics. It is an uncommon myoproliferative disorder confined to females of reproductive age. The lesion consists of one or more nodules of tumorlike proliferation of smooth muscle fascicles divided from each other by lymph channels. The smooth muscle meshwork involves the walls of preexisting lymphatic channels and replaces sinusoids of lymph nodes. Lymphatic obstruction leads to distended collateral vessels and small and large lymph cysts. Ultrasound demonstrates cystic structures of various sizes lying along the course of the aorta and IVC (Fig. 12-83). The cyst walls are thick and often continuous with the walls of the nearby cyst, giving a septated appearance. There are low-level internal echoes.[131]

Lipoblastomatosis. Abdominal lipoblastomatosis is a rare benign tumor of embryonal adipose tissue.[132] Most of these tumors are found superficially in the upper and lower extremities; occasionally they are found in the neck, trunk, mediastinum, and retroperitoneum. Ninety percent occur in infants less than 3 years of age. The

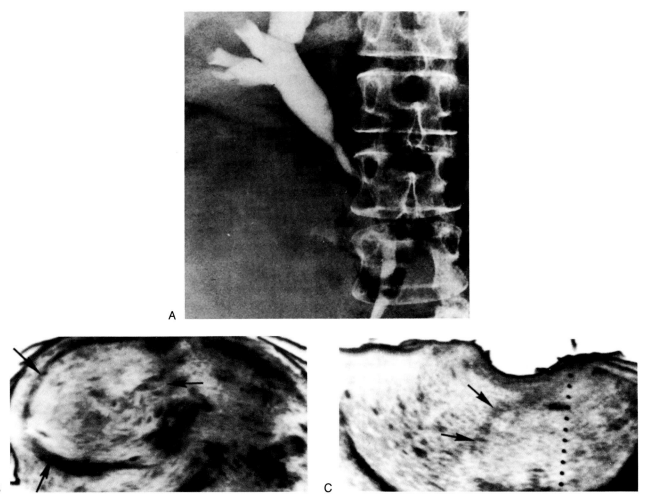

Fig. 12-81. Musculoskeletal tumor. Giant cell tumor of the fifth lumbar vertebra. (A) Intravenous urogram demonstrating destructive bony changes and a large soft tissue mass. Note the upward rotation of the kidney and the marked medial displacement of the right ureter. (B) Transverse scan 1 cm below the umbilicus defining a large intra-abdominal mass on the right (arrows). (C) Longitudinal scan 8 cm to the right of midline. A large mass is seen extending to the right hepatic margin. The interface at the mass-liver junction (arrows) indicates an extrahepatic location of the mass. (From deSantos and Goldstein,[129] with permission.)

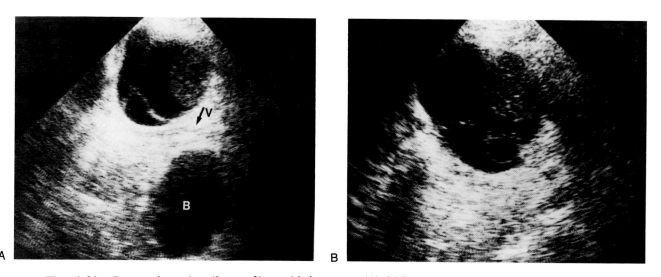

Fig. 12-82. Retroperitoneal malignant fibrous histiocytoma. (A) Oblique sonographic section of the tumor anterolateral to the left iliac vessels. (B, bladder; V, iliac vessels.) (B) Detail. The cystic central parts with marked septations as well as the more peripheral solid parts are clearly seen and there is posterior acoustic enhancement. (From Schut and van Imhoff,[130] with permission.)

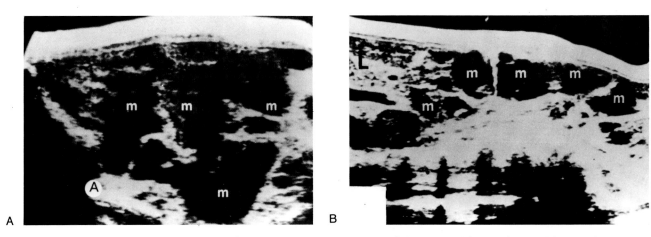

Fig. 12-83. Lymphangiomyomatosis. **(A)** Transverse sonogram of the true pelvis showing multiple cystic masses *(m)*. **(B)** Longitudinal parasagittal section through the liver *(L)* at the level of the inferior vena cava showing multiple masses *(m)* extending from the interior portion of the liver to the true pelvis. Note the thick septae between the masses. Some masses are anechoic, while others have low-level echoes within them. (From Walsh et al,[131] with permission.)

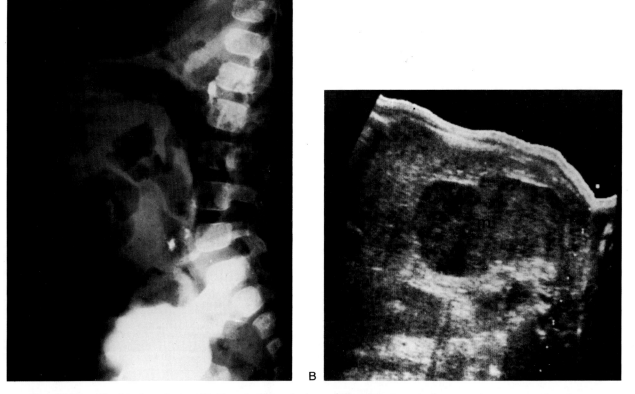

Fig. 12-84. Lipoblastomatosis. **(A)** Case 1. Lateral view of the abdomen during excretory urography. An apparently bilobed mass is seen inferior to the right kidney, surrounded by a lucent rim of fat. The difference between the fatty and solid tumor tissue is accentuated by total body opacification. There is a small amount of residual barium anterior to L5. **(B)** Longitudinal scan. There is clear differentiation in echogenicity between the central myxoid masses *(m)* and the adjacent fat. *(Figure continues.)*

tumor consists of lobules of immature adipose tissue with myxoid stroma separated by richly vascularized connective tissue septa. Ultrasound has delineated a myxoid mass embedded within highly echogenic fat[132] (Fig. 12-84).

Vascular Tumors. *Hemangiopericytoma.* Hemangiopericytomas are unusual and uncommon vascular neoplasms that arise from the pericytes of Zimmermann, contractile spindle cells that surround capillaries and postcapillary venules.[133] These cells are found in close apposition to capillaries and are thought to have some contractile capabilities. Hemangiopericytomas typically comprise uniform elongated cells surrounding a rich, branching network of thin-walled vessels of various sizes and shapes. These lesions can occur anywhere in the body but are most common in the lower extremity and pelvic retroperitoneum. In one series, 35 percent affected the lower extremity with 25 percent in the pelvis or retroperitoneum.[133] Hemangiopericytomas account for less than 2 percent of soft tissue sarcomas.[133] The

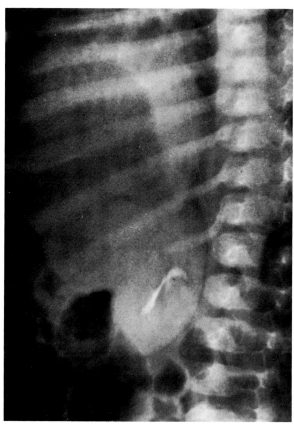

C

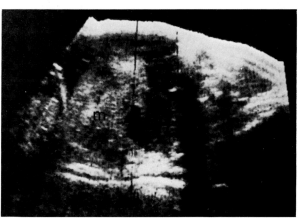

D

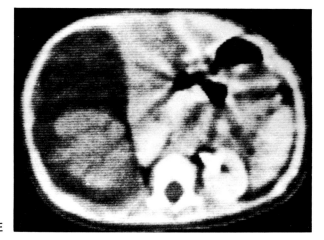

E

Fig. 12-84 *(Continued).* **(C)** Right posterior oblique 10-minute radiograph from an excretory urogram. The intact right kidney is displaced caudally by an avascular radiolucent mass in the right upper quadrant. **(D)** Longitudinal scan demonstrating a large, highly echogenic mass of fatty tissue *(m)* with a smaller, hypoechoic mass of myxoid tissue inferiorly. **(E)** CT scan 5.3 cm below the xyphoid. A large fat-containing mass is seen in the right abdomen, within which is a smaller, denser area subsequently shown to be myxoid tissue. The lateral border of the right lobe of the liver is markedly displaced but was separate from the tumor. (From Fisher et al,[132] with permission.)

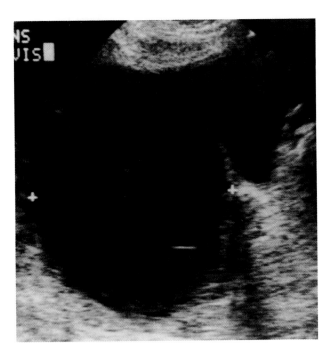

Fig. 12-85. Pelvic hemangiopericytoma in an 81-year-old woman. Transverse sonogram shows well-circumscribed hypoechoic mass with inhomogeneous internal echopattern. The bladder was compressed externally. (From Lorigan et al,[133] with permission.)

peak incidence is in the fifth to sixth decades, with equal sex distribution.[133,134]

This tumor usually presents as a painless mass, but pressure on adjacent viscera may cause symptoms. The signs and symptoms are insidious, so the mass is quite large before symptoms present. Various paraneoplastic syndromes have been described in association with this tumor, including hypoglycemia, hypophosphatemic osteomalacia, and hypertrophic pulmonary osteoarthropathy. Since it is a highly vascular tumor, it occasionally causes clinically significant arteriovenous shunting.[133] Most are considered benign, and the 5-year survival rate is high.[134]

The ultrasound pattern of hemangiopericytomas may be varied. In one reported series, all of the patients had lesions that were well circumscribed and hypoechoic.[133] One may see a well-defined predominantly cystic mass, a mixed solid and cystic mass, or a solid mass with acoustic shadowing[134] (Figs. 12-85 and 12-86). Ultrasound can be used to define the limits of the mass and to monitor the mass while the patient is undergoing therapy.[134] These lesions must be distinguished from the more common sarcomas such as malignant fibrous histiocytoma, liposarcoma, and synovial sarcoma. This tumor should be considered in the differential diagnosis of hypervascular soft tissue masses arising in the retroperitoneum, pelvis, or lower extremity.

Lymphangioma. Lymphangioma of the retroperitoneum occurs in patients of all ages.[135] Its cause has not been clearly established, but it is thought to be a developmental malformation in which lymphangiectasia follows the failure of developing lymphatic tissue to establish normal communication with the remainder of the lymphatic system.[135,136] As a result, the abnormal lymphatic channels dilate to form a cystic mass that may be uni- or multilocular.[135] These lymphangiomas have been classified into three histologic types: (1) simple lymphangiomas with capillary-size lymphatic channels; (2) cavernous lymphangiomas that contain dilated lym-

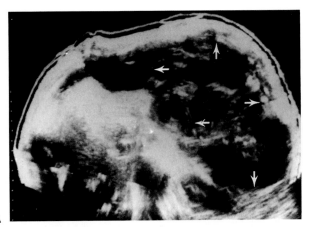
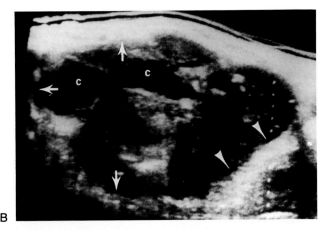

Fig. 12-86. Hemangiopericytoma. **(A)** Transverse scan at 3 cm inferior to the xyphoid. A large mixed solid and cystic mass is seen occupying the entire left abdomen (arrows). **(B)** Longitudinal scan at 4 cm to left of midline. A mixed solid and cystic mass (arrows) is seen extending into the left iliac fossa (arrowheads). Note the internal cystic region with ragged border *(c)*. (From Grant et al,[134] with permission.)

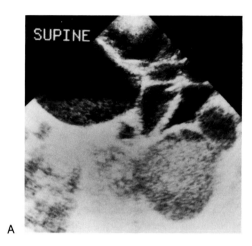
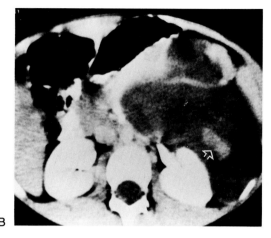

A   B

Fig. 12-87. Lymphangioma. Images of lymphangioma with multiple, thickly septated locules that contain evidence of recent and prior hemorrhage. At surgery, the tumor was located in the anterior pararenal space and adhered to the pancreas. **(A)** Sonogram in the transverse plane demonstrating multiple locules containing echogenic debris. Fluid-debris levels have formed in some locules. **(B)** Contrast-enhanced CT scan demonstrating the same findings as in Fig. A. The high-attenuation material within one locule is compatible with clot found in the specimen (arrow). (From Davidson and Hartman,[135] with permission.)

phatics and fibrous adventitia; and (3) cystic hygromas that are macroscopic multilocular cystic masses with cysts of various sizes lined with a single layer of endothelium and containing serous or milky fluid.[136] In this location, chyle and mural calcification are very uncommon.[135]

In one series, the ultrasound features of the lymphangiomas were predominantly those of anechoic fluid-filled masses; if septa were present, they were thin. Ultrasound showed a multilocular fluid collection in 61 percent of cases and a unicameral mass in 39 percent[135] (Figs. 12-87 and 12-88). The most characteristic appear-

ance is a multiloculated cystic mass with septa of variable thickness that contains solid components arising from the cyst wall or the septa. Pathologically, this echogenic component corresponds to a cluster of abnormal lymphatic channels, too small to be resolved by ultrasound. The fluid is uncomplicated in 56 percent of lymphangiomas, with the remainder containing debris that sometimes layer. The most characteristic finding is that of an elongated tumor containing uncomplicated fluid with or without septa. Complete surgical removal may be difficult since the cysts tend to form along tissue planes.[136]

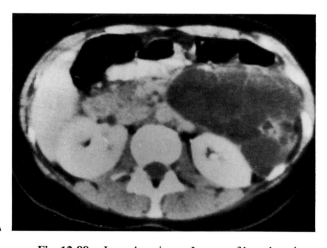
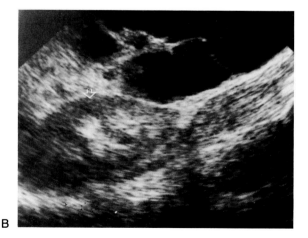

A   B

Fig. 12-88. Lymphangioma. Images of lymphangioma anterior to the left kidney with multiple locules separated by thin septa. **(A)** Contrast-enhanced CT scan. **(B)** Coronal sonogram. The kidney (arrow) is superior and posterior to the lymphangioma. (From Davidson and Hartman,[135] with permission.)

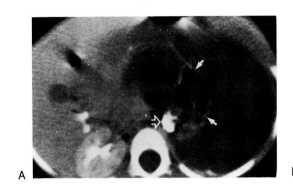
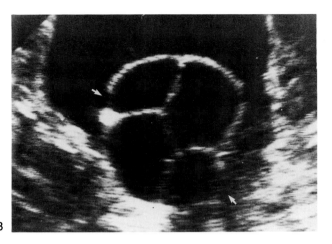

Fig. 12-89. Mature teratoma. **(A)** Contrast-enhanced CT scan and **(B)** transverse sonogram showing a mature teratoma in a 1-year-old girl. The teratoma is composed predominantly of uncomplicated fluid. A soft tissue and loculated cystic component is located eccentrically in the mass (white arrows). Calcification (open arrow in Fig. A) has the pattern classified as congealed. (From Davidson et al,[140] with permission.)

Neurogenic Tumors. Neurogenic tumors are common in the paravertebral region, where they arise from nerve roots or sympathetic chain ganglia (Fig. 12-79).

Tumors of Sympathetic Nerve Origin. *Paraganglioma.* Paragangliomas in the retroperitoneum arise from paraganglia, collections of specialized neural crest cells symmetrically distributed along the aorta in close association with the sympathetic chain.[137] Most patients are between the ages of 30 and 45 years, with men affected more frequently than women.[137] These tumors are close to the aorta, which may help differentiate them from other primary retroperitoneal tumors[137] (Fig. 12-79). It may

be difficult to differentiate them from para-aortic lymph node involvement by lymphoma or from metastases of a variety of primary neoplasms to retroperitoneal nodes.[137]

Germ Cell Tumors. *Teratoma.* Teratomas are usually differentiated tumors containing tissues from the three germ layers. The retroperitoneal space is the fourth most frequent site of origin; they most commonly occur in the ovaries, testes, anterior mediastinum, retroperitoneum, and sacrococcygeal region.[138,139] Most occur in the vicinity of the upper pole of the left kidney. There is a predi-

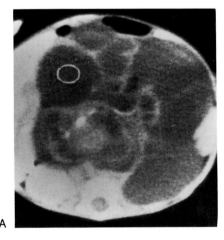
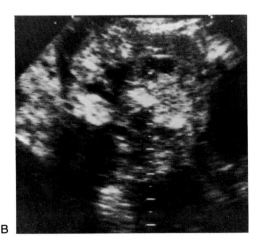

Fig. 12-90. Mature teratoma. **(A)** Unenhanced CT scan and **(B)** transverse sonogram showing a mature teratoma in a 2-month-old girl. Fluid and soft tissue components of the tumor are approximately equal. On CT scan, the measured attenuation value of the tumor was −18 HU. (From Davidson et al,[140] with permission.)

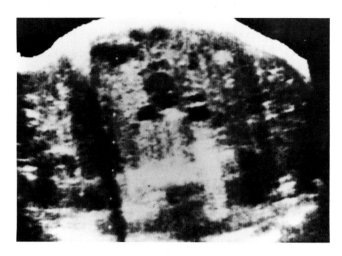

Fig. 12-91. Mature teratoma. Longitudinal sonogram demonstrating a solid teratoma in a 5-day-old girl. Note the specular echoes and acoustic shadows produced by calcium in the tumor. (From Davidson et al,[140] with permission.)

lection for the left side, for the midline, and for a suprarenal location.[140]

There appears to be a female predominance of 3.4:1 in patients with mature teratomas of the retroperitoneum.[140] There is a peak incidence in the first 6 months of life and a second peak in early adulthood. The incidence of malignancy is 6 to 10 percent (90 percent are benign); 50 percent of teratomas occur in the pediatric age group.[138,139] In one series, all of the lesions were well circumscribed, showed no evidence of invasion, and affected adjacent organs simply by virtue of their bulk.

The benign teratomas exhibit a spectrum from predominantly fluid-filled to completely solid masses.[140] They are characteristically heterogeneous with solid areas, calcification, and cystic spaces[1,138] (Figs. 12-89 to 12-91). They can appear cystic.[139] In slightly fewer than 50 percent of cases in one series, an eccentric protrusion into a cyst of either solid or solid and cystic tissue, the so-called dermoid plug or Rokitansky body, was detected on ultrasound.[140] On ultrasound, 76 percent exhibit uncomplicated fluid and calcium is present in 50 percent of cases. Fat is not reliably distinguished from other soft tissue components on ultrasound. A complex mass containing a well-circumscribed fluid component of variable volume, adipose tissue and/or sebum in the form of a fat-fluid level, and calcification in either a congealed or linear strand pattern is the most characteristic finding.[140] CT is thought to be superior to ultrasound in the localization and characterization of retroperitoneal teratomas and permits unequivocal identification of fat as adipose tissue and the characterization of fluid as sebum, serous, or complex.[140]

REFERENCES

1. Koenigsberg M, Hoffman JC, Schnur MJ: Sonographic evaluation of the retroperitoneum. Semin Ultrasound CT MR 1982;3:79

2. Yeh H-C: Ultrasound and CT of the adrenals. Semin Ultrasound CT MR 1982;3:97

3. Sample WF: Adrenal ultrasonography. Radiology 1978;127:461

4. Sample WF: A new technique for evaluation of the adrenal gland with gray scale ultrasonography. Radiology 1977;124:463

5. Yeh HC: Adrenal gland and nonrenal retroperitoneum. Urol Radiol 1987;9:127

6. Kangarloo H, Diament MJ, Gold RH et al: Sonography of adrenal glands in neonates and children: changes in appearance with age. J Clin Ultrasound 1986;14:43

7. Yeh H-C: Adrenal sonography. p. 101. In Leopold GR (ed): Clinics in Diagnostic Ultrasound: Ultrasound in Breast and Endocrine Disease. Vol. 12. Churchill Livingstone, New York, 1984

8. Gunther RW, Kelbel C, Lenner V: Real-time ultrasound of normal adrenal glands and small tumors. J Clin Ultrasound 1984;12:211

9. Yeh HC: Ultrasonography of the adrenals. Semin Roentgenol 1988;23:250

10. Cubberley DA, Gosink BB, Forsythe J: Coronal sonography: a review of abdominal applications. J Ultrasound Med 1985;4:35

11. Goldberg BB, Pollack HM, Bancks NH: Retroperitoneum. p. 188. In Resnick MI, Sanders RC (eds): Ultrasound in Urology. Williams & Wilkins, Baltimore, 1979

12. Zappasodi F, Derchi LE, Rizzatto G: Ultrasonography of the normal adrenal glands: a study using linear-array real-time equipment. Br J Radiol 1986;59:759

13. Krebs CA, Eisenberg RL, Ratcliff S, Jouppi L: Cava-suprarenal line: new position for sonographic imaging of left adrenal gland. J Clin Ultrasound 1986;14:535

14. Sample WF: Ultrasonography of the adrenal gland. p. 73. In Resnick MI, Sanders RC (eds): Ultrasound in Urology. Williams & Wilkins, Baltimore, 1979

15. Marchal G, Gelin J, Verbeken E et al: High-resolution real-time sonography of the adrenal glands: a routine examination? J Ultrasound Med 1986;5:65

16. Callen PW, Filly RA, Sarti DA, Sample WF: Ultrasonography of the diaphragmatic crura. Radiology 1979;130:721

17. Ritchie WGM: Sonographic demonstration of abdominal visceral lymph node enlargement. AJR 1982;138:517

18. Pardes JG, Auh YH, Kneeland JB et al: The oblique coronal view in sonography of the retroperitoneum. AJR 1985;144:1241

19. Pardes JG, Kazam E, Kneelard JB et al: Sonography of the retroperitoneum: value of the oblique coronal view. Proceedings of the American Institute of Ultrasound in Medicine. J Ultrasound Med 1983;2:3

20. Dodds WJ, Darweesh RMA, Lawson TL et al: The retroperitoneal spaces revisited. AJR 1986;147:1155

21. Raptopoulos V, Kleinman PK, Marks S et al: Renal fascial pathway: posterior extension of pancreatic effusions within the anterior pararenal space. Radiology 1986;158:367

22. Bernardino ME, Goldstein HM, Green B: Gray scale ultrasonography of adrenal neoplasm. AJR 1978;130:741

23. Yeh H-C, Mitty HA, Rose J et al: Ultrasonography of adrenal masses: usual features. Radiology 1978; 127:467

24. Ghorashi B, Holmes JH: Gray scale sonography appearance of an adrenal mass: a case report. J Clin Ultrasound 1976;4:121

25. Oppenheimer DA, Carroll BA, Yousem S: Sonography of the normal neonatal adrenal gland. Radiology 1983;146:157

26. Scott EM, Thomas A, McGarrigle HHG, Lachelin GCL: Serial adrenal ultrasonography in normal neonates. J Ultrasound Med 1990;9:279

27. Menzel D, Hauffa BP: Changes in size and sonographic characteristics of the adrenal glands during the first year of life and the sonographic diagnosis of adrenal hyperplasia in infants with 21-hydroxylase deficiency. J Clin Ultrasound 1990;18:619

28. Silverman PM, Carroll BA, Moskowitz PS: Adrenal sonography in renal agenesis and dysplasia. AJR 1980; 134:600

29. McGahan JP, Myracle RR: Adrenal hypertrophy: possible pitfalls in the sonographic diagnosis of renal agenesis. J Ultrasound Med 1986;5:265

30. Sample WF, Sarti DA: Computed body tomography and gray scale ultrasonography: anatomic correlation and pitfalls in the upper abdomen. Gastrointest Radiol 1978;3:243

31. Marchal G, Oyen R, Verschakelen J et al: Sonographic appearance of normal lymph nodes. J Ultrasound Med 1985;4:417

32. Callen PW, Filly RA, Marks WM: The quadratus lumborum muscle: a possible source of confusion in sonographic evaluation of the retroperitoneum. J Clin Ultrasound 1979;7:349

33. Auh YH, Rubenstein WA, Schneider M et al: Extraperitoneal paravesical spaces: CT delineation with US correlation. Radiology 1986;159:319

34. Auh YH, Rubenstein WA, Markisz JA et al: Intraperitoneal paravesical spaces: CT delineation with US correlation. Radiology 1986;159:311

35. Gore RM, Callen PW, Filly RA: Displaced retroperitoneal fat: sonographic guide to right upper quadrant mass localization. Radiology 1982;142:701

36. Graif M, Manor A, Itzchak Y: Sonographic differentiation of extra- and intrahepatic masses. AJR 1983; 141:553

37. Lim JH, Ko YT, Lee DH: Sonographic sliding sign in localization of right upper quadrant mass. J Ultrasound Med 1990;9:455

38. Yeh H-C, Mitty HA, Rose J et al: Ultrasonography of adrenal masses: unusual manifestation. Radiology 1978;127:475

39. Pery M, Kaftori JK, Bar-Maor JA: Sonography for diagnosis and follow-up of neonatal adrenal hemorrhage. J Clin Ultrasound 1981;9:397

40. Mittelstaedt CA, Volberg FM, Merten DF, Brill PW: The sonographic diagnosis of neonatal adrenal hemorrhage. Radiology 1979;131:453

41. Nissenbaum M, Jequier S: Enlargement of adrenal glands preceding adrenal hemorrhage 1988;16:349

42. Heij HA, van Amerongen AHMT, Ekkelkamp S, Vos A: Diagnosis and management of neonatal adrenal haemorrhage. Pediatr Radiol 1989;19:391

43. Mineau DE, Koehler PR: Ultrasound diagnosis of neonatal adrenal hemorrhage. AJR 1979;132:443

44. Cohen EK, Daneman A, Stringer DA et al: Focal adrenal hemorrhage: a new US appearance. Radiology 1986; 161:631

45. Dunnick NR: Adrenal imaging: current status. AJR 1990;154:927

46. Sarnaik AP, Sanfilippo DJ, Slovis TL: Ultrasound diagnosis of adrenal hemorrhage in meningococcemia. Pediatr Radiol 1988;18:427

47. Murphy BJ, Casillas J, Yrizarry JM: Traumatic adrenal hemorrhage: radiologic findings. Radiology 1988; 169:701

48. Sivit CJ, Hung W, Taylor GA et al: Sonography in neonatal congenital adrenal hyperplasia. AJR 1991;156:141

49. Bryan PJ, Caldamone AA, Morrison SC et al: Ultrasound findings in the adreno-genital syndrome (congenital adrenal hyperplasia). J Ultrasound Med 1988;7:675

50. Cehreli C, Gokcin A, Toktas FR et al: Detection of adrenal gland hyperplasia by abdominal ultrasonography in a patient with primary hyperaldosteronism. J Clin Ultrasound 1991;19:39

51. Atkinson GO Jr, Kodroff MB, Gay BB Jr, Ricketts RR: Adrenal abscess in the neonate. Radiology 1985;155:101

52. Wilson DA, Nguyen DL, Tytle TL et al: Sonography of the adrenal glands in chronic disseminated histoplasmosis. J Ultrasound Med 1986;5:69

53. Barki Y, Eilig I, Moses M, Golcman L: Sonographic diagnosis of a large hemorrhagic adrenal cyst in an adult. J Clin Ultrasound 1987;15:194

54. Scheible W, Coel M, Siemers PT, Siegel H: Percutaneous aspiration of adrenal cysts. AJR 1977;128:1013

55. Robbins SL, Cotran RS (eds): The endocrine system adrenal cortex. p. 1387. In Pathologic Basis of Disease. WB Saunders, Philadelphia, 1979

56. Derchi LE, Rapaccini GL, Banderali A et al: Ultrasound and CT findings in two cases of hemangioma of the adrenal gland. J Comput Assist Tomogr 1989;13:659

57. Musante F, Derchi LE, Zappasodi F et al: Myelolipoma of the adrenal gland: sonographic and CT features. AJR 1988;151:961

58. Behan M, Martin EC, Muecke EC, Kazam E: Myelolipoma of the adrenal: two cases with ultrasound and CT findings. AJR 1977;129:993

59. Vick CW, Zeman RK, Mannes E et al: Adrenal myelolipoma: CT and ultrasound findings. Urol Radiol 1984;6:7

60. Bowerman RA, Silver TM, Jaffee MH et al: Sonography of adrenal pheochromocytomas. AJR 1981;137:1227

61. Robbins SL, Cotran RS (eds): The endocrine system: ad-

renal medulla. p. 1402. In Pathologic Basis of Disease. WB Saunders, Philadelphia, 1979

62. Hamper UM, Fishman EK, Hartman DS et al: Primary adrenocortical carcinoma: sonographic evaluation with clinical and pathologic correlation in 26 patients. AJR 1987;148:915

63. Prando A, Wallace S, Marins JLC et al: Sonographic findings of adrenal cortical carcinoma. Pediatr Radiol 1990;20:163

64. Bousvaros A, Kirks DR, Grossman H: Imaging of neuroblastoma: an overview. Pediatr Radiol 1986;16:89

65. Forman HP, Leonidas JC, Berdon WE et al: Congenital neuroblastoma: evaluation with multimodality imaging. Radiology 1990;175:365

66. Rosenfield NS, Leonidas JC, Barwick KW: Aggressive neuroblastoma simulating Wilms tumor. Radiology 1988;166:165

67. Jasinski RW, Samuels BI, Silver TM: Sonographic features of retroperitoneal ganglioneuroma. J Ultrasound Med 1984;3:413

68. White SJ, Stuck KJ, Blane CE, Silver TM: Sonography of neuroblastoma. AJR 1983;141:465

69. Dershaw DD, Helson L: Sonographic diagnosis and follow-up of abdominal neuroblastoma. Urol Radiol 1988;10:80

70. Amundson GM, Trevenen CL, Mueller DL et al: Neuroblastoma: a specific sonographic tissue pattern. AJR 1987;148:943

71. Berger PE, Kuhn JP, Munschauer RW: Computed tomography and ultrasound in the diagnosis and management of neuroblastoma. Radiology 1978;128:663

72. Day DL, Johnson R, Cohen MD: Abdominal neuroblastoma with inferior vena caval tumor thrombus: report of three cases (one with right atrial extension). Pediatr Radiol 1991;21:205

73. Crade M, Taylor KJW, Rosenfield AT: Discovery of an adrenal tumor by ultrasound: case report. J Clin Ultrasound 1978;6:191

74. Cunninghan JJ: Ultrasonic findings in "primary" lymphoma of the adrenal area. J Ultrasound Med 1983;2:467

75. Antoniou A, Spetseropoulos J, Vlahos L, Pontifex G: The sonographic appearance of adrenal involvement in non-Hodgkin's lymphoma. J Ultrasound Med 1983;2:235

76. Forsythe JR, Gosink BB, Leopold GR: Ultrasound in the evaluation of adrenal metastases. J Clin Ultrasound 1977;5:31

77. Gooding GAW: Ultrasonic spectrum of adrenal masses. Urology 1979;13:211

78. Vicks BS, Perusek M, Johnson J, Tio F: Primary adrenal lymphoma: CT and sonographic appearances. J Clin Ultrasound 1987;15:135

79. Abrams HL, Siegelman SS, Adams DF et al: Computed tomography versus ultrasound of the adrenal gland: a prospective study. Radiology 1982;143:121

80. Sample WF, Sarti DA: Computed tomography and gray scale ultrasonography of the adrenal gland: a comparative study. Radiology 1978;128:377

81. Gerzof SG: The role of ultrasound in the search for intra-abdominal and retroperitoneal abscesses. p. 101. In Taylor KJW, Viscomi GN (eds): Clinics in Diagnostic Ultrasound: Ultrasound in Emergency Medicine. Vol. 7. Churchill Livingstone, New York, 1981

82. Wicks JD, Silver TM, Thornbury JR: Complementary use of radiography, ultrasonography and gallium-67 scintigraphy in the diagnosis of a retroperitoneal abscess. Urol Radiol 1979;1:25

83. Kumari S, Pillari G, Phillips G, Pochaczevsky R: Fluid collections of the psoas in children. Semin Ultrasound CT MR 1982;3:139

84. Laing FC, Jacobs RP: Value of ultrasonography in the detection of retroperitoneal inflammatory masses. Radiology 1977;123:169

85. Gerzof SG, Gale ME: Computed tomography and ultrasonography for diagnosis and treatment of renal and retroperitoneal abscess. Urol Clinic North Am 1982;9:185

86. Hoffer FA, Shamberger RC, Teele RL: Ilio-psoas abscess: diagnosis and management. Pediatr Radiol 1987;17:23

87. Graif M, Martinovitz U, Strauss S et al: Sonographic localization of hematomas in hemophilic patients with positive iliopsoas sign. AJR 1987;148:121

88. Shirkhoda A, Mauro MA, Staab EV, Blatt PM: Soft-tissue hemorrhage in hemophiliac patients: computed tomography and ultrasound study. Radiology 1983;147:811

89. Kumari S, Fulco JD, Karayalcin G, Lipton R: Gray scale ultrasound: evaluation of iliopsoas hematoma in hemophiliacs. AJR 1979;133:103

90. Fagan CJ, Amparo EG, Davis M: Retroperitoneal fibrosis. Semin Ultrasound CT MR 1982;3:123

91. Fagan CJ, Larrieu AJ, Amparao EG: Retroperitoneal fibrosis: ultrasound and CT features. AJR 1979;133:239

92. Sanders RC, Duffy T, McLoughlin MG, Walsh PC: Sonography in the diagnosis of retroperitoneal fibrosis. J Urol 1977;118:944

93. Center S, Schwab R, Goldberg BB: The value of ultrasonography as an aid in the treatment of idiopathic retroperitoneal fibrosis. J Ultrasound Med 1982;1:87

94. Jacobson JB, Redman HC: Ultrasound findings in a case of retroperitoneal fibrosis. Radiology 1974;113:423

95. Bowie JD, Bernstein JR: Retroperitoneal fibrosis: ultrasound findings and case report. J Clin Ultrasound 1976;4:435

96. Fried AM, Williams CB, Litvak AS: High retroperitoneal lymphocele: unusual clinical presentation and diagnosis by ultrasonography. J Urol 1980;123:583

97. Spring DB, Schroeder D, Babu S et al: Ultrasonic evaluation of lymphocele formation after staging lymphadenectomy for prostatic carcinoma. Radiology 1981;141:479

98. Doust BD, Thompson R: Ultrasonography of abdominal fluid collections. Gastrointest Radiol 1978;3:273

99. Robbins SL, Cotran RS (eds): Lymph nodes and spleen. p. 757. In Pathologic Basis of Disease. WB Saunders, Philadelphia, 1979

100. Smeets AJ, Zonderland HM, van der Vorde F, Lameris JS: Evaluation of abdominal lymph nodes by ultrasound. J Ultrasound Med 1990;9:325

101. Rubaltelli L, Proto E, Salmaso R et al: Sonography of abnormal lymph nodes in vitro: correlation of sonographic and histologic findings. AJR 1990;155:1241

102. Carroll BA, Ta HN: The ultrasound appearance of extranodal abdominal lymphoma. Radiology 1980; 136:419

103. Carroll BA: Ultrasound of lymphoma. Semin Ultrasound CT MR 1982;3:114

104. Carroll BA: Lymphoma. p. 52. In Goldberg BB (ed): Clinics in Diagnostic Ultrasound: Ultrasound in Cancer. Vol. 6. Churchill Livingstone, New York, 1981

105. Rochester D, Bowie JD, Kunzmann A, Lester E: Ultrasound in the staging of lymphoma. Radiology 1977;124:483

106. Brascho DJ, Durant JR, Green LE: The accuracy of retroperitoneal ultrasonography in Hodgkin's disease and non-Hodgkin's lymphoma. Radiology 1977;125:485

107. Kaude JV, Joyce PH: Evaluation of abdominal lymphoma by ultrasound. Gastrointest Radiol 1980;5:249

108. Asher WM, Friemanis AK: Echographic diagnosis of retroperitoneal lymph node enlargement. AJR 1969; 105:438

109. Neiman HL: Retroperitoneum. p. 90. In Goldberg BB (ed): Clinics in Diagnostic Ultrasound: Ultrasound in Cancer. Vol. 6. Churchill Livingstone, New York, 1981

110. Kobayashi T, Takatani O, Kimura K: Echographic patterns of malignant lymphoma. J Clin Ultrasound 1976;4:181

111. Leopold GR: A review of retroperitoneal ultrasonography. J Clin Ultrasound 1973;1:82

112. Creed H, Reger K, Pond GD, Aapro M: Potential pitfall in CT and sonographic evaluation of suspected lymphoma. AJR 1982;139:606

113. Schnur MJ, Hoffman JC, Koenigsberg M: Gray scale ultrasonic demonstration of peripancreatic adenopathy. J Ultrasound Med 1982;1:139

114. Mueller PR, Ferrucci JT Jr, Harbin WP et al: Appearance of lymphomatous involvement of the mesentery by ultrasonography and body computed tomography: the "sandwich sign." Radiology 1980;134:467

115. Dunnick NR, Reaman GH, Head GL et al: Radiologic manifestation of Burkitt's lymphoma in American patient. AJR 1979;132:1

116. Shawker TH, Dannick NR, Head GL, Magrath IT: Ultrasound evaluation of American Burkitt's lymphoma. J Clin Ultrasound 1979;7:279

117. Hillman BJ, Haber K: Echographic characteristics of malignant lymph nodes. J Clin Ultrasound 1980;8:213

118. Townsend RR, Laing FC, Jeffrey RB, Bottles K: Abdominal lymphoma in AIDS: evaluation with US. Radiology 1989;171:719

119. Yee JM, Raghavendra BN, Horii SC, Ambrosino M: Abdominal sonography in AIDS: a review. J Ultrasound Med 1989;8:705

120. Radin DR, Baker EL, Klatt EC et al: Visceral and nodal calcification in patients with AIDS-related *Pneumocystis carinii* infection. AJR 1990;154:27

121. Bach DB, Vellet AD: Retroperitoneal sarcoidosis. AJR 1991;156:520

122. Deutch SJ, Sandler MA, Tankanow LB: Abdominal lymphadenopathy in sarcoidosis. J Ultrasound Med 1987;6:237

123. Zornoza J, Jonsson K, Wallace S, Lukeman JM: Fine needle aspiration biopsy of retroperitoneal lymph node and abdominal masses: an updated report. Radiology 1977;125:87

124. Zornoza J, Cabranillas FF, Altoff TM et al: Percutaneous needle biopsy in abdominal lymphoma. AJR 1981;136:97

125. Neumann CH, Robert NJ, Rosenthal D, Canellos G: Clinical value of ultrasonography for the management of non-Hodgkin's lymphoma patients as compared with abdominal computed tomography. J Comput Assist Tomogr 1983;7:666

126. Derchi LE, Rizzatto G, Banderali A et al: Sonographic appearance of primary retroperitoneal cysts. J Ultrasound Med 1989;8:381

127. Chung W-M, Ting YM, Gagliardi RA: Ultrasonic diagnosis of retroperitoneal liposarcoma. J Clin Ultrasound 1978;6:266

128. Karp W, Hufstrom LO, Jonsson PE: Retroperitoneal sarcoma: ultrasonographic and angiographic evaluation. Br J Radiol 1980;53:525

129. deSantos LA, Goldstein HM: Ultrasonography in tumors arising from the spine and bony pelvis. AJR 1977;129:1061

130. Schut JM, van Imhoff WL: Retroperitoneal malignant fibrous histiocytoma: an unusual echographic presentation. J Clin Ultrasound 1987;15:145

131. Walsh J, Taylor KJW, Rosenfield AT: Gray scale ultrasonography in retroperitoneal lymphangiomyomatosis. AJR 1977;129:1101

132. Fisher MF, Fletcher BD, Dahms BB et al: Abdominal lipoblastomatosis: radiographic, echographic and computed tomographic findings. Radiology 1981;138:593

133. Lorigan JG, David DL, Evans HL, Wallace S: The clinical and radiologic manifestations of hemangiopericytoma. AJR 1989;153:345

134. Grant EG, Gromvall S, Sarosi TE et al: Sonographic findings in four cases of hemangiopericytoma: correlation with computed tomographic, angiographic, and pathologic findings. Radiology 1982;142:477

135. Davidson AJ, Hartman DS: Lymphangioma of the retroperitoneum: CT and sonographic characteristics. Radiology 1990;175:507

136. Sheth S, Nussbaum AR, Hutchins GM, Sanders RC: Cystic hygromas in children: sonographic-pathologic correlation. Radiology 1987;162:821

137. Hayes WS, Davidson AJ, Grimley PM, Hartman DS: Extraadrenal retroperitoneal paraganglioma: clinical, pathologic and CT findings. AJR 1990;155:1247

138. Aston JK: Ultrasound demonstration of retroperitoneal teratoma. J Clin Ultrasound 1979;7:377

139. Weinstein BJ, Lenkey JL, Williams S: Ultrasound and CT demonstration of a benign cystic teratoma arising from the retroperitoneum. AJR 1979;133:936

140. Davidson AJ, Hartman DS, Goldman SM: Mature teratoma of the retroperitoneum: radiologic, pathologic, and clinical correlation. Radiology 1989;172:421

13

Kidney

Carol A. Mittelstaedt

NATIVE KIDNEY

In the past decade ultrasound of the kidney has become a valuable and common examination. Initially ultrasound was used to evaluate renal masses to determine whether they were cystic or solid. However, the more common applications of renal ultrasound have been expanded to include (1) evaluation for hydronephrosis, (2) evaluation of the nonvisualized kidney on excretory urography, (3) evaluation of a flank mass in a neonate or child, and (4) evaluation for a renal abscess, among others. Although the sonogram is best performed with direct reference to a previous intravenous urogram when a mass is present, it may be performed without the aid of the urogram when radiation exposure is unwarranted, such as during pregnancy, when the patient is allergic to radiographic contrast material, or when poor renal function precludes an adequate intravenous urographic study.

In more recent years, urinary tract ultrasound has been expanded to include evaluation of the bladder and ureters (see Ch. 14), as well as the renal transplant and Doppler ultrasound of the urinary tract. The clinical usefulness of this modality depends to a significant degree on how well the urinary tract structure and its surroundings are visualized. This, in turn, is dependent on the sonographic technique and the examiner's knowledge. As with other organ systems, the use of the newer high-resolution real-time systems has vastly improved and facilitated ultrasound examination of the urinary tract.

TECHNIQUE

Preparation

No specific preparation is required for a renal ultrasound examination. For a Doppler examination of the renal vessels, it is best to have the patient fasting for at least 6 hours; an overnight fast is preferred. Occasionally, sedation is necessary in very young patients. The requirement for sedation is much less frequent than in former years because the examination is performed primarily by real-time systems that can allow more patient movement without compromising the study. However, with the Doppler examination, it is essential that the patient is cooperative—able to hold still and to hold a breath when required.

Ultrasound Examination

Evaluation of the kidneys is a real-time examination. It is much faster to find the kidney, determine its long axis, and complete a satisfactory study with real-time systems than with the previously used static systems. There is more flexibility using the real-time transducer, and the system is portable, enabling the performance of high-quality studies out of the ultrasound laboratory.

The right kidney is best visualized with the patient supine or in the left lateral decubitus position, using the liver as an acoustic window (Fig. 13-1). The left kidney is best scanned in the right lateral decubitus position, with the spleen or fluid-filled stomach as an acoustic window.[1] The right kidney may be best visualized by scanning in the anterior axillary line, whereas the left may be best seen by scanning in the posterior axillary line[2] (Fig. 13-1). In the decubitus position, the true frontal plane of the kidney is viewed so that lesions in the kidney and perirenal and pararenal spaces can be easily located.[3] The coronal view also has the advantage of allowing easier differentiation between a parapelvic cyst and hydronephrosis.[4] The medial and lateral borders of the kidneys are better visualized in the decubitus position.[5]

Although it is possible to evaluate the kidneys with the patient prone, there are more problems associated with optimal visualization in this position than in the decubitus position. In the prone position, the paraspinal muscles may attenuate much of the sound beam and the lower ribs cast acoustic shadows, lending to a suboptimal examination.[1] If the patient can be scanned only in the prone position, a pillow or rolled sheet placed under the anterior abdomen at the level of the kidneys will improve the renal image because the compression reduces the thickness of the soft tissues overlying the kidneys, thus lessening the sound attenuation.[6] Also, the scattering and absorption of the sound beam will be reduced.[6] Similarly, in the decubitus position there is less interference from adjacent tissue and closer correlation with the functional anatomy of the kidney.[7] In the prone or supine position the dorsal and ventral borders of the kidneys are better visualized.[5]

Scans are generally obtained with the patient in the position that allows optimal visualization. The primary positions are described above. If the patient cannot be examined in the decubitus position, coronal scans through each flank can be obtained in the supine position. It is often helpful to examine the kidney in more than one position.

As with all ultrasound studies, the highest-frequency transducer that allows adequate visualization of parenchymal detail in each projection should be used. For adults, this is generally a 3- to 5-MHz transducer; in children, a 5- to 7.5-MHz scanhead may be used.

Optimal demonstration of renal parenchymal anatomy and renal mass lesions requires appropriate gain settings. The gain setting will vary with the kind of machine and transducer used; determination of the correct gain setting therefore requires significant experience with the equipment.[8] The ultrasound beam is attenuated exponentially during its passage through tissue. To compensate for the attenuation, selective amplification of the distant echoes compared with the proximal ones is obtained by the time gain compensation (TGC). The operator must set the proper TGC to achieve even-sized echoes throughout the homogenous tissue.[9] The gain

should be high enough to fill the cortex but low enough that the medulla is not obliterated[8] (Fig. 13-1).

There are several components to a complete renal ultrasound examination. Each kidney should be scanned carefully in the sagittal and transverse planes. The maximum superior-inferior length of the kidney should be obtained during held inspiration. (Fig. 13-1). Several measurements should be taken and averaged. The renal cortical echodensity should be compared with that of the liver at a comparable level and evaluated for uniformity (Fig. 13-1). The renal medullary pyramids should be identified in most patients, and in many cases a cortical thickness measurement can be obtained by measuring from the corticomedullary junction (Fig. 13-1). The corticomedullary junction is identified by the arcuate vessel interface. The renal sinus should be identified with an evaluation for signs of hydronephrosis. The renal artery and renal vein are often seen during real-time examination, with the artery being the posterior vessel (Fig. 13-2). Whether there is respiratory motion of the kidney should be noted. Generally, the examination is concluded if there is no solid mass or hydronephrosis. If hydronephrosis is present, the examiner must try to identify the ureter. If the bladder is distended, the kidney can be rescanned for evidence of hydronephrosis after voiding. If a solid renal mass is present, the examination is not complete without evaluation of the renal vein and the inferior vena cava, as well as the liver.

Doppler Examination

Hilar Vessels

To adequately evaluate the renal arteries, it is necessary to use a low-frequency (2- to 3.5-MHz) transducer with a focal point in the vicinity of the depth of the renal artery.[10] The sample volume must also be varied. By using a minimal sample volume size, the angle is adjusted to achieve the optimum Doppler signal; accurate measurement of the angle is not always possible.[11] The patient may be scanned supine first in the sagittal plane for identification of the renal arteries. The aorta and inferior vena cava should be identified along with the right renal artery, which is seen coursing posterior to the inferior vena cava[11] (Fig. 13-2). The velocity in the aorta adjacent to the renal arteries may be recorded.[10] The transducer is turned to the transverse plane at the level of the right renal artery, and the lateral branches of the aorta are sought[11] (Fig. 13-2C). When possible, the renal arteries are scanned over their entire length.[11] To interrogate the right renal artery, the transducer is moved slightly to the left in the abdomen; it is angled toward the right to achieve an angle with the vessel of less than 60 degrees[11] (Fig. 13-2). For more frequent visualization of

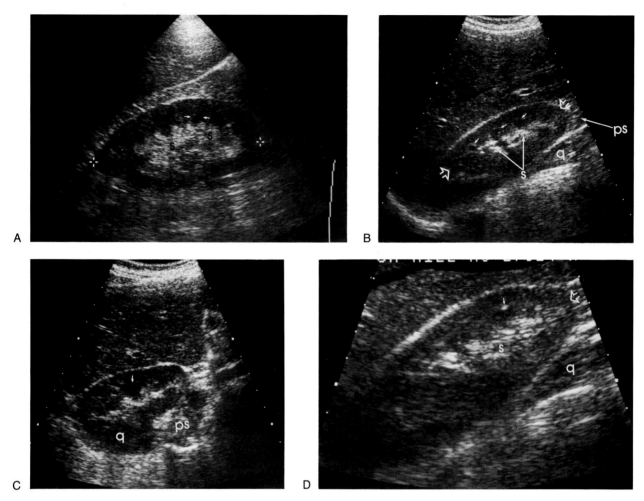

Fig. 13-1. Normal right kidney. **(A & B)** Sagittal scans in two different patients with the transducer in the anterior axillary line. **(C)** Transverse view of the kidney from Fig. B. The renal pyramids (small arrows) are seen as triangular, poorly defined hypoechoic areas in the region of the medulla. **(D)** By magnifying the view of the lower pole in Fig. B, the pyramids are better visualized. The arcuate artery may be seen as an echodense dot (arrow) at the corticomedullary junction on Fig. D. The renal cortex, between the medulla and renal capsule, is slightly less dense than liver. The renal sinus *(s)* is the echodense central area. The renal length (calipers, open arrows) can be determined by measuring from the superior to the inferior pole. (*q,* quadratus lumborum muscle; *ps,* psoas muscle.)

the laterally arising renal arteries, the patient may be placed in the left lateral decubitus position to obtain a coronal view of the major vessels (Fig. 13-2F).

Other investigators use a translumbar approach with the examined side slightly elevated.[12] The kidneys are imaged in the transverse or coronal projection, positioning the range gate in the renal hilum. In this position, measurements can be performed in the distal renal artery and/or the proximal part of the segmental artery.[12]

Evaluation for Parenchymal Disease

Proper technique is crucial for obtaining useful information in any Doppler examination. In most Doppler studies of the kidney, 2.25- to 3.5-MHz transducers are used and color Doppler is not required.[13] The patient may be examined in the right and left anterior oblique positions. The Doppler sample volume (set to 2 at 5 mm) is placed at the corticomedullary junction of the kidney (arcuate arteries) or along the border of medullary pyramids (interlobar arteries)[13,14] (Fig. 13-3). These are extremely small vessels, which have relatively low velocities with associated small frequency shifts. If the wrong Doppler settings are used, only slight deflections from the baseline will be produced, making accurate resistance measurement more difficult. The lowest wall filter for the particular machine should be used to offset this problem.[13] The Doppler examination should be done by using the scale with the smallest possible frequency range (minimum pulse repetition frequency)

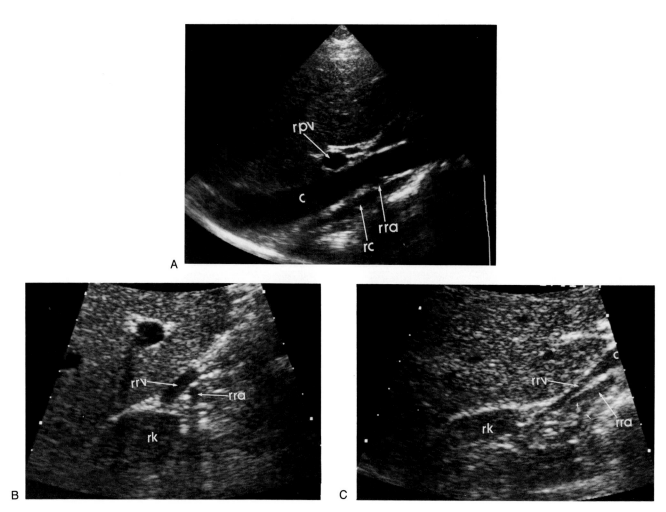

Fig. 13-2. Normal right renal vessels. **(A)** The right renal artery *(rra)* is localized on a sagittal view of the inferior vena cava *(c)*. *(rpv,* right portal vein; *rc,* right crus.) **(B)** By moving the transducer slightly to the right, the right renal artery *(rra)* and vein *(rrv)* can be seen within the renal hilum. *(rk,* right kidney.) **(C)** The transducer is turned almost transversely to visualize the right renal artery *(rra)* and vein *(rrv)* in long axis. In this case, there are two renal arteries (small arrows) in the renal hilum. *(rk,* right kidney.) *(Figure continues.)*

that does not produce aliasing. With this, the highest sensitivity to low flow is produced and a spectrum that fills as much of the scale as possible is generated.[13]

Intrarenal impedance may be characterized by the resistive index (RI), which is an easily calculated, commonly used Doppler parameter.[13] The RI represents the peak systolic shift minus the minimum diastolic shift divided by the peak systolic shift.[13] Sampling must be done from at least three different sites within the kidney for most renal examinations to obtain a mean intrarenal arterial RI. The proper technique is not difficult, although it is operator-dependent, and a full renal Doppler study (both kidneys) may be obtained within 15 minutes.[13]

Hydronephrosis versus Vessels

Doppler ultrasound may be used to help differentiate true collecting system dilatation and hilar vessels.[15] First, duplex ultrasound or color Doppler may be used to assess the lucent area in the region of the collecting system to ensure that it is indeed the collecting system (no signal, no flow) rather than renal hilar vessels (positive flow).[15] In 43 percent of patients (61 percent of patients 12 years or younger) in one series, it was shown that vascular structures accounted for the separation of the renal sinus echoes.[15] By performing this simple procedure, the false-positive diagnosis of hydronephrosis should be kept to a minimum.

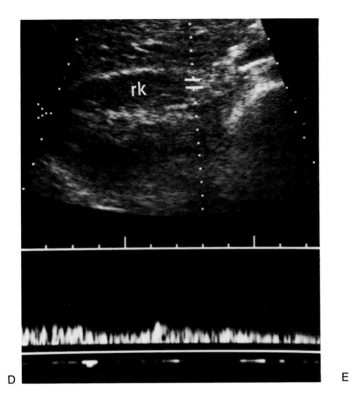

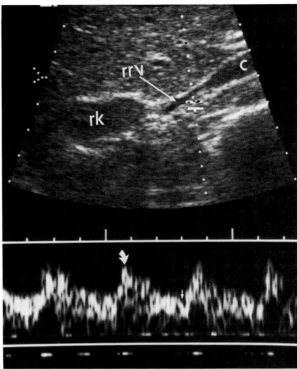

D

E

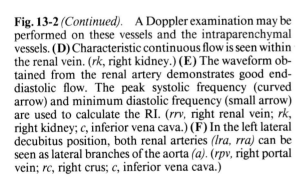

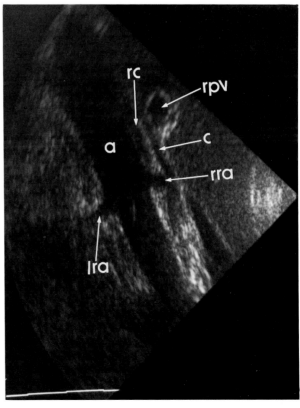

Fig. 13-2 *(Continued).* A Doppler examination may be performed on these vessels and the intraparenchymal vessels. **(D)** Characteristic continuous flow is seen within the renal vein. (*rk,* right kidney.) **(E)** The waveform obtained from the renal artery demonstrates good end-diastolic flow. The peak systolic frequency (curved arrow) and minimum diastolic frequency (small arrow) are used to calculate the RI. (*rrv,* right renal vein; *rk,* right kidney; *c,* inferior vena cava.) **(F)** In the left lateral decubitus position, both renal arteries *(lra, rra)* can be seen as lateral branches of the aorta *(a).* (*rpv,* right portal vein; *rc,* right crus; *c,* inferior vena cava.)

F

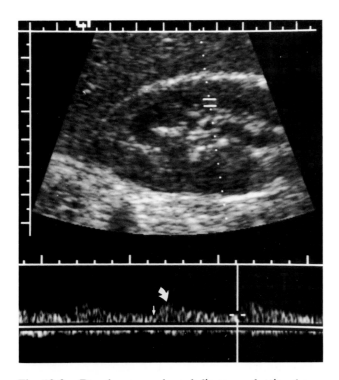

Fig. 13-3. Doppler, parenchymal disease evaluation (same patient as in Fig. 13-2). The RI, which is determined at the corticomedullary junction, is 0.53. This is determined by using the peak systolic frequency (curved arrow) and the minimum diastolic frequency (small arrow). This value is within normal limits.

Obstructive versus Nonobstructive Pyelocaliectasis

Doppler ultrasound may also be used to assist in the differentiation of obstructive versus nonobstructive pyelocaliectasis.[16,17] For this examination, pulsed Doppler evaluation of the intrarenal arteries may be performed on each kidney. This examination may be performed on the arcuate arteries at the corticomedullary junction and/or interlobar arteries along the border of the medullary pyramids (Fig. 13-4). Gray-scale images of the kidney are obtained along with multiple Doppler signal tracings. The RI (peak systolic frequency shift minus the minimum diastolic frequency shift divided by the peak systolic frequency shift) is obtained. A nonobstructive kidney should have an RI of less than 0.70.[16] This technique may also be used to assess adequate therapy (percutaneous nephrostomy, internal stent, etc.), since the RI should decrease if adequate therapy has been achieved.

Diuretic Examination

Besides using Doppler ultrasound to assist in the differentiation of obstructive versus nonobstructive pyelocaliectasis, a diuretic ultrasound examination may be performed.[18,19] To perform this test, a baseline renal ultrasound is done first to obtain a clear measurement of the degree of collecting system dilatation. After the ini-

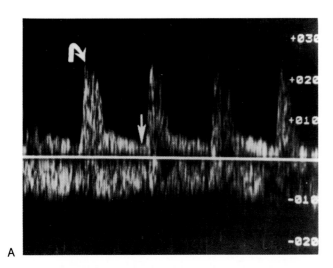

A

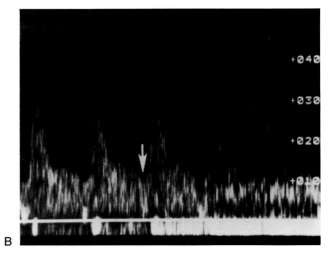

B

Fig. 13-4. Doppler, obstructive versus nonobstructive pyelocaliectasis. **(A)** Doppler tracing obtained from the intrarenal artery of the kidney with a dilated, obstructed collecting system. Representative points where peak systolic flow (curved arrow) and lowest diastolic flow (straight arrow) were measured are indicated. Flow beneath the baseline is venous (RI = 0.81). **(B)** Doppler tracing obtained from the intrarenal artery 4 days after nephrostomy. End-diastolic flow has increased (arrow), and the RI has decreased to 0.65. (From Platt et al,[17] with permission.)

tial scan, 250 ml of physiologic saline and 40 mg of furosemide are injected intravenously (over 15 to 20 minutes) and renal scans are obtained at 5, 10, and 15 minutes.[18] Alternatively, patients with renal pelvis dilatation of 10 mm may be given 20 to 40 mg of furosemide orally or 0.3 mg/kg intravenously with scans repeated at 30, 60, and 90 minutes.[19] After the patient voids, further renal scans are obtained at 30, 45, 60, 90, 120, and 150 minutes in both the upright and supine positions.[18] The procedure is performed similarly in young children, with the infusion of physiologic saline being related to the patient's weight (5 ml/kg) and the furosemide dose being 0.5 to 1 mg/kg.[18] The relative increase in the pelvicalyceal diameters and the time taken for the renal collecting system to return to its initial dimensions are assessed.[18] This dynamic diuretic ultrasound technique has a sensitivity of 94 percent, a specificity of 94 percent, a positive predictive value of 91 percent (obstructive), a negative predictive value of 96 percent (nonobstructive), and a total diagnostic capacity of 94 percent.[18]

Pediatric

The renal ultrasound examination of the child does not differ greatly from the adult examination. However, it is critical to maintain body temperature, so heaters and warm gel are used. With the real-time systems, this examination can be performed in the neonatal intensive care unit. Sedation is rarely indicated. At times it is advantageous to examine the neonatal kidneys by using a coronal approach.[20] With this technique there is little manipulation of the infant, less hindrance from monitoring devices or tubes, and improved visualization of the retroperitoneal structures as a result of less interference by bowel gas.

When evaluating a neonate with a renal mass, it is important to examine the contralateral kidney because there is a high incidence of abnormalities, as well as implications of bilateral disease.[21] The enlarged kidney may function as a sonic window through which to view the contralateral one. With the patient in an anterior oblique position with the enlarged kidney anteriorly, longitudinal oblique scans via a flank approach can be performed.[21]

NORMAL ANATOMY

The kidney is covered by a fibrous capsule closely applied but not adherent to the parenchyma. Surrounded by fat, the kidney is bounded anteriorly and posteriorly by the fibrous sheath, Gerota's fascia; laterally and anterior and posterior leaves fuse to form the lateroconal fascia, which becomes continuous with the peritoneum along the abdominal wall.[2] The perirenal space is closed superiorly and laterally and does not communicate across the midline. It is open or potentially open inferiorly. As such, inflammation could track inferiorly or track back superiorly into the posterior pararenal space.

Adult

Cortex

The normal adult renal cortex has been described as homogeneously echogenic with low-level echoes similar in density to that of liver parenchyma[8] (Fig. 13-1). Alternatively, the cortex may be less echogenic than the liver (in the absence of hepatic disease), spleen, or renal sinus.[22] Although, in the past, a density similar to that of the liver was described as abnormal, it has been shown that 72 percent of such patients have normal renal function.[23]

In a normal kidney, the renal vascular bed has low impedance to blood flow, which is reflected by continuous forward flow in diastole[13] (Figs. 13-2 and 13-3). A mean RI of 0.58 ± 0.05 with a maximum normal value of 0.67 has been reported in a larger series of normal subjects.[13]

Medulla

The normal medullary pyramids are hypoechoic and are usually 1.2 to 1.5 cm thick[24] (Figs. 13-1 and 13-5). The medulla and cortex can be differentiated in approximately half of adult patients depending on the patient's body habitus and the frequency of the transducer.[22] This corticomedullary differentiation is best demonstrated with a high-frequency transducer.[22] There may be a change in medullary detection with patient hydration, becoming more prominent with diuresis.[22] The arcuate vessels at the corticomedullary junction are recognized as discrete high-level echoes; they serve as a marker for evaluation of cortical thickness[8,9,25,26] (Figs. 13-1 and 13-5). These arcuate vessels can be identified in 25 percent of patients.[8,22] Renal columns of Bertin consist of cortical tissue extending into the space between adjacent pyramids[24] (Figs. 13-5 and 13-6).

The finding of a compound renal pyramid has been described.[27] This compound calyx is generally found at the poles of the kidney and occurs in a high percentage of patients.[27] There is at least one compound papilla in 70 percent of kidneys, with 50 percent in the upper pole, 30 percent in the lower pole, and 20 percent in the midpole.[27] A compound pyramid is associated with a com-

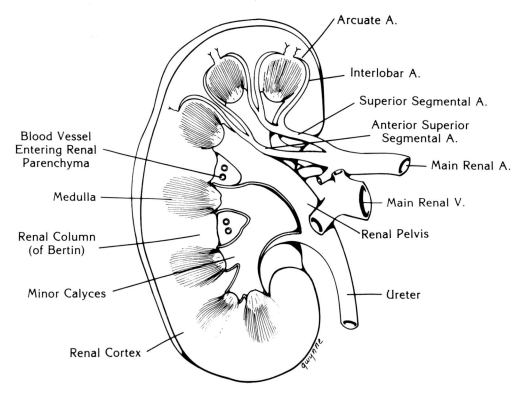

Fig. 13-5. Kidney section. Cut section through the right kidney showing the internal anatomy.

pound calyx. It is more evident on a pediatric sonogram since these patients tend to be thinner, allowing the use of a high-frequency transducer. This complex gives rise to a hypoechoic area, which may mimic abnormalities such as obstruction of the upper pole of a duplex system, focal caliectasis, simple cyst, hydrocalyx due to infundibular stenosis from a crossing vessel, or a hypoechoic mass.[27] This hypoechoic area is a well-defined, irregular, hypoechoic region without calyceal distortion, especially in the upper pole, and should not be misinterpreted[27] (Fig. 13-7).

Sinus

The renal sinus contains the collecting system, renal vessels, lymphatics, fat, and fibrous tissue (Fig. 13-5). The renal sinus appears as an ovoid intense echo collection in the kidney in the longitudinal plane and as a rounded echodense area in the transverse plane[28,29] (Figs. 13-1 and 13-2). If the collecting system is bifid, two lobulations of echodensity may be seen[2] (Fig. 13-8). If there is an infiltrative process such as edema, fibrosis, or cellular infiltration, a change in the appearance of the sinus will be produced that usually renders it inhomogeneous or less echogenic with less distinction between the renal sinus and parenchyma.

Collecting System

Duplication. It may be difficult to identify a nondilated duplicated collecting system on imaging studies (Fig. 13-8). Its identification is usually straightforward when it is dilated and/or associated with either an ectopic ureter or an ectopic ureterocele (Fig. 13-9). A duplex system should be suspected "whenever duplication occurs on the contralateral side regardless of the (ipsilateral) radiographic appearance."[30] The ultrasound signs may be absent when there is a diminutive nonfunctioning upper moiety.[30]

Artifacts secondary to sound beam refraction are common. Such a renal duplication artifact has been described. This artifact appears as a duplication of the collecting system, as a suprarenal mass, or as upper-pole cortical thickening[31] (Figs. 13-10 and 13-11). This artifact has been shown to be due to sound beam refraction between the lower pole of the spleen or liver and adjacent fat. When sound waves pass obliquely through an interface between tissues with different sound transmission rates, they are bent.[31] This refraction has a magnitude proportional to the difference in the speed of sound in the two tissues.[31] These refraction artifacts occur to a greater degree between soft tissue-fat interfaces.[31]

When sound travels totally in the fat below the spleen, it is not refracted; therefore renal tissue positioned below

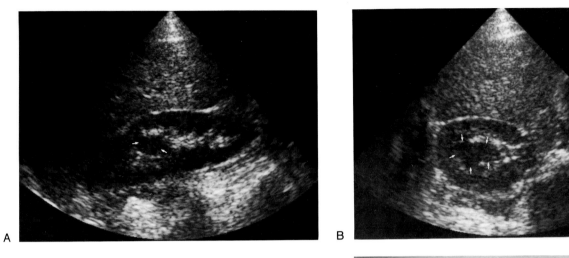

A

B

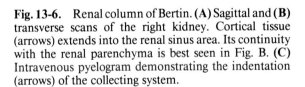

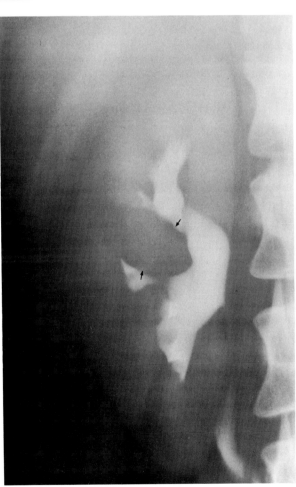

Fig. 13-6. Renal column of Bertin. **(A)** Sagittal and **(B)** transverse scans of the right kidney. Cortical tissue (arrows) extends into the renal sinus area. Its continuity with the renal parenchyma is best seen in Fig. B. **(C)** Intravenous pyelogram demonstrating the indentation (arrows) of the collecting system.

C

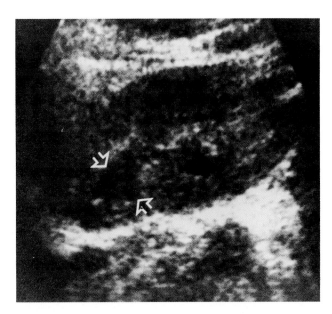

Fig. 13-7. Compound renal pyramid. Sagittal scan of the right kidney of a 3-year-old boy with hematuria demonstrating a large, irregular, hypoechoic area in the upper pole (arrows), representing a normal compound pyramid. The low-level echoes and the lack of through transmission distinguish this from a focal hydronephrosis. However, this appearance was mistaken for a hypoechoic mass. (From Jones et al,[27] with permission.)

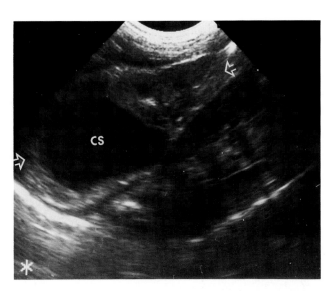

Fig. 13-9. Duplicated collecting system, dilatation. Sagittal view of the right kidney (arrows) demonstrating a large anechoic area *(cs)* in the upper pole. This represents a dilated upper pole collecting system.

the spleen is localized correctly on the image.[31] The sound that enters and exits the convex lower pole of the spleen is refracted inferiorly, and so the upper pole of the kidney is localized incorrectly on the image. This produces the duplication of the portion of the upper pole

that has been crossed by the unrefracted sound traveling below the spleen and refracted sound passing through the lower pole of the spleen.[31] It is visualized much more commonly in the left kidney and occurs more frequently in the obese patient.[31]

To avoid this duplication artifact, the transducer may be moved more superiorly on the patient such that the sound beam is traveling completely through the spleen and does not encounter an interface between the spleen and fat.[31] It is more likely for refraction at the splenic tip to cause artifacts in the upper pole of the left kidney than for refraction at the liver tip to cause artifacts in the upper pole of the right kidney.[31] The increased frequency of this artifact within obese patients may be due to the amount of perisplenic fat, which may affect either the magnitude of refraction or the positions of the spleen and kidney so that the refraction results in a more obvious artifact.[31] It is important to recognize the appearance and cause of this artifact to avoid diagnostic errors.[31]

Wall Thickening. As a rule, the collecting system is not normally distended and its walls are not defined (Figs. 13-1 and 13-2). It has been only recently, with the advent of high-resolution ultrasound, that visualization of the abnormal wall of the collecting system has been described. This thickening is best seen on the surfaces perpendicular to the ultrasound beam, most often in the renal pelvis but also in some calyces and ureters[32] (Fig. 13-12). The TGC curve must be set at a low level to minimize the background echoes that could create a false image of thickening. Thickening of the wall of the

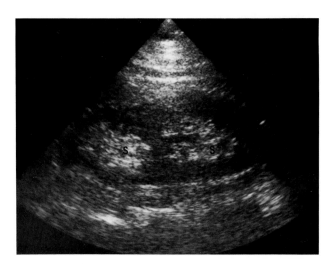

Fig. 13-8. Bifid collecting system. Sagittal scan of the left kidney demonstrating two separate echodense areas *(s)* in the region of the renal sinus.

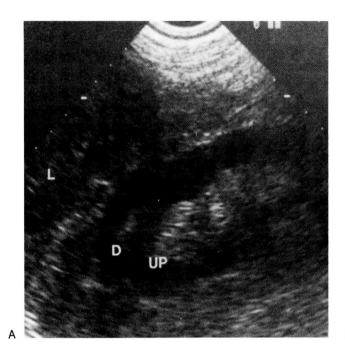
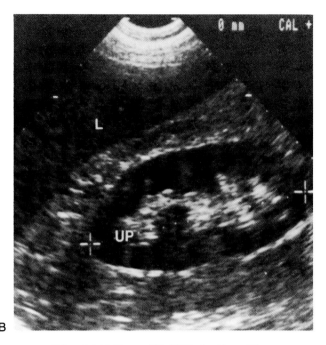

A   B

Fig. 13-10. Renal duplication, artifact. Longitudinal sonograms of the right kidney. **(A)** With the liver *(L)* positioned over the upper pole *(UP)* of the kidney, there is artifactual duplication *(D)* of that pole. **(B)** With the transducer repositioned superiorly, the liver *(L)* completely covers the kidney and the artifactual duplication is eliminated. *(UP,* upper pole.) (From Middleton and Melson,[31] with permission.)

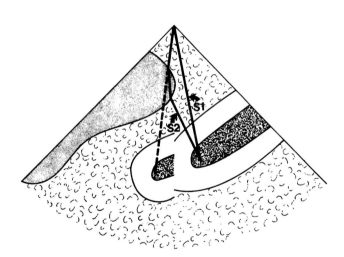

Fig. 13-11. Renal duplication, artifact. Production of the renal duplication artifact. Sound traveling entirely in fat below the spleen *(S1)* is not refracted, and therefore the infrasplenic portion of the kidney is accurately displayed on the image. Sound traveling through the tip of the spleen *(S2)* is refracted inferiorly as it enters and exits the spleen, allowing it to reflect off the upper pole of the kidney in a location similar to S1. Because localization of reflecting interfaces assumes a straight path for the sound (dotted line), the upper pole is duplicated in a more superior location. (From Middleton and Melson,[31] with permission.)

collecting system has been evaluated and identified as a nonspecific finding associated with urinary tract infection, reflux, or chronic obstruction.[32] Others have reported this finding in association with acute tubular necrosis, urinary tract infection complicating hydronephrosis, congenital hydronephrosis after pyeloplasty, congenital hydronephrosis due to reflux, and total parenteral nutrition.[33] In renal transplant patients, this thickening has been found to represent submucosal edema in those with acute rejection; it has also been associated with inflammatory cell infiltrate, fibrosis, muscular hypertrophy, or hemorrhage into the submucosal space, although these findings are speculative.[33] It has been seen to resolve after therapy.[32,33] Very slight thickening (<2 mm) is of uncertain significance.[32] Its increasing recognition may be secondary to the improved resolution of modern ultrasound equipment and increased awareness by the sonologist.[33] As such, this finding should be correlated with the clinical and laboratory findings.[32]

Parenchyma Variations

Junctional Defect. The kidney is thought to develop by fusion of an upper and a lower parenchymatous "mass."[34] The superior mass lies posteriorly with its

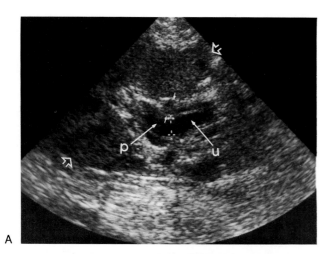

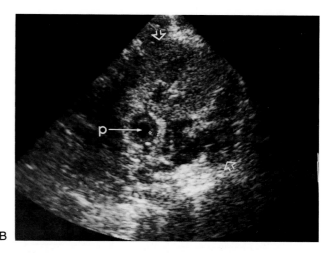

A   B

Fig. 13-12.   Collecting system, wall thickening. **(A)** Sagittal and **(B)** transverse scans through the renal pelvis *(p)* and ureter *(u)* of a renal transplant (open arrows) showing thickening (4 mm, arrows) of the wall of the collecting system. This renal transplant was undergoing rejection.

sinus opening anteriorly or anteromedially, with the inferior mass lying anteriorly and overlapping the superior mass.[34] The sinus of the inferior mass is directed medially or posteromedially.[34] In the region where the two masses overlap, the cortices often form an oblique coronal plane corresponding to the "intermediate cortical mass."[34] The renal pelvis exits medially from the inferior mass, with the renal vein usually emerging from the kidney anteriorly from the sinus of the superior mass.[34] Fat within the sinus from the superior mass may cause an impression, on a sagittal scan, of an echogenic mass bordered cranially by parenchyma of the superior mass and caudally by parenchyma of the inferior mass, which overlies its more horizontally directed sinus.[34]

This echogenic parenchymal defect, which assumes a triangular appearance on slightly more lateral parasagittal images, may have a small tongue of fat extending from the sinus laterally and superiorly along a slight depression in the parenchyma that marks the anterior junction of the superior and inferior masses (Fig. 13-13A – C). This junctional parenchymal defect is usually oriented more horizontally than vertically and is best depicted on sagittal scans.[34] It is frequently demonstrated as an echogenic area in the anterior aspect of the upper-pole parenchyma of the right kidney. Similarly, one may be visualized on the left in the posterior aspect. The visualization on the left depends on the availability of an anterior acoustic window, such as with splenomegaly.

The triangular echogenic focus of perirenal tissue in the anterosuperior or posteroinferior margin of the kidney, the junctional parenchymal defect, and an oblique echogenic line (the interrenicular septum) connecting the junctional defect to the renal hilum are normal ultrasound findings in children[35] (Fig. 13-13D). In a series of children, either the junctional defect or the interrenicular junction defect has been demonstrated in 46 percent of right kidneys and 19 percent of left kidneys.[35] The junctional defect was seen in 47 percent of right kidneys and 18 percent of left kidneys, with the interrenicular junction defect seen in 39 percent of right kidneys and 12 percent of left kidneys.[35] The incidence of these defects appears to be unrelated to age.[35] There is a lower incidence in the first year of life, which may be related to the lack of echogenic fat in the perirenal and hilar spaces.[35]

A spectrum of fusion defects may be identified. To differentiate these junctional parenchymal defects from a pathologic abnormality, the examiner must rely on the lesion's characteristic anterior and superior location and trace it medially and slightly inferiorly into the renal sinus.[34] The examiner must be aware of these so as to not confuse them with an abnormality.

Column.   A renal column represents cortical tissue, which runs between papillae and separates them. Within each renal lobe is a central mass of medullary tissue enveloped by a cortical layer. The "cloison" of Bertin is thought to be formed by the fusion of two layers of septal cortex of two adjacent lobes.[36] When these renal columns hypertrophy, they become a diagnostic challenge to radiologists. Many synonyms have been used for this, including renal pseudotumor, focal nodular hyperplasia, cortical invagination with prominent column of Bertin, lobar dysmorphism, benign cortical rest, cortical nodule, and more, recently, cloisons.[36]

There is an increase in both incidence and size of the cloison in the middle third of the kidney.[36] By ultrasound, renal columns are visualized in 47 percent of

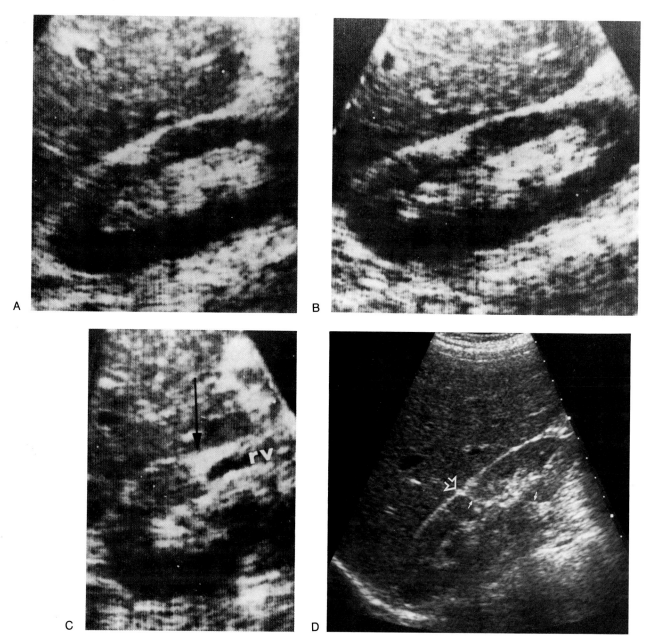

Fig. 13-13. Junctional parenchymal defect (JPD) and interrenicular septum (IRS). Case 1. JPD. **(A)** Sagittal sonogram of the right kidney demonstrating a triangular echogenic focus in the anterior renal parenchyma. **(B)** Sagittal scan slightly medial to this showing the defect becoming more rotund as it approaches the renal sinus. **(C)** Transverse image at the level of the renal vein *(rv)* demonstrating the echogenic defect (arrow) to be continuous with the anteriorly directed renal sinus. Case 2. IRS. **(D)** Parasagittal view of the right kidney somewhat medially. The echogenic IRS (small arrows) runs obliquely from the anterosuperior JPD (open arrow) through the hilum. (Figs. A–C from Carter et al,[34] with permission.)

healthy subjects, with bilaterality in 18 percent and a 4 percent incidence of two columns in one kidney.[22] These hypertrophied columns of Bertin are usually seen less frequently on the right than the left.[36]

Ultrasound has the advantage of imaging the kidney in various planes. The axillary view is especially reveal-

ing in the search for large columns of Bertin.[36] The following signs have been identified as associated with a hypertrophied renal column: (1) it indents the renal sinus laterally; (2) it is clearly defined from the renal sinus; (3) its largest dimension is less than 3 cm: (4) it is contiguous with the renal cortex; and (5) its echogenicity is close to that of the cortex[37,38] (Fig. 13-6). Others describe the following additional descriptions: (1) the sinus may engulf it in a clawlike fashion and (2) the renal contour is smooth.[36] A focal mass that meets all these criteria should be considered a renal column. It may be best seen by scanning the patient in the decubitus position because the column would be in profile.[37] If there is any question, a renal nuclear medicine study may be performed to confirm that the "mass" is composed of functioning tissue.[38]

Length and Volume

The renal dimensions on ultrasound are smaller than those noted by radiography because there is neither geometric magnification nor change in size related to an osmotic diuresis from contrast.[39] At autopsy, the average adult kidney is 11 to 12 cm long and 6 cm wide; on radiography, the average length is 12.5 to 13.5 cm with a width of 6 cm.[39] The normal renal size on ultrasound has been reported to be 10 cm long, 5 cm wide, and 2.5 cm thick[40] (Fig. 13-1). Others report an ultrasound length of 9 to 13 cm for a person of average height.[22] The normal size depends on a number of variables: age, sex, body habitus, and state of hydration.

Various investigators have evaluated the sonographic renal size. One study found the right mean length in the prone position to be 10.74 cm (standard deviation, 1.35 cm), with the left 11.10 cm (standard deviation, 1.15 cm).[39] Another study correlated the renal length (RL) to the distance between the first four lumbar transverse processes (4TP). To determine the lumbar length, a sagittal scan in the paraspinal location is performed with the patient prone.[41] The RL/4TP ratio was found to be 1.04 ± 0.22 on ultrasound.[41] Ninety-five percent of normal patients fall within this range.[41]

There are pitfalls in using ultrasound to measure renal size. Scanning must be done carefully to obtain the longest axis possible.[39] In addition, the renal inclination (the angle the kidney makes with the horizontal plane) must be taken into account when measuring the maximum renal length[42] (Fig. 13-14).

Determination of renal volume is a more sensitive means of detecting renal size abnormalities than is any single linear measurement of the kidney.[43,44] The formula for calculating the renal volume is based on a three-dimensional ellipsoid formula adjusted by a correction factor for the magnitude of difference compared with renal volume estimated by water displacement:[45]

$$V = 0.49 \times L \times W \times AP$$

where L is renal length; W is the average measurement from the widths at the hilum and 1 cm above and 1 cm below the hilum; and AP is the anteroposterior dimension.

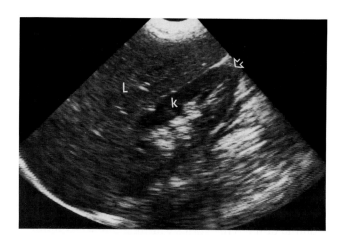

Fig. 13-14. Renal inclination. Sagittal supine scan, right. Note the severe anteroposterior angulation of this right kidney *(k)*. The inferior pole (open arrow) is quite anterior. (*L*, liver.)

Pediatric

Neonate

Cortical Echopattern. In the normal neonate, accentuated corticomedullary differentiation is demonstrated up to 6 months of age[46] (Fig. 13-15). The enhanced corticomedullary differentiation can be explained by an in-

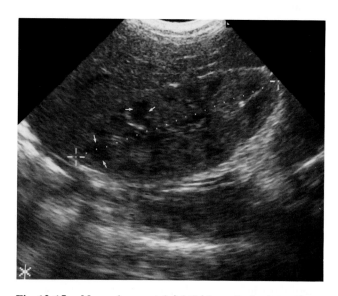

Fig. 13-15. Normal neonatal right kidney. Sagittal scan demonstrating the renal pyramids (small arrows), which are much more prominent in the neonate than in the adult. The pyramids can be differentiated from dilated collecting system in that they do not connect together and they are not as sharply defined as the dilated collecting system. The renal pelvis cannot be identified as such. No real renal sinus fat is visualized. The renal margins (calipers) are much more difficult to define on the freeze-frame image than in the adult. The renal parenchyma blends with the liver parenchyma.

crease in renal cortical echo production possibly combined with a slight decrease in echo production from the renal pyramids. The variation in size and maturity of individual nephrons and glomeruli may contribute to the increased echogenicity of the renal cortex in the neonatal kidney. In the neonatal period, the glomeruli occupy 18 percent of the volume of the cortex compared with 8.6 percent in the adult.[47] Histologically, the glomerular loops are matted together, invaginated, and surrounded by high, columnar epithelium; as they mature, this epithelial layer is lost and the loops expand.[46] The increased echogenicity of the renal cortex is due to the glomeruli, which occupy a proportionately greater volume of the renal cortex during the first 2 months of life.[47]

Studies have been performed to assess the normal echopattern of the cortex in neonates.[48-50] An increased renal cortical echogenicity has been seen in 29 percent of babies.[49] Age appears to be the most important factor associated with the increased echogenicity, with the infant's immaturity the most important determinant.[49] The cortical echogenicity of the newborn kidney decreases with increasing infant weight and maturity.[48] With infant growth and weight gain, the echogenicity of the renal cortex progresses from higher than that of the adjacent liver/spleen to equal to or lower than that of the liver/spleen.[48] The increased echodensity in the newborn may occur because, during the first 2 months of life, the glomeruli occupy a proportionally greater volume of the renal cortex than in the adult kidney, resulting in an increased echogenicity as a result of the increased cellular interfaces.[48] The kidney grows rapidly during the first 2 months of life, mainly because of disproportionate growth of the renal tubules as they increase in length.[47] By 7 months of age, the renal parenchyma demonstrates the adult pattern.[50]

Medulla. The pyramids are triangular and are arranged with their apices pointing toward the central collecting system (Fig. 13-15).[51] The prominent and hypoechoic renal pyramids can be explained by the larger volume of the medulla in the neonate, which results in a ratio of cortex to medulla of 1.64 : 1 in the neonate compared with 2.59 : 1 in the adult.[47] All neonates and 62 percent of infants up to 6 months of age have prominent and anechoic medullary pyramids with accentuation of corticomedullary definition.[50] The arcuate artery, which is seen as a bright reflective dot at the base of the pyramid denoting the corticomedullary junction, serves as a marker for assessment of parenchymal thickness.

Sinus. The echodensity of the urothelial surface of the collecting system calyces and infundibula is less marked than typically seen in the adult kidney, probably representing the paucity of renal sinus fat in the neonate.

Fetal Lobation. The definitive kidney develops both from repeated branching of the ureteric bud and from differentiation of its surrounding primitive mesenchyma.[52] These lobes are well demarcated by sulci as early as 10 weeks gestation in the human fetus.[52] This future kidney may be termed the renunculus. With fusion of renunculi during the late second trimester, the opposing portions of the cortex of two adjacent renunculi or lobes form the cloisons, septa, or columns of Bertin.[52] The renal surface becomes smoother and interlobar grooves less prominent as fusion of the lobes progress in infancy.[52] Sometimes, one or more of these interlobar grooves persist throughout childhood and into adulthood, extending through the renal cortex, partly or completely to the hilum.[52] The most prominent of these are the interrenicular junction defect and the junctional parenchymal defect[52] (Fig. 13-13).

On ultrasound, these interlobar grooves are sharply defined markings, linear on sagittal and triangular on cross-sectional cuts of the kidney[52] (Fig. 13-13). They are seen in the center of a cloison of Bertin and are surrounded on both sides by cortex of normal thickness and echogenicity.[52] These interlobar grooves should not be mistaken for renal scars, which are thicker, less sharply defined, and always accompanied by loss of cortex or hyperechogenic cortical angiomyolipomas that are rounded as opposed to the linear grooves of persistent fetal lobation.[52]

Hilar Vessels. In 98 percent of neonates, the renal hilar arteries and veins may be imaged bilaterally.[48] However, vascular flow within the renal vessels may be documented by Doppler in only 69 percent of the hila examined.[48] This failure to detect vascular flow is frequently attributed to patient motion and at times to lack of tissue penetration in larger infants.[48]

Length and Volume. Various investigators have evaluated the renal length in neonates.[48,50,53,54] One group has correlated neonatal renal length and body weight[48] (Fig. 13-16). A second group has evaluated infants from 2 to 56 weeks, assessing age, weight, length, head circumference, abdominal circumference, and C7-to-coccyx length.[53] In this second series, the net kidney length appeared to correlate best with a combination of infant length and weight[53] (Fig. 13-17). Other groups have measured renal length and volume, correlating them with age, body weight, height, and total body surface area, permitting preparation of nomograms with predicted means and 95 percent prediction intervals.[50]

To determine whether kidney sizes are within normal limits, three scans of each kidney should be obtained.[53] An average length is obtained for each kidney with the best correlate of the left kidney and of the right kidney.[53] Comparison of kidney length with four parameters

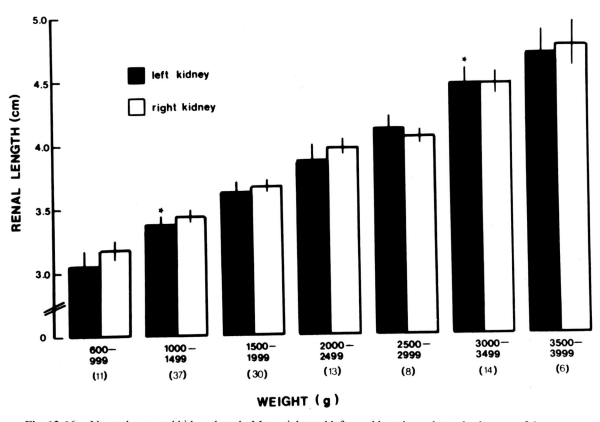

Fig. 13-16. Normal neonatal kidney length. Mean right and left renal lengths and standard errors of the mean (vertical lines) are plotted against infant weight. Asterisks denote the two cases for which left renal lengths were not obtained secondary to overlying chest tube dressings. (From Erwin et al,[48] with permission.)

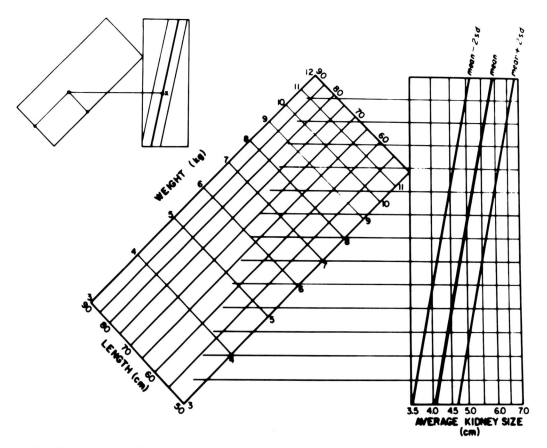

Fig. 13-17. Normal infant kidney length. Nomogram for determination of normal infant kidney lengths. (From Blane et al,[53] with permission.)

(body weight, body length, body surface area, and gestational age) shows that a graph of kidney length versus body weight can yield a linear distribution with a high correlation coefficient[54] (Fig. 13-18).

Renal volume can be calculated as follows: volume (V) = length (L) × thickness (T) × width (W) × 0.5233.[50]

Child

Cortex and Medulla. The echopattern of the renal cortex and medulla in the older child should be similar to that in the adult.

Collecting System. A variation in the ultrasound appearance of the renal pelvis in the pediatric patient has been noted with positional change.[55] When patients were studied in both the supine and prone positions, 30 percent had dilatation of a previously normal renal pelvis in the prone position and 3 percent had increasing dilatation in the prone position.[55] This positional change may be due to a shifting of urine from the normal-sized calyces (when supine) to the distensible renal pelvis (when prone).[55] Additionally, there may be elevation of bladder pressure in the prone position, which may impede urine flow and produce the observed changes.[55] As such, it is important to recognize this positional change and to understand that slight dilatation of the renal pelvis does not necessarily imply a pathologic condition.[55]

The size of the renal pelvis in children has been evaluated by ultrasound.[56] It was found that a 10-mm diameter (maximum anteroposterior measurement) can be considered the upper limit of the normal renal pelvis[56]; only 1.7 percent of normal renal pelvis have been found to exceed 10 mm.[56] Measuring the renal pelvis size by

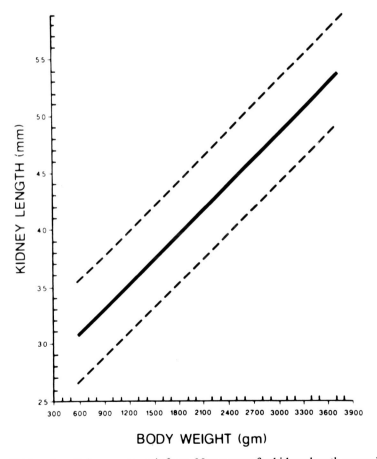

Fig. 13-18. Normal kidney length in premature infants. Nomogram for kidney length versus body weight. The solid line represent the mean, and the dotted line denotes the 95 percent confidence limits. (From Schlesinger et al,[54] with permission.)

ultrasound is highly reliable in diagnosing obstructive uropathy (100 percent sensitivity, 90.3 percent specificity).[56] However, when the 10-mm criterion is used as the sole diagnostic measurement, many nonobstructive hydronephrosis cases may be misdiagnosed.[56] Many factors influence the size of the renal pelvis, yielding false results: (1) bladder distension, (2) increased urine outflow (e.g., from diuretics, contrast agents, diabetes insipidus, overhydration), (3) "floppy" collecting systems caused by infections (e.g., urinary tract infection, pyelonephritis), and (4) cystic renal disease that mimics hydronephrosis.[56] False-negative results may be caused by (1) dehydration, (2) acute obstruction due to the not yet dilated system, (3) obstruction of the distal urinary tract, (4) rupture of the collecting system, and (5) misinterpretation.[56]

Length. Correlation of the ultrasound renal length versus the patient's age is a useful screening tool if the patient is specifically referred for renal ultrasound. As with the adult, the radiographic technique yields some variability in the apparent size of the kidney as a result of differences in centering of the tube and its distance from the patient, phase of respiration, and osmotic effect of iodinated contrast. The neonatal kidney (see above) ranges in length from 3.3 to 5.0 cm (the left being 2 to 5 mm longer) with a width of 2 to 3 cm and a sagittal diameter of 1.5 to 2.5 cm.[51,57] Investigators have found the following formula and Table 13-1 useful in calculating normal renal length[58]:

$$> 1 \text{ yr} - \text{Renal length (cm)} = 6.79 + 0.22 \times \text{age (years)}$$

$$< 1 \text{ yr} - \text{Renal length (cm)} = 4.98 + 0.155 \\ \times \text{age (months)}$$

Ultrasound renal volume correlates better with urologic volume than with urographic renal length. It may therefore be important in monitoring growth patterns in children. The ultrasound length is more accurate than the urographic length. Renal length is defined as the maximum midsagittal length.[59]

Investigators have evaluated the normal renal size in children with myelodysplasia.[60] These patients undergo periodic assessment of the upper urinary tract anatomy, and renal size is an important component of the management of these children. The mean renal length for each age group was found to be below the mean values for normal children.[60] This may reflect a relative decrease in lower body mass that occurs in many, but not all, children with spina bifida.[60] There is development of progressive scoliosis, frequently associated with hyperlordosis or kyphosis with increasing age of the patients.[60] Although the ultrasound measurement of renal length in

TABLE 13-1. Summary of Grouped Observations— Mean Renal Length

Mean Age[a]	Interval[a]	Mean Renal Length (cm)	SD	n
0 mo	0–1 wk	4.48	0.31	10
2 mo	1 wk–4 mo	5.28	0.66	54
6 mo	4–8 mo	6.15	0.67	20
10 mo	8 mo–1 yr	6.23	0.63	8
1.5	1–2	6.65	0.54	28
2.5	2–3	7.36	0.54	12
3.5	3–4	7.36	0.64	30
4.5	4–5	7.87	0.50	26
5.5	5–6	8.09	0.54	30
6.5	6–7	7.83	0.72	14
7.5	7–8	8.33	0.51	18
8.5	8–9	8.90	0.88	18
9.5	9–10	9.20	0.90	14
10.5	10–11	9.17	0.82	28
11.5	11–12	9.60	0.64	22
12.5	12–13	10.42	0.87	18
13.5	13–14	9.79	0.75	14
14.5	14–15	10.05	0.62	14
15.5	15–16	10.93	0.76	6
16.5	16–17	10.04	0.86	10
17.5	17–18	10.53	0.29	4
18.5	18–19	10.81	1.13	8

[a] Years unless specified otherwise.
(From Rosenbaum et al,[58] with permission.)

such patients may be somewhat limited, ultrasound is better able to measure the true renal length when the renal axis is altered by spinal curvature deformity than is an intravenous pyelogram. These authors developed a normal renal growth curve, based on sonographic renal measurements, for children with spina bifida.[60]

Ultrasound is frequently used to evaluate for renal growth in children, especially in those with renal abnormalities. It has been shown that the mean interobserver variation between any two imagers ranges from 3.87 to 5.49 mm, with a mean intraobserver variation of 0.87 to 3.61.[61] This observed variability in ultrasound measurement of renal length is comparable to the expected annual increase in length of the kidneys during childhood (2.2 to 5.7 mm/yr).[61] As such, caution is suggested when using ultrasound to evaluate renal growth in children over a 1-year period.[61]

RENAL ABNORMALITIES

Congenital

In the general population, the reported incidence of urinary tract abnormalities varies widely from 0.7 percent on clinical grounds to 4.5 percent in urogram studies to 9.6 percent in postmortem studies.[62] In a reported series evaluating children with documented congenital heart disease, an 11.9 percent incidence of urinary tract abnormalities was found; these abnormalities included hydronephrosis, duplication, ectopia, agenesis, and dysplasia of kidneys.[62] In patients with associated extracardiac anomalies, there is a significantly higher incidence of renal tract anomalies (39.1 percent) compared with that in patients with isolated congenital heart disease (4.7 percent).[62] Screening renal sonography of apparently healthy infants has shown a 1.4 percent incidence of silent but significant urinary tract abnormalities.[62] Therefore a routine ultrasound evaluation of the urinary tract is recommended to screen for previously undetected or silent but potentially serious abnormalities in children with congenital heart disease, especially when angiographic screening is not performed or is unsuccessful.[62]

Renal Cystic Disease

Ultrasound provides the initial diagnostic basis in patients with cystic kidney disease, distinguishing solid from cystic lesions and defining the type of cystic disease. Because these cysts are nonfunctional, they are not directly visualized on excretory urography, which is dependent on renal function. Ultrasound is an anatomic study and does not depend on renal function.[63] Real-time ultrasound is particularly suitable for renal imaging since it is noninvasive, lacks ionizing radiation, and can be performed portably.[64]

Multicystic Dysplastic Kidney. Several theories have been proposed for the production of a multicystic kidney.[65-67] This kidney may represent hydronephrosis secondary to atresia of the ureter, pelvis, or both during the metanephric stage of intrauterine development.[63,66,67] There is a spectrum from unilateral multicystic kidney, through segmental and focal multicystic dysplasia, to bilateral multicystic kidney disease.[66] In the classic multicystic kidney there is complete ureteral obstruction (atresia) early in fetal life (8 to 10 weeks' gestation).[67] Ureteral branching is interfered with, and there is decreased branching of the collecting tubules and inhibition of induction and maturation of the nephron. The collecting tubules enlarge, and the terminal portions develop into cysts. The cysts do not communicate, and a reniform shape is maintained. If obstruction is incomplete, occurring after nephrogenesis is complete (36 weeks' gestation), the pelvis and calyces are dilated and the normally developed nephrons and ducts may be dilated but without dysgenesis.[67] The glomeruli and tubules continue to function, resulting in hydronephrosis; the altered excretory function inhibits cellular development of the renal parenchyma. In incomplete obstruc-

tion (10 to 36 weeks' gestation) there are various degrees of cystic and dysplastic changes and pelvis and calyceal dilatation.[67] If the upper ureter alone is atretic, the proximal hydronephrotic pelvis may communicate with the multiple cysts. This is indistinguishable from hydronephrosis. If there is atresia of the pelvis as well, the usual form of pelvoinfundibular atresia results.[65]

The multicystic dysplastic kidney is the most common cause of an abdominal mass in the newborn.[63] Although this lesion is usually unilateral, a significant number of infants (15 percent) have abnormalities in the other kidney.[68] The left kidney is affected twice as often as the right.[68] The ultrasound findings of the classic multicystic kidney include (1) cysts of various shapes and sizes with the largest peripheral (nonmedial location of largest cyst, 100 percent accurate),[65] (2) absence of connection between adjacent multiple cysts (93 percent accurate),[65] (3) presence of interfaces between cysts (100 percent accurate),[65] (4) absence of identifiable renal sinus (100 percent accurate),[65] (5) absence of renal parenchyma surrounding cysts (74 percent accurate),[65] and (6) presence of eccentric echogenic areas (tiny cysts)[65,67] (Fig. 13-19). The septa separating the cysts and cores of rudimentary tissue (renal) may contain dysplastic glomeruli with tubular atrophy.[63]

A variation in the classic pattern may be seen, with only a solitary cyst, a large cyst and daughter cyst combination, or any of numerous other pattern combinations.[69] In the hydronephrotic form of multicystic dysplastic kidney, small peripheral cysts, budding from a

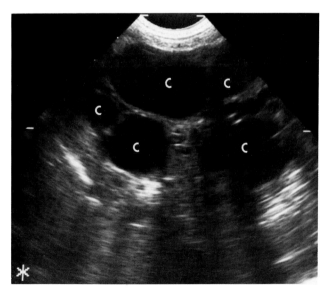

Fig. 13-19. Classic multicystic kidney. Sagittal scan of a flank mass in a newborn. A large structure containing multiple cysts (c) (anechoic areas) is seen in the left renal fossa. No renal parenchyma or sinus is identified. There is no communication between the cysts.

large central cyst, may be seen.[69] The lesion may not be identified until childhood or adulthood (Fig. 13-20). Ultrasound followed by nuclear medicine appears to be a logical diagnostic sequence in the evaluation of neonates with a flank mass. The differentiation between hydronephrosis and multicystic kidney is important clinically because the therapeutic approach and indications for surgery differ. Usually no function is seen in a multicystic kidney on a nuclear medicine scan in either early or delayed images.[65]

Unilateral hydronephrosis is a differential diagnosis of the ultrasound findings described for multicystic kidney.[20] Ultrasound is accurate in differentiating classic multicystic kidney from moderate hydronephrosis, but it is often difficult to differentiate severe hydronephrosis from the hydronephrotic form of multicystic kidney.[67] The severity of the dysplastic changes depends on the completeness of the obstruction and the gestational age at the time of obstruction. The ultrasound criteria helpful in the diagnosis of hydronephrosis include (1) visible

renal parenchyma surrounding the central cystic component, (2) small peripheral cysts (calyces) budding off a large central cyst, (3) cystic spaces of uniform size that are confluent with each other and with the renal pelvis, (4) visualization of a dilated ureter, and (5) the presence of a single large cyst[63,67] (Fig. 13-21).

The term *renal dysplasia* has been used to describe the presence of "primitive" tubules and mesenchymal tissue in the kidney, with the glomeruli, tubules, and collecting ducts decreased in number.[70] This abnormality is thought to be due to a diminished branching of the ampullary portion of the collecting ducts derived from the ureteric bud.[70] Multicystic kidney represents a variant of this condition. As described above, there is a spectrum of findings depending on the time and level of the urinary tract obstruction. With the obstruction at the level of the ureteropelvic junction (UPJ), the typical appearance of the multicystic kidney is seen (Fig. 13-19). With the obstruction at the level of the distal ureter, a smaller kidney containing few cysts of variable sizes is usually seen[70]

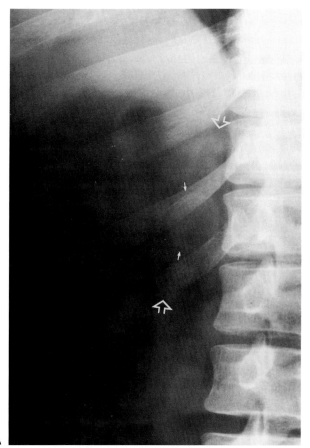

A

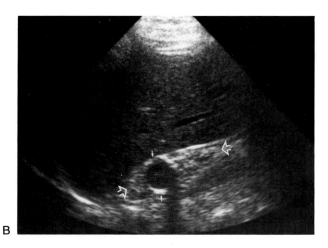

B

Fig. 13-20. Multicystic kidney. Adolescent boy with a calcific density (arrows) seen on **(A)** oblique radiograph of the right renal area. The kidney is outlined by the open arrows. **(B)** Sagittal sonogram of the right renal fossa showing an echogenic ring (arrows), which was seen as the calcific density in Fig. A. It is difficult to outline the renal margins (open arrows). This represented the residua of a multicystic kidney.

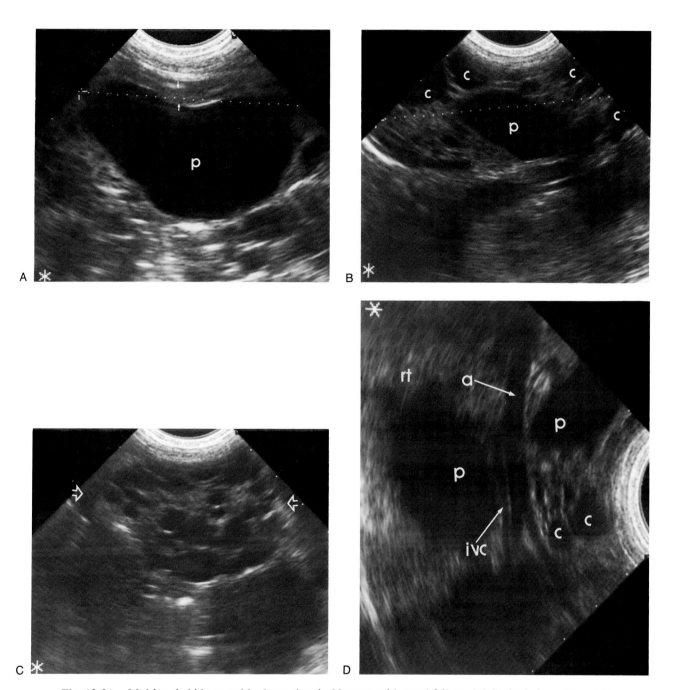

Fig. 13-21. Multicystic kidney and hydronephrosis. Neonate with renal failure. (A) Sagittal view of the right renal fossa demonstrating a large anechoic area *(p)* consistent with a dilated renal pelvis secondary to ureteropelvic junction obstruction. The entire renal length could not be displayed on this image. The parenchyma is noted between the two small arrows. (B) Sagittal medial and (C) lateral views of the left kidney demonstrating a dilated renal pelvis *(p)* centrally with multiple small cystic areas *(c)* in the region of the renal parenchyma. These cystic dysplastic changes are best demonstrated on the lateral view (Fig. C); they did not connect. (open arrows, renal length.) (D) Coronal sagittal view of the abdomen showing both dilated renal pelves *(p)*, as well as the cystic areas *(c)* within the left renal parenchyma. (*a*, aorta; *ivc,* inferior vena cava, *rt,* right.)

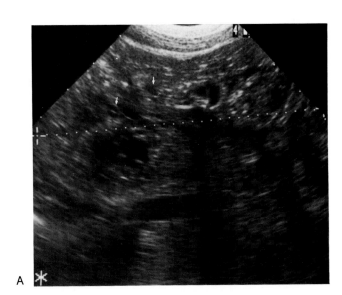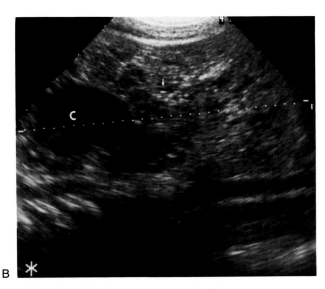

Fig. 13-22. Infantile polycystic kidney disease. Case 1. Sagittal scans of the **(A)** left and **(B)** right kidneys. The kidneys are markedly enlarged (calipers, open arrows, length, 8 cm) for a newborn. There are multiple tiny cystic areas (arrows) within both kidneys. There was a large cystic area *(c)* within the upper pole of the right kidney. *(Figure continues.)*

(Fig. 13-21). With the obstruction at the level of the urethra, the kidney is typically small with few or no cysts.[70] The ultrasound features are dominated by the presence of cysts; the more proximal the level of the obstruction, the more likely that cysts will be visible on ultrasound.[70] It has been postulated that if the obstruction is at a higher level, the calyces distend more and the cystic form of dysplasia develops; if the obstruction is at the level of the urethra, the pressure effects are more generalized and less severe, so the calyces do not distend to the same extent, although the kidney does become dysplastic.[70] The milder pressure increase appears to be the reason why urethral and distal ureteric obstructions are more frequently associated with focal dysplasia than are higher-level obstructions.[70] The identification of dysplasia is significant because it indicates permanent renal damage.[70]

At times, these dysplastic changes produce focal masses.[71] With dysplasia, there are abnormally developed and immature nephronic and ductal structures producing histologic disorganization of the renal parenchyma with abundant fibrous tissue and metaplastic cartilage.[71] Cancer has been detected in well-documented cases of renal dysplasia, so careful examination is imperative in patients with evidence of renal dysplasia and with a concomitant renal mass.[71]

Patients with multicystic dysplastic kidneys have been monitored to assess the natural history of this lesion.[72] The multicystic kidney may increase in size in utero and then shrink.[72] There is a high incidence of lethal contralateral anomalies (bilateral multicystic dysplastic kidney or contralateral renal agenesis) and involution of a unilateral multicystic dysplastic kidney, leading to the erroneous diagnosis in the neonate of unilateral renal agenesis.[72] There are contralateral kidney abnormalities in 57 percent, with most being hypertrophy of the contralateral kidney (65 percent).[72] This lesion may not be removed unless it grows during the first year of life.[72] Most patients with classic pelvoinfundicular multicystic dysplastic kidney do not have problems related to the size of the kidney.[72] Taking all multicystic dysplastic kidneys into account, 73 percent will not change in size, 13.5 percent will shrink or disappear, and 13.5 percent are removed because they grow.[72] The multicystic kidney therefore appears to be an evolving and progressive disorder.[73] The associated cysts start to involute either in utero or after birth, resulting in a small noncystic mass, called the "aplastic" kidney, or even in complete disappearance[73] (Fig. 13-20). This kidney appears to be vulnerable to anoxia or infection, and necrosis may supervene.[73] It has been demonstrated that 9 percent of these lesions will disappear within the first 3 years of follow-up, and as such, a longer period of follow-up is recommended.[72] These findings support the nonoperative approach to this abnormality.[72]

Infantile Polycystic Kidney Disease. *General.* Blyth and Ockenden have subdivided infantile polycystic disease into four groups: (1) perinatal (Potter I), in which more than 90 percent of the renal tubules are involved with minimal periportal fibrosis; (2) neonatal; (3) infantile; and (4) juvenile, in which 10 percent or less of the

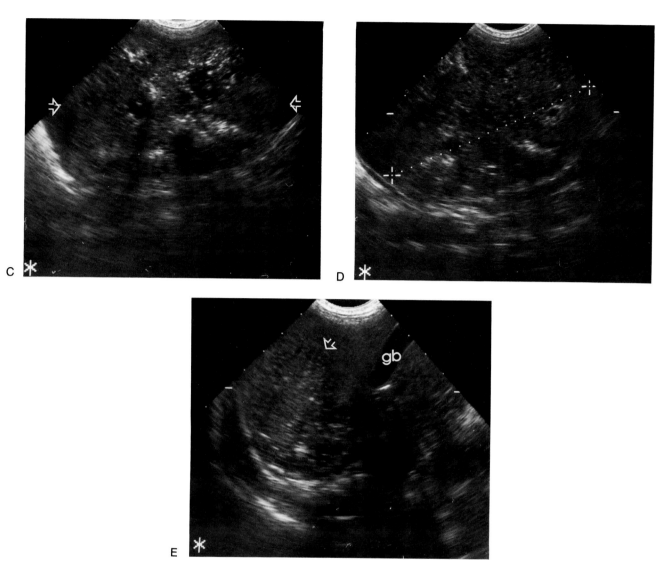

Fig. 13-22 *(Continued).* Case 2. Sagittal scans of the **(C)** right and **(D)** left kidneys with **(E)** transverse view of the right kidney demonstrating nephromegaly (8.5 cm); both kidneys contained multiple tiny cystic areas similar to Figs. A and B. (*gb*, gallbladder; open arrows, border between kidney and liver.)

renal tubules are involved with hepatic fibrosis and portal hypertension.[74] This form of cystic disease is uncommon and is inherited in an autosomal recessive fashion. The infant presents with organomegaly secondary to the large kidneys, which are enlarged because of the ectatic tubules that are 1 to 2 mm in diameter. On microdissection, these collecting tubules have cystic dilatation and hyperplasia.

In previous reports, the ultrasound appearance of kidneys affected by infantile polycystic kidney disease was that of enlarged echogenic kidneys. There was poor definition of the renal sinus, medulla, and cortex[74] (Fig. 13-22). The echogenicity and irregular cortical surface make it difficult to discern the border of the kidney.[74,75] The ectatic tubules, which were very small, were not seen

by ultrasound, but the interfaces produced by the walls of the tubules caused increased echogenicity throughout the parenchyma.[63,75] In the normal newborn there is increased echogenicity of the cortex, with sharply delineated hypoechoic medullae (Fig. 13-15). In infantile polycystic disease, the increased echoes from the tubules in the cortex and medulla lead to a loss of the corticomedullary junction definition.[63]

With newer, high-resolution, real-time equipment, a distinctive ultrasound appearance may now be defined.[69] Although the large kidneys are predominantly echogenic, there is a prominent central lucency and a lucent rim.[69] One series believed that the demonstration of a relatively thick rim of renal cortex with normal echogenicity was a good predictor of concurrent normal renal clearance and prolonged survival[76] (Fig. 13-23). As before, the increased echogenicity is thought to be secondary to the infinite number of interfaces produced by this multitude of ectatic tubules being cut at different angles by the sonic beam.[69] The renal pelvis and calyces are the central lucent area, with the peripheral lucent rim possibly representing the remnant of the peripherally compressed renal cortex.[69]

Three ultrasound patterns have been described with infantile polycystic kidney: (1) classic picture, with diffusely enlarged and echogenic kidneys with poor definition and distortion of the cortex, medulla, and sinus echoes and indistinct borders between the kidneys and the surrounding structures; (2) enlarged kidneys with normally echoic prominent rim of renal cortex with moderately echogenic medulla, poorly separated from the renal sinus; and (3) enlarged kidneys with resolvable cysts and an isoechoic thin rim of renal cortex.[77] On intravenous urogram, the recessive type manifests as bilaterally enlarged kidneys with prolonged and/or delayed nephrogram characterized by radiopaque/radiolucent striations going from the cortex to the medulla; contrast media also may be seen in the renal pelvis if renal failure is minimal.[77]

Other sonographic patterns described with infantile polycystic kidney disease are the specific "pepper-and-salt" and "striped" patterns.[78] Provided that the medullary pyramids have not undergone cystic degeneration, they show a normal conical shape.[78] The medullary pyramids and renal cortex are interspersed with innumerable small cysts whose diameters are a few millimeters only, resulting in a spongelike appearance[78] (Fig. 13-22). These are baglike dilated collecting ducts, microscopi-

cally, which extend radially towards the renal capsule.[78] On high-resolution real-time sonography, radially arranged minute cysts (down to 2 mm in diameter) may be detected in the newborn.[78] The "pepper-and-salt echoes" refer to the diffusely interspersed high-amplitude echoes.[78] The morphologic correlation of the high-amplitude echoes is unknown but may represent fibrotic tissue changes or the numerous interfaces of multiple minute cysts.[78] With the "white-and-black stripes" pattern, the white stripes appear behind high-amplitude echoes and are probably secondary to reverberation echoes,[78] whereas the black stripes may be "edge-shadowing effects" associated with larger cysts.[78] The renal function does not appear to correlate with either the size of the cysts or their distribution within the cortex or the medulla.[78]

A strikingly lucent band at the periphery of the kidney has been recognized in some cases and has been attributed to relative cortical sparing or fluid in the perirenal space.[79] This cortical rim was found to be minimal at 5 days of age, well-developed at 2 months, and even more pronounced at 7 months.[79] On histologic examination it corresponded to a zone of the kidney more severely involved by tubular dilation than the rest of the kidney, suggesting that the large amount of fluid present in these extremely thin-walled cystic spaces, rather than compression of normal cortex, may be the cause of the finding.[79]

Several diagnoses besides infantile polycystic kidney disease must be considered when ultrasound demonstrates enlarged, echogenic kidneys with loss of distinct pelvocalyceal echoes; these include acute glomerulonephritis, bilateral renal vein thrombosis, and nephroblas-

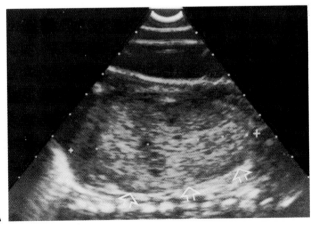
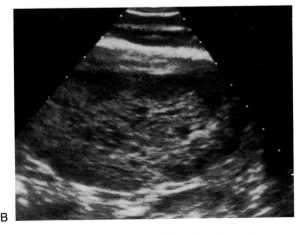

A   B

Fig. 13-23. Infantile polycystic kidney disease. Sonolucent rim. **(A)** Renal ultrasound at 5 days, longitudinal section of the left kidney (5 MHz). The kidney is enlarged and hyperechoic. Tiny cysts are seen in the medulla. A very thin sonolucent cortical rim is present (arrows). **(B)** Renal ultrasound at 2 months, longitudinal sections of the left kidney (5 MHz). A sonolucent rim approximately 0.5 cm wide is now clearly identified. (From Currarino et al,[79] with permission.)

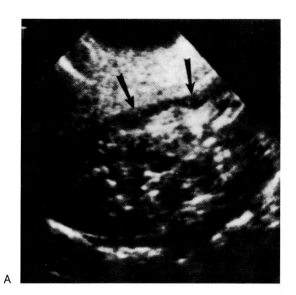 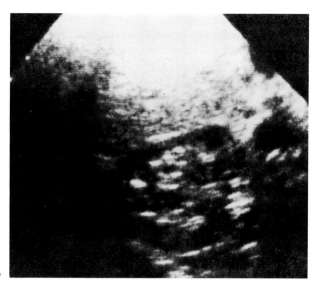

A   B

Fig. 13-24. Juvenile polycystic kidney disease. (A) Longitudinal sonogram through the right kidney demonstrating an enlarged kidney, which is predominantly echogenic but has a sonolucent rim (arrows). (B) Transverse sonogram through the right kidney demonstrating similar findings. (From Hayden et al,[69] with permission.)

tomatosis.[77] With acute glomerulonephritis and bilateral renal vein thrombosis, there is usually diffusely hypoechoic enlargement of the kidneys with preservation of the pelvocalyceal echoes.[77] With nephroblastomatosis, there is usually diffuse renal enlargement and disruption of the intraparenchymal echotexture; the masses are more commonly hypoechoic than echogenic and the infants are usually not in renal failure.[77]

Juvenile Polycystic Disease. Juvenile polycystic disease is part of the spectrum of infantile polycystic kidney diseases. The degree of involvement of the kidney relative to the liver and the rapidity of progression are determined by the age at which the disease presents. In the infant, there is kidney failure; the older child may have systemic hypertension or portal hypertension with varices. The ultrasound pattern depends on the clinical course and pathologic condition. All sonograms demonstrate increased echogenicity to the cortex and medulla of the kidney owing to the ectatic tubules leading to an indistinct corticomedullary junction (Figs. 13-24 and 13-25). There may be a lucent rim of compressed cortex.[69] The liver findings are variable. Periportal involvement of the liver seen with this disease may lead to hepatic fibrosis and portal hypertension.[74] The echogenicity of the liver may be increased if there is significant periportal fibrosis and if bile duct ectasia is present.[63]

Renal Tubular Dysgenesis. Renal tubular dysgenesis is a newly reported entity thought to be inherited as an autosomal recessive trait.[80] It may be associated with oligo-

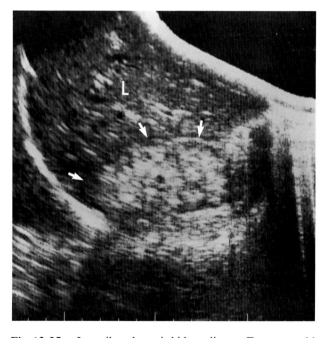

Fig. 13-25. Juvenile polycystic kidney disease. Four-year-old child with hematemesis due to esophageal varices; a biopsy of liver was diagnostic for infantile polycystic kidney disease of the liver and kidney. On a longitudinal scan of the right kidney (arrows), there is increased echogenicity throughout the parenchyma compared with the liver *(L)* and loss of corticomedullary junction (similar findings in left kidney). (From Grossman et al,[63] with permission.)

hydramnios in later pregnancy, although ultrasound before 22 weeks' gestation may show an adequate amount of amniotic fluid.[80] Potter syndrome is present, with flexion or extension deformity of the joints, rocker-bottom feet, and simian creases of the hand.[80] The most common cause of death is respiratory failure due to pulmonary hypoplasia.[80]

The kidney is normal or occasionally enlarged but never small.[80] The lobar structure is usually preserved, with the corticomedullary margin well demarcated, but the corticomedullary rays are usually indistinct.[80] The presence of immature and poorly differentiated tubules in the cortex with absence of proximal tubules is the most striking abnormality.[80] There is an increase in the amount of interstitial tissue in the medulla. The reported ultrasound findings correspond to the pathologic abnormalities. Normal-sized kidneys are seen, with no macroscopic renal cysts but with abnormal parenchyma. There is lack of corticomedullary differentiation, giving the appearance of a thick cortex, corresponding to the crowded glomeruli, very immature tubules, and small medullary pyramids found histologically[80] (Fig. 13-26). Included in the differential diagnosis are the recessive-type polycystic kidneys, acute corticomedullary necrosis, renal vein thrombosis, and renal dysplasia.

Glomerulocystic Disease. As a rare condition that may occur in otherwise normal infants or in association with multiple malformations such as oral-facial-digital syndrome, renal retinal dysplasia, trisomy, and Zellweger syndrome, glomerulocystic disease is always bilateral, consisting of cystic dilatation of Bowman's space, confined to the renal cortex, usually most severely affecting the more peripheral cortex.[81] There may be a variable degree of dilatation of the collecting tubules, with some having an inflammatory infiltrate or fibrosis in the interstitium.[81] The reniform shape is usually maintained, but the kidneys are frequently enlarged. An autosomal dominant pattern of inheritance has been suggested, although cases may be sporadic.[81]

The ultrasound findings associated with glomerulocystic disease may be confused with those of infantile polycystic kidney. Both conditions are characterized by small cysts in enlarged kidneys. The cysts are limited to

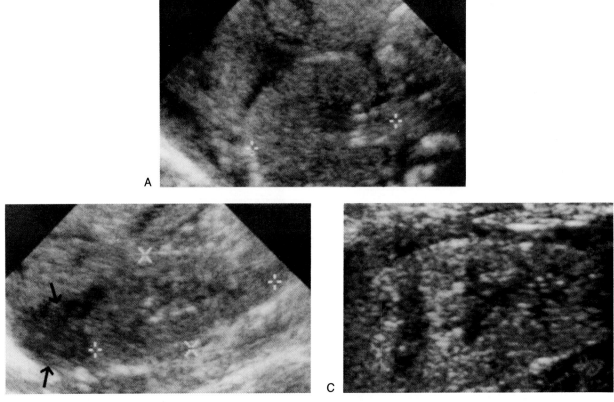

Fig. 13-26. Renal tubular dysgenesis. **(A)** Transverse and **(B)** longitudinal sonograms of the right kidney. Note the poor corticomedullary differentiation, giving the appearance of homogeneity of the renal parenchyma and a thickened cortex. No cysts are evident. The size of the kidney is normal. Arrows (Fig. B) mark the normal adrenal gland. **(C)** Close-up longitudinal sonogram of the left kidney showing the same finding. (From Luisiri et al,[80] with permission.)

the distal nephron in infantile polycystic kidney disease; however, the predominant finding in glomerulocystic disease is dilatation of Bowman's capsule.[81] Both conditions show bilateral nephromegaly, indistinct renal margins, increased echogenicity of the renal cortex, and loss of definition of the corticomedullary junction[81] (Fig. 13-27). With glomerocystic disease, the renal size may diminish as the child grows.[81] The natural history of this disease is uncertain because of the rarity of clinical recognition; renal function may be normal.

Histologic confirmation is required when clinical examination and family screening studies fail to determine the diagnosis, because of the importance of a correct diagnosis for genetic counseling and, perhaps, patient management.[81] Both parents should be carefully examined and investigated with renal and liver ultrasound when a child is found to have bilateral renal enlargement with macrocysts and/or increased echogenicity.[81] When there is no evidence of a multiple malformation syndrome and no histologically confirmed diagnosis of a cystic renal disease in a sibling, a renal and liver biopsy should be performed to determine a definitive diagnosis, especially when neither parent has evidence of adult polycystic kidney disease or tuberous sclerosis.[81]

Adult Polycystic Kidney Disease. This form of polycystic disease is inherited as autosomal dominant trait with a high degree of penetrance. The penetrance of the gene is such that morphologic evidence of the disease is seen in most patients by 80 years of age.[82,83] It has become apparent that the adult type of polycystic kidney disease

can occur in the neonate[69] (Fig. 13-28). It occurs in 1 of 500 persons, with 5 to 8 percent of patients requiring dialysis or transplantation.[24] The disease usually becomes clinically apparent in the fourth decade, although children sometimes present with symptoms.[63] In this type of cystic disease, there are cystic dilatations of the proximal convoluted tubules and Bowman's capsule as well as the collecting tubules. Classically, the cysts enlarge with age such that the patient presents when renal function begins to decrease.[75]

The most frequent complication of this disease is infection and renal calculi.[84] In addition, there may be cyst rupture, hemorrhage, and ureteric obstruction.[85] There can be calcification associated with the cysts, but it is not distinctive. It may appear as a thin rim, ringlike, curvilinear, or small flecks, or as irregular amorphous concretions.[85] The most common cause of death associated

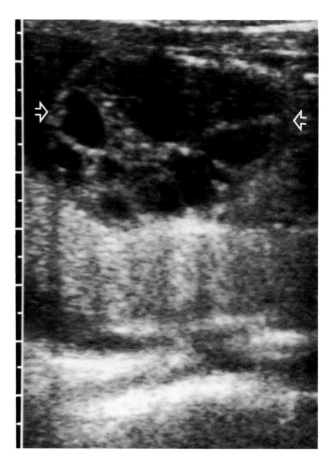

Fig. 13-28. Adult polycystic kidney disease, fetus. This fetus had bilateral renal enlargement with multiple large cysts, as seen on a sagittal view of one kidney (open arrows). Fluid was visualized within the fetal urinary bladder. The amniotic fluid volume was slightly decreased. The fetus, which also had a large encephalocele, was aborted and was found to have polycystic kidney disease, adult type, associated with Meckel syndrome.

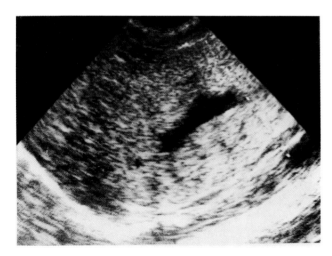

Fig. 13-27. Glomerulocystic disease. Renal ultrasound at 1 month of age demonstrating an enlarged right kidney with diffuse increased echogenicity, loss of the corticomedullary junction, ill-defined renal margins, and mild dilatation of the renal pelvis. The left kidney (not shown) demonstrated similar findings. (From Fitch and Stapleton,[81] with permission.)

with this disease is uremia (59 percent), with cerebral hemorrhage (13 percent) and cardiac disease being less frequent causes.[84] In 25 to 50 percent of patients there are liver cysts; occasionally cysts are also seen in the pancreas (9 percent), lungs, spleen, ovaries, testes, epididymis, thyroid, uterus, and bladder.[84-87]

On ultrasound kidneys affected with polycystic disease are enlarged with discrete cysts in the cortical region[63,86,87] (Figs. 13-29 to 13-31). The renal contour is poorly demarcated from surrounding tissue and may be secondary to multiple peripheral cysts that distort the renal capsule, to perirenal fibrosis, or to an organized hemorrhage in peripheral cysts that cause a decrease in specular reflections from the renal capsule[24] (Fig. 13-31). When involvement of the kidneys is identified by ultrasound, one should carefully scan the liver, pancreas, and spleen for evidence of cystic involvement (see Figs. 5-51 and 7-16). In addition, ultrasound can be used to screen family members to diagnose polycystic disease that is not clinically manifested.[82,83,86] This would also help to provide genetic counseling prior to procreation and to learn more about the natural history of the disease.

Although polycystic kidney disease is described as a bilateral process, there have been reports of unilateral disease and of segmental disease.[88-90] Both of these would be difficult to diagnose by ultrasound alone. The differential diagnosis would have to include segmental polycystic disease (very uncommon), localized hydronephrosis, and multilocular cyst.[88]

The adult type of polycystic kidney disease can occur in the neonate.[91] On ultrasound the kidneys are noted to be normal in shape but markedly enlarged and homogeneously echogenic.[69,91] Corticomedullary junction differentiation is absent, and no clear-cut calyces or papillae are identified. The clue is the absence of impaired renal function.

Medullary Cystic Disease. Two forms of medullary cystic disease may be encountered in the pediatric patient; both produce collecting tubule abnormalities confined to the medullary zone of the kidney.[69] Patients with juvenile nephronophthisis usually present with azotemia, in contrast to patients with medullary sponge kidney, which in itself does not alter function, but its complications (stone formation, infection) bring the patient to the physician.[69]

The pathogenesis of medullary cystic disease or nephronophthisis is obscure, as is its mode of inheritance. It is familial, with both dominant and recessive modes of transmission. Clinically, patients present with renal failure, polyuria, thirst, renal salt wasting, hyposthenuria, severe anemia, and a positive family history with a normal urinary sediment but no edema or hypertension.[92,93] The onset of clinical symptoms is usually at age 3 to 5 years to early adulthood, with progressive renal insufficiency over the next 5 to 10 years.[93] Pathologic examination gives variable results, with renal biopsies showing interstitial fibrosis and cellular infiltration, tubular atrophy and dilatation, and periglomerular fibrosis. As such, a needle biopsy is not really diagnostic. At postmortem, the kidneys are found to be small with cysts less than 1 mm to greater than 1 cm in the medullary and corticomedullary regions.[92]

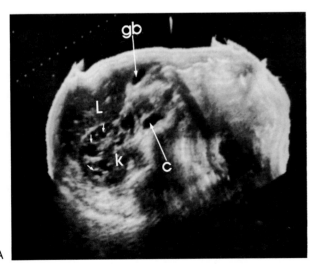
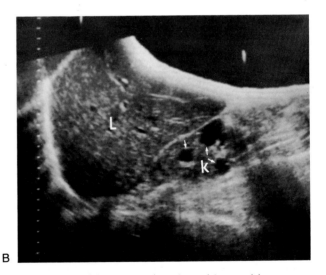

A   B

Fig. 13-29. Adult polycystic kidney disease. Twenty-year-old patient without symptoms but with a positive family history for the disease. **(A)** Transverse and **(B)** longitudinal supine scans showing multiple cysts (arrows) within the right renal cortex. The left kidney appeared similar. (*L*, liver; *k*, right kidney; *c*, inferior vena cava; *gb*, gallbladder.)

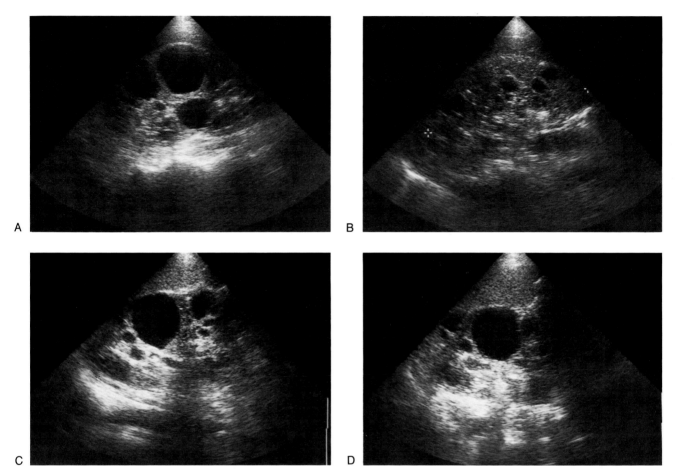

Fig. 13-30. Adult polycystic kidney disease. Twenty-one-year-old man with a positive family history for the disease. **(A & B)** Sagittal scans of the right kidney (with Fig. A more lateral than Fig. B) and **(C)** sagittal and **(D)** transverse views of the left kidney demonstrating enlarged kidneys containing multiple cysts, seen as well-defined anechoic areas. The renal margins are very poorly defined.

Radiographic diagnosis is difficult if renal function is poor and the cysts are small. Most frequently, there is poor opacification of the renal collecting system. On high-dose nephrotomography, sometimes the diagnosis can be made by the identification of well-defined corticomedullary lucencies in association with a thin cortex. The retrograde pyelogram findings are variable in demonstrating communication between the collecting system and cysts.[92] With medullary sponge kidney the intravenous urogram is usually normal, whereas with juvenile nephronophthisis little if any excretion is demonstrated.[69]

The ultrasound findings represent a spectrum of irregularly widened central echoes with small cysts and well-defined cystic structures when larger medullary cysts predominate[94] (Fig. 13-32). The most characteristic ultrasound findings are small cysts confined to the medullary portions of both kidneys.[63,92] There may only be irregular widening of the central echoes with small cysts.[94] The presence of a few small medullary or corticomedullary cysts in a normal-sized or moderately small kidney, coupled with loss of corticomedullary differentiation and increased parenchymal echogenicity, should suggest the diagnosis of juvenile nephronophthisis in a child with severe uremia.[93] In children with juvenile nephronophthisis with severe uremia, the ultrasound typically demonstrates a few medullary or corticomedullary "cysts" in normal or moderately small kidneys, coupled with loss of corticomedullary differentiation and increased parenchymal echogenicity[69] (Fig. 13-33).

With medullary sponge kidney, there is characteristic renal tubular ectasia characterized by cystic dilatation of renal collecting ducts.[95] These patients may be asymptomatic or may present with hematuria. The most common complications are infection and stones.[95] The ultrasound scan may be normal in cases of medullary

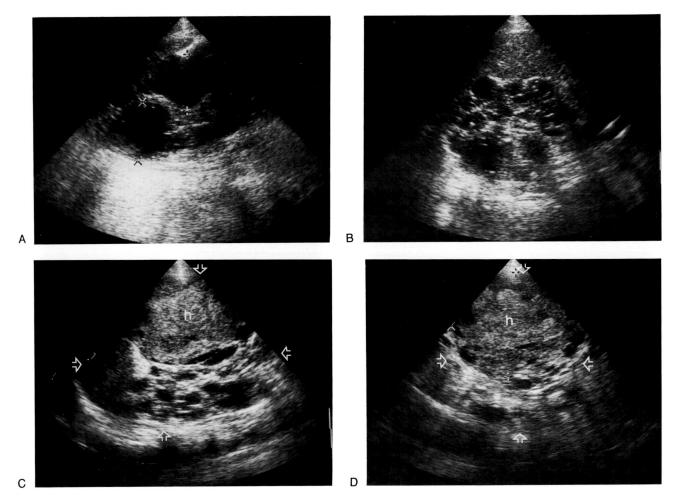

Fig. 13-31. Adult polycystic kidney disease. **(A)** Sagittal and **(B)** transverse scans of the right kidney in this pretransplant patient demonstrating multiple large and small cysts within the kidneys. The kidney is so large that it is difficult to get an accurate measurement. **(C)** Sagittal and **(D)** transverse scans through the left kidney showing a large echogenic mass (*h*, 10 × 8 cm) within the large polycystic kidney. This patient had hemorrhaged into one of the cysts. (open arrows, left renal margins.)

sponge kidney, but occasionally hyperechogenic pyramids due to calcium deposition are seen[69] (Figs. 13-34 to 13-36). Ultrasound may reveal hyperechogenic pyramids, at first at the periphery, later generalized.[95] It is postulated that the calcium concentration is normally greatest in the medulla and is removed by lymphatic flow.[95] Calcium is first deposited in the interstitum about the collecting ducts and may become the nidus for stone growth if the calcium load should exceed the lymphatic transport capacity. In childhood, the differential diagnosis should include the form of infantile polycystic disease characterized by tubular ectasia with hepatic fibrosis.

The differential diagnosis for medullary cysts is limited, including abnormalities containing fluid that may or may not communicate with the pelvocalyceal system. Those abnormalities with collecting system communication should be visualized on excretory urography and include pyogenic cysts, abscesses, diverticula, papillary

necrosis, and medullary sponge kidney. Those without communication would include simple cyst and medullary cystic disease, as well as parapelvic cysts, which are usually not multiple. In polycystic kidney disease, the cysts are variable in size and location and are associated with enlarged kidneys with irregular cortical outlines.[92] The simplicity and reliability of ultrasound make it superior to other modalities in such cases, particularly when a positive family history is lacking or medullary cysts are not seen in biopsy samples.[93]

Congenital Nephrosis. This entity is sometimes termed microcystic disease of the kidney. It is inherited in an autosomal recessive fashion. The infant presents with a low birth weight, associated with a large placenta, failure to thrive, proteinuria, and edema. The kidneys are diffusely enlarged, and microscopy shows dilatation of the

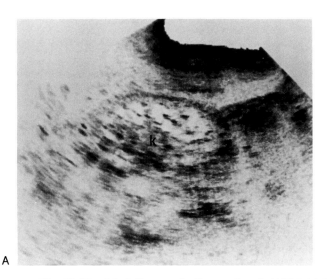
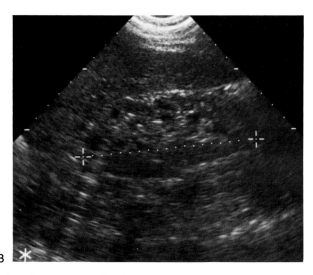

A

B

Fig. 13-32. Medullary cystic disease. Case 1. **(A)** Multiple 1- to 2-cm cysts confined to the medullary portion of the kidney *(k)* are seen. The kidneys are small (6 cm), with a regular cortical outline. Case 2. **(B)** Sagittal view of the right kidney (calipers), which is small (8 cm), showing several very small cysts confined to the medullary portion of the kidney. (Fig. A from Rego et al,[92] with permission.)

proximal tubules and widening of Bowman's spaces. On ultrasound, the kidneys are enlarged with marked echogenicity and loss of a distinctive cortex, medulla, and renal sinus[96] (Fig. 13-37). The differential diagnosis would have to include infantile polycystic kidney disease.[96]

Multilocular Renal Cyst. There are several theories for the etiology of a multilocular cyst, and the condition has several names including benign cystic nephroma, cystic Wilms' tumor, cystic hamartoma, cystic lymphangioma, and Perlmann's tumor. Generally, the Wilms' tumor is relatively benign. This lesion is rare, nonheredi-

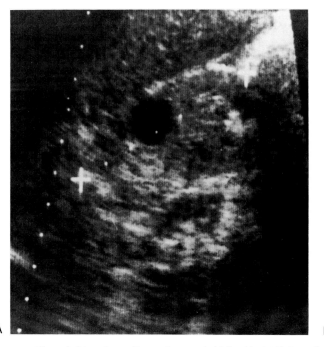
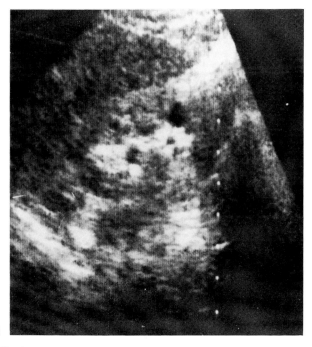

A

B

Fig. 13-33. Juvenile nephronophthisis. **(A & B)** Longitudinal sonograms demonstrating a moderately small kidney with loss of corticomedullary differentiation, increased parenchymal echogenicity, and associated medullary and corticomedullary "cysts." (From Hayden et al,[69] with permission.)

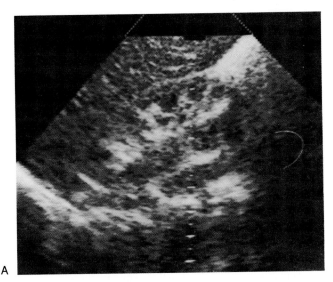
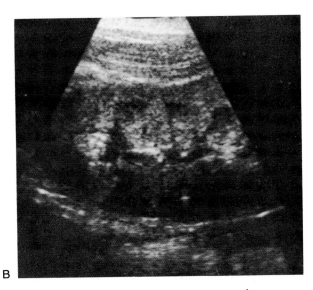

A   B

Fig. 13-34. Medullary sponge kidney. The diagnosis was established at age 2 months by excretory urography. **(A)** Supine longitudinal sonogram of the right kidney at 6 years. Pyramids are surrounded at the tips and sides by a band of hyperechogenicity. **(B)** Longitudinal sonogram 3 years later. Hyperechoic pyramids have become more prominent. (From Patriquin and O'Regan,[95] with permission.)

tary, and limited to one area of the kidney, with normal functioning tissue elsewhere in the kidney. The involved part of the kidney is bulky and well encapsulated, consisting of multiple noncommunicating cysts that are sharply separated from surrounding normal tissue. This lesion represents a well-encapsulated benign tumor consisting of multiple noncommunicating cysts.[69]

On ultrasound, a large tumor with multiple fluid-filled masses is seen separated by highly echogenic septations with normal renal tissue in the rest of the kidney[63] (Fig. 13-38; see Fig. 13-128). The ultrasound typically dem-

onstrates highly suggestive findings of multiple cysts separated by highly echogenic septae that displace and compress the remaining normal kidney.[69] On excretory urography, the mass is nonfunctional, with the rest of the kidney normal but with distortion or hydronephrosis.[63] (See also Multilocular Cystic Nephroma, and Wilms' Tumor, both under Primary Renal Tumor.)

Simple Cyst. This lesion arises in the renal cortex and is more often single than multiple. The etiology is unknown, and the condition is not hereditary. The highest

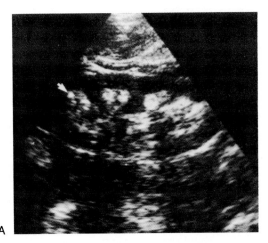
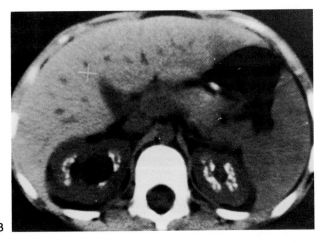

A   B

Fig. 13-35. Medullary sponge kidney with nephrocalcinosis (age 8 years). **(A)** Prone longitudinal sonogram of the left kidney. Pyramids are highly echogenic (arrow), especially at the periphery. Several acoustic shadows are seen. **(B)** Unenhanced CT scan 2 weeks later. Calcium surrounds the calyces and pyramids. Right hydronephrosis secondary to ureteral stone was noted. (From Patriquin and O'Regan,[95] with permission.)

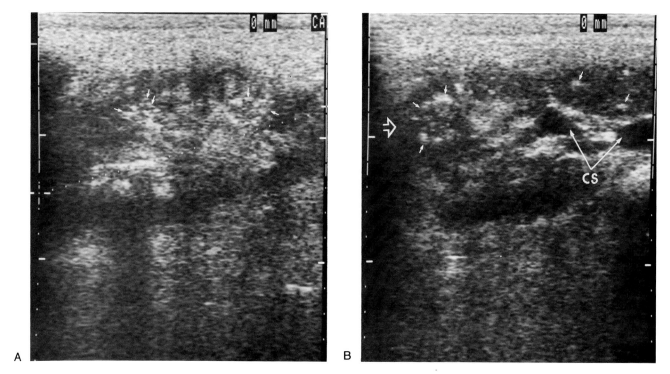

A B

Fig. 13-36. Medullary sponge kidney. **(A)** Sagittal and **(B)** transverse linear-array real-time scans demonstrating multiple tiny echogenic foci (small arrows) within the region of the pyramids. They appear to be particularly prominent in the periphery of the pyramids. (open arrow, renal border; *cs*, collecting system.)

incidence is after age 30, but it can be seen in children. These simple serous cysts of the kidneys are uncommonly diagnosed in children, except at autopsy.[69] On ultrasound the characteristic cyst is anechoic and well-defined and exhibits acoustic enhancement[63] (see Figs. 13-101 to 13-103). (See also Renal Masses.)

Miscellaneous Cortical Cysts. There are a number of syndromes such as Conradi's disease, Zellweger syndrome, and Turner syndrome that may be associated with small cortical cysts.[69] These cysts may also be seen in association with certain of the trisomies, and they may be seen with tuberous sclerosis (see under Renal Masses);

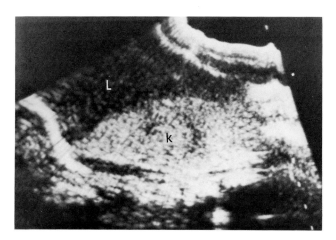

Fig. 13-37. Congenital nephrosis. Longitudinal scan of the right abdomen showing an enlarged kidney (7 to 8 cm in length) with a strikingly increased echogenicity and a coarse granular pattern. (*k*, kidney; *L*, liver.) (From Graif et al,[96] with permission.)

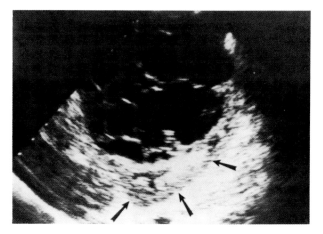

Fig. 13-38. Multilocular renal cyst. Longitudinal sonogram demonstrating multiple cysts separated by highly echogenic septa. The lesion displaces and compresses the remaining normal portion of the kidney (arrows). (From Hayden et al,[69] with permission.)

the cysts may be quite large in these conditions[69] (see Fig. 13-109). These cysts must be differentiated from the normal neonatal or infantile kidney, which is characterized by very prominent lucent renal pyramids.[69]

Parapelvic Cyst. These cysts arise in the hilum of the kidney and do not communicate with the collecting system. Their pathogenesis is uncertain. They are usually seen in adults as incidental findings, but they sometimes present as a mass on excretory urography. On ultrasound, a medially placed cystic mass is seen with echogenic walls (Fig. 13-39). The mass may displace the pelvocalyceal complex and must be differentiated from hydronephrosis by its noncommunication.[63] (See also Renal Masses.)

Ureteropelvic Junction Obstruction. At times, a neonate, infant, or child may be referred to ultrasound for evaluation of a palpable mass that represents a UPJ obstruction. This lesion is frequently diagnosed on an antenatal ultrasound, and the neonate is referred to ultrasound on that basis. These infants often do not have a palpable mass.

There are a number of reported causes for congenital UPJ obstruction. These include extrapelvic adhesions, an abnormally situated junction between the renal pelvis and ureter, aberrant vessels to the lower pole of the kidney, folds of mucosa in the upper ureter, and intrinsic and functional abnormalities of the pelvoureteral junction.[97]

The diagnosis is made on ultrasound by identifying a large, dilated, anechoic renal pelvis that communicates with the calyces without a dilated ureter[68] (Figs. 13-21A and 13-40 to 13-42). At times the renal pelvis is so enormous that the calyces cannot be identified (Figs. 13-40 to 13-42). Still, the diagnosis of UPJ obstruction should be considered. Functional data concerning the affected kidney may be obtained by excretory urography or nuclear medicine. With nuclear medicine, differential function curves can be obtained for each kidney so that the clinician may know the amount of renal function contributed by the affected kidney. If the diagnosis of

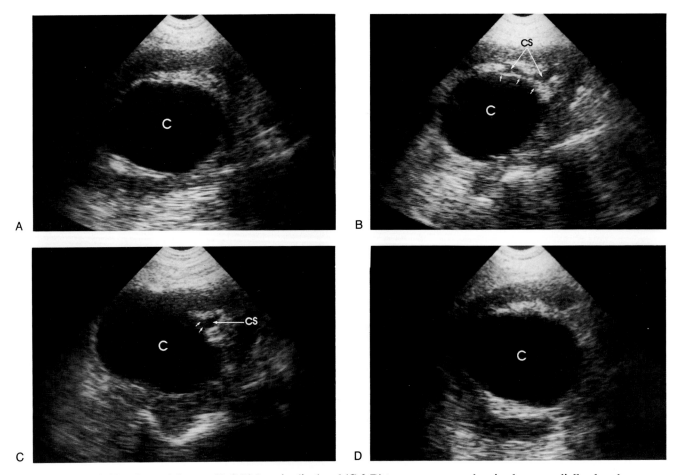

Fig. 13-39. Parapelvic cyst. **(A & B)** Longitudinal and **(C & D)** transverse scans showing large, medially placed cystic *(C)* mass. It does not communicate (small arrows) with the collecting system *(cs)* but does compress it.

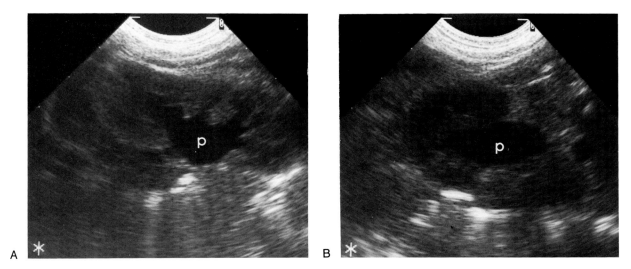

Fig. 13-40. Ureteropelvic junction obstruction. Neonate noted to have a dilated renal pelvis on a perinatal ultrasound. **(A)** Sagittal and **(B)** transverse scans of the right kidney demonstrating dilatation of the renal pelvis *(p)* with little caliectasis. A dilated ureter was not seen.

UPJ obstruction can be made early in life and corrective surgery performed, a great deal of renal function can be saved. Generally function decreases with increasing age at diagnosis.

Congenital Megacalyces. With congenital megacalyces or megacalicosis, there is considered to be a nonobstructive dilatation of the calyces as a result of a congenital underdevelopment of the pyramids.[98] This condition may be unilateral or bilateral and can be an incidental finding or can be associated with some complications

such as infection or stone formation due to urinary stasis in the dilated calyces.[98] An association with hypertension and hematuria has also been found.[98] The condition is usually associated with normal renal function and is nonprogressive.

At urography, the findings are usually very suggestive and are characterized by a prompt nephrographic phase with delayed opacification of the entire collecting system because of the large volume of contrast needed to fill the dilated calyces.[98] There may be enlargement of the calyces, which may be increased in number with flattened papillae with short and broad infundibula.[98] The in-

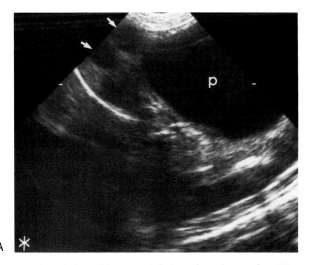

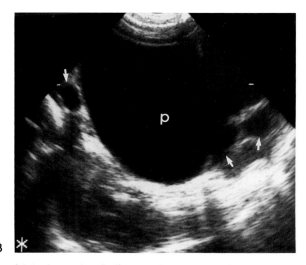

Fig. 13-41. Ureteropelvic junction obstruction. Neonate with hydronephrosis diagnosed on an obstetric sonogram. **(A)** Sagittal and **(B)** transverse scans through the right abdomen demonstrating a very large cystic area *(p,* renal pelvis) with small cystic areas (arrows) representing calyces. A dilated ureter was not seen.

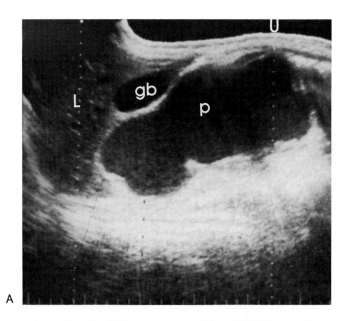

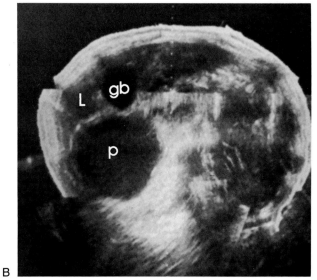

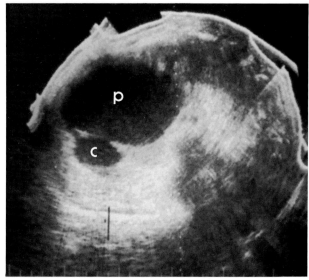

Fig. 13-42. Ureteropelvic junction obstruction. Sixteen-year-old pregnant patient, presenting too large for dates for her 8-week pregnancy. **(A)** Sagittal scan 6 cm to right of midline. A large anechoic *(p)* structure is seen in the renal fossa. (*L*, liver; *gb*, gallbladder; *U*, level of umbilicus.) Transverse scans **(B)** 12 cm and **(C)** 4 cm above the umbilicus showing an anechoic area *(p)* in the right renal fossa and dilated calyces *(c)* posteriorly on Fig. C. Although there is acoustic enhancement, there are many internal echoes. The patient later developed pyonephrosis. (*L*, liver; *gb*, gallbladder.)

volved kidney may be normal in size or mildly enlarged with smooth borders. The renal pelvis and ureter are usually normal.

At ultrasound, the associated findings are nonspecific and must be differentiated from refluxing hydronephrosis, chronic pyelonephritis, distal ureteral obstruction, and postobstructive atrophy.[98] With all of these, the calyces may be more dilated than the pelvis[98] (Fig. 13-43).

As such, the diagnosis should be suggested by the presence of multiple small fluid-filled spaces, usually of uniform size, without evidence of significant pelvic dilatation in a normal-sized or mildly enlarged kidney with a diffuse and uniform decrease in the parenchymal thickness and smooth borders. With obstructive hydronephrosis, there is usually significant pelvic dilatation on ultrasound.[98] Vesicoureteral reflux should be suggested

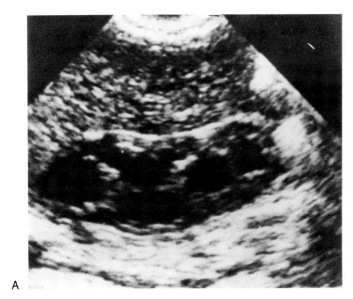
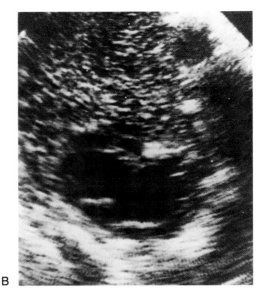

A

B

Fig. 13-43. Congenital megacalyces. (**A**) Longitudinal and (**B**) transverse sonograms of the right kidney demonstrating caliceal dilatation and a decrease in the parenchymal thickness. (From Garcia et al,[98] with permission.)

if there are changes in the degree of calyceal dilatation during the examination and especially after voiding. With chronic pyelonephritis and reflux nephropathy, there is commonly associated focal parenchymal scarring. A voiding cystourethrogram and excretory urogram should be done to rule out these other diagnoses.

Bardet-Biedl Syndrome. The Bardet-Biedl syndrome (previously called the Laurence-Moon-Biedl syndrome) is characterized by obesity, pigmentary retinopathy, hypogonadism, polydactyly, and mental retardation.[99] Renal abnormalities associated with this syndrome have been demonstrated, with some degree of renal abnormality present in all cases.[99] The abnormalities appear to be dysplastic rather than due to reflux. There is a wide variety of histologic changes, including periglomerular and interstitial fibrosis, cystic dilatation of tubules, cortical and medullary cysts, and glomerular changes.[99] The most characteristic findings include calyceal abnormalities (clubbing and pronounced diverticula) and fetal-type lobation.[99] The diagnosis might be particularly useful in the younger patient in whom eye changes are not yet advanced and the diagnosis is still in doubt.[99] Ultrasound is not as successful in identifying the communicating cysts/diverticula as is intravenous urogram. As such, the intravenous urogram may still be the best modality for defining the calyceal and cystic changes, with ultrasound revealing the cortical lobation, renal cortical changes, and coincidental genital abnormalities.[99]

Collecting System Duplication

The occurrence of collecting system duplication has been reported to be 0.5 to 10 percent of live births, with an incidence on urography of 6 percent. The diagnosis is usually made by excretory urography. However, ultrasound may be done in the place of excretory urography to evaluate for presence of kidneys and to exclude hydronephrosis and a duplication anomaly.[100]

The ureters develop from separate ureteric buds that have grown from a single wolffian duct. The ureter to the lower pole enters the bladder at the trigone. The ureter draining the upper pole enters the bladder below this point. Occasionally, the upper-pole ureter ends ectopically outside the bladder. In males, the ureter end that is proximal to the external urinary sphincter may enter the vesical neck, prostatic urethra, seminal vesicle, vas deferens, or ejaculatory duct. An ectopic ureter is much more common in females and usually drains into the vesical neck or beyond the sphincter into the urethra, vagina, or uterus. The upper-pole ureter frequently ends in the internal sphincter or in association with a ureterocele. This results in hydroureteronepehrosis of the upper pole. The renal cortex of the upper pole is usually a functionless shell of dysplastic tissue. The excretory urogram is diagnostic in only 50 percent of cases[101] (see also Ch. 14).

Ultrasound can be helpful in the diagnosis of a duplicated collecting system by identifying two echodensities in the area of the renal sinus (Figs. 13-8, 13-9, and 13-

44). If dilatation is present, the system affected would have the sonographic characteristics of hydronephrosis. The presence of an associated dilated ureter should be determined and its course followed. If dilated ureters are seen within the pelvis, a search for a ureterocele should be made (see also Ch. 14). At times, the ultrasound signs of duplication will be absent if there is a diminutive nonfunctioning upper moiety.[30]

Abnormalities of Amount of Renal Tissue

If agenesis is bilateral and total, death will result. If agenesis is unilateral, there may be adequate renal function. Agenesis is presumed to be due to unilateral absence of the nephrogenic primordium or to failure of the wolffian duct to make contact with the mesodermal mass. Occasionally, a small undifferentiated mass is present. The renal artery and vein may be absent or rudimentary. With hypoplasia, the kidney fails to develop to normal size. This entity is most commonly unilateral. There are a reduced number of renal lobules and calyces.[24]

It is extremely difficult for ultrasound to diagnose agenesis. If no identifiable kidney is seen in the renal fossa, an ectopic kidney cannot be excluded. This diagnosis is better made by a renal nuclear medicine study. On the other hand, if a very small kidney is identified in the renal fossa, with hypertrophy of the contralateral kidney, one may suspect hypoplasia on the basis of ultrasound (Fig. 13-45). It is important to note that if only one kidney is visualized, there is a 69.9 percent incidence of genital abnormalities in the female.[102]

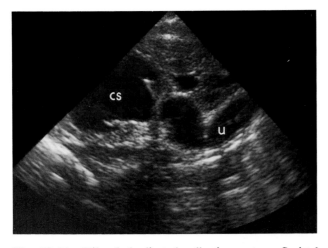

Fig. 13-44. Dilated duplicated collecting system. Sagittal scan of the left kidney demonstrating dilatation of the upper pole collecting system *(cs)* with a dilated ureter *(u)*.

Anomalies of Position, Form, and Orientation

The kidneys may not lie in the normal renal fossa. A kidney may lie either just above the pelvic brim or sometimes within the pelvis (Fig. 13-46). Rarely, a kidney is even intrathoracic, with the left hemithorax being the most common location.[103] The theory for the cause of the intrathoracic location is related to the abnormally high ascent of the embryonic kidney, which comes in contact with the diaphragm and affects its development.[103] The kidney may resemble a Bochdalek hernia; a neurogenic mass including neuroblastoma, ganglioneuroma, neurofibroma, neurogenic cyst, and meningocele; or a pericardial cyst or sequestration. The congenitally high ectopic kidney characteristically has a thin membrane diaphragm layer above the superior pole, in contrast to a thoracic kidney in association with either traumatic or Bochdalek hernia[103] (Fig. 13-47). Patients with a pelvic kidney may be referred to ultrasound for evaluation of a pelvic mass. If the mass seen by ultrasound resembles a kidney, ectopia should be suspected and both renal fossae should be scanned for confirmation. If the primary question is one of renal ectopia, the patient is better served by a renal nuclear medicine study.

Crossed renal ectopia is relatively uncommon, with the fused ectopic kidney being more common than the unfused variety.[104,105] Crossed-fused renal ectopia occurs in approximately 1 of 7,500 autopsies.[106] It is most often right-sided, with fusion of the two renal units eight times more common than nonfusion.[107] The aberrant vascular supply may show great variability and can arise from either side of the lower aorta or from the common or external iliac arteries.[107] Anomalies of renal fusion can be complex, which reflects the complicated embryologic development of the urinary tract.[106] With the unfused type, one kidney is in the normal position and the other is most often located at or below the level of the sacral promontory. With both kidneys on the same side of the abdomen, one of the two ureters crosses the midline to the vesical orifice on the contralateral side.[105] These abnormalities have been attributed to faulty development of the ureteral bud, vascular impediments, and teratogenic factors.[106] The various forms of fusion anomalies include unilateral fused, cake, disc, sigmoid, L-shaped, and solitary crossed ectopia.[106] The lesion itself produces no symptoms and typically comes to the attention of the physician during workup of a patient for other problems, so the examiner should be aware of its appearance. Because ultrasound is used frequently as an initial imaging technique, failure to recognize the abnormality an cause misdiagnosis.

A crossed-fused kidney may mimic a single kidney with a duplicated system or a kidney with a renal mass[105]

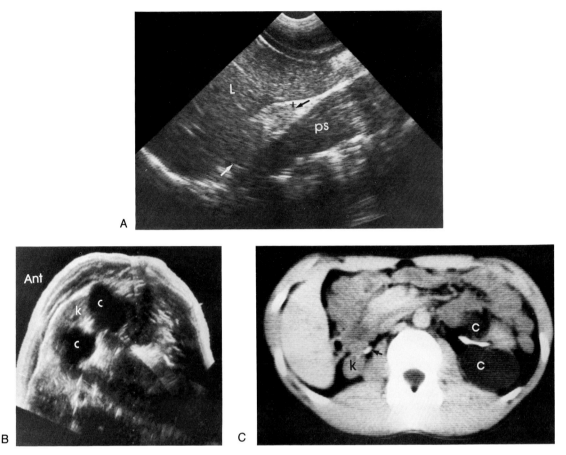

Fig. 13-45. Hypoplastic kidney. Sixteen-year-old patient with hypertension. **(A)** Longitudinal scan showing a very small structure (arrows) in the right renal fossa. (*ps*, psoas muscle; *L*, liver.) **(B)** Right lateral decubitus position, transverse scan of the left kidney showing multiple anechoic areas (*c*, cysts) in the area of the left kidney *(k)*. (*Ant*, anterior.) **(C)** Enhanced CT scan. A very small kidney *(k)* is seen on the right, with contrast in the ureter (arrow). The left kidney demonstrates multiple low-density areas (*c*, cysts).

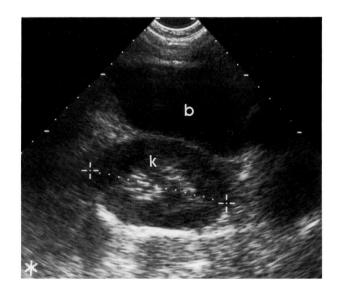

Fig. 13-46. Pelvic kidney. Sagittal transabdominal scan through the distended urinary bladder *(b)* with a pelvic kidney *(k)* located posteriorly.

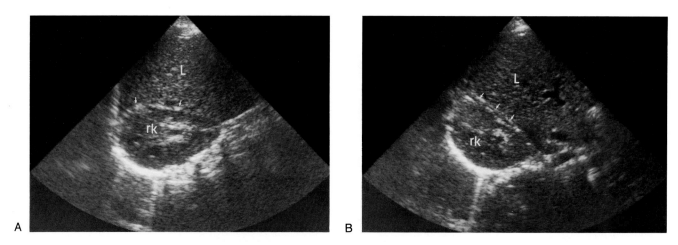

Fig. 13-47. Thoracic kidney. **(A)** Sagittal and **(B)** transverse scans showing the right kidney *(rk)* above the hemidiaphragm (arrows). The relationship of the kidney to the hemidiaphragm was most dramatic at real-time. *(L, liver.)*

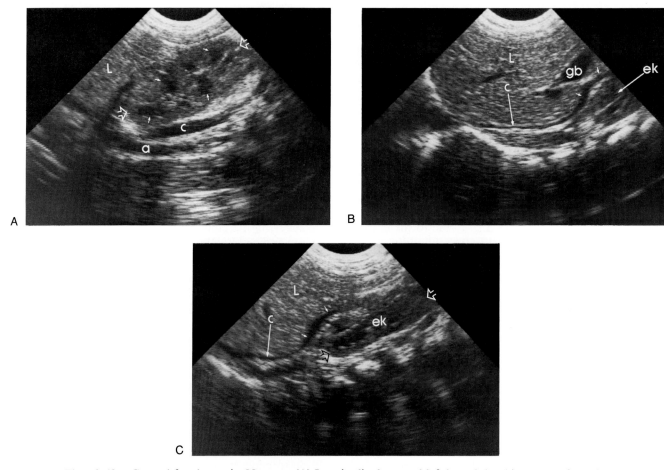

Fig. 13-48. Crossed-fused ectopia. Neonate. **(A)** Longitudinal coronal left lateral decubitus scan of the right kidney. The kidney (open arrows) is identified in the renal fossa anterior to the inferior vena cava *(c)* and aorta *(a).* (small arrows, pyramids; *L*, liver.) **(B & C)** Longitudinal scans with Fig. B more superior than Fig. C. The inferior vena cava *(c)* is displaced (small arrows) anteriorly and to the left by the crossed-fused kidney *(ek,* open arrows). *(gb,* gallbladder; *L*, liver.) *(Figure continues.)*

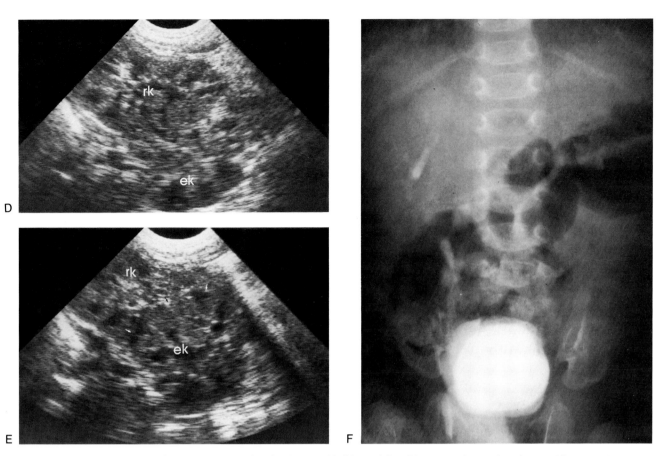

D

E

F

Fig. 13-48 *(Continued).* **(D & E)** Longitudinal coronal left lateral decubitus scans lower than the renal fossa, and more medial. A mass *(ek,* arrows, crossed-fused kidney) is seen continuous with the right kidney *(rk).* **(F)** Intravenous pyelogram documenting the finding.

(Figs. 13-48 to 13-51). The characteristic anterior and/or posterior notch provides the major clue to the correct diagnosis[105] (Figs. 13-49 and 13-50A). In addition, the kidney will be much too long for a single kidney. Other ultrasound findings described when there is a complicated ipsilateral fused kidney include (1) echoic texture of the renal "mass," (2) differential orientation of the renal pelves, (3) the content of the contralateral renal fossa, (4) the size of the ipsilateral kidney, (5) extension of the isthmus medially anterior to the spine, and (6) the presence of a deep anteroposterior notch.[106] In cases of renal agenesis or ectopia, colonic flexure and small bowel may occupy the contralateral renal fossa, mimicking a mass or a hydronephrotic kidney.[105,108] Colon filled with stool or fluid may simulate a kidney or a mass.[108]

The sonographer/sonologist should be aware that fused renal units are quite different in appearance from the usual "duplex" systems encountered.[106] In these situations, when the examiner encounters a "mass" connected to the kidney, fusion, duplication, and neoplasm

must be considered. To differentiate these possibilities, the following parameters may be of value: (1) echoic texture and architecture of the mass, (2) orientation of the pelves of the fused elements with respect to each other, (3) contralateral renal fossa for the presence and normality of the contralateral kidney, (4) size of the ipsilateral kidney, (5) extension medially anterior to the spine, and (6) deep anteroposterior notch.[106]

Occasionally there is multicystic renal dysplasia in a cross-fused or nonfused ectopic kidney, which may produce unusual findings.[107] The cause of the multicystic kidney associated with crossed-fused ectopia may be secondary to obstruction created by the renal fusion.[107] The anomalous blood supply may cause constriction of the renal pelvis or ureter.[107] With marked dilatation of the crossed ureter, cystic dysplasia is usually caused by the obstruction that occurs with ureteral ectopia and the associated ureterocele. The diagnosis should be considered if the following are identified: (1) multicystic mass of variable size that is contiguous with the lower pole of a hydronephrotic, malrotated kidney; (2) ureteral dis-

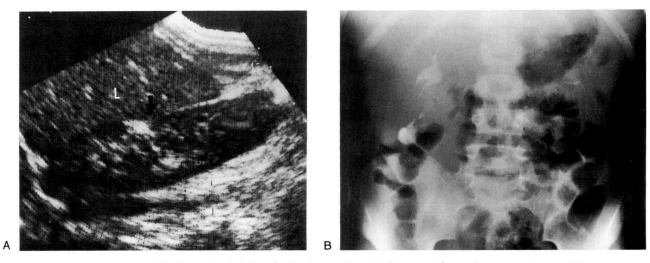

Fig. 13-49. Crossed-fused ectopia. **(A)** Longitudinal scan through right renal fossa, demonstrating a reniform structure with a notch (arrow). (*L*, liver.) **(B)** Abdominal radiograph after a contrast CT, showing crossed-fused ectopia. (From McCarthy and Rosenfield,[105] with permission.)

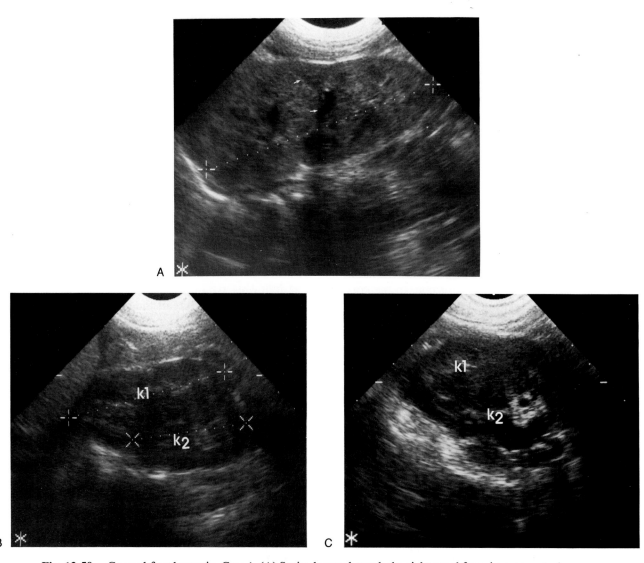

Fig. 13-50. Crossed-fused ectopia. Case 1. **(A)** Sagittal scan through the right renal fossa in a neonate demonstrating a reniform structure with a notch (arrows) noting the place of fusion. Case 2. **(B)** Sagittal coronal and **(C)** transverse lateral decubitus scans demonstrating a mass in the region of the right renal fossa representing the two fused kidneys. One (*k1*, 52 mm) is more posterior and inferior to the other (*k2*, 72 mm).

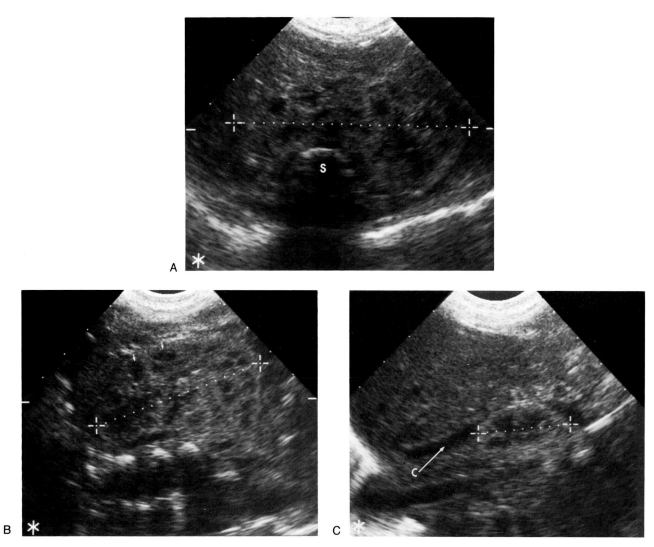

Fig. 13-51. Crossed-fused ectopia. **(A)** Transverse scan in the midline showing a large mass which is 7 cm wide (calipers). (*S*, spine.) **(B)** Sagittal scan slightly to the left showing a reniform mass (calipers, 5.5 cm). Renal pyramids are seen as hypoechoic areas (arrows). **(C)** Sagittal scan slightly to the right of midline showing reniform tissue (calipers) posterior to the inferior vena cava *(c)*. Most of the renal mass is to the left of midline.

placement and/or dilatation; and (3) contralateral absence of the kidney and its renal artery.[107]

A horseshoe kidney occurs in 0.2 to 1 percent of autopsies and, as such, represents a commonly anomaly.[24,109,110] Most of these kidneys are fused at the lower pole, with 10 percent fused in the upper pole. The bridge at the lower poles has the ureters passing anteriorly. This anomalous kidney is not more prone to disease. However, renal calculi are slightly more frequent.[24] These kidneys can also be associated with ectopia (i.e., they can be in a pelvic location).[109]

The patient with a horseshoe kidney is often referred to ultrasound for evaluation of a pulsatile mass. On the sonogram, a mass is seen anterior to the abdominal aorta (Figs. 13-52 and 13-53). Instead of immediately consid-ering pancreatic enlargement or lymphadenopathy, the examiner should consider a horseshoe kidney. The renal axes should be obtained by using real-time ultrasound. The lower poles can be followed into the mass by oblique scanning. The isthmus across the lower poles usually is seen at the fourth to fifth lumbar area[111] (Figs. 13-52 and 13-53). It appears as solid renal tissue.

A patient may have an exaggerated anteroposterior axis to the kidney such that the lower pole is very superficial (Figs. 13-14 and 13-54). This patient is often referred to ultrasound for evaluation of a palpable abdominal mass.[112] The kidney is embedded in perirenal fat and lies on the anterior surface of the paravertebral and psoas muscles. The fat is most abundant behind and inferior to the lower pole of the kidney.[112] The normal axis is paral-

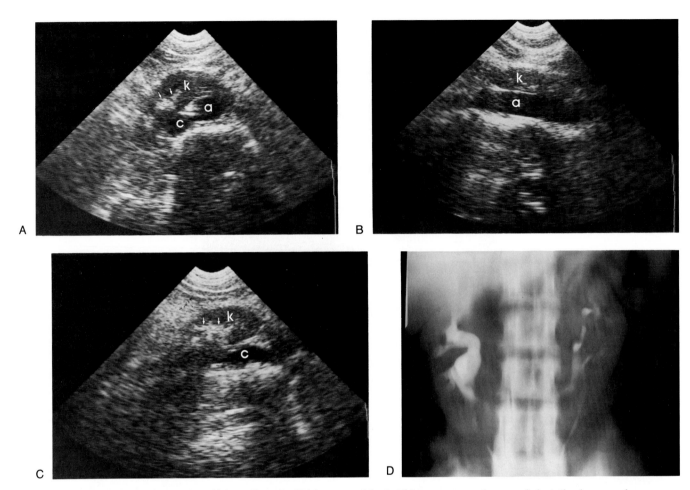

Fig. 13-52. Horseshoe kidney. Longitudinal scans of both kidneys appeared normal, but the lower poles appeared to be oriented medially. **(A)** Transverse scan demonstrating a mass *(k)* anterior to the aorta *(a)* and inferior vena cava *(c)*. The transducer is angled slightly oblique. Echodense renal sinus echoes (arrows) can be seen. **(B & C)** Longitudinal scans showing a mass *(k)* anterior to the aorta *(a)* and inferior vena cava *(c)*. Renal sinus echoes (arrows) are seen in Fig. C. **(D)** Intravenous pyelogram confirming the ultrasound findings of a horseshoe kidney.

lel to the spine, with the lower pole slightly more anterior than the upper pole. Using real-time scanning, one can quickly establish that the mass is indeed the normal lower pole of the kidney (Fig. 13-54). However, careful scanning of the renal fossa should be performed to exclude a mass that is displacing the kidney anteriorly.

Obstructive Uropathy

Hydronephrosis represents dilatation of the renal pelvis and calyces associated with progressive atrophy of the kidney owing to obstruction of the outflow of urine. The high pressure in the renal pelvis is transmitted back through the collecting ducts into the cortex, causing renal atrophy, and compressing the renal vasculature of the medulla, causing a decrease in the inner medullary plasma flow.[24]

There are numerous causes of hydronephrosis. In addition to identifying the presence of hydronephrosis, it is necessary to investigate the cause. The congenital anomalies include posterior urethral valves, urethral strictures, meatal stenosis, bladder neck obstruction, UPJ narrowing or obstruction, and severe vesicoureteral reflux. The acquired organic causes of obstruction include calculi, benign prostatic enlargement, tumors (bladder or prostate tumors, contiguous malignant disease, carcinoma of the cervix or uterus), inflammation (prostatitis, ureteritis, or urethritis), sloughed papillae or blood clot, normal pregnancy, and functional disorders (neurogenic).[24] Intrinsic causes may include calculus, blood clot, tumor, stricture, ureterocele, pyelonephritis, or

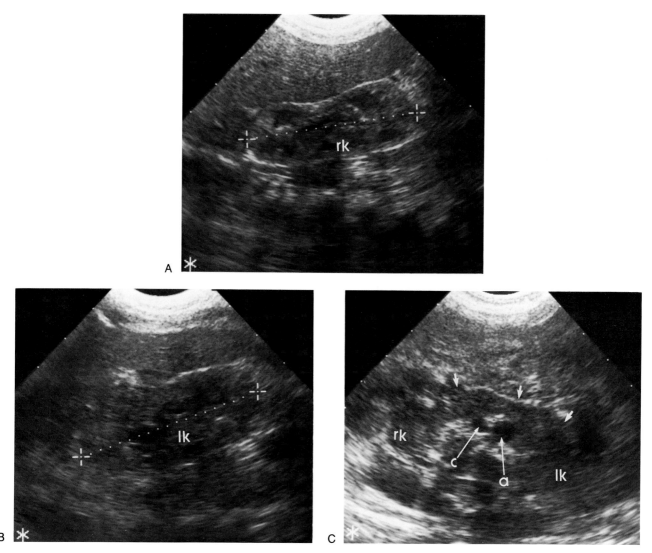

Fig. 13-53. Horseshoe kidney, neonate. Sagittal scans of the **(A)** right *(rk)* and **(B)** left *(lk)* renal fossae demonstrating somewhat low kidneys with the inferior pole more anteriorly located than usual. **(C)** Transverse view through the midline of the abdomen showing tissue (arrows) anterior to the aorta *(a)* and inferior vena cava *(c)* connecting the two kidneys *(rk, lk)*.

congenital conditions such as UPJ obstruction, posterior urethral valves, or ectopic ureterocele.[84] Extrinsic causes are multiple and include neoplasm, trauma, postoperative, neurogenic bladder, retroperitoneal fibrosis, pregnancy, gynecologic problems (endometrioma, tuboovarian abscess, etc.), and bladder outlet obstruction (caused by neoplasm, prostatic enlargement, and/or urethral problems).[84]

Ultrasound is an accurate modality to screen for hydronephrosis.[113,114] Normally, there is no separation of the dense echo collection in the region of the renal sinus (Fig. 13-1). With mild hydronephrosis, there is slight separation with a lucency noted[101] (Fig. 13-55). With moderate hydronephrosis, there is further separation of the echoes by lucency (Fig. 13-56). In severe hydronephrosis, there is a huge lucent sac with marked thinning of the renal parenchyma[115] (Fig. 13-57). The degree of collecting system dilatation depends on parameters such as duration of obstruction, renal output, and presence or absence of spontaneous collecting system decompression.[116] The amount of residual renal cortex identified is of more prognostic significance than the size of the hydronephrotic sac.[84]

There have been reports concerning the influence of hydration and bladder distension on the sonographic diagnosis of hydronephrosis. Findings of moderate bi-

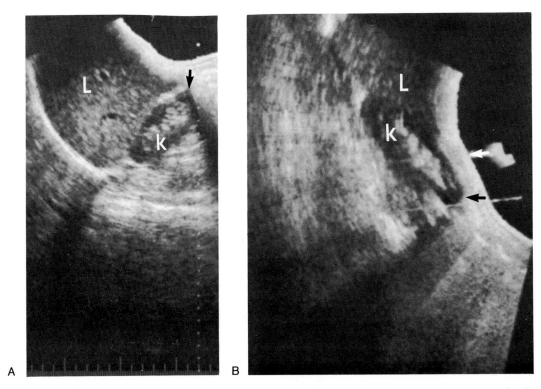

Fig. 13-54. Palpable kidney. Thin, young woman with a palpable right abdominal mass. **(A)** Longitudinal supine scan, right kidney *(k)*. Note how anterior (arrow) the inferior pole of kidney is. (*L*, liver.) **(B)** longitudinal upright scan. The kidney *(k)* is even more superficial. The level (white arrow) of the lower pole in the supine position was marked. In the upright position, the lower pole (black arrow) of the kidney has moved downward. (*L*, liver.)

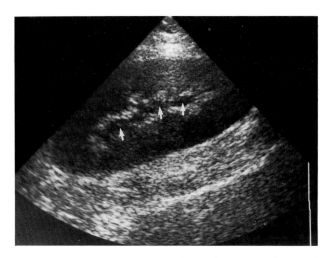

Fig. 13-55. Mild hydronephrosis. Sagittal scan of a renal transplant demonstrating mild dilatation of the collecting system (arrows).

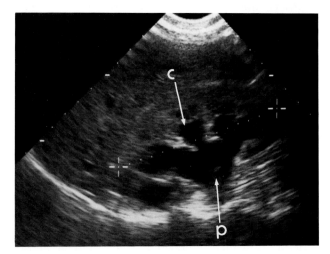

Fig. 13-56. Moderate hydronephrosis. Sagittal scan of the right kidney in an adult demonstrating moderate dilatation of the collecting system (*p*, pelvis; *c*, calyces). There is a moderate amount of parenchyma. The dilated collecting system makes up half the kidney.

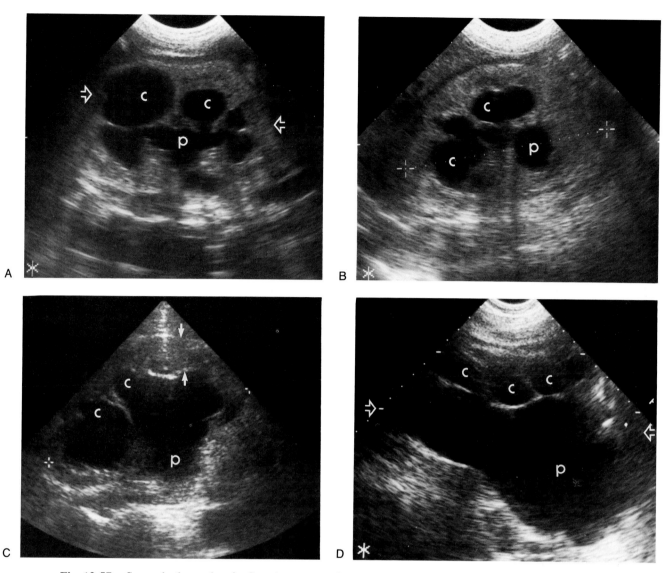

Fig. 13-57. Severe hydronephrosis. Case 1, neonate with posterior urethral valves. **(A)** Sagittal and **(B)** transverse scans of the left kidney. The collecting system is markedly dilated, filling more than half the kidney. (calipers, open arrows, renal margin; *p*, renal pelvis; *c*, calyces.) Cases 2 and 3, adults. **(C & D)** Sagittal views of the right kidneys showing severe dilatation of the collecting system. Although there is parenchyma (arrows) in Fig. C, it is not identified in Fig. D. (*p*, renal pelvis; calipers, open arrows, renal margin; *c*, calyces.)

lateral hydronephrosis may be encountered in a dehydrated patient undergoing rehydration. In addition, the filled bladder in a patient undergoing hydration may result in the ultrasound appearance of hydronephrosis. The differentiation between volume depletion and obstructive uropathy is difficult clinically. The ultrasound should be done with an empty bladder and before initiation of rehydration.[117] It should be remembered that dilatation of the collecting system does not always equate with obstruction[8]; it can also be seen with retroperitoneal fibrosis, diabetes insipidus, previous obstruction, ureterovesical reflux, and infection.

The renal sinus is composed of the collecting system structures, vessels, lymphatics, and fibrofatty tissue. Nonhydronephrotic fragmentation of the central renal complex is usually attributed to nephrolithiasis, renal sinus lipomatosis, and some forms of cystic disease. There are certain entities associated with false-negative diagnoses of hydronephrosis. These include staghorn calculus filling the collecting system (the acoustic shadow obscures the dilatation) (Figs. 13-58 and 13-59); acute renal obstruction (the system is not dilated); spontaneous decompression of an obstructive system; numerous cysts with superimposed hydronephrosis; misin-

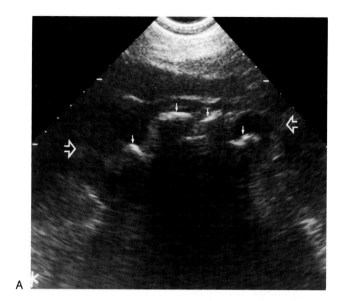
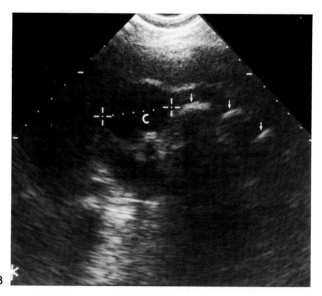

Fig. 13-58. Staghorn calculus. **(A)** Sagittal and **(B)** transverse scans of the right kidney showing multiple echogenic foci (arrows) within the region of the collecting system; these are associated with acoustic shadowing and represent portions of a staghorn calculus. In Fig. B dilatation of some of the calyces *(c)* is seen, along with portions of the stone (arrows). (open arrows, renal outline.)

terpretation of hydronephrosis or cystic disease; retroperitoneal fibrosis; misinterpretation of calyectasis as large, lucent pyramids; a fluid-depleted patient with partial obstruction; intermittent obstruction; and technical factors (obesity, adjacent gas, uncooperative patient).[116]

There are also causes of a false-positive diagnosis of hydronephrosis. These include normal variants (distensible collecting system, extrarenal renal pelvis [Fig. 13-60], full bladder, congenital megacalyces [Fig. 13-43], calyceal diverticulum); increased urine flow (overhydration, medications, osmotic diuresis during or immediately after urography, diabetes insipidus, diuresis in nonoliguric azotemia); inflammatory disease (acute pyelonephritis, chronic pyelonephritis, tuberculosis); renal cystic disease (single cyst, parapelvic cyst [Fig. 13-39], adult polycystic kidney disease [Figs. 13-28 to 13-31], medullary cystic disease [Fig. 13-32], multicystic dysplastic kidney); and other causes such as postobstructive or postsurgical dilatation, vesicoureteral reflux, papillary necrosis, and renal sinus lipomatosis.[29,84,116]

Grade I Hydronephrosis

The minimally dilated renal collecting system has been evaluated by ultrasound.[118] By ignoring the grade I hydronephrosis, the false-positive rate of diagnosis of obstruction will be decreased, but this is at the expense of an unacceptable increase in the false-negative rate.[118]

When the clinical question of renal obstruction is raised, however, it appears that grade I hydronephrosis (minimally dilated renal collecting system) is significant.[118] It seems unlikely to be of any significance when it is discovered as an incidental finding.[118] As such, renal ultrasound findings must be considered in conjunction with the overall clinical situation.

Doppler Evaluation

Studies have been performed to evaluate the capability of duplex ultrasound to differentiate obstructive from nonobstructive pyelocaliectasis.[16,17,119,120] In animal studies, it has been shown that renal obstruction causes an increase in renal vascular resistance, which falls after release.[16] To perform this study, pulsed Doppler evaluation is carried out on the intrarenal arteries of each kidney (see under Technique).[16] These signals are usually obtained from arcuate arteries at the corticomedullary junction and/or interlobar arteries along the border of the medullary pyramids (Fig. 13-3; see Fig. 13-191). The RI is calculated from the duplex waveform. The mean RI for obstructed kidneys is 0.77 ± 0.05, with that for the nonobstructed kidney being 0.63 ± 0.06.[16,17] Using an RI of 0.70 results in a sensitivity of 92 percent, a specificity of 88 percent, and an accuracy of 90 percent for distinguishing between obstructive and nonobstructive pyelocaliectasis.[16] However, obstruction is not the only abnormality that can elevate the RI; in cases of

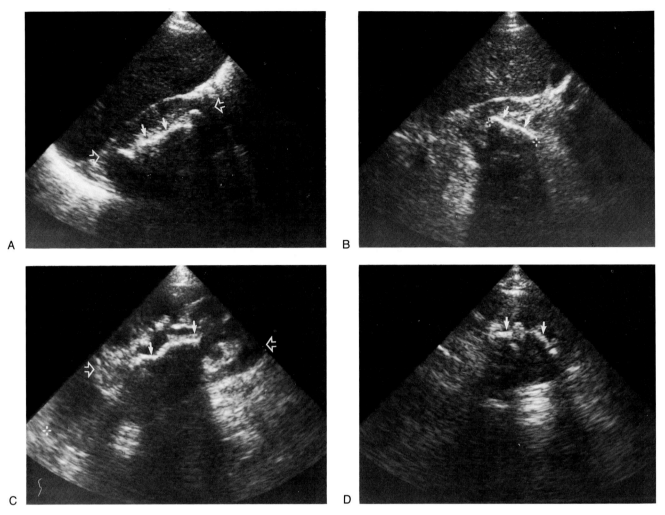

Fig. 13-59. Bilateral staghorn calculi. **(A)** Sagittal and **(B)** transverse scans of the right kidney and **(C)** sagittal and **(D)** transverse scans of the left kidney showing echogenic foci (stones, arrows) within the region of the collecting system. No definite dilatation of the collecting system is noted. Since there is extensive posterior acoustic shadowing, posterior dilatation could be overlooked. (open arrows, renal margins.)

underlying renal disease, an elevated RI may be demonstrated.[16] As such, in the setting of known renal disease and bilateral pyelocaliectasis, an elevated RI may be due to the renal disease with or without true obstruction, which may limit the value of a finding of an abnormal RI.[16] The use of duplex ultrasound should improve the specificity and accuracy of ultrasound in the noninvasive diagnosis of obstruction; therefore duplex ultrasound should be used when a dilated collecting system is visualized.[16,17]

Besides being used to differentiate obstructive from nonobstructive pyelocaliectasis, duplex ultrasound can be used to evaluate the kidney after intervention (e.g., surgery, nephrostomy tube) for effectiveness in relieving the obstruction.[17] In most patients in one series, the relief of obstruction resulted in a reduced RI with the RI becoming less than 0.70.[17] Identifying this change in Doppler waveform (decreased RI) indicates that the renal obstruction is being properly relieved by a functioning tube or stent, despite persistent dilatation of the collecting system, as is often observed.[17] This test is particularly helpful in clinical conditions in which dilatation is usually present. Such conditions include previous surgery that predisposes the patient to reflux (ileal loop, ureterosigmoidostomy, bladder augmentation), a history of chronic reflux, or known postobstructive dilatation of the collecting system.[17]

Another situation that might be ameniable to Doppler evaluation would be the evaluation of the patient with grade I hydronephrosis.[15] It is known that the presence of blood vessels in the region of the renal sinus or hilum may mimic the appearance of hydronephrosis on the

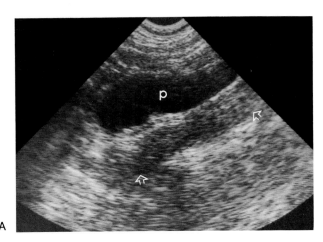
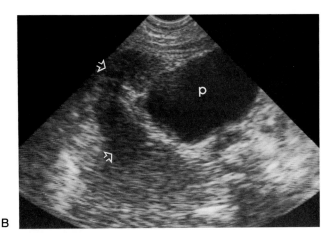

Fig. 13-60. Extrarenal pelvis. **(A)** Sagittal and **(B)** transverse scans of the right kidney showing a large anechoic area *(p)*, which is the dilated extrarenal pelvis. It is seen anterior to the renal parenchyma (open arrows) on the medial longitudinal view (Fig. A) and medial on the transverse view (Fig. B). The calyces were not dilated, and the patient was asymptomatic.

real-time image.[15] By using Doppler assessment of the area of greatest separation of the central renal sinus echoes, true dilatation can be distinguished from vessels mimicking hydronephrosis. In 43 percent of patients, vascular structures account for the separation of the sinus echoes.[15] This frequency rises to 61 percent in patients 12 years of age or younger.[15] As such, pulsed Doppler may be useful in differentiating true dilatation from vessels and should decrease the frequency of false-positive diagnoses of hydronephrosis.[15]

Diuretic Ultrasound

As described above, ultrasound by itself (without Doppler) may have a low specificity in differentiating between obstructive and nonobstructive pyelocaliecta-sis. To further increase its specificity, the study may be performed in conjunction with administration of a diuretic.[18] (For the procedure, see under Technique.) The relative increase in the pelvicalyceal diameters and the time taken for the renal collecting system to return to its initial dimensions are assessed.[18]

It is known that correct management of upper tract obstruction depends on its diagnosis and the degree of obstruction. An accuracy rate of 95 percent may be achieved with any two of the following three tests: diuretic intravenous urogram, diuretic renography, and the Whitaker test.[18] This test, diuretic ultrasound, is particularly helpful to determine whether upper tract stasis, detected on a standard intravenous urogram, is due to obstruction. With this technique, the largest number of correct diagnoses (99 percent) may be found in the normal group, with a high sensitivity (94 percent) and a high negative predictive value (96 percent.)[18] In the presence

of obstruction, the reliability of the test is high with a specificity of 94 percent and a positive predictive value of 91 percent.[18] The test may be useful in the investigation of suspected obstructive uropathy, with additional advantages including its noninvasive nature, the absence of contraindications, its technical ease, its repeatability, and its wide applications.[18]

Others have evaluated ultrasound in conjunction with a forced diuresis, namely diuretic renography and/or diuretic urography with furosemide.[19] As is known, ultrasound has a false-positive diagnosis of 8 to 40 percent.[19] This series recorded a false-negative rate of 14 percent, which is much higher than previously reported.[19] It was thought that the most important reason for this was an insufficient state of hydration of the patient.[19] If ultrasound showed a dilatation of the renal pelvis of 10 mm or more, the patient was given 20 to 40 mg of furosemide orally or 0.3 mg intravenously.[19] The ultrasound was then repeated at 30, 60, and 90 minutes. It is important to perform the renal ultrasound examination after a standardized fluid intake and, in equivocal cases, to use the diuretic urography with furosemide.[19] Normally, the normal central echodense renal complex does not split even during water loading or the furosemide test.[19]

Obstructive Uropathy Follow-up

Studies have been performed to evaluate the effectiveness of preoperative and follow-up ultrasound in patients with obstructive uropathy or vesicoureteral reflux.[121] The most reliable morphometric criteria for objective sonographic staging and follow-up of urinary tract obstruction appear to be the renal volume and anteroposterior diameter of the renal pelvis.[121] Within 4 weeks of ureteral reimplantation, kidneys with transient postoperative ureterovesical junction obstruction were found to revert to normal on ultrasound.[121] It took 6 months for most kidneys to present almost normal ultrasound findings in cases of UPJ obstruction.[121] The most severe size changes were noted with kidneys with UPJ obstruction, which had a mean renal volume of about 300 percent and a marked dilatation of the renal pelvis.[121] The knowledge of the sonographic biometry and the uncomplicated postoperative course makes postsurgical monitoring easier and more reliable.[121]

Congenital Causes

Ureteropelvic Junction Obstruction. UPJ obstruction is a common cause of severe pyelocaliectasis in the child.[122,123] The patient may present with a flank mass or urinary tract infection. On ultrasound the dilated renal pelvis without ureteral dilatation would be seen[123] (Figs. 13-40 to 13-42). With severe UPJ obstruction, the calyces and pelvis become one large, lucent mass.[122] (See also Congenital section under Renal Abnormalities.)

Duplex Collecting System. With a duplex system, hydronephrosis involving either or both systems is visible (Figs. 13-8, 13-9, and 13-44; see Figs. 14-68 and 14-71 to 14-73). Dilatation of a duplex collecting system is fairly common, with the upper system more often dilated. Occasionally, there is hydronephrosis of the lower pole system, resulting in nonvisualization of the lower pole, simulating a mass, on intravenous pyelogram.[124] With ultrasound, the typical hydronephrosis pattern is seen. Dilatation of the upper or lower pole system may be caused by reflux. There is significant dilatation of the ureter and upper system in 85 percent of those with ureteroceles[101] (see Figs. 14-68 and 14-71 to 14-73). With real-time imaging, churning of urine within the ureter or within the calyces may be visible.[125] There may be UPJ obstruction of either system if a dilated ureter is not seen. The examiner should search for a ureterocele when dilatation of an upper duplicated system is seen.

Infundibulopelvic Stenosis. Infundibulopelvic stenosis is characterized by calyceal dilatation, infundibular stenosis, and hypoplasia or stenosis of the renal pelvis.[126] It is a rare congenital form of hydrocalicosis in which dilated calyces drain through a stenotic infundibulum into a variably hypoplastic or stenosed renal pelvis. It belongs to a spectrum of obstructive dysplastic renal diseases, from generalized pyelocaliectasis secondary to ureteral or ureteropelvic stenosis at one end to functionless dysplastic kidney at the other.[126] Hydrocalicosis denotes dilatation of one or more calyces secondary to infundibular stenosis, which may be intrinsic or extrinsic. The extrinsic variety is usually congenital and in most cases results from vascular compression of the infundibulum draining the calyces. The acquired type is caused by trauma or a space-occupying lesion. Hydrocalicosis secondary to intrinsic stenosis may be congenital or secondary to an acquired lesion such as infection, tumor, or trauma. On the sonogram a variable degree of caliceal dilatation without associated pelvic dilatation is seen (Fig. 13-61). The differential diagnosis of infundibular stenosis must include the usual type of hydronephrosis as well as megacalicosis and any space-occupying lesion of the renal hilum, such as a parapelvic cyst or tumor.

Renal Cystic Disease. At times, it is difficult to differentiate severe hydronephrosis from severe renal cystic disease. The identification of a dilated renal pelvis is the most reliable indicator of hydronephrosis.[127] If no dilated renal pelvis is seen, the diagnosis is more probably cystic disease. When there is end-stage hydronephrosis, the differentiation may be particularly difficult. With severe hydronephrosis there is often less normal renal parenchyma. To differentiate the two entities one should look for the following: (1) hepatic cysts, bilateral involvement, calculi, and uniform size of cysts, suggestive of cystic disease; or (2) central circular lucency with small interconnecting lucencies (collecting system), suggestive of hydronephrosis.[127]

Miscellaneous Causes of Hydronephrosis. Hydronephrosis may be secondary to ureteral obstruction. Ureterovesical obstruction is most commonly secondary to extrinsic compression. This may be due to pelvic lymphoma, pelvic abscess, ovarian mass, or large abdominal mass. The dilated ureters are seen as tubular lucencies extending from the kidney to the bladder (see Fig. 14-3). On a transverse scan, they are seen as circular lucencies posterior to the bladder (see Fig. 14-76). If ureteral dilatation is seen proximal to an adynamic narrowed segment of the distal ureter, primary megaureter may be the diagnosis. With a stenotic ureteral orifice, there may be ballooning of the submucosal segment such as a ureterocele, which may prolapse into the bladder outlet, causing the obstruction. In most cases of ureteral obstruction, ultrasound is not capable of locating the exact site of the obstruction.[123]

Bladder outlet, urethral obstruction, or nonobstructive dilatation is usually bilateral. The bladder outlet may be obstructed by congenital anomalies such as duplication, septation, or tumor. Urethral obstruction may be due to an anatomic lesion such as posterior urethral valves or post-traumatic urethral stricture. Functional urethral obstruction may be produced by spasm of the

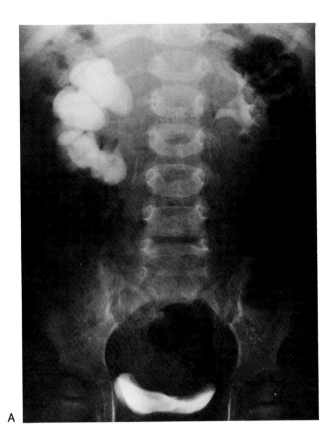

A

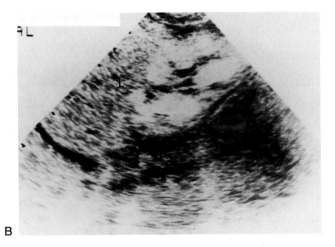

B

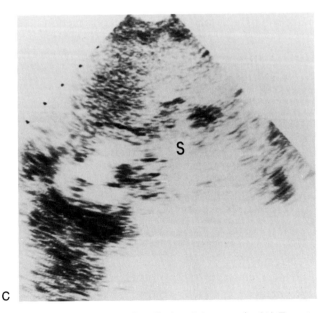

C

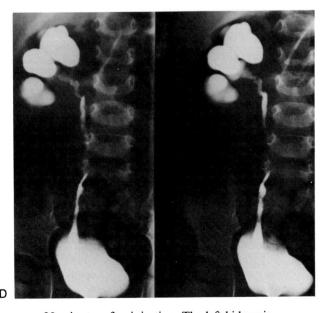

D

Fig. 13-61. Infundibulopelvic stenosis. **(A)** Excretory urogram 20 minutes after injection. The left kidney is normal. There is severe dilatation of all calyces of the right kidney. Part of the right ureter is seen, but the right pelvis is not seen. **(B)** Longitudinal and **(C)** transverse scans of the right kidney showing severe caliceal dilatation. The renal pelvis is not identified. (*L,* liver; *S,* spine.) **(D)** Retrograde ureteropyelogram showing a hypoplastic renal pelvis and severe caliceal dilatation. (From Lucaya et al,[126] with permission.)

external urinary sphincter (neurogenic bladder).[123] (For further discussion of the lower urinary tract, see Ch. 14.)

There may be some degree of hydronephrosis associated with other congenital abnormalities not previously mentioned. With renal dysmorphism and dysplasia, there may be some dilatation with obstruction. In congenital megacalyces, there are congenital, abnormally dilated, blunted supernumerary calyces that may be associated with a nonobstructive, nonreflux dilatation (Fig. 13-43). In Eagle-Barrett syndrome (prunebelly syndrome or abdominal muscle deficiency), there is dilatation of the calyces, ureters, bladder, posterior urethra, and (occasionally) anterior urethra. The degree of dilatation is variable but often is marked. Seventy percent of these patients have vesicoureteral reflux that contributes to the dilatation.[123]

Reflux. Ultrasound can be a valuable screening procedure in evaluating the first urinary tract infection in children to detect congenital abnormalities of the urinary tract and, in particular, obstructive lesions.[128,129] Ultrasound alone can miss major reflux, although it can detect reflux at times.[128] As such, in the very young child (younger than 5 years of age) who is at risk for reflux nephropathy, the ultrasound examination should be accompanied by a voiding cystourethrogram or an isotope cystourethrogram.[128] The most accurate and reliable method of detection of reflux is conventional voiding cystourethrography, and it should be the first diagnostic study.[130] If the child is older than 5 or 6 years and the ultrasound is normal, it may be sufficient as the only investigation of a noncomplicated first-documented urinary tract infection.[128]

Investigators have evaluated the use of ultrasound instead of the excretory urogram as the imaging modality in evaluation of urinary tract infection in children.[129,130] When compared with urography, the sensitivity and specificity of ultrasound are 100 and 51 percent, respectively, provided that it was of good technical quality.[130] As such, in the absence of vesicoureteral reflux in children with urinary tract infection, the evaluation may be performed by ultrasound.[130] In the presence of reflux or a suspicious or abnormal ultrasound, an excretory urogram appears to be necessary.[130]

Vesicoureteral reflux, which can be a congenital anomaly, has been seen in the fetus; it decreases in frequency with age.[128] This abnormality may be acquired as a result of intrauterine or postnatal obstruction, neurogenic causes, or infection.[128] In most cases of reflux in infants and children, the abnormality is primary and is due to a number of anatomic and physiologic factors.[131] Detection of hydronephrosis at perinatal ultrasound has the benefit that there may be prompt evaluation and treatment of the asymptomatic term infant after delivery.[131] The younger the child, the greater the risk of significant parenchymal damage and possible reflux nephropathy.[128] Whenever possible, reflux nephropathy must be prevented since it is a significant cause of endstage renal disease, leading to dialysis and renal transplant.[128] The reflux is capable of delivering infected urine from the bladder to the renal collecting system (and, in the presence of intrarenal reflux, into the renal parenchyma itself) and is the main contributing factor to reflux nephropathy.[130] Renal damage may be prevented or minimized by antibiotic prophylaxis and/or surgical treatment in such infants[131] (see also Ch. 14).

Miscellaneous Causes

Pregnancy. Hydronephrosis is often seen in pregnancy. The incidence of right hydronephrosis is greater (90 percent) than that on the left (67 percent).[132,133] The calyceal diameter of both kidneys is found to increase gradually through pregnancy, with the right increasing more rapidly than the left. There is less likely to be pathologic dilatation when minimal dilatation is seen in an asymptomatic patient.[132] As such, the finding of dilatation should be interpreted with caution because there are sequential variations. Neither parity nor a history of urinary tract problems is relevant to the degree of dilatation.

The etiology of hydronephrosis in pregnancy is controversial. Mechanical pressure of the gravid uterus is thought to be the most important pressure on the ureter as it crosses the pelvic brim.[132] This is thought to cause partial obstruction of urine flow, increasing the pressure in the proximal ureter and subsequent ureteral and pelvic dilatation. Other theories for the production of the hydronephrosis are hormonal. The high progesterone level of pregnancy produces smooth muscle relaxation of the ureteral walls that is analogous to progesterone-induced smooth muscle relaxation of the uterus.[133]

Renal Colic. One group of investigators has evaluated the role of ultrasound in patients with renal colic.[134,135] For adequate assessment, these patients are hydrated to emphasize mild early caliectasis and ureterectasis and to fill the bladder. The kidneys are evaluated for calculi, hydronephrosis, and perinephric fluid; the pelvis is evaluated for the distal ureter, hydroureter, ureterovesical junction calculi, ureterovesical junction edema, and the presence of ureteral jets (see Ch. 14). The criterion for a positive examination is visualization of a urinary tract calculus or unilateral hydronephrosis with or without ureterectasia[135] (Figs. 13-62 and 13-63). This has a sensitivity of 100 percent with a specificity of 95 percent.[135]

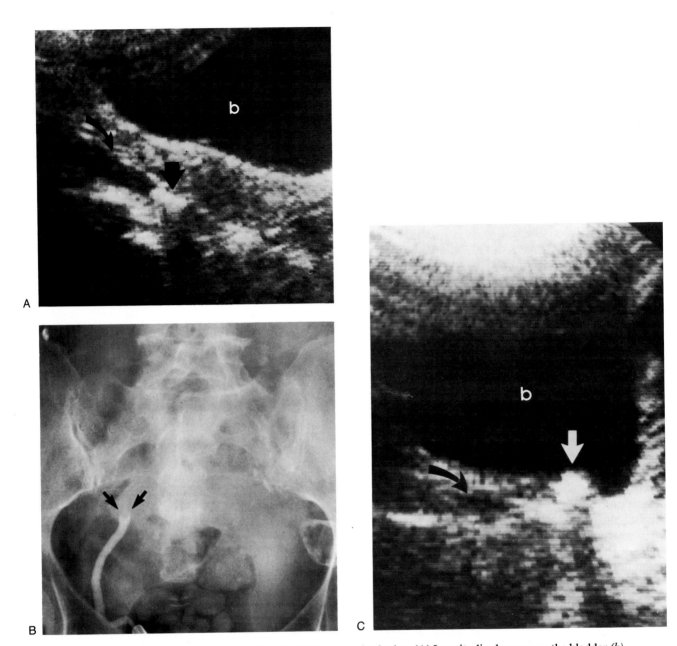

Fig. 13-62. Ureterovesical calculus. Case 1. Distal ureteral calculus. **(A)** Longitudinal scan near the bladder *(b)* demonstrating an echogenic calculus (large arrow) with posterior shadowing within the distended ureter (curved arrow). **(B)** Retrograde ureterogram confirming the presence of a nonopaque calculus (arrows) within the distal right ureter. **(C)** Longitudinal scan taken 1 week later demonstrating the calculus (straight arrow), which has moved to the ureterovesical junction. Note the dilated ureter (curved arrow). (*b*, bladder.) *(Figure continues.)*

Eighty-nine percent of those with proven calculi have unilateral hydronephrosis, and 17 percent have perirenal fluid.[135] Ultrasound detects stones that are not visualized by radiography. The use of ultrasound in the initial evaluation of renal colic is recommended.

Other investigators have also evaluated the role of ultrasound in evaluating acute flank pain.[136] Abdominal radiography can detect approximately 90 to 99 percent of suspected ureteral calculi.[136] It does not appear to be as useful for evaluating patients with acute flank pain in whom acute obstruction may be present.[136] It is not as sensitive as excretory urography for diagnosing hydronephrosis, for detecting ureteral or renal calcification, or for diagnosing forniceal rupture.

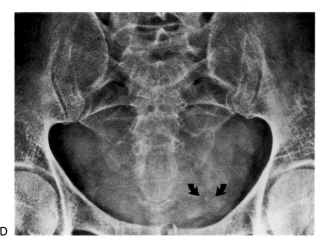
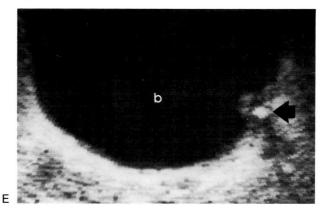

Fig. 13-62 *(Continued).* Case 2. Ureterovesical junction calculus. **(D)** Abdominal radiograph showing a small, left-sided pelvic calcification (curved arrows). **(E)** Transverse scan demonstrating an echogenic calculus (arrow) with posterior acoustic shadowing. Note the mound of edematous tissue at the ureterovesical junction. (*b*, bladder.) (From Erwin et al,[135] with permission.)

Diverted Kidneys. Ileal loop is one of the most frequently used bladder substitutes, and it is associated with numerous short- and long-term problems.[137] The most frequent complication is obstruction at the ureteroileal anastomosis; a less frequent problem is the progressive deterioration of previously insulted upper tracts, occurring in the absence of obstruction.[137] Obstruction is the only reversible condition when renal function appears to be deteriorating.[137]

Ultrasound may be effective in excluding the diagnosis of renal obstruction in patients with loops, although the number of false-positive results in one series was very high — 40 percent.[137] As such, in these patients the detection of a dilated collecting system has less than the usual significance. As the grade of hydronephrosis progresses from grade 1 to grade 3, the association between hydronephrosis and renal obstruction increases.[137] A specificity of only 65 percent has been demonstrated when obstruction was specifically addressed.[137] This might be another use for Doppler evaluation; however, since in many of these cases there is underlying chronic renal disease, the evaluation of the RI may not be as specific. Further imaging studies may be required to differentiate nonobstructive from obstructive hydronephrosis.

Imaging and Accuracy

Real-time ultrasound is the preferred method for scanning because of the greater flexibility and shorter scan time. In one series comparing the accuracy of real-time versus static scanning, real-time scanning demonstrated an overall accuracy of 94 percent, as opposed to 93 percent for static scanning.[115] Other authors have reported a sensitivity of 98 percent for ultrasound when compared with urography.[114,138] Ultrasound is most accurate (100 percent) in detecting moderate to severe hydronephrosis.[114] The inaccuracies are in the area of minimal hydronephrosis. This pattern may be seen normally without hydronephrosis with a full renal pelvis. It may also be seen with multiple parapelvic cysts.

How accurate is ultrasound in diagnosing hydronephrosis in the patient with chronic renal disease and decreased renal output? Whenever there is obstruction of the urinary outflow, the hydrostatic pressure proximal to the obstruction is elevated and is eventually transmitted through the renal tubules to the glomerulus. The ultimate effect on the glomerular filtrate rate is variable, depending on a balance among blood flow, filtration pressure and intratubular pressure, site of the obstruction, degree and duration of the obstruction, and rapidity of onset. This is reflected in the extent of the dilatation of the collecting system. Whatever the cause, the precipitous effect of all these variables coupled with dehydration and sepsis apparently results in a markedly decreased urinary output and thus little or no dilatation. As such, minimal dilatation in a patient with chronic renal disease may actually represent significant hydronephrosis.[139,140]

To aid the evaluation of acute renal failure, ultrasound appears to be the imaging method of choice.[141] However, in cases of complete and long-term obstruction of the urinary tract, there may not necessarily be dilatation of the upper part of the tract.[141] The cause of the absence of dilatation is a matter of conjecture — there may be either

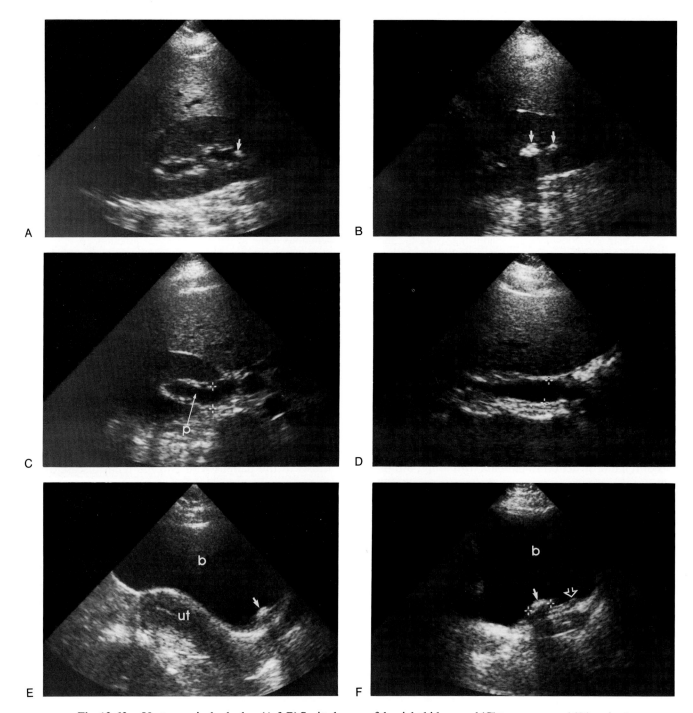

Fig. 13-63. Ureterovesical calculus. **(A & B)** Sagittal scans of the right kidney and **(C)** transverse and **(D)** sagittal views of the renal pelvic area demonstrating echogenic foci (stones, arrows) within the minimally dilated upper-pole collecting system. The dilated renal pelvis *(p)* is seen in Fig. C with the proximal dilated ureter (calipers, 16 mm) seen in Fig. D. **(E)** On sagittal and **(F)** transverse views of the pelvis, a stone (echogenic foci, arrow) is seen in the region of the right ureterovesical junction. (*ut*, uterus; *b*, bladder; open arrow, left ureterovesical junction.)

an absence of increased pressure inside the cavities or a modification in the physical properties of the urinary tract wall.[141] With experimental studies, it has been shown that the glomerular filtration and transtubular reabsorption are never totally abolished in cases of complete obstruction of the ureter.[141] Absence of dilatation, despite the increased pressure, could be due to a modification of the physical properties of the parietal layer.[141] Alternatively, it is possible that this absence of dilatation is due to a particular morphology of the renal pelvis.[141] Notwithstanding, the sonographer/sonologist should be aware of this possibility. These investigators believed that ultrasound was losing some of its specificity as a diagnostic tool since their results contradicted the current belief that a urinary tract obstruction necessarily induces dilatation of the collecting system.[141]

Ultrasound appears to be more accurate than nuclear medicine in detecting hydronephrosis. In one study, ultrasound demonstrated a sensitivity of 90 percent with a specificity of 98 percent and an accuracy of 97 percent.[142] Nuclear medicine had a specificity of 89 percent with an accuracy of 88 percent.[142] Nuclear medicine was less sensitive in detecting obstruction, particularly in the presence of chronic renal disease, but offered additional information regarding relative blood flow, total effective renal plasma flow, and interval change in renal parenchymal function. Although each technique had its advantages, ultrasound was highly sensitive and specific regardless of the degree of renal function impairment.[142]

Evaluation of the Nonfunctioning Kidney

Since ultrasound is independent of renal function, it is the ideal modality for evaluation of the kidney not visualized on excretory urography.[143-146] Ultrasound can confirm the presence of a kidney and evaluate its size and configuration regardless of renal function.[143] In the child, the differential diagnosis would include UPJ obstruction (Figs. 13-40 to 13-42), multicystic kidney (Figs. 13-19 to 13-21), unilateral renal vein thrombosis, and Wilms' tumor. In the adult, 75 percent of cases are due to hydronephrosis, with tumor also included in the differential.[145] The differential diagnosis of a nonvisualized kidney includes chronic infarction, unilateral polycystic kidney disease, agenesis, ectopia, fractured kidney, replacement lipomatosis, and xanthogranulomatous pyelonephritis.[102] (Many of these entities are discussed elsewhere in this chapter.)

If the nonvisualized kidney is normal-sized or enlarged, tumor should be considered. A renal mass may produce nonvisualization by extensive destruction of the parenchyma or obstruction of either blood flow or urine flow[147] (Fig. 13-64). Renal cell carcinoma is the most common mass that produces nonfunction by parenchymal infiltration, obstruction of the collecting system, vascular thrombosis, or compression, with the most common mechanism that of renal vein occlusion by tumor extension into the lumen[147] (Fig. 13-64). Other masses that produce nonfunction include transitional cell carcinoma, an inflammatory mass, and adult polycystic kidney disease (Figs. 13-28 to 13-31).

There are other causes of nonvisualization of a normal or enlarged kidney. These include primary cortical disease, medullary involvement, and disease processes affecting the pyelocalyceal region.[147] Disease processes such as leukemia and amyloid can affect any portion of the kidney (see below.)

With a small nonvisualized kidney, the offending process may be unilateral or bilateral. The most common mechanical causes of a small nonfunctioning kidney are infarction, ischemia, infection, glomerulonephritis, and nephrosclerosis.[147]

Urinoma

The possibility of urinary extravasation (urinoma) should be considered if a lucent lesion is seen around a hydronephrotic kidney and a renal nuclear medicine scan confirms the finding. A urinoma (perirenal pseudocyst) is defined as a loculated urine collection formed when urine extravasates into the perirenal space, through either rupture of a calyceal fornix or a tear in the renal parenchyma.[148] The fluid within this lesion can be contained within the perirenal space between Gerota's fascia and the renal capsule or can enter the peritoneal cavity through direct communication or transudation, presenting as urinary ascites.[148,149] Such urinary leaks are caused by renal injuries, an operation, infection, tumor, calculous erosion, or ureteral obstruction of acute or gradual onset. When the urinary tract is obstructed acutely by a pathologic process or abdominal compression or both, the resultant increase in intraluminal pressure, augmented by a sudden diuretic load of urographic contrast, may lead to a rupture at the weakest point. In an otherwise healthy upper urinary tract, the point of rupture is at the calyceal fornices and extravasation of urine dissects into the loose connective tissue of the renal sinus and is absorbed by the lymphatics. This extravasation is transient and relatively innocuous. The most common cause in the neonatal period is usually posterior urethral valves.[148]

Extravasation of urine from a tear in the collecting system affected by chronic obstruction, infection, calculous erosion, or tumor usually has grave consequences and requires surgery. This urinary extravasation may cause retroperitoneal fibrosis, stricture of the upper ure-

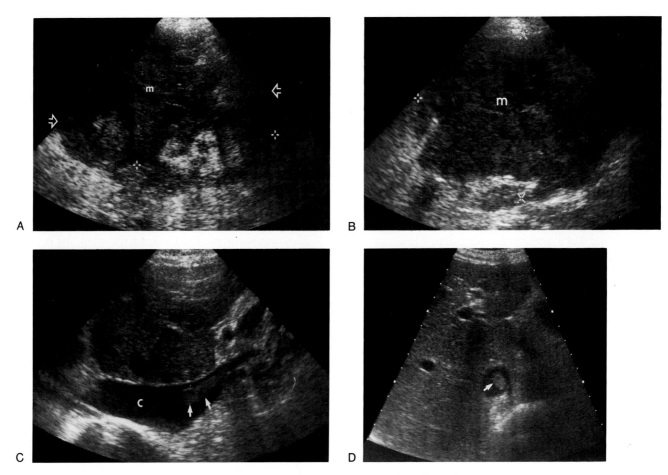

Fig. 13-64. Nonvisualized kidney, renal cell carcinoma. In the region of the left kidney, a large solid inhomogeneous mass (*m*, calipers, open arrows, $10 \times 14 \times 9.5$ cm) is seen on **(A)** sagittal and **(B)** transverse views. The mass has an echogenic pattern. A reniform shape (calipers) is seen in Fig. A; this may represent the remainder of the left kidney. **(C)** Sagittal and **(D)** transverse views of the inferior vena cava *(c)* showing the tumor thrombus (arrows), which has extended from the left renal vein.

ter, or perinephric abscess. The urine infiltrates the retroperitoneal perirenal area, producing a fibroblastic cavity that confines the urine in about 5 to 12 days and produces dense connective tissue encapsulation in 3 to 6 weeks.[150]

Ultrasound is a sensitive method for demonstrating such collections of urine or urinomas. A urinoma is elliptical and orients inferomedialy, often displacing the adjacent kidney upward. A hypoechoic or anechoic mass is seen associated with the kidney (Figs. 13-65 to 13-67). However, the ultrasound diagnosis of a urinoma is not specific. The differential diagnosis of such an ultrasound pattern must include lymphocele, hematoma, abscess, cyst, pancreatic pseudocyst, or even ascites. The diagnosis of urinoma may be confirmed by nuclear medicine, excretory urography, or ultrasound-guided aspiration of the fluid. A negative nuclear medicine study or excretory urography does not exclude urinoma. The aspirated

fluid should be sent for biochemical analysis. At times it is difficult to differentiate the above entities by this method in the poorly functioning kidney when the urea concentrations in the urine and serum are similar.[150]

There have been reported cases of urinomas containing numerous septations[148] (Fig. 13-68). These septations may be composed partially of blood and proteins extravasated into the perirenal space at the time of renal parenchyma rupture.[148] This renal rupture is most likely to occur at birth but may occur in utero.[148] It is possible that the fascia around the kidney also contributes to the septations if it becomes disrupted at the time of renal rupture.[148] Blood products forming layers in the loculations may also account for the solid appearance of the regions of the mass.[148]

At times, the mass effect created by the urinoma causes diagnostic confusion.[148] In such cases, the kidney may be distorted and markedly displaced from the renal

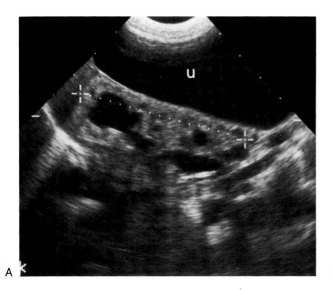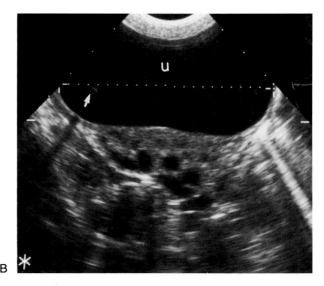

Fig. 13-65. Urinoma. Newborn with posterior urethral valves who developed bilateral urinomas in utero. **(A)** Sagittal and **(B)** transverse views of the right kidney showing a large cystic mass *(u)* anterior to the right kidney (calipers, Fig. A). The collecting system is moderately dilated (lucent areas). A dilated urinary bladder with a thickened wall was seen (not shown). The tip (arrow) of a percutaneous drainage catheter, which was placed within the urinoma after birth, is seen within the urinoma in Fig. B.

fossa, making it difficult to identify.[148] Urinary ascites may be simulated on plain films when bilateral urinomas displace bowel gas centrally.[148]

Percutaneous Nephrostomy

Percutaneous nephrostomy has become a well-established technique for permanent or temporary urinary diversion.[151-159] The application of ultrasound and percutaneous puncture techniques in the diagnosis of

various fluid-filled renal anomalies permits rapid delineation of anatomic detail, more definitive physiologic evaluation, and when necessary, drainage in a safe and cost-effective manner. The indications for the procedure are multiple.[160,161] In the azotemic patient with bilateral obstruction or obstruction of a single functioning kidney, this procedure is the initial treatment of choice for severe obstructive renal failure. The treatment of pyonephrosis (see under Inflammatory Disease) by percutaneous drainage provides the most gratifying setting for

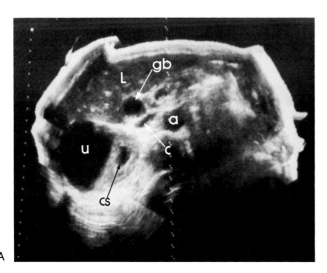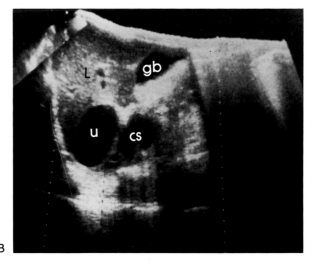

Fig. 13-66. Urinoma. Adult with prostatic carcinoma and hydronephrosis. Supine **(A)** transverse and **(B)** longitudinal scans demonstrating an anechoic mass *(u)* that is superior and lateral to the hydronephrotic right kidney. (*cs*, dilated collecting system; *gb*, gallbladder; *L*, liver; *c*, inferior vena cava; *a*, aorta.)

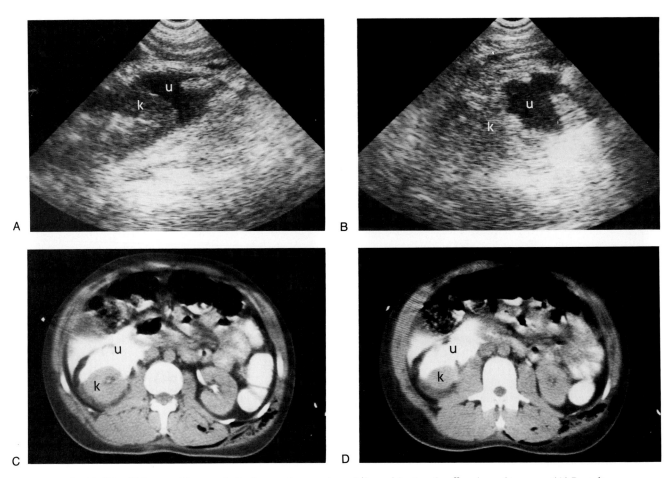

Fig. 13-67. Urinoma. Young adult who was in an automobile accident and suffered renal trauma. **(A)** Longitudinal and **(B)** transverse supine scans demonstrating an anechoic mass *(u)* inferior and medial to the right kidney *(k)*. Fig. B is just below the lower pole of the kidney. No hydronephrosis is noted. **(C & D)** CT scans with Fig. D at the level of the lower pole of the kidney *(k)*. Extravasation *(u)* of contrast can be seen anterior and medial to the right kidney.

this procedure. The septicemic patient with gram-negative shock shows prompt clinical improvement and develops clear urine within 24 to 48 hours. Other indications for percutaneous nephrostomy include uncertain functional capacity of an obstructed kidney; contraindications to immediate surgery; and expected brief duration of the obstruction. A ureteral fistula may close if a percutaneous catheter drains the urine. This catheter can be used for calculus irrigation and possibly even calculus extraction and/or an antegrade pyelogram.[151] Additionally, it can be used for ureteral stent insertion. A stent is a catheter that extends from the pelvocalyceal system across the ureteral narrowing to provide internal drainage into the bladder or an intestinal conduit.[157] A stent is seen on ultrasound as a tubular structure within the collecting system (Fig. 13-69). Ultrasound can be used to evaluate for hydronephrosis following stent placement.

The indications for percutaneous nephrostomy in neonates, infants, and children include preservation of renal function while awaiting growth of the infant, preservation of renal function in anticipation of relief of transient obstruction, drainage of pyonephrosis, and assessment of reversibility of the impaired renal function.[162]

The procedure itself may be performed with guidance by ultrasound alone, by a combination of ultrasound and fluoroscopy, or by fluoroscopy alone.[157] By using the combined approach, there is less radiation and fewer needle sticks.[156,163] The choice of guidance method is influenced heavily by the background and biases of the operator and to a lesser extent by the imaging equipment available. Establishing a functioning nephrostomy requires three basic steps: (1) a needle or trocar puncture of the pelvocalyceal system; (2) replacement of the needle or trocar by a catheter with or without the aid of intermediary instruments; and (3) optimal positioning of the

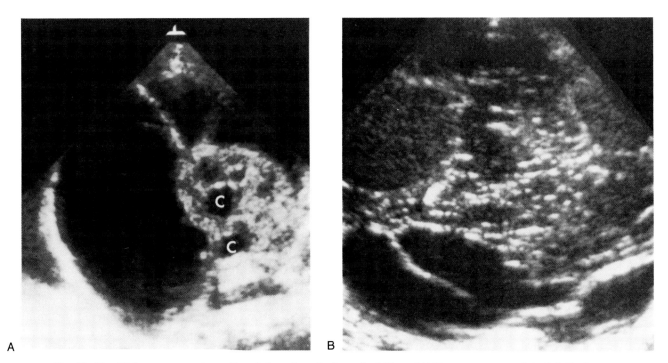

Fig. 13-68. Urinoma, septations. Case 1. Imaging of a 5-week-old boy. **(A)** Transverse scan of the left flank. A fluid collection with few septa surrounds the anterior and lateral aspects of the left kidney. Although the kidney is compressed, renal medullary pyramids are identified peripheral to mildly dilated, more lucent calyces *(c)*. On voiding cystourethrography (not shown), a delayed abdominal film at the conclusion of fluoroscopic study showed left-sided grade V reflux and extravasation of contrast material into the subcapsular space and into the less dense perirenal space. Case 2. Imaging of an 8-day-old girl. **(B)** Transverse scan through the left flank showing multiple septa in this complex mass with a significant hyperechoic component. The kidney is not seen on this view. The left kidney, which was displaced across the midline, was identified on other views. (From Feinstein and Fernbach,[148] with permission.)

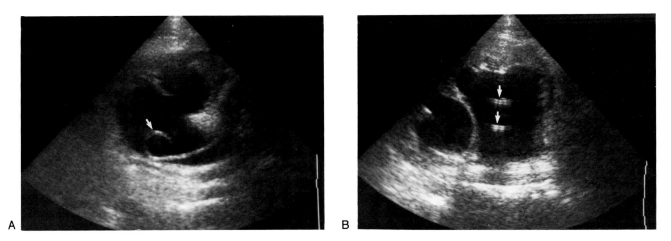

Fig. 13-69. Ureteral stent. Severe dilatation of the collecting system is seen on **(A & B)** sagittal views. The coil (arrow) of the ureteral stent is seen in Fig. A. In Fig. B, several echogenic double lines (arrows) are seen, representing the catheter or stent.

catheter within the system.[157] (See Ch. 19 for a more detailed description.)

The success rate of the procedure has been reported to be 97 to 100 percent[157]; it depends on the placement and the maintenance of adequate drainage. There is a 4 percent incidence of significant complications and a 0.2 percent incidence of mortality (surgical mortality is 6 percent). The only relative contraindication is bleeding diathesis.[157]

Inflammatory Disease

Ultrasound is a rapid, noninvasive, and relatively inexpensive modality for evaluating the renal collecting system, parenchyma, and adjacent retroperitoneum for evidence of infection.[164] It can be a valuable screening procedure in evaluating the first urinary tract infection in children to detect congenital abnormalities of the urinary tract and, in particular, obstructive lesions.[128,129] (See Obstructive Uropathy and Ch. 14 for further discussions of reflux.)

A nonspecific sign of urinary tract infection has been identified: a thickened renal pelvic mucosa/submucosa.[32,33,165] This thickening of the wall of the renal collecting system is seen as a marginal, intraluminal hypoechoic rim (see Fig. 13-12). It has been found in renal transplants with rejection, in native kidneys in patients with urinary tract infection, reflux, or chronic obstruction,[32,33,165] and in patients with acute tubular necrosis, urinary tract infection complicating hydronephrosis, congenital hydronephrosis after pyeloplasty, congenital hydronephrosis due to reflux, and one patient on total parenteral nutrition.[33] With chronic obstruction, reflux, and calculi, there may be direct trauma to the collecting system wall, producing edema and inflammatory infiltration but also fibrosis and muscle hypertrophy.[32] The thickening may also be caused by inflammatory cell infiltrate, fibrosis, muscular hypertrophy, or hemorrhage into the submucosal space.[33] Although it is a nonspecific finding, it should be correlated with the clinical and laboratory findings; it can be seen in a variety of renal diseases and may be taken as a nonspecific sign of upper urinary tract infection.[32,33,165] The finding has been seen to resolve after therapy.[33,165] In one report, it appeared to be present in cases of *Candida* infection and resolved with therapy.[165] It was postulated that the yeast infection may cause more severe and diffuse mucosal edema than bacterial infections.[165]

Acute Diffuse Bacterial Infection

Acute Pyelonephritis. Infection is the most common disease of the urinary tract and constitutes 75 percent of problems requiring urologic evaluation.[166] Most cases of bacterial pyelonephritis occur via an ascending route beginning at the level of the bladder and ascending to the kidney. The avenue for such spread is via the subepithelial lymphatic channels of the bladder and ureter and then the renal interstitium. The spread is facilitated by the presence of obstruction, ureteric reflux, or a deformed urinary tract.[166] The most common organism is *Escherichia coli* (in more than 85 percent of cases), which usually responds well to therapy with antibiotics.[164,167] Patients with such conditions as neurogenic bladder, bladder cancer, a history of debilitating disease, chemotherapy or intravenous drug abuse, prolonged catheter drainage and reflux, altered host resistance, trauma, diabetes, and urinary tract infection, as well as pregnancy, have an increased incidence of this disease process.[167,168]

As a diffuse renal infection, acute pyelonephritis initially primarily involves the urothelium of the collecting system and the renal interstitium.[164] The combination of parenchymal, caliceal, and pelvic inflammation constitutes pyelonephritis. The kidney is enlarged by inflammatory edema and contains foci of intense inflammation with microabscess formation and infiltration by polymorphonuclear cells throughout the involved interstitial tissue. This results in purulent casts in the collecting tubules and often in an inflammatory reaction in the pelvic and caliceal epithelium.[168] The upper urinary tract infection may first involve only the lining membranes of the renal pelvis. Then infection spreads through the pyramids to the cortex to produce pyelonephritis. Focal areas of inflammation that progress to suppuration, forming microabscesses, may coalesce to form carbuncles. This may extend to the perinephric space.[166]

On ultrasound, the affected kidney may appear normal or may demonstrate either subtle or dramatic changes.[164] It may be noted to be enlarged with an increased anechoic corticomedullary area and multiple scattered low-level echoes[166-171] (Fig. 13-70). Enlargement, which is the most consistent ultrasound finding, is due to inflammation and edema.[164] There may be decreased echogenicity of the corticomedullary areas in a relatively diffuse pattern, accentuating the distinction between the renal sinus and parenchyma.[164] This pattern is produced by the multiple small abscesses and necrosis in the outer part of the medulla and cortex.[169] The backwall of the affected kidney may be stronger than that of the corresponding normal kidney because the infected kidney has an increased fluid content[169] (Fig. 13-70).

Children. Ultrasound is also useful in differentiating upper from lower urinary tract infection in children; this is important because of therapeutic and prognostic consequences.[172] In the children studied, the increase in renal volume and asymmetry in kidney size determined

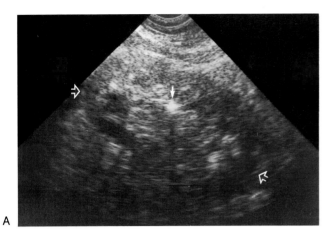
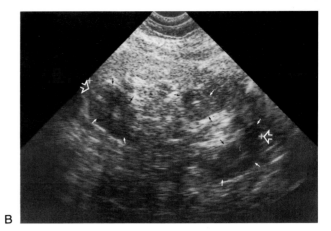

Fig. 13-70. Acute pyelonephritis. **(A & B)** Longitudinal scans of the left kidney. The kidney is enlarged (open arrows) with poor definition between the renal sinus and parenchyma. There appears to be a calculus (arrow) with shadowing within the collecting system in Fig. A. In Fig. B there are increased anechoic corticomedullary areas (small arrows) with multiple scattered low level echoes.

by ultrasound was a valuable diagnostic criterion for differentiation between infections of the upper and lower urinary tracts.[172] In this study, there was an average 175 percent increase in kidney volume associated with acute pyelonephritis; this occurred in 76 percent of the kidneys in the acute phase of pyelonephritis.[172] This renal enlargement was most impressive during the first year of life; the mean increase in volume was 300 percent in infants and toddlers.[172] There was a bilateral increase in renal size and/or distinct volume asymmetry in 50 percent of cases[172] Patients with lower urinary tract infections had a mean renal volume of 99.68 percent and a physiologic volume asymmetry comparable to that of normal kidneys.[172] The most important indication of pyelonephritis, whether or not renal asymmetry was present, was unilateral or bilateral renal enlargement.[172] If renal morphometry revealed enlargement to at least 140 percent of normal, the specificity for acute upper urinary tract infection was 98 percent and the sensitivity was 76 percent.[172] When a cutoff of 120 percent was used, the sensitivity increased to 98 percent but the specificity dropped to only 82 percent.[172]

When using ultrasound to monitor children with acute pyelonephritis, there appears to be a time-dependent volume decrease after the onset of therapy; it is expected to take at least 4 to 6 days until almost complete normalization of kidney volume can be found.[172]

Other groups have investigated the use of ultrasound in the evaluation of acute pyelonephritis in children.[173] In 24 percent of the entire group studied, changes consistent with acute pyelonephritis were demonstrated on ultrasound; of those who demonstrated abnormalities on scintigraphy, only 39 percent showed abnormalities on ultrasound.[173] The ultrasound findings included in-creased cortical echogenicity, decreased echogenicity and renal abscesses, and, in a lesser number, dilatation of the renal collecting system and renal enlargement.[173] This group of investigators concluded that ultrasound was a relatively insensitive test for the detection of acute inflammatory changes of the renal cortex.[173]

Emphysematous Pyelonephritis. Emphysematous pyelonephritis is a life-threatening disease, usually occurring in middle-aged or elderly diabetic patients or females with urinary tract obstruction.[174] At least one-third of patients have associated urinary tract infections.[164] It has also been described in immunocompromised individuals, particularly in immunosuppressed renal transplant recipients.[164] It is most often caused by *E. coli* infection; other offending organisms, which are facultative anaerobes, are *Klebsiella, Proteus,* and *Aerobacter.*[164,174] It is characterized by anaerobic gas production within the renal parenchyma and is usually unilateral.[164]

The most reliable diagnostic test is the plain abdominal film, which demonstrates gas collection in the renal parenchyma as mottled radiolucent shadows.[174] However, this intraparenchymal gas may be seen on plain film in only 33 percent of patients.[174] Ultrasound allows the identification of intraparenchymal gas as strongly echogenic structures with sharp and usually flat anterior margins and distal, dirty acoustic shadows[164,174] (Fig. 13-71). This dirty shadow is caused by the high acoustic impedance difference between the soft tissue (including kidney) and the gas, the so-called reverberation artifact.[174] There may also be associated retroperitoneal and renal sinus gas.[164]

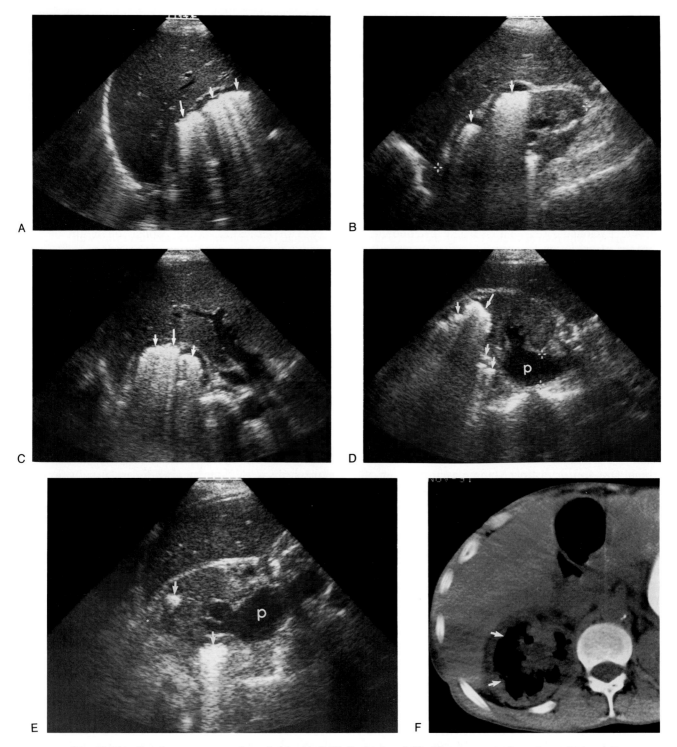

Fig. 13-71. Emphysematous pyelonephritis. **(A & B)** Sagittal and **(C–E)** transverse views through the right renal fossa showing a highly echogenic focus (arrows) in the region of the anterior aspect of the right renal parenchyma. This is associated with a "dirty" shadow, consistent with air. The dilated collecting system is seen in Figs. D and E, as is air extending out to the region of the renal cortex. (*p*, renal pelvis.) **(F)** CT scan showing a massive amount of air (arrows) within the right kidney. After right nephrectomy, the patient's critical status markedly improved.

Chronic Infection

With the availability of effective antibiotics and the early detection and treatment of acute urinary tract infections and the conditions that predispose a patient to chronic infection, chronic renal infections are becoming increasingly rare.[175] Most cases of chronic infection involve host factors that decrease the ability to resist or eradicate infection; they are not the result of a specific organism.[175] Other predisposing conditions to chronic infection include vesicoureteral reflux, obstruction, urinary calculi, diabetes mellitus, congenital anomalies of the urinary tract, analgesic abuse, gout, urinary diversion, and neurogenic bladder.[175]

Chronic Pyelonephritis. With chronic pyelonephritis (chronic atrophic pyelonephritis, reflux neuropathy) there is a chronic interstitial nephritis caused by infection and there may be some damage due to autoimmune mechanisms.[175] This condition has the same bacteriologic cause as acute pyelonephritis, and in most cases, it is the result of scarring from prior infections.[175]

With chronic pyelonephritis, scarring most often results from lower urinary tract infection and vesicoureteral relux, usually in childhood.[175] It can also occur in the presence of calculi and chronic obstruction.[175] In adults, most pyelonephritis scarring is the result of renal calculi and recurrent infection.[175]

The urographic findings with this disorder are caused by focal damage of an entire ray, producing loss of medullary and cortical tissue.[175] As a result, there is a discrete, deep cortical scar overlying a blunt calyx.[175] More than one ray may be involved, and the exact appearance of the kidney depends on the severity and distribution of damage.[175] There is less involvement of the midpoles than of the poles.[175]

This process may involve the full thickness of the kidney with retraction of the papilla, dilatation of the surrounding calyx, depression of the surface and loss of renal parenchyma, and, most commonly, vesicoureteral reflux. There may be a focal or multifocal process with loss of renal parenchyma, retraction of one or more calyces, decrease in renal size, and increased echoes from fibrosis.[176] With ultrasound, the diagnosis may be diffi-

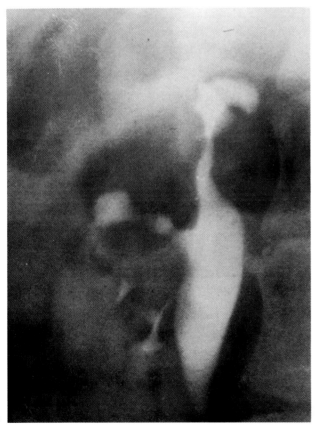

A

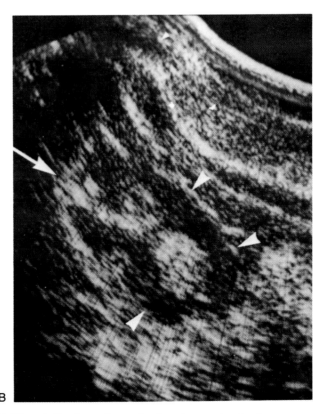

B

Fig. 13-72. Chronic atrophic pyelonephritis. Case 1. **(A)** There is focal scarring and calyceal retraction in the upper pole of the right kidney, typical of chronic atrophic pyelonephritis. **(B)** Right kidney (arrowheads) with the patient prone. There is focal loss of parenchyma, extension of a calyx from the renal sinus to the renal margin, and associated focal increased echogenicity due to fibrosis (arrow) in the upper pole. *(Figure continues.)*

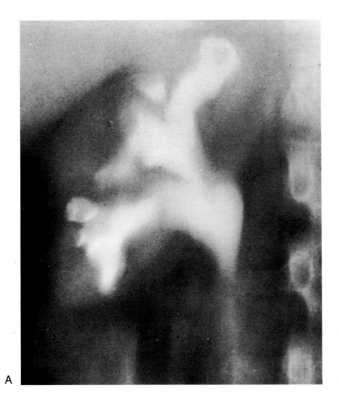

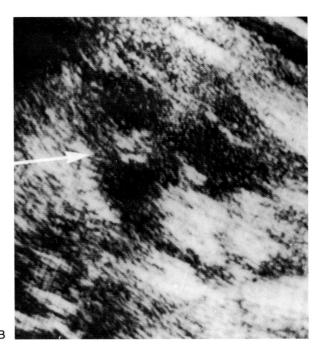

A   B

Fig. 13-72 *(Continued).*   Case 2. **(C)** There is focal scarring in both upper and lower poles of the right kidney with associated caliceal blunting. **(D)** Right kidney, prone. Focal scarring and extension of the renal sinus to the renal margin in the upper pole of the right kidney (arrow) and increased echogenicity and loss of parenchyma in the lower pole are apparent. (From Kay et al,[176] with permission.)

cult.[175] The focal fibrosis produces increased echoes in the involved area of the medulla and cortex (Fig. 13-72). With retraction of a calyx, if it is not distended, an echogenic zone is seen to extend beyond the normal area of the renal sinus[176] (Fig. 13-72). It is easier to recognize the focal scars and blunted calyces by urography than by ultrasound.[175] Focal abnormalities associated with other disease processes such as acute or chronic glomerulonephritis, diabetic glomerulosclerosis, acute tubular necrosis, and Alport's disease usually produce a generalized increase in cortical echoes and preserve the lucent medulla, leading to accentuated normal anatomy.

Xanthogranulomatous Pyelonephritis. Xanthogranulomatous pyelonephritis, characterized by destruction and replacement of normal parenchyma by sheets of lipid-laden histiocytes, is a rare form of chronic inflammatory disease in patients with obstructive uropathy secondary to long-standing calculi.[164,175,177,178] As such, the most common etiologies include chronic infection and obstruction of the UPJ, generally by a staghorn calculus. This disease may also follow inadequate response to antibiotic therapy.[164] As a rule, there is a long history of urinary tract infections, with *Proteus mirabilis* and *E. coli* the most common organisms.[164,178,179] There are

renal calculi in 50 to 80 percent of cases, with resultant hydronephrosis.[164,177,180] The patients generally have signs and symptoms of malaise, flank pain, mass, weight loss, and urinary tract infection.[178,180] The disease has a higher incidence in diabetics and is rare in blacks.[180] There is a slight female predominance.[177] The disease can occur at any age; there is a peak incidence in the fourth and fifth decades.[178]

Pathologically, this disease is characterized by abscess formation surrounded by inflammatory foam cells, plasma cells, and multinucleated giant cells that give the abscess the characteristic yellow color.[180] The pathologic spectrum is variable depending on the chronicity of the disease process.[177] Pus-filled dilated calyces may predominate, with less extensive xanthogranulomatous tissue. Alternatively there may be replacement of the kidney with xanthogranulomatous tissue that may predominate, with less of a purulent component.[177] The process begins within the calyces and pelvis; later there are mucosal destruction and extension into the adjacent medulla and cortex. The distended calyces compromise the medullary perfusion, leading to papillary necrosis.[178]

There are two forms of xanthogranulomatous pyelonephritis: diffuse and segmental. With the diffuse form, there is usually an association with a staghorn calculus or stone at the UPJ; with the segmental form, the mass involves either one pole of a duplicated system or an obstructed portion of a single system and the contiguous parenchyma.[164] Regardless of the form, the inflammatory process begins within the pelvocalyceal system with pyonephrosis and progressive mucosal destruction.[164]

The ultrasound pattern of xanthogranulomatous pyelonephritis varies with the pattern of involvement (diffuse or segmental).[178] In the typical diffuse pattern, the parenchyma is replaced by multiple circular, apparently fluid-filled masses that surround the central echocomplex[175,177-179,181] (Figs. 13-73 to 13-76). These

masses correspond to the debris-filled dilated calyces and/or foci of parenchymal destruction.[178] The kidney is enlarged, but the reniform shape is maintained with a smooth contour.[164,178] The central echocomplex is usually highly reflective, with distal shadowing associated with the calculi present.[164] The echogenicity of the masses depends on the amount of debris and necrosis within them. The central echogenic stone may be difficult to define, as may its associated acoustic shadow.[178] In segmental disease, one or more masses surround a single calyx that contains a calculus.[178] The masses may be hypoechoic or anechoic, with the echogenicity correlating with the amount of necrosis and debris.[178]

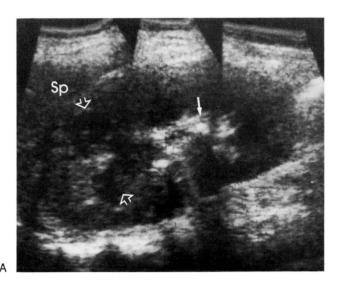

A

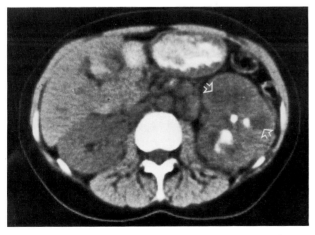

B

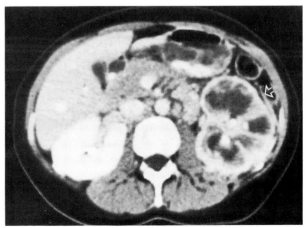

C

Fig. 13-73. Xanthogranulomatous pyelonephritis. **(A)** Coronal longitudinal scan through the spleen *(Sp)* showing an enlarged left kidney, a central echogenic focus with shadowing (arrow), and a central mixed echopattern (open arrows). Note the apparent thickening of the renal parenchyma. **(B)** CT scan through the midportion of the kidney (nonenhanced) showing multiple calculi in the enlarged left kidney. Areas of diminished attenuation (open arrows) are seen measuring −5 to +5 HU in various locations. **(C)** CT scan, enhanced (same level as Fig. B). Areas of diminished attenuation are now better seen and are only minimally enhanced. Surrounding rims of tissue are greatly enhanced, indicative of vascular inflammatory tissue associated with the remaining parenchymal areas. Note the thickening of Gerota's fascia surrounding the kidney (open arrow). (From Subramanyam et al,[177] with permission.)

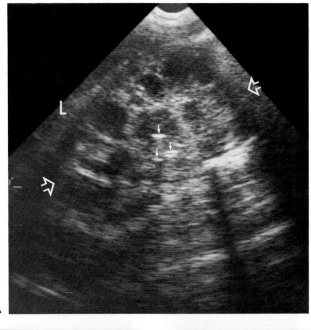

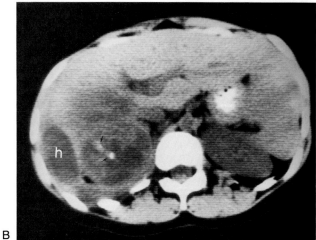

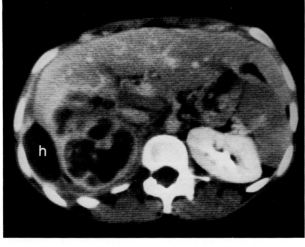

Fig. 13-74. Xanthogranulomatous pyelonephritis. **(A)** Left lateral decubitus longitudinal real-time scan of the right kidney. The kidney is diffusely enlarged with poorly defined margins (open arrows), central echogenic areas (small arrows), and scattered parenchymal anechoicities. (*L*, liver.) **(B)** Unenhanced CT scan showing multiple calculi (small arrows) within the enlarged right kidney. There are multiple areas of low density within the renal parenchyma. There is a low-density area *(h)* lateral to the kidney, which represents a hematoma that developed after a percutaneous drainage procedure performed after Fig. A was taken. **(C)** Enhanced CT scan showing multiple areas of diminished attenuation surrounded by rims of enhancing tissue, representing inflammatory tissue. At surgery, there was xanthogranulomatous pyelonephritis as well as abscess formation. (*h*, hematoma.)

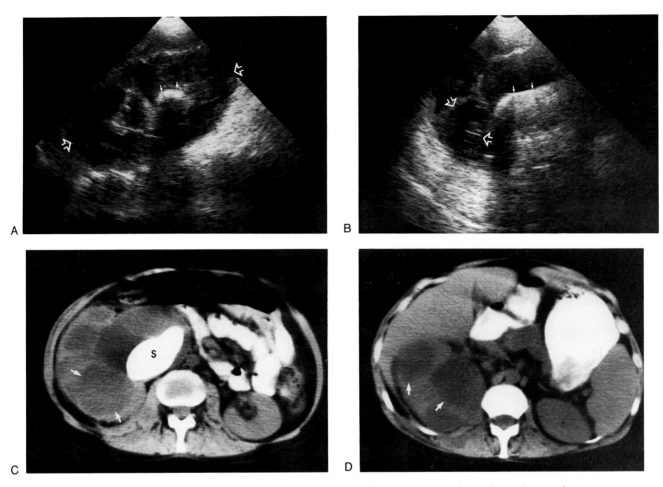

Fig. 13-75. Xanthogranulomatous pyelonephritis. Paraplegic young male patient with a history of recurrent infectious urologic problems. He presented with fever and right flank pain. Supine **(A)** longitudinal and **(B)** transverse scans. The right kidney (open arrows, renal length in Fig. A) is markedly enlarged and hypoechoic, but a reniform shape is maintained. There is an echogenic focus (small arrows, calculus) in the region of the renal pelvis. The parenchyma appears to be replaced by multiple hypoechoic areas (open arrows in Fig. B). **(C & D)** Unenhanced CT scans showing a large, dense calculus *(s)* within the renal pelvis. Multiple poorly defined low-density areas (arrows) are seen within the renal parenchyma. The ultrasound pattern is consistent with xanthogranulomatous pyelonephritis.

The ultrasound differential diagnosis of the findings described with xanthogranulomatosis pyelonephritis would include pyonephrosis, neoplasm, and extensive papillary necrosis.[164] Lymphoma may appear very similar.

Parenchymal Malakoplakia. As an uncommon chronic inflammatory disease that usually involves the urinary tract collecting system, malakoplakia produces lesions within the renal parenchyma in approximately 16 percent of cases.[164] It is a rare granulomatous inflammatory disease associated with chronic *E. coli* infection.[175] The lower urinary tract is affected most often, but the kidney may be involved as well.[175] The typical patient is a middle-aged woman with recurrent urinary tract infec-

tions.[175] The malacoplakia occurs because of abnormal monocyte function.[175] A chronic inflammation results, characterized by 5- to 10-μm basophilic intracellular inclusions called Michaelis-Gutmann bodies, which represent incompletely destroyed bacteria surrounded by concentric lipoprotein membranes and crystalline calcium phosphate.[175]

Malakoplakia occurs in two forms: unifocal and multifocal.[164] The multifocal form occurs in 75 percent of cases and is bilateral in 50 percent.[164] This abnormality has a close association with gram-negative urinary tract infections, the vast majority being due to *E. coli*.[164]

In most cases, there is unilateral renal involvement with multifocal disease.[175] Although the ultrasound findings of malakoplakia are nonspecific, the paren-

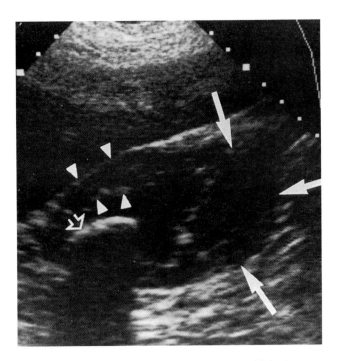

Fig. 13-76. Xanthogranulomatous pyelonephritis in 67-year-old woman. Excretory urography showed calculus in the non-visualized right kidney. Sonogram shows thin upper-pole parenchyma (arrowheads), calculus (open arrow), and nearly isoechoic mass in the lower pole (solid arrows), suggesting xanthogranulomatous pyelonephritis. Pathologic examination showed xanthogranulomatous pyelonephritis in the lower pole and diffuse chronic pyelonephritis. (From Kenney,[175] with permission.)

chyma appears hypoechoic.[175] Enlarged kidneys with multiple poorly defined hypovascular cortical masses may be seen[175] (Fig. 13-77). When there is diffuse disease, ultrasound may show distortion and compression of the central echocomplex by poorly defined masses of variable echogenicity. A nonspecific echogenic mass may be seen if the disease is unifocal.[175]

Megalocystic Interstitial Nephritis. Megalocystic interstitial nephritis is a very rare condition, similar to renal malacoplakia, which involves mainly the renal cortex and to some extent the medullary region. The precise etiology is not completely understood, but it does appear to be an immunoresponse to certain strains of bacteria, mainly *E. coli* and *Aerobacter aerogenes*. In the absence of obstruction, the excretory urogram shows decreased or normal function depending on the stage of the disease. On ultrasound, an enlarged kidney is seen with an overall increased transonic response (Fig. 13-78). The calyceal echoes are splayed and compressed centrally by peripheral, ill-circumscribed masses that contain low-level echoes.[182]

Pyonephrosis. Pyonephrosis is a serious complication of hydronephrosis that develops as a direct consequence of urinary stasis and secondary infection. It is defined as the presence of pus in a dilated collecting system.[183] It is seen with a spectrum of disease processes from infected hydronephrosis to xanthogranulomatous pyelonephritis. Acute infections may occur in an obstructed system, but true pyonephrosis is a chronic process, as evidenced by pathologic change.[175] With pyonephrosis, there is infection with accumulation of pus proximal to an obstructive urinary tract lesion such as calculus, congenital anomaly, stricture, or tumor.[164] Stasis and collecting system dilatation develop secondary to the obstruction, which promotes infection.[164] As renal function decreases, bacteria and pus fill the collecting system.[184] In most instances, the offending organism is *E. coli.*[164] Pathologically, there is purulent exudate composed of sloughed urothelium and a variety of inflammatory cells. The amount of tissue and cellular debris varies and is determined by the type and severity of the inflammatory process.[185]

Prompt and reliable diagnosis of this entity and its differentiation from hydronephrosis is of the utmost im-

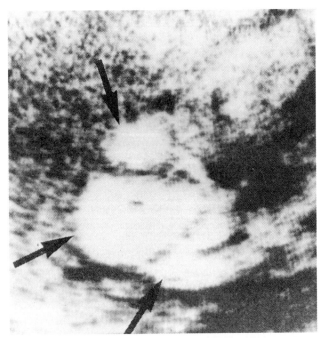

Fig. 13-77. Malacoplakia. Renal parenchymal malacoplakia in a patient with symptoms of chronic urinary tract infection. An excretory urogram revealed an inhomogeneous upper pole mass. Longitudinal sonogram shows multiple hypoechoic masses (arrows) in the right upper pole. These findings are not specific but are consistent with focal parenchymal malacoplakia. Pathologic examination of the nephrectomy specimen proved the diagnosis. (From Kenney,[175] with permission; courtesy of R. B. Jeffrey, San Francisco, CA.)

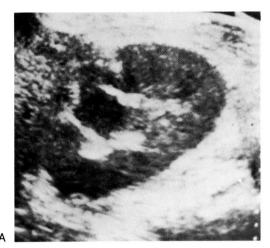
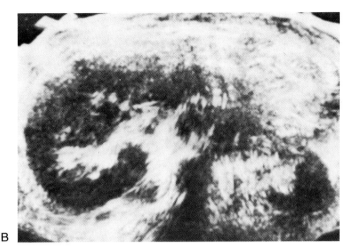

Fig. 13-78. Megalocystic interstitial nephritis. **(A)** Supine longitudinal scan, right kidney. No focal cystic components are seen. Note the enhanced sonic transmission by the kidney. **(B)** Transverse views of both kidneys showing massive uniform enlargement of the right kidney and thickening of the capsular area. (From Gonzalez et al,[182] with permission.)

portance in clinical practice because the medical implications and therapeutic management of the two diseases differ. The diagnosis of pyonephrosis should be suspected in the presence of fever and flank pain, combined with radiographic evidence of hydronephrosis. The ultrasound diagnosis is based on the presence of internal echoes dispersed or dependent within a dilated pelvocalyceal system with a shifting urine-debris level within the obstructed pyelocalyceal system[167,183,185] (Figs. 13-79 to 13-81). Specific ultrasound findings with pyonephrosis include (1) dependent echoes within the collecting system, (2) a shifting fluid-debris level, (3) gas within the collecting system, and (4) echoes throughout the pelvocalyceal system[164,175] (Figs. 13-79 to 13-81). Additional ultrasound findings with pyonephrosis include persistent dependent echoes, a shifting urine-debris level, dense peripheral echoes with shadowing secondary to gas-forming organisms, and poor transonicity with echoes completely filling the pelvis and calyces.[183,184]

Ultrasound has been shown to be 90 percent sensitive and 97 percent specific in the diagnosis of pyonephrosis when abnormal echoes within the renal collecting system were required for this diagnosis.[164,185] However, there have been reports describing pyonephrosis in which the collecting system was completely echofree or contained very low-level echoes that were believed to represent artifact.[186,187] In these reports, although the specificity for diagnosing pyonephrosis was 100 percent, the sensitivity was only 62 to 66.7 percent.[186,187] These groups of investigators recommend ultrasound-guided diagnostic needle aspiration in patients with urosepsis and significant hydronephrosis.[186,187] With ultrasound guidance, aspiration of the collecting system fluid may

be performed to make a definitive diagnosis. If pus is obtained, a percutaneous catheter may be inserted to drain the infected urine and evaluate residual kidney function before surgery. The catheter can be used for diagnostic nephrostogram, ureteral perfusion, therapeutic dissolution of stones, and indefinite drainage of the kidney.[183]

Tuberculosis. Most commonly, renal tuberculosis (TB) spreads hematogeneously from other foci, usually from the lungs.[164,175] However, only 30 percent of patients with renal TB have an abnormal chest radiograph and only 10 percent show signs of active pulmonary TB.[175] Constitutional symptoms may or may not be present.[175] Bilateral disease is usually present, although unilateral disease may occur. In the presence of a nonfunctioning kidney, a normal ultrasound is considered typical of TB, although parenchymal infiltration usually causes loss of corticomedullary definition.[164]

Pathologically, tubercle bacilli lodge in the periglomerular capillaries during hematogeneous seeding that occurs after inhalation.[175] There are cortical granulomas that may remain stable for years, and then, when reactivation occurs, the organisms spread into the medulla causing a papillitis that may extend into the collecting system.[175] In the end, there is diffuse disease with destruction, loss of function, and calcification of the entire kidney (autonephrectomy).[175] The process may spread beyond the kidney, with perinephric and retroperitoneal involvement with fistulas that may extend into the gastrointestinal tract or the skin.[175]

Radiographically, the earliest recognizable abnormality is irregularity of the caliceal contour as a result of

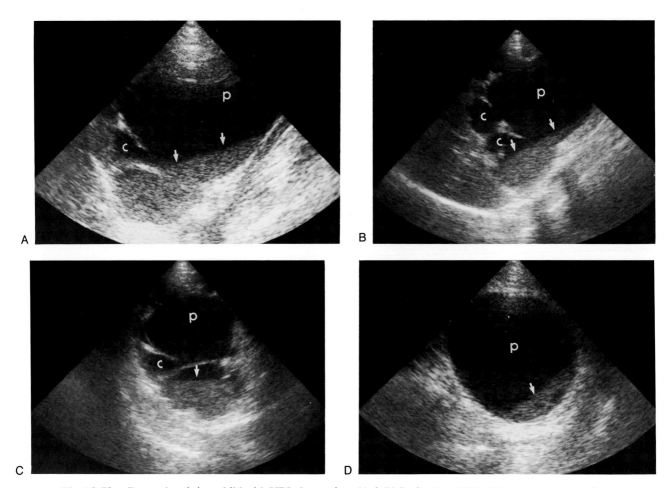

Fig. 13-79. Pyonephrosis in a child with UPJ obstruction. **(A & B)** Sagittal and **(C & D)** transverse views of the right kidney showing a markedly dilated collecting system. The renal pelvis *(p)* is very large, and the calyces *(c)* are barely identifiable. Echogenic layering material (arrows) is seen within the dependent portion of the renal pelvis. The patient was febrile.

necrotizing papillitis.[175] There may be single or multiple calyces involved in one or both kidneys.[175] Cavities communicate with the collecting system with further necrosis.[175] The parenchymal masses that can develop may be calcified.[175] A common finding is the development of infundibular, pelvic, or ureteral strictures, which is nearly pathognomonic for TB.[175]

Ultrasound most frequently shows focal renal lesions[188] (Figs. 13-82 to 13-86). The small lesions (5 to 15 mm) may be echogenic or may have an echogenic border with a central area of low echogenicity.[188] With the larger lesions (> 15 mm), a lesion of mixed echogenicity is seen as a focal lesion with a poorly defined border.[188] There may be focal calcification (highly echogenic areas) with distal shadowing.[188] Other ultrasound findings may include (1) hydronephrosis with debris, (2) strictures of the urinary tract leading to dilatation and infection of a portion of the collecting system (focal pyonephrosis), and (3) a focally dilated collecting system containing debris.[164] With papillary involvement, there

may be echogenic nonshadowing masses localized to a few of the calyces and sloughed calyceal wall.[188] Calyceal filling defects similar to those caused by blood clot, fungus ball, or debris may be seen.

In one series, ultrasound was shown to be less accurate than CT or urography in the detection of advanced urinary tuberculosis.[189] Ultrasound may be less revealing than CT or urography because of (1) difficulties in detecting the subtle calyceal, pelvic, or ureteral changes; (2) difficulties in recognizing isoechoic parenchymal masses; (3) lower sensitivity to calcifications; (4) inability to identify cavities that communicate with the collecting system; and (5) inability to evaluate the function of the kidney.[175]

Candidiasis. *Candida* is the most common cause of upper urinary tract fungal infections; less frequently implicated fungi include *Aspergillis, Actinomyces, Cryptococcus, Phycomycetes, Torulopsis, Coccidioides,* and

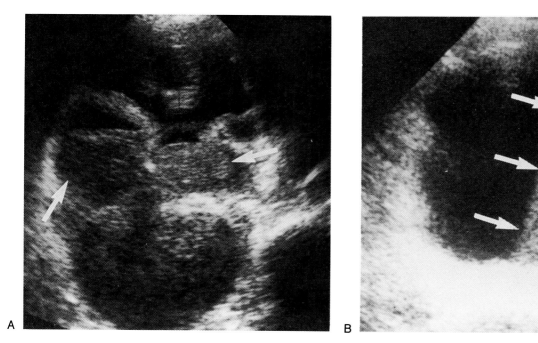

A   B

Fig. 13-80. Pyonephrosis. Case 1. **(A)** Pyonephrosis in a 22-year-old woman with pain in the right upper quadrant and fever. An excretory urogram revealed no excretion of contrast material by the right kidney. Transverse sonogram of the right kidney shows a dilated collecting system with echogenic material in the pelvis and calyces (arrows). Because of the severity of hydronephrosis with the absent renal parenchyma, diagnosis of congenital UPJ obstruction and pyonephrosis was made and confirmed at nephrectomy. Case 2. **(B)** Pyonephrosis in a 72-year-old woman with left flank pain and fever. Sonogram of the left kidney shows severe hydronephrosis with a layer of echogenic material (arrows), indicating pyonephrosis. Subsequent percutaneous aspiration yielded frank pus and *E. coli*. Nephrostomy was placed; a subsequent nephrectomy revealed congenital UPJ obstruction and chronic pyonephrosis. (From Kenney,[175] with permission.)

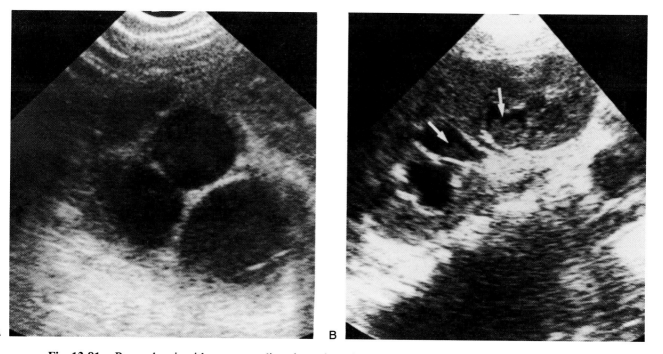

A   B

Fig. 13-81. Pyonephrosis with coarse medium-intensity echoes. **(A)** Echoes are dispersed throughout the dilated collecting system. **(B)** Clumps of medium-intensity echoes are seen (arrows). (From Jeffrey et al,[186] with permission.)

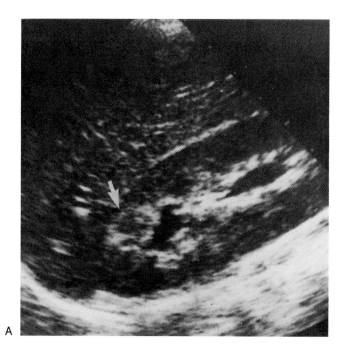

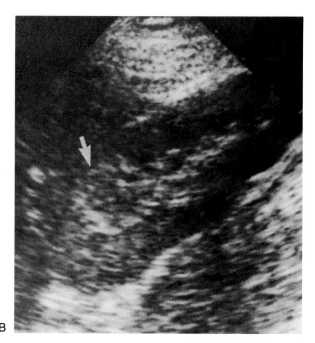

A   B

Fig. 13-82.   Tuberculosis. **(A)** Focal renal lesion in a 12-year-old boy with renal tuberculosis who had intermittent fever and hematuria. Sagittal sonogram of kidney showing an echogenic focal lesion in the upper-pole area (arrow), occupying the cortex and medulla. Results of a fine-needle aspiration cytologic examination were positive for tuberculosis. **(B)** Large tuberculous focal lesion in a 34-year-old woman with pain in the right kidney. Sagittal sonogram of right kidney showing an echogenic focal lesion (arrow), which resembles a tumor, occupying the cortex, medulla, and central sinus area. Results of a fine-needle aspiration cytologic examination were positive for tuberculosis. (From Das et al,[188] with permission.)

Blastomyces.[164,175] As a saprophytic human fungus, *Candida* can become pathogenic under certain predisposing conditions. *Candida albicans* is a normal inhabitant of the skin and the mucous membranes of the mouth, vagina, and GI tract. *Candida* infection can be local (e.g., oral thrush, vulvovaginitis) or become disseminated.[190]

Premature infants (in whom prolonged hyperalimentation long-term indwelling catheters are used) are particularly likely to be ideal hosts for overwhelming *Candida* sepsis.[190] These premature infants with renal candidiasis can have a fulminant course with rapid development of hydronephrosis and destruction of the renal parenchyma.[191] Renal candidal infection occurs, as a rule, in the setting of blood-borne disseminated candidiasis, although primary renal candidiasis constitutes a distinct clinicopathologic entity.[164]

Renal fungus balls are most commonly due to *Candida* in patients with altered host resistance, diabetes, cancer (especially leukemia or lymphoma), indwelling foreign bodies, chronic illness, premature birth, or a history of intravenous drug abuse; in those receiving prolonged antibiotic, corticosteroid, or immunosuppressive therapy; and in those immunocompromised from acquired immune deficiency syndrome (AIDS), steroid

therapy, or immunosuppression for organ transplants.[175,191,192] In reviewing cases of deep organ involvement, it was found that 80 percent had renal involvement, while 72 percent had genitourinary tract involvement, and 52 percent had central nervous system (CNS) involvement.[190]

Pathologically, the affected kidney is enlarged with multiple microabscesses in the renal cortex, interstitium, and tubules.[190] With further involvement, necrotizing papillitis and fungus balls are found within the collecting system.[190] There may be resultant papillary necrosis, particularly in premature infants.[175] With renal pelvis and ureter involvement, there may be urothelial thrush, with formation of a white membrane made up of fungal growth and inflammatory cells invading the mucosa and submucosa.[175] The clinical signs are nonspecific and include flank pain, fever, and chills. They can be confused with bacterial septicemia, making an early diagnosis difficult.[191]

Ultrasound may indicate (1) changes in renal size, (2) abnormal renal cortical echogenicity, and (3) renal fungus balls[175,190] (Figs. 13-87 and 13-88). When there is chronic renal or pelvic involvement, fungus balls, made up of fragments of fungi with mycelia (and occasionally yeast forms) and necrotic debris, may form in the renal

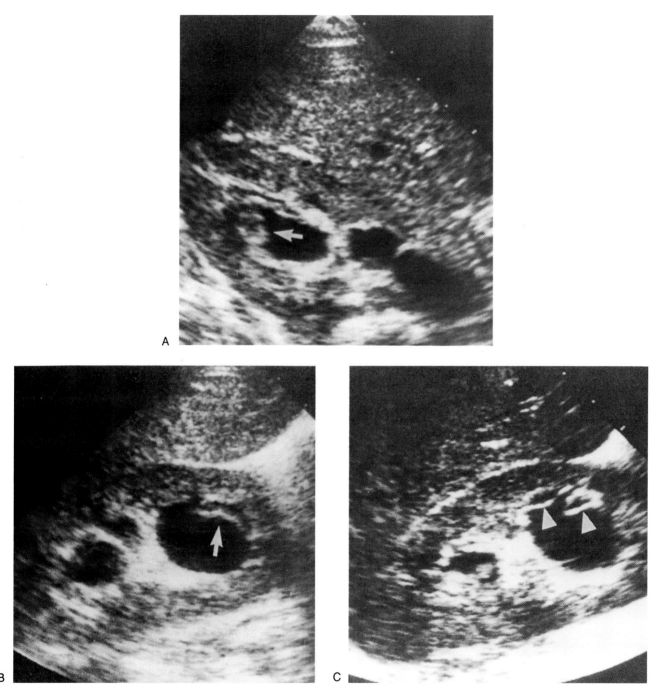

Fig. 13-83. Tuberculosis. Papillary mass and sloughed caliceal wall in a 30-year-old woman with pain in the right loin. **(A)** Sagittal sonogram of right kidney showing dilated calyx with an echogenic nonshadowing filling defect caused by the papillary mass (arrow). **(B)** Oblique sonogram showing the sloughed calyceal wall as a double-outlined calyceal wall (arrow). **(C)** Sagittal sonogram showing overhanging flaps of sloughed wall attached to the wall of the calyx (arrowheads). (From Das et al,[188] with permission.)

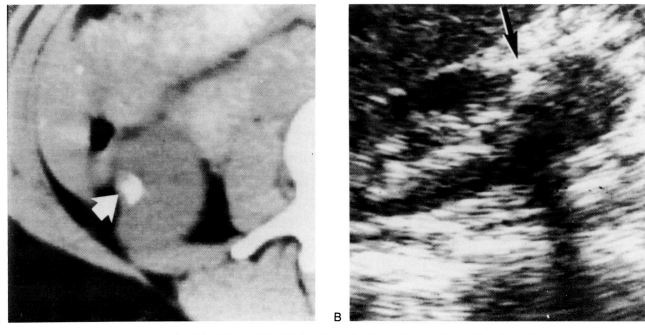

Fig. 13-84.   Tuberculosis, right kidney. **(A)** CT showing a focal scar (arrow) in small region of homogeneous calcification. **(B)** Sonogram also showing focal parenchymal thinning (arrow). Calcification is very echogenic and casts a shadow. (From Premkumar et al,[189] with permission.)

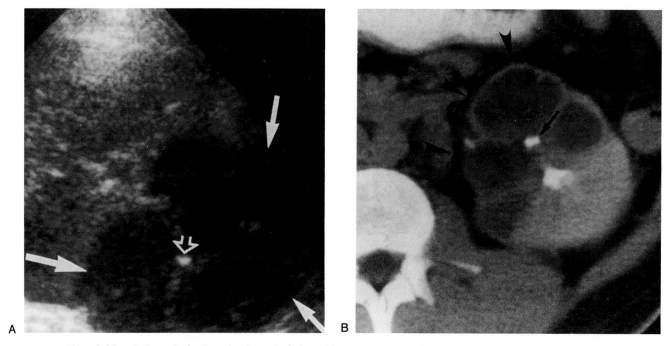

Fig. 13-85.   Tuberculosis. Renal tuberculosis in a 33-year-old man with symptoms of chronic urinary tract infection that did not respond to routine antibiotics. Subsequent imaging diagnosis and urine cultures proved positive for tuberculosis. **(A)** Longitudinal sonogram showing a mass in the left lower pole (solid arrows) that is hypoechoic and contains calcification (open arrow). **(B)** CT scan showing a low-density mass (arrowheads) in the lower pole; calcifications (arrow) are again seen. (From Kenney,[175] with permission.)

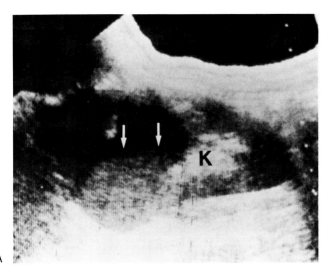
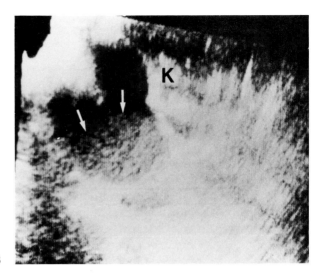

Fig. 13-86. Tuberculosis, renal. **(A)** Longitudinal sonogram of the right kidney *(K)* demonstrating severe focal dilatation of the upper-pole collecting system, which contains layering debris (arrows). **(B)** Transverse sonogram demonstrating a shift in position of the dependent debris (arrows). (*K*, kidney.) There was nonvisualization of the upper-pole collecting system on the right on excretory urography, resulting from infundibular stricture. (From Piccirillo et al,[164] with permission.)

pelvis[175] (Figs. 13-87 and 13-88). These fungus balls may be seen as echogenic (more echogenic than surrounding renal parenchyma) nonshadowing masses in the collecting system[164,175,192] (Fig. 13-88). These fungus balls can be found incidentally during radiologic investigation of debilitated or immunocompromised patients suspected of having infection.[175] Furthermore there may be diffuse

bacterial nephritis, pyonephrosis, intra- and extrarenal abscess, and fungus ball formation within the collecting system.[164]

The differential diagnosis in such an instance would include tumor, blood clot, or pyogenic debris within the collecting system. In addition, there has been a report of normal renal papillae simulating caliceal filling defects

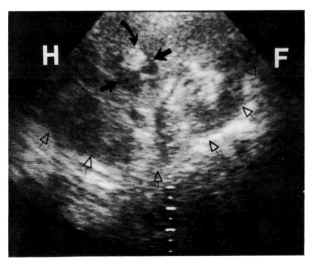
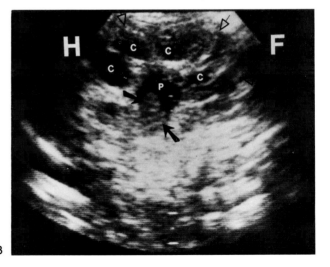

Fig. 13-87. Renal fungus ball. Case 1. **(A)** Unilateral renal fungus ball in an adult diabetic. Real-time coronal scan, with the patient in a right lateral decubitus position, showing a hyperechoic, nonshadowing mass (curved arrow) within the mildly dilated left upper-pole collecting system (straight black arrows) (*H*, patient's head; *F*, patient's feet; open arrows, renal outline.) Case 2. **(B)** Bilateral renal pelvis fungus balls in a neonate. Real-time coronal scan of the right kidney showing an echogenic nonshadowing mass (black arrows) within the renal pelvis *(P)* and mild hydronephrosis. (*C*, dilated calyces; *H*, patient's head; *F*, patient's feet; open arrows, renal outline.) (From Stuck et al,[192] with permission.)

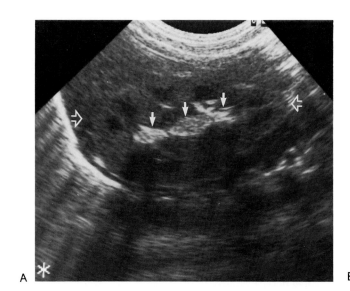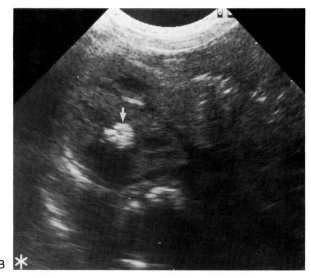

Fig. 13-88. Renal candidiasis, neonate. **(A)** Sagittal and **(B)** transverse views of the right kidney (open arrows) demonstrating echogenic material (arrows) within the region of the collecting system. The collecting system progressively dilated secondary to the echogenic debris caused by candidiasis.

on ultrasound.[193] In these cases, there was hydronephrosis with abnormal papillae; with necrosis in situ, where the papilla remained attached, the attached papillary tips became more echogenic and projected as filling defects within the dilated calyces.[193] Careful scanning technique should enable the examiner to distinguish true filling defects from normal papillae by showing continuity of normal papillae with the surrounding renal parenchyma.[193] In the absence of hematuria or pyuria and in the presence of candidemia, the calyces and the nonshadowing echodense material in the renal pelvis should suggest renal candidiasis even without hydronephrosis.[191] The parenchymal lesions are less specific but, in the presence of candidemia, should suggest candidiasis.[191] When echodense areas are seen within the medulla, acute tubular necrosis and nephrocalcinosis must be considered.[191] With a strong clinical suspicion of sepsis and abnormal-appearing kidneys, a rapid ultrasound evaluation of other organ systems should be performed.[190]

Acute Focal Bacterial Infection

Acute Focal Bacterial Nephritis. Acute focal bacterial nephritis (acute lobar nephronia) is an inflammatory mass without drainable pus.[154,194-196] The offending organism is usually a gram-negative bacterium that probably ascends through ureteral reflux.[194,196] The most common organism is *E. coli.*[164] The patient generally presents with fever, chills, and flank pain.[197] Most affected individuals are female, and many are diabetic.[164]

Excretory urography during the acute renal infection often is normal but may show diffuse enlargement, delayed calyceal filling, dilatation, or distortion of the collecting system.[194,197] Focal renal enlargement is a rare urographic abnormality with acute pyelonephritis.[194]

The ultrasound appearance of acute focal bacterial nephritis is characteristic and consists of (1) a poorly defined hypoechoic mass, (2) absence of corticomedullary definition, and (3) no enhanced through transmission[164,166,168,171,194-197] (Figs. 13-89 and 13-90). When the lesion is monitored by ultrasound during antibiotic therapy, anechoic areas may be seen, representing liquefaction. With further follow-up, the mass should resolve. If the mass becomes progressively more lucent, the diagnosis of an abscess must be entertained and an aspiration may be performed. An abscess is an anechoic mass with irregular margins and good acoustic enhancement; the number of internal echoes depends on the debris[197] (Fig. 13-91). Ultrasound cannot absolutely differentiate acute focal bacterial nephritis from abscess or even tumor. If there is a question of an abscess, a needle aspiration may be performed.[197,198]

As a rule, the typical CT appearance of acute lobar nephronia is that of a mass with the same or slightly decreased density on noncontrast images.[196] There have, however, been reports that these lesions may appear as high density on CT.[196] These particular lesions then appeared as wedge-shaped echogenic areas on ultrasound[164,196] (Fig. 13-92). This echogenic appearance may represent hemorrhagic focal bacterial nephritis without signs of liquefaction.[190]

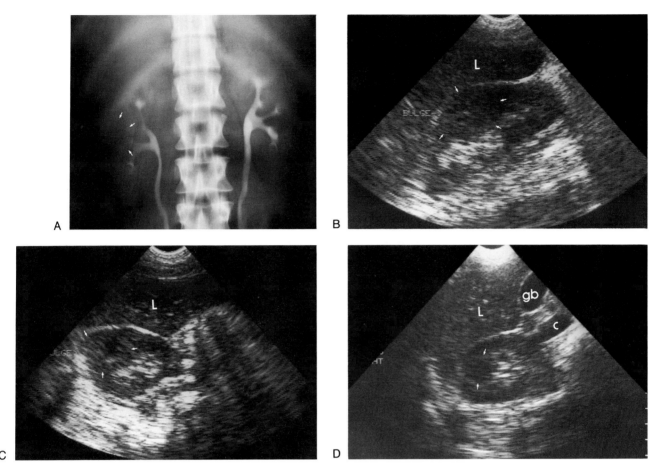

Fig. 13-89. Acute focal bacterial nephritis. **(A)** Intravenous pyelogram showing a mass effect (arrows) on the right. **(B)** Longitudinal and **(C)** transverse scans of the right kidney showing a mass effect (arrows). It is similar in echodensity to the remainder of the kidney. (*L,* liver.) **(D)** Transverse follow-up scan. The mass effect (arrows) in the right kidney has decreased in size after antibiotic therapy. (*L,* liver; *gb,* gallbladder; *c,* inferior vena cava.)

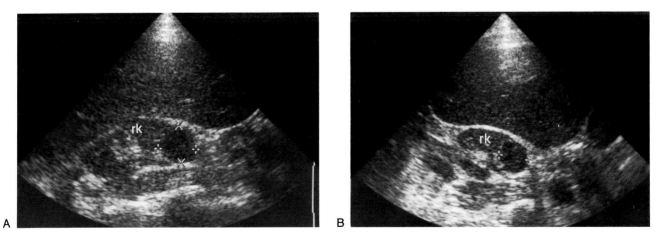

Fig. 13-90. Acute focal bacterial nephritis (AFBN). **(A)** Sagittal and **(B)** transverse scans of the right kidney *(rk)* showing a slightly hypoechoic mass (calipers, 20 × 21 × 17 mm) within the anteroinferior midportion of the kidney. The patient was febrile with right flank pain. Although a tumor could not be excluded by the ultrasound alone, the clinical picture fit more closely with AFBN. On a follow-up scan after antibiotic therapy, the mass was seen to resolve.

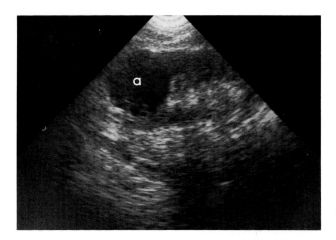

Fig. 13-91. Renal abscess. Longitudinal right lateral decubitus scan of the left kidney showing a well-defined hypoechoic rounded mass *(a)* in the upper pole of the kidney. No acoustic enhancement is seen.

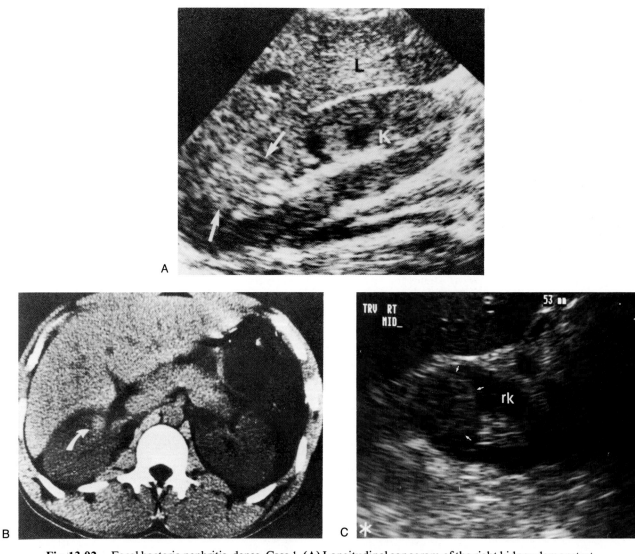

Fig. 13-92. Focal bacteria nephritis, dense. Case 1. **(A)** Longitudinal sonogram of the right kidney demonstrating a wedge-shaped area of increased echogenicity in the upper pole (arrows). (*K*, normal lower pole of kidney; *L*, liver.) **(B)** Noncontrast CT image showing a focal area of increased density in right kidney (curved arrow) corresponding to the sonographic abnormality. (On a postcontrast CT image, a nephrographic defect was seen in the same area.) Case 2. **(C)** Transverse view of the right kidney *(rk)* showing a relatively echogenic mass (arrows, 3.3 cm) within the lateral aspect of the kidney. The patient was febrile with flank pain. On unenhanced CT scan, the mass was noted to have increased density consistent with hemorrhage. (Figs. A & B from Rigsby et al,[196] with permission.)

Abscess. The most common organism found in renal abscesses in the past has been hematogeneously disseminated *Staphylococcus aureus.*[164] More recently, gram-negative organisms disseminated via either the hematogeneous or ascending route have become dominant.[164,175] Patients with abscesses usually present acutely, but these lesions may follow a chronic indolent course.[175] These abscesses occur less frequently now than in the past because of the early institution of antibiotic therapy for acute infections; most renal abscesses result from an inadequately treated acute infection.[175] Up to 20 percent of patients with renal abscess have a negative urinalysis and culture.[167]

Renal abscesses may be intrarenal (within the renal parenchyma) or extrarenal (within the perirenal and pararenal space).[164] Intrarenal abscesses may result from hematogeneous dissemination from distant sources or from progression of an ongoing renal suppurative process.[164] An intrarenal abscess may decompress into the collecting system or perforate the renal capsule to form a perinephric abscess.

On ultrasound an intrarenal abscess appears as a well-marginated anechoic mass that is round to oval with a wall that is irregular and fine[164,166,167,199,200] (Figs. 13-91, 13-93, and 13-94). There may be debris within the lesion, producing increased echoes. The ultrasound ap-

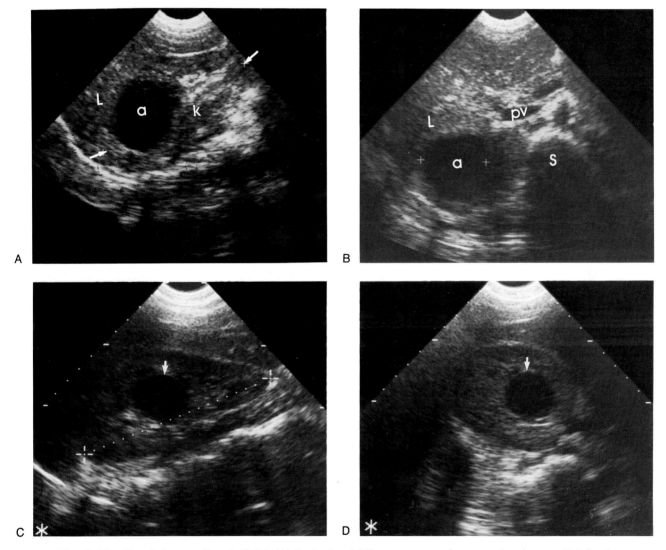

Fig. 13-93. Renal abscess. Case 1. Child. **(A)** Sagittal and **(B)** transverse supine scans showing a well-defined anechoic area *(a)* in the upper pole of the right kidney *(k,* arrows). No acoustic enhancement is seen. The abscess was drained percutaneously. *(L,* liver; *S,* spine; *pv,* portal vein.) Case 2. Adolescent. **(C)** Sagittal and **(D)** transverse views of the left kidney (calipers) in this febrile patient showing an anechoic mass (arrow, 3 cm) in the midportion of the kidney. It is well-defined, but there is no acoustic enhancement. It was drained percutaneously.

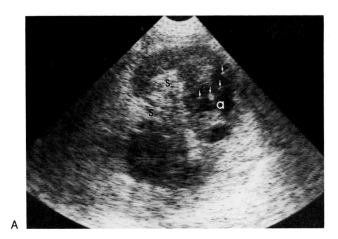
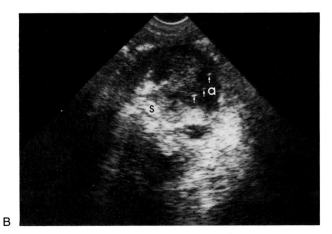

Fig. 13-94. Renal abscess. Air. **(A & B)** A reflective pattern (arrows) is seen in the area of the poorly defined hypoechoic renal mass *(a)* on right lateral decubitus transverse scans of the enlarged left lower pole (*s*, renal sinus).

pearance may be variable, ranging from anechoic to an echogenic mass, depending on the thickness of the contents.[175] Characteristically, there is acoustic enhancement.[200] The abscess may be highly echoic as a result of bright echoes caused by microbubbles of gas, implying infection by gas-forming organisms[166] (Fig. 13-94). Abscesses smaller than 2 cm may be missed by ultrasound.[201] If debris is present within a renal cyst, calyceal diverticulum, or abscess, infection should be strongly considered, although other lesions (such as hemorrhagic cysts) and neoplasms may have similar patterns.[164] CT can better define associated fascial thickening or detect subtle alterations in perinephric fat.[201]

On ultrasound extrarenal abscesses may be visualized in the peri- or pararenal spaces as similar echofree or debris-containing collections[164] (see Figs. 12-59 and 12-61 to 12-63). They may arise either from underlying lesions or from lesions of contiguous structures.[164]

To establish a definitive diagnosis, an ultrasound-guided aspiration of the lesion may be performed.[198] If pus is obtained, the patient may be referred for percutaneous catheter drainage. When the aspiration is performed, only a small amount of fluid is withdrawn for Gram stain and culture. The remainder of the fluid is left to facilitate catheter placement.[199]

Abscess Drainage. This percutaneous procedure is very similar to that for percutaneous nephrostomy. Indications for the procedure include ultrasound diagnosis of a renal abscess with an aspiration yielding pus. This is a rapid, reliable, and safe means of distinguishing abscess from noninflammatory collections.[166,200,202] The basis of effective treatment of intrarenal abscess is early diagnosis and drainage. Percutaneous catheter drainage in combination with antibiotic therapy can be definitive in

the treatment of intrarenal abscesses even with perinephric extension.[198] If the patient's condition does not improve or deteriorates, open surgical drainage can be performed.[198] (See Ch. 19 for further discussion of drainage.)

Hemorrhage

Trauma

Epidemiology and Symptoms. Injuries of the kidney rank at or near the top in frequency among all abdominal injuries.[203] Blunt trauma is responsible for most renal injuries (80 percent), but the number attributable to penetrating wounds increased dramatically in urban settings with a high rate of violent crime.[203,204] Trauma may be blunt, penetrating, or secondary to operative intervention. The automobile is the major offender, with contact sports, falls, fights, and assaults responsible for most of the rest of injuries.[203] Renal trauma, whatever the mechanism of injury, is often accompanied by damage to other important structures. This is more common with penetrating injuries, in which associated damage to the liver, intestine, stomach, or chest is encountered in 80 percent of cases.[203]

The single most important finding suggesting urologic injury is hematuria.[204] Although there is no positive correlation between the degree of hematuria and the degree of urologic injury, it is found in 90 percent of cases.[204]

Associated Conditions. Preexisting renal abnormalities such as ectopia, anomalies, or tumor predispose to significant renal damage even when the traumatic event is mild.[104] Disruptions of a hydronephrotic renal pelvis, ruptures of renal cysts and tumors, lacerations of poorly protected ectopic or horseshoe kidneys, or fracture of fragile infected kidneys may be the first manifestation of these and other underlying disorders.[203]

Classification of Injuries. Renal injuries should be classified by severity to provide a guide to both treatment and prognosis.[203] Four categories have been defined: (1) category I—lesions, including contusions and corticomedullary lacerations, that do not communicate with the collecting system (accounting for 75 to 85 percent of injuries); (2) category II—lesions consisting of parenchymal lacerations that communicate with the renal collecting system, with extravasation of urine; (3) category III—catastrophic injuries with shattered kidneys or injuries to the renal vascular pedicle (5 percent of cases); and (4) category IV—uncommon entities of UPJ avulsion and laceration of the renal pelvis.[203] Subcapsular or perinephric hematomas may be present with any of the categories; their size is usually proportional to the extent of the underlying injury.[203]

Management. Renal trauma is generally managed conservatively, with indications for surgery being on a clinical basis. Most category I lesions (renal contusions and minor lacerations) heal spontaneously, and this category is treated without surgery. Surgical intervention is used for category III and IV lesions.[203] The management of category II injuries is controversial.[203]

Imaging. The goal of the imaging modality is to define the extent of renal injury so that the maximum amount of functioning renal parenchyma can be preserved and predictable complications can be held to a minimum.[203] The workup will depend not only on the needs of the individual patient but also, to an extent on existing trauma protocols already in place in a given institution.[203]

Excretory Urography. In the past, excretory urography was the radiologic modality most commonly used to evaluate trauma to the upper urinary tract. The radiologic classification of renal trauma has been as follows: (1) minor—normal urogram or one showing diminished renal concentration of contrast, a decreased nephrogram, minimal distortion of the calyces, or blood clots in the pelvis; (2) major—extravasation of contrast; and (3) catastrophic—nonvisualization of the kidney or marked deformity of the pelvocalyceal system with extravasation of contrast (the kidney may or may not be damaged in the presence of significant surrounding retroperitoneal injury).[205] Excretory urography is a satisfactory screening procedure but may fail to provide in-

formation on the full extent of the renal injury. Nuclear medicine yields rapid assessment of the extent of parenchymal damage and reveals any significant injury to the renal pedicle.[205]

Ultrasound. The information available on ultrasound is anatomic, not functional. Bleeding into the retroperitoneal space may be seen as a lucency or a density (primarily depending on how soon after the injury the ultrasound is performed) (Figs. 13-95 to 13-98; see Figs. 12-61 to 12-63). With subcapsular hematoms a small sickle-shaped lucent area may be seen inside the renal capsule, whereas perirenal or pararenal and retroperitoneal hematomas are similarly sickle-shaped or crescent-shaped but lie outside the renal capsule or in the retroperitoneal space[206] (Figs. 13-95 to 13-98; see Figs. 12-61 to 12-63). Focal areas of internal hemorrhage and edema may be seen as hypoechoic areas (Fig. 13-99). With renal contusions and hematomas, the ultrasound appearance may vary.[203] With a fresh hematoma, a hypoechoic mass may be seen; older hematomas may become more echogenic.[203] In a limited number of cases, no findings may be seen on renal ultrasound, with the exception of blood clots in the renal pelvis. Blood clot may be seen in the collecting system as a mass containing low-level echoes, separating the walls of the affected system[205] (see Fig. 13-193). A linear reproducible absence of echoes is seen in the area of a traumatized kidney, suggesting a renal fracture[205,207] (Fig. 13-100). This must be differentiated from rib artifact, in which anechoic areas are seen anterior and posterior to the kidney and from a bifid collecting system.[205] With lacerations, a linear defect may be seen; with a shattered kidney, multiple mobile fragments may be seen.[203] Urinomas produced by the trauma can be seen as anechoic masses in a perirenal location (Fig. 13-67). Doppler examination may be performed to assess the patency of the main renal vessels.[203]

The utility of ultrasound as a free-standing method of evaluating renal trauma is limited by its lack of physiologic information.[203] Bloody and urinous collections cannot be well differentiated by ultrasound.[203] However, ultrasound is easily transportable and may be used as an alternative in patients who cannot receive contrast. Ultrasound may also be limited by technical difficulties in the acutely injured patient with broken ribs, bandages, ileus, and immobility.[203]

In some parts of the world (e.g., Europe), ultrasound is used more extensively for evaluation of renal trauma.[203] A high correlation has been demonstrated between the results of ultrasound and those of surgery or other imaging modalities in 88 patients with renal injury.[206] That group of investigators endorsed ultrasound as the most useful initial study in renal trauma; if the ultrasound findings were normal and hematuria was minimal, no

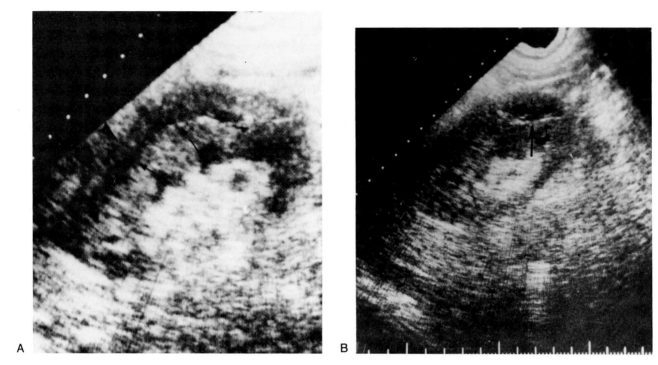

Fig. 13-95. Renal trauma, subcapsular and retroperitoneal hematoma. **(A)** Longitudinal scan demonstrating a perinephric fluid collection around the left kidney (arrows, arrowhead). Increased cortical echoes may be due to acoustic enhancement through the hematoma. **(B)** Transverse scan showing a collection indenting the margin of the left kidney (arrows) consistent with a subcapsular collection. (From Kay et al,[205] with permission.)

other studies were needed.[206] When a more serious injury was suspected, excretory urography was done concurrently or when the ultrasound was abnormal.[206]

Serial ultrasound may be used to monitor an injury identified on ultrasound.[205] Ultrasound has been re-

ported to be 100 percent accurate if performed with a urogram if minimal lesions are disregarded.[208] In most instances, its role is in monitoring patients for reapproximation of separated renal fragments and for resolution of urinous or bloody perinephric collections.[203]

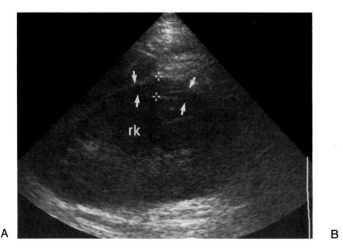

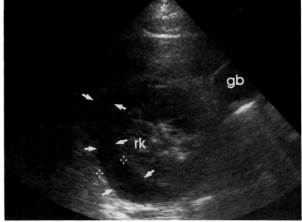

Fig. 13-96. Renal trauma, perinephric hematoma. **(A)** Sagittal and **(B)** transverse scans of the right kidney *(rk)* showing a hypoechoic mass effect (calipers, arrows) surrounding the kidney (in a perinephric location), measuring 12 to 16 mm in width. The borders of the fluid collection are difficult to define. *(gb,* gallbladder.)

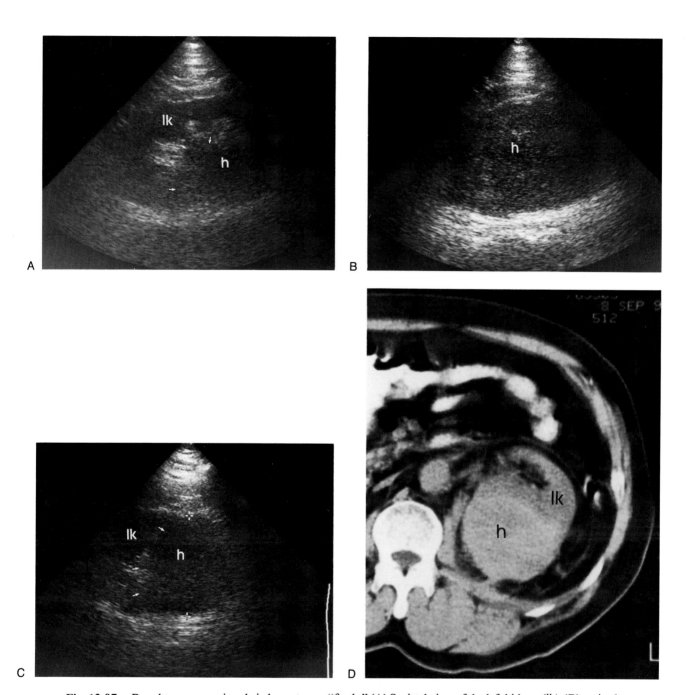

Fig. 13-97. Renal trauma, perinephric hematoma, "fresh." **(A)** Sagittal view of the left kidney *(lk)*, **(B)** sagittal view lateral to the left kidney, and **(C)** transverse view of the left kidney showing a large echogenic mass (*h*, calipers, arrows, 14 × 7.5 cm) that extends posterior and lateral to the left kidney. The mass (hematoma) is similar in echopattern to that of renal parenchyma, and its borders are ill-defined. The borders of the kidney are poorly defined. **(D)** Unenhanced CT scan showing a dense mass *(h)* posterior to the kidney *(lk)*. This is an acute hematoma.

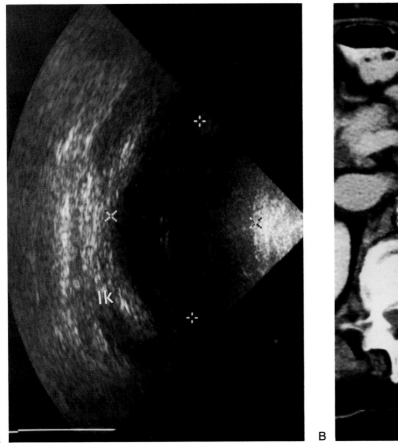
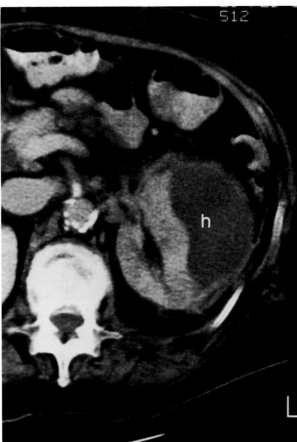

Fig. 13-98. Renal trauma, perinephric hematoma, "old." **(A)** Sagittal (coronal) view of the left kidney *(lk)* demonstrating a large hypoechoic mass (calipers, 92 × 75 × 97 mm) lateral to the kidney. This represented an older hematoma than in Fig. 13-97. **(B)** Unenhanced CT scan (similar in projection to Fig. A) showing a low-density mass *(h)* lateral to the kidney but within Gerota's fascia. This would be consistent with an older hematoma than in Fig. 13-97.

Computed Tomography. As a modality for evaluation of abdominal trauma, CT has many advantages: (1) contusions are clearly identified; (2) the location and extent of lacerations are more precisely pinpointed; (3) extrarenal hematomas are more easily detectable; and (4) small amounts of urinary extravasation are more readily appreciated.[203] CT has the additional advantage that in an emergency setting it can also evaluate all of the abdominal and pelvic viscera. It is the most informative of the radiologic modalities and is the examination of choice in patients suspected of having serious renal injuries or associated injuries amenable to CT evaluation.[203] As such, CT is usually the preferred modality for evaluation of renal trauma since it is capable of accurately defining virtually the entire panorama of renal injuries from simple contusions to devastating arterial occlusions.[203]

Pediatric. Renal injuries in children differ from those in adults in several ways: (1) the child's kidney is relatively

large with little protective perinephric fat, and it is therefore more vulnerable to injury; (2) the ratio of blunt to penetrating injuries is greater in children; (3) the renal injuries in children are more severe; (4) associated nonrenal injuries are more common; and (5) preexisting renal abnormalities are more common in children.[203] Therefore, despite the small size of the child, the imaging modality of choice is usually CT.

Spontaneous Subcapsular and Perirenal Hemorrhage

Although spontaneous renal hemorrhage into the subcapsular and perinephric space is rare, it is an important clinical problem that heralds a variety of kidney abnormalities.[209] The clinical history should enable one to exclude the following conditions associated with perirenal bleeding: (1) trauma; (2) anticoagulation medica-

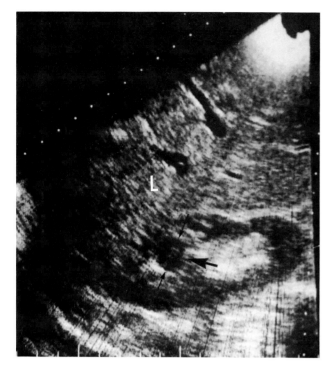

Fig. 13-99. Renal trauma. Blood clot. Longitudinal scan. A mass containing low-level internal echoes is seen in the upper pole (arrows). This mass was also seen on an intravenous pyelogram. (*L*, liver.) (From Kay et al,[205] with permission.)

ruptured cyst[210] (Fig. 13-31). In reviews of the literature it has been shown that malignant tumors are responsible for about 30 to 35 percent of cases with benign tumors (usually angiomyolipomas) responsible for 24 to 30 percent; vascular diseases are responsible for 18 to 20 percent, inflammatory disease for 5 to 10 percent, and miscellaneous conditions for the remainder.[209,210]

As a rule, CT of the abdomen will demonstrate the subcapsular hemorrhage and perinephric hemorrhage and in most cases will also enable a correct diagnosis of its cause.[210] Even though the CT may not demonstrate a tumor, one may still be present, having been "hidden" by the hemorrhage. As such, a follow-up CT scan is recommended. In a reported study, CT suggested the correct diagnosis in 78 percent of cases, demonstrating that it was the most valuable examination for patients with spontaneous renal hemorrhage.[209] In most cases surgical exploration is unnecessary, since with the current imaging technology there is an increased ability to diagnose the cause of the spontaneous hematoma.[210]

In these patients, ultrasound is highly sensitive to the presence of an abnormality but nonspecific as to its cause.[209] In the study reported, there appeared to be no consistent, reliable ultrasound pattern that could be used to differentiate among carcinoma, tumor necrosis, clotted blood, or fatty tissue.[209]

tion; (3) bleeding diathesis; (4) arteritis; (5) tuberous sclerosis; and (6) long-term hemodialysis.[210] Conditions associated with spontaneous renal hematoma include (1) renal cell carcinoma; (2) angiomyolipoma; (3) arteriovenous malformation; (4) renal artery aneurysms (including arteritis); (5) renal infarction; (6) abscess; and (7)

Renal Masses

Cyst

Simple Cyst. Almost all renal cysts are found by chance when an imaging study is performed to evaluate a patient for a urinary tract or other abdominal process.

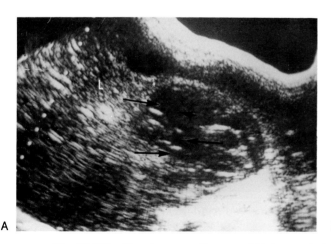

A

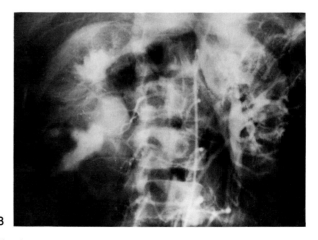

B

Fig. 13-100. Renal trauma. Fracture. **(A)** An anechoic line is seen through the upper half of the right kidney (arrows). (*L*, liver.) **(B)** Aortogram confirming the fracture of the kidney (arrowhead) with associated leakage of contrast material (arrow). (From Kay et al,[205] with permission.)

Simple cysts occur in 50 percent of patients over 55 years old.[211-214] The cysts demonstrated range in size from less than 1 cm to 10 to 15 cm.[214] They are uncommon in children but become more common with increasing age.[215] They are usually unilocular with an epithelial lining and can be located anywhere in the kidney.

On ultrasound the classic cyst meets the following criteria: (1) clear wall demarcation; (2) spherical or slightly ovoid; (3) absence of internal echoes; and (4) acoustic enhancement beyond the cyst[26,211-213,215-218] (Figs. 13-101 to 13-103). An additional finding is a narrow band of acoustic shadowing just beyond the outer margin of the cyst at each border of the acoustic enhancement[213] (Fig. 13-102). This shadowing is secondary to refraction and deflection of the echoes around the curved surface of a cystic mass.[213] Each renal cyst examined by ultrasound should be carefully evaluated for irregularity and/or tex-

tural changes that might suggest an atypical appearance.[219]

Several technical factors can interfere with the recognition of the true anechoic nature of cysts. Reverberation and effects of the beam width can interact with adjacent acoustic reflectors to produce artifactual echoes. Sonic enhancement in the distal tissues varies with TGC, frequency, and position of the focal zone. The operator who is aware of these problems can compensate for them and thereby improve diagnostic accuracy.[220]

The reverberation from the skin-transducer interface and from the specular reflectors lying anterior to the cyst are recognized as a source of artifact. In a large cyst, such artifacts are usually restricted to the anterior portion of the fluid and rapidly decrease in amplitude after several reflective cycles. They can be suppressed by having the

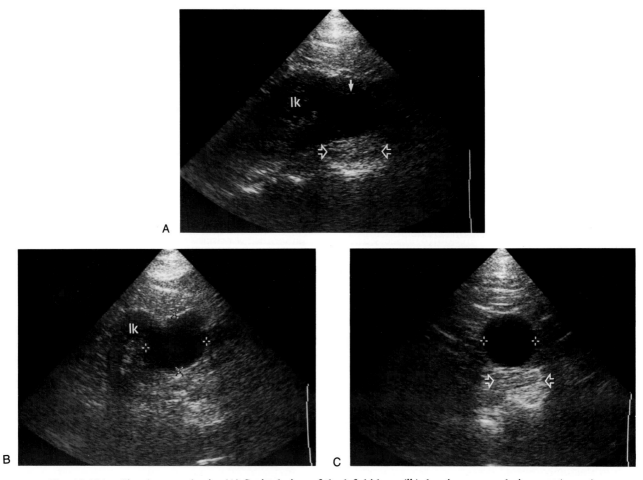

Fig. 13-101. Simple cyst, classic. **(A)** Sagittal view of the left kidney *(lk)* showing an anechoic mass (arrow) within the lower pole. The borders appear well-defined, and there is slight posterior acoustic enhancement (open arrows). **(B & C)** Transverse views. By changing the patient's position slightly and moving the "mass" into a more optimal zone for evaluation, a very well-defined anechoic mass (calipers, 37 × 44 × 39 mm) is seen (the kidney *[lk]* is not seen in Fig. C). The outline of the lesion is much better defined in Fig. C, and its relationship to the kidney can be seen in Fig. B. Posterior acoustic enhancement is also best visualized on Fig. C (open arrows).

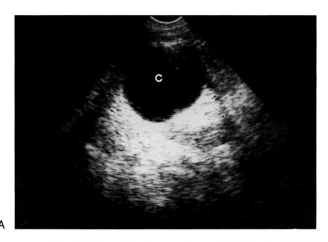
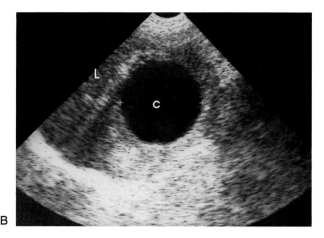

A   B

Fig. 13-102.   Simple cyst. Acoustic shadowing. **(A)** Transverse and **(B)** longitudinal scans of a right renal cyst *(c)* showing acoustic shadowing (arrows) paralleling the borders of the mass and on either side of the acoustic enhancement. (*L,* liver.)

beam strike the reflector at different angles as the cyst can be scanned from an opposite approach through the body. Small cysts are most resistant to artifactual off-axis signals when they lie within the focal zone. These larger changes in transducer output are least likely to result in echo fill-in, especially if there are no specular reflectors in the surrounding media.[220]

The distal sonic enhancement sign is a nonattenuation characteristic of a cystic lesion caused by the TGC and is most visible with greater slopes used with high-frequency transducers. The effect is amplified when the tissue distal tal to the cyst lies in the intensity peak created by focusing the transducer beam[220] (Figs. 13-101 to 13-103).

If all the criteria for a simple cyst are demonstrated on ultrasound, this diagnosis can be made with confidence and no further studies need be done.[214] To keep the diagnostic errors to a minimum, the following potential pitfalls should be remembered: (1) when evaluating a mass seen on excretory urogram or CT, the scan should be available when the ultrasound is interpreted; (2) clustering malformations closely adjacent to one another may harbor a small carcinoma that could be missed on the ultrasound examination; (3) vascular malformations or aneurysm, although rare, could be mistaken for cystic disease if real-time studies do not demonstrate pulsations or large feeding vessels; (4) because of their location adjacent to (and often interspersed between) the structures of the collecting system, parapelvic cysts often contain artifactually created echoes and require confirmation by CT; and (5) lesions that contain calcium, septations, irregular margins, or any suspicious area should be studied further by CT.[214]

The unequivocal ultrasound diagnosis of a cyst is 95 to 98 percent accurate, with 2 percent of inaccurate diag-noses due to hematomas, localized hydronephrosis, or septa in cysts.[211–213,216,221] The causes of incorrect diagnoses include lesions less than 2 cm masses in the left upper pole, diffusely infiltrating urothelial tumors, echogenic fatty lesions, and acute abscesses and hematomas.[37] To maintain this high degree of accuracy, one must adhere strictly to the criteria listed for a cyst. If a lesion meets only a portion of the criteria, it is indeterminate for a cyst and further diagnostic tests, such as CT or a cyst puncture, are warranted. Some authors recommend the use of ultrasound with or without aspiration for all cystlike renal masses that are indeterminate on CT.[222] If, however, the lesion meets all the criteria for a classic cyst on ultrasound, no further investigation is needed.[211] Diagnoses to be considered if the mass does not meet all the criteria for a cyst include complicated cyst, abscess, hematoma, renal artery aneurysm, hydronephrosis, and homogeneous or cystic tumor.[217]

Simple Cysts in Children.   There have been several reports in the literature of simple renal cysts in children.[223,224] In one series, the overall frequency of simple renal cysts was 0.22 percent with a roughly similar prevalence in all age groups.[223] It has been found that 45 percent of simple renal cysts in children are located in the upper pole of the kidney.[224] Forty-three percent of the cysts occur in the right upper pole, with 11 percent in the upper pole of the left kidney.[223] These cysts varied from 0.3 to 7.0 cm in maximum diameter, with an average diameter of approximately 1 cm in all age groups.[223] The natural history of simple renal cysts in infants is not known, but limited experiences with children suggest that the cysts do not change in size during a brief period of follow-up.[224] When a simple renal cyst appears on an

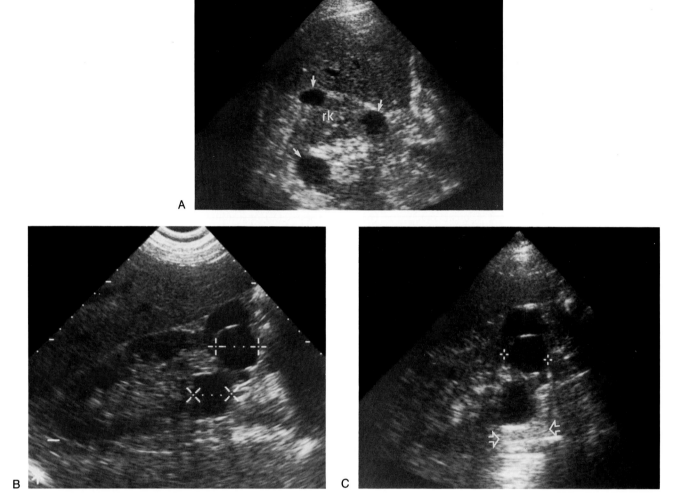

Fig. 13-103. Multiple simple cysts. Case 1. **(A)** Transverse view of the right kidney *(rk)* in an elderly patient, showing multiple small cysts (arrows, largest 1 cm) within the cortex of the kidney. The smaller the cyst, the more difficult it is to assess for acoustic enhancement. This is also the case when there are multiple cysts close together. Case 2. **(B)** Sagittal view of the right kidney demonstrating multiple cysts (anechoic masses) in the lower pole. The largest cyst was 27 mm. **(C)** Transverse view throughout the lower pole showing the multiple cysts and demonstrating acoustic enhancement (open arrows).

abdominal ultrasound in a pediatric patient with normal renal function and echogenicity, no intervention beyond symptomatic treatment is warranted.[223]

Hemorrhagic Cyst. There is a 1 to 11.5 percent incidence of hemorrhage in simple cysts.[213,225] The incidence is even greater in polycystic kidney disease. On ultrasound, one may see internal echoes and/or lack of acoustic enhancement (Figs. 13-31 and 13-104). Because these cysts do not meet the classic criteria for a cyst on ultrasound, they should be subject to further investigation by aspiration or CT.[226] On a CT scan, these lesions may appear hyperdense.[225-227]

Infected Cyst. As with the hemorrhagic cyst, the infected cyst does not meet the classic ultrasound criteria for a cyst. It often contains internal echoes, and the patient is symptomatic. Again, this lesion should be subject to further studies, primarily aspiration under ultrasound guidance. Even if the cyst appears classic for a simple cyst, infection should be considered in a symptomatic patient.

Atypical Cyst. Septation may be seen within a simple cyst as a linear echodensity (Figs. 13-105 and 13-106). The septa should be evaluated to ensure that they are

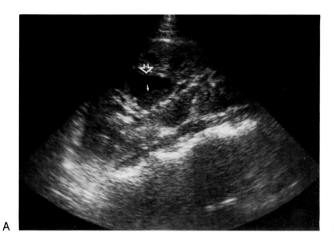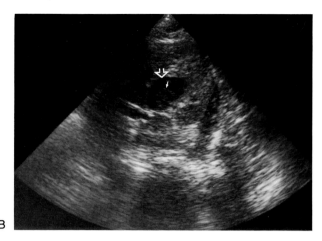

A   B

Fig. 13-104. Hemorrhagic cyst. **(A)** Sagittal and **(B)** transverse right lateral decubitus scans demonstrating a cystic mass (open arrow) within the parapelvic region of the left kidney. The mass is noted to contain a fluid-fluid level (small arrow), which was secondary to blood. This fluid-fluid level may also be seen within an infected cyst or even a complicated mass.

thin. In one reported series, the addition of a septation with no other variation in the criteria could be considered benign.[218] If the mass contains multiple and/or thick septations, the lesion should be viewed with suspicion and multilocular cystic nephroma, abscess, hematoma, and complicated cyst should be considered.[218] Additionally, multiple septa may produce a multilocular mass. A solid component within the cystic mass is the most worrisome of features.[218]

Besides septation, there may be cysts that contain calcification in their wall (Fig. 13-107). The calcification diminishes the sound transmission and may cause the mass to appear solid.[213] This calcification in a renal lesion is always a troubling sign because a solid-appearing mass may be malignant, but small plaques of fine linear

calcium can occur in the wall of benign cysts, so the pattern and amount of the calcium are important.[214] The presence of a small amount of calcium or a thin, fine area of calcium in the wall or septa of a lesion without evidence of associated soft tissue density or contrast enhancement can be consistent with a complicated cyst and may not be a sign of cancer provided all other ultrasound and CT criteria for a cyst are present.[214]

A cyst containing milk of calcium may have a confusing appearance. This cyst usually represents a calyceal diverticulum that has lost its communication with the calyceal system[192] (see also under Renal Medical Disease). Ultrasound shows a cystic mass containing a layering linear band of echoes with a shadow[213] (similar to Fig. 13-178).

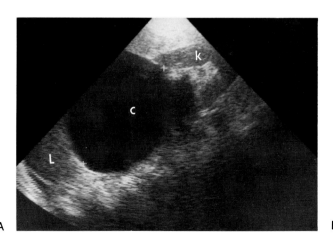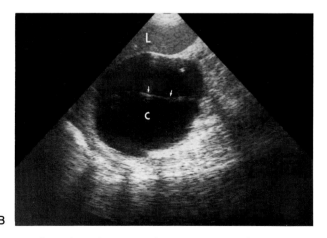

A   B

Fig. 13-105. Atypical cyst. Septation. **(A)** Longitudinal scan of the right kidney showing a large well-defined anechoic mass *(c)* in the upper pole of the right kidney *(k)*. *(L*, liver.) **(B)** Left lateral decubitus longitudinal view showing a septum (arrows) within the cyst *(c)*. *(L*, liver.)

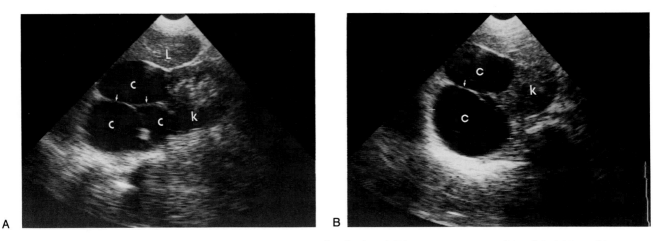

Fig. 13-106.   Atypical cyst. Septation. Right **(A)** longitudinal and **(B)** transverse scans of the right kidney *(k)* demonstrating a multiseptated (arrows) renal cyst *(c)*. *(L,* liver.)

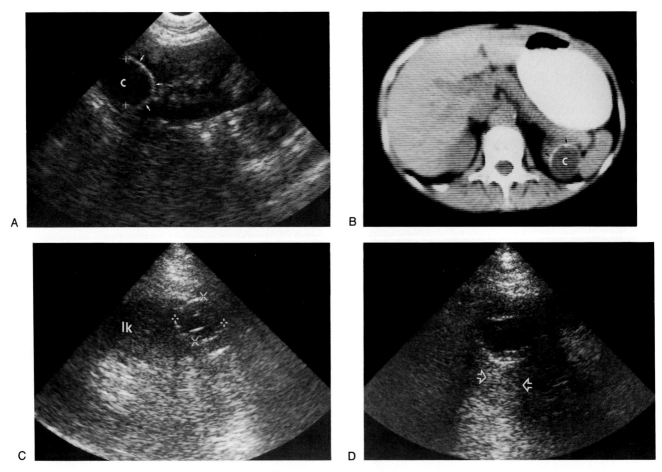

Fig. 13-107.   Atypical cyst. Calcification. Case 1. **(A)** Longitudinal prone scan of the left kidney demonstrating a well-defined round, anechoic mass *(c)* in the upper pole. The mass has very echodense walls (arrows) without acoustic enhancement. **(B)** Unenhanced CT scan showing a low-density mass *(c)* in the upper pole of the left kidney. The walls contain calcification (arrows). Case 2. **(C)** Sagittal and **(D)** transverse images in the right lateral decubitus position demonstrating a complicated mass (calipers, 23 × 26 mm) within the lower pole of the left kidney *(lk)*. It is relatively anechoic but has a thickened wall (calipers) best seen in Fig. C. In Fig. D there appears to be subtle acoustic enhancement (open arrows). The findings in this mass would be worrisome. On a CT scan, the mass was found to contain calcification within the wall and proved to be a complicated cyst.

Parapelvic Cyst. Parapelvic cysts are not true cysts but may be lymphatic in origin or may develop from embryonic rests with no communication with the collecting system. They represent 6 percent of cysts.[228,229] Patients with these cysts are usually asymptomatic but may have hypertension, hematuria, or hydronephrosis or may become secondarily infected. Real-time ultrasound is especially helpful in their evaluation to determine whether the cysts communicate with the calyces. At times, these cysts may be difficult to distinguish from hydronephrosis[229,230] (Figs. 13-39 and 13-108).

Tuberous Sclerosis. Classically, patients with tuberous sclerosis present with the triad of mental retardation, epilepsy, and adenoma sebaceum.[231] The presentation may vary with age: the newborn may have intracranial hamartomas and cardiac rhabdomyomas, whereas the older child may have the typical skin lesions, as well as renal lesions.[231] This condition is secondary to an auto-somal gene, although only 50 percent of patients have a family member with any feature of tuberous sclerosis.[231] Tuberous sclerosis is an inherited neurocutaneous disorder in which the characteristic renal lesion is an angiomyolipoma, presenting in 40 to 80 percent of patients. Less common manifestations of this disease are cysts (Fig. 13-109). The cysts in tuberous sclerosis have a hyperplastic eosinophilic epithelial lining that projects into the lumen of the cyst. The etiology of the cysts in this disease is unclear. The cysts do not usually cause severe renal impairment, but some do. When a child is noted to have the pattern of adult polycystic kidney disease on ultrasound, the examiner should also consider the diagnosis of tuberous sclerosis[232] (Fig. 13-109).

Coexistent Cyst and Tumor. The incidence of coexistent tumor and cyst is 2.1 to 7 percent[219,233,234] (Fig. 13-110). It is most commonly thought that the tumor plays an etiologic role in cyst formation.[219]

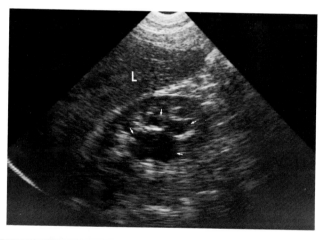

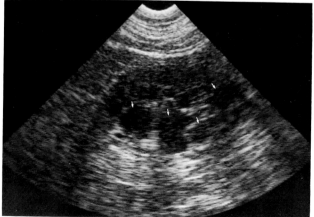

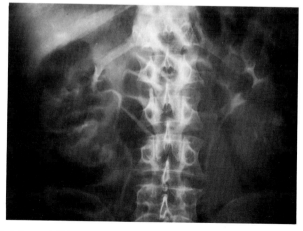

Fig. 13-108. Parapelvic cysts. Longitudinal scans of the **(A)** right and **(B)** left kidneys. Multiple anechoic areas (arrows) are seen in the region of the renal sinus. They appeared to connect at real-time, suggesting hydronephrosis. (*L,* liver.) **(C)** Intravenous pyelogram. No hydronephrosis is seen. Instead, the mass effect of multiple parapelvic cysts is visible.

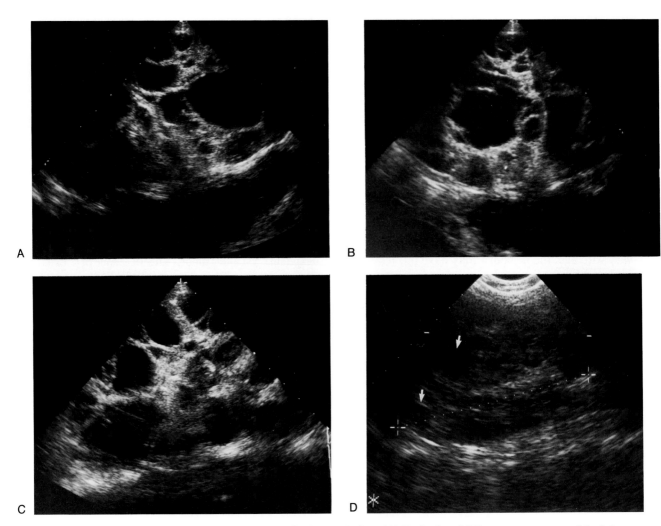

Fig. 13-109. Multiple cysts, tuberous sclerosis. Case 1. Infant. **(A)** Sagittal and **(B)** transverse scans of the left kidney and **(C)** sagittal scan of the right kidney showing markedly enlarged kidneys (12 and 13 cm long) with multiple cysts. It is difficult to define the normal renal parenchyma. By the ultrasound pattern alone, it would be difficult to differentiate this from adult polycystic kidney disease. However, the patient had known tuberous sclerosis, and therefore the cysts were thought to be secondary to that disease process. Case 2. Adolescent. **(D)** Sagittal view of the right kidney (11.3 cm) in a patient with known tuberous sclerosis. The renal margins are poorly defined, and there are poorly defined anechoic areas (arrows) within the parenchyma. The left kidney appeared similar.

Cyst Puncture. The indications for cyst puncture in the past included (1) a cystic lesion that did not meet the ultrasound criteria for a cyst (indeterminate); (2) a cyst that did meet the criteria but presented in a patient suspected of infection; and (3) a classic cyst on ultrasound of a patient less than 40 years old with hematuria or with a high index of suspicion for tumor. More recently, cyst punctures have been less frequently performed and were performed only for specific indications; opacification was only occasionally performed after puncture, with cytology the laboratory procedure of choice for aspirated fluid.[235] The specific indications for the procedure now include (1) diagnosis of an infected cyst; (2) diagnosis of

lesions that might be malignant in high-risk patients; (3) therapy of painful or obstructing cysts; and (4) lesions considered indeterminate on CT and ultrasound.[214,218] The reason for the decreased frequency of cyst puncture has been the use of more sophisticated imaging techniques.[235] Most investigators consider CT the gold standard in evaluating cystic masses in the kidney and mandatory in all cases in which there is any clinical or radiologic suspicion of cancer of an apparent renal cyst.[235]

The diagnosis of a cyst by aspiration approaches 100 percent. Clear fluid has occasionally been found in cases of cystic or necrotic renal cell carcinomas (RCCs), as

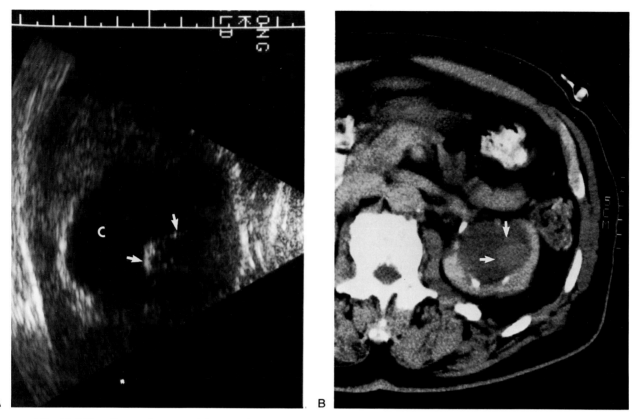

Fig. 13-110. Cyst and tumor. **(A)** Magnified (coronal, sagittal) view of a cystic mass *(c)* within the left kidney. This mass contains a solid mass effect (arrows) within its lateral wall. **(B)** This was confirmed on enhanced CT scan. At surgery, the mass (arrows) was found to be a renal cell carcinoma (tubopapillary type) with involvement of the cortex.

well as when RCC occurs in the wall of a cyst.[218] Not only may the fluid be clear, but also the cytologic test results in such cases may be negative.[218] As such, one should be aware of the procedure's shortcomings. The incidence of major complications is 1.4 percent.[236] Most complications seen on ultrasound include perirenal hemorrhage; the most common minor complication is hematuria.

To begin the procedure of cyst puncture, the patient is usually placed in a prone or semiprone position with a pillow or rolled sheet under the stomach. The kidney is scanned in held-respiration, and the cyst is localized. A point in the center of the lesion is selected. If the lesion is large, the aspiration procedure may be performed without direct ultrasound visualization. If the cyst is small or if several cysts must be punctured (such as in the polycystic patient), the patient is scanned in a sterile fashion while the puncture is performed. After the usual sterile preparation of the skin and administration of local anesthesia, a 22-gauge needle is inserted to the premeasured depth in one swift movement. A pop is felt when the needle enters the cyst. Fluid is aspirated and sent for cytologic testing. As a rule, clear yellow fluid (that looks

like urine) is obtained from a simple cyst. If the fluid is hemorrhagic or turbid, the lesion becomes suspicious. If there is any question of infection, the fluid should be Gram stained and sent for cultures (see also Ch. 19).

Abscess

Abscesses are discussed under Inflammatory Disease.

Infarction

Not all focal parenchymal lesions are tumors. Renal infarction may appear as an area of hyperechogenicity (Figs. 13-111 and 13-112). The increase in echoes is probably secondary to an admixture of fibrosis with acoustically dissimilar tissues within the affected region. A focally increased area of parenchymal echoes in association with thinning of the involved cortex has been found in chronic atrophic pyelonephritis as well as renal infarction.[237] Other lesions in the differential diagnosis of a focal area of increased echogenicity would include

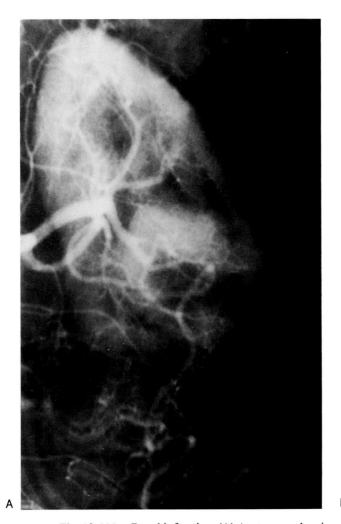

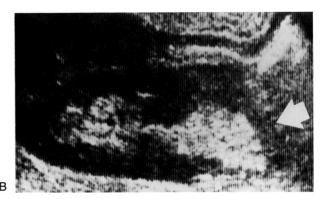

Fig. 13-111. Renal infarction. **(A)** Aortogram showing an avascular region involving the lower pole of the left kidney. **(B)** Longitudinal scan of the left kidney showing an echogenic wedge-shaped lower pole renal mass (arrow). (From Erwin et al,[237] with permission.)

solitary and diffuse angiomyolipomata, cavernous renal hemangioma, RCC, angiosarcoma, undifferentiated sarcoma, oncocytoma, and metastatic neoplasm.[237]

Some investigators have evaluated experimentally the sonographic pattern of renal infarction[238] (Fig. 13-112). Within 24 hours after arterial occlusion, a focal hypoechoic mass is seen. Within 7 days, echoes begin to appear within the mass such that it becomes echogenic by 17 days, and total renal arterial occlusion produces no appreciable change in cortical echogenicity. As such, when being evaluated specifically for renal infarction, the patient may be best served by a physiologic study.

No significant change in size, echogenicity, or corticomedullary definition has been reported with global renal infarction.[239] It is postulated that Doppler ultrasound should be able to detect global or major segmental renal infarction by demonstrating the absence of blood flow.[239] A normal ultrasound examination with Doppler evaluation probably cannot exclude segmental infarction.[239] In one reported case, demonstration of lack of blood flow in the vessels of the affected kidney supported the diagnosis of infarction.[239]

With segmental renal infarction, a spectrum of ultrasound findings may be visualized; these include a normal appearance, a focal hypoechoic mass, a focal echogenic mass, and an echogenic area of cortical thinning.[239] In the appropriate clinical setting the diagnosis should be suggested, but confirmation may require correlative imaging or follow-up studies.[239]

Vascular Lesions

See Vascular Abnormalities under Renal Medical Disease; see also Chapter 11.

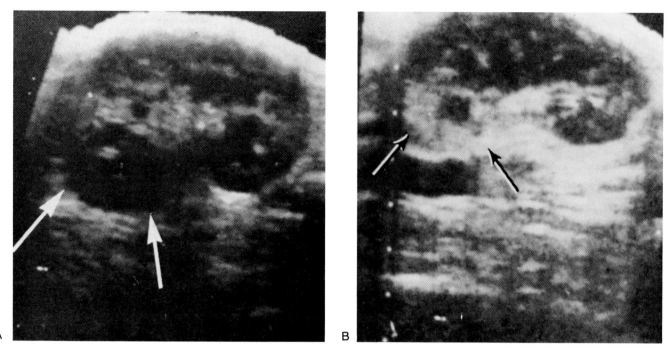

Fig. 13-112. Renal infarction. Experimental arterial occlusion. Sequence of changes in segmental infarction 27 days after arterial occlusion. **(A)** Scan 8 hours after segmental arterial occlusion showing bulging along the superoposterior aspect of the kidney (arrows). The infarcted area demonstrates decreased echogenicity. **(B)** Longitudinal scan 27 days later showing thinning of the renal cortex and increased cortical echogenicity (arrows) in the area of the infarction. (From Spies et al,[238] with permission.)

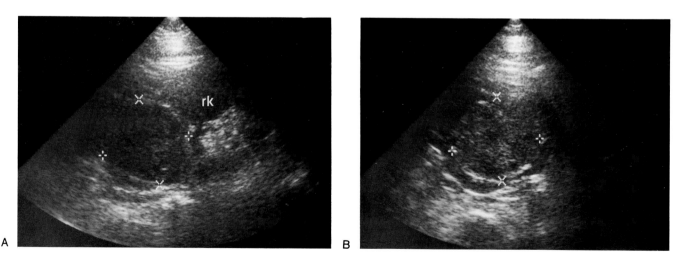

Fig. 13-113. Renal cell carcinoma, clear cell type. **(A)** Sagittal and **(B)** transverse views of the right kidney *(rk)* showing a large mass (calipers, 59 × 61 × 63 mm) within the upper pole. It is similar in echopattern to the renal parenchyma but does contain well-defined margins.

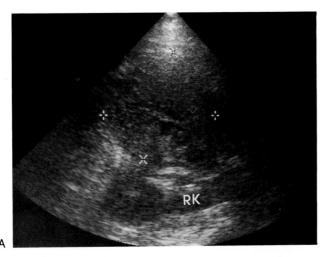

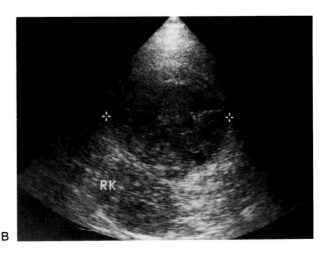

Fig. 13-114. Renal cell carcinoma, clear cell type. **(A)** Sagittal and **(B)** transverse scans showing a relatively well-defined mass (calipers, 56 × 57 × 66 mm) within the anterior aspect of the right kidney *(RK)*. The mass is similar in echopattern to the renal parenchyma.

Primary Renal Tumors

Renal neoplasms are being detected earlier with increased frequency.[240] In a 5-year period in the 1980s, a fivefold increase in the number of small (≤ 3.0 cm) renal neoplasms were detected and removed with the use of high-resolution CT and ultrasound, compared with a similar period in the 1970s.[240] There has been a considerable increase in the number of individuals in the general population who undergo kidney imaging because of the widespread use of CT and ultrasound.[240] The kidneys are imaged as part of every abdominal ultrasound as well as every abdominal CT.

Regardless of lesion size, the imaging findings that differentiate benign from malignant lesions are basically the same, although small lesions can be even more problematic because the findings can become smaller and this requires more detailed and more sensitive imaging studies.[240] Ultrasound has become the initial technique in the discovery of a large number of these incidentally found tumors when the kidney is studied in the course of abdominal imaging, although it is not as sensitive as contrast-enhanced CT in depicting these small masses.[240] Its major use is to help differentiate small cysts from small solid tumors.[240]

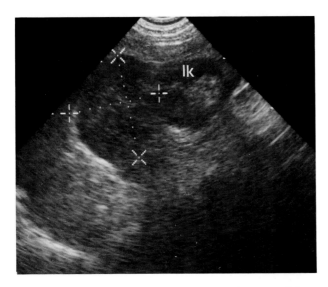

Fig. 13-115. Renal cell carcinoma. Sagittal right lateral decubitus view showing a large mass (calipers, 67 × 74 mm), which appears to be originating from the upper pole of the left kidney *(lk)*. The mass is somewhat mixed in its texture.

Renal Cell Carcinoma. RCC represents 1 to 3 percent of all visceral cancers and 80 to 90 percent of renal cancers in adults.[24] The lesion is seen in the sixth to seventh decade, with a 3:1 male/female ratio.[24] Classically, the patient presents with costovertebral angle pain, mass, and hematuria (hematuria is the most reliable presentation). These lesions commonly metastasize widely before they produce local symptoms. Fifty percent go to the lungs and 33 percent to bones, followed by nodes, liver, adrenals, and brain.[24] From 10 to 15 percent metastasize to the opposite kidney. The average 5-year survival is 45 percent, with 70 percent if there are no distant metastases.[24] The prognosis is poor even though the tumor grows slowly, with an overall survival rate of approximately 20 to 25 percent 10 years after nephrectomy.[241] There is a 60 percent 5-year survival if the cancer is confined to the kidney, with a 50 percent 10-year survival.[241]

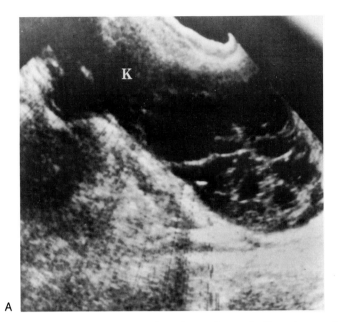

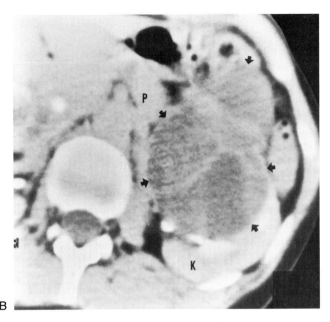

A   B

Fig. 13-118. Multilocular cystic renal cell carcinoma. **(A)** Prone longitudinal scan of the left kidney *(K)* showing multiple fluid-filled cysts separated by thick, echogenic septa. **(B)** CT scan showing a large multicystic mass originating from the left kidney *(K)* compressing the kidney dorsally and extending vertically (arrows). (*P*, pancreas.) (From Feldberg and van Waes,[248] with permission.)

masses.[247] There are one or more RCCs in approximately 50 percent of cases of von Hippel-Lindau syndrome, and these are frequently multiloculated.[247] The diagnosis of RCC is favored in the presence of intravascular extension or distant metastases.[247] Multiloculated RCC is composed of multiple noncommunicating fluid-filled cystic spaces of various sizes.[247] Usually the mass is sharply marginated by a pseudocapsule, and the locules often contain variable amounts of both new and old blood.[247] The complex cysts are separated by highly echogenic areas, also seen infrequently in necrotic and cystic RCCs[248] (Fig. 13-118). Cyst aspiration and cytologic examination might confirm the diagnosis.

Papillary Pattern. From 5 to 10 percent of RCCs are papillary, which is a microscopic subclassification that is characterized by slower growth, less extensive involvement at the time of diagnosis, and a better prognosis than the nonpapillary renal parenchymal cancer.[249,250] It represents 5 to 15 percent of all malignant tumors in the kidney.[246] There is a high frequency of internal calcifications (about 30 percent of cases).[246,250] Papillary RCC may appear as a unilocular mass.[246] On ultrasound, 64 percent of papillary tumors and 23 percent of nonpapillary tumors have been reported to be hypoechoic[249] (Fig. 13-119). Data suggest that the papillary carcinomas tend to be hypoechoic as a result of the large central area of cystic necrosis in the tumor. Another study reported no

consistent ultrasound pattern associated with papillary RCC.[250] In this series, 85 percent of the papillary tumors were confined within the renal capsule (stage I) whereas more than 50 percent of the nonpapillary tumors had extended beyond the limits of the kidney.[249]

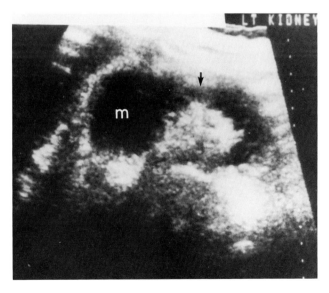

Fig. 13-119. Papillary renal cell carcinoma. Longitudinal scan of the left kidney showing a 5-cm mass *(m)* that is less echogenic than the adjacent renal cortex (arrow). (From Blei et al,[249] with permission.)

Cholesterol. All histologic types of RCC characteristically contain large amounts of cholesterol.[251] They may contain an average of 378 mg percent cholesterol compared with 0.25 mg percent for fresh normal kidney.[251] The cholesterol is predominantly in the form of intracellular crystalline ester, which can be seen as birefringent spheroidal droplets with Maltese cross markings within viable portions of renal tumors.[251] An unusual ultrasound appearance has been described with this finding. It appears that the very high concentration of extracellular cholesterol crystals within the necrotic portions of the renal tumor produces the unusual pattern on ultrasound. As such, if dense acoustic shadowing is seen arising from a noncalcified renal mass, the possibility of a cholesterol-laden RCC should be considered.[251]

Mass Evaluation. When a solid renal mass is identified on ultrasound, the study is not complete. The contralateral kidney must be examined carefully. In addition, the inferior vena cava and renal vein should be examined for evidence of tumor extension[252,253] (Figs. 13-64 and 13-120). The prognosis is poorer with tumor extension into the inferior vena cava.[253] The para-aortic area should be evaluated for the presence of nodes, and the liver should also be evaluated for metastases.[253] In staging RCC ultrasound is correct in 70 percent of cases, with CT correct in 91 percent.[254]

Ultrasound Accuracy. Ultrasound has been shown to have an accuracy of 90 percent in diagnosing solid masses. The causes of incorrect diagnoses have been at-

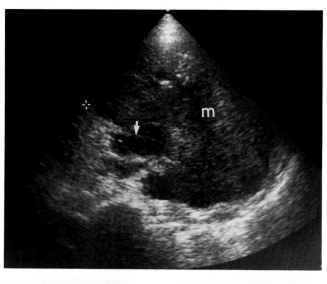

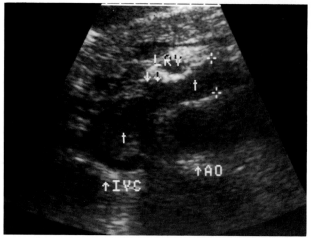

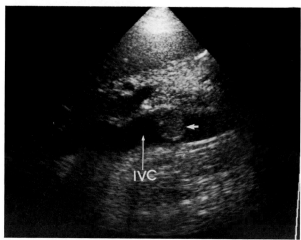

Fig. 13-120. Renal cell carcinoma with vascular invasion. **(A)** Transverse view of the left renal fossa showing a large, poorly defined mass *(m)*. The left kidney as such could not be identified. Echogenic material could be seen within the dilated vein (arrow) within the hilum of the mass. **(B)** Transverse midline view showing the dilated left renal vein *(LRV)*, as well as the inferior vena cava *(IVC)*. Echogenic material *(t)* is noted within both vessels. *(AO, aorta.)* The globular tumor thrombus (arrow) is also seen on the **(C)** sagittal view of the inferior vena cava *(IVC)*.

tributed to lesions of less than 2 cm, masses in the left upper pole, diffusely infiltrating urothelial tumors, echogenic fatty lesions, or acute abscess and hematoma. Angiography in the same series was correct in 88 percent of solid lesions.[37]

Oncocytoma. Oncocytomas are uncommon benign tumors that usually occur in middle to old age, with males affected more than females (male/female ratio, 1.7:1).[255] They account for 2 to 14 percent of renal tumors that were preoperatively thought to be cancer.[256] These tumors are usually asymptomatic, although some patients present with pain or hematuria. Although they are usually single, they may be multiple and bilateral.

Oncocytomas have distinct clinical and pathologic characteristics. They are not associated with vascular invasion, local recurrence after surgery, or distant metastases.[255] Typically, they range from 0.3 to 26 cm in diameter; are well-defined, smooth, and homogeneous; and often have a central stellate scar.[255,256] Thus, as the mass enlarges, it may outstrip its blood supply with concomitant infarction, hemorrhage, and necrosis. The central stellate fibrotic scar may form after the central hemorrhage undergoes organization and healing.[256] A comparable RCC will often be well-defined but will not contain a central scar but, instead, hemorrhage and necrosis.

On ultrasound on oncocytoma appears as a sold renal mass with low-level echoes similar to an RCC[257] (Fig. 13-121). If a central, echogenic scar is seen in an otherwise homogeneous mass on ultrasound or CT, an oncocytoma should be suspected[255,256] (Figs. 13-121 and 13-

122). This criterion appears to apply only if the mass is greater than 3 cm.[255] If the tumor is greater than 6 cm with necrosis or calcification, it cannot be differentiated by ultrasound.[256] The radiologic differentiation of oncocytoma and RCC prior to surgery is important because an oncocytoma is treated by local resection or heminephrectomy without chemotherapy or radiation therapy. If no central scar is seen by ultrasound or CT, an angiogram may be performed. In a typical oncocytoma a spoke-wheel arterial supply or dense tumor blush is extremely suggestive.[255]

Angiomyolipoma. An angiomyolipoma (renal hamartoma) is an uncommon benign renal tumor composed of fat cells intermixed with smooth muscle cells and aggregates of thick-walled blood vessels. This lesion is usually unilateral, although it may be multiple. The female/male ratio is 2.3:1 to 12.5:1. Eighty percent occur in females, with 80 percent on the right side.[258] Twenty-five percent are extrarenal, including the renal sinus.[258] The size varies from 1 cm to greater than 20 cm (mean, 9.4 cm). From 60 to 80 percent of patients with tuberous sclerosis have these lesions, which are usually bilateral and multiple.[258-260] Others have reported the association of angiomyolipoma with tuberous sclerosis to be decreasing.[261] In 1969, the reported frequency was found to be 50 percent as opposed to 80 percent reported in 1932.[261] Solitary lesions are not associated with tuberous sclerosis and typically present in the fourth to sixth decade.[258,259]

The clinical presentation of angiomyolipoma is varied.[260] Most are asymptomatic; the symptomatic lesions

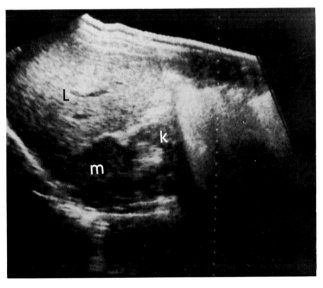
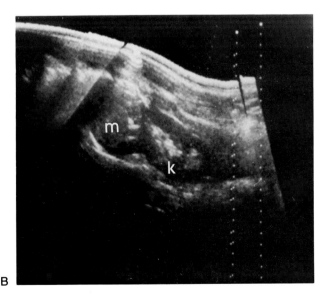

A　　　　　　　　　　　　　　　　　　　　　　　B

Fig. 13-121.　Renal oncocytoma. Longitudinal **(A)** supine and **(B)** prone scans of the right kidney *(k)* showing a solid mass *(m)* in the upper pole. It is similar in density to renal parenchyma. *(L, liver.)* At angiography, a rounded, well-defined mass was seen with a spoke-wheel pattern of vascularity.

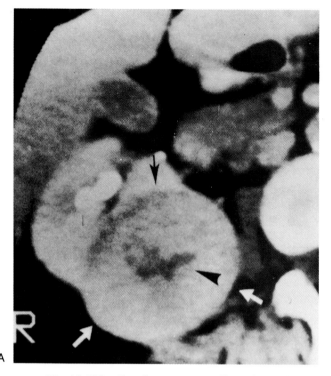
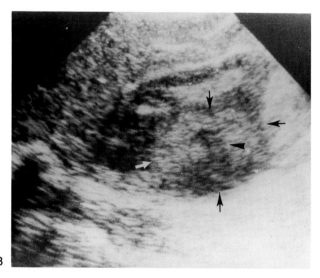

Fig. 13-122. Renal oncocytoma. Central scar. **(A)** CT scan demonstrating a well-defined mass (arrows) with a central stellate area of low density (arrowhead) that corresponds to the central scar. **(B)** Longitudinal scan showing a well-defined solid mass (arrows). The central scar is recognized as a small central hypoechoic zone (arrowhead). (From Quinn et al,[255] with permission.)

tend to be much larger and are more likely to contain angiomatous tissue.[262] Hemorrhage within the lesions or within the retroperitoneum is common; it often presents with acute onset of flank or abdominal pain and/or shock. The small lesions have no known malignant potential, and nonoperative management is suggested.

The most characteristic ultrasound pattern is a hyperechoic lesion (more dense than the renal parenchyma)[221,257-265] (Figs. 13-123 and 13-124). One series evaluated small (0.5 to 2.5 cm) hyperechoic nodules of the renal parenchyma.[265] All the lesions in this series had a homogeneous hyperechoic structure (round with sharp margins) and echogenicity equal to or higher than that of the renal pelvicaliceal complex.[265] Lesions with a dense pattern appear to have a more myomatous or vascular element. The marked echogenicity is due to the high fat content, multiple nonfat interfaces, heterogeneous cellular architecture, and/or numerous vessels often present within the angiomyolipoma. The less echogenic areas within this tumor may be due to the nonfatty portions of the tumor adjacent to dilated calyces, or they may be due to hemorrhage and necrosis. Those with a mixed pattern demonstrate spontaneous hemorrhage and necrosis.[260] Some have a hypoechoic pattern, less dense than the renal sinus.

Although the echodense pattern is the most common, it is not pathognomonic for angiomyolipoma.[260] Some investigators believe that if the well-defined feature of small lesions is observed, as a serendipitious finding without clinical symptoms, other diagnostic procedures would not be needed.[265] In rare cases, tumor extension within the inferior vena cava is seen.[266] Other lesions to be considered in the differential diagnosis of echogenic renal nodules include (1) malignant tumors such as adenocarcinoma, liposarcoma, and lymphoma; (2) benign tumors such as lipoma, oncocytoma, and cavernous hemangioma; (3) infarctions; and (4) renal sinus lipomatosis.[261]

CT is highly specific when adipose tissue is demonstrated within the lesion; however, when the lesion is smaller than 2 cm, determination of attenuation may be unreliable because of partial volume effect.[261,267] The CT detection of fat within a renal lesion should establish the diagnosis of angiomyolipoma and may be the only radiologic finding that can differentiate the lesion from RCC.[267]

At present, treatment may be more conservative if the diagnosis can be confirmed by ultrasound, CT, or biopsy.[261] If the lesion is larger or symptomatic (and possibly hypervascular), it may be treated by partial ex-

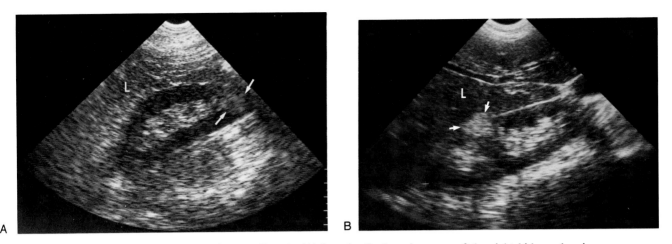

Fig. 13-123. Renal angiomyolipoma. Case 1. **(A)** Longitudinal supine scan of the right kidney showing a well-defined echogenic mass (arrows) in the lower pole. (*L*, liver.) Case 2. **(B)** Longitudinal scan of the right kidney demonstrating an echodense mass (arrows) extending anteriorly from the midportion of the kidney. (*L*, liver.)

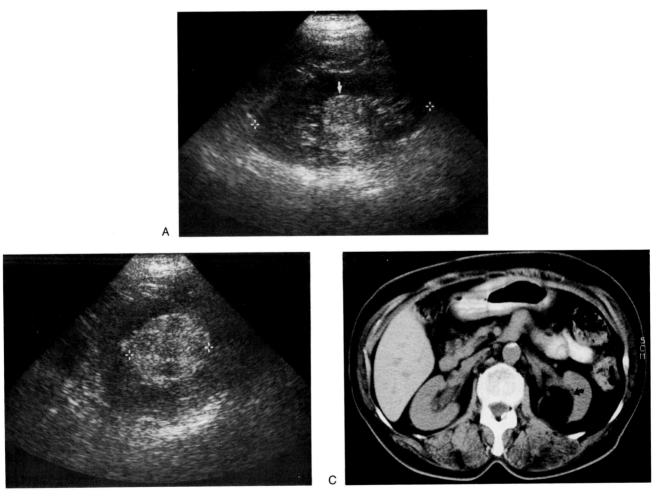

Fig. 13-124. Renal angiomyolipoma. Middle-aged woman undergoing evaluation for urinary tract infections. **(A)** Sagittal and **(B)** transverse views of the left kidney (calipers, Fig. A) showing a very echogenic mass (calipers, arrow, 43 mm) in a parapelvic location. This pattern was thought to be most consistent with an angiomyolipoma. **(C)** Unenhanced CT showing a mass (arrow) of fat density within the left kidney.

cision or embolization.[261] Follow-up alone may be proposed if the lesion is small and the patient is asymptomatic.[261]

A similar echopattern to that of angiomyolipoma has been reported with fat-filled postoperative renal cortical defects.[268] With surgical filling of renal cortical wedge resection defects with vascularized retroperitoneal fat, an echogenic mass results in a postoperative ultrasound and CT appearance that simulates a focal renal mass.

Liposarcoma. A case of primary renal liposarcoma has been reported.[269] It is a rare neoplasm with no distinct symptomatology; however, the most common presentation is that of an abdominal mass with or without colicky pain due to hemorrhage into the tumor.[269] Of the cases reported, one-third have been in patients with tuberous sclerosis; again, 40 to 80 percent of all angiomyolipomas also occur in association with tuberous sclerosis.[269]

These lesions may represent sarcomatous changes in angiomyolipoma and lipoma but this is unknown.[269] In the reported case, this tumor was seen as a hyperechoic, fat-containing tumor confined to the kidney.[269]

Juxtaglomerular Tumors. The finding of a hypovascular solid renal mass in a patient with elevated renin but no renal arterial lesion should suggest a juxtaglomerular tumor. These patients present with hypertension; the tumors are more frequent in females (mean age, 31 years). The renin-producing tumor (reninoma) is a rare but curable cause of hypertension.[270] These patients frequently present with symptoms of moderate to severe

headaches, polydipsia, polyuria including enuresis, and intermittent neuromuscular complaints.[270]

These tumors are usually small, solitary, and confined to the kidney, with an average size of 2 to 3 cm; most are just beneath the renal capsule. Pathologically, there is a pseudocapsule and small foci of hemorrhage within the tumor. On ultrasound these lesions are usually echogenic, possibly because of the numerous interfaces between the juxtaglomerular cells and the abundant small vascular channels within the tumor[270] (Fig. 13-125). If hemorrhage and necrosis are present, the lesion may be hypoechoic.

Lymphangiomyoma. Lymphangiomyomas are rare lesions, which arise from the proliferation of smooth muscle in the walls of lymphatics.[271] More than half usually occur in lymphangiomyomatosis syndrome and are usually seen in association with characteristic pulmonary involvement.[271] In the chest, there is characteristic smooth muscle proliferation along pulmonary channels, producing honeycombing, chylous effusions, and spontaneous pneumothoraces.[271] With or without pulmonary involvement, these lesions have been found exclusively in women.[271]

At ultrasound, such a lesion may appear as a multilocular mass[271] (Fig. 13-126). The other diagnostic considerations for such a mass in a middle-aged adult would include multilocular cystic nephroma, RCC, localized renal cystic disease, and echinococcal cyst.[271]

Carcinoid. Carcinoid of the kidney is rare.[272] These lesions have been seen as moderate-sized to large tumors ranging from 7 to 30 cm in greatest dimension.[272] Of six

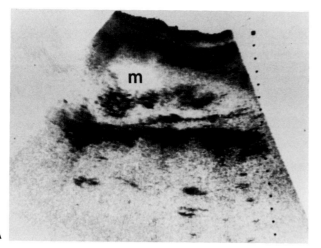

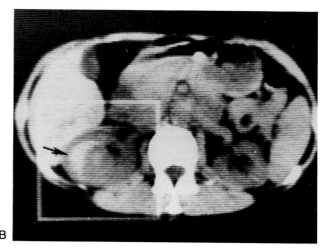

A   B

Fig. 13-125. Renal juxtaglomular tumor. **(A)** Longitudinal scan showing a 5-cm solid hypoechoic mass *(m)* in the upper pole of the right kidney. **(B)** Unenhanced CT scan. The periphery of the mass is isodense with the normal renal parenchyma. A crescent-shaped area of increased attenuation (arrow) is seen representing hemorrhage within the central portion of the mass. (From Dunnick et al,[270] with permission.)

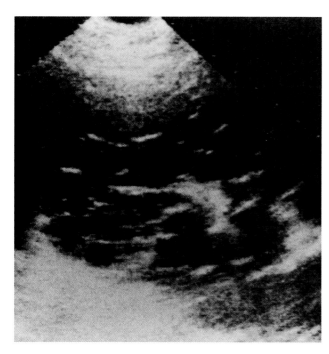

Fig. 13-126. Lymphangioma. Sagittal renal sonogram showing multiple clustered cystic masses with echogenic septa replacing the normal renal parenchyma. (From Jacobs et al,[271] with permission.)

reported, five were solid and one was cystic with tumor in soft polypoid projections from the cyst wall. Tumor margination by a fibrous capsule is frequently noted, with both central and peripheral calcification described.[272]

In the cases reported, this lesion was seen to be hyperechoic in texture, reflecting the angiographically hypovascular nature of the tumor (Fig. 13-127). RCC is the other tumor to be considered. Although RCC is uncommon, it should be included in the differential diagnosis of such a lesion.

Multilocular Cystic Nephroma. This lesion is an uncommon nonfamilial neoplasm that predominantly affects boys and women. It is seen in both males and females but with remarkably different modalities (i.e., males during infancy, up to age 4 years, and women from 50 to 60 years); the female/male ratio ranges from 2 : 1 to 6 : 1.[246] In most of the children with this tumor, the condition is detected within the first 4 months of life because of a palpable flank mass.[273] Seventy-three percent of affected children younger than 4 years are boys; 89 percent of patients older than 4 years are females.[274] It is usually solitary. It commonly occurs as an asymptomatic mass, occasionally with hematuria. The mass is usually seen on a plain radiograph, and occasionally there are curvilinear calcifications. The excretory urogram and retrograde

pyelogram are helpful when there is pelvic herniation of the tumor or when septa are noted with total-body opacification. On an angiogram, the lesion may be avascular, hypovascular, or hypervascular.[274]

The lesion is an uncommon neoplasm characterized by a well-circumscribed encapsulated mass that contains multiple noncommunicating fluid-filled locules with thick internal septations.[246,257,274,275] It is composed of multiple cysts of various sizes that are separated by connective tissue septa.[247] At times, the mass herniates into the renal pelvis and extends into the renal space.[247] Fibrous tissue, mature or immature tubular elements, or immature blastemal tissue may be in the intervening septa.[276] This lesion has many names: benign multilocular cystic nephroma, multilocular cyst, cystic nephroma, cystic adenoma, benign cystic differentiated nephroblastoma, cystic partially differentiated nephroblastoma, polycystic nephroblastoma, differentiated nephroblastoma, cystic nephroblastoma, well-differentiated polycystic Wilms' tumor, lymphangioma, and partially polycystic kidney.[274,275] The pathogenesis of this lesion is controversial. The findings of local recurrence, distant metastases, growth of the lesion, and presence of embryonic mesenchyme support the thesis that it is a neoplasm, but it is not always benign.[274] Because of the frequency of microscopic foci of nephroblastoma in multilocular nephroma and because of an occasional case of nephroblastoma with focal features of multilocu-

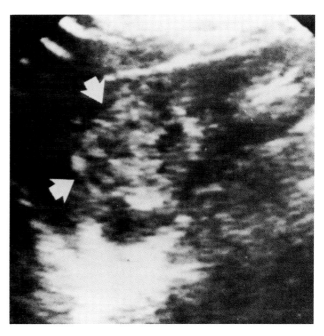

Fig. 13-127. Carcinoid. Longitudinal sonogram showing a round hyperechoic mass (arrows) incompletely marginated by a thin, anechoic rim. (From McKeown et al,[272] with permission.)

lar nephroma, it is believed that these two tumors probably develop along separate lines from a common ancestor, metanephric blastoma.[274]

The ultrasound findings are related to the amount of stroma and size of the locules. When the cysts are large enough, ultrasound will demonstrate a cluster of echo-free masses separated by intense echoes (connective tissue septa), and this pattern is suggestive of multilocular cystic nephroma[274] (Figs. 13-38 and 13-128). A finely cystic structure with jellylike contents plus solid components of embryonic tissue give it a solid character at times.[275] If cyst aspiration is performed, clear to yellow fluid is obtained, similar to serum. If contrast is injected, only the lobule directly punctured by the needle will fill.[274] The treatment is nephrectomy and occasionally removal of the mass.

Clear Cell Sarcoma. Clear cell sarcoma occurs in the same age group (3 to 7 years) as Wilms' tumor, with Wilms' tumor being the most common neoplasm in this age group.[277] It has a peak incidence between 3 and 5 years of age.[276] It accounts for up to 6 percent of renal tumors in children.[276-278] Although it is rare, it accounts for a disproportionately high percentage of combined total deaths in the National Wilms' Tumor Study, reflecting its highly malignant nature.[277] It has an additional feature of predilection for bone metastasis and a worse prognosis than Wilms' tumor.[277] There is a re-

ported incidence of 42 to 76 percent for a predilection to form bone metastases.[278]

The tumors reported were unilateral and large (8.5 to 16 cm in diameter), and all but one were predominantly solid, containing some well-defined portions of low attenuation of hypoechogenicity that represented tumor necrosis.[277] Many may contain uncomplicated fluid-filled cysts, with diameters ranging from a few millimeters to 5 cm.[277] No definite pattern that would permit discrimination between clear cell sarcoma with Wilms' tumor has been identified.[276,277] The survival rate for clear cell sarcoma is less than 50 percent, and survival is common only if the tumor is detected in the early stages.[278]

The CT and ultrasound features are those of a focal expansile mass, usually with a dominant soft tissue component, although necrotic areas may be seen[277] (Fig. 13-129). With most, cysts were common but were small, and only a few were present.[277] In this group, 58 percent had a cystic component of varying size and multiplicity. A well-established feature of clear cell sarcoma of the kidney is uncomplicated cysts.[277] In 25 percent there was radiologic evidence of calcification.[277] All the tumors in this series were unilateral, and extension into the inferior vena cava was absent.[277]

Malignant Rhabdoid Tumor. Originally described as a sarcomatous variant of Wilms' tumor, malignant rhab-

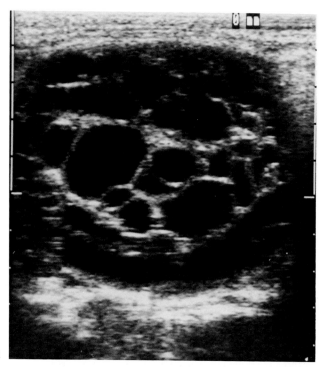

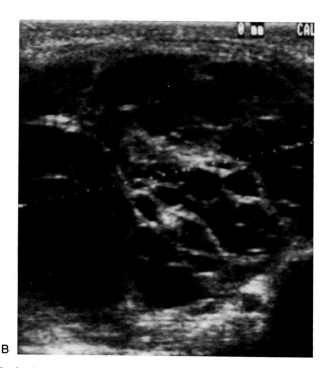

A   B

Fig. 13-128. Multilocular cystic nephroma. Child. **(A)** Sagittal and **(B)** transverse images of the left renal fossa demonstrating a multicystic mass. The cysts are of various sizes and do not communicate.

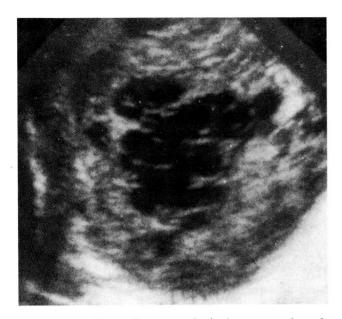

Fig. 13-129. Clear cell sarcoma. Sagittal sonogram through the middle of tumor showing multiple anechoic septated cysts surrounded by solid tumor. (From Glass et al,[277] with permission.)

doid tumor of the kidney is now recognized as a separate entity with distinct clinical and pathologic features.[279] It is a highly malignant tumor, accounting for 2 percent of the malignant renal neoplasms entered into the National Wilms' Tumor Study.[276,279] The age range at the time of diagnosis is 3 months to 4.5 years (mean, 13 months), and there is a 2:1 male/female ratio.[276] This rhabdoid tumor infiltrates the renal parenchyma; this is different from the classic Wilms' tumor, which has a well-defined fibrous pseudocapsule.[279]

Children with this tumor usually present with a palpable abdominal mass and less frequently with increased intracranial pressure or hematuria.[279] Rhabdoid tumor may be one component of a multiple primary tumor syndrome since it may be seen concomitantly with primary tumors of the posterior cranial fossa, soft tissues, and thymus.[279] On ultrasound, the solid nature and renal origin of the mass may show either a homogeneous or complex pattern[276] (Fig. 13-130).

This tumor has a poor prognosis, with a mortality of 90 percent within 2 years of diagnosis.[279] Even with aggressive treatment, the poor prognosis persists and may reflect the presence of other tumors or the embryonal nature of the renal tumor and its proclivity for metasta-

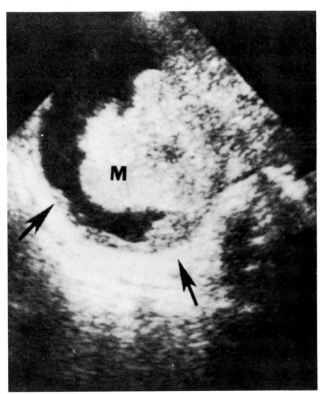

A

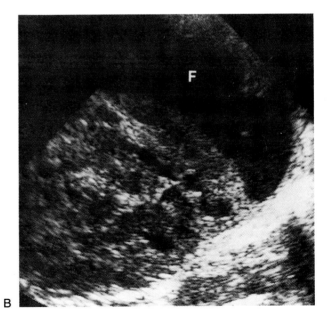

B

Fig. 13-130. Rhabdoid tumor of the kidney. Case 1. **(A)** Transverse sonogram of the right kidney demonstrating an irregular echogenic mass *(M)* replacing the renal parenchyma. A subcapsular fluid collection with numerous tumor nodules (arrows) surrounds the mass. Case 2. **(B)** Transverse sonogram demonstrating an inhomogeneous solid mass with small hypoechoic areas. A subcapsular fluid collection *(F)* with peripheral echogenic masses is present. (From Sisler and Siegel,[279] with permission.)

sis.[279] The frequent sites of metastatic disease include the lungs (76 percent), liver (26 percent), brain (14 percent), and heart (10 percent).[279]

Wilms' Tumor. Wilms' tumor (nephroblastoma) arises from the metanephric blastoma, the normal fetal precursor of the kidney parenchyma. It is the most common solid renal tumor in patients 1 to 8 years old, with a peak at 3 years.[280] Ninety percent of patients are less than 5 years old, and 70 percent are less than 3 years old.[281] It may be associated with congenital anomalies such as hemihypertrophy and hamartomas, as well as Beckwith-Wiedemann syndrome. The most common associated anomalies are cryptorchidism (2.8 percent), hypospadias (1.8 percent), and hemihypertrophy (2.5 percent).[276] It may also be associated with the rarer Drash syndrome (male pseudohermaphrodism, glomerular disease, and Wilms' tumor).[276] Affected patients present with a large asymptomatic flank mass; less frequently there is abdominal pain, fever, hematuria, or anorexia. Hypertension is seen in 47 to 90 percent of cases.[123]

Ultrasound. Ultrasound can be used to confirm the organ of the mass, identify large blood vessel involvement and metastases, and define the status of the contralateral kidney. The mass varies from hypoechoic to moderately echogenic; irregular anechoic areas may be seen corresponding to central necrosis and hemorrhage[123,221,281,282] (Figs. 13-131 and 13-132). The tumor may be seen as a sharply demarcated, large mass with echogenicity slightly greater than that of the liver.[276] Although the tumor is predominantly solid, areas of cystic necrosis and hemorrhage are frequently found within the mass.[276] Seventy-one percent of tumors are necrotic at surgery.[281] Necrotic degeneration and decreased tumor size are ultrasound features that correlate with a positive response to therapy.[283] There is no initial correlation between the ultrasound patterns and clinical presentation or prognosis. Ultrasound can correctly predict the internal consistency of the tumor in 94 percent of cases.[281] The contralateral kidney should be carefully examined because there is a 5 to 10 percent incidence of bilateral tumors; bilateral tumors are evident at the time of clinical presentation in two-thirds of cases.[123] Other diagnoses must be considered (multilocular cystic nephroma, multicystic dysplastic kidney, and hydronephrosis) if the mass is predominantly cystic.[276]

By the time of diagnosis, up to 40 percent of Wilms' tumors may have invaded the renal vein, with vena caval or atrial thrombus less common.[284] There may be pulmonary metastases in up to one-fourth of cases at the time of initial diagnosis, with pulmonary emboli being exceedingly rare as a first manifestation of Wilms' tumor.[284] It is rare to have massive tumor emboli as a cause of acute respiratory distress in children.[284] Ultrasound may be useful in showing the cranial extent of tumor thrombus, allowing proper intraoperative approach.[284]

In some circumstances, Wilms' tumor will have only a minimal parenchymal component, with the bulk occupying the renal pelvis instead.[285] When Wilms' tumor arises in the parenchyma, it can extend to the renal pelvis or be associated with a separate renal pelvic mass.[285] It is important to realize the possibility of this type of appearance with Wilms' tumor when planning the preoperative workup and the surgical approach in a child with a renal pelvic filling defect.[285]

Multicystic Variation. The multicystic variant of nephroblastoma is infrequently recognized.[286] It presents clinically much as a typical Wilms' tumor and in the same age group. Pathologically, it is truly a distinct variant of the ordinary nephroblastoma and has no etiologic relationship to infantile multicystic dysplastic kidney or other benign multilocular renal cysts. On ultrasound, a multicystic mass is seen[286] (see Figs. 13-38 and 13-128). The cysts are of different sizes. The prognosis of multicystic Wilms' tumor is considered more favorable than that of its solid counterpart. (This is thought to be the same entity as multilocular cystic nephroma, discussed above, and multilocular renal cyst [see under Renal Abnormalities, Congenital].)

Computed Tomography. CT may be more sensitive in assessing perinephric extension, lymph node involvement, and bilateral tumors of Wilms' tumor than ultrasound is.[287] Additionally, tumor necrosis and a pseudocapsule are more often detected by CT.[287] In one series, ultrasound was correct in 23 percent of cases in determining the extent of a suspected tumor, whereas CT was correct in 77 percent.[287] Both CT and ultrasound are useful methods for diagnosing Wilms' tumor in children.[287] Ultrasound should be the initial screening procedure in children with a suspected abdominal mass. CT scanning is superior to ultrasound in defining the extend of the tumor and its relationships to surrounding structure, information that has therapeutic and prognostic significance.[287]

Nephroblastomatosis. Nephroblastomatosis is the name given to a group of pathologic entities characterized by persistent metanephric blastema in the kidneys in infants and children.[288,289] It bears a close relationship to, but is not synonymous with, bilateral Wilms' tumor. Nephroblastomatosis is thought to occur as a result of arrest in normal nephrogenesis, with persistence of residual blastema. It is a condition in which multifocal or diffuse nephrogenic rests (NRs) are present.[276,289] These

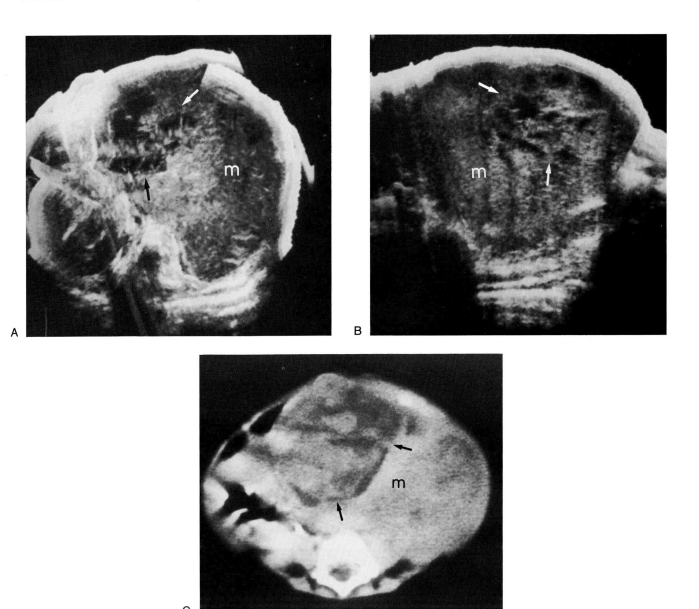

Fig. 13-131. Wilms' tumor. **(A)** Transverse and **(B)** longitudinal static supine scans showing a large, predominantly echodense mass *(m)* filling the left abdomen. There are some anechoic internal spaces (arrows). The left kidney is not seen. **(C)** Enhanced CT scan showing a large mass *(m)* of mixed density. Low-density areas (arrows) are seen with enhancement of the mass. (Fig. A from Mandell et al,[503] with permission.)

NRs represent abnormal persistence of nephrogenic cells that retain the potential for malignant induction to Wilms' tumor.[276] Patients with known nephroblastomatosis are considered at high risk for the development of Wilms' tumor.[289] This condition is found in 12 to 33 percent of kidneys with Wilms' tumor. It is also found frequently in conditions associated with a high incidence of Wilms' tumor, such as hemihypertrophy, Beckwith-Wiedemann syndrome, and major chromosomal anomalies. The relationship of the various types of nephroblastomatosis and Wilms' tumor, is unknown, but

nephroblastomatosis may be a precursor of Wilms' tumor. The prognosis of this disease process is undetermined.[288]

The individual lesions with nephroblastoma have variable histologic findings and distribution in the kidney.[289] The findings described on ultrasound include (1) subcapsular and parenchymal hypoechoic areas, (2) cysts, and (3) nephromegaly with decreased parenchymal echoes (Figs. 13-133 and 13-134). Although lesions may be isoechoic or hyperechoic to normal renal parenchyma, ultrasound typically reveals hypoechoic nodules

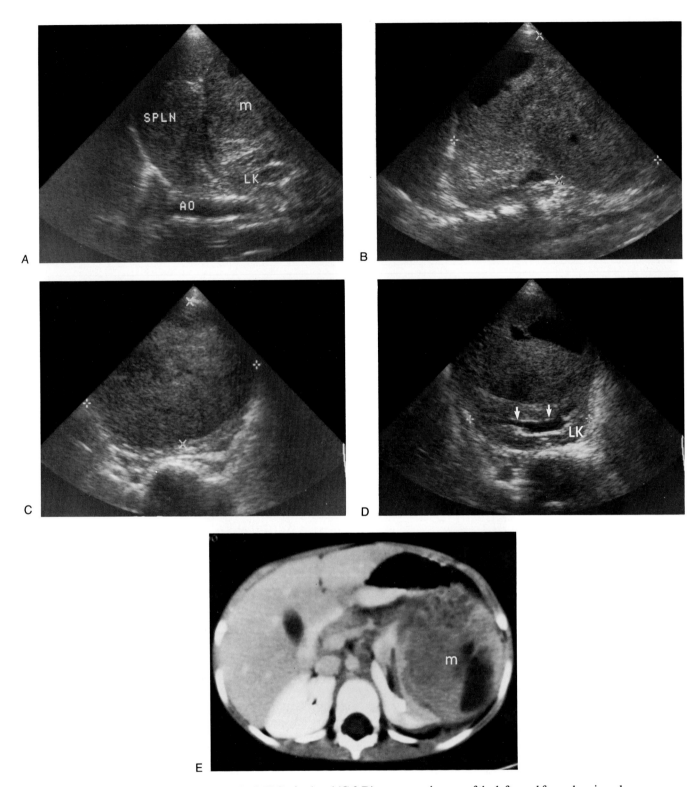

Fig. 13-132. Wilms' tumor. **(A & B)** Sagittal and **(C & D)** transverse images of the left renal fossa showing a large mass (*m*, calipers, 73 × 72 × 63 mm). It is predominately echogenic but does contain some cystic areas. Its relationship to the spleen *(SPLN)* and aorta *(AO)* can be seen in Fig. A. In Fig. C there is a structure posterior to the mass, which was believed to represent the left kidney *(LK)* with a dilated collecting system (arrows). This image appears very similar to the enhanced CT scan. **(E)** The mass *(m)* involves the left kidney and extends laterally. It has a mixed pattern on CT similar to that on ultrasound. The mass does not appear to cross the midline.

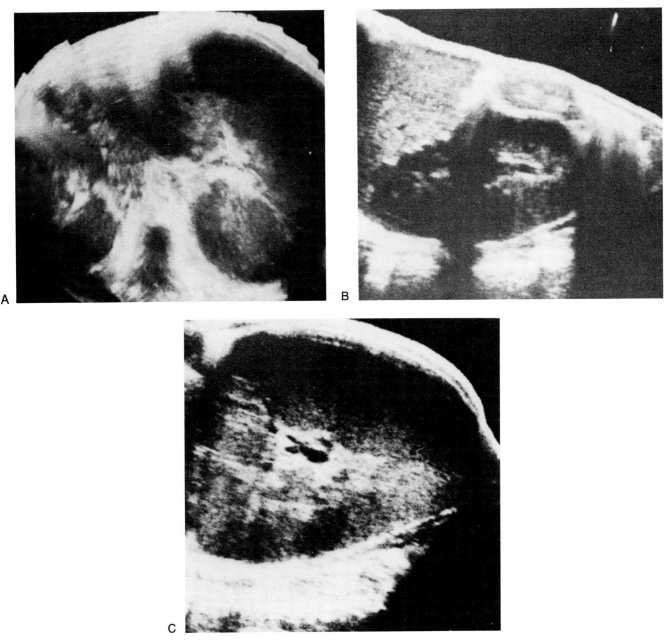

Fig. 13-133. Nephroblastomatosis. **(A)** Transverse and longitudinal scans of **(B)** the right and **(C)** the left kidneys. Both kidneys are enlarged, particularly the left. There is considerable reduced echogenicity of the cortical region. (From Franken et al,[288] with permission.)

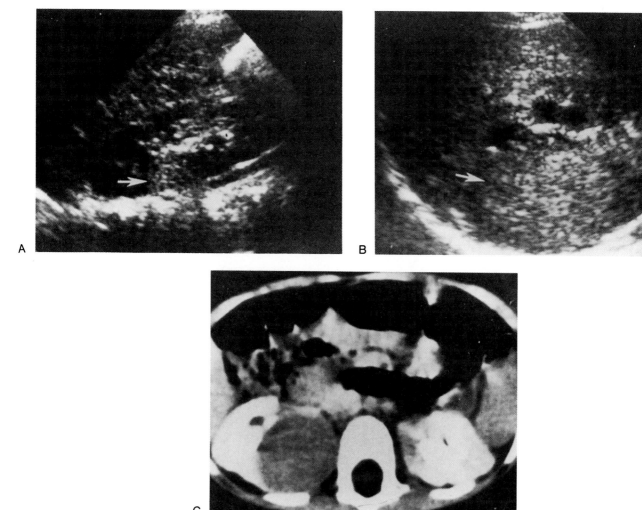

Fig. 13-134. Nephroblastomatosis. **(A)** Longitudinal renal ultrasound of a patient with sporadic aniridia and chromosome 11p13, showing a hyperechoic focus in the renal parenchyma (arrow) consistent with a nephrogenic rest. **(B)** Sonogram and **(C)** CT scan obtained 6 months later showing marked enlargement (arrow, Fig. B) of the previously noted lesion. Findings at surgical resection confirmed neoplastic transformation of this nephrogenic rest to Wilms' tumor. (From White et al,[289] with permission.)

in the kidney.[289] Enlargement is the hallmark of neoplastic transformation of a benign NR.[289] If an NR becomes rounded, expansile, and mass like, it should be removed to rule out neoplastic change.[289]

Adults. Wilms' tumor is rare in adults; it represents a primary renal neoplasm containing primitive blastema and embryonic glomerulotubular structures.[290] Reported cases in adults have been reviewed, revealing a mean age of 30 years, with 80 percent of these patients less than 35 years old.[290] Patients present with a large, rapidly growing abdominal mass, have no constitutional symptoms, and are otherwise healthy (80 percent).[290]

Women are more commonly affected than men.[290] This neoplasm commonly appears as an exophytic mass because the most common location of nephrogenic blastema is the subcapsular portion of the renal cortex.[290] At ultrasound, Wilms' tumor is typically a large, complex mass with large cystic components.[290] As such, an adult Wilms' tumor is suggested when a young patient (< 35 years old) presents with a rapidly growing renal mass that is shown to be complex and cystic by CT or ultrasound and is hypovascular with fine, wavy neovascularity on arteriography.[290] Being aware of this constellation of findings may be useful in diagnosing this unusual tumor in an adult before surgery.[290]

Differential Diagnosis. At times it is difficult to differentiate Wilms' tumor from neuroblastoma. Ultrasound shows relatively distinctive patterns for the two tumors based on textural differences; it is probably most useful in the equivocal cases in which the site of the tumor origin is uncertain.[291] Wilms' tumor may extend through the renal capsule rather than distort the kidney and mimic the appearance of neuroblastoma.[292] Ultrasound can correctly differentiate the two tumors on the basis of the echopattern in 88 percent of cases.[291] Typically, Wilms' tumor is sharply marginated, with compressed renal tissue forming the pseudocapsule. It is fairly evenly echogenic or evenly echogenic with discrete holes corresponding to areas of cystic necrosis. Neuroblastoma is usually quite heterogeneous with irregular hyperechoic areas intermixed with less echogenic areas[291] (see Figs. 12-51 to 12-54).

Mesoblastic Nephroma. Mesoblastic nephroma (fetal renal hamartoma, mesenchymal hamartoma of infancy, congenital Wilms' tumor, fibromyxoma, fibrosarcoma, congenital fibrosarcoma) is a rare tumor but is the most common renal neoplasm diagnosed in the early postnatal period.[68,293-297] Most patients present at less than 3 months old with an asymptomatic abdominal mass. Occasionally hematuria and/or hypertension is present. Many of these infants have been the product of a pregnancy complicated by prematurity and polyhydramnios. Characteristically, a mesoblastic nephroma is a solid tumor with rare cysts or focal areas of hemorrhage and necrosis. The lesion is mixed with smooth muscle or fibroblastic elements and with scattered embryonic tubules and glomeruli. On excretory urography, a mass effect may be seen (Fig. 13-135). Ultrasound shows a solid lesion that cannot be differentiated from Wilms' tumor by ultrasound alone[296] (Fig. 13-135A). It is similar to a noncalcified uterine fibroid, a solid mass with low-level echoes.[297] The prognosis after complete excision is excellent, and adjunctive therapy is unnecessary.[297]

Urothelial Tumors: Transitional Cell Carcinoma. Transitional cell carcinoma (TCC) originates in the renal pelvocalyceal system and represents 7 percent of all renal

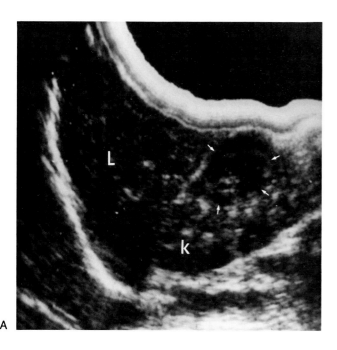

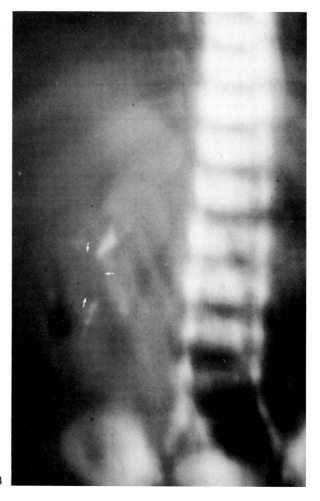

Fig. 13-135. Mesoblastic nephroma. **(A)** Longitudinal scan of the right kidney *(k)* showing a poorly defined hypoechoic mass (arrows) in the lower pole anteriorly. (*L,* liver.) **(B)** Excretory pyelogram showing a mass effect (arrows) on the right.

neoplasms.[298] It constitutes 85 percent of primary renal pelvic tumors.[299,300] Of the urothelial neoplasms, 90 to 92 percent are TCC, with the remainder squamous cell carcinoma (about 10 percent) and rarely adenocarcinoma (about 1 percent).[301,302] Eighty-five percent of TCCs are papillary; the rest are nonpapillary.[302] The male/female ratio is 1.8 : 1 to 3.5 : 1, with a mean age of diagnosis of 61.4 years.[301] The most common presenting symptom is painless hematuria.[300,303]

Etiologic Agents. A number of chemical agents and other factors may be important in the development of urothelial neoplasms. Occupational exposure to such carcinogens as β-naphthylamine, 4-aminobiphenyl, 4-nitrobiphenyl, or 4,4-diaminobiphenyl (used in the synthesis of azo dyes and pigments used in the textile, printing, and plastic industries) has been implicated.[302] With stasis in the upper tracts, there is an increased exposure time, and therefore upper tract tumors result.[302] There may be an association between hydronephrosis, renal calculi, renal infection, and renal pelvic tumors.[302] Al-

though no clear-cut relationship has been found, it may be postulated that metaplasia is a response to calculi or inflammation that may progress to carcinoma.[302]

Ultrasound. The lesion is usually first suspected by seeing a defect on an excretory urogram.[298] It is often small at the time of diagnosis and is usually easily detected radiographically.[301] Several patterns of this lesion on ultrasound have been described: (1) splitting or separation of the central renal echocomplex in a fashion similar to hydronephrosis; and (2) a bulky, hypoechoic mass lesion[298,299,302,304,305] (Figs. 13-136 to 13-139). Some describe the mass as a zone in the renal sinus that is less echogenic than the normal sinus and that corresponds to the extent of the tumor.[303] The echogenicity of the tumor may be similar to that of the renal parenchyma.[257,299] A specific diagnosis of TCC can be made when amputation of the central echocomplex is present along with preservation of the renal pyramids.[300] Once a TCC becomes large, it is nearly impossible to differentiate from other neoplastic processes, especially RCC and lymphomas[301]

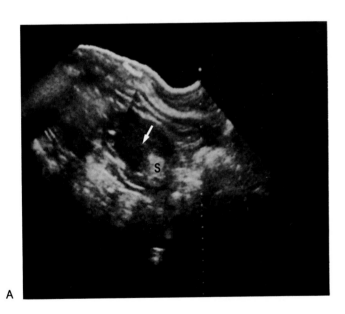

A

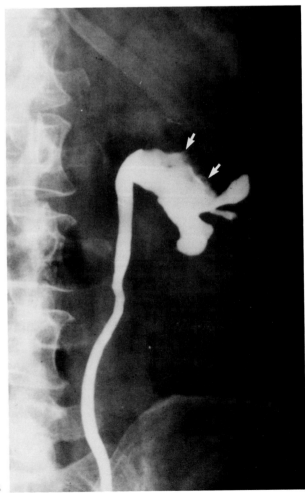

B

Fig. 13-136. Urothelial tumor: transitional cell carcinoma. **(A)** Sagittal scan of the left kidney showing a poorly defined, solid-appearing mass (arrow) in the upper pole. The echopattern is similar to that of the renal parenchyma. (*s,* renal sinus.) **(B)** Retrograde pyelogram showing irregularity (arrows) of the upper collecting system.

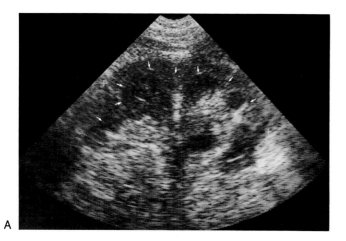

A

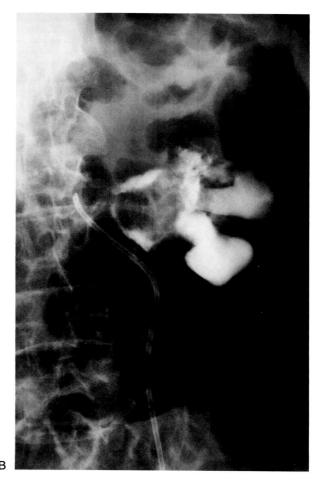

B

Fig. 13-137. Urothelial tumor: transitional cell carcinoma. Patient with transitional cell carcinoma of the bladder metastatic to the left renal pelvis. **(A)** Sagittal scan of the left kidney demonstrating a dilated collecting system (arrows) filled with echoes. This represented metastatic tumor. **(B)** Retrograde pyelogram showing dilatation of the collecting system with filling defects.

(Fig. 13-140). At times, these lesions occupy 30 to 90 percent of the kidney.[301] A central location may help in the differentiation from other tumors.

Transitional cell carcinoma has a propensity for multicentricity, with both synchronous and metachronous lesions.[302] In 20 to 40 percent of patients, TCC of the upper tract is multicentric.[302] There is a high prevalence (10 to 40 percent) of ipsilateral recurrence after partial ureterectomy for TCC.[302] Since metachronous TCC of the bladder occurs after renal and ureteral TCC in 20 to 55 percent of patients, close follow-up evaluation of the lower urinary tract is necessary.[302]

There have been reports of cases in which a renal TCC mimicked a stone.[302,305] In one report, there was a hypoechoic mass replacing the central renal sinus echoes without showing sharp delineation. On some views, a small reflective layer with a weak acoustic shadow could be seen covering the entire surface of the mass.[305] These ultrasound findings were secondary to uric acid incrustations of a renal TCC.[305]

Differential Diagnosis. Ultrasound is helpful in clarifying the nature of a filling defect seen on urograms. Stones should be dense, with an associated acoustic shadow[306] (Figs. 13-58, 13-59, and 13-63; See Figs. 13-174 and 13-175). Tumors and blood clots (see Fig. 13-193) appear as echogenic masses without acoustic shadowing.[29] Urothelial tumors are seen as low-level echoes that separate the walls of the renal sinus (Figs. 13-136 to 13-139). Blood clots may appear similar to this tumor but should change in their echopattern with time; they should show resolution on follow-up examination[29] (see Fig. 13-193).

Urothelial Tumors: Squamous Cell Carcinoma. Squamous cell carcinoma accounts for 15 percent of all urothelial tumors with the remainder (85 percent) being TCC.[307] Squamous cell carcinoma is rare and highly malignant with an insidious onset and a tendency to metastasize early; therefore it is associated with a poor prognosis. Pathologically, a flat, ulcerating mass with extensive indurated infiltration is noted. From 25 to 60 percent of cases are associated with previous chronic renal infection and calculi. UPJ obstruction is common. The presence of faceted calculi and marked hydronephrosis should suggest the diagnosis of squamous cell carcinoma[307] (Fig. 13-141).

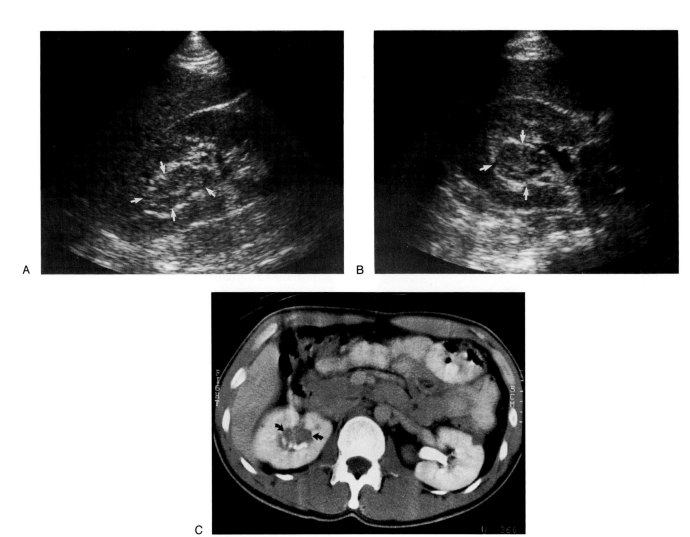

Fig. 13-138. Urothelial tumor: transitional cell carcinoma, papillary type. **(A)** Sagittal and **(B)** transverse view of the right kidney demonstrating a mass (arrows) within the region of the collecting system. The mass has an echopattern similar to that of renal parenchyma. The bright echogenic borders are thought to represent the collecting system margins. **(C)** This was confirmed on an enhanced CT scan showing a soft tissue mass (arrows) within the collecting system of the right kidney.

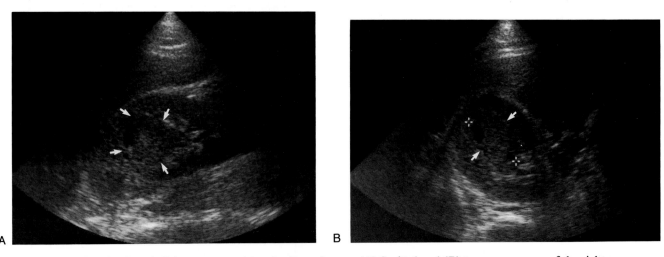

Fig. 13-139. Urothelial tumor: transitional cell carcinoma. **(A)** Sagittal and **(B)** transverse scans of the right kidney showing a mass (calipers, arrows) that appears to be within the center of the collecting system in Fig. A with extension into the parenchyma in Fig. B. The mass is isoechoic to the renal parenchyma.

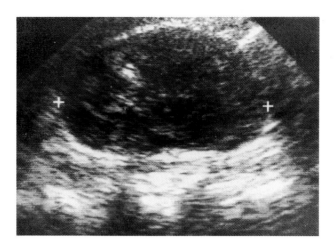

Fig. 13-140. Urothelial tumor: diffusely infiltrating transitional cell carcinoma. Ultrasound examination of the right kidney in longitudinal plane demonstrating preservation of the reniform shape of the kidney, which is diffusely hypoechoic and infiltrated with neoplasm. (From Bree et al,[301] with permission.)

Secondary Renal Tumors

Because a large volume of blood flows through the kidneys they are frequently the sites of metastases from carcinomas and sarcomas.[24] Even though renal blood flow forms 25 percent of the cardiac output, the kidneys are less frequently affected by metastatic disease than are the adrenals.[308] At autopsy, the reported incidence of renal metastases is between 2 and 20 percent.[309] Renal metastases are often detected late in the course of the cancer.[309] The only specific tumor that selectively metastasizes to the kidney is a tumor from the contralateral kidney[24] (Fig. 13-116). In most cases, renal metastases are clinically silent, although in one series 17 percent of patients had azotemia and 24 percent had hematuria.[309] Others may present with albuminuria.[305]

Metastatic lesions can have various patterns. They are usually multifocal, although those from the colon, lung, and breast have been reported as sometimes large, solitary, and otherwise indistinguishable from primary RCC[309] (Fig. 13-142). The lesions are small and multiple with lung, breast, head, and neck and undifferentiated metastases of unknown primary in 67 percent of cases.[309] Lesions from melanoma and lung cancer tend to involve the kidney and perinephric space contiguously.[309] Most metastases are small, multicentric, and bilateral, but up to 2 percent of primary RCCs may also display this pattern.[309] Metastases are often hypoechoic.[221] RCC may mimic large, unilateral exophytic metastases, although invasion of the renal vein and inferior vena cava is less likely with metastases.[309] CT is the most sensitive modality for depicting renal metastases.[309] In a patient with

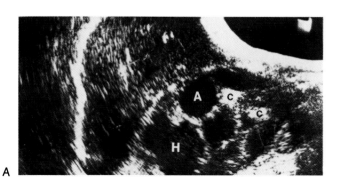

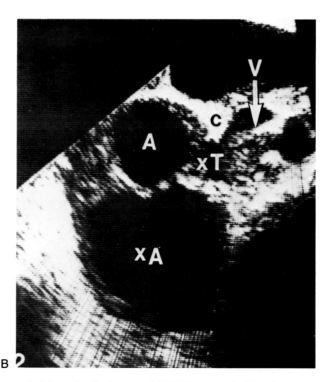

A   B

Fig. 13-141. Urothelial tumor: squamous cell carcinoma. **(A)** Longitudinal scan, right. (*A*, anechoic dilated renal calyx; *H*, hypoechoic renal calyx containing debris; *c*, calculus.) **(B)** Transverse scan, right. (*A*, dilated calyces; *T*, tumor filling renal pelvis and surrounding a dilated calyx; *c*, calculus; *V*, elevation of the inferior vena cava by tumor areas biopsied.) (From Wimbish et al,[307] with permission.)

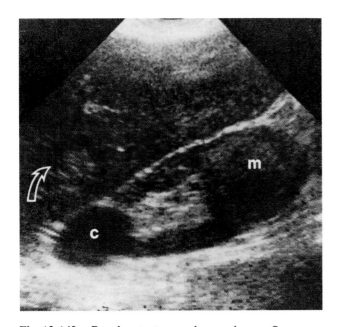

Fig. 13-142. Renal metastases, colon carcinoma. Sonogram demonstrating that the lower-pole mass *(m)* is solid and exophytic while the upper-pole lesion is a cyst *(c)*. A hepatic metastasis is also present (curved arrow). (From Choyke et al,[309] with permission.)

advanced, incurable cancer, the lesion is more likely to be metastatic than primary, and biopsy in this setting is unlikely to be of aid.[309]

Lung Cancer. Although in an autopsy series metastatic disease from the lung was found in 19.4 percent, it is seldom diagnosed or suspected antemortem.[308] The kidney is the most frequent site of metastatic lung cancer, followed by the liver, adrenals, brain, and bone.[308] In 75 percent, unilateral disease is on the right; in 60 percent of cases are bilateral.[308] At ultrasound, these metastases have been described as echopoor, reflecting their hypovascularity, unless they have undergone necrosis or hemorrhage or unless the primary tumor was extremely heterogeneous[308] (Fig. 13-143).

Choriocarcinoma. Choriocarcinoma, a trophoblastic tissue neoplasm and a disease of women in the childbearing years, has a 10 to 50 percent incidence of renal metastases.[310] The most frequent sites of metastases are the lungs and vagina. Once the abdominal viscera, kidneys, and brain are involved, the prognosis is fatal. The metastases are characteristically hemorrhagic and necrotic and spread primarily by the hematogenous route, but lymphatic spread and direct extension are seen. On ultrasound a solid heterogeneous mass is seen with sound attenuation[310] (Fig. 13-144). In a young woman with hematuria and a renal mass, one should consider

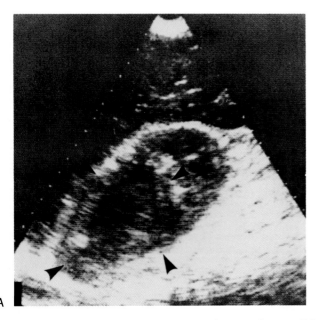

A

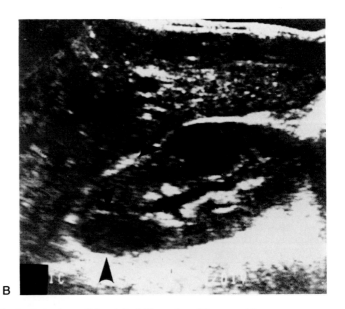

B

Fig. 13-143. Renal metastases, lung carcinoma. **(A)** Sagittal section of the right kidney in a 29-year-old man with adenocarcinoma of the lung. A poorly defined, mixed echopattern metastasis (arrowheads) occupies the upper pole. **(B)** Sagittal section of the right kidney in a 53-year-old woman with adenocarcinoma of the lung. Two hypoechoic metastases (arrowheads) are present in the renal parenchyma. A large metastasis is also seen in the right lobe of the liver. (From Dershaw and Bernstein,[308] with permission.)

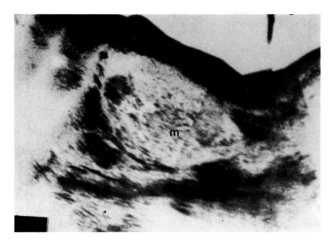

Fig. 13-144. Renal metastasis. Choriocarcinoma. Longitudinal prone scan showing the left kidney replaced by a mass *(m)* that has a heterogeneous echopattern and is sound attenuating. (From Kutcher et al,[310] with permission.)

choriocarcinoma and screen with human chorionic gonadotropin titer.[310]

Melanoma. Renal metastases from melanoma are usually seen in patients with widespread disease.[311] The incidence at autopsy has been reported to be 38 to 77 percent.[311] Metastatic melanoma to the kidney usually

produces multiple microscopic nodules in the renal parenchyma and rarely produces large masses.[311]

These renal metastases are usually multiple and bilateral but may be solitary when metastases are quite large.[311] Except when metastases are quite large, the renal contour is usually preserved.[311] Most renal metastases demonstrate homogeneous hypoechoic areas, although mixed patterns of hypoechoic and echoic areas occur[311] (Fig. 13-145).

Lymphoma. Excluding the hematopoietic and reticuloendothelial systems, the urinary tract is the most common site of involvement by lymphoma at autopsy. Only lung and breast cancers metastasize to the kidneys more often than lymphoma does.[312] Rarely are the kidneys the predominant site of disease at the initial diagnosis. There is renal involvement in 2.7 to 6 percent of cases.[313] Most patients evaluated have known lymphoma and are studied for nodal mass size, flank pain, and/or deteriorating renal function.[313] The discrepancy between the incidence of clinical recognition of renal lymphoma and postmortem findings in the past may be because the infiltration of the kidneys infrequently causes renal insufficiency or failure. The earliest symptoms are nonspecific, with flank pain or mass, weight loss, and hematuria.[312] Rarely, hypertension and renal failure result from vascular or ureteral compression, extensive parenchymal infiltration by tumor, or superimposed artifact.

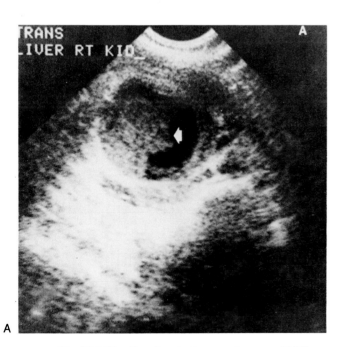

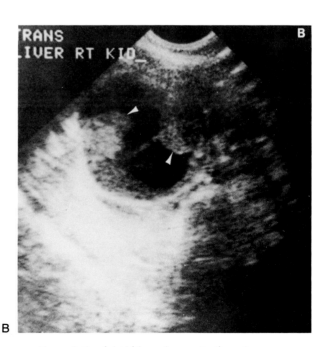

Fig. 13-145. Renal metastases, melanoma. **(A)** Transverse scan through the right kidney demonstrating a large cystic mass with a large bilobar mural nodule (arrow) and thickening of the wall, comparable to the CT appearance. **(B)** Section through the same cystic mass at a different level showing two mural nodules (arrowheads) joined by a linear septumlike structure. (From Tipton et al,[311] with permission.)

The most common form of involvement is that of multiple intraparenchymal nodules, with direct invasion from contiguous retroperitoneal lymph node masses observed somewhat less frequently. The gross morphology and consequent radiographic images depend on (1) the mechanism of renal involvement (hematogenous or direct extension); (2) the pattern of intrarenal growth (interstitial or expansile); (3) the size, number, and distribution of lesions; and (4) the presence of extension beyond the kidney.[312] Lymphoid tissue is not normally present in the kidney; it occurs secondary to hematogenous or contiguous extension. Initially the lymphoma grows between the nephrons, which continue to function, and because this interstitial proliferation preserves gross morphology, radiographic detection is difficult. Later the growth becomes expansile and the lymphomatous mass resembles other neoplasms that enlarge by appositional growth. Continued growth and coalescence of small foci result in progressive parenchymal replacement and rarely in the destruction of the entire kidney. Perinephric extension with subsequent vascular and arterial encasement is common.[312] There is sometimes diffuse infiltration.

There have been various reports on the incidence and pattern of renal involvement with lymphoma. In one series, 61 percent of the kidneys were involved with lymphoma with multiple nodules, 11 percent showed invasion from retroperitoneal disease, 7 percent showed solitary nodules, and 6 percent demonstrated a bulky single tumor.[314] Another series reported lymphomatous involvement in 48 percent with solitary masses, 29 percent with multiple nodules, and 19 percent with almost complete parenchymal replacement by tumor.[312] Renal lymphoma usually occurs late in the disease. In an autopsy

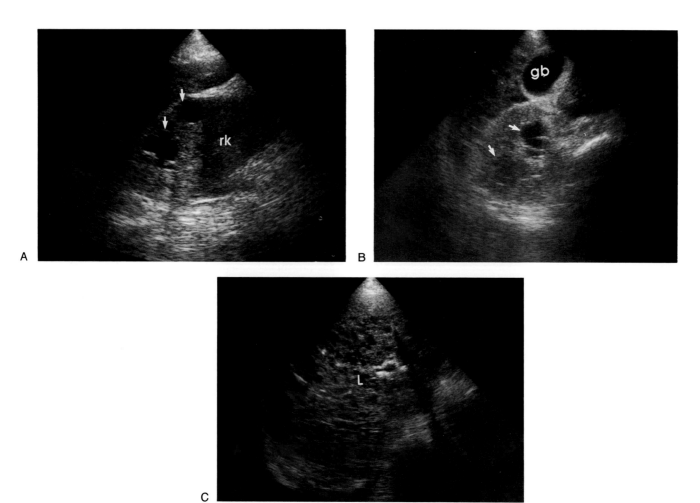

Fig. 13-146. Renal lymphoma, poorly differentiated lymphocytic lymphoma. **(A)** Sagittal and **(B)** transverse views of the right kidney *(rk)* showing well-defined cystic-appearing areas (arrows). Some acoustic enhancement is noted. The left kidney appeared similar. These appear very similar to cysts by ultrasound. (*gb*, gallbladder.) **(C)** Transverse view of the liver *(L)* showing an appearance similar to kidney. This was proved to represent diffuse lymphoma.

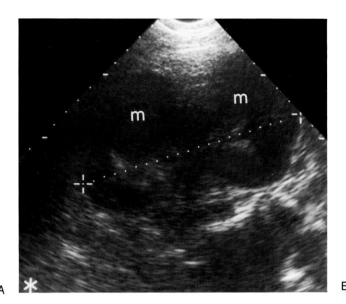

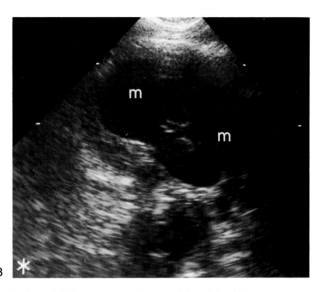

Fig. 13-147. Renal lymphoma, non-Hodgkin's. (A) Sagittal and (B) transverse views of the right kidney demonstrating renal enlargement with poorly defined hypoechoic masses *(m)* within the renal parenchyma. The patient had a known diagnosis of lymphoma. On a follow-up scan after the therapy, the masses were found to have decreased in size.

series of patients with Hodgkin's disease, there was a 13 percent renal involvement.[313] Renal involvement is more common in non-Hodgkin's lymphoma, although the pathologic pattern of renal involvement is similar. There appears to be less common renal involvement with Hodgkin's disease than with non-Hodgkin's lymphoma, although the radiologic findings are similar.[315] From 7.5 to 14 percent of patients with non-Hodgkin's lymphoma have clinically suspected renal involvement, with 42 to 65 percent demonstrating involvement at autopsy.[314] Some investigators report renal involvement in 33.5 percent of malignant lymphomas with the kidneys involved rather late in the disease.[316]

The typical ultrasound appearance of kidneys involved by lymphoma is that of single or multiple anechoic or hypoechoic masses[221,312,313,316,317] (Figs. 13-146 to 13-149). The anechoic masses may even meet all the criteria for a renal cyst, including acoustic enhancement[312,316] (Figs. 13-146 to 13-149). As such, the diagnosis of a cyst should be questioned in a lymphoma patient; further investigation involving cyst puncture or gallium scan should be undertaken. In addition to the focal mass pattern, there may be diffuse renal involvement producing renal enlargement and decreased parenchymal echoes[317] (Figs. 13-146 to 13-149). Lymphomatous involvement may be diagnosed more frequently

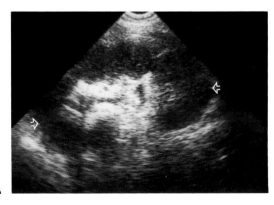

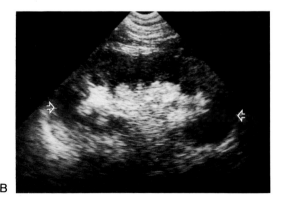

Fig. 13-148. Renal lymphoma. Non-Hodgkin's lymphoma, diffuse. Longitudinal scans of (A) the right (15.7 cm) and (B) the left (16.7 cm) kidneys. The kidneys (open arrows) are markedly increased in length and in anteroposterior dimension. No focal masses are seen.

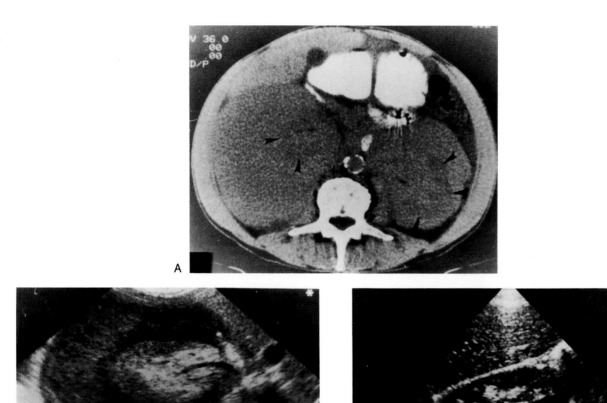

Fig. 13-149. Renal lymphoma. Perirenal lymphoma engulfing the kidney, simulating nepromegaly. **(A)** Non-contrast CT scan showing the hyperdense normal renal parenchyma (arrowheads) embedded in the lymphomatous mass. **(B)** Ultrasound of the right kidney. The hypoechoic mass of perirenal lymphoma is better differentiated from the normal parenchyma. **(C)** Follow-up ultrasound examination 18 months after treatment. The perirenal tumor has resolved. (From Charnsangavej,[318] with permission.)

if an ultrasound examination is performed on the lymphoma patient who develops flank pain, a palpable flank mass, decreased renal function, or lymphocyturia.[316] Contrast-enhanced CT appears to be superior to ultrasound for detection of renal involvement by non-Hodgkin's lymphoma in children.[315]

One group of investigators report various patterns with lymphoma involvement of the kidney.[318] The most common pattern was perirenal involvement[318] (Fig. 13-149). With perirenal involvement there may be perirenal strands or perirenal mass. The renal masses may be bulky parenchymal masses, renal sinus involvement with or without parenchymal invasion, or multiple parenchymal nodules.[318]

Burkitt's lymphoma is a type of non-Hodgkin's lymphoma; it occurs in North American and African forms.[319] The tumor is a very aggressive neoplasm of B-cell origin.[319] With American Burkitt's lymphoma, there appears to be a particular affinity for renal involvement.[319] The following range of abnormalities may be seen: renomegaly, diffuse increase in cortical echogenicity, and focal renal mass.[319] Some focal infiltrations were hypoechoic and some hyperechoic.[319]

Leukemia. The most common cancers of childhood are the acute leukemias; they represent the second leading cause of death in children.[320] There is an initial peak incidence of acute lymphoblastic leukemia among children aged 3 to 5 years.[320] The incidence of renal infiltration in all forms of leukemia is 63 percent based on an

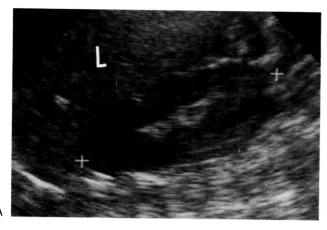
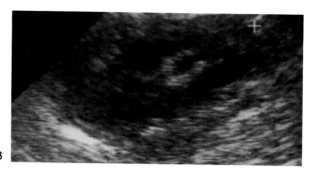

A B

Fig. 13-150. Renal leukemia. Acute lymphocytic leukemia in a child with renal failure. Longitudinal scans of **(A)** the right and **(B)** the left kidneys showing enlarged kidneys with a relatively hypoechoic parenchymal pattern. (*L*, liver.)

autopsy series.[321] In acute lymphocytic leukemia, renal involvement has been reported to occur in 41 to 95 percent of pathologic cases.[320] The clinical signs of renal impairment do not necessarily indicate leukemic infiltrates but may be related to other conditions such as hyperuricemia, septicemia, and hemorrhage.[321,322]

Leukemic infiltrates should be suspected when there is elevated blood pressure. The affected kidneys may or may not be palpably enlarged. The following ultrasound patterns have been described: (1) variable degrees of renal enlargement; (2) loss of definition and distortion of the central sinus echo complex; (3) diffuse coarse echoes throughout the renal cortex with preservation of the renal medullae; and (4) focal renal mass[321] (Figs. 13-150 to 13-153). Multiple nodular areas of anechoicity within enlarged kidneys may be seen; this pattern may revert to normal when the patient is in remission but then recur during a relapse.[322] One group describes enlarged kidneys with multiple nodules of increased echogenicity with leukemia[320] (Fig. 13-153). In this case, it was theorized that the number of acoustic interfaces available to the ultrasound beam is related to how tightly packed the leukemic cells are within an infiltrated area.[320] Ultrasound appears to be more sensitive than urography in delineating the extent of the parenchymal involvement.[320]

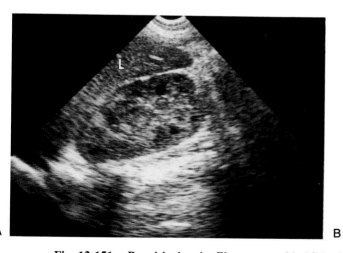
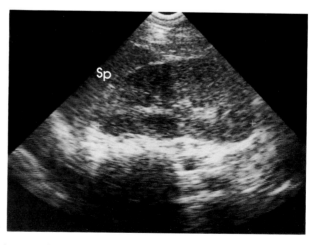

A B

Fig. 13-151. Renal leukemia. Eleven-year-old child with acute lymphocytic leukemia and abnormal renal function. Longitudinal scans of **(A)** the right and **(B)** the left kidneys showing nephromegaly, with the right being 13.3 cm and the left 12.8 cm. The parenchyma is not lucent, but the renal sinus is not well distinguished. After therapy the patient's renal function improved, and on the 2-week follow-up examination the right kidney measured 9.5 cm with the left 10 cm. (*L*, liver; *Sp*, spleen.)

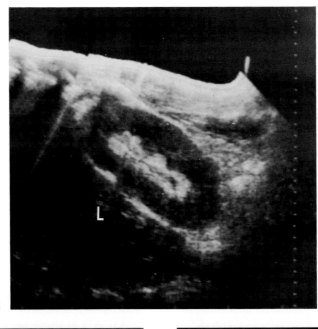

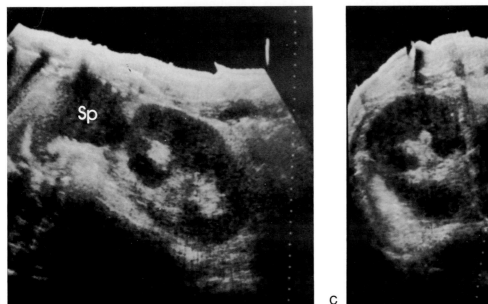

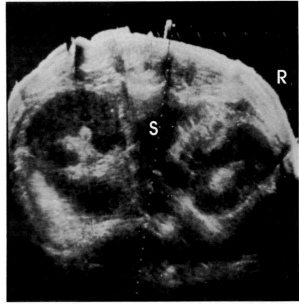

Fig. 13-152. Renal leukemia. Chronic lymphocytic leukemia. Longitudinal prone scans of **(A)** the right and **(B)** the left kidneys with **(C)** transverse scan. The kidneys are enlarged, more so in the anteroposterior dimension than in length. The echopattern is unchanged from normal. (*L*, liver; *Sp*, spleen; *R*, right; *S*, spine.)

Differential Features

Small Renal Mass. At times, small renal masses have an indeterminate density on CT. Ultrasound may be particularly valuable in assessing such masses, as well as in evaluating renal masses when intravenous contrast cannot be given.[323] Mass size may be a limiting factor in the usefulness of ultrasound in evaluating small renal cysts,

since factitious internal echoes and lack of acoustic enhancement are more frequently encountered than with large cysts[323] (Fig. 13-154). Additionally, reverberation, slice thickness, and side lobe and/or range ambiguity artifacts account for the occasional noncystic appearance.[323] Advances in real-time technology with higher frequency and variable-focus transducers have enhanced the ability of real-time equipment alone to

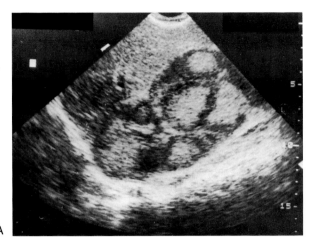
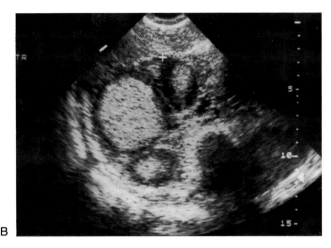

A   B

Fig. 13-153. Acute lymphoblastic leukemia, renal involvement. Ultrasonic appearance of the right kidney in **(A)** longitudinal and **(B)** transverse sections showing enlargement with focal areas of hyperechogenicity causing contour deformities. (From Jayagopal et al,[320] with permission.)

demonstrate the fluid-filled properties of these small cysts.[323]

Over the years, renal neoplasms have been detected earlier and with increased frequency, as is well documented in the literature.[240,324-326] There has been a five-fold increase in the number of small (≤ 3.0 cm) renal neoplasms detected and removed in a 5-year period in the 1980s as a result of the use of high-resolution CT and ultrasound compared with a similar period in the 1970s in one reported series.[240] The kidneys are visualized on most ultrasound examinations of the abdomen, so the radiologist has the opportunity to visualize the kidneys in many more patients.[240] Another reason for the increased detection is that these imaging techniques are

able to detect lesions of the kidney not seen on urography.[240] Some investigators believe that CT is the best overall imaging procedure for the detection of small RCCs, with ultrasound providing useful information by documenting the solid or complex nature of a renal mass.[324] It may be difficult, even with CT, to differentiate benign from malignant lesions when the lesions are very small.

Regardless of the size of the renal lesion, the imaging findings that differentiate benign from malignant renal lesions are basically the same; however, smaller lesions can be very problematic because the findings are also smaller, requiring more detailed and more sensitive imaging studies.[240] A RCC should be considered if the small renal lesion is not a cyst, pseudotumor, angiomyolipoma, lymphoma, or metastatic carcinoma[240] (Figs. 13-154 to 13-156). The detection of these small lesions will surely improve the cure rate of RCC. Small RCCs may be removed by partial nephrectomy.[240] Early detection and removal of these tumors should permit many patients to be saved who would ordinarily not have had their cancer diagnosed until the disease was past the possibility of cure.[240]

Small RCCs usually are low-stage lesions, which may be managed by partial nephrectomy; however, a radical nephrectomy is generally the preferred method for managing small renal carcinomas.[326] In the past, partial nephrectomy was usually reserved for patients who had renal functional impairment or coexisting disorders that might cause progressive functional impairment of the kidney in the future.[326]

The ideal way to treat these small renal carcinomas may be simple surgical enucleation.[324] However, the traditional role of nephrectomy as the preferred method of

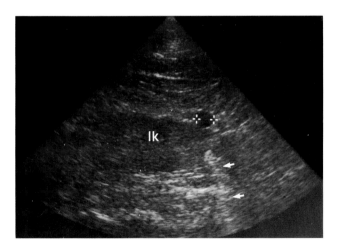

Fig. 13-154. Small renal tumor, cyst. Sagittal view of the left kidney *(lk)* in an elderly patient showing a tiny (12-mm) cystic mass (calipers) that is exophytic to the renal outline. Despite its very small size, it exhibits acoustic enhancement (arrows).

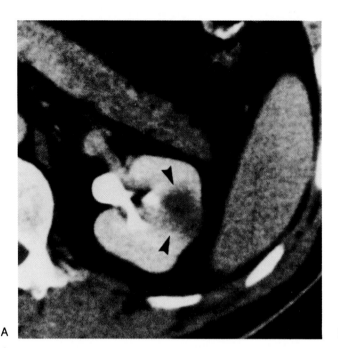
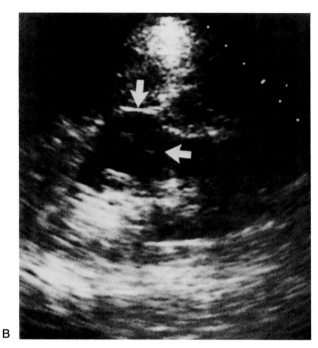

Fig. 13-155. Small renal cell carcinoma. **(A)** Contrast-enhanced CT scan in a 42-year-old man with abdominal pain showing poorly defined 2.7-cm mass (arrowheads) in the midregion of the left kidney. **(B)** Real-time coronal sonogram through the midaxillary line shows an inhomogeneous mass (arrows) with internal echoes and no posterior acoustic enhancement. (From Levine et al,[326] with permission.)

treatment for both small and large RCCs may be indicated because of the unusually high frequency of satellite nodules (15 percent) in one series.[324]

One group of investigators compared their RCC imaging results over the years.[325] Between 1974 and 1977, only 5.3 percent of RCCs were 3.0 cm or smaller, whereas between 1982 and 1985, 25.4 percent were 3.0 cm or smaller, indicating an almost fivefold increase.[325] The major difference between these two periods was the increased availability of CT and ultrasound.[325] During the period from 1982 to 1985, 96.7 percent of the small lesions were detected incidentally and 77.4 percent were initially detected by CT or ultrasound.[325] In this group of patients, 48.4 percent of the small renal tumors were treated with partial nephrectomy.[325] At the time of publication, there were no reports of recurrence in these patients.[325] This group of authors believe that partial nephrectomy may be used increasingly in the management of these small tumors when one considers that these tumors are in a very early stage, that they are well marginated and circumscribed, and that to date no patient with a small tumor in this series has developed metastatic disease or tumor recurrence regardless of the extent of surgical removal of the tumor.[325] Undoubtedly, the use of CT and ultrasound of the abdomen has increased the earlier detection of small RCC in

the general population, which will lead to an overall improvement in the cure rate of this neoplasm.[325]

The prognosis of RCC depends on the size, stage, and grade of the tumor at diagnosis.[325] As expected, the survival rate for patients with tumor contained in the capsule of the kidney is better than for patients with perinephric involvement.[325] There is a positive straight-line relationship between the size of the RCC and the frequency of extension of the tumor into the renal vein and mestastes demonstrated.[325]

Doppler Evaluation. Investigators have evaluated renal masses with pulsed Doppler.[241,245] Most malignant renal tumors are characterized by abnormal vascular structures that can be recognized by angiography.[245] By using Doppler ultrasound, noninvasive assessment of the vascular signals from neovascular tissue may be performed.[245] To evaluate tumors with Doppler, the cursor is placed around the periphery of the mass.[245] While searching for Doppler shifts, a wide sample window is used; once a signal is detected, the sample window is reduced to 4 mm and the transducer is repositioned so that the line of sight is more parallel to the direction of blood flow.[245]

Two types of Doppler signals have been reported in tumors: (1) a high-frequency signal with a large systolic-

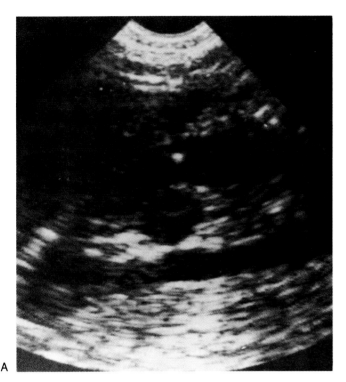

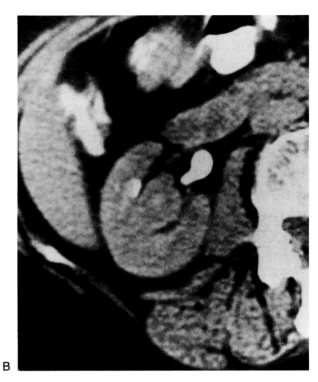

A   B

Fig. 13-156. Renal pseudotumor (caused by anomalous parenchymal lobe) in a 64-year-old woman who underwent sonography to evaluate the gallbladder. **(A)** Sonogram showing a mass in the central portion of the right kidney. CT was advised for further evaluation. **(B)** CT scans were obtained with and without contrast medium (only the contrast-enhanced scan is shown). The "mass" proves to enhance identically to renal tissue and represents an anomalously placed renal parenchymal lobe (lobar dysmorphism). (From Bosniak,[240] with permission.)

diastolic gradient and originating from arteriovenous shunting; and (2) a relatively high-frequency, almost continuous signal with little systolic-diastolic fluctuation (these low-impedance signals are related to muscular walls, a characteristic commonly found in tumors)[245] (Fig. 13-117). Seven of nine carcinomas in one series had Doppler shifts of 4 kHz or more and were hypervascular or vascular.[245] As such, high-frequency Doppler signals are associated with arteriovenous shunts.[245] If no signal is found or there is a small Doppler shift, a hypovascular mass would be expected.[245]

One series found tumor signals (the Doppler-shifted frequency of the lesion exceeded the frequency shift in the ipsilateral main renal artery) in 83 percent of untreated RCCs.[241] These tumor signals were also found in three of four Wilms' tumors and in two patients with metastases.[241] None of the benign renal masses in this series demonstrated tumor signals.[241] As such, the abnormal, high velocity, Doppler-shifted signals can help in the differential diagnosis of renal masses.[241]

Another group of authors evaluated renal masses by Doppler.[327] A 70 percent sensitivity was demonstrated, with the use of the criterion of a peak-systolic Doppler

shift frequency of 2.5 kHz or greater as evidence of neovascularity; 26 of 37 malignant lesions demonstrated tumor signals.[327] A 94 percent specificity was demonstrated with benign lesions, with 31 of 33 benign lesions lacking tumor signals.[327] The false-positive results in this series were associated with inflammatory masses with peak frequencies of 3.0 and 3.7 kHz.[327] As in other reports, tumor vascularity in most malignant renal mass lesions gives rise to abnormal high-frequency Doppler-shifted signals that can aid in the differential diagnosis of renal masses.[327]

Infiltration Patterns. A number of tumors demonstrate an infiltrative growth pattern.[328] These imaging findings include (1) poorly defined margins of the mass; (2) trapped, nondisplaced infundibulae; and (3) calyces with occasional caliectasis, diminished contrast enhancement, occasional nephrographic striations, replacement of central sinus fat, loss of central sinus echoes, and variable renal parenchymal echogenicity.[328] On ultrasound, the most characteristic features of infiltrative growth are enlargement of the kidney with preservation of the reniform shape and abnormal echogenicity of the parenchyma[328] (Fig. 13-157). Additionally, there may be loss of the renal sinus echoes.[328] The tumors that have exhibited this pattern at times include invasive TCC, renal lymphoma, metastasis to the kidney, acute bacterial nephritis, mesoblastic nephroma, squamous cell carcinoma of the renal pelvis, and RCC.[328] Although TCC grows by expansion while it is confined to the collecting system, it converts to an infiltrative growth pattern when it invades the renal parenchyma.[328] As such, an invasive TCC is suspected when an infiltrating renal mass coexists with a pelvic filling defect or irregular narrowing or amputation of the collecting system is seen.[328]

Cystic Renal Tumors. Cystic renal tumors are seen with a variety of lesions in which solid and liquid components coexist.[246] Such lesions may be benign or malignant; they include multilocular cystic nephroma, RCC, and papillary adenocarcinoma.[246] CT may be more helpful than ultrasound; ultrasound is confined to the evaluation of the thickness of the septa, but this does not give useful information to discriminate multilocular cystic nephroma from RCC in this group's experience.[246] Again, although both CT and ultrasound identify cystic renal tumors, CT appears to be superior in discriminat-

ing between benign and malignant tumors, owing to a superior evaluation of the septa and vegetations; this superiority is due to the contrast, which considerably enhances the visualization of the septa in malignant tumors compared with benign ones[246] (Fig. 13-110).

Renal Medical Disease

When a patient presents with renal insufficiency, ultrasound is performed to exclude hydronephrosis and to evaluate for renal medical disease.[22] A diagnosis of renal parenchymal disease is based on renal size and contour, cortical echogenicity, distinctness of the corticomedullary junction, detectability and size of the renal pyramids, and appearance of the renal sinus.[22]

Use of the current ultrasound equipment permits the identification of three distinct anatomic regions: cortex, medulla, and renal sinus. The corticomedullary junction can be identified by the interface produced by the arcuate vessels. All of the following can be assessed by ultrasound when evaluating a kidney for medical disease: renal length, appearance of the renal sinus, detectability and size of the renal pyramids, distinctness of the corticomedullary junction, and cortical echogenicity (by

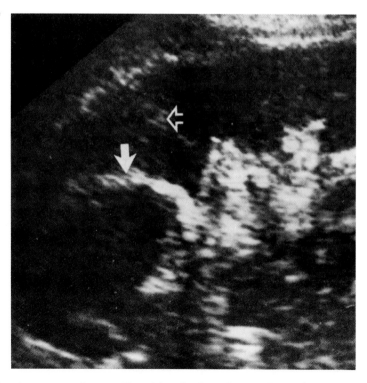

Fig. 13-157. Infiltrative pattern of tumor. Transitional cell carcinoma. Expansile growth is seen within collecting system, and infiltrating growth is seen within parenchyma. Longitudinal sonogram of left kidney showing focal displacement of renal sinus fat by pelvic tumor (solid arrow). Poorly defined increased echogenicity in the upper pole (open arrow) corresponds to parenchymal invasion. (From Hartman et al,[328] with permission.)

comparing the density with that of the liver at a comparable depth and with that of the renal sinus).[329] The pyramids are considered enlarged if their height exceeds or their width is thicker than the overlying cortex.[116] The clarity of the corticomedullary junction does not correspond to any histopathologic finding. There is no correlation between the nature and severity of the glomerular lesion on renal biopsy and the ultrasound findings.[330] However, there is a definite relationship between the nature and severity of interstitial changes on biopsy and the echointensity of the cortex.[330]

Parenchymal Disease

The hallmark of parenchymal disease is a diffuse increase in echogenicity throughout the parenchyma of both kidneys.[22] The ability of ultrasound to detect the corticomedullary junction and pyramids may be affected by these histopathologic changes. The pyramids may become hypoechoic with medullary congestion. They may become less distinct and more difficult to differentiate from the cortex in other instances.[22] A correlation has been shown between the number of hyaline casts per glomerulus and the loss of visualization of the pyramids.[22]

The sinus echogenicity may be altered with parenchymal disease. There may be an increase in septal thickness, rendering the sinus echoes inhomogeneous and patchy with any infiltrative process.[22] In fibrosis and atrophy, the loss of patchy adipose tissue results in further loss of distinction between the renal sinus and parenchyma.[22]

With early renal medical disease, the histologic changes may be isolated to one of the three primary components of the renal parenchyma: the nephron, vessels, or interstitium. Early changes isolated to the glomeruli may not change cortical echogenicity, since the glomeruli occupy only 8 percent of the cortex in the adult.[22] Cortical echogenicity and corticomedullary differentiation may not correlate with the renal biopsy.[22] A noticeable increase in renal parenchymal echogenicity has been reported in cases in which the renal biopsy shows active interstitial changes.[22] With interstitial disease, the prominent increase in echogenicity probably occurs because most of the cortex is composed of tubules and interstitial tissue.[22] With further progression of renal disease, histologic changes spread among the three primary parenchymal components. As such, increased parenchymal echogenicity results from combined changes within the glomeruli, tubules, and interstitium.[22]

In the past, it was thought that the renal parenchymal echogenicity was abnormal if it was equal to that of the liver or spleen (Fig. 13-1). The normal echogenicity of the parenchyma was thought to be lower than that of liver. A recent study has found that the echogenicity of the kidneys is often equal to that of the liver in patients with no evidence of renal disease.[23] The accepted ultrasound criterion for abnormal renal echogenicity (kidney echogenicity $\geq$ liver echogenicity) was neither sensitive (62 percent) nor specific (58 percent) for renal disease, and it had a positive predictive value of 35 percent[23] (Fig. 13-158). Many of the inaccuracies occur because 72 percent of patients in whom the renal echogenicity was equal to that of the liver had normal renal function.[23] By

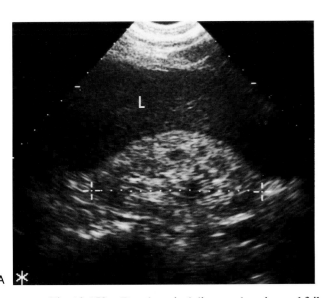

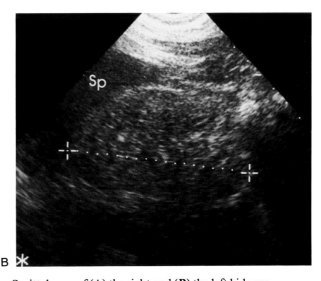

Fig. 13-158. Renal cortical disease, chronic renal failure. Sagittal scan of **(A)** the right and **(B)** the left kidneys. The renal parenchyma is more dense than the liver *(L)* or spleen *(Sp)*. The kidneys are small, and their borders are poorly defined (calipers).

using a stricter criterion for abnormality (kidney echogenicity > liver echogenicity), a specificity of 96 percent and a positive predictive value of 67 percent can be achieved; however, the sensitivity was only 20 percent.[23] As such, the criterion of renal echogenicity equal to liver echogenicity is not a good indicator of disease. A more specific but insensitive test is the use of a stricter criterion: kidney echogenicity greater than liver echogenicity.[23]

The echogenicity of the kidney may be altered in the presence of ascites.[331] The echogenicity is directly proportional to the amount of fluid interposed between the clinically normal kidney and the transducer.[331] The cause of this finding is probably related to the acoustic enhancement behind a collection of liquid very much like the acoustic enhancement seen beyond a cyst or behind a urine-filled bladder.

Doppler Evaluation. A number of investigators have evaluated Doppler ultrasound and its relationship to parenchymal disease.[14,332] Kidneys with active disease in the tubulointerstitial compartment have a mean RI of 0.75 ± 0.07[332] (Fig. 13-159). This is statistically significantly different from the RI in kidneys with disease lim-

ited to the glomeruli (mean RI, 0.58 ± 0.05). With acute tubular necrosis, there is an elevated RI (mean RI, 0.78 ± 0.03); with vasculitis/vasculopathy, there is also an elevated RI (mean RI, 0.82 ± 0.05).[332] In patients with hypertension, proteinuria, or hematuria, the kidneys do not have a significantly higher RI than do those in patients without these clinical factors.[332] This study found a weak correlation between the creatinine level and RI value, reflected by the linear correlation coefficient of 0.34.[332] It may be concluded that some forms of obstructive renal disease can produce changes in the Doppler waveform detectable by RI measurements.[332] The Doppler waveform changes are strongly influenced by the site of the main disease within the kidneys.[332] Disease limited to the glomeruli, no matter how severe, does not appear to significantly alter the RI, whereas active disease within the tubulointerstitial compartment or vasculitis/vasculopathy generally results in a elevation of the RI.[332]

Other investigators found the RI to correlate significantly with the prevalence of arteriolosclerosis, glomerular sclerosis, arteriosclerosis, edema, and focal interstitial fibrosis.[14] In this series, no difference in the RI was found in the five groups of different renal parenchymal

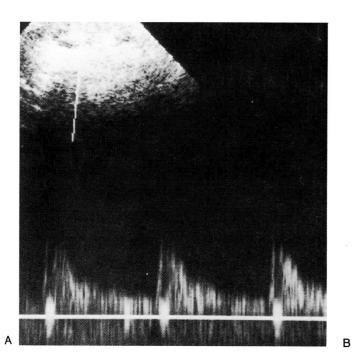

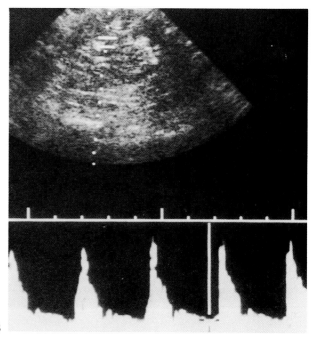

A   B

Fig. 13-159.   Parenchymal disease, Doppler. Case 1. **(A)** Renal Doppler of a patient with acute tubular necrosis. The patient had a rapid rise in creatinine level from 1.4 to 3.1 mg/dl in 2 weeks. Standard real-time sonography of kidneys was normal. Doppler signal from intrarenal artery shows reduced end-diastolic flow resulting in an elevated RI of 0.78. Renal biopsy was consistent with acute tubular necrosis. Case 2. **(B)** Renal Doppler of patient with vasculopathy. Creatinine level became elevated after a cardiac transplant. Standard real-time sonography was normal. Doppler signal obtained from intrarenal artery shows a significant reduction in end-diastolic flow compared with peak systolic flow, resulting in an elevated RI of 0.83. Biopsy revealed changes consistent with cyclosporine vasculopathy. (From Platt et al,[332] with permission.)

diseases. In renal parenchymal disease, the renal vascular resistance and the RI were influenced predominantly by nonspecific vascular and glomerular abnormalities.[14] A normal range of less than 0.70 was found. The RI was noted to increase as the patient aged, as a result of the higher incidence of arteriosclerosis.[14] This group concluded that quantitative duplex ultrasound using the RI does not reliably distinguish different types of renal medical disease.

Cortical Disease

Two parenchymal patterns have been described on ultrasound of patients with renal disease.[8,9,26,330] The type I pattern involves a diffuse increase in echogenicity of the cortex with preservation of the corticomedullary junction; the echointensity in the cortex is equal to or greater than that in the adjacent liver or spleen and equal to that in the adjacent renal sinus[8,9] (Fig. 13-158). The increased cortical echoes are seen in disease processes in which there is deposition of collagen or calcium and in some acute processes.[8] Diseases that demonstrate a type I pattern include acute and chronic glomerulonephritis, renal transplant rejection, lupus nephritis, hypertensive nephrosclerosis, renal cortical necrosis, methemoglobinuric renal failure, Alport syndrome, amyloidosis, diabetic nephrosclerosis, and some chronic diseases. With chronic disease, the kidney becomes smaller, the cortex has increased echogenicity, and eventually the medulla becomes equally echogenic. The type II pattern involves focal or diffuse loss of the corticomedullary junction definition.[8,9] It is seen with such focal lesions as cysts, calyceal diverticuli, renal artery aneurysm, some abscesses, and hematomas.[26]

Echogenic kidneys are associated with medical renal disease in 94 percent of pediatric patients (excluding neonates). In one series, the cause was glomerular in 30 percent, tubointerstitial in 48 percent, and end-stage in 16 percent.[333] Patients with end-stage disease had small, dense (echogenic) kidneys). The severity of the renal parenchymal disease in neonates could not be correlated because the normal neonatal kidney is echogenic.[334]

Abnormalities Causing an Increased Density. The etiology of nephrocalcinosis is quite variable. Calcifications in the cortex are associated with a number of abnormalities: oxalosis, metastatic tumors, islet cell neoplasms, chronic glomerulonephritis, renal cortical necrosis, and Alport syndrome.[22] They can also be seen with renal tubular disease, enzyme disorders, hypercalcemic states, parenchymal renal disease, and vascular phenomena, and they may be idiopathic.[335,336] Cushing syndrome is the least common cause.[335] The most common cause of hypercalcemia in the general population is malignant

neoplasm.[336] This may be due to the direct lytic effect on bone by the metastatic tumor. In the absence of bone metastases, tumor-related hypercalcemia may be mediated by the ectopic production of parathyroid hormone, prostaglandins, or osteoid. Hypercalcemia leads to nephrocalcinosis by overloading the renal resorptive mechanism.[336] The high calcium load causes cellular damage followed by calcium salt deposition in the tubular cells, in the basement membrane, and within the loops of Henle.[336]

The classic distribution of nephrocalcinosis is along the corticomedullary junction, but the calcium salts may be deposited elsewhere in the renal parenchyma. There is diffusely increased cortical echogenicity without acoustic shadowing, and there is sparing of the renal pyramids with accentuation of the corticomedullary junction[22] (Fig. 13-160). The observed cortical calcifications may not always be detected on plain radiographs or digital electronic radiographs; CT often shows diffuse cortical nephrocalcinosis or renal cortex Hounsfield unit readings of 70 to 145 on a noncontrast scan, which is well above that for soft tissue or collagen.[22]

In the cortical type of nephrocalcinosis, there are focal or diffuse, punctate or confluent densities in the cortex of the kidney, producing, in the most severe form, a dense outline of the kidney[335,336] (Fig. 13-160). The ultrasound pattern may resemble other forms of parenchymal disease.[337,338] CT would be more sensitive in detecting this pattern of nephrocalcinosis.[335,337]

Preeclampsia. Occurring during pregnancy after the 20th week of gestation, preeclampsia is a syndrome complex characterized by hypertension, with or without proteinuria or edema.[339] Preeclampsia is primarily a dis-

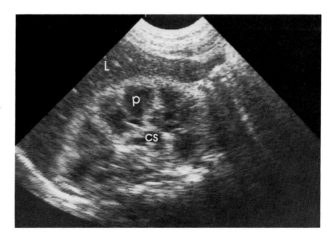

Fig. 13-160. Renal cortical calcification. Left lateral decubitus longitudinal scan of the right kidney in an infant showing that the density of the renal parenchyma is higher than that of the liver *(L)* and the hypoechogenicity of the renal pyramids *(p)* is accentuated. (*cs*, collecting system.)

order of primigravida, occurring frequently in adolescents and in women in their late 30s and early 40s.[339] It occurs in approximately 6 percent of pregnant women, usually in the third trimester. In a case report, the kidneys were evaluated serially. Marked cortical echogenicity with prominent pyramids was noted. After delivery, the kidneys decreased in size and the echogenicity of the cortex improved. One month following delivery, the kidneys appeared normal.

When renal biopsy specimens of preeclamptic patients are evaluated microscopically, there is swelling of the endothelial cells with vacuolization and deposition of amorphous material within the cytoplasm.[339] Cortical microinfarctions are produced by mesangial cell hyperplasia and cortical capillary fibrin thrombi. The change in the ultrasound pattern may be secondary to the reversibly of this condition.

Primary Hyperoxaluria. Primary hyperoxaluria is a rare hereditary autosomal recessive disorder resulting in an inborn error of glyoxalate metabolism (type I) or hydroxypyruvate metabolism (type II).[340-342] It is characterized by hyperoxaluria, calcium oxalate, nephrolithiasis, widespread renal and extrarenal deposits of calcium oxalate crystals (oxalosis), and progressive renal failure, leading to death usually before adulthood. The highly insoluble calcium oxalate crystals are deposited in extrarenal tissues including the bone, blood vessels, heart, and male urogenital system.[342] Renal parenchymal injury is caused by the calcium oxalate deposits, which lead to progressive renal failure.[340] The renal tubules, especially the cortical convoluted tubules, contain many pale, doubly refractile crystals arranged in rosettes in affected infants and minimally involved renal allografts.[342] Sixty-five percent of the patient's symptoms are due to renal calculi prior to the age of 5.

On ultrasound an increase in the echogenicity of the renal parenchyma in normal-sized kidneys is evident[341] (Fig. 13-161). The abnormalities described include nephrolithiasis, nephrocalcinosis, dense vascular calcifications, abnormal bone density, and characteristic metaphyseal abnormalities.[342] These findings, combined with the urinalysis and ophthaloscopic examination, can be diagnostic and may eliminate the need for biopsy.[341] It is imperative to diagnose the disease process early so that appropriate therapy may be instituted to alter the natural history of the process.

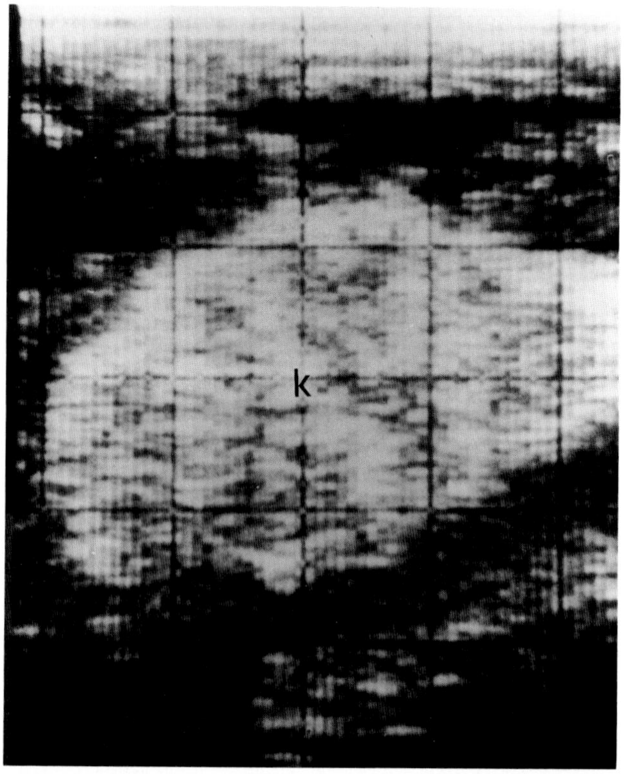

Beckwith-Wiedemann Syndrome. In Beckwith-Wiedemann syndrome, the kidneys are grossly enlarged with smooth cortical margins. There is increased echogenicity of the cortex, with accentuation of the cortical medullary definition reflecting the micropathology (Fig. 13-162). The increased cortical echoes are directly related to the degree of the interstitial abnormality. The pathologic finding of glomeruloneogenesis presumably accounts

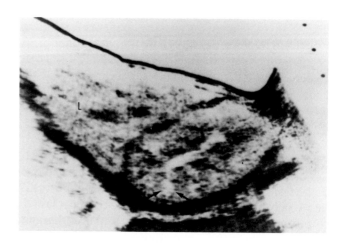

Fig. 13-161. Primary hyperoxaluria. Longitudinal scan of intensely echogenic kidney *(k)* of normal size demonstrating corticomedullary distinction. The gain has been turned down, causing the liver to appear anechoic. (From Brennan et al,[341] with permission.)

Fig. 13-162. Beckwith-Wiedemann syndrome. Longitudinal scan demonstrating nephromegaly. The renal cortex is of higher echogenicity than the liver *(L)*, and the pyramids (arrows) are prominent. Increased central lucency reflects a slightly dilated collecting system. (From McCarten et al,[343] with permission.)

for the increased interstitial density, which causes increasing echoes on ultrasound. On ultrasound, the kidneys may be normal or bilaterally enlarged.[343]

Amyloidosis. Reactive systemic amyloidosis is associated with chronic infection, inflammation, or nonimmunocyte-derived dyscrasias or neoplastic disorders.[344] Juvenile rheumatoid arthritis (Still's disease) is the most common predisposing illness associated with reactive systemic amyloidosis in the pediatric patient.[344] The kidneys that are involved may be normal-sized, small, or enlarged. The echogenicity may be equal to or greater than that of the liver and equal to that of the renal sinus, with prominence of the corticomedullary junction and obscuration of the arcuates.[344] Markedly pronounced renal cortical echoes may reflect deposition of amyloid in the glomeruli and interstitium.[344]

Medullary Disease

Abnormalities Causing an Increased Density. Increased medullary echogenicity relative to normal cortical echogenicity is seen in many types of parenchymal abnormalities (Fig. 13-163). This pattern has been reported in patients with gouty kidney, hypokalemia, and medullary nephrocalcinosis.[22,345,346] A specific diagnosis may be made in a patient with hyperechoic pyramids by using a systematic clinical approach that includes evaluation of patient age, serum and urine calcium concentration, and renal function.[346]

The causative abnormalities may be classified by the age of patient. With the adult, increased medullary density has been found with gout, medullary sponge kidney, primary hyperaldosteronism, hyperparathyroidism, glycogen storage disease, Wilson's disease, and Sjögren syndrome.[346] Causes of medullary nephrocalcinosis in the adult include renal tubular acidosis, hyperparathyroidism, hypervitaminosis D, primary hypercalciuria, and sarcoidosis.[346] Nephrocalcinosis and medullary density in children have been associated with cretinism, Bartter syndrome, oxalosis, Cushing syndrome, immobilization hypercalciuria, idiopathic hypercalciuria, hyperparathyroidism, and steroid therapy.[346] Correlation of urine and serum calcium levels and renal function tests has shown that hyperechoic renal pyramids revealed clinical entities associated with hypercalciuria to be a factor in 69 percent of cases.[346]

Iatrogenic nephrocalcinosis has been found by one group to be the single most frequent cause of increased renal medullary echogenicity.[347] Once nephrocalcinosis is excluded as a cause, a large differential diagnosis remains. The ultrasound findings may be secondary to anatomic abnormalities of the renal pyramids (medullary tubular ectasia), deposits of proteins in the collecting tubules, deposits of urates, fibrosis of the pyramids, or simple vascular congestions.[347]

Gout. When gout affects the kidneys, there are urate deposits in the collecting system and interstitial changes, which are thought to cause the hyperechoic renal pyramids.[22,345] In cases of hyperuricemia associated with Lesch-Nyhan syndrome, xanthine crystal deposits in the medulla have been seen.[346]

Hypokalemia. Patients with primary aldosteronism and pseudo-Bartter syndrome with persistent hypokalemia have had the ultrasound appearance of increased medullary echogenicity.[22] The cause of the hyperechoic pyramids has been postulated to be secondary to disturbances in renal concentrating ability with resulting

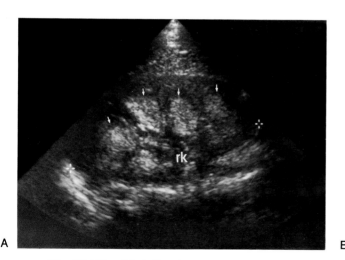
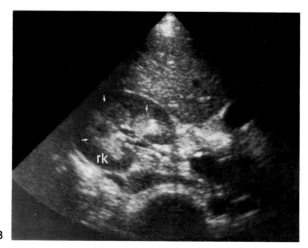

A   B

Fig. 13-163. Medullary hyperechogenicity. **(A)** Sagittal and **(B)** transverse views of the right kidney *(rk)* in a neonate showing markedly increased echogenicity of the renal pyramids (arrows).

tubular damage from interstitial lymphocytic infiltration and fibrosis.[22] Other investigators postulate that the hyperechoic medulla in patients with primary aldosteronism is due to changes in the renal tubules, collecting tubules, and interstitial tissue as a result of hypokalemia.[345]

Anderson-Carr Progression. On the basis of cadaver studies, the Anderson-Carr progression of renal stone formation was developed. This postulates that the aggregation of calcium begins at the tips and margins of the renal pyramids; with progressive calcium deposits, there

is formation of calcium plaques, which may perforate the calyx and form a nidus for further stone growth[348] (Fig. 13-164). The calcium level in fluids about the renal tubules is high, and calcium is normally removed from this area by lymphatic flow. If, however, the calcium load exceeds the lymphatic capacity, microscopic calcium aggregates occur in the medulla, mainly at the tips of the fornix and at the margins. These may fuse to form plaques ("Randall's plaque") and migrate toward the calyceal epithelium, finally perforating it. As such, nidus for urinary tract stones is formed. Ultrasound evaluation of children appears to support this progression.

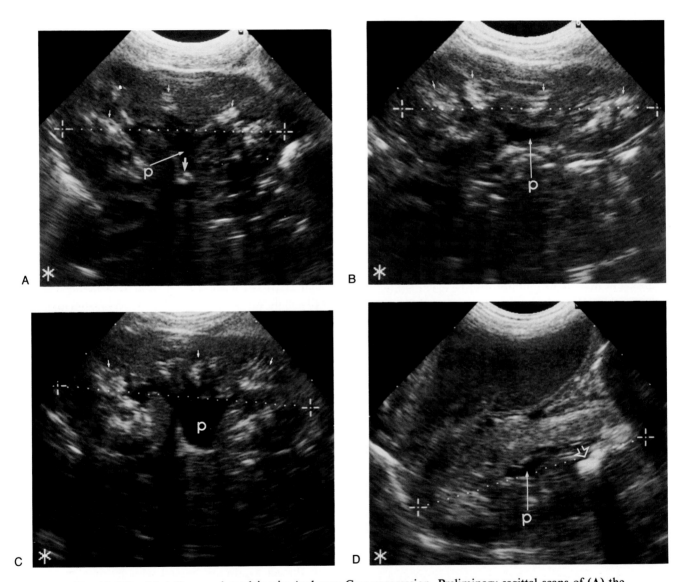

Fig. 13-164. Medullary nephrocalcinosis: Anderson-Carr progression. Preliminary sagittal scans of (**A**) the right and (**B**) the left kidneys showing multiple echogenic foci (small arrows) in the region of the renal pyramids. The renal pelves *(p)* are slightly prominent. There is a small calculus (larger arrow) in the right renal pelvis. Sagittal scans of (**C**) the right and (**D**) the left kidneys obtained 2 months later demonstrating dilatation of the right renal pelvis *(p)*. There are collecting system calculi (open arrow) now seen on the left. The medullary hyperechogenicities have progressed.

Medullary Nephrocalcinosis. A number of causes of medullary nephrocalcinosis have been described, including distal tubular acidosis, furosemide therapy (in infants), medullary sponge kidney, prolonged adrenocorticotropic hormone (ACTH) therapy, secondary hyperparathyroidism, Cushing syndrome, oral pharmacologic doses of vitamin E and calcium, Bartter syndrome, hyperparathyroidism, sarcoidosis, malignant neoplasms (bony metastasis, production of a parathyroid hormone-like substance), milk-alkali syndrome, Lesch-Nyhan syndrome, and steroid administration.[22,335,345,346,349-354]

With medullary nephrocalcinosis, the cortical echogenicity is normal but there are focal areas of increased echogenicity corresponding to the renal pyramids[22,335,338,349,351,355] (Figs. 13-163 to 13-165). The calcification is often not revealed by radiography.[352,355] There may or may not be an associated acoustic shadow with these densities, which suggests that macroscopic aggregates of calcium are necessary to produce an acoustic shadow posterior to the echogenic pyramids.[22,352] The calcifications can be unequivocally localized to the medulla if the arcuate vessels are seen capping the base of the echogenic wedge-shaped area.[352]

One group of authors has found a pattern of echogenic rings, the earliest sign of nephrocalcinosis.[356] These rings have been seen in the periphery of the renal pyramids. This finding may be demonstrated without biochemical abnormalities or plain radiography changes. Others have described echogenic "rings" in the periphery of the pyramids as a sign of renal disease.[357] In two cases, this corresponded to fibrosis with and without calcification.

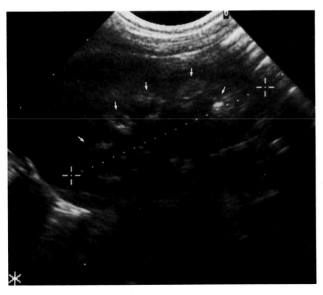

Fig. 13-165. Medullary nephrocalcinosis. Sagittal scan of the right kidney (calipers, 4.6 cm) in a neonate demonstrating multiple echogenic foci (arrows) in the region of the pyramids.

Long-term Furosemide Therapy. Both nephrocalcinosis and nephrolithiasis have been documented in low-birth-weight infants treated with furosemide, a potent diuretic.[346] In the neonatal intensive care unit, continuous furosemide therapy is used to reduce lung congestion in infants with hyaline membrane disease, patent ductus arteriosus, and bronchopulmonary dysplasia and in neonates with congestive heart failure, neonatal asphyxia, and idiopathic edema.[346] The exact mechanism for this production of nephrocalcinosis is uncertain, but it appears to be multifactorial. Furosemide therapy can cause alkalosis and hypercalciuria and, as such, has been implicated as a cause of nephrocalcinosis.[353] The hypercalciuria that accompanies increased sodium excretion in preterm infants is increased 10-fold by the administration of furosemide.[358] It appears to increase the urine calcium excretion. An average daily dose of 2 mg/kg/day of furosemide for as little as 2 weeks has been found to be associated with radiographic evidence of renal calcification.[359] As such, infants receiving an average dose of as low as 1 mg/kg/day should be monitored by ultrasound.

Both parenchymal and collecting system renal calcification can be seen with furosemide therapy.[359] For infants on furosemide therapy, the following guidelines can be used for the diagnosis of renal calculi: (1) rounded or elliptic echogenic foci greater than 3 mm in smallest diameter; (2) gravity-dependent location of focal echogenic structures or layering of calcium within the collecting system; and (3) changing size and intensity of echogenic foci compared with earlier scans.[359] The associated renal calcifications are best detected by ultrasound with either a parenchymal or collecting system pattern[359] (Fig. 13-164).

Bartter Syndrome. Bartter syndrome is characterized by hypokalemic alkalosis, hyperaldosteronism, hyperreninemia, hypertrophy of the juxtaglomerular apparatus, and normotension.[346,351,360,361] Some investigators believe that the pathogenesis of this syndrome is uncertain, but it is thought to be related to either a proximal or distal tubular sodium reabsorption defect.[361] The level of prostaglandin E_2 increases, which may stimulate conversion of an inactive metabolite of vitamin D to the active form. This may cause an increase in the absorption of calcium from the gastrointestinal tract, resulting in increased urine excretion of calcium and leading to precipitation of calcium aggregates in the medulla.[346]

One group of investigators have evaluated patients with Bartter syndrome treated with indomethacin.[360] Hypercalciuria is uniformly associated with an increase in levels of urinary prostaglandin E_2 and serum 1,25-$(OH)_2D$, the active metabolite of vitamin D. Indomethacin acts by inhibiting cyclooxygenase, which blocks excessive prostaglandin production.[360] It was shown that indomethacin effectively reduces urinary calcium excretion.[360] Significant improvement but incomplete resolution of nephrocalcinosis occurred in two-thirds of the infants studied.[360] It is thought that early diagnosis and treatment with indomethacin may result in correction of the hypercalciuria, decreasing the nephrocalcinosis and preserving renal function.

William Syndrome. Idiopathic hypercalcemia of infancy (William syndrome) is a heritable syndrome characterized by typical facies, cardiovascular abnormalities (supravalvular aortic stenosis/peripheral pulmonic stenosis), and a variable degree of mental retardation.[362] With ultrasound, a pattern of striking medullary echogenicity predominantly peripapillary in location is found.[362] The factors causing the hypercalcemia and hypercalciuria are unknown.[362]

Renal Tubular Acidosis. The clinical syndrome of renal tubular acidosis is caused by various defects in renal tubular secretion of hydrogen ions.[346] There is a wide spectrum of associated diseases. Distal tubular acidosis has been reported associated with Sjögren syndrome and glycogen storage disease.[345] The most common type to be associated with medullary nephrocalcinosis is distal (type I) renal tubular acidosis.[346] With this type, secretion of hydrogen ions is impaired in the collecting tubules and metabolic acidosis results.[346]

Transient Renal Insufficiency. It has been proposed that the increased medullary echogenicity associated with transient renal insufficiency may represent transient tubular blockade caused by protein precipitation that forms aggregates and blocks the tubules.[346] One series reports cases of "benign" transient acute tubular disease that had similar clinical presentations with oliguria and a similar ultrasound appearance.[363] As such, echogenic pyramids may be seen with oliguria.[363]

Sickle Cell Hemoglobinopathy. A variety of papillary abnormalities have been associated with sickle cell disease. The associated papillary necrosis is thought to be due to medullary ischemia that results from sickling in the straight vessels of the kidney.[346] The medullary portion can become necrotic and slough into the collecting system, where the cells become encrusted with calcium.[346]

Vascular Causes. With neonatal vascular insults, there may be hyperechoic areas within the kidney resembling hyperechoic medullary pyramids.[346]

Papillary Necrosis. Renal papillary necrosis may complicate a variety of pathologic conditions including diabetes, obstructive uropathy, sickle cell hemoglobino-pathies, acute or chronic pyelonephritis, acute tubular necrosis, renal vein thrombosis, severe infantile diarrhea, and chronic alcoholism. Pathologically, necrotic papillae are seen within the kidney or in the tissue sloughs passed in the urine. The patient initially presents with flank pain, dysuria, and fever. There may be acute oliguric renal failure, hematuria, and hypertension.[364]

The urographic demonstration of renal papillary necrosis is hindered by subtlety or absence of discernible changes in early or less severe cases or by poor opacification of the collecting system. Ultrasound reveals multiple round to triangular cystic spaces in the medulla, arranged about the renal sinus (Fig. 13-166). Echo reflections of the arcuate vessels are noted at the periphery of the lucent spaces, helping to distinguish this entity from hydronephrosis.[364]

One group of authors has described the early findings of papillary necrosis.[365] Bilateral highly echogenic foci were found in the medullary pyramids (Fig. 13-167). From the larger echogenic focus, irregular inhomogeneous acoustic shadowing was noted. Internally, the echogenic areas were lucent. It was postulated that the intense, elliptic, echogenic foci associated with irregular acoustic shadowing were due to ischemic necrosis of pyramidal tissue with fibrofatty degeneration. The lucent areas around the echogenic foci represented fluid dissection into and around necrotic papillae, equivalent to the ring shadow on urography.

Sinus Disease

Sinus Lipomatosis. This entity is common in older patients (in the sixth to seventh decade) as the normal parenchyma atrophies. Its etiology is linked to obesity, parenchymal atrophy, or destruction, and it can be a normal variant.[228] Replacement lipomatosis can be seen with atrophy, and it can be a sequela of chronic calculous disease and inflammation. Renal sinus lipomatosis indicates an increase in nontumorous fatty tissue linked to obesity, parenchymal atrophy or destruction, and normal variation.[22] Renal calculi are found in 70 percent of cases, and the resultant hydronephrosis leads to associated infection and hence to renal parenchymal atrophy.

The renal sinus, which is a potential space between the parenchyma and collecting system, is a bed of fatty tissue through which course the artery, vein, and lymphatics. It is in direct continuity with the hilus and perirenal fat.[366] In replacement lipomatosis, the void created by ongoing parenchymal atrophy may be filled by an abundant amount of fatty tissue within the renal sinus, hilum, and perinephric space.[367] Pathologically, the kidney may be enlarged and have a gross fibroadipose appearance with a thin renal parenchyma.[367] The renal sinus and hilum contain hyperplastic fat.

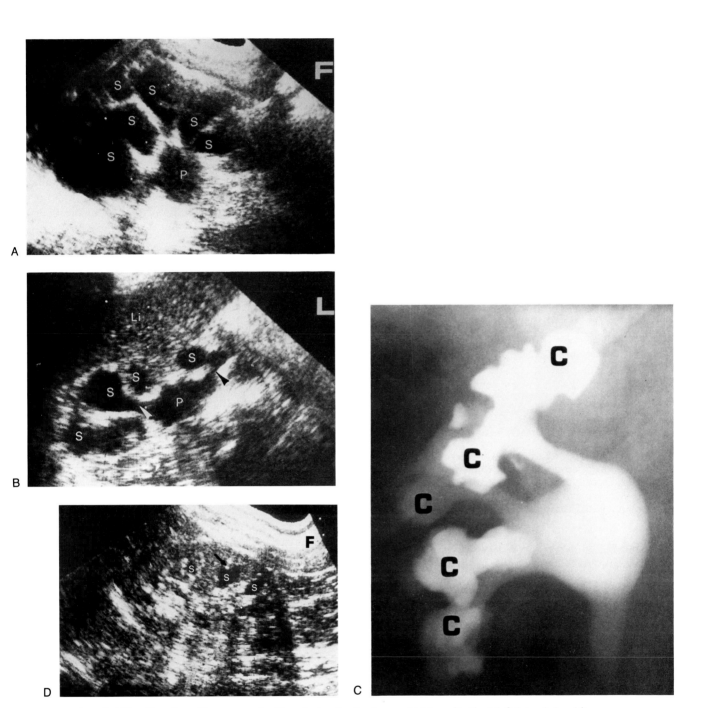

Fig. 13-166. Renal papillary necrosis. Case 1. Analgesic abuser. **(A)** Longitudinal left lateral decubitus scan showing multiple large fluid-filled spaces *(S)* within the kidney arranged in a spokewheel fashion about the renal pelvis *(P),* which is mildly distended. *(F,* toward patient's feet.) **(B)** Transverse scan in the same position demonstrating the narrow infundibuli (arrowheads) between the fluid-filled clubbed "calyces" *(S)* and the renal pelvis *(P). (Li,* liver; *L,* toward patient's left.) Case 2. Unilateral disease. **(C)** Right retrograde urogram demonstrating blunted clubbed calyces *(C).* **(D)** Longitudinal left lateral decubitus scan showing triangular fluid-filled spaces *(S)* about the renal sinus echoes that correlate with the retrograde findings. Note the echo reflection of the arcuate vessels (arrow) at the periphery of the blunted calyx. *(F,* toward patient's feet.) (From Hoffman et al,[364] with permission.)

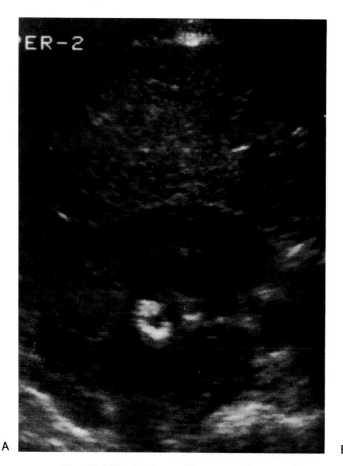

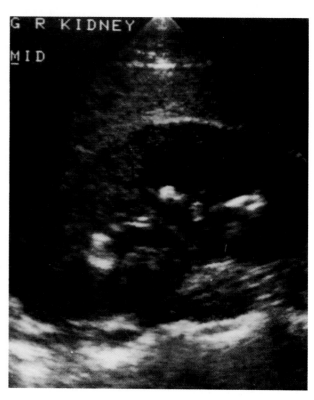

A

B

Fig. 13-167. Early papillary necrosis. **(A)** Transverse sonogram of the right upper pole demonstrating an elliptical echogenic focus with irregular shadowing in a medullary pyramid; the center of the focus is less echoic and is surrounded by an echolucent space. These findings represent papillary necrosis. **(B)** Sagittal sonogram of the right kidney showing echogenic foci in several medullary pyramids. Hydronephrosis was not present. (From Braden et al,[365] with permission.)

On ultrasound, the kidney with lipomatosis may be enlarged, with preservation of the reniform shape, and outlined by the hypoechoic rim representing the residual parenchyma, renal capsule, and the thick Gerota's fascia. The fat in the renal sinus appears similar to but larger than the usual renal sinus.[367] (Fig. 13-168). The renal sinus fat causes predominantly pelvocalyceal echoes.[368] In the past, renal sinus lipomatosis was described as a relatively hypoechoic area resembling a mass.[369] Unlike cysts, though, the fat is ill-defined and has weak internal echoes.[369] The amount of renal parenchyma decreases with increasing age, whereas the amount of renal sinus fat increases.[22]

Abnormalities with Acquired Immunodeficiency Syndrome

The AIDS spectrum may range from Kaposi sarcoma and infection to such general symptoms as lymphadenopathy, fever, and weight loss; or, there may be no symptoms at all.[370] This abnormality is thought to be due to a defect in cell-mediated immunity in a patient with no history of or cause for immune dysfunction; associated risk factors, in decreasing order of frequency in the United States, include homosexuality (in men), intravenous drug abuse, Haitian descent, and possibly hemophilia.[370]

There are many causes of renal failure in AIDS. It may be prerenal secondary to vomiting and diarrhea, or it may be postrenal secondary to hydronephrosis from obstructive abdominal or pelvic lymphomatous lymphadenopathy.[22] AIDS-related nephropathy and the use of nephrotoxic drugs (such as pentamidine) are renal causes.[22] The dominant morphologic pattern is focal and segmental glomerulosclerosis (referred to as AIDS-associated nephropathy).[22] There are other glomerular causes of AIDS nephropathy, including focal to diffuse mesangial hypercellularity, diffuse proliferative glomerulonephritis, and membranoproliferative glomerulonephritis.[22] Besides focal segmental glomerulosclerosis,

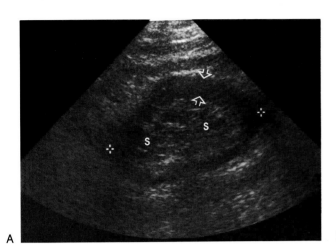
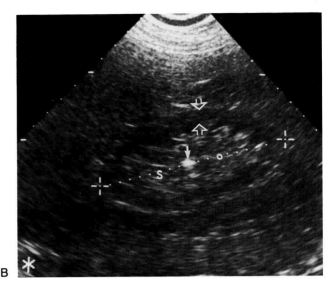

Fig. 13-168. Renal sinus lipomatosis. **(A & B)** Sagittal scans of the kidney (calipers) in two different patients. Note the large renal sinus *(s)* denoted by the echodense area related to the fat in that region. The renal parenchyma (open arrows) is very thin. (arrow, stone, Fig. B)

pathologic examination may show different degrees of tubular abnormalities.[371] There may be striking, irregularly dilated, infolded tubules with flattened epithelium and intratubular deposits of proteinaceous material and sometimes cystlike formation involving the medulla and cortex seen with grade III (cortex and sinus isoechoic) kidney disease, whereas mild dilatation of the tubules may be seen in patients with grade I (cortex and liver isoechoic) disease.[371]

At ultrasound, the affected kidneys are seen to be either normal in size or enlarged, with a normal or increased cortical echogenicity and preservation of the corticomedullary junction (Fig. 13-169). One series has reported the following: (1) normal-sized or enlarged kidneys with grade I cortical echogenicity in 36 percent; (2) grade II (cortex > liver echogenicity) echogenicity in 8 percent; and (3) grade III echogenicity in 14 percent.[371] In 42 percent of those studied, the renal echodensity was normal.[371] The main factors that appear to affect the increased echogenicity in AIDS nephropathy are the striking tubular abnormalities seen in these patients.[371]

Even if a patient has no laboratory evidence of renal disease, a baseline renal ultrasound might be useful for comparison if the patient ultimately presents with proteinuria or uremia.[370] Increasing cortical echogenicity on serial scans may indicate progressive renal impairment.[370] However, no definite correlation between the degree of echogenicity and the severity of renal disease was observed in this series.[370]

There has been a report of an unusual pattern of nephrocalcinosis in association with AIDS-related *Mycobacterium avium-intracellulare* (MAI) infection involving the kidney.[22,372] There was asymmetric involvement of the cortex and medulla, with parenchymal calcifications distributed inhomogeneously[22,372] (Fig. 13-170). This pattern has been termed partial nephrocalcinosis.[372] On ultrasound, focal areas of increased echogenicity were seen in the cortex, septa, and pyramids, with intervening areas of spared parenchyma. Besides MAI infection, diffuse punctate renal calcifications have been described with AIDS-related disseminated *Pneumocystis carinii* infection not only in the kidneys but also, more commonly, in the liver, spleen, and lymph nodes.[22]

Pediatric Renal Medical Disease

Renal parenchymal abnormalities found in infancy and childhood are different from those encountered in the adult. Vascular and cystic abnormalities are the predominant form of renal parenchymal disease in the neonate and young infant. Renal vein thrombosis (see Ch. 11), renal corticomedullary necrosis, and renal artery thrombosis secondary to dehydration, sepsis, blood loss, and severe hypoxia are the most common renal vascular diseases in infancy.[22] Nephrotic syndrome, which is uncommon in neonates and young infants, has been reported and is usually secondary to infection such as syphilis, rubella, toxoplasmosis, or cytomegalovirus or a familial form of congenital nephrotic syndrome known as the Finnish type.[22] The most frequent renal parenchymal disease found later in childhood is secondary to acute glomerulonephritis and the nephrotic syndrome.[22]

When an increased cortical echogenicity is shown in the pediatric patient, it is very sensitive in detecting parenchymal renal disease.[22] There is no correlation between the ultrasound appearance and histologic type of

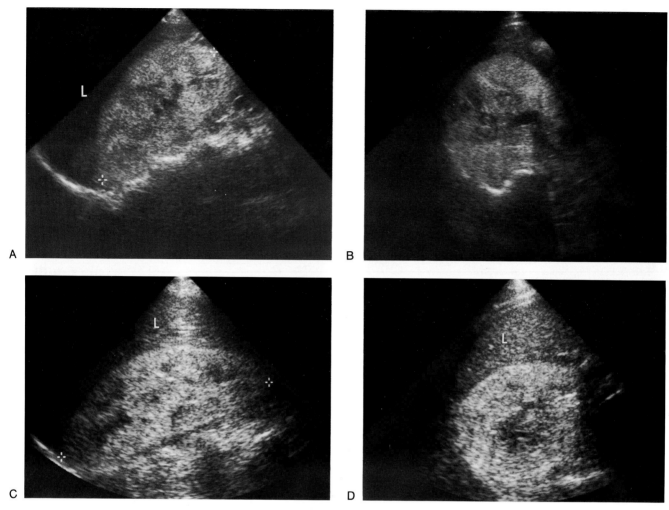

Fig. 13-169. AIDS nephropathy. Case 1. **(A)** Sagittal and **(B)** transverse images of a very echogenic (enlarged) right kidney (calipers). (*L,* liver.) Case 2. **(C)** Sagittal and **(D)** transverse scans of an enlarged, very echogenic right kidney. In both cases, the kidneys are markedly dense compared with the liver *(L).* Both had a tissue diagnosis of focal segmental glomerulosclerosis.

renal disease. A relationship has been found between the degree of cortical echogenicity and severity of histopathologic change on renal biopsy.[22] This is limited in the very young infant, since the normal appearance of the neonatal kidney does not permit the gradation of cortical echogenicity possible in older patients. Other investigators studying renal disease in pediatric patients have found a positive correlation between an increase in renal cortical echoes and interstitial infiltration, as well as glomerular obsolescence, tubular atrophy, and vascular changes.[373] As such, ultrasound cannot act as a prognostic index of the type or severity of disease in the pediatric patient.[373]

Juvenile Glomerulonephritis. Juvenile glomerulonephritis is an immune complex-mediated condition of children.[22,374] The most common by far is the acute

poststreptococcal form, which develops at an average age of 6 to 7 years.[22] Regardless of the cause of the disease, the ultrasound pattern is variable. The kidneys may appear normal or enlarged with acute glomerulonephritis, whereas they may be small and echogenic with chronic disease.[22]

Nephrotic Syndrome. Usually presenting at a younger age, nephrotic syndrome can be associated with any progressive glomerulonephritis (90 percent) and a number of systemic conditions including collagen vascular disease, toxic nephropathy, amyloidosis, and neoplasms (10 percent). Patients present with proteinuria, hypoproteinemia, edema, and hyperlipidemia.[374] The histologic diagnosis is minimal-change nephrotic syndrome or a variant in most cases.[22] Pathologically, there is an increase in glomerular capillary permeability, causing

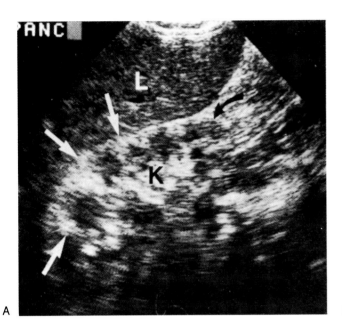

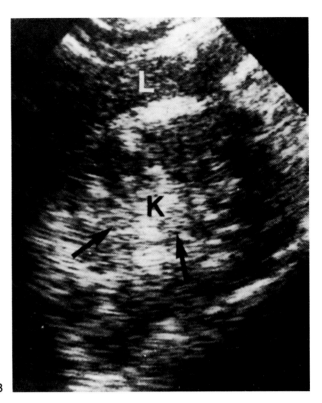

Fig. 13-170. AIDS, partial, combined pattern. **(A)** Longitudinal sonogram of the right kidney *(K)* showing high-level echoes throughout portions of the cortex (straight arrows), whereas spared areas of cortex have normal echogenicity (curved arrow). *(L,* liver.) **(B)** Transverse sonogram of the right kidney *(K)* showing medullary pyramids with increased echogenicity (arrows) interspersed with uninvolved pyramids. *(L,* liver.) (From Falkoff et al,[372] with permission.)

proteinuria. At ultrasound, the affected kidneys appear normal or may be enlarged with increased parenchymal echogenicity.[22]

The Finnish type of congenital nephrotic syndrome is caused by a rare, autosomal recessive gene and presents in infancy.[22,375] This type presents in early life with proteinuria, peripheral edema, and hypoalbuminemia.[375] On ultrasound, the kidneys may be markedly enlarged with diffusely increased parenchymal echogenicity and a thin, relatively hypoechoic subcapsular cortex layer.[22,375] The increased echogenicity may be secondary to the marked dilatation of the proximal tubules, and the thin subcapsular layer that normally lacks glomeruli is visible as a result of patient size, which allows the use of high-resolution ultrasound.[22,375] The major lesions are confined to the cortex, sparing the medullary pyramids, which are partially recognizable.[375] With progression, the kidneys may lose volume, appearing small and echogenic.[22]

Hemolytic Uremic Syndrome. Hemolytic uremic syndrome consists of a group of entities that have in com-

mon a direct toxic injury to the endothelium of glomerular capillaries.[376] It is characterized by a microangiopathic hemolytic anemia that causes thrombocytopenia, renal failure, and hypertension, and it occurs principally in children.[22,376] From 70 to 80 percent of cases in children occur in those less than 5 years of age, with a peak prevalence in the summer and early fall.[376] Often, it is preceded by diarrhea, which is commonly bloody.[376] The syndrome is secondary to endothelial damage to the microvasculature of the renal cortex, presumably by an endovascular toxin.[376] The resultant endothelial damage promotes red blood cell lysis, fibrin deposition, and platelet consumption.[376]

The ultrasound findings may be normal initially, or nephromegaly may be seen. There may be increased cortical echogenicity with more severe involvement (Fig. 13-171). The degree of cortical echogenicity on the initial ultrasound examination has been shown to correlate with the clinical outcome in 80 percent of patients.[22] The accentuation of the normal corticomedullary differentiation is caused by a relative increase in cortical echogenicity, with preservation of the normally hypoechoic renal medulla.[376]

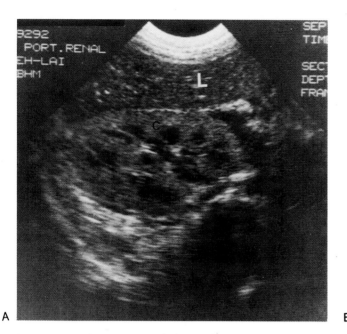
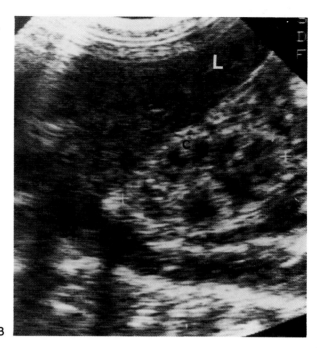

Fig. 13-171. Hemolytic uremic syndrome. Case 1. **(A)** Grade II, moderate disease. The renal cortex *(c)* is slightly more echoic than the liver *(L)*. Case 2. **(B)** Grade III, severe disease. The renal cortex *(c)* is hyperechoic compared with the liver *(L)* and approaches the echogenicity of the perinephric fat. (From Choyke et al,[376] with permission.)

The associated ultrasound findings may have multiple causes. They probably result from swelling of the glomerular endothelial and meseangial cells and from the presence of platelet aggregates and fibrin thrombi in the lumen of glomerular capillaries.[22] This abnormality may represent the one situation in which the increased echogenicity correlates better with the interstitial processes of the kidney.[22]

In the initial evaluation, ultrasound may be very useful. As graded by ultrasound, cortical echogenicity correlates with the severity of the illness at its onset in 80 percent of cases.[376] As such, ultrasound may be helpful in defining patients at increased risk for permanent renal damage, who would be most likely to benefit from early intensive medical care.[376]

Hypertension. Ultrasound may show a striking increase in the intrarenal vascular echoes in children with hypertension, resulting in a dotted pattern at the corticomedullary junction[22,377] (Fig. 13-172). This pattern may be caused by a diffuse calcifying process involving the lamina elastica of the interlobar and arcuate arteries.[22,377] This calcification was not visible on the radiograph. Hypertension in children is frequently secondary to renal disease. Therefore, when evaluating a child with renal disease the examiner should look for hypertension.

Nephrocalcinosis. In children, nephrocalcinosis is rare and is usually associated with hypercalcemic states (treated hereditary rickets), renal tubular diseases, vascular causes, enzyme disorders, Cushing syndrome, homozygous familial hypercholesterolemia, prolonged furosemide therapy, and Tamm-Horsfall proteinuria in infants.[22]

Other. There are a number of other causes of increased renal cortical echogenicity in children. These include type I glycogen storage disease, acute multifocal pyelonephritis, sickle cell anemia, primary polycythemia, glomerulosclerosis with renal hypertrophy, oculocerebrorenal syndrome, renal dysplasia, oxalosis, and renal amyloidosis.[22]

Idiopathic arterial calcification of infancy is a rare disease of unknown cause. It is characterized by patchy destruction and disruption of the internal elastic membrane, with deposition of calcium hydroxyapatite in this layer.[378] Although the process affects both systemic and pulmonary arteries of all sizes, myocardial ischemia due to coronary artery involvement usually leads to death before 1 year of age.[378] In this case report, ultrasound revealed intense echogenicity of the aorta and its branches, with striking acoustic shadowing from the vessel walls. The kidneys were not enlarged but were dif-

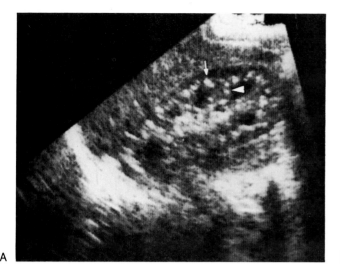
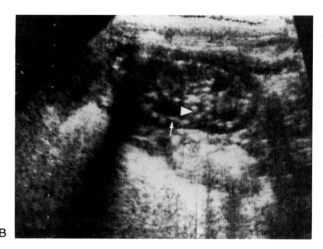

A

B

Fig. 13-172. Renal vascular calcification. Hypertensive child. Longitudinal scans of the **(A)** right (supine) and **(B)** the left (prone) kidneys. The arcuate arteries (arrow) and interlobar arteries (arrowhead) are abnormally visible. (From Garel et al,[377] with permission.)

fusely hyperechoic.[378] At autospy, there was microscopic calcification of the renal tubules and glomeruli.

Nephrolithiasis

Nephrolithiasis refers to a pathologic condition of calcium salts in the renal parenchyma.[339] They occur in 0.1 to 6 percent of the general population and are more common in males than females.[24] Most (65 to 70 percent) are calcium-containing stones such as calcium oxalate, or calcium oxide with calcium phosphate. Stones can form at any level of the urinary tract, but most arise in the kidney. The most important determinant of stone formation is an increase in the urine concentration of the stone constituents. A variety of conditions are associated with nephrolithiasis, including hyperparathyroidism, hypervitaminosis D, milk alkali syndrome, renal tubular acidosis, medullary sponge kidney, and hyperoxaluria.[75] To be detected by radiography, the calculi must be quite large.[337,355] Radiography often fails to show early renal calcification.[337,355] Ultrasound can reveal calculi as echogenic structures regardless of chemical composition.[379]

Renal Vascular Calcification. Calcification in the renal arterial network should be considered when echogenic foci with shadowing are seen in the area of the renal sinus (Fig. 13-173). This diagnosis should be considered in the sonographic differential diagnosis, especially in patients with long-standing diabetes, hypertension, or other systemic disease associated with accelerated atherosclerotic vascular disease.[380] Real-time scanning can help differ-

entiate these echodensities from calculi, since they are seen to pulsate.

Collecting System Calcification. Ultrasound has potential value in the investigation of opaque and nonopaque filling defects within the renal pelvis and in patients with urologic nonvisualization who are at high risk for uric acid lithiasis. The nonopaque stone may be formed of uric acid or urate, although there is the rare instance of xanthine and mucoid matrix stones. Uric acid calculi account for 8 percent of all renal stones.[381] Patients at

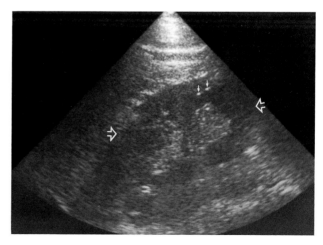

Fig. 13-173. Renal vascular calcifications. Adult diabetic with hypertension and chronic renal failure. Longitudinal scan of the right kidney (open arrows) showing multiple linear echodensities (small arrows) in the area of the renal arterial network. These were seen to pulsate at real-time examination.

risk for uric acid stones include ileostomy patients and those with myeloproliferative disorders (especially those being treated with cytotoxic agents), gout, and other disorders of uric acid metabolism.[381] By radiography it is difficult to distinguish nonopaque stones from TCC in the renal pelvis and calyces.

On ultrasound, all stones, regardless of composition, appear echodense with acoustic shadowing[379] (Figs. 13-58, 13-59, 13-63, 13-174, and 13-175). The intensity of the shadow does not depend on either the size or composition of the stone.[382] At times, the echodensity of the collecting system stone may be difficult to distinguish from the echoes of the renal sinus. The key is the acoustic shadow. For optimal visualization of this shadow, the following should be undertaken: (1) careful control of the overall gain setting (usually lower) to demonstrate the shadow; and (2) use of a transducer with the narrow part of its focal zone in the region of the suspected stone.[29]

The ultrasound detection of renal stones may be affected by transducer and scanning parameters.[383] At times, the ultrasound detection of renal calculi is disappointing. The need to show posterior acoustic shadowing may be the most problematic of the factors that contribute to the lack of specificity of ultrasound. With or without posterior shadowing, stones smaller than 5 mm in diameter are difficult to detect. Low-contrast images are best for detection of the associated posterior shadows. Echogenic foci in the kidneys that have posterior shadowing can be diagnosed correctly as renal stones 81 percent of the time; detection of the absence of a stone is more likely to vary with reinterpretation. A sensitivity of 80 percent and specificity of 86 percent have been achieved in the detection of renal stones. It is difficult to rule out renal stones in highly echogenic kidneys. By decreasing the contrast, either by increasing the dynamic range or by selecting a linear gray-scale map, this effect may be reduced. If focal zones may be varied, they

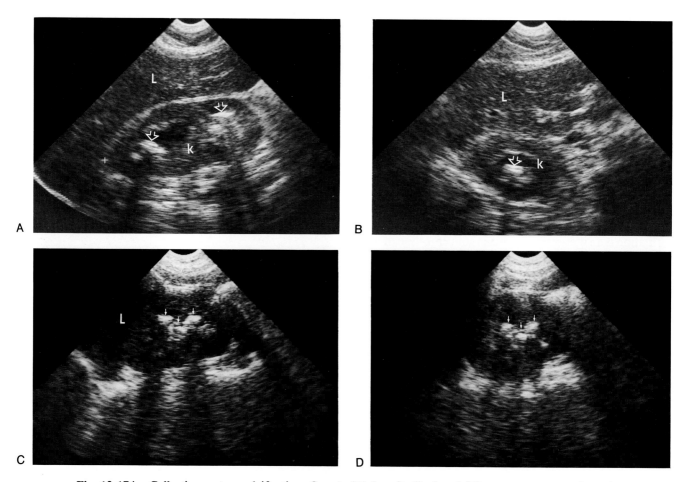

Fig. 13-174. Collecting system calcification. Case 1. **(A)** Longitudinal and **(B)** transverse scans of the right kidney *(k)* demonstrating collecting system calculi (open arrows) in both the upper and lower poles. There is dilatation of the collecting system. *(L,* liver.) Case 2. **(C)** Longitudinal and **(D)** transverse views of the right kidney. Multiple echodense collecting system stones (arrows) are seen. *(L,* liver.)

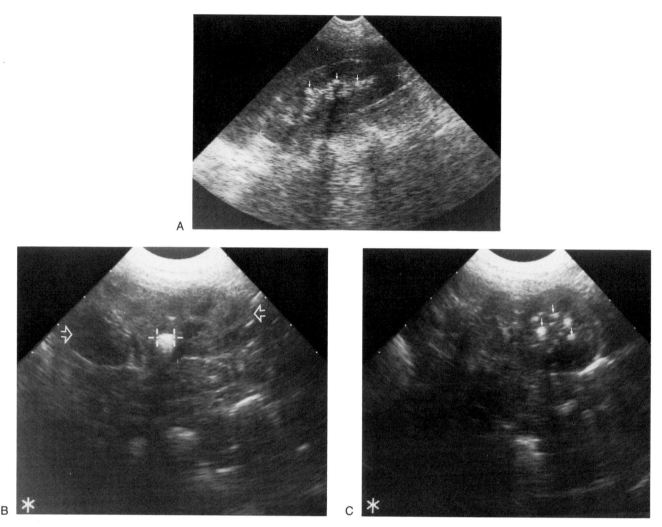

Fig. 13-175. Collecting system calculi. Case 1. Patient with acute monomyelocystic leukemia and urate nephropathy. **(A)** Longitudinal scan of the right kidney showing echodensities (arrows, calculi) in the region of the collecting system with associated shadowing. These were urate stones. Case 2. Neonate. **(B)** Sagittal and **(C)** transverse scans of the left kidney (open arrows) demonstrating an echogenic stone (calipers) in the region of the renal pelvis in Fig. B and several (arrows) in the lower collecting system in Fig. C.

should be placed at the depth of or slightly deeper than the suspected stone. By placing the focal zone at or slightly below the echogenic focus representing the stone, the posterior shadowing is sharper and there is less noise in the shadow. When comparing the various transducers, the annular-array transducer depicted stone shadowing with less ambiguity than mechanical sector transducers did 81 percent of the time.[383]

The sensitivity of ultrasound in the evaluation of renal calculi has been assessed.[384] It was found that the ability to detect renal stones by ultrasound was dependent on stone size but was independent of stone location or patient size.[384] There was similar sensitivity between the right and left kidneys. As such, ultrasound is believed to

be an effective means of detection of kidney stones in patients with suspected nephrolithiasis.

Extracorporeal Shock Wave Lithotripsy. Extracorporeal shock wave lithotripsy (ESWL) is the preferred treatment of renal calculi in more than 70 percent of patients.[385] After ESWL, patients with retained fragments require periodic radiographic follow-up.[385] Stone fragments act as a nidus for stone growth, and there is a greater prevalence of recurrent symptoms after ESWL in patients with retained fragments. The traditional means of following up patients with renal calculi is plain radiography.[385] It is important to have an accurate knowledge of number and size of fragments to determine the likelihood that they will be excreted spontaneously or require additional therapy.[385] Ultrasound tends to overestimate fragment diameter by a mean of 1 mm.[385] Even under ideal circumstances, ultrasound may fail to detect fragments as large as 2 mm. In determination of size, transducers of 5 and 7.5 MHz were more accurate than those of 3.5 MHz.[385]

After ESWL, ultrasound is not necessarily recommended. However, it is important to determine stone size to predict whether residual fragments will pass spontaneously. Ultrasound estimation of stone size in this instance was frequently inaccurate.[384] Additionally, ultrasound does not allow differentiation of intact stones from fragmented stones and cannot resolve closely spaced stones as separate. As such, it may be inappropriate for determining the success of ESWL.[384]

Other investigators found that the ability of ultrasound to detect renal calculi related not only to stone size but also to location.[386] In this series, 35 percent of calculi were not detected by ultrasound. Accounting for 28 percent of the undetected stones were stones less than or equal to 5 mm in diameter.[386] Taking into account the stones greater than 5 mm that were not detected, only a few were within a calyx or the renal pelvis. A total of 90 percent of the stones greater than 5 mm within a calyx or renal pelvis were delineated by ultrasound. Although ultrasound may be helpful pre-ESWL, its variable findings following ESWL indicate that it is less useful in evaluating the effectiveness of therapy.[386]

Calyceal Diverticulum Calcification. Calyceal diverticula are uncommon parenchymal cystic lesions that are believed to be wolffian duct remnants secondary to failure of regression of the ureteric bud. They are connected to the system by the renal pelvis, infundibulum, or minor calyx. They may develop stones and are a site of recurrent infection or rupture. Gravity-dependent echogenic debris within a cystic structure is seen with milk of calcium or stones in a calyceal diverticulum[387-389] (Fig. 13-176). Alternatively, an echogenic structure with associated shadowing may be seen with stones.[389] This may simulate calcification within the wall of a cystic mass.[389] As such, one should obtain scans with the patient in various positions to demonstrate movement.

At times, calyceal calculi are confused with gallstones on the radiograph[390] (Fig. 13-176). If calcifications are multiple, closely grouped, and faceted, the diagnosis of cholelithiasis is thought to be certain; however, they may represent calyceal calculi. Using physiochemical models for stone formation, investigators have shown that if more than one nidus for stone formation is in a saccular structure, the surfaces of the adjacent stones form unusual flattened rings of crystals in the plane of contact.[390] It is this flattening at the plane of contact when multiple stones are developing that leads to the formation of

faceted stones and can develop in either a hydronephrotic calyx, renal pelvis, or large calyceal diverticulum.[390]

Matrix Calculus. Matrix calculi of the urinary tract are rare.[391] This matrix is a mucoprotein that constitutes less than 5 percent of the dry weight of crystalline stones and between 42 and 85 percent of matrix calculi.[391]

Occurring more frequently in women, matrix calculi present with symptoms of renal or ureteral colic. Less commonly there are hematuria and dysuria. There may be coexistence of crystalline calculi, and they usually occur in the presence of infection with urea-splitting bacteria, typically *Proteus mirabilis* or *Proteus vulgaris*.[391] They form a cast of the collecting system and are puttylike in consistency.

If urinary matrix calculi are pure, they are entirely radiolucent; impurities may impart a faintly opaque, stippled appearance on plain film.[391] At ultrasound, such a matrix calculus is seen as a predominantly echopoor mass in the renal pelvis (Fig. 13-177). There was no associated acoustic shadow even when the focal zone of the transducer was selectively placed at the level of the mass. It was postulated that matrix calculi may have an absorption coefficient and acoustic impedance more closely approximating those of renal parenchyma owing to their low crystalline content. This might explain the lack of acoustic shadowing.

Milk of Calcium. Milk of calcium in the urinary tract is rare.[392] It is associated with primary hyperparathyroidism and possibly milk alkali syndrome.[388] The milk of calcium represents primarily small crystals of calcium carbonate, although calcium phosphate, calcium oxalate, ammonium phosphate, and calcium hydroxyapatite are also seen.[388,393] As a viscous colloidal suspension of various calcium salts, milk of calcium is chiefly carbonate, phosphate, and oxalate.[392] It may form relatively quickly and at an early age.[392] In most cases, obstruction and low-grade inflammation occur in a calyceal diverticulum, proximal to a partial urinary obstruction.[392] At least partial obstruction to urine flow with stasis seems to be a requirement for the formation of milk of calcium.[393] It is less commonly associated with UPJ obstruction, hydronephrosis, and/or a nonfunctioning kidney[393] (Fig. 13-178). Most patients are asymptomatic, although there may be coexistent pain and hematuria.[392] Ultrasound appears to be the most sensitive detector of this abnormality.[392]

Vascular Abnormalities

Color Doppler is potentially very useful in the detection and diagnosis of renal vascular lesions and has several advantages over conventional duplex ultrasound.[394] With duplex ultrasound, more active evaluation is re-

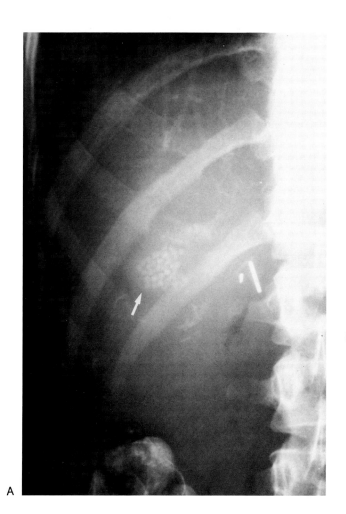

A

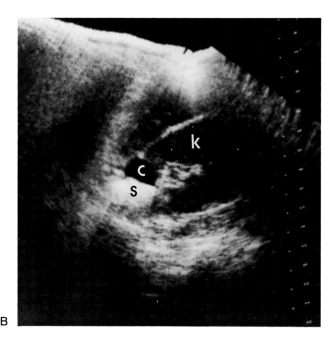

B

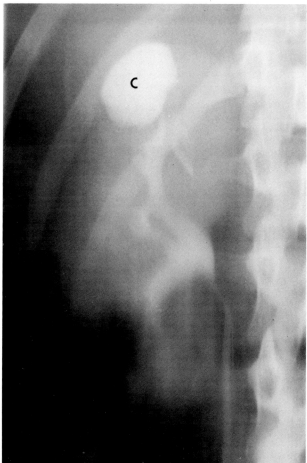

C

Fig. 13-176. Calyceal diverticulum calcifications. Stones. Patient who was postoperative cholecystectomy. **(A)** Plain film showing that gallstones (arrow) still appear to be present. **(B)** Longitudinal scan of the right kidney *(k)* showing an anechoic upper-pole mass (*c*, calyceal diverticulum) with echodense material (*s*, stones) layering within it. **(C)** Intravenous pyelogram showing a calyceal diverticulum *(c)* in the right upper pole.

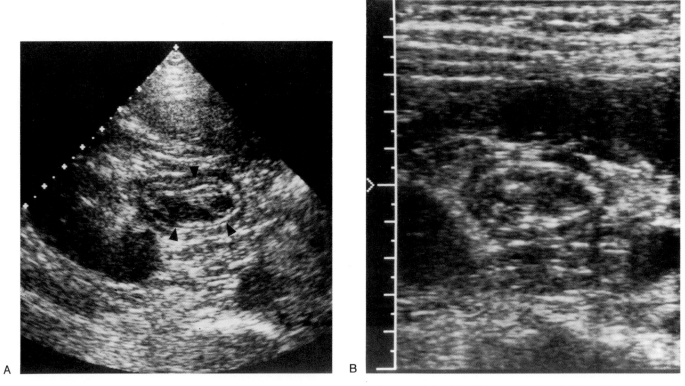

Fig. 13-177. Matrix calculus. **(A & B)** Transverse sonographic images of the right kidney at the level of the right pelvis. In Fig. A a predominantly echopoor mass (arrowheads) fills the right renal pelvis. Fig. B is a view using a 5-MHz linear phased array transducer. A mass 3.7 cm in diameter fills the renal pelvis. The margins of the mass are echogenic, but there is no posterior shadowing. (From Zwirewich et al,[391] with permission.)

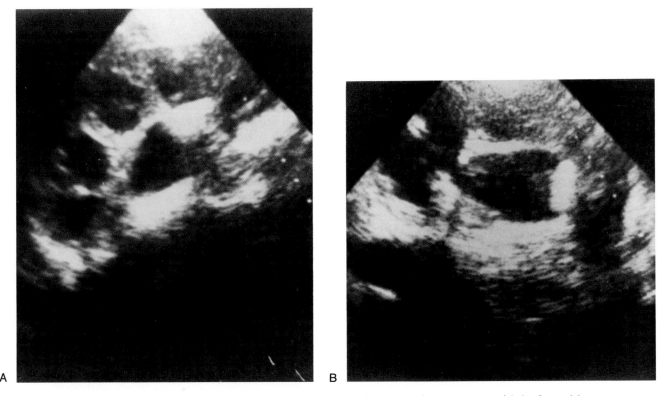

Fig. 13-178. Milk of calcium. Ureteropelvic junction stenosis. **(A)** Supine sonogram with horizontal beam showing urinary milk of calcium (UMC) levels in the dependent part of the dilated calyces. **(B)** Upright sonogram showing movement of UMC with changes in patient position. (From Patriquin et al,[392] with permission.)

quired by the examiner. For subtle lesions, considerable skill and persistence are required to asses flow. An area of unsuspected blood flow it is more likely to be detected by color Doppler than duplex ultrasound.[394] A color Doppler preliminary diagnosis can lead to a more tailored and efficient angiogram and, if possible, embolization.[394] More cases are needed to determine the sensitivity of color Doppler.

Hypertension. With renal artery disease, there may be fibromuscular hyperplasia and atherosclerosis.[10] In up to 80 percent of cases, the proximal renal artery is involved in atherosclerosis.[10] With fibromuscular hyperplasia, the involvement may be at all levels of the renal artery, but it is unusual for the orifice of the renal artery to be the site of narrowing.[10] The diagnosis of renal vascular hypertension requires (1) documentation of narrowing of one or both renal arteries, (2) evidence that the lesions are hemodynamically significant, and (3) evidence that the demonstrated lesions are compatible with the clinical picture for a renal cause for the elevation in blood pressure.[10] In patients with essential hypertension, there may be a loss of relative renal artery diastolic velocity corresponding to an increase in renal vascular resistance.[395]

Renal Artery Stenosis. Hypertension is a very common disease in the United States, but it has a definable cause in only 5 to 10 percent of cases.[13] The most common correctable cause of hypertension is renal artery stenosis (RAS).[396] RAS is present in 2 percent of adults with hypertension.[396] Several techniques for screening for RAS have been evaluated. Screening is most important in young hypertensive patients and patients with accelerated hypertension. Doppler has been evaluated over the past 10 years as a possible screening technique for RAS. Since it is a noninvasive technique and its cost is relatively low, it is a popular choice for the study.[13] Duplex ultrasound may have a possible role in the demonstration of normal renal artery flow pattern and the alteration of these blood flow patterns by vascular stenosis.[11] Renal arterial flow is affected not only by the vessel of supply but also by the physiology and pathology of the end organ.[11]

The main renal artery waveform has been evaluated. A peak systolic velocity (> 100 cm/s) is a useful criterion for indicating a 50 percent or greater stenosis of the renal artery.[13] A subsequent study showed that this threshold value resulted in a 31 percent false-positive rate and suggested the use of a higher threshold velocity (125 cm/s).[13] More recently, disappointing results have been noted when trying to apply a peak systolic velocity criterion to patients with different degrees of RAS.[13]

The ratio of peak systolic velocity in the main renal artery to peak systolic velocity in the aorta (renal/aortic ratio) has been described as a second major Doppler criterion for RAS.[13] When applying this ratio to significant (≥ 60 percent) RAS, a high sensitivity and specificity has been reported.[13] Other investigators have found it disappointing.

One promising method is the acceleration index (AI), a measurement of the tangent of the pulse inclination during systole that is corrected for the frequency of the transducer.[397] A sensitivity of 100 percent and a specificity of 93 percent have been reported.[397] This AI is angle-dependent, and this may cause problems in some patients.[398]

Some investigators have evaluated the pulsatility flow index (PFI) in the assessment of RAS.[12] The PFI is calculated by dividing the area (A) by the cycle time (T) and the maximum frequency shift $(Y_{max}: PFI = A/(Y_{max} \times T)$. In normal subjects the values range from 0.48 to 0.71. In individuals with RAS the PFI range is 0.72 to 0.79.[12] In the normal subjects with normal angiograms, the PFI is normal. The PFI may prove to be a fast method for the detection of RAS in hypertensive patients and a sensitive follow-up technique to track success after percutaneous transluminal angioplasty.

Color Doppler assessment of RAS has been evaluated as a screening examination for the detection of significant RAS.[396] The peak systolic velocity (PSV) in the renal artery, the renal/aortic ratio (RAR) (ratio of the PSV in the renal artery to the PSV in the aorta), and the renal artery RI were assessed and compared with those demonstrated at angiography.[396] In this study, ultrasound criteria for RAS were an RAR of 3.5 or greater and/or a renal artery PSV of greater than 100 cm/s.[396] Both RAR and PSV demonstrated a sensitivity of 0 percent in the diagnosis of RAS.[396] In this study, technically adequate examinations were achieved in only 51 percent of kidneys (69 percent of kidneys with a patent single renal artery, 9 percent of kidneys with two renal arteries). This group of investigators concluded that with the current technical capability, color Doppler is not an adequate screening method for the detection of RAS. Continued prospective studies with color Doppler are needed.

There has been little attention in the literature to the intrarenal Doppler study of peripheral renal vessels (arcuate/interlobar) with regard to screening of hypertensive patients.[13] Intrarenal arterial Doppler might prove potentially useful since even with the most experienced sonographers, unlimited time available, and the presence of a single renal artery, Doppler examination of the main renal artery will still be technically suboptimal owing to gas, obesity, prior surgery, or other factors in many patients.[13] However, a recent study has reported the intrarenal RI to have no significant correlation to the degree of RAS in patients with hypertension.[13]

Technical and anatomic bases may explain the discrepancy between the results of different reports of

Doppler examinations.[13] Renal artery examinations are highly operator-dependent, and the accurate performance of these studies with reproducible results requires a skilled sonographer with considerable experience in this type of examination.[13] A complete examination may be very time-consuming, often taking 60 minutes or more just for the Doppler evaluation. Success rates of slightly greater than 50 percent have been reported by some; others report a 10 percent success rate.[13] Another problem with these studies is the presence of multiple renal arteries, which occur in 22 to 24 percent of hypertensive patients.[13] Doppler examinations in most of these patients are technically unsatisfactory.

Aneurysms. Renal arterial aneurysms are relatively uncommon abnormalities, with an incidence of 0.73 percent in a selected group undergoing renal arteriography.[399] These renal aneurysms may be true or false, with the false pseudoaneurysms (PAs) resulting from laceration of the renal artery or its branches secondary to penetrating, blunt, or iatrogenic trauma.[399] With duplex ultrasound, pulsatile blood flow may be demonstrated within the echofree lesion.[399] Others have shown swirling, bidirectional blood flow in the area of abnormality with a large renal PA.[394] As such, Doppler may provide an noninvasive diagnosis of renal aneurysm and may obviate the need for angiography or needle aspiration[394] (see also Ch. 11).

Arteriovenous Fistula and Malformation. Renal arteriovenous fistulas (AVF) are pathologic abnormalities that have markedly increased in frequency in recent years owing both to better diagnostic evaluation of the kidney through widespread use of angiography and to a real increase in frequency of the disease as a complication of renal biopsy, abdominal trauma, or certain urologic surgical procedures.[400] There are three types based on etiology; congenital, idiopathic, and post-traumatic. Congenital renal AVFs are rare.[401] Small lesions with no apparent origin are considered congenital, with large fistulas having a crisoid appearance probably representing true congenital abnormalities.[396] Acquired fistulas are usually the result of trauma and surgical or biopsy procedures or associated with RCC, but inflammation has been reported as a possible etiologic factor.[247,400]

In most cases, AVFs are asymptomatic. When symptoms are present, they include hematuria, hypertension, abdominal bruit, and high-output cardiac failure.[247,396,401] The most common complaint is hematuria.

At ultrasound, a cluster of dilated, blood-filled arteries and veins may be detected as a multiloculated mass[247] (Fig. 13-179 and Plate 13-1). Alternatively, a cystlike structure in the renal pelvis associated with dilatation of the inferior vena cava and renal veins may be seen.[396] Often associated with a saccular aneurysm, the fistula is frequently complicated by peripheral mural thrombus.[247] At ultrasound, this may be recognized by an anechoic central lumen surrounded by the solid irregular thrombus.[247] The use of Doppler allows both identification of the vascular nature of the disease process through demonstration of flow within the cystlike structures surrounding the renal pelvis and the correct diagnosis of AVF through analysis of the characteristics of the waveforms. Within the lesion, turbulent high-velocity flow may be seen by Doppler and high-velocity flow may be seen within the renal vein.[394]

By using color Doppler, a large frequency-shift range (55 cm/s) of maximum average flow velocity at zero Doppler angle) is used to depict high-velocity blood flow in the arteriovenous malformation (AVM). These abnormalities can be seen as focal areas of flow, portrayed as a mixing of light colors[402] (Plate 13-1). When considering the flow rate alone, only slightly or markedly high-velocity flow of the AVM is shown by flow of lighter colors.[402] The hue depends on the angle of insonation between the ultrasound beam and the moving blood as well as on the frequency shift, which is determined by the velocity of the moving reflectors.[402] Not only may color Doppler detect AVM, but also it may be used to monitor patients who have transcatheter arterial embolization or ablation as well as conservative therapy.[402] Successful therapeutic intervention is implied by the disappearance or diminution of flow shown as mixing of lighter colors.[402] In conclusion, color Doppler may be used to diagnose and monitor AVMs (see also Ch. 11).

Renal Vein Thrombosis. In most cases, Doppler assessment of renal vein thrombosis (RVT) has concentrated on the identification of flow within the renal vein itself.[13] The real-time findings of acute RVT are nonspecific.[13] There may be enlargement of the renal vein or thrombus within it.[403] Doppler interrogation of the renal vein may be difficult because of problems such as bowel gas, patient obesity, or excessive patient motion.[13] There may be increased renal impedance as a result of compromise of venous drainage and perhaps intrarenal edema in acute RVT. There should be an expected reduction of diastolic flow, detectable as an elevated intrarenal arterial RI.[13] The diagnosis of RVT may be suggested by the diastolic arterial damping in the renal parenchyma.[403]

The intrarenal arterial Doppler examination may be useful as a secondary sign of RVT, particularly in patients in whom renal vein examination is not feasible[13] (see also Ch. 11).

Renal Biopsy

The renal biopsy is the singular most important instrument in the diagnosis of renal medical disease. Satisfactory categorization of the biopsy specimen requires light microscopy, electron microscopy, and immunofluorescence studies. The success rate of a percutaneous renal biopsy depends on the ability to accurately localize the kidney.[404] Ultrasound has helped immensely with this.[405] The lower pole is usually chosen for the biopsy because this area contains the smallest number of large blood vessels and is the least vascular portion of the parenchyma. Real-time ultrasound has not only increased the speed of the procedure but has also led to a decreased number of passes by the biopsy needle. This procedure is usually done by both the nephrologist and sonologist. The sonologist monitors the sterile ultrasound, while the nephrologist performs the biopsy by using a real-time needle guide (see also Ch. 19).

The complication rate for the renal biopsy procedure has been reported to be 0.7 to 8.1 percent. Complications include oliguria, decreased hematocrit, hematuria, AVF, and abscess. More than 50 percent of patients have hematomas on CT, but most of these hematomas are small and are not clinically apparent.[329,406]

Obtaining enough tissue for diagnosis while causing the minimum morbidity and mortality is the ultimate goal of the renal biopsy.[161] In one series, surgical and percutaneous biopsies were compared. Adequate tissue was obtained in 100 percent of surgical biopsies and in 82.5 percent of closed biopsies.[161] Other investigators report an accuracy of 93 to 96 percent when using ultrasound to guide the renal biopsies.[407,408] A 100 percent accuracy has been described in obtaining renal tissue, with an 88.6 percent rate of obtaining glomeruli.[404] After the initial diagnosis is made by biopsy, there is good correlation between cortical echogenicity and the sever-

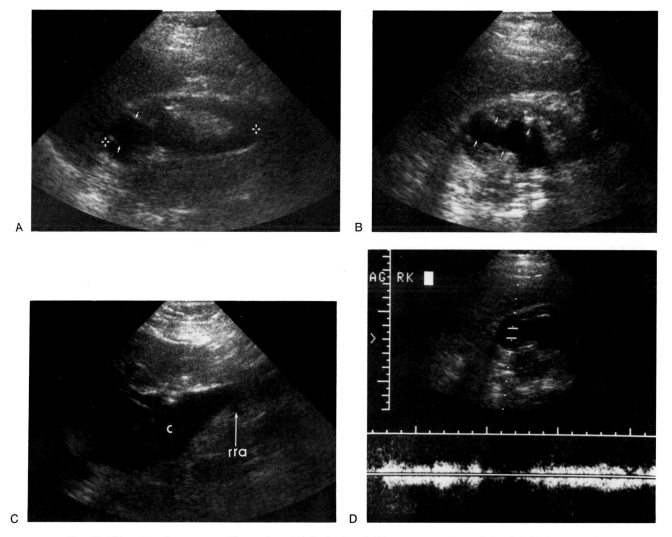

Fig. 13-179. Arteriovenous malformation. **(A)** Sagittal and **(B)** transverse views of the right kidney showing a tubular lucent area (arrows) in the region of the collecting system. **(C)** Sagittal view of the inferior vena cava *(c)* showing that the vessel is more dilated above the level of the right renal artery *(rra)*. **(D)** Duplex ultrasound showing turbulent flow within the lucent area. (See also Plate 13-1.)

ity of histopathologic changes, providing a promising noninvasive method for monitoring the progression of renal disease.[329]

The optimal needle size for renal biopsy has been assessed.[409] Both 16- and 18-gauge needles were evaluated both in vitro and in vivo; their use permitted a definitive histologic diagnosis in 86 and 75 percent of patients, respectively. The complication rate for the 16-gauge needle was 3.5 percent for major complication and 5.8 percent for minor complication. The 18-gauge needles of the same design have no major complications. The retrieval rate of glomeruli with these smaller (18-gauge) needles was insufficient.[409]

Investigators have evaluated the use of the Biopty gun in the pediatric renal biopsy.[410] With this gun, an 18-gauge needle is used, which is smaller than traditionally used. The use of the gun eliminates the more complicated movements needed to obtain samples by conventional manual biopsy techniques. There were no major complications and only one minor complication in this series. The time needed to obtain the tissue samples was decreased with this technique. These authors recommend the use of the gun in native pediatric biopsies.[410]

Renal Failure

Renal failure is defined as a degree of renal insufficiency causing substantial alteration of plasma biochemistry. Some investigators define it as acute reduction in renal function associated with a rise in the serum creatinine level of greater than 2.5 mg/dl.[411] It is termed acute if it develops over days or weeks and chronic if it develops over months to years. As has been described above, there is significant correlation between the cortical echopattern and the severity of the histopathologic changes, especially with prevalence of global sclerosis, focal tubular atrophy, hyaline casts, and leukocyte infiltration. Early in the process, the histologic changes may be isolated within the nephron, vessel, or interstitium. Tubular and interstitial alterations usually follow glomerular changes, so the degree of involvement in all three compartments is similar. Increased cortical echoes in advanced-stage disease result in combined changes within the glomeruli, tubules, and interstitium.[406]

Characteristic changes in the medulla have been noted in response to diuretic states. With increasing diuresis, the pyramids become prominent, anechoic, and easily identified. With increased edema encompassing the peritubular capillaries in the medullary region with medullary congestion, and with increased blood flow through the kidney, the medullary pyramids are easily identified, prominent, and anechoic. Although detection of the medullary pyramids appears to correlate with the histopathologic changes in the cortex, there appears to be a relationship between the number of hyaline casts per glomerulus and nonvisualization of the pyramids. By contrast, the pyramids are echogenic and nephrocalcinosis.[406]

On ultrasound the renal sinus is characteristically echodense, primarily as a result of the hilar adipose tissue, whereas the blood vessels and collecting structures make a secondary contribution. The high-amplitude pattern is secondary to the inherent scattering properties of the fat cells and is not due to coexisting fibrous tissue septa. Minor cellular infiltration causes partitioning of the fat cells. With increased septal thickness, the spatial design of the renal sinus is altered. The sinus echoes evolve into a inhomogeneous, patchy, coarse pattern. As the infiltrative process proceeds, fibrosis follows and atrophy and loss of adipose tissue cells are noted. In the advanced stage, fibrous tissue predominates, with a few widely spaced fat cells. Therefore, as the renal sinus is replaced by fibrous tissue, the fat cells are rarely seen and the echogenicity of the renal sinus decreases with loss of a distinct renal sinus.[406]

Renal size is another parameter that can be evaluated in renal failure. The long axis is inclined and the kidney rotated with its hilum facing forward and medial. The upper pole is posterior and the lower pole anterior. The decubitus coronal scan provides the long dimension of the kidney, and the renal hilum is best displayed. Renal lengths obtained on prone or supine views are inaccurate. If the adult kidney is less than 10 cm long, it is considered small.[406]

Acute Renal Failure

Acute renal failure (ARF) may be prerenal (renal hypoperfusion secondary to a systemic cause), renal (as a result of medical disease), or postrenal (as a result of outflow obstruction). The prerenal form may be distinguished from the others by laboratory and clinical data. Since the postrenal etiologies (5 percent incidence) are surgically repairable, the diagnosis should be made rapidly with a high degree of accuracy. The renal medical diseases are the most common causes of ARF, with the most common being acute tubular necrosis (ATN) (Table 13-2). In infants, ARF may be caused by the precipitation of Tamm-Horsfall proteins in the tubules.[13] Other causes of ARF include acute interstitial nephritis (often drug-induced), cortical necrosis, and a varied group of disease that affect glomeruli and small blood vessels, including acute portstreptococcal glomerulonephritis, systemic lupus erythematosus, polyarteritis nodosa, and the hemolytic uremic syndrome.[13] In rare cases, ARF is seen with rhabdomyolysis,

TABLE 13-2. Medical Cause of Acute Renal Failure

Acute tubular necrosis
    Ischemic disorders
        Major trauma
        Massive hemorrhage
        Compartmental syndrome
        Septic shock
        Transfusion reaction
        Myoglobinuria
        Postpartum hemorrhage
        Cardiac, aortic, and biliary surgery
        Pancreatitis
        Gastroenteritis
    Nephrotoxicities
        Heavy metals
        Radiographic contrast
        Organic solvents
        Pesticides, fungicides
        Antibiotics
Cortical necrosis
Acute interstitial nephritis
Diseases of the glomeruli and small vessels
    Acute poststreptococcal glomerulonephritis
Systemic lupus erythematosus
Polyarteritis nodosa
Subacute bacterial endocarditis
    Goodpasture syndrome
    Schönlein-Henoch purpura
Serum sickness
Malignant hypertension
Hemolytic uremic syndrome
Drug-related vasculitis
Abruptio placentae
Rapidly progressing glomerulonephritis

(Data from Huntington et al[22] and Chan et al.[405])

acute pyelonephritis, or major blood vessel diseases such as RVT or RAS, dissection, or thrombosis.[13]

The ultrasound findings in ARF are usually unremarkable. The main role of the ultrasound examination is to exclude hydronephrosis.[13,406] The kidneys may be normal-sized or enlarged. Usually, the cortical echogenicity is normal but may be low secondary to edema or hemorrhage.[13] In interstitial nephritis, the cortical echogenicity may be increased by cellular infiltration of the interstitium.[13] Usually, the corticomedullary boundary is well preserved; in some it may be accentuated by edema and congestion associated with increased medullary blood flow.[13] The medulla may be readily visible, probably as a result of congestion and edema. There may be compression of the renal sinus, or there may be pelvoureteral atony, with slight distension of the pelvicalyceal system.[13]

The causes of acute ARF in the neonate include bilateral renal agenesis, renal dysplasia, infantile polycystic kidney disease, congenital nephrotic syndrome, congenital nephritis, trauma, hypotension, hemorrhage, hypovolemia, perinatal hypoxia, congestive heart failure, dehydration, septicemia, disseminated intravascular coagulopathy, renovascular accident, drugs, toxins, and obstruction.[412]

Azotemic Patients and Obstruction. Studies have been performed to evaluate urinary obstruction in azotemic (creatinine level > 1.8 mg/dl) patients or those with worsening renal function.[413] Once patients with known obstructive uropathy, renal calculi, renal mass, or hematuria were excluded, only 9 percent had hydronephrosis. The authors concluded that in patients without a clinical history that suggests obstruction (such as calculi, bladder outlet obstruction, or pelvic mass), the likelihood of finding bilateral hydronephrosis by ultrasound is small.[413]

Another group of investigators evaluated azotemic patients who were at high risk for obstruction and those who were at low risk.[414] In the high-risk group, 29 percent were found to have obstruction, whereas 1 percent of those in the low-risk group did so. It was concluded that ultrasound be performed in these two groups only if temporization and standard medical treatment did not resolve the azotemia.[414]

Role of Doppler. Patients with ARF have been studied by Doppler to evaluate for distinction between acute prerenal failure and ATN.[415] Prerenal disease and ATN together account for 75 percent of ARF cases and are more common when ARF develops in the hospital.[415] It is certainly important clinically to distinguish between ATN and prerenal disease because volume status changes and optimization of cardiac output will generally restore renal function in patients with prerenal disease but will be ineffective or potentially harmful in those with ATN. The mean RI for those with ATN was 0.85 ± 0.06, which was significantly higher than the mean RI of 0.67 ± 0.09 in patients with prerenal ARF[415] (Fig. 13-180). An elevated RI was seen in 91 percent of patients with ATN but in only 20 percent of patients with prerenal azotemia.[415] Most of the patients in the prerenal azotemic group with elevated RIs appear to be in the group of patients with severe liver disease. This study showed that intrarenal Doppler allows detection of changes associated with ARF far more often than does standard ultrasound and may be helpful in distinguishing ATN from prerenal azotemia.[415]

Acute Tubular Necrosis. There are three different entities associated with ATN, and they have different echopatterns.[416] The most common cause of ATN is renal ischemia, followed in frequency by exposure to nephrotoxic substances.[13] Different patterns have been shown on ultrasound correlating with distinct clinical entities.[13] In ischemic renal damage, the kidney most commonly appears normal at ultrasound, with no change in cortical echogenicity or in the appearance of the pyramids.[13,416] When ATN is secondary to nephrotoxicity, there may be an increase in cortical echogenicity with preservation of

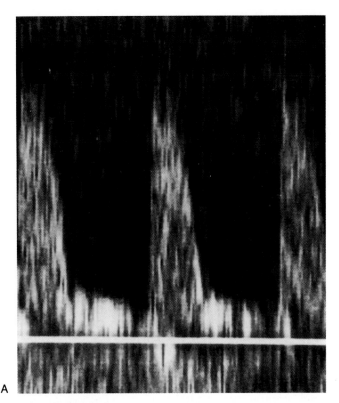
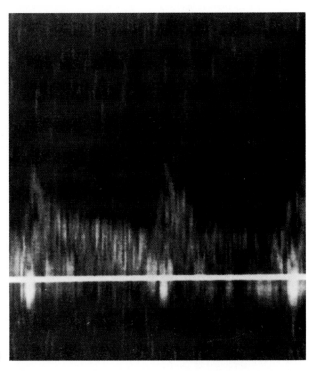

A   B

Fig. 13-180. Doppler in acute renal failure. Case 1. Acute tubular necrosis causing acute renal failure. **(A)** Doppler spectrum obtained from an intrarenal location in the right kidney is markedly abnormal with an elevated RI of 0.88. Case 2. Acute prerenal failure. **(B)** Doppler spectrum obtained from the right kidney is normal despite a markedly elevated creatinine level of 7.3 mg/dl (645 μmol/L). (From Platt et al,[415] with permission.)

the corticomedullary junction, and these findings show excellent correlation with decreased cortical blood flow.[13,416] With precipitated Tamm-Horsfall protein in the renal tubules, increased echogenicity of the renal pyramids is also seen.[13,416]

Some investigators describe several prominent findings with ATN: (1) increased renal size (especially the anteroposterior diameter, with the normal anteroposterior dimension being 4.26 ± 0.37 cm) and (2) sharp delineation of the swollen pyramids[411] (Fig. 13-181). The kidney with ATN is enlarged as a result of interstitial edema and increased water content; the degree of enlargement depends partly on the severity of functional or histologic damage.[411] The kidneys with an increased anteroposterior diameter/length (H/L) ratio may have a longer recovery time (mean, 32.4 days), with most requiring hemodialysis, whereas those with a normal H/L ratio may require less recovery time (mean, 15.5 days), with few requiring hemodialysis.[411]

Renal Cortical Necrosis. Renal cortical necrosis is a rare form of ARF usually associated with shock, sep-

sis, myocardial infarction, postpartum hemorrhage, and burns.[13,417] Ischemia may be due to intravascular thrombosis, toxin production causing capillary endothelium damage, or vasospasm of small vessels. The tubular cells of the cortex undergo necrosis, and interstitial fluid and leukocytes infiltrate the periphery of the involved area. The glomeruli may be necrotic, and thrombosis of arterioles can be seen. The medulla and the thin rim of subcapsular tissue are preserved. Calcification is often seen at the interface of the necrotic and viable tissue, with its earliest appearance at 6 days after the insult.[13,417]

On ultrasound, a distinctive pattern has been described.[13,417] There is loss of the normal corticomedullary region,[13,417] with a hypoechoic outer rim of cortex without calcification. (Fig. 13-182). The hypoechoic rim is thought to be the histologic zone of cortical necrosis. Both kidneys are of normal size.

Myoglobinuric Renal Failure. Myoglobin causes 5 to 7 percent of all cases of ARF, with renal failure occurring in 33 percent of patients with myoglobinuria. This pro-

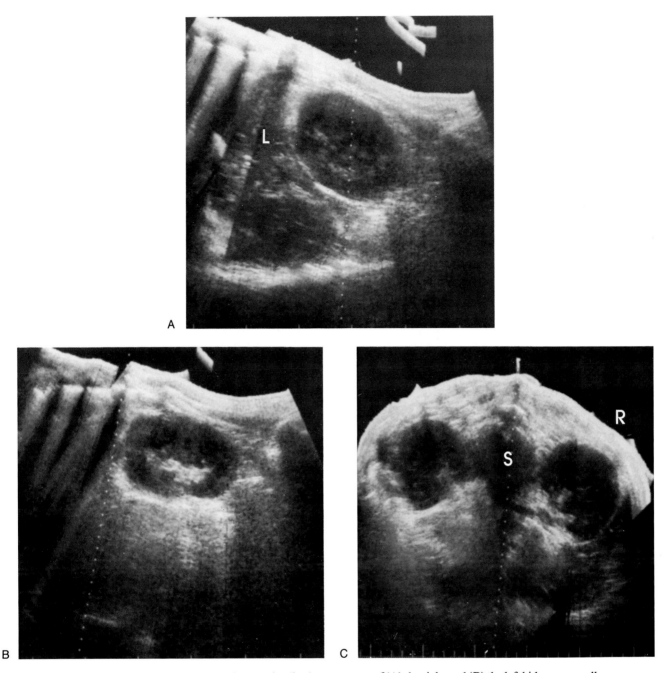

Fig. 13-181. Acute tubular necrosis. Longitudinal prone scans of (**A**) the right and (**B**) the left kidneys, as well as (**C**) a transverse prone scan. The kidneys have not increased in length but have markedly increased in their anteroposterior dimension. (*S*, spine; *R*, right; *L*, liver.)

cess results from rhabdomyolysis, which can occur in a variety of conditions. It is seen in drug and alcohol abusers. Ethanol and heroin have a direct myotoxic effect.[418] It can lead to ATN and renal failure that can be recurrent and can result in permanent renal damage. The theories for the pathogenesis of myoglobinuric renal failure are vascular, nephrotoxic, and tubular destruction.[418] On ultrasound there may be a spectrum of findings. The kidneys may appear normal, or they may be enlarged with increased echoes in the cortex with prominent pyramids[418] (Fig. 13-183). Making the correct diagnosis has prognostic significance.

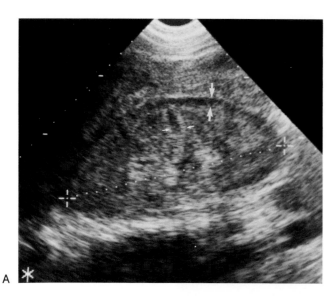 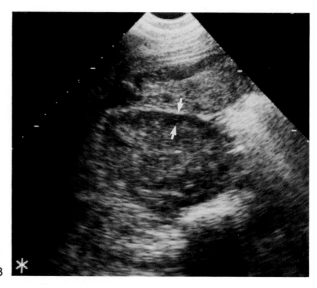

Fig. 13-182. Renal cortical necrosis. **(A)** Sagittal and **(B)** transverse scans of the right kidney in a sickle cell patient. Bilateral cortical necrosis developed. There is a circumferential hypoechoic band (arrows). Additionally, there are hypoechoic areas (small arrows) extending between the pyramids. At CT scan, these areas were lucent.

Ethylene Glycol Poisoning. Clinically, with ethylene glycol poisoning, there is a history of antifreeze ingestation with CNS, cardiopulmonary, renal, and metabolic manifestations. Ethylene glycol is metabolized in the liver to several intermediary forms, producing oxalic acid, which is deposited as microscopic calcium oxalate crystals in various organs including the brain, liver, and kidneys. The renal manifestations are potentially reversible renal failure and widespread deposition of calcium oxalate crystals within the tubules and their epithelial lining. On ultrasound the affected kidney is enlarged with increased echogenicity and partial obliteration of the definition of the corticomedullary junction (Fig. 13-184). Once the renal failure resolves, the kidney returns to normal size and echopattern; this may take 66 days.[419]

Chronic Renal Failure

There are three main types of chronic renal failure: nephron, vascular, and interstitial abnormalities (Table 13-3). After the kidney has been injured for a long period in the chronic stage, pathologic changes are seen in all three compartments, since they are interrelated. Multiple causes of chronic failure have been described, including glomerulonephritis, chronic pyelonephritis, renal vascular disease, diabetes, gout, sarcoidosis, dysproteinemias, and hereditary or congenital conditions such as polycystic renal disease and chronic tubular acidosis.[13]

With the exception of cystic disease, the ultrasound findings are not specific for a diagnosis.[406,420] There is no definite correlation between the echogenicity of the kidney, kidney size, and degree of decreased renal function.[420] However, if the kidney is more echogenic than normal liver, chronic renal parenchymal disease is probably present[420] (Fig. 13-158). The ultrasound appearance of the renal parenchyma corresponds to the degree of the histopathologic changes, and the advanced changes in the glomeruli, interstitium, and tubules cause an increase in the echoes in the cortex. In the end-stage kidney, there is loss of distinction between the cortex and the medulla (Fig. 13-185). When correlating kidney length with severity of the pathologic changes, a relationship is noted between length and prevalence of global sclerosis, focal tubular atrophy, and the number of hyaline casts per glomerulus.[406] In cases of renal failure, ultrasound is usually performed to exclude obstruction. Fifty-seven percent of kidneys are small, or there is a size difference of more than 1.5 cm between the two kidneys.[420] In 43 percent of cases, the kidneys are of normal size.[420]

Dialysis Patients

In patients with end-stage kidney disease, especially those treated with dialysis, proliferative processes develop in their native kidneys that result in the formation of multiple acquired renal cysts, renal adenomas, and carcinomas.[421] Dialysis appears to fail to clear unknown bioactive substances, possibly polyamines, which exert renotropic or mitogenic effects on the native kidneys,

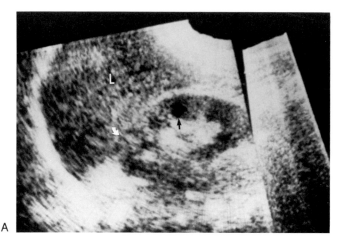
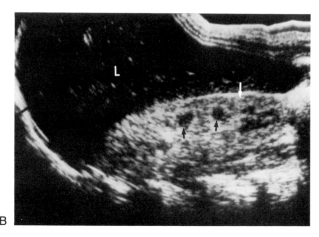

Fig. 13-183. Myoglobinuric renal failure. **(A)** Longitudinal scan of the right kidney through the right lobe of the liver *(L)* showing an enlarged kidney (14 cm). The renal pyramids are prominent (black arrow). Renal cortical echogenicity is equal to or greater than that of the liver (white arrow). **(B)** Longitudinal scan of an enlarged right (15-cm) kidney with increased cortical echogenicity (white arrow) and prominent renal pyramids (black arrows). Renal cortical echogenicity is much greater than liver *(L)* echogenicity. (From Pardes et al,[418] with permission.)

nducing smooth muscle, glomerular, or tubular proliferative processes.[422] Lined by low cuboidal or columnar epithelium, cysts are thought to develop as fusiform dilatations of the proximal tubules.[422] The solid neoplasms that develop (adenomas or RCCs) are almost always superimposed on antecedent acquired kidney disease and arise in some cases from papillary projections from the cyst wall.[422] In prospective study over a 7-year period, acquired cysts were seen in 87 percent of patients at the end of the study compared with 57 percent at the study's onset and there was a significant increase in mean renal volume with time.[421] In 17 percent there were large hemorrhagic renal cysts, and in 13 percent there were large perinephric hematomas.[421] With renal symptoms, 7 percent developed renal cell carcinomas.[421]

Uremic Renal Cystic Disease

There is a high incidence of bilateral cystic disease in patients who have uremia of chronic renal disease that is being treated by intermittent hemodialysis. Seventy-nine percent of patients have cysts when hemodialysis is continued for longer than 3 years.[406,423,424] Some report a 90 percent incidence after 3 years of long-term dialysis.[422] Ninety percent of patients on dialysis for 10 years or more develop acquired renal cystic disease.[421] After

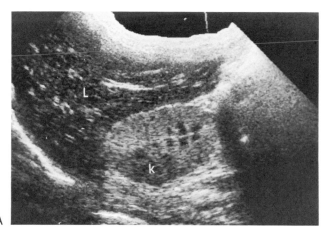
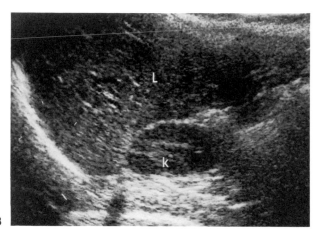

Fig. 13-184. Ethylene glycol poisoning. **(A)** Longitudinal scan of the right kidney *(k)* showing intensely echogenic parenchyma with incomplete obliteration of the corticomedullary junction. The kidney is grossly enlarged. *(L,* liver.) **(B)** Longitudinal scan of right kidney *(k)* obtained after full recovery of renal function demonstrating a normal size and echopattern. *(L,* liver.) (From Walker et al,[419] with permission.)

TABLE 13-3. Medical Cause of Chronic Renal Failure

Glomerulonephritis
Chronic pyelonephritis
Renal vascular disease
Metabolic
    Diabetes
    Gout
    Hypercalcemia
    Hyperoxaluria
    Cystinosis
    Fabry's disease
Nephrotoxins
Tuberculosis
Sarcoid
Dysproteinemia
    Myeloma
    Amyloidosis
    Mixed IgA-IgM cryoglobinemia
    Waldenström's macroglobinemia
Hereditary or congenital
    Polycystic kidney disease
    Medullary cystic disease
    Alport syndrome
    Cystinosis
    Hyperoxaluria
    Chronic tubular acidosis
    Infantile nephrotic syndrome
    Dysplastic kidney
Radiation
Major blood vessel disease
    Renal artery
        Thrombosis
        Embolism
        Stenosis
    Bilateral renal vein thrombosis
Hepatorenal syndrome
Acute pyelonephritis

(Data from Huntington et al[22] and Chan et al.[405])

less than 3 years of dialysis, 43 percent of patients are affected.[406,423,424] The mean age of such a patient is 40 years.[425]

These cysts are located throughout the kidney and may be multiple, 0.5 to 2 cm in diameter, and bilateral.[424] They are lined by flattened cuboidal or papillary epithelium. Proposed etiologies for their production includes altered compliance of the tubular basement membrane and an obstructive lesion caused by focal proliferation of the tubular epithelium. Other theories imply that the ducts become obstructed by surrounding interstitial fibrosis or oxalate crystals.[424–426] Still other causes include vascular insufficiency and direct toxicity by circulating metabolites.[426]

The kidneys involved are generally low-normal in size or atrophic. The renal volume is decreased when there is parenchymal destruction. With cyst development, the kidneys may increase in size[423] (Fig. 13-186). In the absence of complications, the cysts do not significantly increase renal size.[426] Complications of these cysts are not uncommon. Hemorrhage into the cysts with macrohematuria and retroperitoneal hemorrhage from cyst rupture are possibilities.[421,423,426] The dialyzed patient is at risk for hemorrhage as result of frequent anticoagulant therapy for dialysis.[426] Bleeding diatheses of uremic patients also contribute to risk, and unsupported sclerotic blood vessels rupture with minor trauma.[425] Increased awareness of the occurrence of uremic cystic disease and its complications should lead to annual screening of patients undergoing hemodialysis.[425] If a patient on

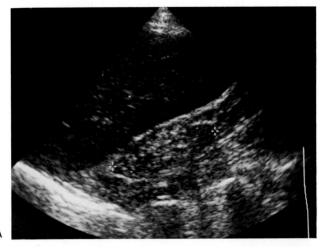
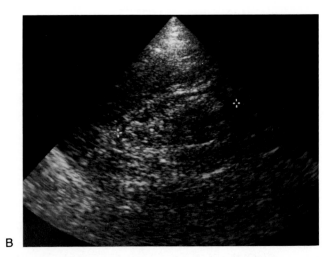

A   B

Fig. 13-185. Chronic renal failure. Sagittal scan of (**A**) the right and (**B**) the left kidneys. The outline of the kidneys can barely be distinguished (calipers). The kidneys are small and more echogenic than the liver or spleen. It was easier to distinguish renal margins on real-time sonography. There is loss of distinction between cortex, medulla, and renal sinus. This hypertensive patient had long-standing chronic renal failure.

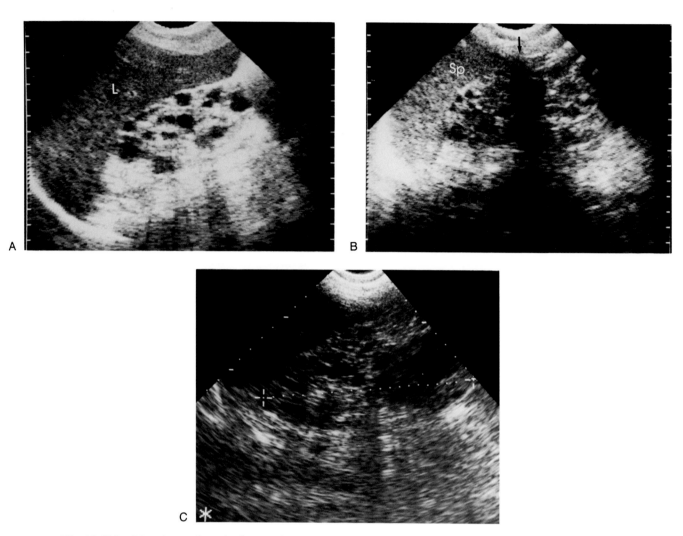

Fig. 13-186. Uremic renal cystic disease. Case 1. Longitudinal scans of the **(A)** right (supine) and **(B)** the left (decubitus) kidneys showing a moderate increase in echogenicity in the right kidney, with a slight increase in the left. Multiple small cysts are present bilaterally. The corticomedullary junction and central medullary echocomplex are lost. An overlying rib (arrow) causes an attenuation artifact on the left. (*L*, liver; *Sp*, spleen.) Case 2. **(C)** Sagittal view of the left kidney (14.2 cm) showing multiple tiny cystic areas as well as several larger ones in the lower pole. (Figs. A & B from Kutcher et al,[425] with permission.)

chronic dialysis develops hematuria, flank pain, and/or a flank mass, the examiner should evaluate for uremic cystic disease.[423]

Renal Cell Carcinoma

Besides the increased incidence of cysts in dialyzed patients, there is also an increased incidence of renal tumors.[421–424,426–428] Forty percent of patients have multiple and bilateral tumors.[423,427] Other authors report a 13.3 percent incidence of tumors.[429] In a multiple series review, a prevalence of 7 percent for tumors was found for solid renal masses; most were benign adenomas.[422] An annual incidence of 0.048 percent has been reported, which is six times greater than the age-adjusted annual incidence of RCC of 0.008 percent among the general population in the United States.[421] RCC is four times common in men than in women, with a mean age in more common in men than in women, with a mean age in dialysis patients with RCC of about 50 years.[421] These tumors may be papillary adenomas and RCC.[426] Usually cysts are already present, especially atypical cysts, when the tumors appear. The neoplastic stimulus may be dialysis-related epithelial proliferation of both glomerulus and tubule. Polyamines, which are biologically active hormonelike substances retained in uremia, have been

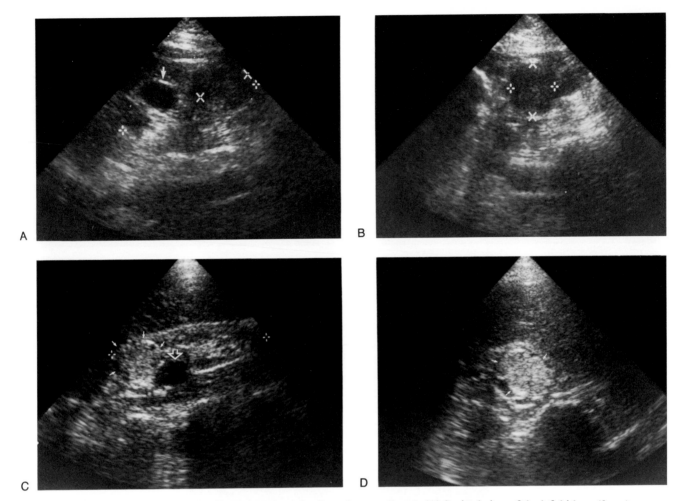

Fig. 13-187.   Uremic cystic disease and renal cell carcinoma. Case 1. **(A)** Sagittal view of the left kidney (9 cm) showing cystic changes (arrow) as well as a solid lower-pole mass (calipers). **(B)** Transverse view showing that this solid mass is outlined; it represented a renal cell carcinoma. Case 2. **(C)** Sagittal view of the right kidney demonstrating a central cyst (open arrow) and an echogenic upper pole mass (small arrows). **(D)** Transverse view showing that this mass (small arrows) is well outlined. It also represented a renal cell carcinoma.

considered responsible for this epithelial proliferation and subsequent tumor formation. These tumors tend to be small renal neoplasms (3 cm or less) and are significantly more common than invasive or metastatic carcinoma in dialysis patients.[421] Therefore, in addition to evaluation of the native kidneys for cysts, solid tumors must be excluded[424] (Fig. 13-187).

Physicians with dialysis patients must be aware of these complications. When such a dialysis patient presents with hematuria, flank pain, or any unexplained fever or systemic illness, this patient should undergo renal imaging studies. The discovery of an RCC in an elderly, unfit patient may have no effect on patient management or prognosis.[421]

Correlative Imaging

Investigators have compared CT and ultrasound in the evaluation of uremic cystic disease and tumors.[428] The two modalities were equivalent in the detection of solid tumors, whereas CT provided the best anatomic image quality and was more accurate in detection of acquired cystic kidney disease.[428] In the long-term dialysis patient, CT is better than ultrasound (59 percent to 18 percent) for detecting acquired cystic kidney disease.[422]

Most investigators recommend screening patients after 3 years of dialysis.[428] Some suggest dynamic contrast-enhanced CT scanning with the supplemental use of ultrasound as the best imaging regimen.[428]

RENAL TRANSPLANT

As a widely applied treatment of renal insufficiency, renal transplantation is a successful procedure secondary to better organ matching, improved surgical techniques, and more effective immunosuppressive drugs.[430] There has been a steady increase in graft survival (1) for patients who receive organs from living-related donors—currently 90 to 95 percent and (2) for patients who receive cadaveric transplants (at 1 year after transplantation)—currently 75 to 85 percent.[430] One-year graft survival rates are 80 percent or greater.[431] Serious surgical and medical complications can develop, which may threaten graft survival and, at times, recipient survival.[431] It has become increasingly important to develop noninvasive techniques that reliably detect and discriminate between such allograft complications as obstruction, perinephric fluid collections, rejection, cyclosporin A toxicity, ATN, vascular insufficiency, and infection in order to guide proper therapy in the large and growing renal transplant patient population.[430,431]

TECHNIQUE

Preparation

It is helpful to examine the transplant patient with some fluid in the bladder since this not only gives an anatomic landmark but also increases sound transmission. If hydronephrosis appears to be present, the patient should be rescanned after voiding. Differentiation between such fluid collections as lymphocele and bladder must be made by having the patient void.

Ultrasound Technique

Because the transplanted kidney is very superficial, a higher-frequency transducer may be used than during an examination of the native kidneys. As a rule, a 5-MHz scanhead will give adequate penetration. As with the routine renal ultrasound, the scan technique must be optimized to obtain parenchymal detail (Fig. 13-188). The sensitivity settings of the receiver unit and output of the transducer should be adjusted for each patient to allow optimal delineation of the renal cortex and medulla.[432]

This examination is especially facilitated by the real-time system because the renal axis is extremely variable. The first step of the examination is to locate the long axis of the kidney; subsequent scans are performed relative to that axis (Fig. 13-188). Besides evaluating the renal parenchyma (echogenicity) and sinus (pelvocaliceal distension), the maximum superoinferior length of the kidney should be measured. At times, the transverse and anteroposterior measurements are also necessary. These measurements are all relative to the kidney's axis, not the patient's position, because the long axis may be in the transverse plane while the transverse scans of the kidney may be performed in the sagittal plane. No study of the renal transplant is complete without evaluating the perirenal and pelvic areas for fluid collections. It is sometimes helpful to have the patient void and rescan the renal sinus if there is a question of hydronephrosis.

A baseline ultrasound should be performed in the early postoperative period, before the patient is discharged, or if there is a problem. The baseline scan is used to assess size, texture, etc.; its greatest value is its use as a comparison if the patient returns with problems.

If the scan is performed in the very early postoperative period, it can be performed by draping the scanhead and cable with a sterile glove and bag and using either sterile gel or sterile antibiotic ointment as an acoustic coupler. A scan performed in the late postoperative period need not be performed with sterile techniques.

Doppler Evaluation

A Doppler examination of the kidney should be performed as a part of every transplant study to screen the graft and associated vascular structures, with color Doppler followed by a duplex examination of detected flow abnormalities[433] (Figs. 13-189 and 13-190 and Plates 13-2 and 13-3). Additionally, color Doppler may

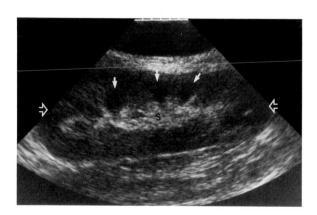

Fig. 13-188. Normal renal transplant. Sagittal scan along the long axis of a transplanted kidney showing the renal pyramids (arrows) as poorly defined hypoechoic areas. The arcuate artery can often be seen as echodense dots at the corticomedullary junction. The width of the cortex is measured between the medulla and the renal capsule. The renal sinus *(s)* appears echodense. The renal length (open arrows) is measured in its long axis.

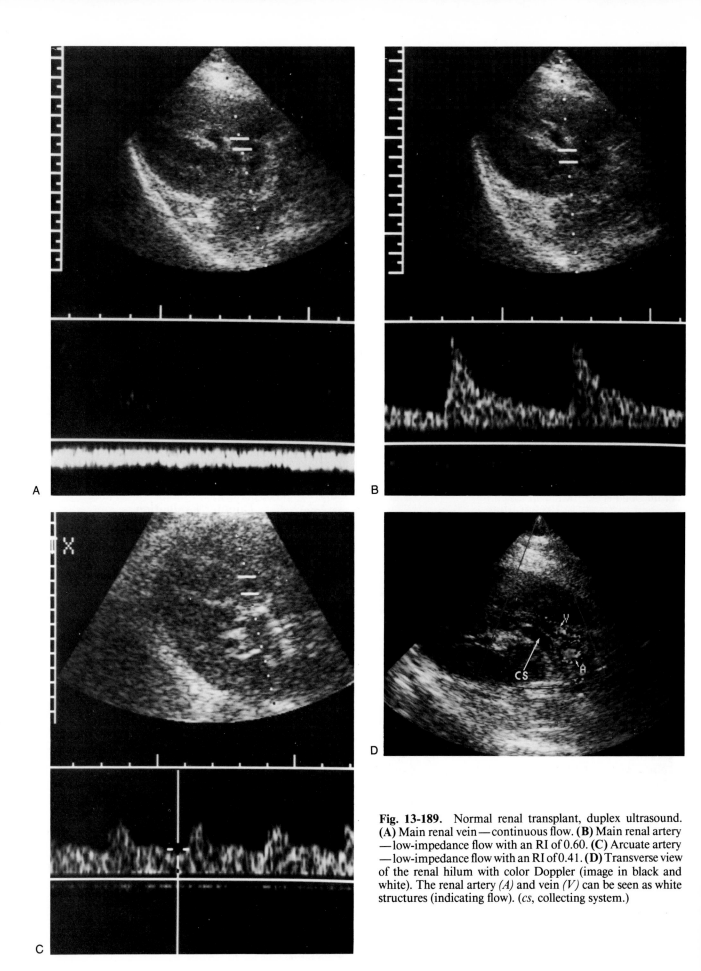

Fig. 13-189. Normal renal transplant, duplex ultrasound. **(A)** Main renal vein—continuous flow. **(B)** Main renal artery —low-impedance flow with an RI of 0.60. **(C)** Arcuate artery —low-impedance flow with an RI of 0.41. **(D)** Transverse view of the renal hilum with color Doppler (image in black and white). The renal artery *(A)* and vein *(V)* can be seen as white structures (indicating flow). (*cs,* collecting system.)

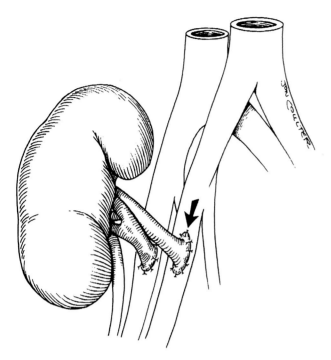

Fig. 13-190. Normal renal transplant, vascular anatomy. Anatomic diagram showing typical end-to-side anastomosis of the main renal artery and vein to the external iliac artery and vein. Note the Carrel patch (arrow). (See also Plate 13-2.) (From Dodd et al,[433] with permission.)

be used to localize the vascular anatomy for duplex evaluation (Figs. 13-190 and Plates 13-2 and 13-3). All four orders of the renal arteries may be examined: the main renal artery at the renal hilum, the segmental branches within the renal sinus, the interlobar branches on either side of the pyramids, and the arcuate vessels at the corticomedullary junction[434,435] (Fig. 13-5). Color Doppler can sample a long segment of one or more vessels at a time and display flow in vessels invisible to gray-scale ultrasound much faster than duplex ultrasound; it is also less likely to miss vascular complications than is duplex ultrasound.[433] Since color Doppler is unable to accurately quantify flow disturbances, all flow abnormalities detected by color Doppler must be quantified by duplex ultrasound.[433] Normally, the arterial Doppler waveform shows antegrade flow throughout the entire cardiac cycle when the renal capillary bed maintains its normal low-impedance state.[436] Information about the resistance of the renal microcirculation is reflected by the amount of diastolic flow in the main, segmental, or arcuate arteries as shown by duplex ultrasound.[436] The RI may be determined.[435]

To perform an adequate screening examination, appropriate adjustment of the Doppler controls must be implemented. Both color Doppler and duplex ultrasound should be performed with the lowest filter setting, maximal gain without background noise, and smallest

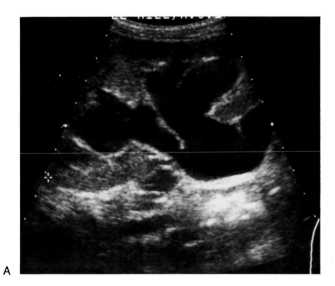

A

Fig. 13-191. Renal transplant, hydronephrosis. **(A)** Sagittal view showing that the collecting system of this transplant is markedly dilated. **(B)** By checking the RI at the junction of the collecting system with the renal parenchyma, the RI was found to be 0.60. This would indicate that this is an example of nonobstructive pelvocaliectasis.

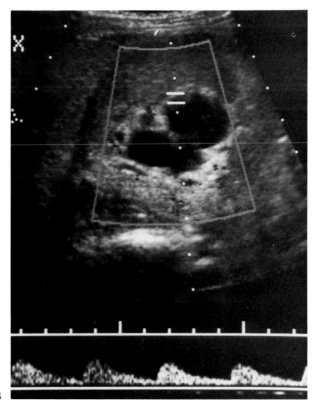

B

scale that will accommodate the highest normal peak velocities without aliasing.[433] The angle of the transducer should be adjusted to provide a small angle between the expected plane of the vessel and the ultrasound beam.[434] The assignment of colors to display vascular flow should conform to the convention that flow toward the transducer be displayed as red and flow away from the transducer be displayed as blue (Fig. 13-190 and Plates 13-2 and 13-3). It is most helpful if the peak velocities of the antegrade and retrograde flows are displayed in colors different from each other and different from the reds and blues used to display slower flow.[433]

It may be most helpful for new recipients of renal allografts to be referred for a baseline ultrasound examination within 24 hours after surgery, usually immediately afterward.[437] With the baseline Doppler scan, the amount of "normal" turbulence at the site of vascular anastomosis can be established.[436] This baseline examination should exclude occlusion of the anastomosed vessels.

Evaluation for Obstructive Hydronephrosis

For evaluation for possible obstructive hydronephrosis, pulsed Doppler examination of the intrarenal (arcuate or intrarenal) arteries are performed (Fig. 13-191). This is similar to the technique used for the native kidney (see above). These Doppler waveforms are made on the narrowest frequency range possible without aliasing, which maximizes the size of the Doppler spectrum and decreases the percentage of error in the measurement.[438] The lowest possible wall filter for the ultrasound machine is used. The Doppler sample volume should be 2 to 5 mm.[438]

NORMAL ANATOMY

Parenchyma

The sonographic features of the renal cortex, medulla, and sinus of the transplant are very similar to those of the native kidney (Figs. 13-1 and 13-188). To evaluate the renal parenchyma, the following should be assessed: cortical echogenicity, distribution of cortical echoes, characteristic corticomedullary junction, and size and appearance of the pyramids[432] (Fig. 13-188). If the medullary pyramids are greater than the height of the overlying cortex, they are judged to be enlarged.[439] Medullary conspicuity and diminution in renal sinus-fat echogenicity are subjective based on comparison with a normal native kidney.[439] Pelvi-infundibular thickening is present if the walls of these structures are perceptible.[439] Normally, the kidney has a smooth contour,

echogenic central sinus, and relatively hypoechoic cortex.[440]

Vascular Anatomy

To be able to accurately diagnose vascular abnormalities, one must be familiar with the postoperative vascular anatomy[433] (Fig. 13-190 and Plates 13-2 and 13-3). The choice of the type of arterial anastomosis undertaken is guided by the type of allograft available. A cadaveric kidney is harvested with an intact main renal artery and an attached portion of the aorta.[433] This aortic piece is made into a circular or oval configuration (Carrel patch) and sutured end-to-side to the external iliac artery of the recipient. When a living donor kidney is used, a portion of the aorta is not obtained.[433] Instead, the main renal artery of the donor is sutured either directly end-to-side to the recipient's external iliac artery or sometimes end-to-end to the recipient's internal iliac artery.[433] Most of the venous anastomoses are performed end-to-side to the recipient's external iliac vein.[433]

The kidney in small children is transplanted intra-abdominally with an anastomosis of the donor renal artery to the distal aorta and an anastomosis of the donor renal vein to the inferior vena cava.[440]

Size

The transplant tends to be longer than the native kidney, averaging around 11 cm. From the time of transplant, the kidney begins to hypertrophy. By the end of the second week, there is a 7 to 25 percent increase in volume (mean, 10 percent) with 14 to 32 percent (mean 22 percent) by the end of the third week.[432] Renal size in terms of volume can be calculated from the formula $V = L \times AP \times W \times 0.49$, where L is length, AP is anteroposterior dimension, and W is width.[432] Renal volumes calculated by using the prolate ellipsoid method ($L \times W \times H \times 0.5233$) correlate well with acute renal mass.[441] For the normal group there is a 24 percent increase in the follow-up versus baseline scan.[441] In the rejection group, there is a 73 percent increase in volume, with only a 27 percent increase in the ATN group.[441] If the anteroposterior diameter of the transplant is equal to its transverse diameter, transplant swelling is diagnosed.[439]

Perirenal Fluid

Normally, no fluid is seen around the kidney or within the pelvis of the transplant patient.

TRANSPLANT ABNORMALITIES

Renal transplantation has become the treatment of choice in the management of chronic renal failure. With improved surgical techniques, the operative mortality and morbidity are significantly lower but the transplant patient still remains at high risk of developing serious, even life-threatening postoperative complications.[442] Because the symptoms of surgical complications such as perinephric and pelvic fluid collections, renal vascular problems, and obstructive uropathy are similar to those associated with transplant rejection and ATN, radiographic imaging techniques are important in the evaluation of the transplanted kidney and its site.[442] The correlation of clinical symptoms, time of presentation of each complication, and diagnostic yield of an imaging technique provides the data for an algorithmic radiologic approach to renal transplant complications.[442]

Acute tubular necrosis, rejection, arterial occlusion, arterial stenosis, and renal vein thrombosis all cause ARF in the early post-transplant period. Differentiation of these entities by clinical and laboratory data is not possible. Radiologic procedures with contrast are not recommended because they contribute to further renal damage and seldom produce a specific answer. Multiple nuclear medicine studies provide functional and anatomic information, allowing specific diagnosis, but are frequently inconclusive. Ultrasound has enhanced the diagnostic armentarium for evaluating the renal transplant patient.

There have been several reports describing a nonspecific finding of renal collecting system wall thickening.[32,33] This thickening requires special attention to ultrasound technique for the accurate detection of this sign.[32] Visible thickening of the wall of the collecting system is seen on ultrasound as a marginal, intraluminal hypoechoic rim, which has been associated with acute rejection in the renal transplant as well as with a variety of other disorders[33] (Fig. 13-12). It has also been associated with urinary tract infection, reflux, and chronic obstruction in both transplanted and native kidneys.[32] Anatomically, the wall thickening correlates with submucosal edema in patients with rejection.[32] It may also be caused by inflammatory cell infiltrate, fibrosis, muscular hypertrophy, or hemorrhage into the submucosal space.[33] A thickening of more than 2 mm has been associated with rejection in grafts with marked thickening due to severe end-stage acute or chronic rejection in several patients who required nephrectomy after no response to medical therapy.[32] This finding resolves after therapy.[33] Since this is a nonspecific finding, it must be correlated with the clinical and laboratory findings.[32]

Urologic Complications

At times it is difficult to differentiate between rejection of the transplanted organ and ATN due to urologic complications, Also, multiple problems may coexist.[430] Urologic complications have been reported to occur in approximately 10 percent of renal transplant patients; they include urinary tract obstruction, extravasation, and pararenal fluid collections. It is very important that these conditions be immediately diagnosed and differentiated from rejection of the graft or recurrence of the patient's primary disease.[430] Delay in treatment of such complications has been associated with mortality rates of up to 22 percent and may result in loss of the transplanted kidney.[430]

Obstructive Uropathy

Compared with normal kidneys, the renal transplant collecting system can be more dilated in the absence of obstruction and the degree of dilatation can be influenced more by the amount of bladder distension. Patients with the greatest bladder distension may show the greatest degree of hydronephrosis, but hydronephrosis is not always seen with a distended bladder. If a distended urinary bladder is noted in conjunction with pelvocaliectasis, the kidney should be rescanned and the collecting system reassessed.

Obstructive versus Nonobstructive Pyelocaliectasis. It may be difficult to differentiate between obstructive and nonobstructive hydronephrosis in the transplant. As has been shown with the native kidney, Doppler may be helpful in this differentiation.[438] It is particularly important to diagnose this condition accurately in the transplant early in the course of disease in order to reduce transplant damage.[438] By performing Doppler evaluation of the intrarenal (arcuate or interlobar) arteries, the RI may be calculated (Fig. 13-191). With obstruction, an elevated RI (≥ 0.75) is seen.[438] Alternatively, a normal RI should argue against obstruction unless a ureteral leak is also present.[438]

Etiologies. The most frequent causes of obstruction in transplants include ureteral strictures, torsion, ureteral necrosis, blood clots, calculi, ureteral kinking, and extrinsic compression from lymphoceles or other masses[430,431,443] (Figs. 13-191 to 13-194). Ureteral obstruction occurs in 1 to 10 percent of transplants. The most common serious cause of obstruction following renal transplantation is ureteral necrosis; this usually presents within the first 6 weeks after operation.[444]

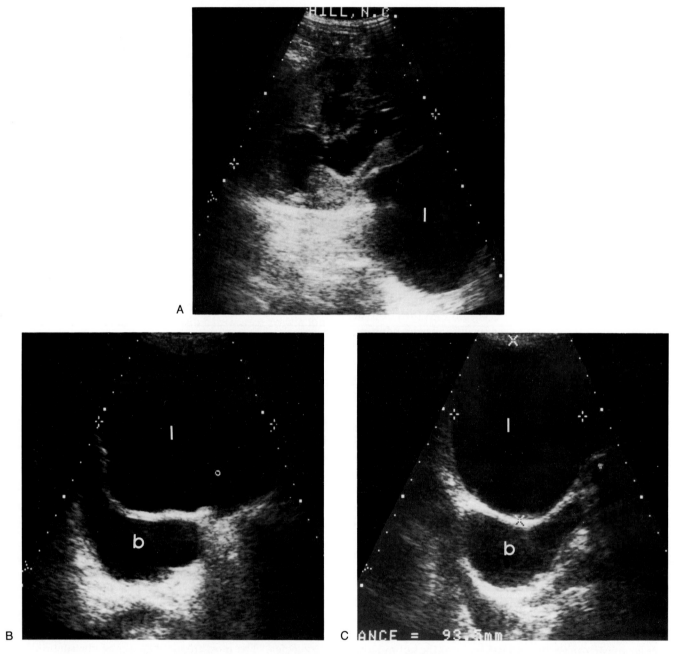

Fig. 13-192. Renal transplant, hydronephrosis and lymphocele. **(A)** Sagittal view showing dilatation of the collecting system of this transplant. A cystic mass (*l*, calipers, 99 × 69 × 94 mm) is identified within the pelvis, separate from the urinary bladder *(b)* on **(B)** sagittal and **(C)** transverse views of the pelvis. This represented a lymphocele; its mass effect was producing the obstruction.

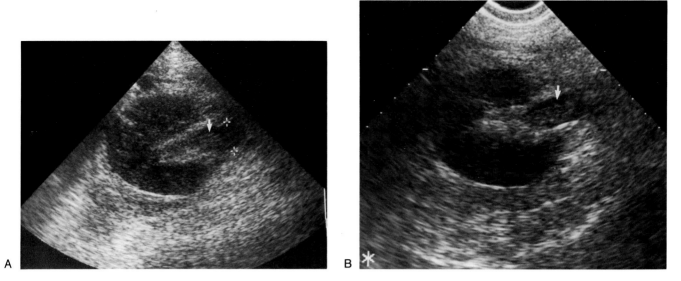

Fig. 13-193. Renal transplant, hydronephrosis and blood clots. This patient, who was recently post-percutaneous renal biopsy, developed hematuria following the biopsy. **(A & B)** Transverse views showing echogenic material (arrow) within the dilated collecting system. This was thought to represent blood clot.

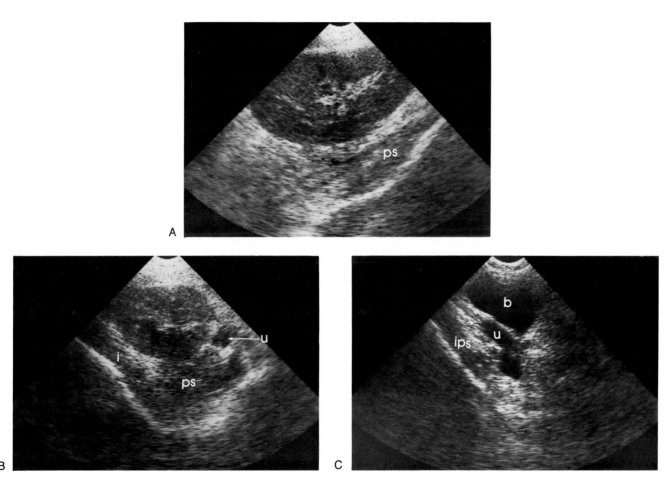

Fig. 13-194. Transplant, hydroureter. No dilatation of the collecting system is seen on **(A)** longitudinal and **(B)** transverse scans of the kidney. The ureter *(u)* is dilated medial to the kidney in Fig. B and posterolateral to the bladder *(b)* on **(C)** transverse scan of the bladder. On a nuclear medicine scan, there was isotope stasis within the ureter. (*ps,* psoas muscle; *i,* iliacus muscle; *ips,* iliopsoas muscle.)

Ureteral strictures are a late complication, in which patients present with a gradual increase in creatinine levels and deterioration in renal function.[444] They more commonly occur distally and are thought to be due to compromise of the tenuous ureteral blood supply, which results in ischemia and subsequent stricture.[430] The transplanted ureter depends on a rather long artery that originates from a lower-pole renal vessel.[444] During the donor surgery, the blood supply that originally arose from the bladder or retroperitoneum was severed.[444] This single long artery or the vein may become thrombosed during surgery, resulting in diminished blood supply to the ureter.[444]

Other causes of ureteral stricture include technical problems at the ureteroneocystostomy, acute rejection with edema at the vascular anastomotic site, and edema at the ureteric implantation site.[431,444] The long continuous blood supply for the ureter may become edematous secondary to rejection, with decreased blood supply again leading to stricture formation.[444] This may be treated by transplant ureteral dilatation.[430] Edema at the ureteric implantation site can cause temporary mild obstruction in the early postoperative period.[431]

Calculi may be another possible cause of obstruction. Calculi are unusual but may become more frequent as renal transplant patients live longer with their allografts.[444] In those reported, calculi presented more than a decade postoperatively.[444] These calculi may be secondary to altered calcium metabolism associated with increasing longevity.[444] The calcifications may be late complications, usually due to biopsy, infection, or alterations in calcium metabolism.[440] Uric acid levels may be quite high in patients treated with cyclosporine, which may also contribute to the increased incidence of stone disease.[444] These stones may serve as a nidus for possible infection.[444] At ultrasound, these calcifications appear as echogenic foci with acoustic shadowing and may be found in the collecting system or the renal parenchyma[440] (Fig. 13-195).

The ureter may be large postoperatively as a result of innervation and possibly relative ischemia. The size of the ureter cannot be used as a criterion for hydroureter (Fig. 13-194). Once hydronephrosis is identified in a transplanted kidney, one must search for a possible extrinsic mass[443] (Fig. 13-192). Optimally, the treatment of obstruction caused by blood clots, debris, or calculi is percutaneous nephrostomy.[430]

Perirenal Fluid Collections

Renal transplant patients are often evaluated by nuclear medicine to assess function. At times, a "halo" or photopenic area is seen around or to the side of the

kidney.[445] The differential diagnosis for such an abnormality would include a perirenal hematoma, a lymphocele, urinoma, or inflammatory edema.[445] These patients are often referred to ultrasound for further evaluation.

In as many as 51 percent of patients post-transplantation, there are perirenal transplant masses.[446] Well-known causes of perirenal transplant masses are hematomas, lymphoceles, seromas, urinomas, and abscesses.[446] Rarely, there is bowel herniation through rents in the peritoneum that occur inadvertently at the time of transplantation during preparation of the iliac fossa or through defects of the peritoneum that occur as anatomic variants.[446] The real-time observation of peristalsis establishes that bowel is present in the perirenal mass.[446]

Urinoma. A urinoma is a serious complication with a 3.23 percent incidence; it requires immediate surgery.[447,448] A urine leak is often followed by a wound infection that may lead to loss of the graft, generalized sepsis, and, ultimately, death. The most common cause of the urinary leak is a defect at the ureteropelvic, ureteroureter, or ureterovesical anastomosis. Ureteropelvic and ureteroureter anastomoses have a high incidence of associated urinomas and so are used less frequently. A less common cause is infarction of the kidney, with resultant necrosis of the parenchyma, and ureteral tip necrosis secondary to vascular compromise.[449] These represent primary leaks from the ureteroneocystostomy or bladder and leaks from the ureter caused by vascular injury.[431]

Patients with urinomas may present with decreased urine output, pain, and swelling over the transplant. These usually occur from 1 day to 3 weeks postoperatively, with less than 3 days most common.[442] On ultrasound, a hypoechoic mass (often with internal septation) usually producing hydronephrosis, is found[450] (Fig. 13-196). The location of the urinoma is variable, with most located near the lower pole.[451,452] Direct percutaneous aspiration and biochemical analysis of the lesion may not help if the graft function is poor, since the urea concentration in the urine can be similar to that in the serum.[431,449] Additionally, an antegrade pyelogram may be performed with percutaneous ultrasound guidance.

Lymphocele. The incidence of lymphoceles is 2 to 18 percent.[447,450] Symptomatic lymphoceles occur in 2 to 8 percent of renal transplant recipients.[430] The cardinal features of a lymphocele include progressive decrease in renal function, painless fluctuant swelling over the kidney, soft tissue shadow around the graft, and absence of demonstration of urinary fistula on excretory urogram or nuclear medicine study.[453] The presenting symptoms

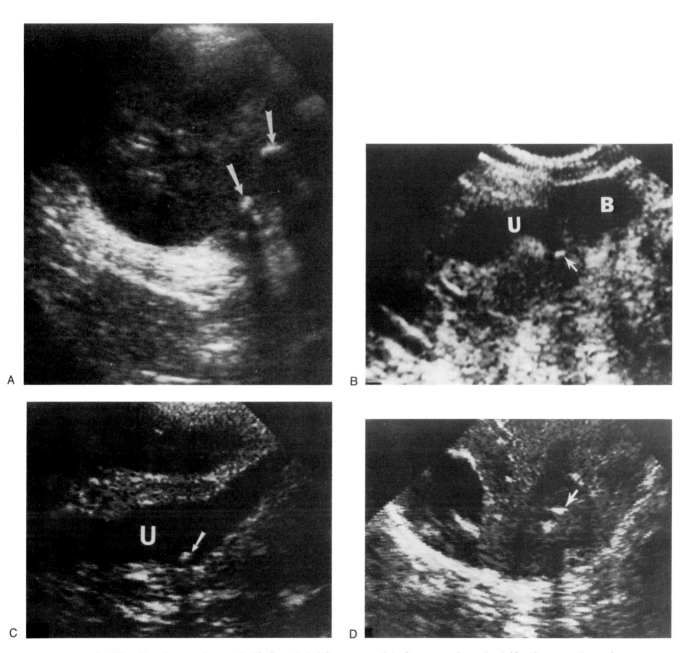

Fig. 13-195. Renal transplant, calculi. Case 1. **(A)** Sonogram showing parenchymal calcifications as echogenic foci (arrows) with acoustic shadowing. Case 2. **(B)** Sagittal scan along the course of the ureter showing hydroureter *(U)* down to the level of a brightly echogenic calculus (arrow). Dilatation of the renal collecting system was shown on other views. (*B*, urinary bladder.) Case 3. **(C)** A brightly echogenic calculus (arrow) is identified adjacent to the dependent wall of the dilated ureter *(U)*. **(D)** Ten minutes after Fig. C was obtained, the calculus was observed to move in retrograde direction up into the kidney (arrow). Other bright echoes within the kidney suggested additional calculi. (Fig. A from Surratt et al,[440] with permission; Figs. B–D from Stuck et al,[444] with permission.)

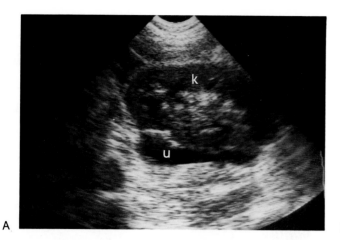
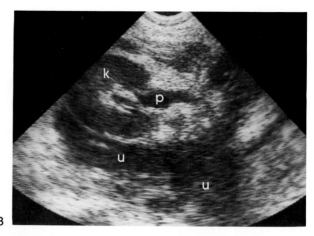

Fig. 13-196. Transplant, urinoma. **(A)** Long-axis and **(B)** cross-sectional views of a transplanted kidney *(k)* in a transverse lie showing fluid *(u)* posterior to the kidney; it extends into the pelvis. (*p*, extrarenal pelvis.)

may include pelvic mass, ipsilateral leg edema, ureteral obstruction, or hypertension.[430] Lymphoceles develop 10 days to 2 years postoperatively, with the average being 2 months.[430,442] Some investigators report their occurrence within 3 weeks of transplantation (although they can be seen later, particularly with acute rejection).[431]

There are two possible causes of lymphoceles. The lymph forming these lesions may result from the operation in which the pelvic lymphatics are divided and from the graft kidney.[447,450,452,454–456] There may be incomplete ligation of the lymphatics along the host iliac artery, permitting lymphatic leakage and accumulation in the surrounding connective tissue.[430] The lymphatic channels are damaged during the preparation of the pelvic area, and the kidney itself leaks from the injured capsular and hilar lymphatics.[454] The source of the lym-

phatic leakage may be from the transplanted kidney, especially during rejection episodes or urinary obstruction.[430] The lymph drains into the peritoneal cavity, provoking a fibrous reaction and becoming walled off. As the lesion gradually expands, there is pressure on the ureter, bladder, and kidney. These lymphoceles may deviate and compress the transplanted ureter or may compress the iliac vein and possibly result in fatal pulmonary embolism.[430] The importance of the lesion lies in its effect on surrounding structures, exerting pressure on the iliac veins (producing leg swelling) and pressure on the graft ureter (producing hydronephrosis).[450]

On ultrasound, a lymphocele appears as a well-defined cystic area that may be anechoic to hypoechoic[430,454,455] (Figs. 13-192, 13-197, and 13-198). They are usually situated medial and/or inferior to the lower

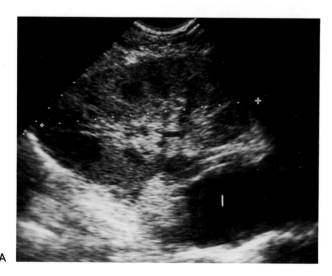
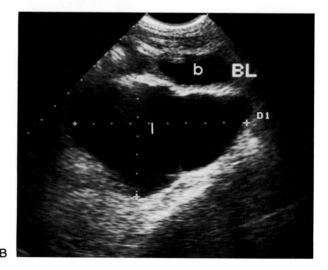

Fig. 13-197. Renal transplant, lymphocele. **(A)** Sagittal view of the renal transplant and **(B)** transverse view of the pelvis demonstrating a cystic pelvic mass (*l*, 92 × 62 mm) posterior to the bladder *(b, BL)*. No hydronephrosis was noted.

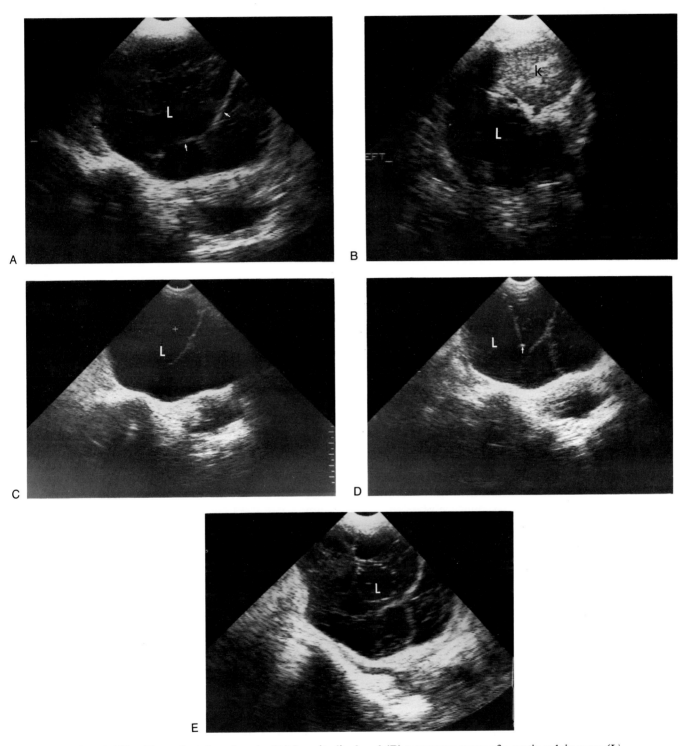

Fig. 13-198. Transplant. lymphocele. **(A)** Longitudinal and **(B)** transverse scans of a cystic pelvic mass *(L)*. Although the mass is cystic, it contains many septations (arrows). In Fig. B, the lower pole of the kidney *(k)* is seen along the lateral aspect of the mass. Because there was hydronephrosis, percutaneous drainage was undertaken. **(C)** Longitudinal scan of the cystic mass *(L)*. A depth was determined (caliper). **(D)** After 92 ml of fluid was removed, the lymphocele was rescanned. The mass *(L)* is smaller, and the needle tip (arrow) can be seen as a bright echo within the mass. The lymphocele was aspirated as dry as possible. **(E)** One day later, the mass *(L)* was rescanned longitudinally. The mass had reaccumulated, and many more septations were present.

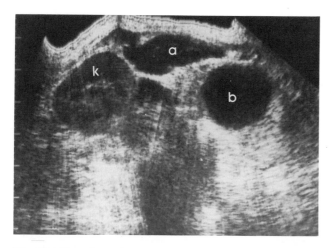

Fig. 13-199. Transplant, abscess. Oblique scan parallel to the inguinal ligament. An irregular complex mass *(a)* is seen between the bladder *(b)* and transplanted kidney *(k)* containing echogenic debris. (From Coyne et al,[442] with permission.)

pole of the transplant, where they can obstruct the ureter and cause graft dysfunction.[431] In one series, 67 percent were located inferomedial to the transplant.[442] They are commonly large and septated.[431] Sixty-seven percent were cystic with septations, 33 percent were cystic, and 55 percent conformed to the anatomic pelvis.[442] Ultrasound is not capable of differentiating lymphoceles from urinomas, hematomas, or abscesses.[430] Although ultrasound-guided aspiration may help exclude a urinoma and make the diagnosis of a lymphocele, it is usually not definitive in the treatment of the abnormality.[430,448] As such, lymphoceles must be observed for recurrence and surgical therapy is recommended if

symptoms recur.[430] Lymphoceles are generally treated by marsupialization into the peritoneum or external drainage with breakdown of all loculi.[450,456]

Abscess. A paratransplant abscess is not a common problem but is often associated with other complications, such as urinary fistula, lymphocele, or hematoma.[430] Since transplant patients are immunosuppressed, abscess formation can rapidly proceed to sepsis and death.[430] Patients with an abscess post-transplant present with elevated temperature, increased white blood cell count, proteinuria, and increased creatinine levels. Steroids may mask the usual signs.[447] These lesions develop from 6 days to 4 months postoperatively, with an average of 2 months.[442] The abscess may be variable in location and echofree to complex in its echopattern[442,448] (Fig. 13-199). Although ultrasound alone may not be able to differentiate abscesses from other fluid collections, a percutaneous aspiration can rapidly help to yield the diagnosis.[430]

Hematoma. The patient with acute hematoma may present with a minimal decrease in hemoglobin and blood pressure, decreased urine output, and pain and/or palpable mass. With a chronic hematoma, an increased creatinine level and temperature are seen. These develop 4 days to 4 months postoperatively, with 67 percent occurring in 4 days or less.[442] They may be variably located, with a complex echopattern (Figs. 13-200 to 13-203). The ultrasound pattern varies with the age of the hematoma, with the acute and chronic ones lucent and the intermediate ones complex[447,448] (Figs. 13-200 to 13-203).

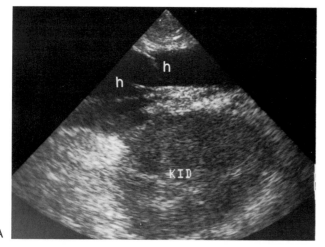

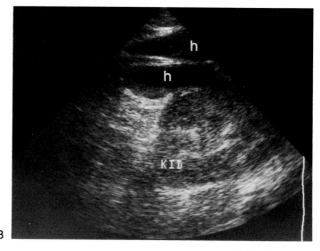

Fig. 13-200. Renal transplant, hematoma. **(A)** Sagittal and **(B)** transverse views of the kidney demonstrating a superficial lucent mass, which represented a hematoma *(h)* anterior to the kidney *(KID)* within the abdominal wall.

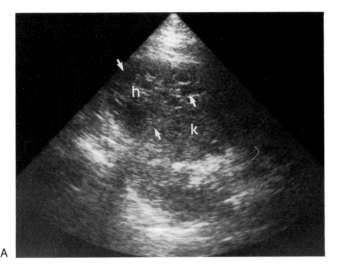
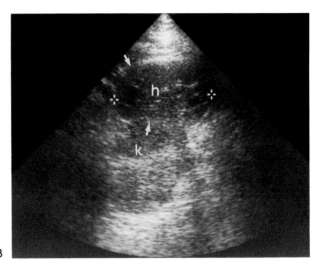

Fig. 13-201. Transplant, hematoma. **(A)** Sagittal and **(B)** transverse views of the kidney *(k)* demonstrating an echogenic mass *(h,* arrows) similar in echopattern to the kidney. This represented a perinephric hematoma secondary to a renal biopsy. This was a more acute hematoma than in Fig. 13-200.

Differentiation of Fluid Collections. As noted above, it appears that all the perirenal post-transplant fluid collections appear similar on sonograms. How does one differentiate the various collections? One group of investigators has evaluated this.[451] These investigators found that 51 percent of their patients had abnormal fluid collections; 43 percent of these were lymphoceles, 30 percent abscesses, 18 percent urinomas, and 9 percent hematomas.[451] Lymphoceles most commonly caused obstruction and were usually septated. Eighty percent of

lymphoceles and 100 percent of hematomas were septated.[451] Lymphoceles were usually larger than abscesses or urinomas. Most urinomas were located near the lower pole. Ultrasound-guided aspiration can provide a diagnosis and facilitate management, but one should be careful to avoid the bowel. Because of the septation in lymphoceles, they may be difficult to aspirate. The patient may be referred to surgery on the basis of deteriorating clinical situation and increasing fluid collection. At times, catheter drainage is possible.

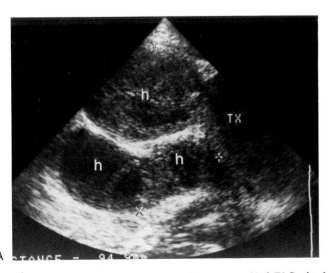
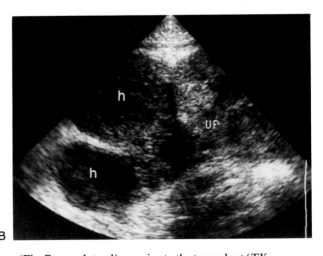

Fig. 13-202. Transplant, hematoma. **(A & B)** Sagittal scans (Fig. B more lateral) superior to the transplant *(TX, UP)* showing a large, solid, multiseptated mass *(h),* which represents a large perinephric hematoma similar in size to the kidney.

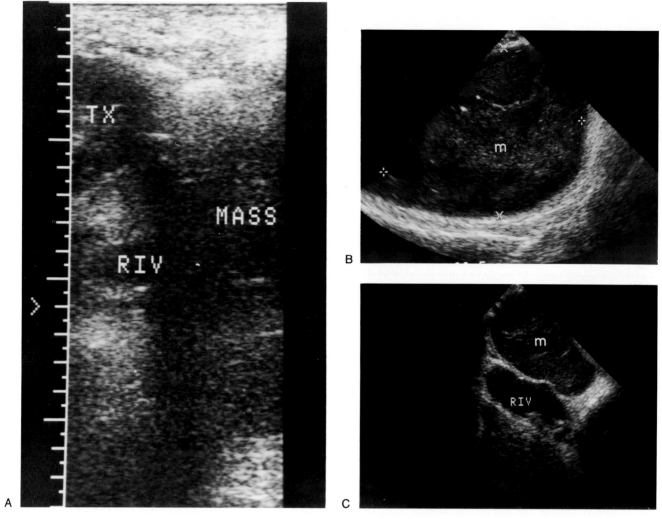

Fig. 13-203. Transplant, hematoma. This patient was scanned to evaluate decreased renal function. With Doppler, normal flow was demonstrated within the transplant. There was no flow within the right iliac vein *(RIV)* below the level of the renal hilum. **(A)** Sagittal view below the lower pole of the transplant *(TX)* showing a poorly defined mass *(MASS),* which appeared to be originating from the pelvis and compressing the right iliac vein. **(B)** Endovaginal sagittal scan showing a large cul-de-sac mass (calipers, *m*), which appeared semisolid. **(C)** Transverse endovaginal scan showing the mass *(m)* to be compressing the right iliac vein. There was echogenic material within the right iliac vein *(RIV),* and no flow was seen with Doppler. The pelvic mass was thought to represent a hematoma (the hematocrit was decreased). The patient was anticoagulated, which restored flow in the right iliac vein and improved renal function. The pelvic mass became more cystic in echopattern with time.

Vascular Abnormalities

A number of vascular abnormalities associated with renal transplantation have been reported, including stenosis of the renal artery or segmental branches, arterial or venous thrombosis, AVF in the kidney or renal pedicle, and pseudoaneurysms.[457] These occur in up to 10 percent of transplant patients, with the most common being arterial and venous stenoses and thromboses and intrarenal and extrarenal AVF, and PAs.[433] In the past,

angiography was used to identify these complications, but it is an invasive technique, which requires the use of nephrotoxic contrast medium.[457] More recently, duplex ultrasound and color Doppler have been used to evaluate these vascular complications. Color Doppler offers the advantage of displaying the deep parenchymal vessels superimposed on the gray-scale image.[457]

The use of color Doppler has obviated many of the problems of duplex ultrasound by adding flow data to the gray-scale image. The identification of vessels and direct analysis of flow patterns according to color encoding facilitate the examination and guide the positioning of the sample window to record frequency spectra along the vascular tree.[457] The use of duplex ultrasound has been shown to be accurate in detection of renal artery thrombosis and AVF, sensitive but not specific for the diagnosis of RAS, and less sensitive for identification of segmental artery thrombosis and stenosis.[457] Most of the false-negative and false-positive results have been due to the lack of direct visualization of the renal vasculature.[457] The presence of acute arterial thrombosis may be definitely established in patients on the basis of an absent Doppler signal.[436]

High Vascular Impedance

There are a number of causes of renal transplant dysfunction, including acute and chronic rejection, ATN, arterial or venous thrombosis, obstruction, infection, and cyclosporin A nephrotoxicity.[436] Experience in renal transplant Doppler has shown that an increased RI (a reflection of increased vascular resistance) is not sufficiently specific to obviate biopsy in most cases of dysfunction.[436] A particularly poor outcome has been noted in patients with extremely high vascular resistance, as evidenced by actual reversal of flow in diastole.[436] In one series, it was found that 30 percent of patients with reversed diastolic flow required transplant nephrectomy.[436] RVT should be suspected in patients with reversed diastolic flow; more specific features (flat retrograde diastolic flow or absence of early diastolic accentuation) should be sought by comparison with scintigraphy.[436] Absent perfusion on a scintigram and this finding on a typical Doppler pattern confirm the diagnosis.

As a rule, the normal renal transplant exhibits low-impedance arterial inflow similar to that seen in the native kidney (Fig. 13-189). The finding of increased vascular impedance resulting in decreased diastolic blood flow and even reversed flow during diastole is most commonly associated with acute vascular rejection (AVR). Other causes include renal vein obstruction, severe tubular necrosis. pyelonephritis, and extrarenal compression of the graft.[434]

Renal Vein Thrombosis

As a rare cause of ARF, acute RVT is predominantly a postsurgical complication due to ischemic alteration of the vessel wall.[458] In one series, all cases occurred within the first 3 postoperative days.[458] In the early postoperative period it has an incidence of 0 to 4 percent.[433] There is no collateral venous drainage in allografts without capsular venous anastomoses to maintain blood circulation or to enable spontaneous recanalization.[458] The imbalance between arterial influx and the decreasing venous outlet leads to an elevation in vascular impedance, and finally the arterial supply of the graft is compromised.[458]

The symptoms of RVT are usually abrupt in onset and consist of graft tenderness, swelling, oliguria, proteinuria, and decreased renal function.[433] Factors that predispose to this complication include hypovolemia, faulty surgical technique, propagation of ipsilateral common femoral or iliac deep venous thrombosis, and renal vein compression by postoperative fluid collections (hematoma, lymphocele, urinoma, abscess).[433]

It is vital to make an early diagnosis of RVT because prompt thrombectomy may restore graft function.[433] In many cases the diagnosis remains undetected, with prolonged venous stasis and thrombosis leading to graft loss.[433]

Real-time ultrasound, which demonstrates only morphologic changes, cannot ensure a sensitive and specific diagnosis because a dilated renal vein occluded by thrombotic material is rarely seen and signs of tissue edema and necrosis are late and nonspecific findings.[458] The renal transplant can appear normal or enlarged, with decreased parenchymal echogenicity and nonvisualized renal veins.[433] The thrombotic material within the vein may not be identified in the acute stages with real-time ultrasound.

The Doppler findings with RVT are more specific, with characteristic findings of acute occlusive RVT including arterial pulsed Doppler patterns of peaked antegrade systolic frequency shift, retrograde plateaulike diastolic frequency shift, and a missing venous Doppler signal[433,458] (Figs. 13-204 and 13-205). Others have described these Doppler findings along with a characteristic arterial pattern, in which the arterial signal shows a sharp systolic peak with a notch on the reverse diastolic component resembling an "inverted M," a previously undescribed finding[459] (Fig. 13-205). This "inverted M" sign may be more specific for RVT in that it may represent nonocclusive thrombus, despite the lack of detectable venous flow, whereas the previously described plateaulike reversed diastolic flow seen in some cases of RVT also occurs in severe allograft rejection and is therefore a nonspecific sign.[459] The specificity of Doppler ultrasound for RVT would be limited by the findings of multiple vessel occlusions in severe, end-stage vascular rejection, in which retrograde diastolic blood flow may also occur and venous signals are absent or weak.[458]

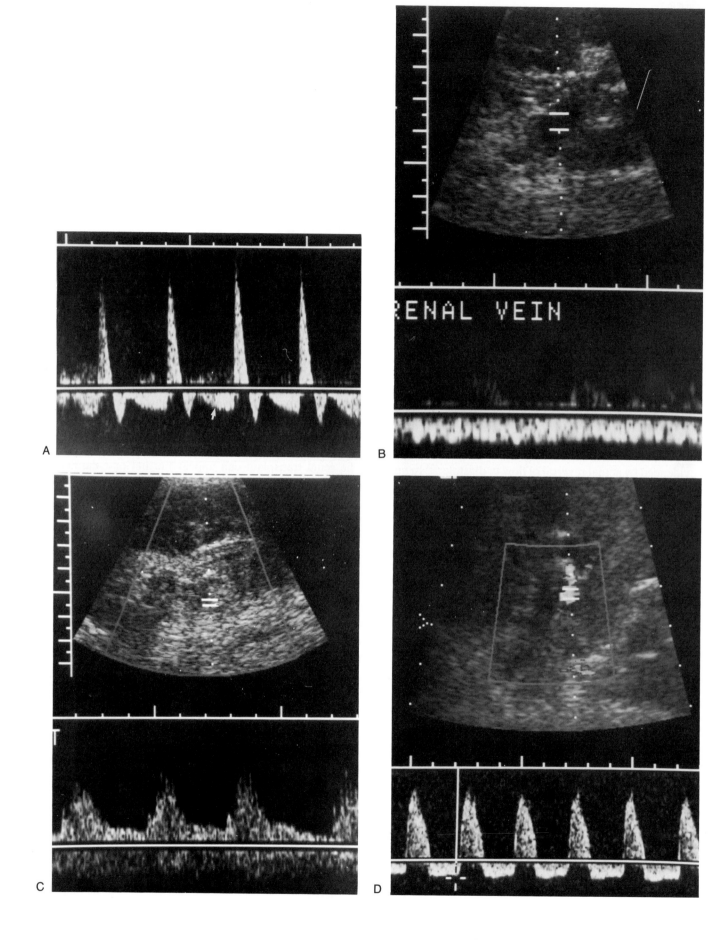

RENAL VEIN

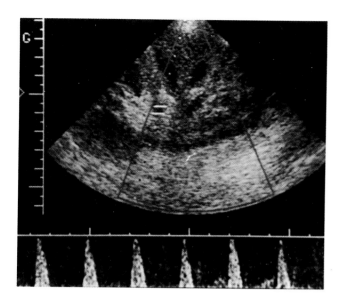

Fig. 13-205. Renal transplant, renal vein thrombosis. Sagittal scan. Doppler arterial waveform obtained at the interlobar artery level, showing a sharp systolic peak and reverse diastolic flow. The diastolic component has an "inverted M" appearance (arrow). (From Baxter et al,[459] with permission.)

Arterial Stenosis

Renal artery stenosis, the most commonly encountered arterial problem, occurs with a 1 to 16 percent incidence with a mean of 10 percent for adults and 3.6 to 12 percent for children.[433,437,457,460,461] A number of factors affect the probability of developing RAS. It may be related to the type of anastomosis, surgical procedure, arterial trauma during harvesting and preservation, and chronic rejection.[460] Distal stenosis may reflect chronic rejection if accompanied by distal intrarenal stenosis or arterial trauma if the distal intrarenal branches are normal; stenosis at the anastomosis may be related to the surgical procedure.[460]

Renal artery stenosis is suggested clinically when there is severe or refractory hypertension, sometimes of sudden onset, and the development of a bruit during the late post-transplant period, but these signs are neither reliable nor specific.[460] The bruit is less common in children than in adults.[460] This complication should be considered a possible cause of early post-transplant hypertension with deteriorating renal function, even though acute rejection may seem clinically more likely. Hypertension is the hallmark of RAS, although up to 80 percent of transplant recipients may exhibit hypertension unrelated to RAS.[433] RAS should be suspected in patients with specific hypertensive profiles, such as newly developed or progressive hypertension, marked hypertension resistant to medical therapy, hypertension with graft dysfunction in the absence of rejection, or hypertension in the presence of a systolic bruit audible over the graft.[433] As a rule, RAS occurs within the first 3 years after transplantation and is more common in grafts from cadavers, especially those of young donors, than in grafts from living donors.[433]

Three types of RAS have been identified: anastomotic, distal donor, and recipient artery.[433] Anastomotic stenoses occur more frequently in the end-to-end anastomoses; distal stenoses occur more frequently in end-to-side anastomoses; and recipient artery stenoses occur equally in both types.[433] Anastomotic stenoses are primarily short-segment stenoses, composed of variable amounts of intimal fibrosis and calcium, that have been ascribed to surgical difficulties such as tight sutures, incomplete intimal approximation, excessive vessel length, twisting of the vascular pedicle, and large discrepancies in donor and recipient arterial size.[398,433,437] There may be single or multiple long-segment stenoses with distal donor stenoses composed primarily of diffuse intimal hyperplasia; these are caused by hemodynamic turbulence distal to the anastomosis, intimal injury due to graft perfusion catheter, or excessive dissection around the main renal artery that results in destruction of the vas vasorum.[398,433,437]

With arterial stenosis, no abnormal echopattern involving the kidney is detected. The only finding is the lack of normal post-transplant hypertrophy.[432] Doppler is a sensitive technique for evaluation of RAS, but is not specific; it cannot differentiate kinking or nonsignificant stenosis in an accessory vessel from significant main RAS.[437]

To evaluate for RAS, both the vessels in the renal hilum and the iliac arteries must be identified.[460] The entire length of the renal artery between the hilum and iliac artery must be evaluated.[460] The stenotic diagnosis

Fig. 13-204. Renal transplant, renal vein thrombosis. Case 1. Using Doppler, no flow could be identified in the region of the renal vein. **(A)** High systolic peaks were associated with the renal arterial vessels with reversed diastolic flow (arrow). The patient was found to have renal vein thrombosis. **(B)** Following the removal of the venous clot, flow could be demonstrated within the renal vein. **(C)** The flow pattern for the renal artery changed. There was no longer reversed diastolic flow; the RI was elevated to 0.84 immediately postoperative. Case 2. **(D)** Using Doppler evaluation of the main renal artery, reversed diastolic flow was demonstrated in this case of renal vein thrombosis immediately postoperative. No flow was visualized within the renal vein.

cannot be based on direct visualization of a stenotic lumen, probably since the vessel is so small.[457] When evaluating for RAS, the vessel must be insonated throughout its entire extent, and abnormally elevated peak velocities and turbulent flow indicative of stenosis must be sought. In most main renal arteries, there is a frequency shift of 2.0 kHz or less, with the smaller vessels having an even lower frequency shift.[460] With 3-MHz transducers, significant stenoses (requiring intervention) are associated with peak Doppler shifts greater than 7 kHz (2 m/s) at the stenosis and turbulence in the immediate poststenotic segment[433,437] (Figs. 13-206 and 13-207 and Plate 13-4). There is a region of marked poststenotic turbulence immediately beyond the stenosis, with blood cells moving at differing speeds (spectral broadening) and in various directions throughout the cardiac cycle (bidirectional flow giving signals above and below the baseline).[460] The blood flow gradually returns to normal distal to the stenosis.[460] There has been a report of kinking of the main renal artery as a cause of high-frequency shifts.[460] The success of this technique depends on directly identifying the area of stenosis. Since the stenosis may occur anywhere, the vessels must be evaluated very thoroughly and meticulously; as such, the duplex examination is a prolonged and tedious procedure in which the arteries are located by a trial-and-error method. Stenoses cannot be excluded if portions of the vessels are skipped.

With the use of color Doppler, the evaluation becomes much faster and a stenosis is less likely to be missed than on a duplex study.[433] The abnormally increased velocities associated with stenoses appear as regions of focal aliasing with properly adjusted color controls.[433] Once the area of concern is located by color Doppler, it may be interrogated by duplex ultrasound.

With color Doppler, the following criteria have been developed for arterial stenosis: (1) direct visualization of a decreased vascular lumen, (2) perivascular artifact or "bruit" around the stenotic segment, (3) spectral broadening, suggesting turbulence, (4) high systolic frequency shift value (215.2 $\pm$ 32 cm/s), and (5) an auditory impression of turbulent flow.[457] The spectral gauges of turbulence are graded as absent, mild, or major[457] (Figs. 13-206 and 13-207 and Plate 13-4). A peak systolic velocity greater than or equal to 190 cm/s is associated with a significant stenosis.[457] As a more subjective criterion, spectral broadening is influenced by system factors such as power output and receiver gain, as well as by turbulence within the insonated vessel.[457] With normal flow, the waveform shows a narrow-frequency bandwidth with a dark window under the systolic peak and a regular upper limit.[457] With mild turbulence, the upper limit of the waveform becomes irregular and the frequency distribution is widened, obscuring the subsystolic clear window without reverse flow.[457] With major turbulence, reverse flow may occur, with most of the points of the

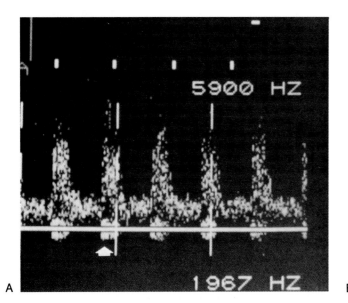

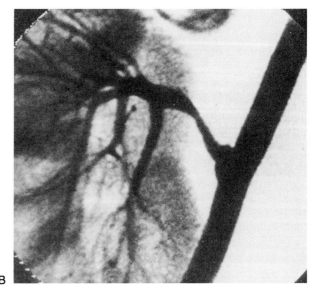

A   B

Fig. 13-206. Renal transplant, renal artery stenosis. **(A)** On duplex ultrasound, renal artery stenosis generally appears as elevated frequency shifts at the stenotic site. In this case, peak frequency shifts are not elevated because the Doppler angle is close to 90 degrees. However, the diagnosis of stenosis was suspected because of the presence of perivascular soft-tissue vibrations, which result from flow turbulence and appear as symetric low-frequency reflections above and below the baseline (arrow). **(B)** Arteriogram helps confirm stenosis near the anastomotic site. (See also Plate 13-4). (From Surratt et al,[440] with permission.)

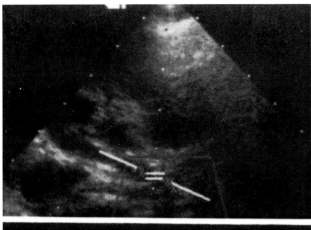

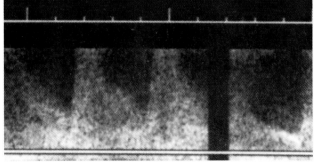

Fig. 13-207. Renal transplant, renal artery stenosis. Duplex ultrasound spectrum at the region of color aliasing showing peak velocities greater than 6 m/s (23 kHz) with marked spectral turbulence consistent with a significant stenosis. (From Dodd et al,[433] with permission.)

spectrum in the low-frequency range.[457] The perivascular artifact may be related to mechanical vibrations transmitted by turbulence.[457] With segmental arterial stenosis, color Doppler may demonstrate major spectral features of turbulence with high systolic frequencies in segmental arteries.[457]

For detection of arterial stenosis within the renal pedicle, the sensitivity and specificity of Doppler reported are 91 and 92 percent, respectively.[457]

Renal Artery Thrombosis

Thrombosis of the main renal artery occurs in less than 1 to 2 percent of renal transplant patients.[433,461,462] This complication usually occurs as an acute event in the early postoperative period (within 1 month) and invariably results in graft loss.[433] The most common causes are hyperacute and acute rejection.[433,462] Other causes that have been cited as precipitators of thrombosis include intraoperative intimal trauma, faulty intimal approximation, wide disparity in vessel size, end-to-end anasto-

moses, vascular kinking, hypotension, hypercoaguable states, cyclosporine, and atherosclerotic emboli.[433]

With renal artery thrombosis, no flow is seen within the renal transplant.[433,457] Absence of flow within the entire kidney or within a portion of the parenchyma can be used as a criterion for renal and segmental artery thrombosis[457] (Fig. 13-208 and Plate 13-5). Additionally, no venous flow is identified.[433] The ischemic parenchymal defects may be quite large (4 to 7 cm in diameter).[457]

Arteriovenous Fistula and Pseudoaneurysm

Arteriovenous fistula and PA are known, but uncommon, complications of renal biopsies, occurring in both native and transplanted kidneys.[433,439,463] As a commonly used method of distinguishing rejection from drug toxicity in a renal allograft, percutaneous needle biopsy is associated with a low morbidity and consists primarily of mild transient hematuria lasting for up to 3 days.[464] In some instances, associated vessel damage may be sufficient to cause arteriovenous (AV) damage; 95 percent of cases resolve spontaneously.[464] There is a greater risk of vascular complications associated with

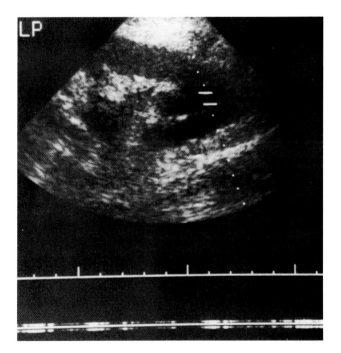

Fig. 13-208. Renal transplant, segmental vascular occlusion. Case 1. On the image obtained on the sixth postoperative day, flow is no longer seen in the lower pole *(LP),* although it was present in the upper pole. The region of the lower pole was not visualized owing to occlusion of the lower-pole artery and resulting infarction. (See also Plate 13-5.) (From Surratt et al,[440] with permission.)

biopsy with an increased number of punctures.[465] PAs result from isolated arterial laceration, whereas AVFs occur with simultaneous laceration of adjacent arteries and veins.[433] These lesions have been reported to have a prevalence of 1 to 18 percent.[433] In angiographic series, these fistulae are reported to occur in 15 to 16 percent of native kidneys.[463]

In most cases, patients with vascular abnormalities are asymptomatic.[465] Since there is a tendency for these vascular complications to heal spontaneously and the patients are usually asymptomatic, there is no need for invasive diagnostic or therapeutic procedures when a vascular lesion is detected by color Doppler in an asymptomatic patient.[465] AVFs may produce symptoms when they become large enough to cause decreased renal perfusion via marked AV shunting or when they communicate with the calyceal system and produce hematuria.[433] These patients with AVFs may present with hypertension, hematuria, or high-output cardiac failure.[439] When a PA ruptures into the perinephric space or collecting system, symptoms are produced.[433]

Both AVFs and PAs develop within and external to the kidney.[462] The incidence and pathogenesis of these lesions vary considerably, although their imaging appearances are similar. As the second most common vascular complication of renal transplantation, intrarenal AVFs and PAs are almost always the result of percutane-

ous biopsies.[462] Extrarenal AVFs and PAs which are due to faulty surgical technique or perivascular infection, are rare. Intrarenal AVFs and PAs are usually self-limiting and resolve spontaneously. The high incidence of spontaneous aneurysm rupture makes extrarenal PAs more ominous.[462]

Intrarenal Arteriovenous Fistula. No matter what the location, AVFs have a classic Doppler waveform, with the feeding artery exhibiting high-velocity, low-resistance flow, whereas the draining vein is pulsatile or "arterialized"[462] (Figs. 13-209 and 13-210 and Plates 13-6 and 13-7). There may be associated decreased RI in all cases when waveform analysis of the supplying artery is evaluated; increased flow velocities may be seen in many cases.[463] In one series, the peak systolic flow velocity in the arteries supplying the fistulas ranged from 55 to 180 cm/s (mean, 92 cm/s), with the range in normal arteries being 20 to 52 cm/s (mean, 32 cm/s).[463] The RIs of the normal arteries ranged from 0.60 to 0.92 (mean, 0.74), and those of the arteries supplying the fistulas ranged from 0.31 to 0.50 (mean, 0.45).[463] With AVFs there are high-velocity, low-impedance arterial waveforms with associated arterialized venous tracings.[433,439,463]

It is much easier to identify and confidently diagnose these abnormalities by color Doppler than by conven-

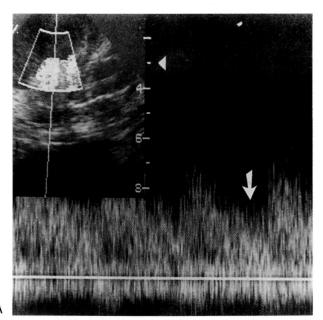

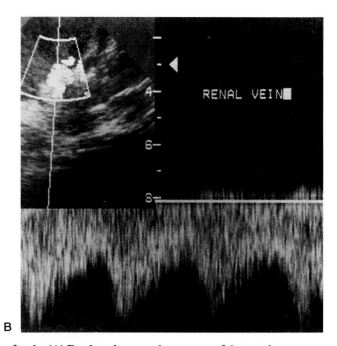

A   B

Fig. 13-209.   Renal transplant, intrarenal arteriovenous fistula. **(A)** Duplex ultrasound spectrum of the arteriovenous fistula feeding artery in the lower pole showing high-velocity, low-impedance flow. Diastolic flow (arrow) is increased. Doppler ultrasound of arterial flow elsewhere in the kidney (not shown) demonstrated normal flow with decreased velocity and lower diastolic flow. **(B)** Duplex ultrasound spectrum of the arteriovenous fistula draining vein showing arterialized venous flow. (See also Plate 13-6). (From Dodd et al,[433] with permission.)

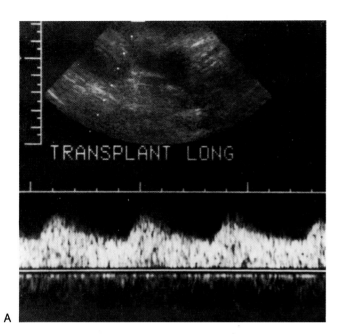
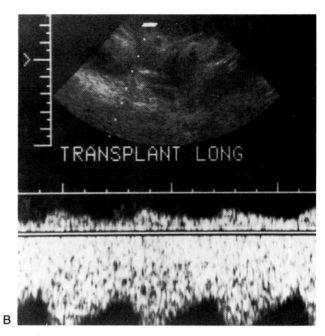

A

B

Fig. 13-210. Renal transplant, arteriovenous fistula. **(A)** A waveform from the artery supplying the arteriovenous fistula demonstrates a high-frequency Doppler shift, generated as a result of the large pressure drop from the artery to the vein. **(B)** On another image, flow within the vein draining the fistula is seen as an arterial waveform below the baseline. (*LONG,* longitudinal.) (See also Plate 13-7.) (From Surratt et al,[440] with permission.)

tional duplex ultrasound since color Doppler can visualize the intrarenal blood flow and the focal hemodynamic alterations caused by the AVF.[463] With color Doppler, exaggerated focal color around an AVF is attributable to perivascular vibration caused by turbulent flow. Direct visualization of the fistula, as well as the feeding artery and draining vein, may be possible with color. Although color Doppler appears to be more sensitive than duplex ultrasound in detection of renal transplant AVF, the actual sensitivity of this method has not been determined.[463] The findings seen on real-time imaging include changes in color saturation of the supplying artery and draining vein, local tissue vibrations from high-flow velocities, and associated turbulence and PA formation.[463]

Intrarenal Pseudoaneurysm. In many cases the perforation in the arterial wall secondary to a biopsy seals off and the hematoma resolves. When the perforation does not seal off, the blood flow from the damaged vessel continuously moves back and forth from the vessel lumen to the surrounding hematoma.[464] Blood is forced through the retracted blood vessel wall into the periarterial tissue during systole.[464] This blood is entrapped by surrounding fascia, forming a focal collection. The center of the hematoma remains liquefied owing to the force of the blood during systole.[464] The blood from the

hematoma returns to the vessel during diastole. The outer wall of the aneurysm is formed from fibrotic tissues secondary to local inflammatory reaction.[464] With continuing blood flow, the cavity undergoes endothelialization.[464] The resultant structure, which does not contain all the normal layers of the arterial wall, is a PA.[464]

In most cases, these PAs heal spontaneously. A number of factors may be responsible for the persistence of a PA: hypertension, bleeding diathesis, and laceration of the larger arteries in the medullary or central portion of the kidney.[464]

At real-time ultrasound, these lesions may be seen as a hypoechoic mass in the vicinity of the arterial anastomosis or within the allograft.[439] The mass may appear to pulsate on real-time imaging.[461] PA can be diagnosed from morphologic criteria on the flow image and "to-and-fro" spectral characteristics[457] (Fig. 13-211 and Plate 13-8). There is highly turbulent pulsatile flow within the central lumen of a PA, with classic "machine-like" to-and-fro flow.[433] PA and AVF may show no difference in the color Doppler and duplex waveforms; however, color Doppler may be superior to duplex ultrasound in diagnosing vascular lesions.[465] The differential diagnosis of PA includes hematomas, AV malformation, and abscesses, all of which occur more frequently than PA.[464] Intrarenal and extrarenal PAs may be difficult to differentiate from benign cortical cyst or small perinephric fluid collections by real-time imaging alone.

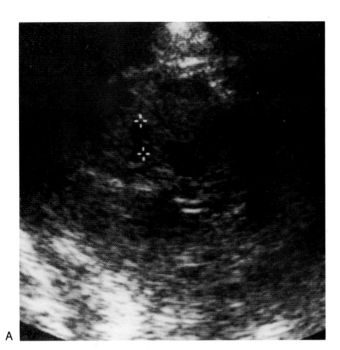

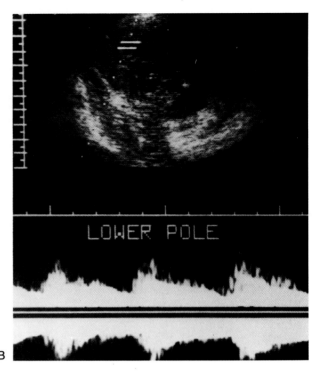

Fig. 13-211. Renal transplant, intrarenal pseudoaneurysm. **(A)** Sonogram demonstrating a typical cystic-appearing mass (calipers). **(B)** Duplex ultrasound image shows pulsatile arterial and venous waveforms within the mass. (See also Plate 13-8.) (From Surratt et al,[440] with permission.)

Extrarenal Arteriovenous Fistulas and Pseudoaneurysm. Less common than the intrarenal variety, extrarenal AVFs and PAs usually have a different cause and a worse prognosis.[433] At times, they cause renal dysfunction by excessive AV shunting or direct compression of the main renal artery.[433] Exsanguination due to spontaneous rupture of a PA is the most serious complication of these lesions.[433]

The most common cause of both extrarenal PA and AVFs is faulty vascular reconstruction.[433] Perigraft infection and erroneous percutaneous biopsies are less common causes.[433]

By using duplex ultrasound and color Doppler, these extrarenal PAs may be diagnosed definitively[433] (Plates 13-9 and 13-10). Extrarenal AVFs may be diagnosed best by angiography but can be suspected by their pattern on duplex ultrasound and color Doppler.[433] The extrarenal AFVs demonstrate Doppler characteristics similar to their intrarenal counterparts.[433] With extrarenal PAs there may be predominantly anechoic, spherical paranephric fluid collections that exhibit Doppler characteristics identical to those of the intrarenal variety.[433] The increased velocity and turbulence in AVF feeding arteries can be mistaken for the abnormal hemodynamics of the more common arterial stenosis in main renal arteries.[433] The diagnosis should be suggested by recognition of the associated increased diastolic flow of an AVF.[433]

Parenchymal Abnormalities

The finding of minimal mucosal thickening of the collecting system (see above) indicates the presence of renal disease even though the cause of the thickening itself is nonspecific.[466] It can occur in acute cellular rejection, chronic vascular rejection, cyclosporin A toxicity, ATN, hypertensive vasculopathy, ischemic necrosis, urinary tract infection, congenital hydronephrosis, and reflux hydronephrosis.[466] With minimal mucosal thickening of the renal pelvis, a circular band of feebly reflective tissue is produced within the central cavity of a transplant[466] (Fig. 13-12). If the two sides of the thickened mucosal surfaces touch each other, a single bright linear echo can be observed in the central cavity of a hollow organ such as a renal graft.[466] At times it is difficult to differentiate between minimal hydronephrosis and minimal mucosal thickening. To help assess this, the transducer should be placed perpendicular to the interface of two opposing surfaces of thickened mucosa to produce a bright, linear echo, which can help distinguish between these two entities.[466]

Acute Tubular Necrosis

With the development of new preservation solutions and transport pump mechanisms, the ischemic insult to the transplant kidney has been decreased.[462] Despite this, all transplants will incur some degree of ischemia and resultant ATN. If a kidney does not function well within 2 to 3 days of transplantation, this is cause for concern.

Acute tubular necrosis is the most common cause of acute post-transplant renal failure, appearing in as many as 50 percent of cadaver kidneys.[394,467,468] Other authors report an occurrence rate of 3 percent for cadaver-donor kidneys and 11 percent for live-related-donor kidneys.[447] The incidence increases with the length of warm ischemia time.[447] Uncomplicated ATN is reversible, and the treatment is maintance of hydration and immunosuppression.

The clinical diagnosis of ATN is most commonly made by exclusion. Clinically, there is an increased creatinine level, and the urine output is low. No demonstrable changes are noted on ultrasound in most patients.[394,448,469,470] One series[471] reported that 77 percent of patients had decreased echogenicity of the renal sinus. A nuclear medicine renal scan will show an intact vascular supply and, in combination with a normal-appearing ultrasound, should suggest the diagnosis of ATN.[394]

Allograft Rejection

Rejection is the most common cause of renal failure after the first post-transplant week. On the basis of clinical and laboratory evidence, the diagnosis is a question. The triad of fever, graft tenderness, and oliguria is considered the hallmark of rejection.[469] The creatinine, blood urea nitrogen (BUN), and creatinine clearance are helpful but lack specificity. Studies with contrast further contribute to renal damage and should be avoided when possible. Nuclear medicine provides functional and anatomic information. Ultrasound demonstrates a spectrum of findings.

Rejection can be divided into acute and chronic on the basis of the nature of the inflammatory lesion on microscopy and not on duration.[470] Rarely is there a hyperacute rejection in less than 48 hours after the transplant. Since rejection is a dynamic process, This spectrum corresponds to the histopathologic changes. Although rejection starts and is most pronounced at the corticomedullary junction, it progresses and involves the entire renal unit.

Ultrasound. Early on there is increased renal size caused by edema, congestion, and mononuclear cell infiltrate.[448,470,472] In 84 percent of cases of acute rejection, there is an abnormal increase in renal volume.[432] An abnormal manifestation of volume includes a sudden increase in volume (> 20 percent increase over 5 days) or renal growth during the second week of greater than 25 percent[432] (Fig. 13-212). The renal size is considered normal if on transverse scans, the anteroposterior diameter is clearly smaller than the transverse diameter.[473] If the anteroposterior diameter is equal to the transverse diameter, it is considered abnormal.[473]

Cortical ischemia results in variably sized parenchymal foci of edema, hemorrhage, or infarction.[470,474] The degree of edema, extent of hemorrhage, and presence or absence of infarction are determined by the severity of the impaired cortical perfusion and vascular occlusion. There is uniform or local decrease in the parenchymal echogenicity, corresponding to areas of hemorrhage, edema, and hemorrhagic infarct.[432] There are focal zones of lucency in the cortex in 20 percent of cases, with patchy lucent areas (cortex and medulla) with coalescence in 16 percent. The cortical echoes may be sparse, probably as a result of abundant mononuclear cell infiltrate in the interstitium.[475] There are increased cortical echoes in 58 percent of patients and decreased echoes in 47 percent.[432]

The pyramids are enlarged in 79 to 88 percent of cases of rejection[432,472] (Figs. 13-212 to 13-214). The pyramids

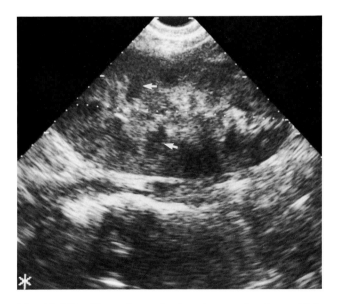

Fig. 13-212. Transplant rejection, increased volume. This transplant kidney is 16 cm long and is increased in its anteroposterior dimension as well. The renal pyramids (arrows) are prominent on this scan, and the renal sinus is inhomogeneous in echotexture.

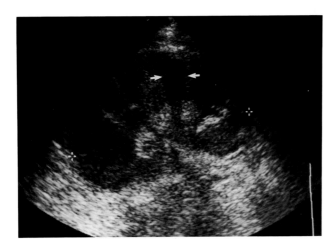

Fig. 13-213. Transplant rejection, enlarged pyramids. Sagittal scan showing markedly enlarged pyramids (arrows). The height of the pyramids exceeds that of the overlying cortex. The renal sinus is barely identifiable.

are considered enlarged if their height exceeds the height of the overlying cortex. The enlargement is due to a combination of edema surrounding the peritubular capillaries and marked congestion of the corticomedullary junction.[406,441,448,470,474,475] The following were evaluated relative to the pyramids: size (corticomedullary ratio), margin sharpness, and conspicuity.[473] The presence of an indistinct corticomedullary junction is strongly indicative of acute rejection[476]; there is loss of corticomedullary junction definition in 58 percent of cases.[432]

Within the hilar adipose tissue, there is early edema that causes uneven widening of the perilobular tissue.

When the changes in the hilar fat are moderate, causing further widening of the intralobular septa, with separation and decrease in size of the fat cells, the ultrasound pattern becomes inhomogeneously dense. With subsequent fibrosis, fat cell atrophy, and fat cell loss, the adipose tissue septation is accentuated. On the sonogram the renal sinus blends with the adjacent parenchyma[406,448,475] (Figs. 13-213 and 13-214). In 74 percent of patients there is a decrease in the amplitude of the renal sinus echoes.[432]

Investigators have evaluated this change in the renal sinus with rejection.[477] There appears to be good correlation between histologic changes and ultrasound changes in rejection, such that ultrasound promises to be a reliable predictor of the severity of rejection via a noninvasive, rapid, simple approach. The intense echoes seen in the renal sinus are primarily due to fat. With acute rejection, changes are minimal to zero in the renal sinus on ultrasound. With moderate rejection, the echoes in the renal sinus are inhomogeneous, patchy, and coarse (Fig. 13-214). With severe rejection, the renal sinus blends with the parenchyma.

In summary, the spectrum of ultrasound findings described with rejection include (1) enlarged pyramids with decreased echogenicity, (2) increased renal volume, (3) increased cortical thickness, (4) decreased or increased echogenicity of the cortex, (5) areas of decreased parenchymal echogenicity, (6) indistinct corticomedullary junction, (7) decreased amplitude of the renal sinus echoes, and (8) perirenal fluid (58 percent).[432,441,468,472] In acute rejection, the following are seen: (1) increased renal size (≤ 20 percent), (2) enlarged pyramids, and (3) indistinct corticomedullary junction.[406] In advanced

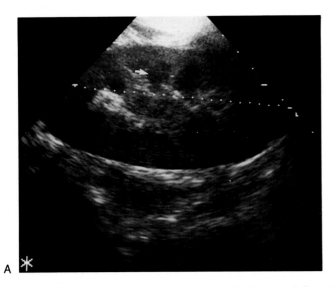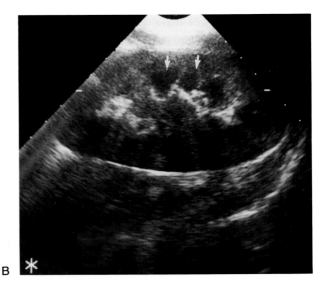

Fig. 13-214. Transplant, severe rejection: renal sinus. **(A & B)** Sagittal scans. The renal sinus blends with the adjacent parenchyma such that it is barely distinguished. The pyramids (arrows) are enlarged.

acute rejection, localized hypoechoic areas may be seen in the cortex and medulla. The spectrum in chronic rejection includes (1) renal enlargement, (2) blending of the cortex and medulla, (3) nondifferentiation of the renal sinus, (4) increased echoes throughout the kidney with a course spatial distribution, (5) small kidney, (6) echogenic kidney, and (7) irregular contour of the kidney owing to scarring[406,470] (Fig. 13-215). The ultrasound findings are most helpful in conjunction with a nuclear medicine study. Although a single ultrasound examination is helpful, it is insufficiently accurate to allow diagnosis of the cause of post-transplant hypofunction. When used in conjunction with other imaging studies (including radionuclide scans), ultrasound can provide valuable adjunctive information.[473]

By using the ultrasound criteria, the study is 84 percent accurate in diagnosing rejection.[406] A high accuracy for detection of acute rejection can result from using a volume increase of 30 to 50 percent combined with at least one of the parenchymal changes.[441] In the group studied, the prevalence of rejection was high (83 percent); the accuracy of a positive prediction of rejection was 83 to 90 percent, but the accuracy of a negative prediction was low (17 to 30 percent).[473] Severe rejection could usually be differentiated from mild or no rejection, but mild rejection was difficult to differentiate from no rejection.[473] There is failure to differentiate acute or chronic rejection in 7 percent of cases.[406]

Pediatric. Investigators have reported problems in evaluating for rejection in the pediatric age group.[478] The ultrasound findings are not helpful if the donor kidney is less than 5 years old. If the donor kidney is more than 5 years old, ultrasound allowed a sensitivity of 97 percent and a specificity of 58 percent when a combination of three or more of the following ultrasound findings is used: (1) increased renal volume of 30 percent over baseline, (2) enlarged broadened rectangular medullary pyramids, (3) reduction or absence of the central sinus echoes, and (4) altered echogenicity in the renal parenchyma.[478]

Other investigators have also encountered problems in evaluating transplants in the pediatric group.[479] There appeared to be a variation of the transplant appearance, with no association between renal function and renal volume, shape, parenchymal echogenicity, or central sinus echoes.[479] A change in size of greater than the usual 90 to 130 percent of baseline volume seen in adults is normal adaptation of the kidney to the recipient body size. This group concluded that ultrasound was not useful in diagnosing chronic rejection or predicting function in the pediatric transplant kidney.[479]

Doppler Evaluation. The specific cause of ARF after renal transplantation may be obscure, although the clinical diagnosis may be obvious.[435] By using various imaging studies, the transplant may be evaluated for obstruction and the presence of peritransplant collections to differentiate them from other causes of failure, such as acute rejection, toxic reactions to cyclosporine, and ATN.[435] There has been less success with differentiation of rejection, toxic reactions to cyclosporine, and ATN.[435]

Cellular and vascular types of acute rejection have been identified.[435] Differences between reported series may be related to the age of the transplant kidney at the time of biopsy; patients who have had transplants for a short time generally have experienced few episodes of rejection.[480] With the interstitial (cellular) type, a reaction of the cellular immune system results in edema of the interstitium and cortical infiltration with mononuclear cells.[435] Although the arteries, arterioles, and glomeruli are usually spared, this infiltration can be found within the intertubular capillaries, venules, and lymphatics.[435] With the vascular type, there is a combination of humoral and cellular immune processes.[435] There is a resultant increase in the downstream impedance when a vascular component of rejection is present.[435] Rejection is the most common cause of increased renovascular impedance in the second postoperative week.[481] If the rejection has a vascular component, this is especially true.[481] The Doppler examination detects this type of rejection most readily.[435] With purely cellular rejection, the Doppler examination may be insensitive.[435] There is poor correlation between the RI and the severity of arterial and arteriolar changes on biopsy.[482]

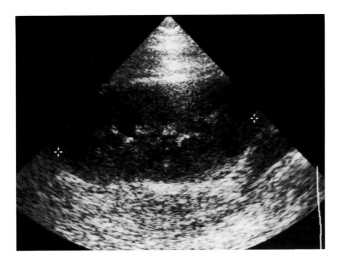

Fig. 13-215. Transplant, chronic rejection. Longitudinal scan. The kidney is small. There is loss of corticomedullary differentiation as well as renal sinus identification.

A number of investigators have evaluated Doppler ultrasound in patients with rejection.[435,480,482,483] Patients with more severe forms of rejection (moderate to severe interstitial with or without vascular rejection) have a higher RI (0.89 ± 0.05)[483] (Fig. 13-216). A 100 percent positive predictive value has been found with an RI greater than 1.00.[435] With an RI of less than 0.70, the likelihood of rejection is lower (negative predictive value of 94 percent).[435] Others have reported a sensitivity of 92 percent with an RI of 0.70 or greater with a specificity of 75 percent in the diagnosis of acute rejection.[484] The sensitivity decreases to 65 percent at an RI of 0.75 or greater with a specificity of 93 percent.[484] Another group found an RI of greater than 0.90 to be 100 percent predictive of acute rejection but with a sensitivity of only 26 percent.[480] Lowering the threshold of abnormality to 0.70 increases the sensitivity in detecting acute rejection to 54 percent but lowers the positive predictive value to 72 percent.[480] An elevated RI is a fairly sensitive al-

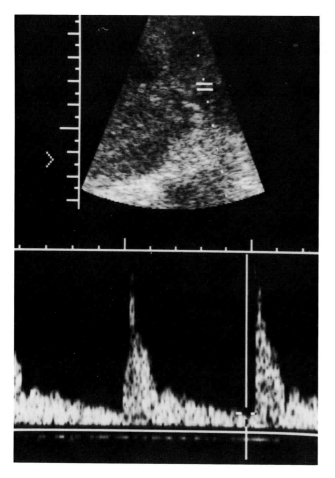

Fig. 13-216. Renal transplant, rejection (same case as Fig. 13-212). The RI is noted to be greater than 0.90, indicative of rejection.

though nonspecific indicator of allograft dysfunction.[484] Elevation of the RI has been found with urinary obstruction and hyperacute, acute, and chronic rejection.[484] Other authors have concluded that the use of RI to assign a diagnosis of acute rejection was no better than establishing this in a random manner.[485]

Doppler ultrasound has shown great promise in differentiating acute rejection from ATN.[435,486] The rejected kidney may have decreased arterial flow with an increase in downstream impedance reflected in the waveform by a decreased diastolic component compared with the systolic component.[435] Other investigators have found no significant differences in the indices for those with rejection versus ATN.[486] If there was a history of either ATN or a previous rejection episode in the same allograft, the sensitivity of the examination was adversely affected.[486] It was thought that scintigraphy was more sensitive in the differentiation of these two diagnoses.[486]

When there is diminished, absent, or reversed diastolic flow in renal allografts, almost always there is pathologically increased renovascular impedance.[481] Increased impedance can be found in rejection, severe ATN, extrarenal compression, obstructive uropathy, renal vein obstruction, and severe pyelonephritis.[481] The presence of high renovascular impedance immediately after surgery should raise the question of RVT. It should be investigated by Doppler. Within the first few days of surgery after a normal postoperative ultrasound, an abnormal renovascular impedance is a highly significant finding. The following should be excluded: obstructive uropathy, severe pyelonephritis, and extrarenal compression by peritransplant fluid.[481] When there has been a very prolonged and severe episode of ischemia, ATN may result in abnormal renovascular impedance.[481]

Some investigators use the pulsatility index (PI) in evaluating renal transplants. The PI is defined as the peak systolic frequency shift minus the minimum diastolic frequency shift, divided by the mean frequency shift.[487] Acute rejection is found to produce a significantly higher PI at each arterial site.[487] The sensitivity of this technique for detection of acute rejection was 75 percent, with a specificity of 90 percent.[487] The same PI yields a sensitivity of 79 percent and a specificity of 90 percent in acute vascular rejection.[487] A specificity of 100 percent may be achieved with a cutoff of 1.8.[487]

Some investigators evaluated the pulsatility of the Doppler waveform.[488] An abnormal study indicating acute rejection was shown by increased pulsatility of the Doppler waveform of intrarenal arterial flow.[488] The sensitivity of this technique varied with the histologic form of rejection, with a 60 percent sensitivity for acute interstitial rejection with or without vascular rejection and an 82 percent sensitivity for acute vascular rejection.[488] The specificity was 95 percent for acute interstitial rejection with or without vascular rejection and 96 percent for acute vascular rejection.[488]

The ability to differentiate between acute transplant rejection and cyclosporine nephrotoxicity would be helpful.[439,489] Duplex ultrasound may be helpful in differentiating these two abnormalities. The peak velocity in systole and the minimum velocity in diastole, using one to three samples from each region, are used to calculate the diastolic/systolic (D/S) ratio.[489] Cyclosporine nephrotoxicity is primarily an abnormality of the tubules, with no significant vascular changes in the early postoperative period.[489] As such, no changes in the D/S velocity ratio would be expected in this period. Arteriolar involvement may develop later.[489] With persistently low D/S ratios, decreased diastolic flow, or diastolic flow reversal, all patients had acute severe vascular rejection with a very poor prognosis.[489] Patients with chronic rejection or cyclosporine toxicity were unlikely to have RIs greater than 0.80.[485] In all the cases of chronic rejection, the RI was less than 0.84.[482]

Investigators have evaluated Doppler in the assessment of renal transplants in children.[490] An RI of less than 0.70 was found in 13 of 14 patients with acute rejection.[490] As such, in this series, it was thought that an RI of less than 0.70 did not exclude acute rejection.[490] The authors hypothesized a number of factors to explain the lack of correlation of the RI with allograft histology: (1) the special circumstances of the adult kidney transplanted into the child; (2) the absence of vascular rejection in this series; and (3) an aggressive approach to biopsy of the allograft in this series, often establishing the diagnosis of rejection before the serum creatinine level became elevated.[490]

The utility of Doppler in transplant rejection appears to be in the area of assessing therapy.[398] An abnormal waveform seems to indicate transplant dysfunction, even though Doppler is neither specific nor sensitive; monitoring changes in waveform seems to be a reasonable way to monitor therapy. In such cases, the Doppler waveform may predate improvements or deterioration in clinical renal function by several days.[398] As such, the clinician who has decided on a particular course of therapy, given a poorly functioning transplant, can evaluate its effectiveness by using the Doppler waveform; decreasing resistance implies improved graft function.[398]

With duplex ultrasound, the underlying pathologic vascular changes do not appear to be reflected.[489] This technique cannot discriminate between the different causes of vascular involvement. A duplex study showing abnormal velocity flow patterns and persistently low D/S velocity ratios is strongly suggestive of severe acute vascular rejection (with a poor prognosis).[489] In a patient with renal dysfunction, a normal Doppler study is suggestive of cyclosporine nephrotoxicity or mild cellular rejection (with a good prognosis).[489]

Doppler may aid in the management of patients with ARF and renal transplant.[435] Therapy may be started immediately depending on the results of the examination. This eliminates delay until after a biopsy is obtained or before histologic diagnosis is confirmed by the pathologist.[435] In many instances, early treatment can salvage a transplanted kidney.[435]

Conclusions. If one or more of the following findings are present on ultrasound, acute rejection may be diagnosed: transplant swelling, increased conspicuity of the medullary pyramids, medullary pyramid enlargement, decreased renal sinus-fat echodensity, and pelvi-infundibular thickening.[439,480] If the anteroposterior diameter of the transplant is equal to its transverse diameter, transplant swelling is diagnosed.[439] If the medullary pyramid is greater than the height of the overlying cortex, it is judged to be enlarged.[439] Pelvi-infundibular thickening is present if the walls of these structures are perceptible.[439] Medullary conspicuity and diminution in renal sinus-fat echogenicity are subjective and are based on comparison with a normal native kidney.[439] Ultrasound may not be used independently to diagnose rejection or to distinguish between cyclosporine nephrotoxicity and rejection.[439] Only with a level of creatinine of 6.9 mg/dl or more is there 100 percent correlation between acute rejection and the presence of abnormal ultrasound findings.[439] As such, ultrasound cannot reliably distinguish cyclosporine nephrotoxicity from acute rejection.[439]

Acute rejection might be predicted with a high accuracy when the RI is greater than 0.90 or all the morphologic features are present.[480] Differences between reported series may be related to the age of the transplant kidney at the time of biopsy; patients with transplants for a short time generally have experienced relatively few episodes of rejection.[480]

Renal allograft rejection has been evaluated by Doppler ultrasound and MRI.[491] Doppler ultrasound was found to be significantly superior to MRI in identifying allograft rejection, demonstrating a higher sensitivity (95 versus 70 percent), specificity (95 versus 73 percent), and accuracy (95 versus 71 percent).[491] Other authors have found MRI to be significantly more accurate, reaching a level of 98 percent.[492] In the same series, ultrasound and scintigraphy had accuracies of 72 and 75 percent, respectively.[492] The role of MRI in evaluating post-transplant renal failure has not been currently established, but because of its high sensitivity in detecting renal abnormalities, MRI may be used for cases when results of ultrasound or scintigraphy are equivocal or contradict clinical impressions or when biopsy cannot be performed for medical reasons.[492]

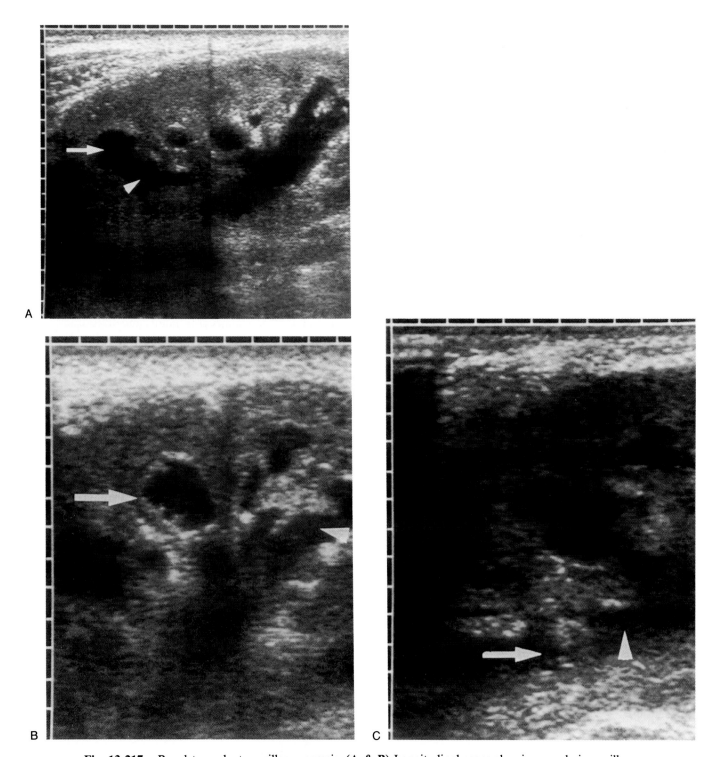

Fig. 13-217. Renal transplant, papillary necrosis. **(A & B)** Longitudinal scans showing anechoic papillary cavities (arrow) with irregular walls connected to the mildly dilated pelvocalyceal system (arrowhead). **(C)** Longitudinal scan showing echogenic sloughed papilla (arrow) in the major upper-pole calyx (arrowhead). (From Shapeero and Vordermark,[493] with permission.)

Papillary Necrosis

Although papillary necrosis in the renal allograft patient is most commonly associated with acute or chronic rejection, it is also seen with S-hemoglobinopathy, ATN, diabetes, and infection such as fulminant candidiasis or acute pyelonephritis.[493] In the allograft, this condition can develop as early as 2 months after transplantation, with medullary ischemia suggested as the final common pathway for the process.[493] When acute rejection is accompanied by decreased perfusion, then stasis, sludging, intravascular thrombosis, and hemorrhage secondary to immunologic damage can produce the papillary necrosis.[493] It can also develop as a part of a long-term rejection and can produce gradual loss of renal function. It is more common in patients receiving a cadaver allograft than in those receiving living-related allografts because of the higher incidence of both diffuse ATN and rejection leading to ischemia in the cadaver allograft.[493] It can happen in a segmental fashion in the area supplied by the last reanastomosed artery, which encountered the longest period of warm ischemia and is at risk for segmental ATN and subsequent papillary necrosis.[493] On intravenous urography of the allograft, the typical findings of papillary necrosis are seen, ranging from clubbing and dilatation of calyces in the milder form to severe deformation with papillary ulcers and extensive loss of papillary tissue.[493]

On ultrasound, multiple round to triangular cystic spaces are seen in the medullary regions, arranged around sinus echoes and the anechoic clubbed "calyx" connected to the pelvis by a narrow infundibulum (Fig. 13-217). It is important to recognize diffuse papillary necrosis in a patient with sudden deterioration of renal function and hematuria, because it can represent the onset of acute rejection, which requires prompt surgical exploration and allograft removal.[493]

Infarction

The process of renal infarction may be related to thrombosis of a small polar artery.[444] With the absence of intrarenal arterial collateral circulation, an infarction may result.[444] Depending on the degree of tissue damage, no tissue loss, scar formation, or formation of a hole in the transplant kidney may result.[444] This abnormality is particularly common after a smaller polar vessel has been anastomosed to a main renal artery.[444]

On ultrasound, the most common appearance of an acute renal infarction is that of a focal hypoechoic mass[444] (Fig. 13-218). Pathologic examination shows that these lesions contain soft, edematous, well-circumscribed areas of hemorrhage.[444] These lesions may extend to and may bulge the capsule.[444] If there is internal coagulative necrosis, the central area may appear more lucent (Fig. 13-218). At ultrasound, it may be difficult to differentiate this lesion from others such as abscess. With segmental infarction, there may be absence of signals in the interlobar arteries.[437]

Rupture

Renal rupture occurs secondary to acute rejection as a serious complication in 3.6 to 6 percent of cases.[406,447,493] Most occur during the early post-transplant period, with

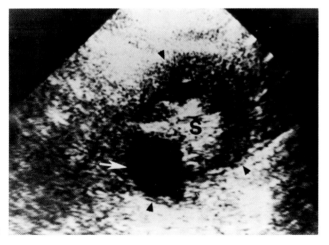
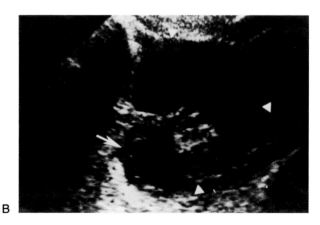

A   B

Fig. 13-218. Renal transplant, infarction. Infarction simulating abscess. **(A)** Transverse scan through the lower pole of the renal transplant showing a round, focal, hypoechoic area (white arrow). (*S*, renal sinus; black arrowheads, renal margin). **(B)** Two days later, the hypoechoic mass (arrow) has developed a thick wall. At surgery, infarction, but no abscess, was confirmed. (arrowheads, renal margin.) (From Stuck et al,[444] with permission.)

80 percent occurring within the first 2 weeks.[406,494] Clinically, it is associated with tachycardia, hypotension, oliguria, decreased hematocrit, pain, tenderness, and swelling.[494] There is no general agreement concerning its pathogenesis. Ischemic necrosis, hypertension, and previous renal biopsy are among the contributing factors.[494]

Renal rupture most commonly occurs along the convex margin of the kidney, with the hematoma developing superior and lateral to the kidney, and it is well demarcated. The hematoma infiltrates the retroperitoneal fat and manifests as a fluid collection containing numerous high-amplitude echoes.[432] On the sonogram there may be gross distortion of the graft contour and a perinephric or parenchymal hematoma[447] (Fig. 13-219).

Infection

Infection is the most common cause of death in the renal transplant patient, and the urinary tract is the most common site of the primary infection.[467] However, it is difficult to diagnose. Not only is the immune system suppressed, but also the signs and symptoms may be masked for quite a time until sepsis is widespread. The most frequent single cause of renal failure in the immediate post-transplant period is ATN, which is associated with a high risk of infection.[467] As an early or late complication of transplantation, infection typically produces few signs unless the collecting system is dilated.[439] The more common infectious agents include cytomegalovirus, herpes simplex virus, *E. coli,* and *C. albicans*[439] (Fig. 13-220). Sepsis is most often secondary to an *E. coli* urinary tract infection.[495] Septic episodes occur in fewer than one-fourth of these, cases with 30 to 60 percent of all allograft recipients treated for urinary tract infections.[495] Among the rarer infectious complications are emphysematous pyelonephritis and genitourinary tuberculosis.[439]

Emphysematous Pyelonephritis. There have been reports of an emphysematous kidney associated with infection.[467,495] Renal allograft infection by gas-producing organisms is rare.[495] Since the clinical signs and symptoms of serious infection are moderated by immunosuppressive drugs, the radiologist can make an early diagnosis of emphysematous pyelonephritis.[495] There is a higher incidence of bacteriuria in diabetics than other

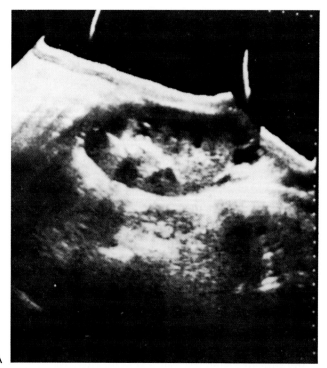
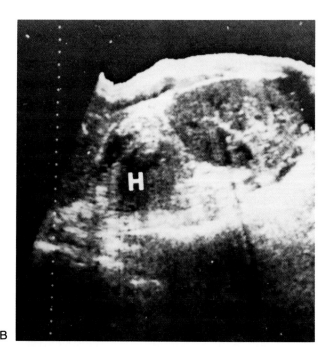

A   B

Fig. 13-219. Transplant rupture, acute rejection. **(A)** Longitudinal scan during acute renal failure. The kidney is globular. There is uneven enlargement of the pyramids. The renal sinus echoes are patchy in distribution. **(B)** Oblique scan on the day of nephrectomy. There is a mixed-echopattern mass hematoma *(H)* inferior to the upper pole of the transplanted kidney. The kidney shows severe changes of rejection, with indistinctness of the corticomedullary boundary and blending of the renal sinus area with remaining parenchyma. (From Hricak,[406] with permission.)

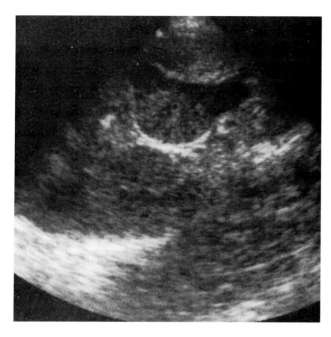

Fig. 13-220. Renal transplant, infection. Sonogram of an allograft in a patient with *C. albicans* infection and deterioration in renal function, showing a debris-fluid level within a dilated pelvis. An antegrade pyelogram (not shown) helped confirm a fungal mass within the pelvis and distal ureter that caused partial obstruction. (From Surratt et al,[440] with permission.)

transplant recipients, but there does not appear to be a significantly increased risk of urinary tract infection complications.[495] There is a marked acoustic impedance mismatch of the gas and renal surfaces, resulting in dense echoes at the acoustic interface with total lack of penetration and the typical reverberation artifacts (Fig. 13-221). Abnormal linear collections of air along the columns of Bertin may be visualized.[495] In such a case, ultrasound can be used to detect the gas and to monitor therapy if indicated. Particular attention should be paid to the insulin-dependent diabetic transplant with acute renal malfunction and clinical signs of renal infection or sepsis.[495]

Tuberculosis. In renal transplant patients, tuberculosis is an uncommon but serious complication.[444] Since renal transplant patients are treated with steroids, they are at increased risk of developing or reactivating tuberculosis.[444] Early on, there is papillary destruction; with progression, there is enlargement to form irregular cavities that communicate with the collecting system.[444] As late sequelae, there may be fibrosis, stricture, and localized or generalized pyonephrosis. The ultrasound findings included distortion of the renal parenchyma without definite hydronephrosis[444] (Fig. 13-222). The transplanted kidney infected with tuberculosis may ap-

pear similar to the native kidney infected with this condition (see Tuberculosis under Native Kidney, above).

Cancer

Patients who are immunosuppressed are at an increased risk of developing de novo tumors.[496,497] Prior to cyclosporine immunosuppression, renal transplant patients had a 6 percent risk of developing a tumor following transplantation, a 100-fold greater incidence than in the general population.[496] Forty percent of the tumors involve the skin and lip; 12 percent are lymphoma in those not receiving cyclosporine.[497] After nonmelanoma skin cancers and in situ cancers of the cervix have been excluded, lymphomas comprise 29 to 38 percent of the post-transplant cancers.[496,497]

In a review series, it was found that of the patients with disseminated post-transplant lymphoma, 33 percent had involvement of the renal allograft.[497] The renal allograft lymphomas are thought to arise from the recipient (host) cells.[497] Since the introduction of cyclosporine immunosuppression, the relative number of lymphomas has increased, with lymphomas comprising 52 percent of tumors compared with 12 percent in patients who have had conventional immunosuppression.[496] Lymphomas develop an average of 8.5 months following transplantation in the cyclosporine group compared with an average of 41 months in patients who have not received cyclosporine.[496]

In the transplant patient, lymphoproliferative disease has been attributed to impaired immune surveillance, chronic antigenic stimulation from the allograft, and oncogenic effects of immunosuppressants.[496] Most of these post-transplant lymphomas are non-Hodgkin's lymphoma, with Hodgkin's disease (the most common lymphoma in the general population) representing only 2 percent of the lymphomas.[496]

The post-transplant lymphomas have a progressive and fatal course; the mortality has exceeded 80 percent in the past.[496] These lesions may be responsive to reduction or suspension of immunosuppression, resulting in improved survival for renal transplant recipients. Because of the highly aggressive nature of many of these tumors, particularly in the setting of cyclosporine immunosuppression, early diagnosis is important for optimal management.[497] As such, recognition of these abnormalities is key to survival.[496] Fine-needle aspiration biopsy may be used if lymphoma is a consideration, but many surgeons would merely opt to reexplore these patients rather than perform a percutaneous biopsy.[497]

There may be involvement of the gastrointestinal tract, liver, lungs, and lymph nodes with the post-transplant lymphoma.[496] Allograft involvement is common and is seen as a hypoechoic mass[496] (Fig. 13-223).

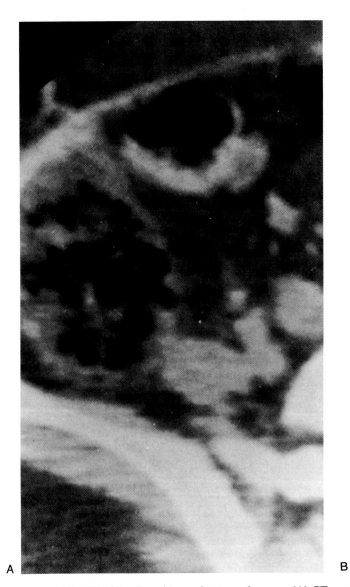

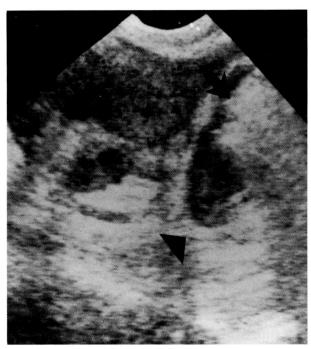

A

B

Fig. 13-221. Renal transplant, emphysema. **(A)** CT section showing the allograft in the right lower quadrant with intrarenal gas in a radial distribution (extrarenal extension not shown). **(B)** Sonogram of the allograft showing normal upper-pole cortex (solid arrowhead) with gas (arrow) shadowing the midpole. (open arrowhead, distended cecum cephalic to the kidney.) (From Potter et al,[495] with permission.)

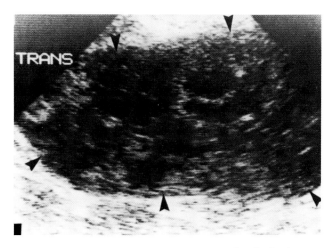

Fig.13-222. Renal transplant, tuberculosis. Sagittal scan through the transplant showing irregular fluid collections and a distorted collecting system, an appearance considered atypical for hydronephrosis. (arrowheads, renal margins). A retrograde pyelogram (not shown) showed a moth-eaten, irregularly marginated collecting system, as well as small cavities adjacent to the papilla. (From Stuck et al,[444] with permission.)

Other ultrasound signs of allograft lymphoma include (1) infiltrative growth traversing tissue planes, resulting in tumor masses with ill-defined margins and coarse trabeculation; (2) central necrosis contributing to nonhomogeneity and increased through transmission; and (3) involvement of the renal pelvis or ureter, resulting in hydronephrosis.[496]

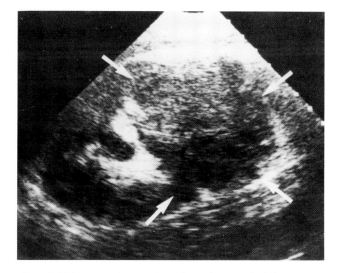

Fig. 13-223. Renal transplant, lymphoma. Ill-defined lymphomatous mass involves the renal allograft. The tumor mass (arrows) appears isoechoic on real-time examination. (From Russ et al,[496] with permission.)

Interventional Procedures

Biopsy

Renal biopsy may be valuable in determining the cause of post-transplant oliguria and differentiating rejection and ATN.[470,498,499] However, it is invasive and could lead to further deterioration of function. The diagnostic difference is based on a paucity or absence of the characteristic features of rejection interstitial nephritis, arteritis, or glomerular lesion. It can sometimes be difficult.

Renal biopsy is generally performed with ultrasound guidance. It is ideal for ultrasound guidance since the kidney lies superficially in the iliac fossa.[445] The superior lateral aspect of the kidney is localized, provided the kidney is placed in a cephalic-caudal orientation. If there is a question about orientation, one should localize the most lateral aspect of the kidney away from the renal hilum (as in a transverse lie). The target area may be localized and marked on the skin, or the nephrologist may be guided directly with real-time visualization and a biopsy needle guide. We have found the latter to be best because it decreases the number of needle sticks, increases the speed of tissue recovery, and decreases the time of the procedure. Once the needle is seen to enter the kidney, the needle is detached from the needle guide and the biopsy is performed "free-handed" (see also Ch. 19).

Other Procedures

Besides renal biopsy, other interventional urologic procedures may be performed on the renal transplant patient. An antegrade pyelogram may be performed if ultrasound shows that hydronephrosis is increasing in severity but no obvious mass is seen. This procedure can be done with ultrasound guidance by using an anterolateral calyx from an angled puncture at the lateral border.[500] A percutaneous nephrostomy may be performed for temporary drainage, to check function, and possibly to remove a calculus.[500] This should be done in a way similar to that described in Chapter 19.

Aspiration and drainage of fluid should be undertaken if the patient's renal function is decreasing or if there is fever, mass, or unilateral leg edema.[500] The fluid aspirated is sent for chemical and bacteriologic analysis. An indwelling catheter and repeated puncture increase the risk of the procedure, so it is recommended that only fluid aspiration be undertaken. With the second recurrence, surgery is recommended. There is a complication rate of 6 percent.[500]

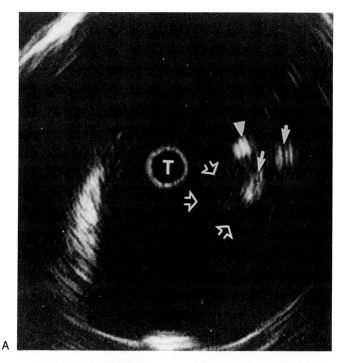

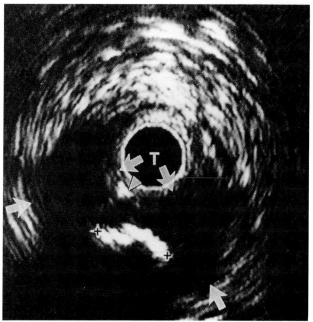

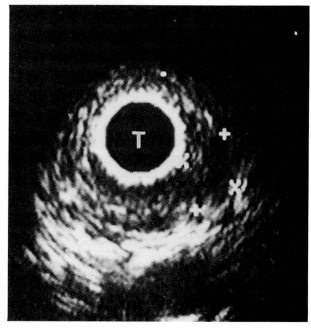

Fig. 13-224. Endoluminal ultrasound of the urinary tract. Case 1. **(A)** Cross-sectional sonogram obtained from within the renal pelvis delineates the renal papilla (open arrows), with two stones identified in the submucosa (solid arrows). Note the bright reflection from the guidewire in contact with the mucosal surface (arrowhead). A portion of another renal papilla is seen between 7 and 10 o'clock. (T, transducer.) Case 2. **(B)** Patient with distal ureteral stone. Cross-sectional sonogram of distal left ureter showing thickened hypoechoic mucosa (arrows). Located within the area of thickened mucosa was a calculus measuring 4.5 mm (calipers) with distal acoustic shadowing. (arrowhead, reflection from guidewire; T, transducer.) Case 3. **(C)** Sonographic transducer (T) located within distal ureter showing area of hypoechoic wall thickening with bulging (calipers) of the outer ureteral wall, measuring 4.1 × 3.0 mm. This was proved to be a low-grade transitional cell carcinoma. (From Goldberg et al,[502] with permission.)

It has been shown that percutaneous procedures can be safely used to help diagnose and treat these urologic complications.[440] The use of percutaneous procedures may obviate or delay surgery while preserving the renal graft and the patient's life.[440]

cause of renal transplant dysfunction.[501] There are two major problems with the Doppler evaluation of transplant dysfunction: (1) both ATN and acute rejection can cause increased vascular resistance, and (2) a significant number of patients with acute rejection have normal (<0.80) RIs.[501]

Real-time ultrasound is needed to assess for parenchymal changes and to evaluate for perirenal fluid collections. Doppler assessment adds unique information about the vascular integrity of the graft and can be used to identify stenosis of the renal artery and other vascular abnormalities.[501] Although an abnormal waveform has been shown to indicate a compromised allograft, this information cannot obviate biopsy.[501]

Conclusions

It has become increasingly evident that renal transplantation has been accepted as the primary treatment for chronic renal failure, and, as such, there has been the need for a reliable noninvasive method of assessing the

NEW DEVELOPMENTS

Endoluminal ultrasound of the urinary tract is a new technique that has been performed by using endoluminal transducers contained within 2-mm-diameter catheters.[502] A variety of lumina including the urethra, urinary bladder, ureters, renal pelvis, endometrial canal, fallopian tubes, bile ducts, and bowel have been evaluated. These specially developed, commercially available 6-French flexible catheters contain transducers of 20 MHz; they have been used in both animal models and humans. With this frequency, an axial resolution of 0.1 mm and a maximum penetration of approximately 2 cm were achieved. The results from this preliminary study suggest that it is a useful procedure (Fig. 13-224). With these flexible transducers, evaluation of the mucosal surface and walls of the bladder, ureters, and renal pelvis, as well as adjacent structures, is permitted. The

images generated allowed the identification of areas of wall thickening or narrowing, calculi, and blood vessels. The flexible nature of these catheters and their small diameters allow their easy passage without the need for urethral dilatation within the bladder. There are limitations to the imaging capabilities. The high frequency used prevents penetration beyond a few centimeters. The small size of the transducer also limits the resolution.

Catheters containing transducers may be guided into the ureter during the course of a cystoscopic or ureteroscopic examination.[502] This technique has proven helpful in detecting stones located beneath the surface of the mucosa in the ureter and kidney. More cases are needed to provide evidence about the long-term use of this technique.

REFERENCES

1. Rosenberg ER, Clair MR, Bowie JD: The fluid-filled stomach as an acoustic window to left kidney. AJR 1982;138:175
2. Finberg H: Renal ultrasound: anatomy and technique. Semin Ultrasound CT MR 1981;2:7
3. Bazzocchi M, Rizzato G: The value of the posterior oblique longitudinal scan in renal ultrasonography. Urol Radiol 1980;1:221
4. Thompson IM, Kovac A, Geshner J: Coronal renal ultrasound: II. Urology 1981;17:210
5. Albarelli JN, Lawson TL: Renal ultrasonography: advantages of the decubitus position. J Clin Ultrasound 1978;6:115
6. Skolnick ML: Enhanced ultrasonic visualization of kidneys via an abdominal compression pillow. J Clin Ultrasound 1978;6:440
7. Thompson IM, Kovac A, Geshner J, Sarma D: Coronal renal ultrasound: I. Urology 1981;17:92
8. Rosenfield AT, Taylor KJW, Crade M, DeGraaf CS: Anatomy and pathology of the kidney by gray scale ultrasound. Radiology 1978;128:737
9. Rosenfield AT, Taylor KJW, Crade M: Renal ultrasound 1979: gray scale, real-time, Doppler. p. 1. In Rosenfield AT (ed): Clinics in Diagnostic Ultrasound. Genitourinary Ultrasonography. Vol. 2. Churchill Livingstone, New York, 1979
10. Strandness DE Jr: Duplex scanning in diagnosis of renovascular hypertension. Surg Clin North Am 1990;70:109
11. Dubbins PA: Renal artery stenosis: duplex Doppler evaluation. Brit J Radiol 1986;59:225
12. Sievers KW, Lohr E, Werner WR: Duplex Doppler ultrasound in determination of renal artery stenosis. Urol Radiol 1989;11:142

13. Platt JF, Ellis JH, Rubin JM: Examination of native kidneys with Duplex Doppler ultrasound. Semin Ultrasound CT MR 1991;12:308

14. Mostbeck GH, Kain R, Mallek R et al: Duplex Doppler sonography in renal parenchymal disease. Histopathologic correlation. J Ultrasound Med 1991;10:189

15. Scola FH, Cronan JJ, Schepps B: Grade I hydronephrosis: pulsed Doppler US evaluation. Radiology 1989;171:519

16. Platt JF, Rubin JM, Ellis JH: Distinction between obstructive and nonobstructive pyelocaliectasis with duplex Doppler sonography. AJR 1989;153:997

17. Platt JF, Rubin JM, Ellis JH, DiPietro MA: Duplex Doppler US of the kidney: differentiation of obstructive from nonobstructive dilatation. Radiology 1989;171:515

18. Rosi P, Virgili G, Di Stasi SM et al: Diuretic ultrasound. A non-invasive technique for the assessment of upper tract obstruction. Br J Urol 1990;65:566

19. Ebel KD, Bliesener JA, Gharib M: Imaging of ureteropelvic junction obstruction with stimulated diuresis. Pediatr Radiol 1988;18:54

20. Magill HL, Tonkin ILD, Badi H, Riggs W Jr: Advantages of coronal ultrasonography in evaluating the neonatal retroperitoneum. J Ultrasound Med 1983;2:289

21. Jacobs NM, Grant EG, Richardson JD: Neonatal renal enlargement as a sonic window. J Clin Ultrasound 1983;11:521

22. Huntington DK, Hill SC, Hill MC: Sonographic manifestations of medical renal disease. Semin Ultrasound CT MR 1991;12:290

23. Platt JF, Rubin JM, Bowerman RA, Marn CS: The inability to detect kidney disease on the basis of echogenicity. AJR 1988;151:317

24. Robbins SL, Cotran RS (eds): The kidney. p. 1115. In Pathologic Basis of Disease. WB Saunders, Philadelphia, 1979.

25. Cook JH III, Rosenfield AT, Taylor KJW: Ultrasonic demonstration of intrarenal anatomy. AJR 1977;129:831

26. Rosenfield AT: Ultrasound evaluation of renal parenchymal disease and hydronephrosis. Urol Radiol 1982;4:125

27. Jones BE, Hoffer FA, Teele RL, Lebowitz RL: The compound renal pyramid. A normal hypoechoic region on the pediatric sonogram. J Ultrasound Med 1987;6:515

28. Sanders RC, Conrad MR: The ultrasonic characteristics of the renal pelvicalyceal echo complex. J Clin Ultrasound 1977;5:372

29. Rosenfield AT, Taylor KJW, Dembner AG, Jacobson P: Ultrasound of renal sinus: new observations. AJR 1979;133:441.

30. Share JC, Lebowitz RL: The unsuspected double collecting system on imaging studies and at cystoscopy. AJR 1990;155:561

31. Middleton WD, Melson GL: Renal duplication artifact in US imaging. Radiology 1989;173:427

32. Nicolet V, Carignan L, Dubuc G et al: Thickening of the renal collecting system: a nonspecific finding at US. Radiology 1988;168:411

33. Babcock DS: Sonography of wall thickening of the renal collecting system: a nonspecific finding. J Ultrasound Med 1987;6:29

34. Carter AR, Horgan JG, Jennings TA, Rosenfield AT: The junctional parenchymal defect: a sonographic variant of renal anatomy. Radiology 1985;154:499

35. Hoffer FA, Hanabergh AM, Teele RL: The interrenicular junction: a mimic of renal scarring on normal pediatric sonograms. AJR 1985;145:1075

36. Lafortune M, Constantin A, Breton G, Vallee C: Sonography of the hypertrophied column of Bertin. AJR 1986;146:53

37. Behan M, Wixson D, Pitts R Jr, Kazam E: Sonographic evaluation of renal masses: correlations with angiography. Urol Radiol 1980;1:137

38. Leekam RN, Matzinger MA, Brunelle M et al: The sonography of renal columnar hypertrophy. J Clin Ultrasound 1983;11:491

39. Brandt TD, Neiman HL, Dragowski MJ et al: Ultrasound assessment of normal renal dimensions. J Ultrasound Med 1982;1:49

40. Bo WJ, Krueger WA: Anatomic concepts of the urogenital system: Gross and cross-sectional anatomy. p. 37. In Resnick MI, Sanders RC (eds): Ultrasound in Urology. Williams & Wilkins, Baltimore, 1979

41. Lewis E, Ritchie WGM: A simple ultrasonic method for assessing renal size. J Clin Ultrasound 1980;8:417

42. Farrant P, Meire HB: Ultrasonic measurement of renal inclinations: its importance in measurement of renal length. Brit J Radiol 1978;51:628

43. Rasmussen SN, Haase L, Kjeldsen H, Hancke S: Determination of renal volume by ultrasound scanning. J Clin Ultrasound 1978;6:160

44. Jones TB, Ruddick LR, Harpen MD et al: Ultrasonographic determination of renal mass and renal volume. J Ultrasound Med 1983;2:151

45. Hricak H, Lieto RP: Sonographic determination of renal volume. Radiology 1983;48:311

46. Haller JO, Berdon WE, Friedman AP: Increased renal cortical echogenicity: a normal finding in neonates and infants. Radiology 1982;142:173

47. Hricak H, Slovis TL, Callen CW et al: Neonatal kidneys: sonographic anatomic correlation. Radiology 1983;147:699

48. Erwin BC, Carroll BA, Muller H: A sonographic assessment of neonatal renal parameters. J Ultrasound Med 1985;4:217

49. Cramer BC, Jequier S, de Chadarevian JP: Factors associated with renal parenchymal echogenicity in the newborn. J Ultrasound Med 1986;5:633

50. Han BK, Babcock DS: Sonographic measurements and appearance of normal kidneys in children. AJR 1985;145:611

51. Scheible W, Leopold GR: High-resolution real-time ultrasonography of neonatal kidneys. J Ultrasound Med 1982;1:133

52. Patriquin H, Lefaivre JF, Lafortune M et al: Fetal lobulation. An anatomo-ultrasonographic correlation. J Ultrasound Med 1990;9:191

53. Blane CE, Bookstein FL, DiPietro MA, Kelsch RC: Sonographic standards for normal infant kidney length. AJR 1985;145:1289

54. Schlesinger AE, Hedlund GL, Pierson WP, Null DM: Normal standards for kidney length in premature infants: determination with US. Work in progress. Radiology 1987;164:127

55. Fernbach SK, Bernfield JB: Positional variation in the ultrasound appearance of the renal pelvis. Pediatr Radiol 1990;21:45

56. Tsai TC, Lee HC, Huang FY: The size of the renal pelvis on ultrasonography in children. J Clin Ultrasound 1989;17:647

57. McInnis AN, Felman AH, Kaude JV, Walker RD: Renal ultrasound in the neonatal period. Pediatr Radiol 1982;12:15.

58. Rosenbaum DM, Korngold E, Teele RL: Sonographic assessment of renal length in normal children. AJR 1984;142:467

59. Moskowitz PS, Carroll BA, McCoy JM: Ultrasonic renal volumetry in children: accuracy and simplicity of the method. Radiology 1980;134:61

60. Gross GW, Boal DK: Sonographic assessment of normal renal size in children with myelodysplasia. J Urol 1988;140:784

61. Schlesinger AE, Hernandez RJ, Zerin JM et al: Interobserver and intraobserver variations in sonographic renal length measurements in children. AJR 1991;156:1029

62. Murugasu B, Yip WCL, Tay JSH et al: Sonographic screening for renal tract anomalies associated with congenital heart disease. J Clin Ultrasound 1990;18:79

63. Grossman H, Rosenberg ER, Bowie JD et al: Sonographic diagnosis of renal cystic diseases. AJR 1983;140:81

64. Sumner TE, Volberg FM, Martin JF et al: Real-time sonography of congenital cystic kidney disease. Urology 1982;20:97

65. Stick KJ, Koff SA, Silver TM: Ultrasonic features of multicystic dysplastic kidney: expanded diagnostic criteria. Radiology 1982;143:217

66. Walker D, Fennell R, Garin E, Richard G: Spectrum of multicystic renal dysplasia: diagnosis and management. Urology 1978;11:433

67. Sanders RC, Hartman DS: The sonographic distinction between neonatal multicystic kidney and hydronephrosis. Radiology 1984;151:621

68. Barth RA, Mindell HJ: Renal masses in the fetus and neonate: ultrasonographic diagnosis. Semin Ultrasound CT MR 1984;5:3

69. Hayden CK Jr, Swischuk LE, Smith TH, Armstrong EA: Renal cystic disease in childhood. RadioGraphics 1986;6:97

70. Sanders RC, Nussbaum AR, Solez K: Renal dysplasia: sonographic findings. Radiology 1988;167:623

71. Gordillo R, Vilaro M, Sherman NH et al: Circumscribed renal mass in dysplastic kidney. Pseudomass vs. tumor. J Ultrasound Med 1987;6:613

72. Vinocur L, Slovis TL, Perlmutter AD et al: Follow-up studies of multicystic dysplastic kidneys. Radiology 1988;167:311

73. Avni EF, Thoua Y, Lalmand B et al: Multicystic dysplastic kidney: natural history from in utero diagnosis and postnatal follow-up. J Urol 1987;138:1420

74. Boal DK, Teele RL: Sonography of infantile polycystic kidney disease. AJR 1980;135:575

75. Babcock DS: Medical diseases of the urinary tract and adrenal gland. p. 113. In Haller JO, Shkolnik A (eds): Clinics in Diagnostic Ultrasound. Diagnostic Ultrasound in Pediatrics. Vol. 8. Churchill Livingstone, New York, 1981

76. Melson GL, Shackelford GD, Cole BR, McClennan BL: The spectrum of sonographic findings in infantile polycystic kidney disease with urographic and clinical correlations. J Clin Ultrasound 1985;13:113

77. Evans JB, Captain MC, Shapeero LG et al: Infantile glomerulonephritis mimicking polycystic kidney disease. J Ultrasound Med 1988;7:29

78. Wernecke K, Heckemann R, Bachmann H, Peters PE: Sonography of infantile polycystic kidney disease. Urol Radiol 1985;7:138

79. Currarino G, Stannard MW, Rutledge JC: The sonolucent cortical rim in infantile polycystic kidneys. Histologic correlation. J Ultrasound Med 1989;8:571

80. Luisiri A, Salinas-Madrigal L, Noguchi A et al: Renal tubular dysgenesis. AJR 1991;157:383

81. Fitch SJ, Stapleton FB: Ultrasonographic features of glomerulocystic disease in infancy: similarity to infantile polycystic kidney disease. Pediatr Radiol 1986;16:400

82. Rosenfield AT, Lipson MH, Wolf B et al: Ultrasonography and nephrotomography in the presymptomatic diagnosis of dominantly inherited (adult-onset) polycystic kidney disease. Radiology 1980;135:423

83. Walker FC Jr, Loney LC, Root ER et al: Diagnostic evaluation of adult polycystic kidney disease in childhood. AJR 1984;142:1273

84. Ralls PW, Halls J: Hydronephrosis, renal cystic disease, and renal parenchymal disease. Semin Ultrasound CT MR 1981;2:49.

85. Kutcher R, Schneider M, Gordon DH: Calcification in polycystic disease. Radiology 1977;122:77

86. Kelsey JA, Bowie JD: Gray-scale ultrasonography in the diagnosis of polycystic kidney disease. Radiology 1977;122:791

87. Lawson TL, McClennan BL, Shirkhoda A: Adult polycystic kidney disease: ultrasonographic and computed tomographic appearance. J Clin Ultrasound 1978;6:297.

88. Kutcher R, Sprayregen S, Rosenblatt R, Goldman M: The sonographic appearance of segmental polycystic kidney. J Ultrasound Med 1983;2:425

89. Lee JKT, McClennan BL, Kissane JM: Unilateral polycystic kidney disease. AJR 1978;130:1165

90. Hantman SS: Unilateral adult polycystic kidney. J Ultrasound Med 1982;1:371

91. Hayden CK Jr, Swischuk LE, Davis M, Brouhard BH: Puddling: a distinguishing feature of adult polycystic kidney disease in the neonate. AJR 1984;142:811

92. Rego JD Jr, Laing FC, Jeffrey RB: Ultrasonographic diagnosis of medullary cystic disease. J Ultrasound Med 1983;2:433

93. Garel LA, Habib R, Pariente D et al: Juvenile nephronophthisis: sonographic appearance in children with severe uremia. Radiology 1984;151:93

94. Rosenfield AT, Siegel NJ, Kappelman NB, Taylor KJW: Gray scale ultrasonography in medullary cystic disease of the kidney and congenital hepatic fibrosis with tubular ectasia: new observations. AJR 1977;129:297

95. Patriquin HB, O'Regan S: Medullary sponge kidney in childhood. AJR 1985;145:315

96. Graif M, Lison M, Strauss S et al: Congenital nephrosis: ultrasonographic features. Pediatr Radiol 1982;12:154

97. Pope TL Jr, Alford BA, Buschi AJ et al: Nuclear scintigraphy and ultrasound in the diagnosis of congenital ureteropelvic junction obstruction. J Urol 1980;124:917

98. Garcia CJ, Taylor KJW, Weiss RM: Congenital megacalyces. Ultrasound appearance. J Ultrasound Med 1987;6:163

99. Cramer B, Green J, Harnett J et al: Sonographic and urographic correlation in Bardet-Biedl syndrome (formerly Laurence-Moon-Biedl syndrome). Urol Radiol 1988;10:176

100. Schaffer RM, Shih YH, Becker JA: Sonographic identification of collecting system duplications. J Clin Ultrasound 1983;11:309

101. Mascatello VJ, Smith EH, Carrera GF et al: Ultrasonic evaluation of the obstructed duplex kidney. AJR 1977;129:113

102. Brown JM: The ultrasound approach to the urographically nonvisualizing kidney. Semin Ultrasound CT MR 1981;2:44

103. Sumner TE, Volberg FM, Smolen PM: Intrathoracic kidney: diagnosis by ultrasound. Pediatr Radiol 1982;12:78

104. Rosenberg HK: Traumatic avulsion of the vascular supply of a crossed unfused ectopic kidney: complementary roles of ultrasonography and intravenous pyelography. J Ultrasound Med 1984;3:89

105. McCarthy S, Rosenfield AT: Ultrasonography in crossed renal ectopia. J Ultrasound Med 1984;3:107

106. Lubat E, Hernanz-Schulman M, Genieser NB et al: Sonography of the simple and complicated ipsilateral fused kidney. J Ultrasound Med 1989;8:109

107. Nussbaum AR, Hartman DS, Whitley N, et al. Multicystic dysplasia and crossed renal ectopia. AJR 1987;149:407

108. Teele RL, Rosenfield AT, Freedman GS: The anatomic splenic flexure: an ultrasonic renal imposter. AJR 1977;128:115

109. Trackler RT, Resnick ML, Leopold GR: Pelvic horseshoe kidney: ultrasound findings and case report. J Clin Ultrasound 1978;6:51

110. Gray BB Jr, Dawes RK, Atkinson GO Jr, Ball TI Jr: Wilms' tumor in horseshoe kidneys: radiologic diagnosis. Radiology 1983;146:693

111. Mindell HJ, Kupic EA: Horseshoe kidney: ultrasonic demonstration. AJR 1977;129:526

112. Bree RL: Anterior position of the lower pole of the right kidney: potential confusion with right upper quadrant mass. J Clin Ultrasound 1976;4:283

113. Hasch E: Ultrasound in the diagnosis of hydronephrosis in infants and children. J Clin Ultrasound 1974;2:21.

114. Ellenbogen PH, Scheible FW, Talner LB, Leopold GR: Sensitivity of gray-scale ultrasound in detecting urinary tract obstruction. AJR 1978;130:731

115. Lee JKT, Baron RL, Melson GL et al: Can real-time ultrasonography replace static B-scan in the diagnosis of renal obstruction? Radiology 1981;139:161

116. Amis ES Jr, Cronan JJ, Pfister RC, Yoder IC: Ultrasonic inaccuracies in diagnosing renal obstruction. Urology 1982;19:101

117. Morin ME, Baker DA: The influence of hydration and bladder distension in the sonographic diagnosis of hydronephrosis. J Clin Ultrasound 1979;7:192

118. Kamholtz RG, Cronan JJ, Dorfman GS: Obstruction and the minimally dilated renal collecting system: US evaluation. Radiology 1989;170:51

119. Gottlieb RH, Luhmann K IV, Oates RP: Duplex ultrasound evaluation of normal native kidneys and native kidneys with urinary tract obstruction. J Ultrasound Med 1989;8:609

120. Bude RO, Platt JF, Rubin JM, Ohl DA: Dilated renal collecting systems: differentiating obstructive from nonobstructive dilation using duplex Doppler ultrasound. Urology 1991;37:123

121. Dinkel E, Dittrich M, Peters H et al: Sonographic biometry in obstructive uropathy of children: preoperative diagnosis and postoperative monitoring. Urol Radiol 1985;7:1

122. Chopra A, Teele RL: Hydronephrosis in children: narrowing the differential diagnosis with ultrasound. J Clin Ultrasound 1980;8:473

123. Markle BM, Potter BM: Surgical diseases of the urinary tract. p. 135. In Haller JO, Shkolnik A (eds): Clinics in Diagnostic Ultrasound. Diagnostic Ultrasound in Pediatrics. Vol. 8. Churchill Livingstone, New York, 1981

124. Nusbacher N, Bryk D: Hydronephrosis of the lower pole of the duplex kidney: Another renal pseudotumor. AJR 1978;130:967

125. Wyly JB, Resende CMC, Teele RL: Ultrasonography of the complicated duplex kidney: further observations. Semin Ultrasound CT MR 1984;1:35

126. Lucaya J, Enriquez G, Delgado R, Castellote A: Infundibulopelvic stenosis in children. AJR 1984;142:471

127. Ralls PW, Esensten ML, Boger D, Halls JM: Severe hydronephrosis and severe renal cystic disease: ultrasonic differentiation. AJR 1980;134:473

128. Jequier S, Forbes PA, Nogrady MB: The value of ultrasonography as a screening procedure in a first-documented urinary tract infection in children. J Ultrasound Med 1985;4:393

129. Kangarloo H, Gold RH, Fine RN et al: Urinary tract infection in infants and children evaluated by ultrasound. Radiology 1985;154:357

130. Leonidas JC, McCauley RGK, Klauber GC, Fretzayas AM: Sonography as a substitute for excretory urography

in children with urinary tract infection. AJR 1985; 144:815

131. Paltiel HJ, Lebowitz RL: Neonatal hydronephrosis due to primary vesicoureteral reflux: Trends in diagnosis and treatment. Radiology 1989;170:787

132. Fried AM, Woodring JH, Thompson DJ: Hydronephrosis of pregnancy: a prospective sequential study of the course of dilatation. J Ultrasound Med 1983;2:255

133. Peake SL, Roxburgh HB, Langlois SLP: Ultrasonic assessment of hydronephrosis of pregnancy. Radiology 1983;146:167

134. Erwin BC, Carroll BA, Sommer FG: Ultrasound in renal colic. Proceedings from the 28th Annual American Institute of Ultrasound in Medicine. J Ultrasound Med 1983;2:14

135. Erwin BC, Carroll BA, Sommer FG: Renal colic: the role of ultrasound in initial evaluation. Radiology 1984;152:147

136. Laing FC, Jeffrey RB Jr, Wing VW: Ultrasound versus excretory urography in evaluating acute flank pain. Radiology 1985;154:613

137. Cronan JJ, Amis ES, Scola FH, Schepps B: Renal obstruction in patients with ileal loops: US evaluation. Radiology 1986;158:647

138. Jeffrey RB, Federle MP: CT and ultrasonography of acute renal abnormalities. Radiol Clin North Am 1983;21:515

139. Curry NS, Gobien RP, Schabel SI: Minimal-dilatation obstructive nephropathy. Radiology 1982;143:531

140. Talner LB, Scheible W, Ellenbogen PH et al: How accurate is ultrasonography in detecting hydronephrosis in azotemic patients? Urol Radiol 1981;3:1

141. Maillet PJ, Pelle-Francoz D, Laville M et al: Nondilated obstructive acute renal failure: diagnostic procedures and therapeutic management. Radiology 1986;160:659.

142. Malave SP, Neiman HL, Spies SM et al: Diagnosis of hydronephrosis: comparison of radionuclide scanning and sonography. AJR 1980;135:1179

143. Shkolnik A: B-mode ultrasound and the nonvisualizing kidney in pediatrics. AJR 1977;128:121

144. Sanders RC: The place of diagnostic ultrasound in the examination of kidneys not seen on excretory urography. J Urol 1975;114:813

145. Marangola JP, Bryan PJ, Azimi F: Ultrasonic evaluation of the unilateral nonvisualized kidney. AJR 1976; 126:853

146. Behan M, Wixson D, Kazam E: Sonographic evaluation of the nonfunctioning kidney. J Clin Ultrasound 1979; 7:449

147. Finberg HJ, Billman B, Smith EH: Ultrasound in the evaluation of the nonfunctioning kidney. p. 105. In Rosenfield AT (ed): Clinics in Diagnostic Ultrasound. Genitourinary Ultrasonography. Vol. 2. Churchill Livingstone, New York, 1979

148. Feinstein KA, Fernbach SK: Septated urinomas in the neonate. AJR 1987;149:997

149. Itoh S, Yoshioka H, Kaeriyama M et al: Ultrasonographic diagnosis of uriniferous perirenal pseudocyst. Pediatr Radiol 1982;12:156

150. Yeh E-L, Chiang L-C, Meade RC: Ultrasound and radio-nuclide studies of urinary extravasation with hydrone-phrosis. J Urol 1981;125:728

151. Sumner TE, Crowe JE, Resnick MI: Ultrasonically guided antegrade pyelography of an obstructed solitary pelvic kidney. J Clin Ultrasound 1978;6:262

152. Pedersen JF, Cowan DF, Kristensen JK et al: Ultrasonically-guided percutaneous nephrostomy: report of 24 cases. Radiology 1976;119:429

153. Barbaric ZL, Wood BP: Emergency percutaneous nephropyelostomy: experience with 34 patients and review of the literature. AJR 1977;128:453

154. Sadlowski RW, Finney RP, Branch WT et al: New technique for percutaneous nephrostomy under ultrasound guidance. J Urol 1979;121:559

155. Baron RL, Lee JKT, McClennan BL, Melson GL: Percutaneous nephrostomy using real-time sonographic guidance. AJR 1981;136:1018

156. Zegal HG, Pollack HM, Banner MP et al: Percutaneous nephrostomy: comparison of sonographic and fluoroscopic guidance. AJR 1981;137:925

157. Stables DP, Johnson ML: Percutaneous nephrostomy: the role of ultrasound. p. 73. In Rosenfield AT (ed): Clinics in Diagnostic Ultrasound. Genitourinary Ultrasonography. Vol. 2. Churchill Livingstone, New York, 1979

158. Burnett KR, Handler SJ, Conroy RM et al: Percutaneous nephrostomy utilizing B-mode and real-time ultrasound guidance: the lateral approach and puncture facilitation with furosemide. J Clin Ultrasound 1982;10:252

159. Stanley P, Bear JW, Reid BS: Percutaneous nephrostomy in infants and children. AJR 1983;141:473

160. Bartone FF, Mazer MJ, Anderson JC et al: Diagnosis and treatment of fluid-filled renal structures in children with ultrasonography and percutaneous puncture. Urology 1980;16:432

161. Bolton WK, Vaughan ED Jr: A comparative study of open surgical and percutaneous renal biopsies. J Urol 1977;117:696

162. Winfield AC, Kirchner SG, Brun ME et al: Percutaneous nephrostomy in neonates, infants, and children. Radiology 1984;151:617

163. Dubuisson RL, Eichelberger RP, Jones TB: A simple modification of real-time sector sonography to monitor percutaneous nephrostomy. Radiology 1983;146: 232

164. Piccirillo M, Rigsby CM, Rosenfield AT: Sonography of renal inflammatory disease. Urol Radiol 1987;9:66

165. Bick RJ, Bryan PJ: Sonographic demonstration of thickened renal pelvic mucosa/submucosa in mixed candida infection. J Clin Ultrasound 1987;15:333

166. Kuligowska E, Newman B, White SJ, Caldarone A: Interventional ultrasound in detection and treatment of renal inflammatory disease. Radiology 1983;147:521

167. Morehouse HT, Weiner SN, Hoffman JC: Imaging in inflammatory disease of the kidney. AJR 1984; 143:135.

168. Gold RP, McClennan BL, Rottenberg RR: CT appearance of acute inflammatory disease of the renal interstitium. AJR 1983;141:343.

169. Edell SL, Bonavita JA: The sonographic appearance of acute pyelonephritis. Radiology 1979;132:683

170. Fiegler W: Ultrasound in acute inflammatory lesions. Eur J Radiol 1983;3:354

171. Ben-Ami T: The sonographic evaluation of urinary tract infection in children. Semin Ultrasound CT MR 1984;5:19

172. Dinkel E, Orth S, Dittrich M, Schulte-Wissermann H: Renal sonography in the differentiation of upper from lower urinary tract infection. AJR 1986;146:775

173. Bjorgvinsson E, Majd M, Eggli KD: Diagnosis of acute pyelonephritis in children: Comparison of sonography and 99mTc-DMSA scintigraphy. AJR 1991;157:539

174. Chou YH, Tiu CM, Chen TW et al: Emphysematous pyelonephritis in a polycystic kidney. Demonstration by ultrasound and computed tomography. J Ultrasound Med 1990;9:355

175. Kenney PJ: Imaging of chronic renal infections. AJR 1990;155:485

176. Kay CJ, Rosenfield AT, Taylor KJW, Rosenberg MA: Ultrasonic characteristics of chronic atrophic pyelonephritis. AJR 1979;132:47

177. Subramanyam BR, Megibow AJ, Raghavendra BN, Bosniak MA: Diffuse xanthogranulomatous pyelonephritis: analysis by computed tomography and sonography. Urol Radiol 1982;4:5

178. Hartman DS, Davis CJ Jr, Goldman SM et al: Xanthogranulomatous pyelonephritis: sonographic-pathologic correlation of 16 cases. J Ultrasound Med 1984;3:481

179. Van Kirk OC, Go RT, Wedel VJ: Sonographic features of xanthogranulomatous pyelonephritis. AJR 1980;134:1035

180. Boutros GA, Athey PA: Ultrasonic demonstration of xanthogranulomatous pyelonephritis. J Clin Ultrasound 1978;6:427

181. Morgan CL, Dempsey PJ, Johnsrude I, Johnson ML: Ultrasound in the diagnosis of xanthogranulomatous pyelonephritis: a case report. J Clin Ultrasound 1975;3:301.

182. Gonzalez AC, Karciogla Z, Waters BB, Weens HS: Megalocystic interstitial nephritis: ultrasound and radiographic changes. Radiology 1979;133:449

183. Yoder IC, Pfister RC, Lindfors KK, Newhouse JH: Pyonephrosis: imaging and intervention. AJR 1983;141:735.

184. Coleman BG, Arger PH, Mulhern CB Jr et al: Pyonephrosis: sonography in the diagnosis and management. AJR 1981;137:939

185. Subramanyam BR, Raghavendra BN, Bosniak MA et al: Sonography of pyonephrosis: a prospective study. AJR 1983;140:491

186. Jeffrey RB, Laing RC, Wing VW, Hoddick W: Sensitivity of sonography in pyonephrosis: a reevaluation. AJR 1985;144:71

187. Schneider K, Helmig FJ, Eife R et al: Pyonephrosis in childhood—is ultrasound sufficient for diagnosis? Pediatr Radiol 1989;19:302

188. Das KM, Indudhara R, Vaidyanathan S: Sonographic features of genitourinary tuberculosis. AJR 1992;158:327

189. Premkumar A, Lattimer J, Newhouse JH: CT and sonography of advanced urinary tract tuberculosis. AJR 1987;148:65

190. Kirpekar M, Abiri MM, Hilfer C, Enerson R: Ultrasound in the diagnosis of systemic candidiasis (renal and cranial) in a very low birth weight premature infants. Pediatr Radiol 1986;16:17

191. Kintanar C, Cramer BC, Reid WD, Andrews WL: Neonatal renal candidiasis: sonographic diagnosis. AJR 1986;147:801

192. Stuck KJ, Silver TM, Jaffe MH, Bowerman RA: Sonographic demonstration of renal fungus balls. Radiology 1981;142:473

193. Dillard JP, Talner LB, Pickney L: Normal renal papillae simulating caliceal filling defects on sonography. AJR 1987;148:895

194. Siegel MJ, Glasier CM: Acute focal bacterial nephritis in children: significance of ureteral reflux. AJR 1981;137:257

195. Rosenfield AT, Glickman MG, Taylor KJW et al: Acute focal bacterial nephritis (acute lobar nephronia). Radiology 1979;132:553

196. Rigsby CM, Rosenfield AT, Glickman MG, Hodson J: Hemorrhagic focal bacterial nephritis: findings on gray-scale sonography and CT. AJR 1986;146:1173

197. Lee JKT, McClennan BL, Melson GL, Stanley RJ: Acute focal bacterial nephritis: emphasis on gray scale sonography and computed tomography. AJR 1980;135:87.

198. Finn DJ, Palestrant AM, DeWolf WC: Successful percutaneous management of renal abscess. J Urol 1982;127:425

199. Gerzof SG, Gale ME: Computed tomography and ultrasonography for diagnosis and treatment of renal and retroperitoneal abscess. Urol Clin North Am 1982;9:185

200. Gerzof SG: Percutaneous drainage of renal and perinephric abscess. Urol Radiol 1981;2:171

201. Hoddick W, Jeffrey RB, Goldberg HI et al: CT and sonography of severe renal and perirenal infections. AJR 1983;140:517

202. Conrad MR, Sanders RC, Mascardo AD: Perinephric abscess aspiration using ultrasound guidance. AJR 1977;128:459

203. Pollack HM, Wein AJ: Imaging of renal trauma. Radiology 1989;172:297

204. Godec CJ: Genitourinary trauma. Urol Radiol 1985;7:185

205. Kay CJ, Rosenfield AT, Armm M: Gray-scale ultrasonography in the evaluation of renal trauma. Radiology 1980;134:461

206. Furtschegger A, Egender G, Jakse G: The value of sonography in the diagnosis and follow-up of patients with blunt renal trauma. Br J Urol 1988;62:110

207. Afschriff M, de Sy W, Voet D et al: Fractured kidney and retroperitoneal hematoma diagnosed by ultrasound. J Clin Ultrasound 1982;10:335

208. Schmoller H, Kunit G, Frick J: Sonography in blunt renal trauma. Eur Urol 1981;7:11

209. Belville JS, Morgentaler A, Loughlin KR, Tumeh SS: Spontaneous perinephric and subcapsular renal hemorrhage: evaluation with CT, US, and angiography. Radiology 1989;172:733

210. Bosniak MA: Spontaneous subcapsular and perirenal hematomas. Radiology 1989;172:601

211. Pollack HM, Banner MP, Arger PH et al: The accuracy of gray-scale renal ultrasonography in differentiating cystic neoplasms from benign cysts. Radiology 1982; 143:741

212. Pollack HM, Banner MP, Arger PH et al: Comparison of computed tomography and ultrasound in the diagnosis of renal masses. p. 25. In Rosenfield AT (ed): Clinics in Diagnostic Ultrasound. Genitourinary Ultrasonography. Vol. 2. Churchill Livingstone, New York, 1979

213. Elyaderani MK, Gabriele OF: Ultrasound of renal masses. Semin Ultrasound CT MR 1981;2:21

214. Bosniak MA: The current radiological approach to renal cysts. Radiology 1986;158:1

215. Bartholomew TH, Slovis TL, Kroovand RL, Corbett DP: The sonographic evaluation and management of simple cysts in children. J Urol 1980;123:732

216. Leopold GR, Talner LB, Asher WM et al: An updated approach to the diagnosis of renal cyst. Radiology 1973;109:671

217. Green WM, King DL, Casarella WJ: A reappraisal of sonolucent renal masses. Radiology 1976;121:163

218. Rosenberg ER, Korobkin M, Foster W et al: The significance of septations in a renal cyst. AJR 1985;144:593

219. Foster WL Jr, Vollmer RT, Halvorsen RA Jr, Williford ME: ultrasonic findings of small hypernephroma associated with renal cyst. J Clin Ultrasound 1983;11:463

220. Jaffe CC, Rosenfield AT, Sommer G, Taylor KJW: Technical factors influencing the imaging of small anechoic cysts by B-scan ultrasound. Radiology 1980; 135:429

221. Sanders RC: Kidneys. p. 68. In Goldberg BB (ed): Clinics in Diagnostic Ultrasound. Ultrasound in Cancer. Vol. 6. Churchill Livingstone, New York, 1981

222. Balfe DM, McClennan BL, Stanley RJ, et al: Evaluation of renal masses considered indeterminant on computed tomography. Radiology 1982;142:421

223. McHugh K, Stringer DA, Hebert D, Babiak CA: Simple renal cysts in children: diagnosis and follow-up with US. Radiology 1991;178:383

224. Steinhardt GF, Slovis TL, Perlmutter AD: Simple renal cysts in infants. Radiology 1985;155:349

225. Sussman S, Cochran ST, Pagani JJ et al: Hyperdense renal masses: a CT manifestation of hemorrhagic renal cysts. Radiology 1984;150:207

226. Curry NS, Brock G, Metcalf JS, Sens MA: Hyperdense renal mass: unusual CT appearance of a benign renal cyst. Urol Radiol 1982;4:33

227. Zirinsky K, Auh YH, Rubenstein WA et al: CT of the hyperdense renal cyst: sonographic correlation. AJR 1984;143:151

228. Cronan JJ, Yoder IC, Amis ES Jr, Pfister RC: The myth of anechoic renal sinus fat. Radiology 1982;144:149

229. Cronan J, Amis ES Jr, Yoder IC et al: Peripelvic cysts: an imposter of sonographic hydronephrosis. J Ultrasound Med 1982;1:229

230. Hidalgo H, Dunnick NR, Rosenberg ER et al: Parapelvic cysts: appearance on CT and sonography. AJR 1982;138:667

231. Narla LD, Slovis TL, Watts FB, Nigro M: The renal lesions of tuberosclerosis (cysts and angiomyolipoma)—

screening with sonography and computerized tomography. Pediatr Radiol 1988;18:205

232. Mitnick JS, Bosniak MA, Hilton S et al: Cystic renal disease in tuberous sclerosis. Radiology 1983;147:85

233. Murphy JB, Marshall FF: Renal cyst versus tumor: a continuing dilemma. J Urol 1980;123:566

234. Ambrose SS, Lewis EL, O'Brien DP III et al: Unsuspected renal tumors associated with renal cysts. J Urol 1977;117:704

235. Amis ES Jr, Cronan JJ, Pfister RC: Needle puncture of cystic renal masses: a survey of the Society of Uroradiology. AJR 1987;148:297

236. Thompson IM Jr, Kovac A, Geshner J: Ultrasound follow-up of renal cyst puncture. J Urol 1980;138:759

237. Erwin BC, Carroll BA, Walter JF, Sommer FG: Renal infarction appearing as an echogenic mass. AJR 1982;138:759

238. Spies JB, Hricak H, Slemmer TM et al: Sonographic evaluation of experimental acute renal arterial occlusion in dogs. AJR 1984;142:341

239. Martin KW, McAlister WH, Shackelford GD: Acute renal infarction: diagnosis by Doppler ultrasound. Pediatr Radiol 1988;18:373

240. Bosniak MA: The small (≤3.0 cm) renal parenchymal tumor: detection, diagnosis, and controversies. Radiology 1991;179:307

241. Ramos IM, Taylor KJW, Kier R et al: Tumor vascular signals in renal masses: detection with Doppler US. Radiology 1988;168:633

242. Coleman BG, Arger PH, Mulhern CT Jr et al: Gray-scale sonographic spectrum of hypernephromas. Radiology 1980;137:757

243. Ladwig SH, Jackson D, Older RA, Morgan CL: Ultrasonic, angiographic, and pathologic correlation of noncystic-appearing renal masses. Urol 1981;17:204

244. Maklad NF, Chuang YP, Doust BD et al: Ultrasonic characterization of solid renal lesions: echographic, angiographic and pathologic correlation. Radiology 1977;123:733

245. Kuijpers D, Jaspers R: Renal masses: differential diagnosis with pulsed Doppler US. Radiology 1989;170:59

246. Dalla-Palma L, Pozzi-Mucelli F, di Donna A, Pozzi-Mucelli RS: Cystic renal tumors: US and CT findings. Urol Radiol 1990;12:67

247. Hartman DS, Davis CJ, Sanders RC et al: The multiloculated renal mass: considerations and differential features. RadioGraphics 1987;7:29

248. Feldberg MAM, van Waes PFGM: Multilocular cystic renal cell carcinoma. AJR 1982;138:953

249. Blei CL, Hartman DS, Friedman AC, Davis CJ Jr: Papillary renal cell carcinoma: ultrasonic/pathologic correlation. J Clin Ultrasound 1982;10:429

250. Press GA, McClennan BL, Melson GL et al: Papillary renal cell carcinoma: CT and sonographic evaluation. AJR 1984;143:1005

251. Katz JF, Nichols L, Kane RA, Balogh K: Renal cell carcinoma: an unusual sonographic appearance. J Ultrasound Med 1986;5:517

252. McDonald DG: The complete echographic evaluation of solid renal masses. J Clin Ultrasound 1978;6:402

253. Green B, Goldstein HM, Weaver RM Jr: Abdominal pansonography in the evaluation of renal cancer. Radiology 1979;132:421

254. Cronan JJ, Zeman RK, Rosenfield AT: Comparison of computerized tomography, ultrasound, and angiography in staging renal cell carcinoma. J Urol 1982;127:712

255. Quinn MJ, Hartman DS, Friedman AC et al: Renal oncocytoma: new observations. Radiology 1984;153:49.

256. Goiney RC, Goldenberg L, Cooperberg PL et al: Renal oncocytomas: sonographic analysis of 14 cases. AJR 1984;143:1001

257. Charboneau JW, Hattery RR, Ernest EC III et al: Spectrum of sonographic findings in 125 renal masses other than benign simple cyst. AJR 1983;140:87

258. Scheible W, Ellenbogen PH, Leopold GR, Siao NT: Lipomatous tumors of the kidney and adrenal: apparent echographic specificity. Radiology 1978;129:153

259. Totty WG, McClennan BL, Melson GL, Patel R: Relative value of computed tomography and ultrasonography in the assessment of renal angiomyolipoma. J Comput Assist Tomogr 1981;5:173

260. Hartman DS, Goldman SM, Friedman AC et al: Angiomyolipoma: ultrasonic-pathologic correlation. Radiology 1981;139:451

261. Bret PM, Bretagnolle M, Gaillard D et al: Small, asymptomatic angiomyolipomas of the kidney. Radiology 1985;154:7

262. Raghavendra BN, Bosniak MA, Megibow AJ: Small angiomyolipoma of the kidney: sonographic-CT evaluation. AJR 1983;141:575

263. Lee TG, Henderson SC, Freeny PC et al: Ultrasound findings of renal angiomyolipoma. J Clin Ultrasound 1978;6:150

264. Duffy P, Ryan J, Aldons W: Ultrasound demonstration of a 1.5 cm intrarenal angiomyolipoma. J Clin Ultrasound 1977;5:111

265. Zappasodi F, Sanna G, Fiorentini G, Frassineti C: Small hyperechoic nodules of the renal parenchyma. J Clin Ultrasound 1985;13:321

266. Kutcher R, Rosenblatt R, Mitsudo SM et al: Renal angiomyolipoma with sonographic demonstration of extension into inferior vena cava. Radiology 1982;143:755.

267. Bosniak MA, Megibow AJ, Hulnick DH et al: CT diagnosis of renal angiomyolipoma: The importance of detecting small amounts of fat. AJR 1988;151:497

268. Papanicolaou N, Harbury OL, Pfister RC: Fat-filled postoperative renal cortical defects: sonographic and CT appearance. AJR 1989;151:503

269. Khan AN, Gould DA, Shah SM, Mouasher YK: Primary renal liposarcoma mimicking angiomyolipoma on ultrasonography and conventional radiology. J Clin Ultrasound 1985;13:58

270. Dunnick NR, Hartman DS, Ford KK et al: The radiology of juxtaglomerular tumors. Radiology 1983;147:321

271. Jacobs JE, Sussman SK, Glickstein MF: Renal lymphangiomyoma—a rare cause of a multiloculated renal mass. AJR 1989;152:307

272. McKeown DK, Nguyen GK, Rudrick B, Johnson MA: Carcinoid of the kidney: radiologic findings. AJR 1988;150:143

273. Fernbach SK: Imaging of neonatal renal masses. Urol Radiol 1991;12:214

274. Madewell JE, Goldman SM, Davis CJ Jr et al: Multilocular cystic nephroma: a radiographic-pathologic correlation of 58 patients. Radiology 1983;146:309

275. Carlson DH, Carlson D, Simon H: Benign multilocular cystic nephroma. AJR 1978;131:621

276. White KS, Grossman H: Wilms' and associated renal tumors of childhood. Pediatr Radiol 1991;21:81

277. Glass RBJ, Davidson AJ, Fernbach SK: Clear cell sarcoma of the kidney: CT, sonographic, and pathologic correlation. Radiology 1991;180:715

278. Kagan AR: Clear cell sarcoma of the kidney: a renal tumor of childhood that metastasizes to bone. AJR 1986;146:64

279. Sisler CL, Siegel MJ: Malignant rhabdoid tumor of the kidney: radiologic features. Radiology 1989;172:211

280. Teele RL: Ultrasonography of the genitourinary tract in children. Radiol Clin North Am 1977;15:109

281. Gates GF, Miller JH, Stanley P: Necrosis of Wilms' tumor. J Urol 1980;123:916

282. Jaffee MH, White SJ, Silver TM, Heidelberger KP: Wilms' tumor: ultrasonic features, pathologic correlation and diagnostic pitfalls. Radiology 1981;140:147

283. Mulhern CB Jr, Arger PH, Coleman BG et al: Wilms' tumor: diagnostic therapeutic implication. Urol Radiol 1982;4:193

284. Bulas DI, Thompson R, Reaman G: Pulmonary emboli as a primary manifestation of Wilms tumor. AJR 1991;156:155

285. Johnson KM, Horvath LJ, Gaisie G et al: Wilms tumor occurring as a botryoid renal pelvicalyceal mass. Radiology 1987;163:385

286. Wood BP, Muurahaihen N, Anderson VM, Ettinger LJ: Multicystic nephroblastoma: ultrasound diagnosis (with a pathologic-anatomic commentary). Pediatr Radiol 1982;12:43.

287. Reiman TAH, Siegel MJ, Shackelford GD: Wilms tumor in children: abdominal CT and US evaluation. Radiology 1986;160:501

288. Franken EA Jr, Yiu-Chiu V, Smith WL, Chiu LC: Nephroblastomatosis: clinicopathologic significance and imaging characteristics. AJR 1982;138:950

289. White KS, Kirks DR, Bove KE: Imaging of nephroblastomatosis: an overview. Radiology 1992;182:1

290. Kioumehr F, Cochran ST, Layfield L et al: Wilms tumor (nephroblastoma) in the adult patient: clinical and radiologic manifestations. AJR 1989;152:299

291. Hartman DS, Sanders RC: Wilms' tumor versus neuroblastoma: usefulness of ultrasound in differentiation. J Ultrasound Med 1982;1:117

292. Fried AM, Hatfield DR, Ellis GT, Fitzgerald KW: Extrarenal Wilms' tumor: sonographic appearance. J Clin Ultrasound 1980;8:360

293. Slovis TL, Perlmutter AD: Recent advances in pediatric urological ultrasound. J Urol 1980;123:613

294. Sty JR, Starshak RJ: Sonography of pediatric urinary tract abnormalities. Semin Ultrasound CT MR 1981;2:71

295. Frank JL, Potter BM, Shkolnik A: Neonatal urosonogra-

phy. p. 159. In Rosenfield AT (ed): Clinics in Diagnostic Ultrasound. Genitourinary Ultrasonography. Vol. 2. Churchill Livingstone, New York, 1979

296. Grider RD, Wolverson MK, Jagannadharao B et al: Congenital mesoblastic nephroma with cystic component. J Clin Ultrasound 1981;9:43

297. Hartman DS, Lesar MSL, Madewell JE et al: Mesoblastic nephroma: radiologic-pathologic correlation of 20 cases. AJR 1981;136:69

298. Arger PH, Mulhern CB, Pollack HM et al: Ultrasonic assessment of renal transitional cell carcinoma: preliminary report. AJR 1979;132:407

299. Subramanyma BR, Raghavendra BN, Mudambra MR: Renal transitional cell carcinoma: sonographic and pathologic correlations. J Clin Ultrasound 1982;10:203

300. Ostrovsky PD, Carr L, Goodman J: Ultrasound of transitional cell carcinoma. J Clin Ultrasound 1985;13:35

301. Bree RL, Shultz SR, Hayes R: Large infiltrating renal transitional cell carcinomas: CT and ultrasound features. J Comput Assist Tomogr 1990;14:381

302. Leder RA, Dunnick NR: Transitional cell carcinoma of the pelvicalices and ureter. AJR 1990;155:713

303. Grant DC, Dee GJ, Yoder IC, Newhouse JH: Sonography in transitional cell carcinoma of the renal pelvis. Urol Radiol 1986;8:1

304. Cunningham JJ: Ultrasonic demonstration of renal collecting system invasion by transitional cell cancer. J Clin Ultrasound 1982;10:339

305. Janetschek G, Putz A, Feichtinger H: Renal transitional cell carcinoma mimicking stone echoes. J Ultrasound Med 1988;7:83

306. Mulholland SG, Arger PH, Goldberg BB, Pollack H: Ultrasonic differentiation of renal pelvic filling defects. J Urol 1979;122:14

307. Wimbish KJ, Sanders MM, Samuels BI, Francis IR: Squamous cell carcinoma of the renal pelvis: case report emphasizing sonographic and CT appearance. Urol Radiol 1983;5:267

308. Dershaw DD, Bernstein AL: Sonography of lung carcinoma metastic to the kidney. Urol Radiol 1985;7:146

309. Choyke PL, White EM, Zeman RK et al: Renal metastases: clinicopathologic and radiologic correlation. Radiology 1987;162:359

310. Kutcher R, Lu T, Gordon DH, Becker JA: Renal choriocarcinoma metastasis: a vascular lesion. AJR 1977;128:1046

311. Tipton A, Goldman SM, Fishman EK, Arnold P: Cystic renal melanoma: CT/ultrasound correlation. Urol Radiol 1987;9:39

312. Hartman DS, Davis CJ Jr, Goldman SM et al: Renal lymphoma: radiologic-pathologic correlation of 21 cases. Radiology 1982;144:759

313. Shirkhoda A, Staab EV, Mittelstaedt CA: Renal lymphoma imaged by ultrasound and gallium 67. Radiology 1980;137:175

314. Heiken JP, Gold RP, Schnur MJ et al: Computed tomography of renal lymphoma with ultrasound correlation. J Comput Assist Tomogr 1983;7:245.

315. Weinberger E, Rosenbaum DM, Pendergrass TW: Renal involvement in children with lymphoma: comparison of CT with sonography. AJR 1990;155:347

316. Kaude JV, Lacy GD: Ultrasonography in renal lymphoma. J Clin Ultrasound 1978;6:321

317. Gregory A, Behan M: Lymphoma of the kidneys: unusual ultrasound appearance due to infiltration of the renal sinus. J Clin Ultrasound 1981;9:343

318. Charnsangavej C: Lymphoma of the genitourinary tract. Radiol Clin North Am 1990;28:865

319. Strauss S, Libson E, Schwartz E et al: Renal sonography in American Burkitt lymphoma. AJR 1986;146:549

320. Jayagopal S, Cohen HL, Bhagat J, Eaton DH: Hyperechoic renal cortical masses: an unusual sonographic presentation of acute lymphoblastic leukemia in a child. J Clin Ultrasound 1991;19:425

321. Kumari-Subaiya S, Lee WJ, Festa R et al: Sonographic findings in leukemic renal disease. J Clin Ultrasound 1984;12:465

322. Goh TS, LeQuesne GW, Wong KY: Severe infiltration of the kidneys with ultrasonic abnormalities in acute lymphoblastic leukemia. Am J Dis Child 1978;132:1204

323. Foster WL Jr, Roberts L Jr, Halvorsen RA Jr, Dunnick NR: Sonography of small renal masses with indeterminant density characteristics on computed tomography. Urol Radiol 1988;10:59

324. Amendola MA, Bree RL, Pollack HM et al: Small renal cell carcinomas: resolving a diagnostic dilemma. Radiology 1988;166:637

325. Smith SJ, Bosniak MA, Megibow AJ et al: Renal cell carcinoma: earlier discovery and increased detection. Radiology 1989;170:699

326. Levine E, Huntrakoon M, Wetzel LH: Small renal neoplasms: clinical, pathologic, and imaging features. AJR 1989;153:69

327. Kier R, Taylor KJW, Feyock AL, Ramos IM: Renal masses: characterization with Doppler US. Radiology 1990;176:703

328. Hartman DS, Davidson AJ, Davis CJ Jr, Goldman SM: Infiltrative renal lesions: CT-sonographic-pathologic correlation. AJR 1988;150:1061

329. Hricak H, Cruz C, Romanski R et al: Renal parenchymal disease: sonographic-histologic correlation. Radiology 1982;144:141

330. Rosenfield AT, Siegel NJ: Renal parenchymal disease: histopathologic-sonographic correlation. AJR 1981;137:793

331. Fontaine S, Lafortune M, Breton G, Vallee C: Ascites as a cause of hyperechogenic kidneys. J Clin Ultrasound 1985;13:633

332. Platt JF, Ellis JH, Rubin JM et al: Intrarenal arterial Doppler sonography in patients with nonobstructive renal disease: correlation of resistive index with biopsy findings. AJR 1990;154:1223

333. Krensky AM, Reddish JM, Telle RL: Causes of increased renal echogenicity in pediatric patients. Pediatrics 1983;72:840

334. Hayden CK Jr, Santa-Cruz FR, Amparo EG et al: Ultrasonographic evaluation of the renal parenchymal in infancy and childhood. Radiology 1984;152:413

335. Foley LC, Luisiri A, Graviss ER, Campbell JB: Nephro-

calcinosis: sonographic detection in Cushing syndrome. AJR 1982;139:610

336. Shuman WP, Mack LA, Rogers JV: Diffuse nephrocalcinosis: hyperechoic sonographic appearance. AJR 1981;136:830

337. Manz F, Jaschke W, Van Kaick G et al: Nephrocalcinosis in radiology, computed tomography, sonography and histology. Pediatr Radiol 1980;9:19

338. Afschrift M, Nachtegacle P, Van Rattinghe R et al: Nephrocalcinosis demonstrated by ultrasound and CT. Pediatr Radiol 1983;13:42

339. Schutz K, Siffring PA, Forrest TS et al: Serial renal sonographic changes in preeclampsia. J Ultrasound Med 1990;9:415

340. Wilson DA, Wenzl JE, Altshuler GP: Ultrasound demonstration of diffuse hyperoxaluria. AJR 1979; 132:659

341. Brennan JN, Diwan RV, Makker SP et al: Ultrasonic diagnosis of primary hyperoxaluria in infancy. Radiology 1982;145:147

342. Day DL, Scheinman JI, Mahan J: Radiological aspects of primary hyperoxaluria. AJR 1986;146:395.

343. McCarten KM, Cleveland RH, Simeone JF, Aretz T: Renal ultrasonography in Beckwith-Wiedemann syndrome. Pediatr Radiol 1981;11:46

344. Subramanyam BR: Renal amyloidosis in juvenile rheumatoid arthritis: sonographic features. AJR 1981; 136:411

345. Toyoda K, Miyamoto Y, Ida M et al: Hyperechoic medulla of the kidneys. Radiology 1989;173:431

346. Shultz PK, Strife JL, Strife CF, McDaniel JD: Hyperechoic renal medullary pyramids in infants and children. Radiology 1991;181:163

347. Jequier S, Kaplan BS: Echogenic renal pyramids in children. J Clin Ultrasound 1991;19:85

348. Patriquin H, Robitaille P: Renal calcium deposition in children: sonographic demonstration of the Anderson-Carr progression. AJR 1986;146:1253

349. Cacciarelli AA, Young N, Levine AJ: Gray-scale ultrasonic demonstration of nephrocalcinosis. Radiology 1978;128:459

350. Sty JR, Starshak RJ, Hubbard AM: Medullary nephrocalcinosis in a newborn: real-time ultrasound evaluation. J Clin Ultrasound 1983;11:326

351. Cumming WA, Ohlsson A: Nephrocalcinosis in Bartter's syndrome: demonstration by ultrasonography. Pediatr Radiol 1984;14:125

352. Glazer GM, Callen PW, Filly RA: Medullary nephrocalcinosis: sonographic evaluation. AJR 1982;138:55

353. Glasier GM, Stoddard RA, Ackerman NB et al: Nephrolithiasis in infants: association with chronic furosemide therapy. AJR 1983;140:107

354. Rausch HP, Hanefeld F, Kaufmann JH: Medullary nephrocalcinosis and pancreatic calcifications demonstrated by ultrasound and CT in infants after treatment with ACTH. Radiology 1984;153:105

355. Alon U, Brewer WH, Chan JCM: Nephrocalcinosis: detection by ultrasonography. Pediatrics 1983;71:970

356. Al-Murrani B, Cosgrove DO, Svensson WE, Blaszczyk M: Echogenic rings—an ultrasound sign of early nephrocalcinosis. Clin Radiol 1991;44:49

357. Paivansalo MJ, Kallioinen MJ, Merikanto JS, Jalovaara PK: Hyperechogenic "rings" in the periphery of renal medullary pyramids as a sign of renal disease. J Clin Ultrasound 1991;19:283

358. Hernanz-Schulman M: Hyperechoic renal medullary pyramids in infants and children. Radiology 1991;181:9.

359. Myracle MR, McGahan JP, Goetzman BW, Adelman RD: Ultrasound diagnosis of renal calcification in infants on chronic furosemide therapy. J Clin Ultrasound 1986;14:281

360. Matsumoto J, Han BK, de Rovetto CR, Welch TR: Hypercalciuric Bartter syndrome: resolution of nephrocalcinosis with Indomethacin. AJR 1989;152:1251

361. Strauss S, Robinson G, Lotan D, Itzchak Y: Renal sonography in Bartter syndrome. J Ultrasound Med 1987;6:265

362. Jantarasami T, Larew M, Kao SCS, Smith W: Ultrasound in demonstration of nephrocalcinosis in William's syndrome. J Clin Ultrasound 1989;17:533

363. Filiatrault D, Perreault G: Transient acute tubular disease in a newborn and a young infant: sonographic findings. J Ultrasound Med 1985;4:257

364. Hoffman JC, Schnur MJ, Koenigsberg M: Demonstration of renal papillary necrosis on sonography. Radiology 1982;145:785

365. Braden GL, Kozinn DR, Hampf FE Jr et al: Ultrasound diagnosis of early renal papillary necrosis. J Ultrasound Med 1991;10:401

366. Ambos MA, Bosniak MA, Gordon R, Madayag MA: Replacement lipomatosis of the kidney. AJR 1981; 130:1087

367. Subramanyam BR, Bosniak MA, Horii SC et al: Replacement lipomatosis of the kidney: diagnosis by computed tomography and sonography. Radiology 1983;148:791

368. Behan M, Kazam E: The echogenic characteristics of fatty tissues and tumors. Radiology 1978;129:143

369. Yeh HC, Mitty HA, Wolf BS: Ultrasonography of real sinus lipomatosis. Radiology 1977;124:791

370. Schaffer RM, Schwartz GE, Becker JA et al: Renal ultrasound in acquired immune deficiency syndrome. Radiology 1984;153:511

371. Hamper UM, Goldblum LE, Hutchins GM et al: Renal involvement in AIDS: sonographic-pathologic correlation. AJR 1988;150:1321.

372. Falkoff GE, Rigsby CM, Rosenfield AT: Partial, combined cortical and medullary nephrocalcinosis: US and CT patterns in AIDS-associated MAI infection. Radiology 1987;162:343

373. Brenbridge AN, Chevalier RL, Kaiser DL: Increased renal cortical echogenicity in pediatric renal disease: histopathologic correlation. J Clin Ultrasound 1986; 14:595.

374. Kraus RA, Gaisie G, Young LW: Increased renal parenchymal echogenicity: causes in pediatric patients. RadioGraphics 1990;10:1009

375. Alkrinawi S, Gradus DBE, Goldstein J, Barki Y: Ultraso-

nographic pattern of congenital nephrotic syndrome of Finnish type. J Clin Ultrasound 1989;17:443

376. Choyke PL, Grant EG, Hoffer FA et al: Cortical echogenicity in the hemolytic uremic syndrome: clinical correlation. J Ultrasound Med 1988;7:439

377. Garel LA, Pariente DM, Gubler MC et al: The dotted corticomedullary junction: a sonographic indicator of small-vessel disease in hypertensive children. Radiology 1984;152:419

378. Rosenbaum DM, Blumhagen JD: Sonographic recognition of idiopathic arterial calcification of infancy. AJR 1986;146:249

379. Stafford SJ, Jenkins JM, Staab EV et al: Ultrasonic detection of renal calculi: accuracy tested in an in vitro porcine kidney model. J Clin Ultrasound 1981;9:359

380. Kane RA, Manco LG: Renal arterial calcification simulating nephrolithiasis on sonography. AJR 1983;140:101

381. Pollack HM, Arger PH, Goldberg BB, Mulholland SG: Ultrasonic detection of nonopaque renal calculi. Radiology 1978;127:233

382. Edell S, Zegel H: Ultrasonic evaluation of renal calculi. AJR 1978;130:261

383. Kimme-Smith C, Perrella RR, Kaveggia LP et al: Detection of renal stones with real-time sonography: effect of transducers and scanning parameters. AJR 1991;157:975

384. Middleton WD, Dodds WJ, Lawson TL, Foley WD: Renal calculi: sensitivity for detection with US. Radiology 1988;167:239

385. Choyke PL, Pahira JH, Davros WJ et al: Renal calculi after shock wave lithotripsy: US evaluation with an in vitro phantom. Radiology 1989;170:39

386. Baumgarter BR, Steinberg HV, Ambrose SS et al: Sonographic evaluation of renal stones treated by extracorporeal shock-wave lithotripsy. AJR 1987;149:131

387. Schabel SI, Rittenberg GM, Moore TE, Lowrance W: Ultrasound demonstration of milk of calcium in a calyceal diverticulum. J Clin Ultrasound 1980;8:154

388. Widder DJ, Newhouse JH: The sonographic appearance of milk of calcium in renal calyceal diverticuli. J Clin Ultrasound 1982;10:448

389. Jacobs RP, Kane RA: Sonographic appearance of calculi in renal calyceal diverticula. J Clin Ultrasound 1984;12:289

390. Hewitt MJ, Older RA: Calyceal calculi simulating gallstones. AJR 1980;134:507

391. Zwirewich CV, Buckley AR, Kidney MR et al: Renal matrix calculus. Sonographic appearance. J Ultrasound Med 1990;9:61

392. Patriquin H, Lafortune M, Filatrault D: Urinary milk of calcium in children and adults: use of gravity-dependent sonography. AJR 1985;144:407

393. Herman RD, Leoni JV, Matthews GR: Renal milk of calcium associated with hydronephrosis. AJR 1978;130:572

394. Sullivan RR, Johnson MB, Lee KP, Ralls PW: Color Doppler sonographic findings in renal vascular lesions. J Ultrasound Med 1991;10:161

395. Friedman DM, Schacht RG: Doppler waveforms in the renal arteries of normal children. J Clin Ultrasound 1991;19:387

396. Desberg AL, Paushter DM, Lammert GK et al: Renal artery stenosis: evaluation with color Doppler flow imaging. Radiology 1990;177:749

397. Hillman BJ: Imaging advances in the diagnosis of renovascular hypertension. AJR 1989;153:5

398. Rubin JM, Platt JF, Adler RS: Applications of Doppler ultrasound in transplant and native kidney disease. Ultrasound Q 1990;8:95

399. Chou YH, Tiu CM, Pan HB et al: Diagnosis of renal pseudoaneurysms by pulsed Doppler ultrasound. J Clin Ultrasound 1985;13:662.

400. Derchi LE, Saffioti S, De Caro G et al: Arteriovenous fistula of the native kidney: diagnosis by duplex Doppler ultrasound. J Ultrasound Med 1991;10:595

401. Macpherson RI, Fyfe D, Aaronson IA: Congenital renal arteriovenous malformation in infancy. The imaging features in two infants with hypertension. Pediatr Radiol 1991;21:108

402. Takebayashi S, Aida N, Matsui K: Arteriovenous malformations of the kidneys: diagnosis and follow-up with color Doppler sonography in six patients. AJR 1991;157:991

403. Parvey HR, Eisenberg RL: Image-directed Doppler sonography of the intrarenal arteries in acute renal vein thrombosis. J Clin Ultrasound 1990;18:512

404. Mets T, Lameire N, Matthys E, Afschrift M: Sonographically guided renal biopsy. J Clin Ultrasound 1979;7:190

405. Chan JCM, Brewer WH, Still WJ: Renal biopsies under ultrasound guidance: 100 consecutive biopsies in children. J Urol 1983;129:103

406. Hricak H: Renal medical disorders: the role of sonography. p. 43. In Sanders RC (ed): Ultrasound Annual 1982. Raven Press, New York, 1982

407. Goldberg BB, Pollack HM, Kellerman E: Ultrasonic localization for renal biopsy. Radiology 1975;115:167

408. Saitoh M: Selective renal biopsy under ultrasonic real-time guidance. Urol Radiol 1984;6:30

409. Mostbeck GH, Wittich GR, Derfler K et al: Optimal needle size for renal biopsy: in vitro and in vivo evaluation. Radiology 1989;173:819

410. Poster RB, Jones DB, Spirit BA: Percutaneous pediatric renal biopsy: use of the Biopsy gun. Radiology 1990;176:725

411. Nomura G, Kinoshita E, Yamagata Y, Koga N: Usefulness of renal ultrasonography for assessment of severity and cause of acute tubular necrosis. J Clin Ultrasound 1984;12:135

412. Jain R: Acute renal failure in the neonate. Pediatr Clin North Am 1977;24:605

413. Stuck KJ, White GM, Granke DS et al: Urinary obstruction in azotemic patients: detection by sonography. AJR 1987;149:1191

414. Ritchie WW, Vick CW, Glocheski SK, Cook DE: Evaluation of azotemic patients: diagnostic yield of initial US examination. Radiology 1988;167:245

415. Platt JF, Rubin JM, Ellis JH: Acute renal failure: possible role of Duplex Doppler US in distinction between acute

prerenal failure and acute tubular necrosis. Radiology 1991;179:419

416. Rosenfield AT, Zeman RK, Cicchetti DV, Siegel NJ: Experimental acute tubular necrosis: US appearance. Radiology 1985;157:771

417. Sefczek RJ, Beckman I, Lupetin AR, Dash N: Sonography of acute renal cortical necrosis. AJR 1984;142:553

418. Pardes JG, Yong HA, Kazam E: Sonographic findings in myoglobinuric renal failure and their clinical implications. J Ultrasound Med 1983;2:391

419. Walker JT, Keller MS, Katz SM: Computed tomographic and sonographic findings in acute ethylene glycol poisoning. J Ultrasound Med 1983;2:429

420. Moccia WA, Kaude JV, Wright PG, Gaffney EF: Evaluation of chronic renal failure by digital gray-scale ultrasound. Urol Radiol 1980;2:1

421. Levine E, Slusher SL, Grantham JJ, Wetzel LH: Natural history of acquired renal cystic disease in dialysis patients: a prospective longitudinal CT study. AJR 1991;156:501

422. Mindell JH: Imaging studies for screening native kidneys in long-term dialysis patients. AJR 1989;153:768

423. Weissberg DL, Miller RB: Renal cell carcinoma and acquired cystic disease of the kidneys in a chronically dialyzed kidney. J Ultrasound Med 1983;2:191

424. Scanlon MH, Karasick SR: Acquired renal cystic disease and neoplasm: complications of chronic hemodialysis. Radiology 1983;147:837

425. Kutcher R, Amodia JB, Rosenblatt R: Uremic renal cystic disease: value of sonographic screening. Radiology 1983;147:833

426. McArdle CR, Grumback K: Sonographic and computed tomographic appearances of acquired renal cystic disease. J Ultrasound Med 1983;2:519

427. Andersen BL, Curry NS, Gobien RP: Sonography of evolving renal cystic transformation associated with hemodialysis. AJR 1983;141:1003

428. Taylor AJ, Cohen EP, Erickson SJ et al: Renal imaging in long-term dialysis patients: a comparison of CT and sonography. AJR 1989;153:765

429. Levine E, Grantham JJ, Slusher SL et al: CT of acquired cystic kidney disease and renal tumors in long-term dialysis patients. AJR 1984;142:125

430. Bennett LN, Voegeli DR, Crummy AB et al: Urologic complications following renal transplantation: role of interventional radiologic procedures. Radiology 1986;160:531

431. Letoruneau JG, Day DL, Ascher NL, Castaneda-Zuniga WR: Imaging of renal transplants. AJR 1988;150:833

432. Hricak H, Cruz C, Eyler WR et al: Acute post-transplant renal failure: differential diagnosis by ultrasound. Radiology 1981;139:441

433. Dodd GD III, Tublin ME, Shah A, Zajko AB: Imaging of vascular complications associated with renal transplants. AJR 1991;157:449

434. Warshauer DM, Taylor KJW, Bia MJ et al: Unusual causes of increased vascular impedance in renal transplants: duplex Doppler evaluation. Radiology 1988;169:367

435. Rifkin MD, Needleman L, Pasto ME et al: Evaluation of renal transplant rejection by Duplex Doppler examination: value of the resistive index. AJR 1987;148:759

436. Kaveggia LP, Perrella RR, Grant EG et al: Duplex Doppler sonography in renal allografts: the significance of reversed flow in diastole. AJR 1990;155:295

437. Taylor KJW, Morse SS, Rigsby CM et al: Vascular complications in renal allografts: detection with Duplex Doppler US. Radiology 1987;162:31

438. Platt JF, Ellis JH, Rubin JM: Renal transplant pyelocaliectasis: role of Duplex Doppler US in evaluation. Radiology 1991;179:425

439. Linkowski GD, Warvariv V, Filly RA, Vincenti F: Sonography in the diagnosis of acute renal allograft rejection and cyclosporine nephrotoxicity. AJR 1987;148:291

440. Surratt JT, Siegel MJ, Middleton WD: Sonography of complications in pediatric renal allografts. RadioGraphics 1990;10:687

441. Raiss GJ, Bree RL, Schwab RE et al: Further observations in the ultrasound evaluation of renal allograft rejection. J Ultrasound Med 1986;5:439

442. Coyne SS, Walsh JW, Tisnado J et al: Surgically correctable renal transplant complications: an integrated clinical and radiologic approach. AJR 1981;136:113

443. Balchunas WR, Hill MC, Isikoff MB, Morillo G: The clinical significance of dilatation of the collecting system in the transplanted kidney. J Clin Ultrasound 1982;10:221

444. Stuck KJ, Jafri SZH, Adler DD et al: Ultrasound evaluation of uncommon renal transplant complications. Urol Radiol 1986;8:6

445. Blumhardt R, Growcock G, Lasher JC: Cortical necrosis in a renal transplant. AJR 1983;141:95

446. Burks DD, Fleischer AC, Richie RE: Sonographic diagnosis of a perirenal transplant bowel hernia. J Ultrasound Med 1985;4:677

447. Johnson ML, Dunne MG, Watts B, Stables D: Ultrasonography in renal transplantation. p. 89. In Rosenfield AT (ed): Clinics in Diagnostic Ultrasound. Genitourinary Ultrasonography. Vol. 2. Churchill Livingstone, New York, 1979

448. Maklad NF: Ultrasonic evaluation of renal transplantation. Semin Ultrasound CT MR 1981;2:88

449. Spigos DG, Tan W, Pavel DG et al: Diagnosis of urine extravasation after renal transplantation. AJR 1977;129:409

450. Brockis JG, Hulbert JC, Patel AS et al: The diagnosis and treatment of lymphoceles associated with renal transplantation. Br J Urol 1978;50:307

451. Silver TM, Campbell D, Wicks JD et al: Peritransplant fluid collections: ultrasound evaluation and clinical significance. Radiology 1981;138:145

452. Koehler PR, Kanemoto HH, Maxwell JC: Ultrasonic "B" scanning in the diagnosis of complications in renal transplant patients. Radiology 1976;119:661

453. Rashid A, Posen G, Couture R et al: Accumulation of lymph around the transplanted kidney (lymphocele) mimicking renal allograft rejection. J Urol 1974;111:145

454. Kurtz AB, Rubin CS, Cole-Beuglet C et al: Ultrasound evaluation of the renal transplant. JAMA 1980; 243:2429

455. Phillips JF, Neiman HL, Brown TL: Ultrasound diagnosis of post-transplant renal lymphocele. AJR 1976; 126:1194

456. Spigos D, Capek V: Ultrasonically guided percutaneous aspiration of lymphoceles following renal transplantation: a diagnostic and therapeutic method. J Clin Ultrasound 1976;4:45

457. Grenier N, Douws C, Morel D et al: Detection of vascular complications in renal allografts with color Doppler flow imaging. Radiology 1991;178:217

458. Reuther G, Wanjura D, Bauer H: Acute renal vein thrombosis in renal allografts: detection with Duplex Doppler US. Radiology 1989;170:557

459. Baxter GM, Morley P, Dall B: Acute renal vein thrombosis in renal allografts: new Doppler ultrasonic findings. Clin Radiol 1991;43:125

460. Stringer DA, O'Halpin D, Daneman A et al: Duplex Doppler sonography for renal artery stenosis in the posttransplant pediatric patient. Pediatr Radiol 1989; 19:187

461. Renigers SA, Spigos DG: Pseudoaneurysm of the arterial anastomosis in a renal transplant. AJR 1978;131:525

462. Pozniak MA, Kalcz F, Dodd GD III: Renal transplant ultrasound: imaging and Doppler. Semin Ultrasound CT MR 1991;12:319

463. Middleton WD, Kellman GM, Melson GL, Madrazo BL: Postbiopsy renal transplant arteriovenous fistulas: color Doppler US characteristics. Radiology 1989; 171:253

464. Weissman J, Giyanani VL, Landreneau MD, Kilpatrick JS: Postbiopsy arterial pseudoaneurysm in a renal allograft. Detection by Duplex sonography. J Ultrasound Med 1988;7:515

465. Hubsch PJS, Mostbeck G, Barton PP et al: Evaluation of arteriovenous fistulas and pseudoaneurysms in renal allografts following percutaneous needle biopsy. Color-coded Doppler sonography versus Duplex Doppler sonography. J Ultrasound Med 1990;9:95

466. Cunningham JJ, Bacani-Faulls M: Sonographic "white line sign" for detection of minimal mucosal thickening in renal transplants. Urology 1990;35:367

467. Brenbridge ANAG, Buschi AJ, Cochrane JA, Lees RF: Renal emphysema of transplanted kidney: sonographic appearance. AJR 1979;132:656

468. Hricak H, Toledo-Pereyra LH, Eyler WR et al: Evaluation of acute post-transplant renal failure by ultrasound. Radiology 1979;133:443

469. Singh A, Cohen WN: Renal allograft rejection: sonography and scintigraphy. AJR 1980;135:73

470. Maklad NF, Wright CH, Rosenthal SJ: Gray scale ultrasonic appearances of renal transplant rejection. Radiology 1979;131:711

471. Barrientos A, Leiva O, Diaz-Gonzalez R et al: The value of ultrasonic scanning in the differentiation of acute posttransplant renal failure. J Urol 1981;126:308

472. Frick MP, Feinberg SB, Sibley K, Idstrom ME: Ultrasound in acute renal transplant rejection. Radiology 1981;138:657

473. Hoddick W, Filly RA, Backman U et al: Renal allograft rejection: US evaluation. Radiology 1986;161:469

474. Conrad MR, Dickerman R, Love IL et al: New observations in renal transplants using ultrasound. AJR 1978;131:851

475. Hricak H, Toledo-Pereyra LH, Eyler WR et al: The role of ultrasound in the diagnosis of kidney allograft rejection. Radiology 1979;132:667

476. Hillman BJ, Birnholz JC, Busch GJ: Correlation of echographic and histologic findings in suspected renal allograft rejection. Radiology 1979;132:673

477. Hricak H, Romanski RN, Eyler WR: The renal sinus during allograft rejection: sonographic and histopathologic findings. Radiology 1982;142:693

478. Slovis TL, Babcock DS, Hricak H et al: Renal transplant rejection: sonographic evaluation in children. Radiology 1984;153:659

479. Babcock DS, Slovis TL, Han BK et al: Renal transplants in children: long-term followup using sonography. Radiology 1985;156:165

480. Townsend RR, Tomlanovich SJ, Goldstein RB, Filly RA: Combined Doppler and morphologic sonographic evaluation of renal transplant rejection. J Ultrasound Med 1990;9:199

481. Taylor KJW, Marks WH: Use of Doppler imaging for evaluation of dysfunction in renal allografts. AJR 1990;155:536

482. Genkins SM, Sanfilippo FP, Carroll BA: Duplex Doppler sonography of renal transplants: lack of sensitivity and specificity in establishing pathologic diagnosis. AJR 1989;152:535

483. Fleischer AC, Hinton AA, Glick AD, Johnson HK: Duplex Doppler sonography of renal transplants. Correlation with histopathology. J Ultrasound Med 1989;8:89

484. Don S, Kopecky KK, Filo RS et al: Duplex Doppler US of renal allografts: causes of elevated resistive index. Radiology 1989;171:709

485. Kelcz F, Pozniak MA, Pirsch JD, Oberly TD: Pyramidal appearance and resistive index: insensitive and nonspecific sonographic indicators of renal transplant rejection. AJR 1990;155:531

486. Allen KS, Jorkasky DK, Arger PH et al: Renal allografts: prospective analysis of Doppler sonography. Radiology 1988;169:371

487. Rigsby CM, Burns PN, Weltin GG et al: Doppler signal quantitation in renal allografts: comparison in normal and rejecting transplants, with pathologic correlation. Radiology 1987;162:39

488. Rigsby CM, Taylor KJW, Weltin G et al: Renal allografts in acute rejection: evaluation using Duplex sonography. Radiology 1986;158:375

489. Buckley AR, Cooperberg PL, Reeve CE, Magil AB: The distinction between acute renal transplant rejection and cyclosporine nephrotoxicity: value of Duplex sonography. AJR 1987;149:521

490. Drake DG, Day DL, Letourneau JG et al: Doppler evaluation of renal transplants in children: a prospective anal-

ysis with histopathologic correlation. AJR 1990;154: 785.

491. Steinberg HV, Nelson RC, Murphy FB et al: Renal allograft rejection: evaluation by Doppler US and MR imaging. Radiology 1987;162:337

492. Hricak H, Terrier F, Marotti M et al: Posttransplant renal rejection: comparison of quantitative scintigraphy, US, and MR imaging. Radiology 1987;162:685

493. Shapeero LG, Vordermark JS: Papillary necrosis causing hydronephrosis in the renal allograft. J Ultrasound Med 1989;8:579

494. Rahatzad M, Henderson SC, Boren GS: Ultrasound appearance of spontaneous rupture of renal transplant. J Urol 1981;126:535

495. Potter JL, Sullivan BM, Flournoy JG, Gerza C: Emphysema in the renal allograft. Radiology 1985;155:51

496. Russ PD, Way DE, Pretorius DH et al: Posttransplant lymphoma. Sonographic characteristics of renal allograft involvement. J Ultrasound Med 1987;6:453

497. Olcott EW, Goldstein RB, Salvatierra O: Lymphoma presenting as allograft hematoma in a renal transplant recipient. J Ultrasound Med 1990;9:239

498. Parker RA, Elliott WC, Muthers RS et al: Percutaneous aspiration biopsy of renal allograft using ultrasound localization. Urol 1980;15:534

499. Spigos D, Capek V, Jonasson D: Percutaneous biopsy of renal transplants using ultrasonographic guidance. J Urol 1977;117:699

500. Curry NS, Cochran S, Barbaric ZL et al: Interventional radiologic procedures in the renal transplant. Radiology 1984;152:647

501. Grant EG, Perrella RR: Wishing won't make it so: duplex Doppler sonography in the evaluation of renal transplant dysfunction. AJR 1990;155:538

502. Goldberg BB, Bagley D, Liu JB et al: Endoluminal sonography of the urinary tract: preliminary observations. AJR 1991;156:99

503. Mandell VS, Mandell J, Gaisie G: Pediatric urologic radiology — intervention and endourology. Urol Clin North Am 1985;12:151

14

Lower Urinary Tract

Carol A. Mittelstaedt

In recent years, the ultrasound examination of the kidneys has been expanded to include an evaluation of the bladder (lower urinary tract) as a part of every examination. More recent has been the addition of the evaluation of the ureters, ureterovesical junction, and urethra. In many situations, the problem identified within the kidney or kidneys is secondary to a problem within the pelvis or lower urinary tract or vice versa.

The clinical usefulness of this modality depends to a significant degree on how well the urinary tract structure and its surroundings are visualized. This, in turn, depends on the sonographic technique and the examiner's knowledge. As with other organ systems, the use of the newer high-resolution real-time systems has vastly improved and facilitated the ultrasound examination of the lower urinary tract.

TECHNIQUE

Preparation

For the bladder to be evaluated adequately, it should be distended with fluid. If this cannot be accomplished with oral fluids, a Foley catheter can be used to fill the bladder in a retrograde fashion. A fluid-filled bladder not only facilitates the evaluation of the bladder wall and its contents but also improves the identification of normal or dilated ureters.

Ultrasound Technique

Bladder

The fluid-filled bladder should be examined with the patient supine, in sagittal and transverse planes angling caudad and cephalad (Fig. 14-1). A high-frequency transducer should be used. The configuration of the bladder on the transverse scans should be symmetric. The bladder wall should be a thin echogenic interface.

In certain situations, an alternative scanning technique may be used. In cases of bladder masses projecting into the bladder lumen, the bladder may be scanned with the patient in the decubitus position (Fig. 14-2). In this position, the mobility of the mass and its relationship to the bladder wall can be assessed and the bladder wall may be evaluated in this new projection. High resolution of the bladder wall and lumen can be achieved with transperineal or endovaginal scans in females. In males (or females), additional high-resolution views of the bladder may be obtained by using a transrectal transducer.

Ureters

Ureters are usually not identified by ultrasound unless dilated. They are certainly easier to follow by using real-time systems than they were with static systems. A fluid-filled bladder facilitates their visualization and serves as an anatomic landmark. The proximal ureter is best seen from the flank (coronal) or prone position, with the dis-

1043

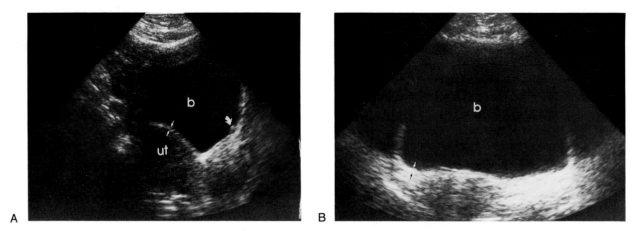

Fig. 14-1. Normal bladder. The normal fluid-filled bladder *(b)* is seen on **(A)** sagittal and **(B)** transverse scans. It has a very thin wall, with the measurement (small arrows) taken at the bladder floor. On the transverse view, the entire portion of the lateral wall is not well-defined. The bladder volume may be calculated by measuring the transverse dimension on the transverse view and the AP dimension and length on the sagittal view. The UVJ (curved arrow) is seen in Fig. A as a raised hypoechoic area. (*ut*, uterus.)

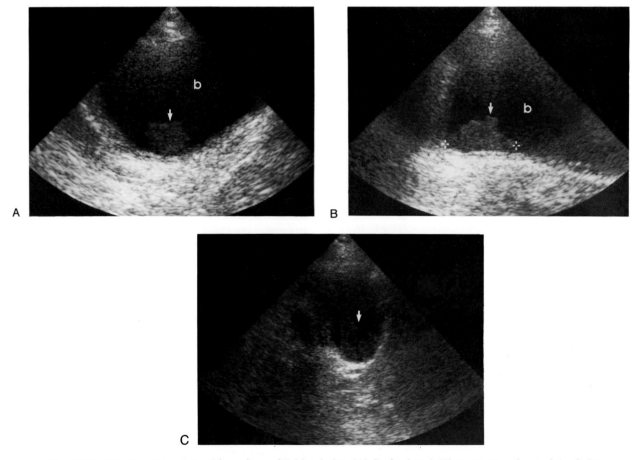

Fig. 14-2. Bladder, lateral decubitus view, with blood clot. **(A)** Sagittal and **(B)** transverse views of the fluid-filled bladder *(b)* demonstrating a heterogeneous intraluminal mass (arrow, 2 to 2.5 cm) with an irregular outline within the posterior bladder on the right. By these images alone, the differential diagnosis would have to include a bladder wall mass, such as tumor. **(C)** This "mass" (arrow) was noted to move and change in configuration with change in patient position on a sagittal left lateral decubitus view, which makes the diagnosis of tumor unlikely.

tal ureter seen through the distended bladder (Fig. 14-3). For best visualization of the normal distal ureter, the examiner should search for the ureterovesical junction (UVJ) transversely and then angle the transducer slightly obliquely (keeping in mind the course of the ureter as seen on intravenous pyelography [IVP]) (Fig. 14-4). The middle portion of the ureter is the most difficult to see because of overlying bowel gas.

Female Urethra

The normal female urethra may be identified transabdominally by scanning a fluid-filled bladder, angling the transducer inferiorly. It is best examined by using a high-frequency transducer (5 to 7 MHz) within the vagina or transperineally.[1] With this technique, the patient is studied in the dorsal lithotomy position with stirrups both before and after voiding. Sagittal and coronal images of the urethra are obtained when scanning transperineally (Fig. 14-5). Only sagittal scans can be obtained endovaginally. The transducer is angled both cephalad and caudad as well as to the right and to the left with this technique. The urethra may also be evaluated by using a transrectal approach.[2] With this method, the transducer is rotated so that the scan plane is posteroanterior, producing an image of the bladder, bladder neck, and urethra.[2] Ultrasound has the advantage of identifying the soft tissue movements during micturition and straining, particularly the periurethral tissue at the bladder neck and neighboring anterior vaginal wall.[2]

Male Urethra

For a discussion of the male urethra, see Chapter 15.

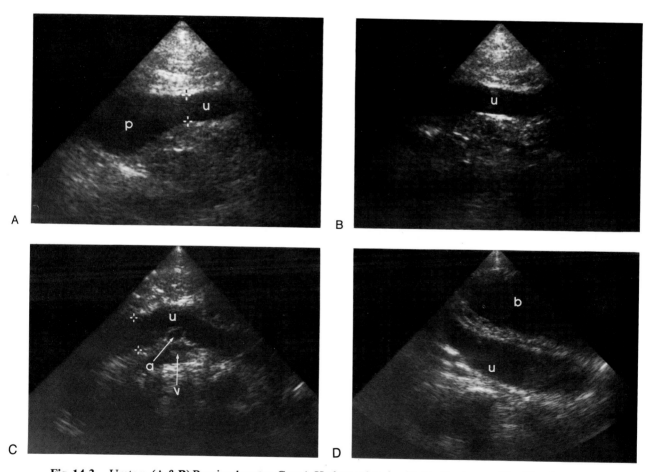

Fig. 14-3. Ureters. **(A & B)** Proximal ureter. Case 1. Hydronephrosis with bladder tumor. The dilated proximal left ureter (*u*, calipers, 12 mm) is seen from the coronal approach on these two sagittal views (p, renal pelvis). **(C & D)** Middle and distal ureter. Case 2. Hydronephrosis with bladder outlet obstruction. The middle portion of this dilated ureter (*u*, calipers, 18 mm) is seen as a tubular lucent structure in Fig. C. It is seen anterior to the iliac vessels (*a*, artery; *v*, vein). In Fig. D the more proximal portion of the distal dilated ureter *(u)* is seen (*b*, bladder). *(Figure continues.)*

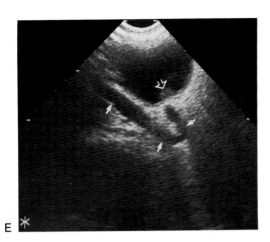 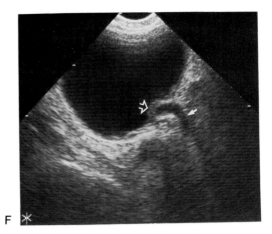

Fig. 14-3 *(Continued).*   **(E & F)** Distal ureter. Case 3. Hydronephrosis with bladder tumor. The distal dilated ureter (arrows) is seen as a tubular lucency posterior to the bladder on these two sagittal views. Fig. E is a true sagittal view, and Fig. F is an oblique view. The UVJ is seen as a raised area (open arrow) within the posterior bladder wall. (The bladder tumor is not shown here.)

NORMAL ANATOMY

Bladder

Shape

The various shapes of the normal bladder have been described.[3] At the neck, it is semilunar, and it is kidney-bean-shaped retropubic and bell-shaped suprapubic. When distended with fluid, the bladder is seen as a symmetric anechoic structure (Fig. 14-1). It has a sausage shape in the sagittal plane, with a somewhat rounded appearance on transverse scan (Fig. 14-1). The seminal vesicles are seen as two small, oval, hypoechoic structures posterior to the bladder and superior to the prostate.[4]

Wall

The wall of the bladder is seen as a thin, smooth, uniform echogenic line that is usually 3 to 6 mm thick.[4] The thickness of the bladder wall as been assessed[5] and found to vary mostly with the state of bladder filling and only minimally with age and gender. A linear relationship has been demonstrated between bladder fullness and bladder wall thickness; the upper limits are 3 and 5 mm for a full and empty bladder, respectively.[5] Mean bladder wall thicknesses of 2.76 and 1.55 mm have been demonstrated when the bladder is almost empty and when it is distended, respectively.[5]

Several factors must be considered when structures as thin as the bladder wall are being measured.[5] Measurements of the wall should be made at the bladder floor by using the correct transducer since the axial resolution is better than the lateral resolution[5] (Fig. 14-1). Also important is the site of measurement. The peritoneal reflection at the dome of the bladder will add 1 mm to the apparent wall thickness. When measuring the bladder floor, one may mistake the wall of the vagina or rectum within the measurement.[5] The anterior bladder wall may be difficult to see as a result of the ring-down artifact of the anterior abdominal wall.

General

During all ultrasound examinations of the bladder, certain factors should be evaluated. The wall thickness and outline should be assessed: wall irregularity will appear as an abnormal density or discontinuity of the wall echoes. Bladder shape should be assessed: with bladder deformity, there is distortion of the normal shape or wall rigidity as a result of tumor infiltration. Bladder capacity should be noted. The bladder volume (V) can be calculated by using the formula $V = $ transverse diameter $\times$ AP diameter $\times$ length[6] (Figs. 14-1 and 14-6). Alternatively, bladder volume can be measured by assuming the bladder to be a sphere and calculating the radius (r) by adding sagittal, transverse, and anteroposterior diameters divided by 8 and using the formula $V = 4/3\pi r^3$. One cannot always obtain a true anteroposterior (AP) diameter and may have to estimate the bladder volume. The normal volume may be up to 500 ml without major discomfort.[7] There may be reduced capacity caused by bladder contraction secondary to tumor infiltration or a large tumor in the lumen.[3]

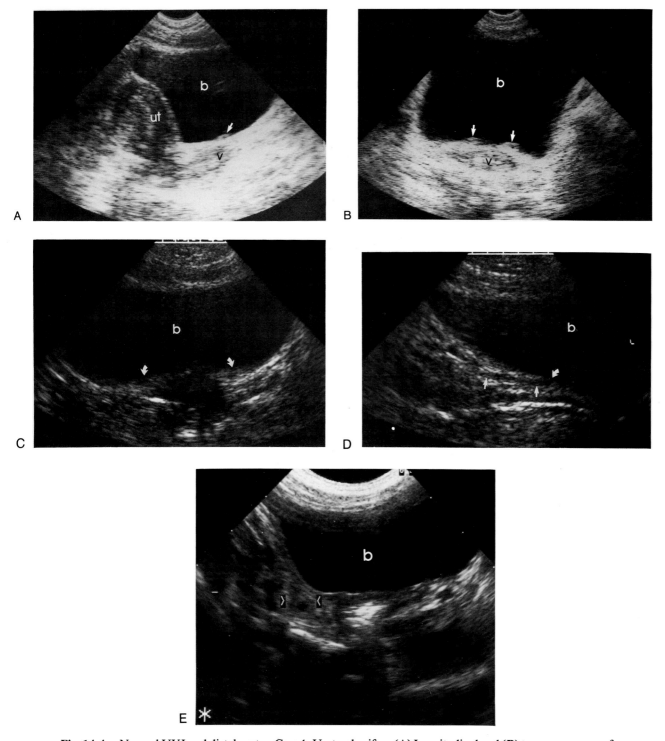

Fig. 14-4. Normal UVJ and distal ureter. Case 1. Ureteral orifice. **(A)** Longitudinal and **(B)** transverse scans of the bladder *(b)* demonstrating the papillae of the orifice of the ureters as mucosal elevations (arrows) in the inferior aspect of the bladder in Fig. A and on either side of the midline in Fig. B. (*ut*, uterus; *v*, vagina.) **(C & D)** Case 2. Normal distal ureter. The UVJ (curved arrows) is localized on a transverse view (Fig. C) of the bladder *(b)* looking for two subtle hypoechoic areas. The UVJ may also be localized by the identification of ureteral jets. Once the UVJ is located, the transducer is angled somewhat obliquely to demonstrate the normal distal ureter (straight arrows in Fig. D. **(E)** Case 3. Normal distal ureter. On this somewhat oblique transverse view of the bladder *(b)*, the normal right ureter (calipers) is seen.

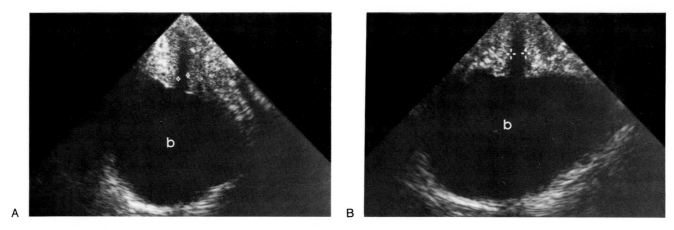

Fig. 14-5. Normal female urethra. The normal urethra is seen as a superficial tubular lucency (calipers) on **(A)** sagittal and **(B)** coronal scans by using a 5-MHz endovaginal transducer with a transperineal approach. The fluid-filled bladder *(b)* is seen posteriorly.

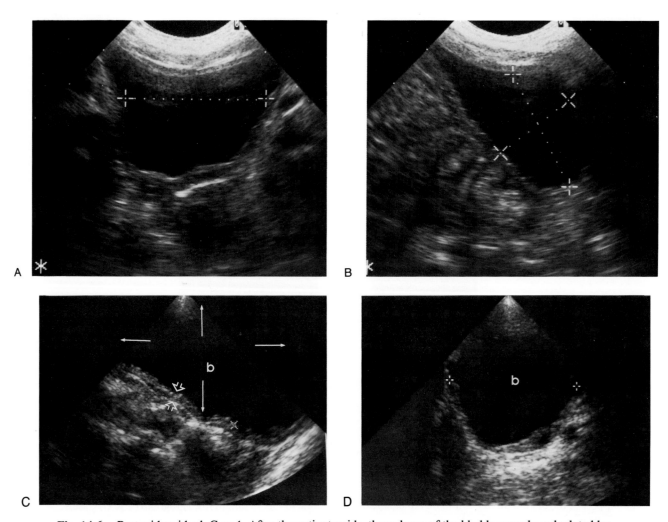

Fig. 14-6. Postvoid residual. Case 1. After the patient voids, the volume of the bladder may be calculated by using the transverse dimension on the **(A)** transverse view (calipers) and the length and AP dimension on the **(B)** sagittal view (calipers). In this case, the postvoid residual (PVR) was 13 ml. Case 2. Older child with posterior urethra valves. The postvoid bladder (*b*, thin arrows) is distended on **(C)** sagittal and **(D)** transverse views with thickening (open arrows) of the wall (trabeculation) and a PVR of 284 ml. On these views, the dilated ureters are not seen. This patient's dilated right ureter was seen in Figs. 14-3C & D.

Ureters

The ureters arise as budlike outgrowths from the mesonephric or wolffian ducts. The buds lengthen to produce a long, definitive tubular structure found in the adult. The average size is 30 cm long with a diameter of 5 mm. The course of the ureter is retroperitoneal. After entering the pelvis, the ureter passes anterior to either the common iliac or external iliac artery.[8]

Although the normal ureters are usually not visualized sonographically, the lower segment of the ureters may be visualized and should not suggest stasis or dilatation[9] (Fig. 14-4). The ultrasound visualization of the lower ureteral segment requires the presence of urine in the lumen. As such, the examination takes time in order to have a peristaltic activity; the amount of time needed varies according to the degree of hydration and bladder filling. Optimal visualization is the observation time extended to include the moment when the ureter is distended during the passage of urine.[9] Hydration is a favoring factor; the degree of fullness of the bladder does not seem to correspond to a greater or lesser ease in visualization.[9] With overdistension of the bladder, there may be reduced urinary flow into the bladder and compression of the ureters.[9] There is indirect visualization of the UVJ by the visualization of jets (Fig. 14-7).

The ureters are identified by following the linear echo-free image of the ureteral lumen down to its outlet in the bladder or by demonstrating on transverse scans two symmetrically prominent mounds corresponding to the intravesical portion of the ureters[9] (Fig. 14-4C–E). This identification of the ureters can facilitate the search for small ureteral calculi in the pelvic area by demonstrating their endoluminal position and their exact distance from the UVJ.[9]

Female Urethra

The normal urethra consists of muscular, erectile, and mucous layers with a central lumen.[10] Just inferior to the bladder, the AP diameter is 1 to 1.5 cm.[10] On transperineal scans, the urethral lumen is seen as a lucent tubular area superficial to the bladder (Fig. 14-5).

Diagnostic Features

Ultrasound can provide many diagnostic features related to the bladder. The capacity of the bladder, volume of residual urine, changes in bladder outline, changes in wall thickness, and elasticity can be evaluated. The bladder capacity decreases in association with large, fixed pelvic masses; in urinary and pelvic inflammatory disease; in patients currently receiving radiation therapy, after radiation therapy, and in advanced stages when the tumor has infiltrated; and after recent surgery. There is increased bladder capacity in bladder neck obstruction and with atonic bladders. Significant residual urine volumes are seen with atonic bladders, bladder neck obstruction, long-standing cystitis, and advanced invasion by carcinoma. Extrinsic lesions can displace the bladder wall, causing changes in bladder shape. Inflammatory changes, tumor infiltration, and recent instrumentation may cause localized loss of elasticity and thickening of the bladder wall with subsequent asymmetry of the blad-

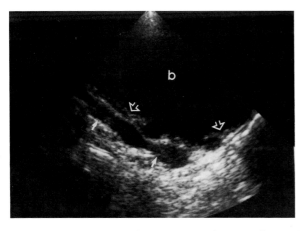
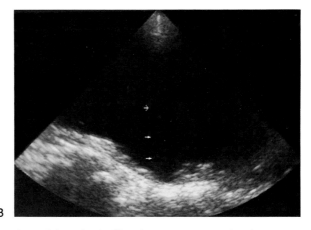

A   B

Fig. 14-7. Dilated distal ureter and jet. Posterior urethral valves. This patient's dilated ureters were seen in Figs. 14-3C & D along with the distended urinary bladder and irregular wall thickening in Figs. 14-6C & D. **(A)** Sagittal view showing the dilated distal left ureter (solid arrows) posterior to the distended urinary bladder *(b)*. The bladder wall is irregularly thickened (open arrows). The UVJ could not be visualized. **(B)** On another sagittal view a jet (arrows) is seen projecting into the bladder as an echodense area.

der outline. Filling defects and irregular bladder wall may be seen with primary bladder tumor, trabeculation, adherent blood clot, granulomatous cystitis, diverticula, benign prostatic hypertrophy and extravesical inflammation, and neoplastic tissue involving the bladder.[7]

Determination of the amount of residual urine in the bladder has improved the therapy of patients with suspected bladder outlet obstruction. Although prostatic enlargement is usually the etiology of bladder residua, chronic cystitis and various systemic disorders produce similar symptoms. The most reliable method of measurement is to catheterize the patient and measure the amount of fluid. This runs the risk of both trauma and infection. With ultrasound, one can simply measure the "empty" bladder by taking the maximum width, height, and depth (longest AP) (Figs. 14-1 and 14-6). This can be applied to the following formula to determine the bladder volume: $V = w \times h \times d$.[11] Alternatively, bladder volumes may be calculated by using the product of the longitudinal, transverse, and sagittal diameters and a correction factor of 0.52.[12] There is good correlation between these methods (ultrasound and catheterized volumes), although large volumes tend to be underestimated by ultrasound.[12]

Ureteral Jets

The term *ureteral jets* has been used to describe the appearance of urine entering the bladder. These jets are seen during bladder filling and are not seen when the bladder is full. They are seen at regular intervals (5 to 20 seconds), with each jet lasting from a fraction of 1 second up to 3 seconds.[13-15] Each ureter functions independently from the other. At the base of the bladder, small elevations of mucosa are noted (Fig. 14-4); the jet echoes emanate from these at a 45-degree angle in a caudal direction. On a sagittal scan, the papilla of the orifice is seen as a mucosal elevation on either side of and at the level of the cervix[15] (Fig. 14-4). At real-time, the jet is seen as a stream of low-strength echoes entering the bladder[16] (Figs. 14-7 and 14-8). The jet starts in the area of the ureteral orifice and flows toward the center of the bladder[13] (Fig. 14-8). The jet extends up to 3 cm and broadens (Fig. 14-8). After a few seconds, the low-intensity echoes become distributed within the bladder and lose their intensity until they are no longer visualized.[13]

There are several theories for the production of the jets and their significance. It has been suggested that the real-time jet and the Doppler shift result from turbulent flow of urine into a static fluid in a closed container (the bladder).[15] It is hypothesized that shear forces between the jets and the adjacent static urine create the interface necessary for imaging the jets. As a result, the continued changes in these shear forces produce turbulent flow in the urine immediately adjacent to the jet, causing a Doppler signal.[15] Other authors have investigated this jet phenomenon and attribute it to acoustic interfaces between fluids of different specific gravities.[13] The clinical importance of the ureteral jet is not yet established. It is impaired in congenital and acquired abnormalities that obstruct the ureter and by abnormal peristalsis.[14]

Other theories proposed to explain this phenomenon include potential sources of reflections from microbubbles or particulate matter in urine, temperature differences between ureteral urine and bladder urine, and development of turbulence or cavitation at the ureteral orifice.[16] Ureteral jets are believed to occur when densely opacified urine from the ureter enters the more dilute or unopacified urine in the bladder and appears as a dense stream exiting the ureteral orifice. Most widely accepted is the explanation that the reflections are generated by differences in density between urine in the bladder and urine exiting the ureter.[16]

To evaluate asymmetry between ureteral jets, a system that is as sensitive as possible for detection of urine flow from the ureteral orifice must be used.[16] Doppler techniques are more sensitive to moving, low-level reflectors than is conventional real-time gray-scale ultrasound.[16] As such, it is better to evaluate the ureteral jets by Doppler techniques than by real-time alone.[16] Color Doppler is more sensitive to fluid flow throughout the field of view and allows for simultaneous visualization of the ureteral jets from both ureteral orifices, whereas duplex ultrasound can be used on only one side at a time.[16]

Investigators have evaluated ureteral jets in healthy subjects and in patients with unilateral ureteral calculi.[16] They found three patterns associated with ureteral calculi: (1) no detectable urine flow from the symptomatic side, (2) low-level continuous flow from the symptomatic side, and (3) periodic ureteral jets on the symptomatic side that were not significantly different from ureteral jets in healthy subjects.[16] It is thought that analysis of ureteral jets by color Doppler can enable detection and qualitative determination of the degree of ureteral obstruction in many patients with unilateral ureteral calculi.[16]

To examine these patients, the bladder is examined in the transverse plane to simultaneous view the left and right ureteral jets at the level of the trigone. Patients should be well hydrated (orally or intravenously), until ureteral jets are easily detected on the asymptomatic side.[16] This may require 600 to 1,000 ml of water prior to the study.[16] Ureteral jets can usually be visualized 15 to 30 minutes after hydration. If the jets are not visualized after initial hydration, the patients are asked to drink more water and delayed scans are obtained.[16] As part of

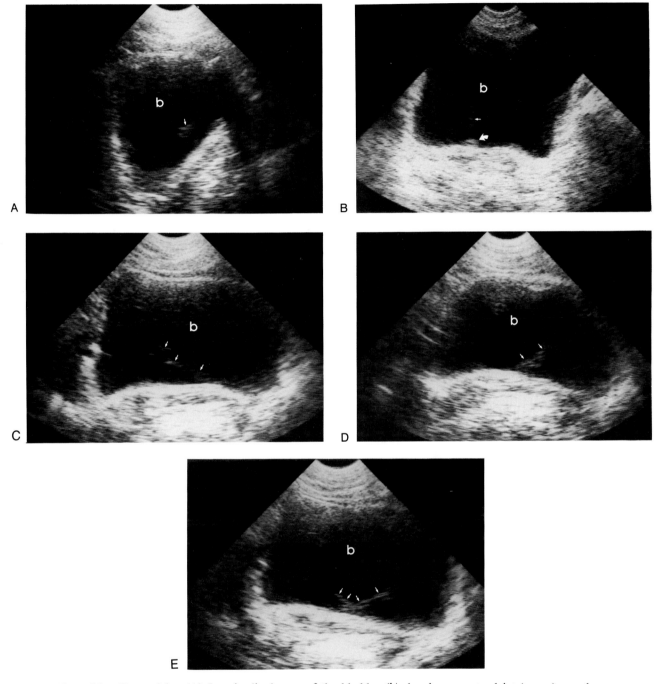

Fig. 14-8. Ureteral jet. **(A)** Longitudinal scan of the bladder *(b)* showing a ureteral jet (arrow) as echoes extending from the ureteral orifice. **(B)** Transverse scan of the bladder *(b)* showing a jet (small arrow) extending straight anterior from the right ureteral orifice (curved arrow). **(C)** Transverse scan of the bladder *(b)* showing a jet (arrows) flowing to the right from the left ureteral orifice. **(D)** Transverse scan of the bladder *(b)* showing a jet (arrows) going to the left from the right ureteral orifice. **(E)** Transverse scan of the bladder *(b)* showing bilateral jets (arrows) crossing.

the study, the kidneys are assessed for any discrepancy in size that might lead the investigator to suspect impaired function.[16] The number of jets from each orifice is tabulated over time to calculate the number of jets per minute.[16] By dividing the difference between those from the left orifice and those from the right orifice by the sum of those from the left and those from the right and multiplying by 100 percent, the percent difference between the number of ureteral jets from the left and right orifices is established.[16]

With lack of normal symmetry between the two ureteral jets, a diagnosis of ureteral obstruction may be possible.[16] There does not appear to be a relationship between the degree of hydronephrosis and the pattern of ureteral jets.[16] This technique has limitations. There may or may not be asymmetry in the ureteral jets in patients with nonobstructing stones or stones producing low-grade obstruction.[16]

Ureterovesical jets in infants and children have been evaluated by both duplex ultrasound and color Doppler.[17] The duration of the jet varies from 0.4 to 7.5 seconds and depends largely on fluid intake.[17] The normal jet is usually directed anteromedially and upward.[17] With severe renal parenchymal scarring, reduced frequency and amplitude of the jets are noted.[17] It is thought that the Doppler analysis of the ureteric jet does not allow diagnosis or exclusion of vesicoureteral reflux.[17] Color Doppler is more sensitive in demonstrating ureteric jets than is gray-scale real-time and does facilitate the study but is equally unable to help predict reflux.[17]

Other investigators have also evaluated vesicoureteral reflux in children to assess prediction with color Doppler.[18] These authors evaluated the measurements of mean urine jet velocity, longitudinal angle, transverse angle, and distance of the origin of the jet from the midline of the bladder in children with proven urinary tract infections.[18] Only the distance of the ureteral orifice from the midline of the bladder was found to correlate with vesicoureteral reflux (mean distance in reflux group, 10.25 mm ± 2.40 mm [SD]; mean distance in nonreflux group, 7.98 mm ± 2.40 mm SD).[18] To obtain the midline-to-orifice distance measurement, a reproducible midline point in the bladder is determined by first measuring the transverse bladder dimension (at the level of the posterior bladder wall).[18] The midpoint of the bladder is defined by placing a cursor at half the measured transverse bladder distance.[18] The origin of the ureteral jet from this defined midline is then measured and recorded.[18] As such, this group concluded that the more laterally positioned the ureteral orifice, the more likely it was to reflux.[18] Color Doppler is useful in the measurement of the laterality of the ureteral orifice and may help predict which children with urinary

tract infection would benefit from voiding cystoure-thrography.

BLADDER ABNORMALITIES

Congenital

The bladder develops from a division of the cloaca by a transverse vertical septum. The fetal bladder extends up to the umbilicus, where it is in continuity with the allantoic stalk. Shortly after birth, the upper half of the bladder narrows as the lower half descends into the pelvis. If a remnant of the allantois remains patent, it presents as a patent urachus that may be an open tube from the bladder to the umbilicus or end as a blind pouch with no connection to the bladder.[3]

The urachus connects the apex of the bladder with the allantois through the umbilical cord. It is situated between the transversalis fascia and the peritoneum within the anterior wall (in the space of Retzius) with extension from the bladder apex to the umbilicus.[19] Normally, it fibroses at birth and atrophies. Rarely, it remains patent in part or whole. The urachus proper is 5 to 6 cm long.[3] If the lower part is patent, a bladder diverticulum or urachal cyst develops.[7]

Urachal Anomalies

Urachal anomalies are rare, with a reported incidence of patent urachus and urachal cyst at autopsies in children reported as 0.13 and 0.2 percent, respectively.[19] In a literature review of urachal anomalies, there were 47.6 percent urachi, 18.4 percent urachal sinuses, 30.8 percent urachal cysts, and 8.2 percent vesicourachal diverticuli.[19]

Urachal cysts or sinuses usually remain clinically silent unless infected or enlarged, when they cause localized or generalized symptoms.[19] The patient often has vague abdominal and/or urinary complaints without classic signs of leakage.[20] With cyst infection, the pressure in the cyst increases, and it usually discharges its contents through the umbilicus or into the urinary bladder, as these two areas represent the weakest sites throughout the urachal canal.[19] Most urachal cysts are located at the lower one-third of the urachus, and 75 percent may be infected.[19]

Depending on the type of defective obliteration during downward progression of the bladder, various types of congenital urachal anomalies can occur[20] (Fig. 14-9). With a patent urachus, a vesicocutaneous fistula persists throughout from the bladder to the umbilicus (Figs. 14-9A and 14-10). A vesicourachal diverticulum represents the caudal segment of the urachus that is patent, opening

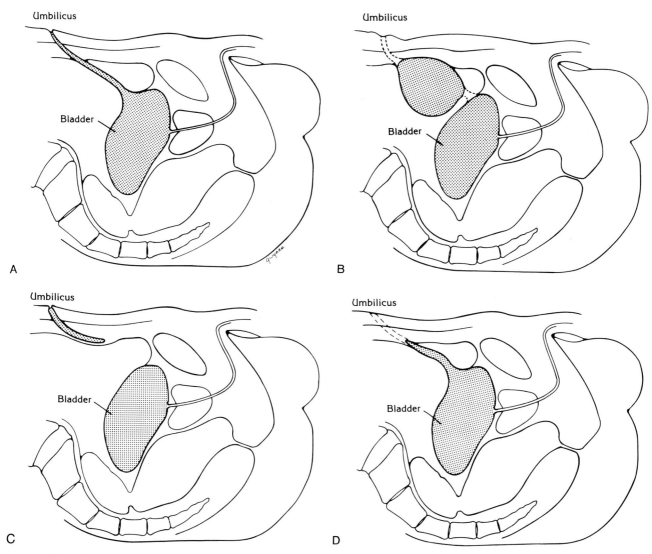

Fig. 14-9. Urachal anomalies. **(A)** Completely patent urachus; **(B)** urachal cyst; **(C)** partially patent urachus, which opens externally but is blind internally (urachal sinus); and **(D)** partially patent urachus. In this instance, it opens internally and is blind externally (vesicourachal diverticulum).

into the bladder (Fig. 14-9D). With a urachal sinus, the cephalic portion of the urachus is patent, opening into the umbilicus (Fig. 14-9C). With a urachal cyst, the midportion of the urachus is patent with both cephalic and caudal ends closed, but the cyst can sometimes spontaneously drain its contents into the bladder and/or the umbilicus with increased pressure (Fig. 14-9B).

As a rule, urachal anomalies are not clinically apparent, except for the congenital patent urachus, unless complicated by infection.[19] On ultrasound, a urachal cyst is seen as an echofree tubular structure in the lower midabdominal anterior wall[20,21] (Fig. 14-11). The upper pole is at the level of the umbilicus, and the duct extends to the bladder.[20] Various configurations associated with urachal abscesses have been reported, including cone-shaped, tubular, curved, club-shaped, oval, and irregular.[19] Complications associated with urachal abscesses include intraperitoneal spread, chronic cystitis, and adhesion to the omentum or the colon; all of these may be suggested by ultrasound.[19] When a lesion is seen within the extraperitoneal fat space of the abdominal wall at the midline below the umbilicus, the diagnosis of urachal abscess should be suggested, especially when there is umbilical discharge and/or when the lesion extends to the umbilicus[19] (Fig. 14-12).

Urachal Remnant. As an allantoic remnant, the urachus is located between the umbilicus and the dome of the bladder. With the lumen obliterated during fetal life, the remnant forms the median umbilical ligament in the

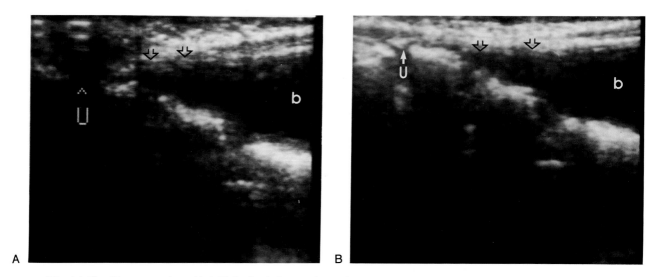

Fig. 14-10. Patent urachus. **(A & B)** Sagittal views, using a linear-array transducer, showing a lucent area (open arrows) extending superiorly from the region of the bladder *(b)* to the umbilicus *(U)*. This infant had a "discharge" from the umbilical area.

fully developed infant; a vestigial small lumen lined with transitional epithelium is often seen.[22] This is also seen in 32 percent of adults.[22]

By using high-frequency transducers, structures in the omphalovesical channel can be visualized by ultrasound.[22] Urachal remnants may be identified normally on scans of bladders of pediatric patients. These appear as small, elliptic, hypoechoic structures on the middle of the anterosuperior surface of the urinary bladder on 62 percent of bladder sonograms[22] (Fig. 14-13). The hypoechoic pattern of this structure may be related to its thick smooth muscle layer.[22] The central echogenic area seen at times within the remnant may correspond to the loca-

tion where one would expect a mucosal lining to occur in the urachal remnant.[22] These should be recognized so as to not be mistaken as a pathologic process unless accompanied by signs and symptoms of infection or bladder obstruction.[22]

Exstrophy

Exstrophy of the bladder represents a developmental failure in the anterior wall of the abdomen and bladder so that the bladder communicates either directly through a large defect with the surface of the body in the

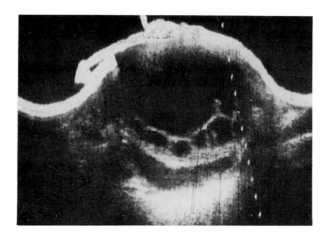
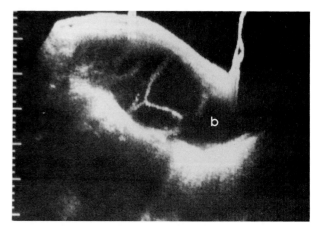

Fig. 14-11. Infected urachal cyst. **(A)** Transverse and **(B)** longitudinal scans showing a predominantly cystic mass superior to the bladder *(b)* in a 5-year-old girl. The septations are the result of fibrosis and adhesions. (From Friedman et al,[81] with permission.)

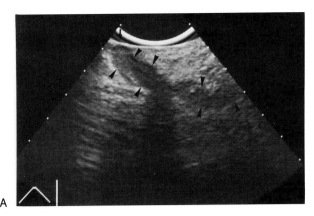

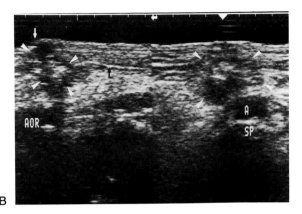

A

B

Fig. 14-12. Urachal abscess. Case 1. **(A)** Midline sagittal sonogram of the lower abdominal wall showing a tubular hypoechoic urachal abscess (arrowheads) with an irregular border. (arrow, umbilical level.) Case 2. **(B)** Sagittal (left image) and transverse (right image) sonograms of the lower abdomen, which was scanned with a 3.5-MHz transducer using a stand-off pad, showing that the peritoneal line (black arrows) is interrupted by the abscess (arrowheads), which is irregular in shape and protrudes into the peritoneal cavity. Surgery disclosed adhesion between the abscess and the colon. (*A, Aor,* aorta; *SP,* spine; white arrow, umbilical level.) (From Wan et al,[19] with permission.)

suprapubic region or as an opened sac. The believed origin is the failure of downgrowth of the mesoderm over the anterior aspect of the bladder; the musculature of the bladder and adjacent abdominal wall never develop, and the bladder ruptures anteriorly to communicate with the skin surface.[8]

Reduplication

Complete reduplication of the bladder is rare. It is difficult to account for replication of the bladder in embryologic terms. The pattern of complete reduplication consists of two separate bladders, each with its own mucosa and muscularis lying side by side, separated by a peritoneal fold. Each bladder receives the ipsilateral ureter and empties into a separate urethra through its own external meatus. There is a common association including reduplication of the genital and distal gastrointestinal system and, less commonly, reduplication or fusion of the lower spine. With reduplication of the bladder, unilateral reflux, obstruction, or infection may occur secondary to stenosis or to atresia of the urethra. Ultrasound can be used initially to diagnose and delineate the anatomy[23] (Fig. 14-14).

Diverticula

A diverticulum is a protrusion of the bladder mucosa through bundles of the detrusor muscle, occurring in areas where the muscle is inadequately formed (i.e., ure-

terovesical junction) or between bundles of hypertrophied muscle.[24,25] It is a pouchlike eversion or evagination of the bladder wall. It may arise as a congenital defect or as an acquired (more frequent) lesion from persistent urethral obstruction. Most bladder diverticula seen in children are associated with reflux, obstructed urethras, or neurogenic bladders. Congenital diverticula, however, do occur independently of these diseases and almost always occur in boys. In approximately 5 to 10 percent of the routine autopsy population of older individuals, diverticula, of both congenital and acquired origins, are common.[25]

Congenital. The congenital form may be due to a focal failure of development of the normal musculature, with resultant herniation of the mucosa at this point, or to some urinary tract obstruction during fetal development that creates increased intravesical pressure and consequent weakening of the wall at one point. Alternatively, diverticula may develop from budlike outgrowths of the fetal bladder. In any event, some musculature is retained within the wall of such diverticula, although it may be thinner than normal. These diverticula may occur as one or (at most) a few defects.

Most (98 percent) congenital bladder diverticula occur in males and are most frequently found in the region of the bladder base.[25] They also are frequently found in the region of the ureteral hiatus, in which case they are known as Hutch's diverticula (Fig. 14-15). Hutch's diverticula are important because they often cause reflux. While distally obstructing lesions such as

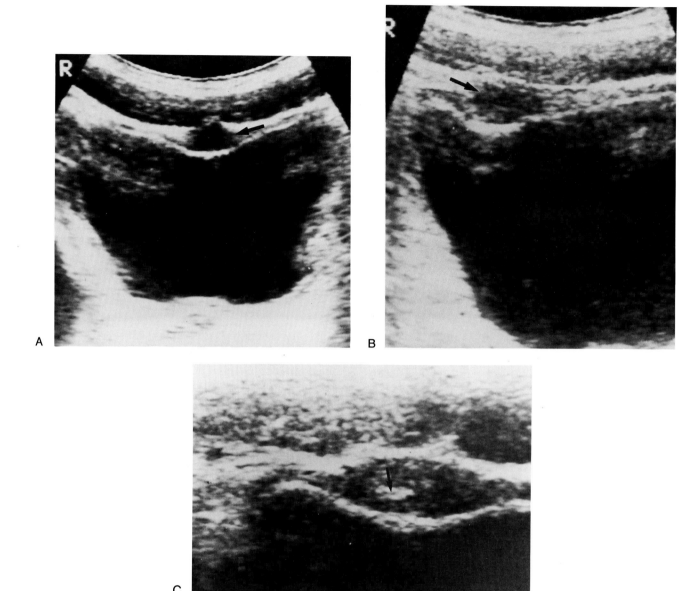

Fig. 14-13. Urachal remnant. Case 1. Ultrasound scans of the bladder of a 9-year-old girl with a urinary tract infection. The urachal remnant (arrow) is seen on the **(A)** transverse and **(B)** sagittal scans. Case 2. **(C)** Ultrasound scan of the bladder of a 7-year-old boy with enuresis. In this case a transverse scan of the urachal remnant shows a small hyperechoic center (arrow), which corresponds to the location of the epithelial lining. (From Cacciarelli et al,[22] with permission.)

urethral valves are found in some cases, most congenital diverticula develop in the absence of outflow obstruction. Congenital diverticula may occur at a point more posterior and lateral to the ureteral hiatus, where they may obstruct the urethra in boys. Because the diverticulum has a wide mouth, more urine may enter it during voiding than passes through the urethra. As a result, the diverticulum may enlarge and press on the posterior wall of the urethra obstructing it.

Acquired. Associated with chronically raised intravesical pressure and usually secondary to anatomic or neuropathic bladder outflow obstruction, acquired diverticula are outpouchings through a focal weakness in bladder muscle occurring in the retrotrigonal region, the posterolateral walls near the ureteral orifices, or the urachal attachment. Cellules or saccules (which are usually multiple, drain satisfactorily, and are of no clinical importance) are small outpouchings between hypertro-

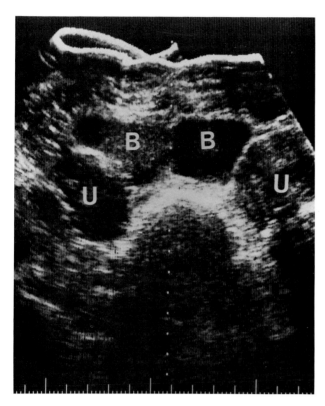

Fig. 14-14. Bladder reduplication. Transverse scan showing a double bladder *(B)*. There is a marked reverberation artifact as a result of obesity, and two widely separated uteri *(U)* are seen. (From Richman and Taylor,[23] with permission.)

ticula. Diverticula measure more than 2 cm in diameter, whereas saccules have diameters of 2 cm or less.

The sequence of events leading to diverticula formation may be urethral obstruction; hypertrophy of the bladder muscle with trabeculation of the wall; formation of small sacculations (cellules) between the muscle trabeculae; and creation of large, saclike pouches, which expand between muscle groups. The diverticula have markedly thinned musculature and, in the more advanced lesions, may have virtually no intrinsic musculature but only a mucosa with tunica propria. In 1 to 6 percent of men with symptoms of prostatism, moderate-sized or large diverticula are reported.

The neck of a diverticulum may be narrow or wide; contractile, wide-mouthed diverticula often produce no clinical difficulties, whereas narrow-necked diverticula tend to retain urine. Large diverticula originating lateral to the ureteral meatus produce a characteristic medial displacement of the adjacent ureter. Less commonly, diverticula arise medially and displace the ureter outward.

Acquired Hutch's (paraureteral) diverticula may occur in benign prostatic hypertrophy and other outlet obstructions. Enlarging diverticula may eventually assimilate the ureteral orifice and may obstruct the ipsilateral or contralateral ureter. Mechanisms that have been proposed to explain the ureteral obstruction include compression of the extravesical ureter against the bladder by a diverticulum; fibrosis from a peridiverticulitis; and deficiency of muscle at the UVJ and distal ureter. Even urethral obstruction may result if the diverticulum dissects below the bladder. Rarely, a diverticulum causes urinary retention in the absence of urethral obstruction when the bladder empties preferentially into the diverticulum rather than the urethra.

phied muscle bands and are anatomically identical to diverticula but smaller. Because there are increasingly severe manifestations of a sustained increase in intravesical pressure, the lesions progress from cellules to diver-

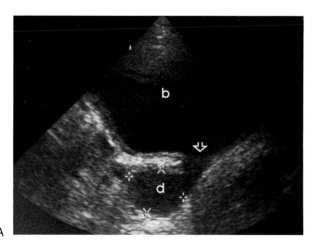

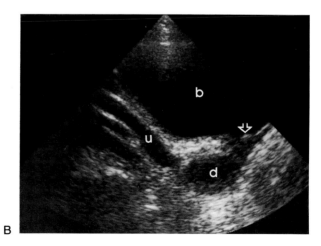

A　　　　　　　　　　　　　　　　　　　　　　　　　B

Fig. 14-15. Bladder diverticulum, Hutch type. **(A & B)** Sagittal views of the urinary bladder *(b)* showing a cystic structure *(d)* in a paraureteral location on the left. In Fig. B the left ureter *(u)* can be seen. The approximate UVJ is seen as a poorly defined lucent area (open arrow).

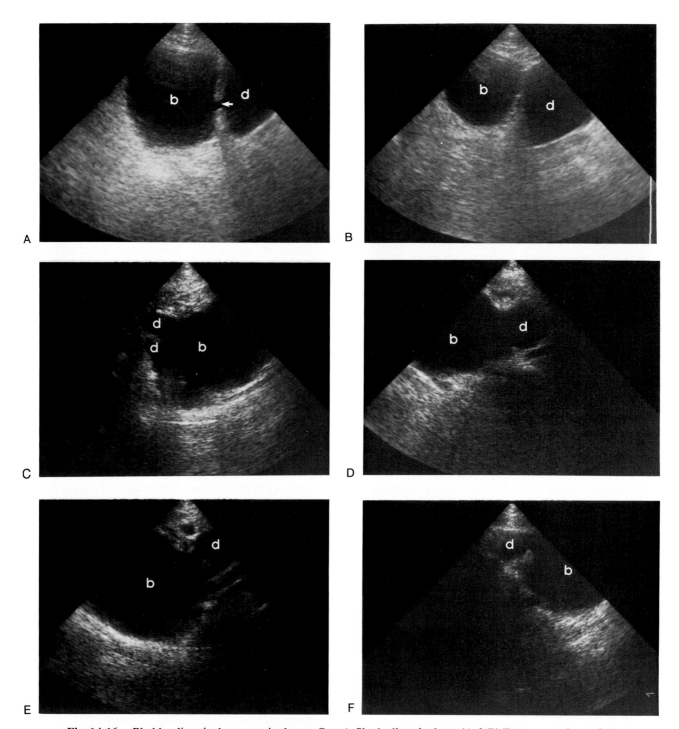

Fig. 14-16. Bladder diverticulum, acquired type. Case 1. Single diverticulum. **(A & B)** Transverse views of the bladder *(b)* showing a cystic mass *(d,* 58 × 68 mm) to the left. In Fig. A, it is seen to communicate (arrow) with the bladder. It was still visualized on postvoid views. Case 2. Multiple cellules and diverticuli. **(C–E)** Transverse postvoid and **(F)** sagittal views of the bladder *(b)* showing multiple cystic masses *(d)* laterally (bilaterally) and superiorly. Those smaller than 2 cm are cellules, and those larger than 2 cm are diverticula. *(Figure continues.)*

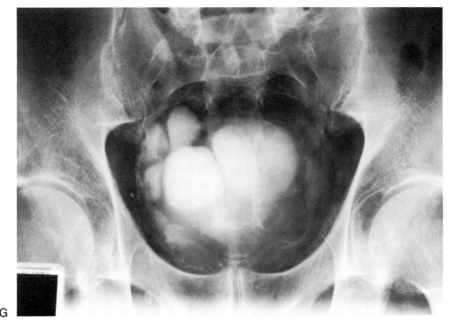

Fig. 14-16 *(Continued).*   **(G)** Cone-down view of the bladder from an IVP demonstrating multiple diverticula and cellules.

Diverticula are easily demonstrated by ultrasound as a lucent mass that may deform and displace the bladder (Figs. 14-15 to 14-17). They vary greatly in size. They are seen as round, well-defined, thin-walled fluid-filled masses with acoustic enhancement[21] (Figs. 14-15 to 14-17). In many, clear demarcation of the communication with the bladder can be seen on the posterior or lateral wall with a straight transverse or sagittal scan.[21] The diverticulum should disappear when the patient voids. The degree of stasis within a diverticulum is best estimated by the postvoid scan (Fig. 14-16).

Bladder ears, which are transitory bladder pouches projecting anteriorly into the inguinal rings in male infants under 6 months of age, must be differentiated from congenital bladder diverticula. Unlike congenital bladder diverticula, bladder ears are in an anterior position and there is no obvious neck connecting the pouching sac to the bladder.

Also to be distinguished from a bladder diverticulum is an outpouching from the bladder posterolateral to the ureteral orifices in girls. This area in girls contains an anatomically thin muscle cover, so that the bladder bulges during voiding. Many investigators regard this as a normal anatomic variation, although some believe that it is a true diverticulum.

Bladder diverticula must be distinguished from wide-mouthed lateral pouches in the bladder with a normal thickness of muscle, which contract when the bladder contracts. Although this is considered a normal anatomic variation, a true diverticulum tends to enlarge as the bladder contracts.

Lastly, bladder diverticula must be distinguished from a disorder in which, after surgery or injury, urine has extravasated and then become walled off. This cavity, which is lined with granulation tissue, remains and communicates with the bladder. To make the diagnosis, the patient's history is necessary.

Complications of diverticula include infection, reflux, ureteral obstruction, and, rarely, rupture. Because they constitute sites of urinary stasis, these bladder diverticula tend to become infected. The thin wall of the diverticulum predisposes to bacterial penetration or perforation and the possible development of perivesical infections or spread of infection into the peritoneal cavity. Reflux has been found in up to 14 percent of patients with benign prostatic hypertrophy. The severity varies from mild to severe. Additionally, urinary stasis in these structures predisposes to precipitation of urinary salts and the formation of bladder calculi. This chronic irritation may further predispose these lesions to the development of carcinomas.

The paraureteral diverticulum is especially important since it may or may not be associated with reflux. These diverticula anatomically occur through the musculature hiatus at the UVJ. If the intramural tunnel of the distal ureter is shorted by the diverticulum, or if the ureter

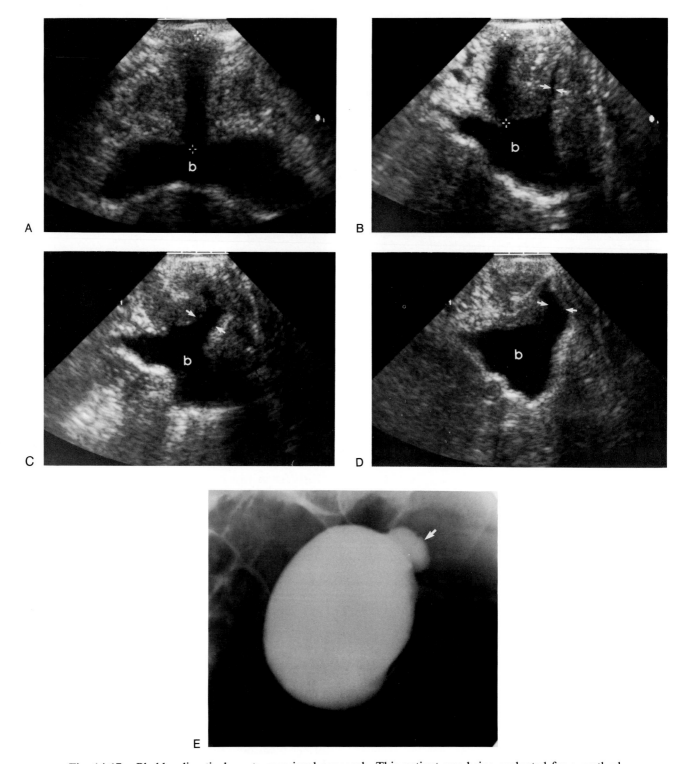

Fig. 14-17. Bladder diverticulum, transperineal approach. This patient was being evaluated for a urethral diverticulum. The urethra (calipers) appeared normal on **(A)** coronal and **(B)** sagittal views. There did appear to be a lucent projection (arrows) on the sagittal view from the inferior bladder *(b)* wall. **(C & D)** Postvoid sagittal views with straining, showing that the defect (arrows) was accentuated (12 mm) *(b, bladder)*. **(E)** Contrast view of the bladder (image oriented similar to Figs. B–D) showing the diverticulum (arrow).

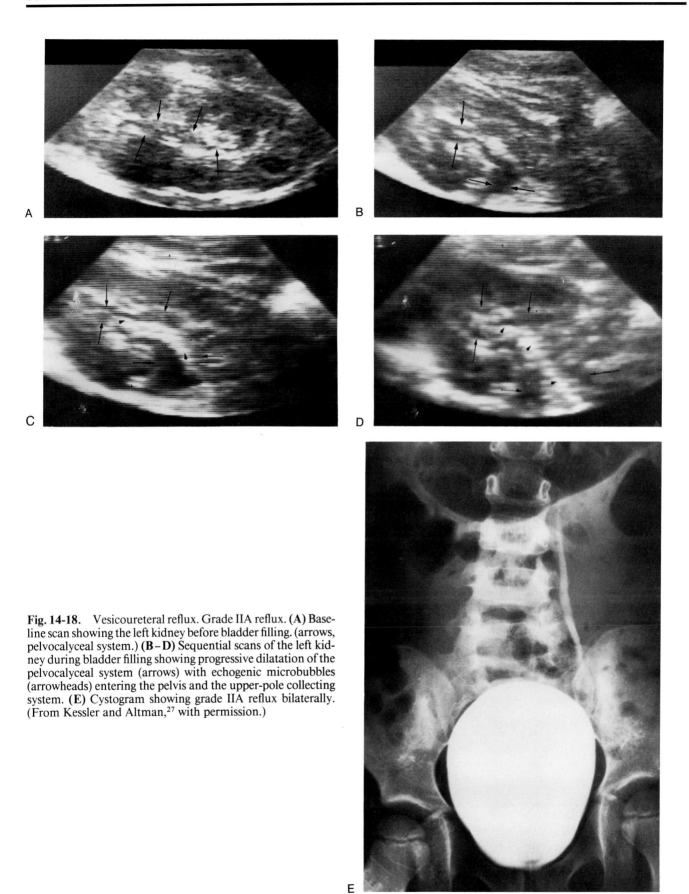

Fig. 14-18. Vesicoureteral reflux. Grade IIA reflux. **(A)** Baseline scan showing the left kidney before bladder filling. (arrows, pelvocalyceal system.) **(B–D)** Sequential scans of the left kidney during bladder filling showing progressive dilatation of the pelvocalyceal system (arrows) with echogenic microbubbles (arrowheads) entering the pelvis and the upper-pole collecting system. **(E)** Cystogram showing grade IIA reflux bilaterally. (From Kessler and Altman,[27] with permission.)

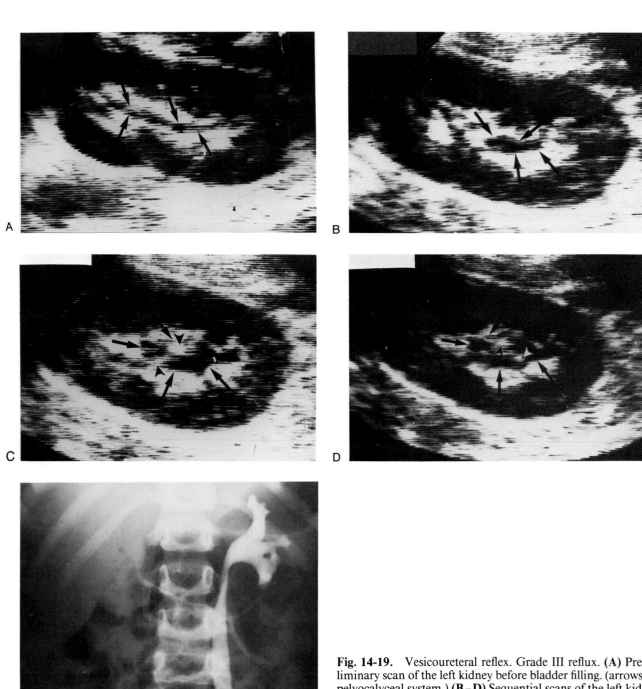

Fig. 14-19. Vesicoureteral reflex. Grade III reflux. **(A)** Preliminary scan of the left kidney before bladder filling. (arrows, pelvocalyceal system.) **(B–D)** Sequential scans of the left kidney during bladder filling showing increased pelvocalyceal dilatation (arrows) and echogenic microbubbles (arrowhead) within the collecting system. **(E)** Cystogram showing grade III reflux on the left. (From Kessler and Altman,[27] with permission.)

enters the diverticulum, reflux will occur. These diverticula are best visualized on voiding cystourethrography as well as by ultrasound.

Vesicoureteral Reflux

Vesicoureteral reflux is a common urinary tract abnormality in children. It may occur as a result of a primary maturation abnormality of the trigone or secondary anomalies such as ectopia, posterior urethral valves, paraureteric cyst, prune belly, and neurogenic bladder. Reflux into the lower system of a duplex collecting system is also often seen.[26] High-pressure reflux (with or without associated urinary tract infection) may be a major cause of chronic renal failure, with marked scarring and atrophic changes in the kidneys. The degree of reflux decreases or disappears in more than 50 percent of children.[27]

The primary diagnostic procedures to evaluate reflux have included voiding cystourethrography, often with excretory urography. Nuclear medicine cystography is a sensitive means of monitoring reflux. Ultrasound may prove valuable in the management of these children, particularly because it provides good visualization of renal size and parenchymal scarring while simultaneously demonstrating reflux.[27]

The ultrasound study for reflux begins with a scan of both kidneys. With the patient supine, an 8F catheter is placed in the bladder of the child (8F straight catheters for boys, and 8F balloon catheters for girls), residual urine is removed, and the patient is returned to the prone position. Cysto-Conray (20 percent) is injected into the bladder after creating turbulence in the contrast by rapidly drawing it in and out of a syringe. Each kidney is scanned while the contrast is injected. The amount of reflux is graded according to the radiographic classification of Dwoskin and Perlmutter[27]:

Grade I: Lower ureteral filling
Grade IIA: Ureteral and pelvocalyceal filling without other changes
Grade IIB: Ureteral and pelvocalyceal filling with mild calyceal blunting without clubbing and without dilatation of the pelvis and tortuousity of the ureter
Grade III: Ureteral and pelvocalyceal filling, calyceal clubbing, and minor to moderate pelvic dilatation with slight tortuousity of the ureter
Grade IV: Massive hydronephrosis and hydroureter

The sensitivity for grade IIA reflux or greater on ultrasound imaging is 87 percent, whereas it is 100 percent for grade IIB or greater in one study.[27] The specificity of this procedure is 100 percent. In each case of reflux, dilata-

tion of the collecting system is preceded by the appearance of microbubbles even in grade IIA reflux when cystograms demonstrate no abnormality (Figs. 14-18 to 14-21). There is greater dilatation with increasing grades of reflux.[27]

Ultrasound has potential value in diagnosing as well as monitoring vesicoureteral reflux.[27] This method may prove valuable in the management of other children, particularly because it provides good visualization of renal size and parenchymal scarring while simultaneously demonstrating reflux. (For further discussion of reflux, see Ureteral Jets above.)

Treatment

Various procedures have been developed for treatment of vesicoureteral reflux. One, the STING procedure, involves the endoscopic injection of Teflon paste under the submucosal portion of the ureter in the bladder.[28] The STING procedure can be used with all grades of reflux.[29] Cessation of reflux after a single STING procedure ranges from 66 to 81 percent.[29] On ultrasound, the Teflon paste at the injection site appears as a hyperechoic focus within the bladder wall with distal shadowing seen postoperatively and on follow-up examinations[28-30] (Figs. 14-22 and 14-23). This has been found in 88 percent of treated ureters.[28] Knowledge of the ultrasound appearance is important to effectively evaluate these children postoperatively.[29] Ultrasound may be useful in determining the location and size of the Teflon mass, in evaluating surrounding soft tissues at various time after injection, and in assessing possible complications such as obstruction.[28] The complications included free fluid in the pelvis, postoperative ureteral dilatation (within the first 4 weeks), and persistent reflux (after the first STING procedure).

Other authors also describe their findings associated with the STING procedure or subureteric injection of Teflon for the treatment of vesicoureteral reflux.[30] As a complication of this injection, Teflon migration may be the result of massive reflux of the Teflon after injection through the ureteral wall.[30] It is important to know the appearance of refluxed Teflon in order to monitor these patients more closely for evaluation of the efficacy of the procedure and disappearance of refluxed material. The refluxed material can be seen as echogenic material within the kidney with posterior shadowing.[30]

Catheters

Catheters can be easily defined within the bladder on ultrasound. The fluid in the Foley balloon is seen as a lucent mass, with the catheter walls identified as echo-

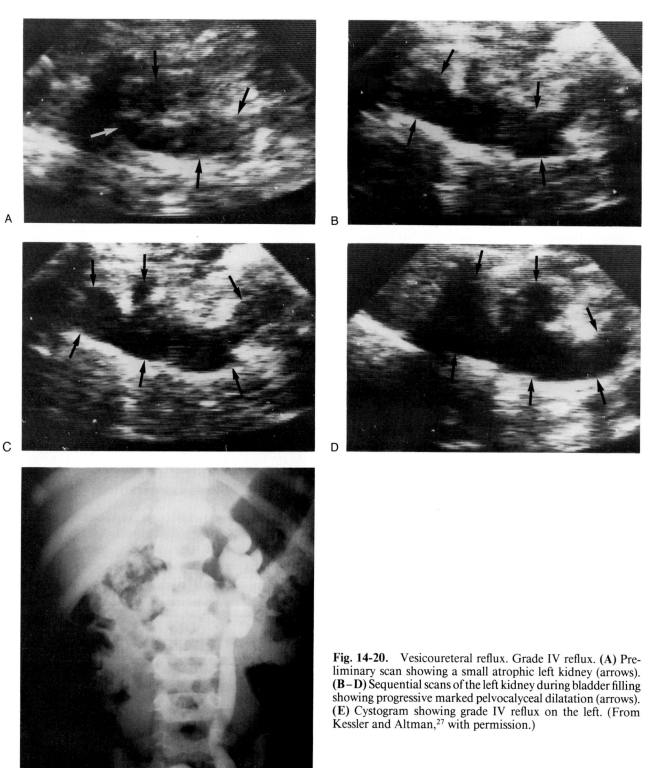

Fig. 14-20. Vesicoureteral reflux. Grade IV reflux. **(A)** Preliminary scan showing a small atrophic left kidney (arrows). **(B–D)** Sequential scans of the left kidney during bladder filling showing progressive marked pelvocalyceal dilatation (arrows). **(E)** Cystogram showing grade IV reflux on the left. (From Kessler and Altman,[27] with permission.)

dense lines (Fig. 14-24). When possible, it is best to examine the bladder without the catheter in place.[7]

Complications related to catheterization of the urinary bladder may be evaluated by ultrasound. Bladder infection is the most common complication, although mechanical problems have been described, including loss of the catheter within the bladder or urethra, knotting of the catheter, hematuria secondary to urethral laceration, and false passages with formation of a urethral fistulae.[31] Other complications include pressure erosion by the catheter with gangrene of the bladder wall and even perforation and bladder rupture.[31]

Ultrasound is an ideal modality for evaluation of the urinary bladder.[31] The examiner may identify the catheter location and alert the clinician to the possibility of improper positioning so that corrective measures may be undertaken.[31]

Blood Clots

When blood clots are adherent to the bladder wall, they may produce an irregularity along the mucosal surface. This appearance may be similar to that of tumor[7] (Figs. 14-2 and 14-25). As a rule, a blood clot is mobile with changes in patient position.

Calculi

A number of causes of bladder stones have been found. These include (1) the presence of an intravesical foreign body; (2) infection with *Proteus* (a urea-splitting organism); (3) exstrophy of the bladder; and (4) the presence of intestinal mucosa in the urinary tract.[32] In humans, the major lithogenic factor for bladder stones

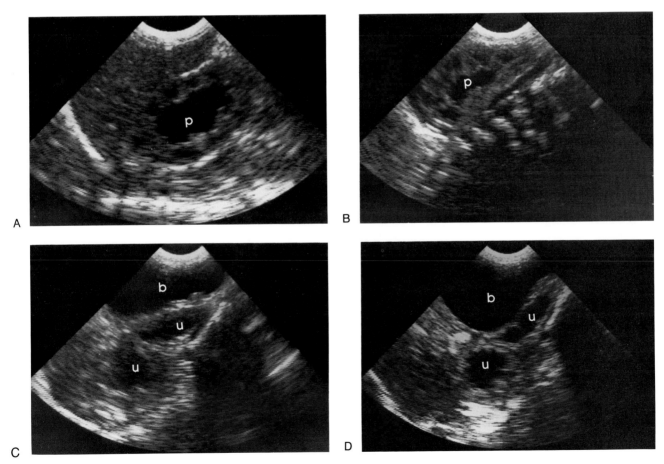

Fig. 14-21. Vesicoureteral reflux. Grade IV reflux. This infant presented with palpable abdominal masses. Longitudinal scans of **(A)** the right and **(B)** the left kidneys showing moderate hydronephrosis on the left and severe hydronephrosis on the right. (*p*, renal pelvis.) **(C)** Right and **(D)** left longitudinal scans of the pelvis demonstrating dilated ureters (*u*) with a fluid-filled bladder *(b)*. Since the ureters are dilated, it is difficult to follow their long axis. *(Figure continues.)*

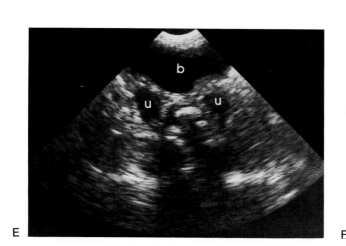

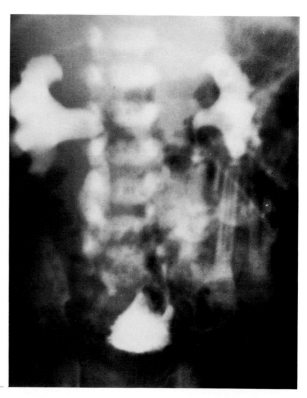

E

F

Fig. 14-21 *(Continued).* **(E)** Transverse scan of the pelvis demonstrating dilated ureters *(u)* with a fluid-filled bladder *(b).* **(F)** Voiding cystourethrogram showing massive bilateral reflux. (From Seeds et al,[98] with permission.)

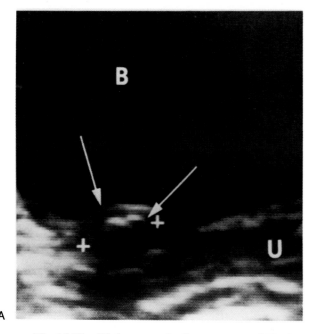

A

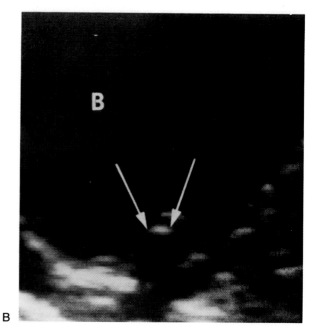

B

Fig. 14-22. Vesicoureteral reflux treatment. STING procedure. A 12-year-old girl with bilateral grade III reflux. Bladder sonogram 12 days after injection of Teflon paste showing an echogenic focus (arrows) with shadowing and surrounding thickening of bladder wall. **(A)** Transverse view. Calipers outline the endoluminal protrusion of the Teflon paste and mucosa; **(B)** sagittal view. (*B*, bladder; *U*, uterus.) (From Mann et al,[28] with permission.)

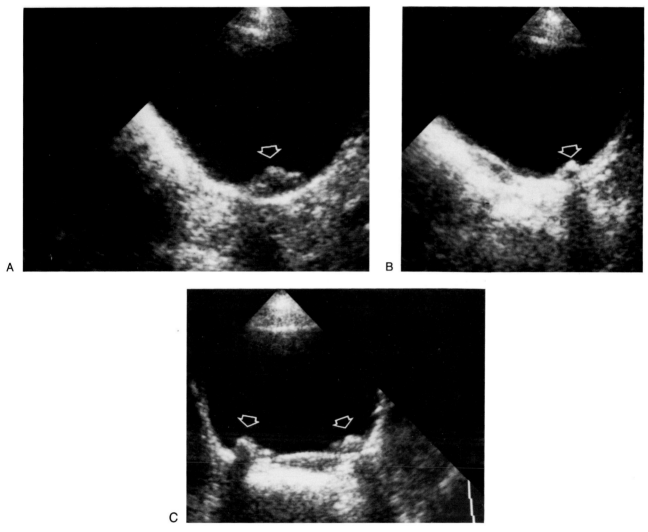

Fig. 14-23. Vesicoureteral reflux treatment. STING procedure. A 5-year-old child studied 1 month after bilateral subureteric Teflon injection. **(A)** Longitudinal sonogram through the left of the bladder showing that the injected material is echogenic and, on this scan, produces almost no shadowing (arrow). **(B)** Longitudinal sonogram through the right of the bladder showing injected material as a small, intensely echogenic focus (arrow) producing marked shadowing. **(C)** Transverse sonogram of the bladder. Both injection sites are visualized as protruding into the bladder lumen (arrows) and as producing acoustic shadowing. (From Gore et al,[29] with permission.)

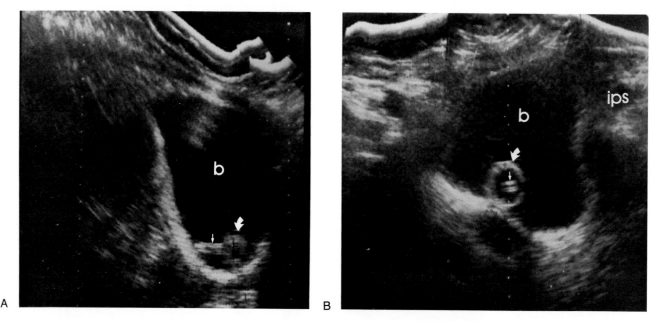

Fig. 14-24. Foley catheter. **(A)** Longitudinal and **(B)** transverse scans of the bladder *(b)* with a Foley catheter. The balloon (curved arrow) is seen as an anechoic circle, with the catheter seen as two parallel lines (small arrow). Note that there is no shadowing associated with the catheter. *(ips,* iliopsoas muscle.)

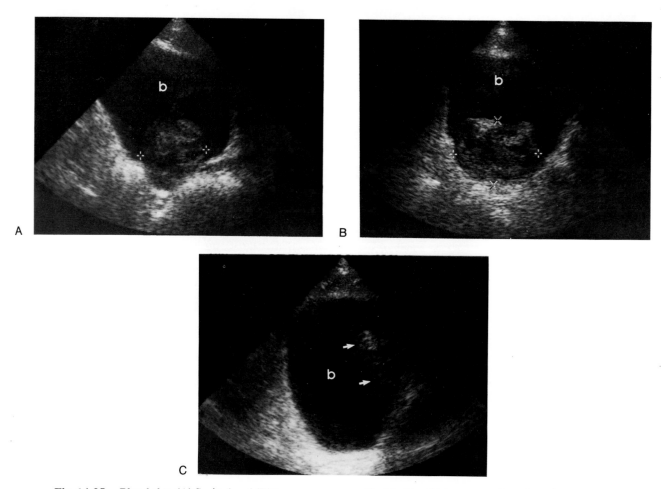

Fig. 14-25. Blood clot. **(A)** Sagittal and **(B)** transverse scans of the bladder *(b)* demonstrating a large inhomogeneous mass (calipers, $50 \times 48 \times 64$ mm) within the posterior bladder. From these views alone, it would be difficult to differentiate this lesion from a tumor. **(C)** Transverse left lateral decubitus view showing that the mass (arrow) moves and changes its configuration, excluding the diagnosis of tumor. *(b,* bladder.)

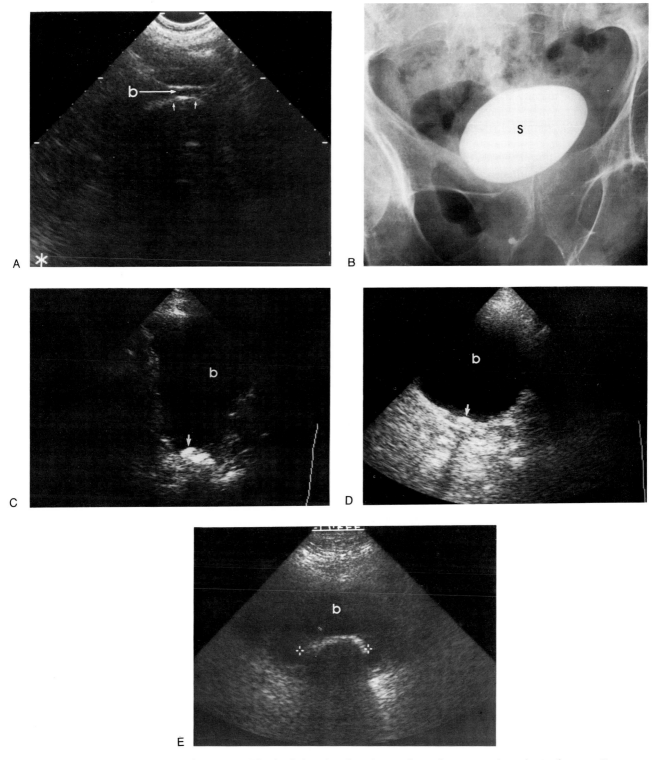

Fig. 14-26. Bladder calculi. Case 1. **(A)** Sagittal view showing a large echogenic structure (anterior surface, small arrows) within the region of the bladder (*b*, bladder lumen) associated with a posterior acoustic shadow. The bladder is not distended, so the lumen is not well visualized. **(B)** Plain film showing the large calculus *(s)*. Case 2. **(C)** Sagittal and **(D)** transverse views showing an echogenic structure (arrow) in the region of the UVJ on the right. The stone did not move with a change in patient position, and there was associated hydronephrosis. (*b*, bladder lumen.) Case 3. **(E)** Transverse view of the urinary bladder *(b)* showing an echogenic stone (calipers, 4 cm) with an associated shadow.

appears to be stasis. The most common presumptive cause of stone formation appears to be the association of an intravesical foreign body with either augmentation of the bladder, exstrophy of the bladder, or ileal dysfunction; the second most common cause is an intravesical foreign body alone. In children, hypercalciuria is a well-known cause of urinary tract calculi.[32] A well-known cause of bladder stones is encrustation of an intravesical foreign body by calcium salts. Catheters and pubic hair (the latter introduced by clean intermittent catheterization [CIC]) have all been shown to be the nidus for formation of a stone.[32] Patients at risk include those with

long-standing intravesical foreign bodies such as catheters, those with intestine incorporated in the urinary tract, and those with extrophy of the bladder on intermittent catheterization.

The role of infection in stone formation appears to be linked specifically to the presence in the urine of urea-splitting organisms, especially *Proteus mirabilis.* These bacteria have been shown to be deeply embedded in the stone and thus are protected from the action of antibacterial agents.[32] Even minute particles left at surgery represent foci of persistent infection that may result in recurrent stones. Encrustation of an intravesical foreign

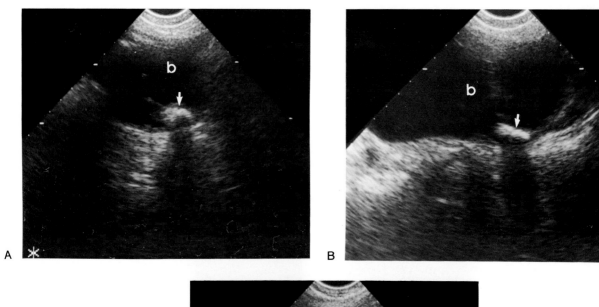

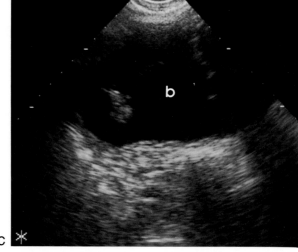

Fig. 14-27.   Bladder stone with infection *(Klebsiella).* This 21-year-old man had spina bifida with a neurogenic bladder and was on intermittent self-catheterization. He presented with fever and decreasing renal function. **(A & B)** Sagittal and **(C)** transverse views showing multiple internal echoes and septations (seen as wavy lines within the bladder *[b]*), as well as a stone (arrow), which is visualized as an echogenic focus with posterior acoustic shadowing. These findings would be most consistent with infection and bladder stone. At surgery, the patient was found to have a fistula between the bladder and small bowel. Additionally, he had a bladder stone associated with a stitch from previous surgery. *Klebsiella* was cultured from the urine.

body by calcium salts is a well-known cause of bladder stones and can be identified by an analysis of the nidus if the specimen is available.

A definite association between ileal dysfunction (such as inflammatory bowel disease or removal of a portion of terminal ileum from the fecal stream for use in the urinary tract) and stone formation has been established.[32] Adenomucosa in the urinary tract probably plays a role in lithogenesis as well. It is assumed that the mucus produced provides a nidus for the formation of calculi. This occurs when the bladder is augmented with intestine, when bowel is used to bridge a ureteral gap, or when there is exstrophy of the bladder and the bladder itself contains rests of bowel mucosa.

Calculi develop primarily in the bladder or pass into the bladder from the upper urinary tract. They are usually single, large, rounded, of homogeneous calcific density, and evident on plain radiography. Patients may be asymptomatic. The stones may cause inflammatory changes or acute bladder neck obstruction. Ultrasound is very helpful in confirming or detecting the stones as seen in this case. The stones are echodense structures producing an acoustic shadow and need not be calcified to be detected by ultrasound[7,33-35] (Figs. 14-26 and 14-27). The calculi shift to the dependent portion of the bladder with changes in the patient's position.[35]

Bladder Neck Obstruction

In the male, bladder neck obstruction most commonly is secondary to benign prostatic hypertrophy or carcinoma. With prolonged obstruction, there is progressive hypertrophy of the muscle coat, which causes thickening and trabeculation of the bladder wall. Ultrasound demonstrates a thickened wall associated with an irregular inner surface in advanced trabeculation[7] (Figs. 14-28 and 14-29).

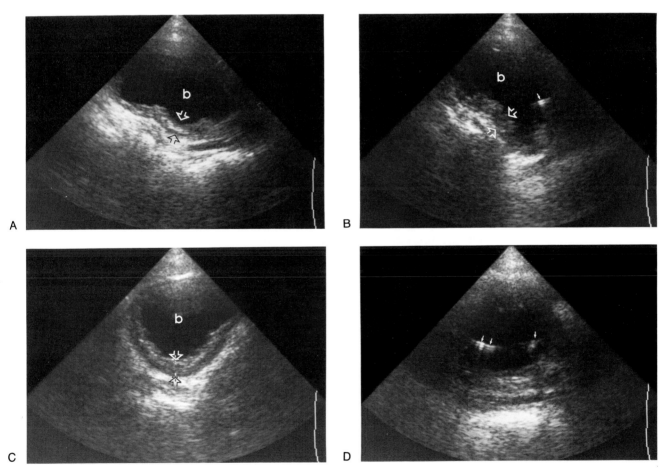

Fig. 14-28. Bladder outlet obstruction with wall trabeculation. This patient had chronic bladder outlet obstruction with bilateral hydronephrosis and internal ureteral stents. **(A & B)** Sagittal and **(C & D)** transverse views of the bladder *(b)* showing wall thickening (open arrows, 10 mm) as well as the tips (small arrows) of the ureteral stents. Views of the kidneys showed marked dilatation of the collecting systems bilaterally.

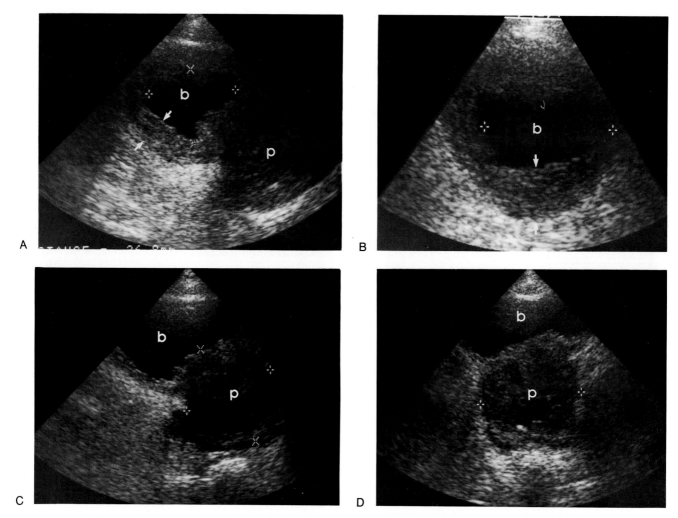

Fig. 14-29. Bladder outlet obstruction with prostatic hypertrophy and wall thickening. **(A)** Sagittal and **(B)** transverse (magnified) views of the bladder *(b)* demonstrating irregular thickening (arrows, 1.8 cm) of the bladder wall. This was found to be secondary to wall trabeculation. *(p, prostate.)* **(C)** Sagittal and **(D)** transverse views with the transducer angled inferiorly, showing a markedly enlarged prostate *(p, 63 × 57 × 24 mm)* with resultant bladder *(b)* outlet obstruction and hydronephrosis. Despite the large size of the prostate, the postvoid residual was only 73 ml.

Cystitis

Infection of the bladder always implies some predisposing factors, including exstrophy, urethral obstruction, fistulas common to the rectum or vagina, catheterization or instrumentation, cystocele, bladder calculi, bladder neoplasm, trauma, debilitating illness, pyelonephritis, pregnancy, and a derangement of bladder innervation. Up to the middle years, it is more frequent in women presumably because of the shorter urethra, pregnancy, and trauma with coitus.[8]

Bacterial pyelonephritis is frequently preceded by bladder infection with retrograde spread. The common etiology is *Escherichia coli,* followed by *Proteus, Klebsiella,* and *Enterobacter.* With chronic infection, there is fibrous thickening of the tunica propria. The symptoms of this disease include frequency, lower abdominal pain localized over the bladder, and dysuria.[8]

There are several distinct types of cystitis. In encrusted cystitis, urinary salts, particularly phosphate, are precipitated on the bladder surface. In bullous cystitis, large vesicles form in the bladder mucosa, which collect large amounts of submucosal edema fluid[8] (Figs. 14-30 and 14-31). The changes with catheter-induced cystitis are consistent with bullous cystitis.[36] The changes include a thickened mucosa that is smooth in the early stages,

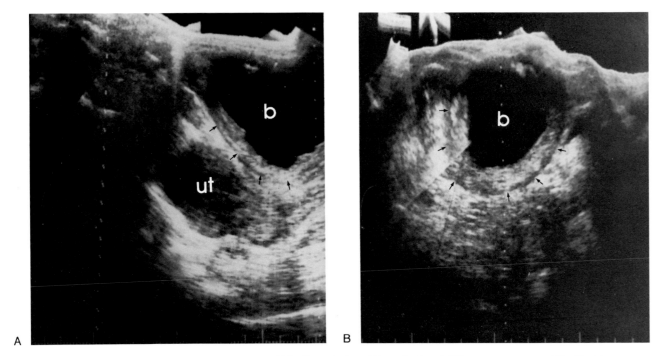

Fig. 14-30. Bullous cystitis. The bladder *(b)* is distended on **(A)** sagittal and **(B)** transverse scans. The bladder wall is thickened (arrows) and is hypoechoic and irregular. (*ut,* uterus.)

becoming redundant and polypoid in later stages. The mucosa is usually hypoechoic, with the lesion localized to the posterior wall, or diffuse and more severe, depending on the length of catheterization.[36]

Cystitis is the most common pathologic lesion in the bladder but is rarely of ultrasound significance. When the process is long-standing, the inflammatory reaction may cause extreme heaping up of the epithelium, fibrous thickening, and loss of elasticity of the bladder wall. This leads to reduced bladder capacity and a rounded, less distensible bladder. Granulation tissue sometimes is seen as an irregular internal bladder surface, and the ultrasound findings are indistinguishable from those of carcinoma.[7,37] With severe purulent cystitis (which may develop secondary to neurogenic dysfunction and urine stasis), a pus-urine fluid level may be formed, with the pus gravitating posteriorly (Figs. 14-32 and 14-33). Mild radiation cystitis is frequently seen producing bladder

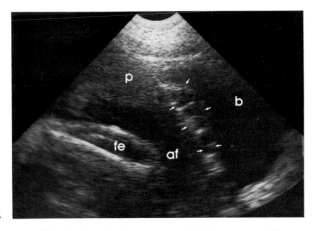
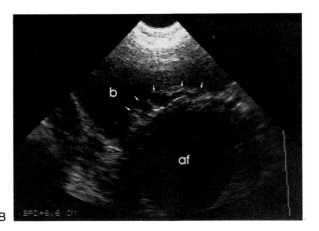

Fig. 14-31. Bullous cystitis. **(A)** Sagittal and **(B)** transverse scans of the bladder *(b)* in a patient who is 27 weeks pregnant. Multiple cystic areas (arrows) are seen within the posterior bladder wall. (*p,* placenta; *fe,* fetal extremity; *af,* amniotic fluid.)

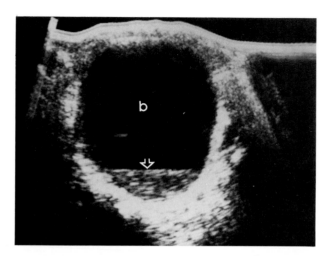

Fig. 14-32. Purulent cystitis. Transverse scan of the bladder *(b)* with a layer of pus (arrow) seen posteriorly. (From Morley,[7] with permission.)

irritability and is associated with decreased capacity. In more severe cases, there may be ulceration and sloughing of the bladder wall that may be seen as mucosal irregularity on ultrasound[7] (Fig. 14-34).

The sonographic appearance of cystitis is variable depending on the severity of the process, and several manifestations of involvement are detectable by ultrasound.[38] With early mild cystitis, there may not be apparent findings at ultrasound. With focal involvement by cystitis, there may be tiny irregular excrescences that cannot be distinguished from early focal transitional cell carcinoma.[38] With further inflammatory involvement, there are thick, bulky vesical wall abnormalities secondary to indwelling catheter with intraluminal or intramural gas at times. A fluid-fluid level within the bladder may be

associated with inflammation but can also be seen with hemorrhage.

Cystitis Cystica

As a nonspecific inflammatory process of the bladder mucosa largely confined to the trigone, cystitis cystica contains thickened irregular mucosa covered with multiple rounded cystlike elevations secondary to localized edema and lymphatic obstruction.[39] The associated intravesical mass is produced by this edematous mucosa and can be visualized by ultrasound.[39] The etiology of this abnormality is unknown, although it is commonly associated with chronic cystitis. It also has been described secondary to chronic Foley catheter placement.[39] With cystitis cystica of the trigone, a localized solid intravesical soft tissue mass that cannot be distinguished from an epithelial tumor may be visualized[39] (Fig. 14-35). This is seen as a broad-based, irregular, solid, nonshadowing soft tissue mass largely localized to the trigone with the mass containing multiple high-intensity echoes that may represent specular reflections from the walls of the multiple small cysts that make up the mass.[39]

Emphysematous Cystitis

Intraluminal gas (primary pneumaturia) and intramural gas (emphysematous cystitis) are considered different manifestations of the same entity.[40] Associated with this condition are diabetes, bacteriuria, and chronic retention.[40] Females predominate (2 : 1) in those over 45 years old.[40] *E. coli* is the most common pathogen, but *Klebsiella, P. mirabilis, Staphylococcus aureus, Streptococcus, Nocardia,* and *Candida albicans* have also been reported.[35] Gas in the bladder wall is the result of bacte-

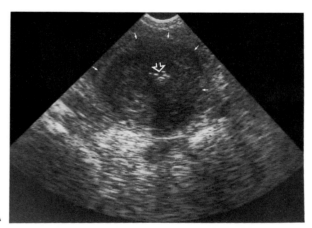

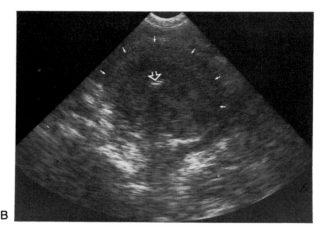

A   B

Fig. 14-33. Purulent cystitis. **(A)** Transverse and **(B)** sagittal real-time images showing a bladder (arrows, bladder outline) completely filled with echoes. Air is seen within the dense fluid collection as linear echodensities (open arrow) that exhibit acoustic shadows.

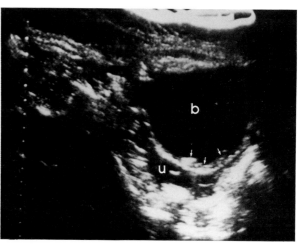

Fig. 14-34. Postradiation cystitis. Mucosal irregularity (arrows) of the posterior bladder *(b)* wall and base is seen. *(u,* uterus.) (From Morley,[7] with permission.)

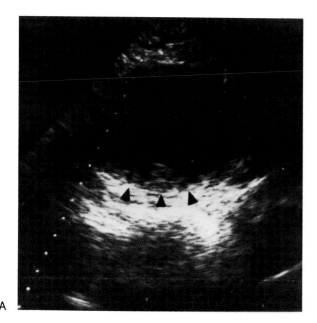

A

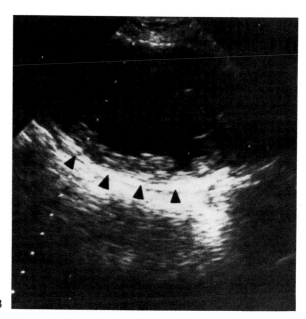

B

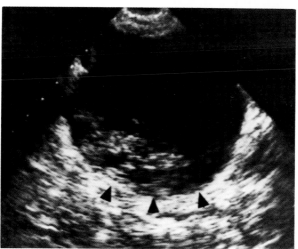

C

Fig. 14-35. Cystitis cystica. Case 1. **(A)** Transverse real-time sonogram of the bladder demonstrating a solid, nonshadowing, irregular soft tissue mass arising from the posterior bladder wall (arrowheads). **(B)** Longitudinal sonogram of the bladder demonstrating the homogeneous strong echogenicity of the mass (arrowheads) superior to a Foley catheter. Case 2. **(C)** Transverse real-time sonogram demonstrating a large, solid, irregular mass involving the posterior bladder wall (arrowheads). Multiple strong echoes are seen throughout this mass. (From Manco,[39] with permission.)

rial fermentation of glucose.[40] When there is reduced urinary oxygen tension caused by dehydration in urinary stasis and diabetes, increased susceptibility to anaerobic infection is considered.[40] The diagnosis may be made by ultrasound when air is demonstrated in the bladder wall or lumen[40] (Fig. 14-36). The wall is diffusely thickened with irregular foci associated with acoustic shadows.

Candida Albicans Cystitis

Candida albicans, which is a normal inhabitant of the oral and intestinal cavities, is the usual source of urinary tract infection with yeast fungus.[41] This infection may occur from a hematogenous source, from lymphatic spread, or by direct inoculation from the anus to the urethra.

C. albicans infections are opportunistic and range from asymptomatic to life-threatening. They may produce a mildly thickened bladder wall and a discrete well-defined dense fluid-fluid interface within the bladder, as well as debris that contains the long threadlike pseudomycelia of the fungus[41] (Fig. 41-37, similar to Fig. 14-32). With a change in patient position, this fluid-fluid interface shifts.[41] This fluid-fluid level can also be seen with blood and other infections, but the possibility of *Candida* infection should be raised.[41] The progress of therapy may be monitored by ultrasound. With con-

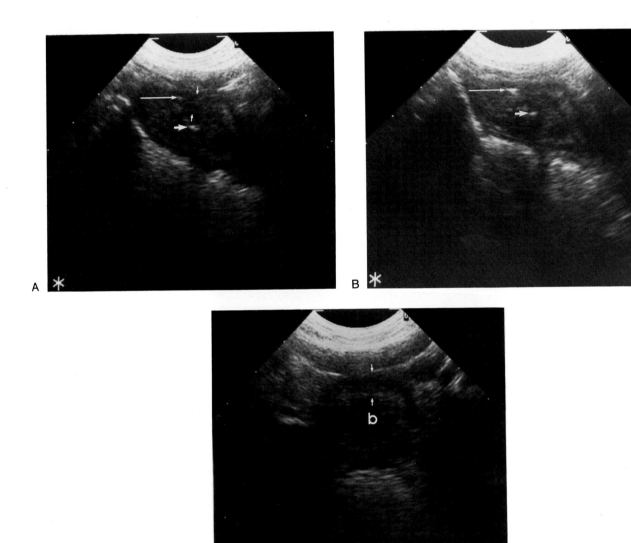

Fig. 14-36. Emphysematous cystitis. **(A & B)** Sagittal and **(C)** transverse views showing that the bladder wall (small arrows) is thickened. There is air (long arrow) within the anterior bladder wall in Figs. A & B. The fluid within the bladder *(b)* is very echogenic, and there is additional air (medium arrow) within that material in Figs. A & B. The patient had an *E. coli* bladder infection.

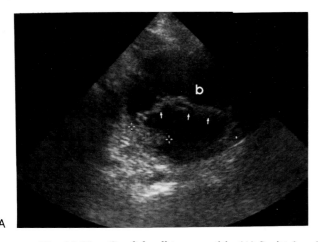 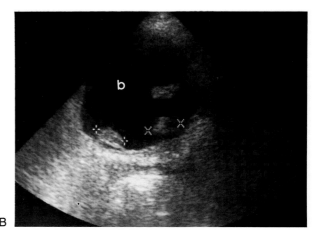

A   B

Fig. 14-37. *Candida albicans* cystitis. **(A)** Sagittal and **(B)** transverse views showing several echogenic masses (calipers) within the bladder *(b)* that were mobile and did not shadow. There is linear density (arrows) within the bladder in Fig. A, as well as bladder wall thickening. The patient was found to have a *Candida* infection with blood clots.

servative successful treatment, there may be clearing of the vesical debris without significant sequelae or the formation of concretions analogous to bezoars and the bladder returns to normal except for minimal residual wall thickening.[41]

Cyclophosphamide Hemorrhagic Cystitis

The cyclic phosphamide of nitrogen mustard (cyclophosphamide) is known to cause nonbacterial hemorrhagic cystitis occasionally.[42] This drug has been widely used for treatment of lymphoma and other solid tumors. This complication is said to occur in 0.5 to 40 percent of patients treated with cyclophosphamide and does not directly correlate with the dosage of the drug.[42] Adults are less frequently affected than children.[42] It is postulated that the cytotoxic effect on the urinary bladder is due to urinary metabolites of cyclophosphamide rather than to the drug itself. Characteristically, there is necrosis of smooth muscles and arteries pathologically.[42]

Patients present with urgency, frequency, hematuria, and pain on urination.[42] Ultrasound shows diffuse thickening of the bladder wall, which is not specific for the diagnosis. The degree of wall thickening correlates with the severity of the clinical symptoms of hemorrhagic cystitis.[42]

Other Cystitides

Crohn's Disease. Crohn's disease (regional enteritis) may rarely produce secondary involvement of the urinary bladder.[43] There may be involvement of the bowel in the proximity of the bladder with associated bladder

wall abnormalities. Cystitis and tumor should also be included in the differential.

Chronic Granulomatous Disease. As a genetically inherited disease of childhood, chronic granulomatous disease is characterized by repeated bacterial and/or fungal infections.[44] It is a disorder of neutrophil function in which phagocytosis occurs but ingested bacteria cannot be killed.[44] Most commonly, the infectious agent is *Staphylococcus*.[44] Only rarely is the genitourinary tract involved with cystitis and pyelonephritis.[44] Bladder wall thickening with nodularity of the bladder wall has been demonstrated.[44]

Cystitis Glandularis. An uncommon cystitis, cystitis glandularis is associated with chronic irritation to the bladder resulting in proliferation of the epithelium and replacement of the submucosa with glandular elements.[45] It is more pronounced at the UVJ, causing ureteral obstruction with subsequent renal failure[45] (Fig. 14-38). It is known to be associated with pelvic lipomatosis, a benign proliferative process that involves the perivesicular retroperitoneum with various effects on the adjacent organs.[45] It is seen in as many as 75 to 80 percent of patients with pelvic lipomatosis.[45] Clinical symptoms may be vague, varying from bladder irritability, recurrent urinary tract infections, hematuria, or back pain to ureteral obstruction. On ultrasound, this type of cystitis may be seen with nodular areas in the trigone with fingerlike projections.[45] Most commonly, there is diffuse bladder wall thickening.[45]

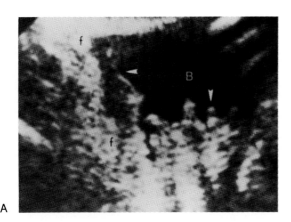
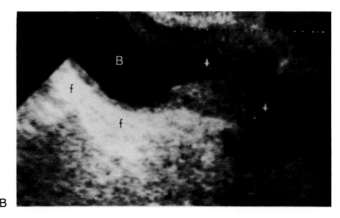

Fig. 14-38.   Cystitis glandularis. **(A)** Transverse scan of the bladder *(B)* showing bladder mucosa thickening with a focal area at the trigone, where nodular fingerlike projections are seen (arrowheads). (*f,* pelvic fat). **(B)** Sagittal scan of the bladder *(B)* showing diffuse mucosal thickening, more extensive at the base of the bladder (calipers). High echogenic tissue, fat *(f)*, is surrounding the bladder. (From Duffis et al,[45] with permission.)

Spinal Cord Injury

It is estimated that there are 0.5 to 1 million Americans with spinal cord injuries and that 20,000 new cases occur each year.[46] These injuries are mainly due to automobile, diving, and gunshot accidents and are much more common in males than females. The leading cause of death in these patients is urinary tract complications that arise where the nerve supply to the bladder is disrupted.

Spinal cord injury patients are subject to lifelong periodic uroradiographic evaluation at intervals of 3 months to 1 year. These patients often undergo excretory urography and voiding cystourethrography to detect calculi, ureterectasia, hydronephrosis, vesicoureteral reflux, and renal parenchymal disease. Ultrasound is capable of circumventing problems of the radiologic procedures that are common to spinal cord injury patients, such as overlying fecal material or bowel gas. In one series, ultrasound yielded significantly more diagnostic information than radiographic procedures in 36 percent of renal studies and 27 percent of bladder studies.[47]

Ultrasound voiding cystourethrography can be performed by filling the bladder with a drip infusion of normal saline through an indwelling Foley catheter.[47] Using real-time ultrasound, one can watch during infusion for reflux. Also, one can scan during voiding to look for reflux.

Ultrasound allows a three-dimensional view of the bladder to assess its size, shape, and volumetric measurements. These patients are subject to bladder calculi (Figs. 14-26 and 14-27). The earliest sign is an acoustic shadow behind the Foley catheter[47] (Fig. 14-39). A calcific crust forms on the Foley catheter and then falls off

into the bladder, forming a nidus for a stone.[42] Ultrasound is reported to have a 100 percent accuracy for detecting bladder stones.[47]

Ultrasound is unable to see normal ureters consistently. In one series, the ureters were seen in 30 percent of cases, with 60 percent of these seen on real-time.[47] Ultrasound is more successful in visualizing ureterectasis (43 percent) than reflux (23 percent).[48] The ureter is best seen with real-time ultrasound, which allows direct observation of peristalsis and/or vesicoureteral reflux. Ureters greater than 8 mm are considered dilated.

Some investigators recommend ultrasound to examine the kidneys and bladder as a replacement for the excretory urogram and voiding cystourethrogram at least at every other periodic examination.[47] Ultrasound has demonstrated 100 percent correlation with excretory urography in parenchymal disease, and for over one-third of patients ultrasound provides information not available on excretory urogram.[47]

Catheter-Induced Hyperreflexia

Spinal cord injury patients may have contractile or noncontractile bladders.[48] The reflex bladder is one type of contractile bladder, which may be defined as having the following features: (1) voiding is completely involuntary, occurring by means of a spinal cord reflex; and (2) the bladder volume required to initiate voiding is smaller than normal.[48]

A healthy person will have a feeling of fullness at a bladder volume of about 100 ml of urine, with a strong urge to void when about 400 to 500 ml of urine is present in the bladder.[48] In cases of a reflex bladder, the bladder

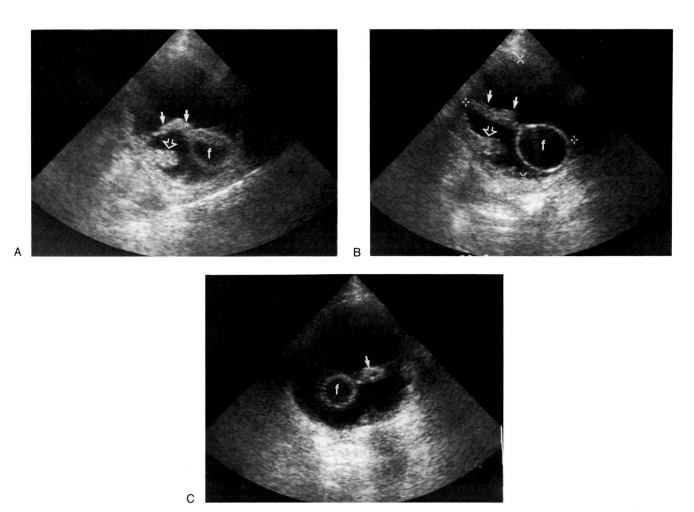

Fig. 14-39. Foley catheter. **(A & B)** Sagittal scans showing that there appears to be much echogenic material (arrows) associated with the Foley catheter tip. The bladder wall is irregular, and there is mobile material (open arrow) within the bladder lumen. This was thought to be related to debris from the catheter. (*f*, Foley balloon.) **(C)** Transverse view showing the echogenic material (arrow) surrounding the lumen of the catheter tip. (*f*, Foley balloon.)

begins to contract involuntarily when about 300 ml of urine or less is present.[48]

The reflex bladder may become very irritable and contract vigorously when it contains 125 ml or less, which is a serious problem for many spinal cord injury patients.[48] Autonomic dysreflexia, which may involve sweating, headache, bradycardia, and hypertension, may occur as this precipitous contraction occurs in all patients with lesions about T5 and in some patients with lesions between T5 and T8.[48] A potentially dangerous precipitous rise in blood pressure may occur, which in an older person might well cause cerebral hemorrhage.[48] As such, it is important to treat these patients with anticholinergic drugs to relax the detrusor.[48]

Several factors can increase the irritability of the detrusor of a reflex bladder sufficiently to lower its thresh-

old for contraction, causing hyperreflexia; these include infection, too rapid an inflow of fluid during urodynamic testing or of contrast material during voiding cystourethrography, or the introduction of a catheter into the bladder.[48]

It is important to determine whether the hyperreflexia is catheter induced. If the hyperreflexia is catheter induced, it is not treated with anticholinergic drugs. To evaluate this, urodynamic studies are performed with the aid of a catheter and ultrasound.[48] When hyperreflexia is encountered, the ultrasound examination is repeated while the bladder is allowed to fill naturally with urine (without the aid of the catheter).[48]

Patients are studied by both urodynamic studies and transrectal ultrasound. For 5 days prior to the combined urodynamic and ultrasound studies, the patient does not receive any drugs, including anticholinergics, so that the natural physiologic state of the bladder may be examined as accurately as possible.[48]

The results show that ultrasound renders a much better picture of the true functional state of the bladder than does urodynamic testing. With catheter-induced hyperreflexia, urodynamic studies give the impression of a small-volume irritable bladder, but when repeat ultrasound is performed on another day without a catheter, the true bladder capacity may be determined.[48]

With the catheter in the bladder in patients with catheter-induced hyperreflexia, the presence of the catheter inflates the bladder pressure to artificially high levels because the detrusor contracts so vigorously, producing misleading high readings.[48] Voiding is so vigorous in patients with catheter-induced hyperreflexia that the catheter can be expelled into the urethra and even out of the body entirely.[48]

Finally, transrectal ultrasound has proved invaluable for diagnosing and preventing catheter-induced hyperreflexia in these patients, and the result has been greatly improved patient care.[48]

Urinary Diversions

As alternatives to the ileal conduit following cystectomy for neoplasm or bladder dysfunction, urinary diversions are gaining wide acceptance.[49] To obviate the inconvenience of wearing an external stomal appliance, clean, intermittent catheterization of the reservoir (pouch) is performed at regular intervals. With these techniques, various portions of the bowel are used — small bowel alone (Camey and Kock techniques) or a combination of cecum and terminal ileum (Indiana, Mainz, Penn, and King techniques). The pouch must protect the upper tracts by preventing reflux, providing urinary continence, and sufficient capacity to require catheterization no more frequently than every 3 to 6 hours.[49]

Bladder augmentation and replacement procedures involving the use of segments of bowel to produce a reconstructed urinary reservoir are being used with increasing frequency. The major types of reconstructive procedures include augmentation, in which a segment of bowel is incorporated into the bladder, and replacement, performed when the entire bladder has been removed.[50] The most popular segment of bowel used is the cecum, ileum, or ileocecal segment. The type of procedure performed and portion of bowel used are tailored to the individual patient.[50]

When bladder augmentation and replacement procedures have been performed, various sonographic findings have been observed.[50] Most common are thick or irregularly shaped bladder walls (96 percent), pseudomasses within the bladder lumen (89 percent), and fine debris or linear strands (47 percent)[50] (Figs. 14-40 and 14-41). The pseudomasses, which are potentially the most confusing, are usually attributable to normal bowel folds, intraluminal mucus collections, or segments of bowel that had been intussuscepted into the bladder to prevent reflux.[50] The contour at the anastomosis of the bowel to the bladder, as well as the shape of the segment of the bowel used in surgery, produces the irregular shape of the reconstructed bladder.[50] As such, the shape of the reconstructed bladder is highly variable.

The preferred method of ureteral reimplantation in many centers is the Cohen transverse (cross-trigonal) ureteral advancement technique of ureteroneocystostomy, which has a success rate of more than 97 percent.[51] Patients who have undergone this procedure may have a characteristic pattern on ultrasound of the bladder — an echogenic, nonacoustically shadowing structure at or just above the trigone that is fixed in position within the bladder wall and covered by intact mucosa[51] (Fig. 14-42). This finding represents the submucosal segment of the reimplanted ureter, producing a "tunnel" sign.[51] The ultrasound appearance of the Cohen ureteral reimplantation is sufficiently specific to permit the examiner to make the correct diagnosis of a reimplanted ureter instead of the incorrect diagnoses of foreign body, ureterocele, hyperplastic polyp or focal cystitis.[51]

Vesicovaginal Fistula

In Western countries, vesicovaginal fistula occurs most often as a complication of gynecologic surgery, especially abdominal hysterectomy.[52] It may also be seen as a complication of urologic procedures such as urethral dilatation, plastic bladder repair, and papilloma fulguration. Less common causes include trauma, sepsis, radiotherapy, and cancer. Although it usually occurs only after 12 to 18 months, vesicovaginal fistula due to radiotherapy occurs in 0.5 to 2 percent of patients with carcinoma of the cervix.[52]

With a clinical history of urine/fluid discharge from the vagina with or without pain (and rarely pneumaturia), a vesicovaginal fistula is suspected.[52] The diagnosis may be made by analysis of the fluid for urea, creatinine, and protein or by cystoscopy. Methylene blue dye may be infused into the bladder, and staining of a vaginal swab or tampon with dye is diagnostic.[52]

Vesicovaginal fistula may be diagnosed radiographically by identification of contrast entering the vagina during an intravenous urogram or cystogram.[52] To visualize the tract, a lateral view is required. Ultrasound identification of a vesicovaginal fistula has been re-

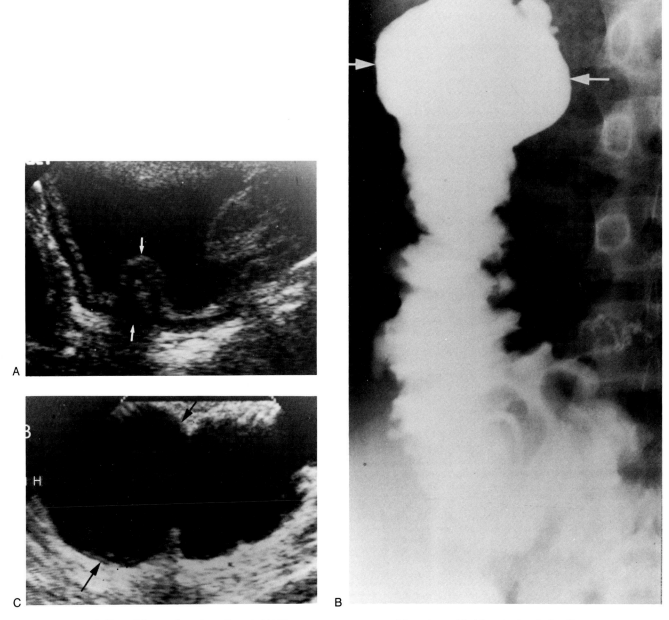

Fig. 14-40. Urinary diversion. Case 1. **(A)** Transverse sonogram of the urinary bladder obtained after ileoceco-cystoplasty showing pseudomasses originating from a thick wall. The echopattern of pseudomass (arrows) is smoothly continuous with that of adjacent bladder wall, indicating that this is a bowel fold. Scattered weak echoes within the bladder represent fine debris, presumably secondary to mucus. Case 2. **(B)** Cystogram obtained after construction of a continent catheterizable ileocecal bladder demonstrating capacious cecal region (arrows) and multiple haustra in ascending colon. Note the correlation with **(C)** the longitudinal sonogram. (*H*, toward patient's head.) (From Hertzberg et al,[50] with permission.)

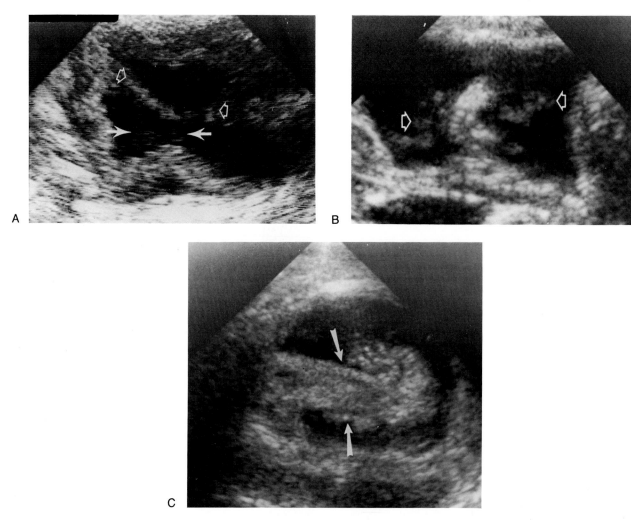

Fig. 14-41.   Urinary diversion. Case 1. **(A)** Longitudinal sonogram obtained after ileocecocystoplasty illustrating the thick bladder wall, pseudomasses due to mucus (solid arrows), and apparent septation due to a mucosal fold (open arrows). Case 2. **(B)** Transverse sonogram obtained after cecocystoplasty showing mucus collections floating freely in the bladder (arrows) and shifted with peristalsis. Case 3. **(C)** Oblique transverse sonogram obtained after ileocecocystoplasty with surgical intussusception of ileum into bladder showing an elongated projection from the bladder wall (arrows) that corresponded to the location of the surgically intussuscepted bowel. (From Hertzberg et al,[50] with permission.)

ported.[52] By using this modality, the fistulous tract may be demonstrated (Fig. 14-43).

Trauma

Rupture

When there is a fracture of the bony pelvis, there may be severe damage to the bladder and urethra. The rupture may be either extraperitoneal (50 to 80 percent) or intraperitoneal (20 to 50 percent).[53,54] Pelvic fractures are the main cause of extraperitoneal bladder rupture, whereas invasive procedures are the main cause of intraperitoneal rupture.[53] Ultrasound may demonstrate a "bladder-within-a-bladder" appearance associated with a ruptured bladder (Fig. 14-44). This may be secondary to the hypoechoic urine within the bladder combined with hypoechoic extraperitoneal extravasated blood and urine surrounding the bladder.[53] The echogenic ring between the two hypoechoic layers represents the thickened muscular wall of the collapsed bladder.[53] Others report a defect of the bladder wall associated with rupture.[55]

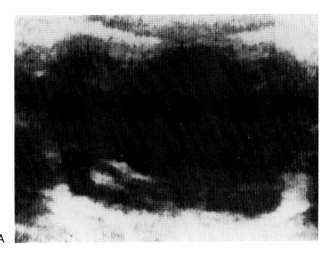

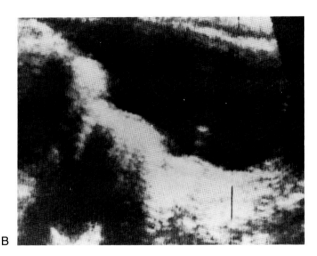

Fig. 14-42. Urinary diversion. **(A)** Transverse sonogram of the pelvis of a 6-year-old boy obtained after Cohen reimplantation of the left ureter, showing the reimplanted ureter traversing the posterior aspect of the bladder. **(B)** Longitudinal scan of the bladder of the same patient demonstrating an echogenic structure arising from the posterior bladder wall. This represents the cross-sectional appearance of the reimplanted ureter. (From Mezzacappa et al,[51] with permission.)

Bladder Flap Hematoma

To obtain access to the uterus, the parietal layer of the peritoneum that reflects over the urinary bladder and the fundus of the uterus is incised, with careful caudal deflection of the urinary bladder.[54] Postoperative hematoma formation predisposing to infection may be secondary to trauma or incomplete hemostasis. The number of significant complications is relatively small, even though the number of hysterectomies and cesarean sections performed is increasing.[54]

A blood collection in a potential space located between the urinary bladder and the lower uterine segment (vesicouterine space) is termed bladder flap hematoma.[54] The sonographic appearance is not specific. If a mass is found in the extraperitoneal pelvic space in the postoperative patient, a bladder flap hematoma may be diagnosed.[54] This mass may be complex and primarily anechoic, with internal septations or debris.[54] An infected hematoma may not be differentiated.

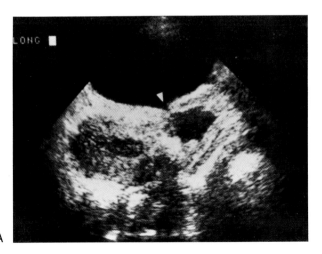

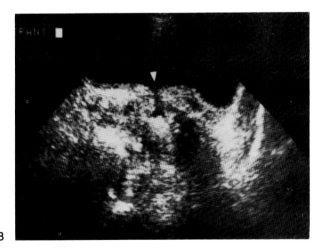

Fig. 14-43. Vesicovaginal fistula. **(A)** Longitudinal and **(B)** transverse images demonstrating vesicovaginal fistula (arrowhead). (From Carrington and Johnson,[52] with permission.)

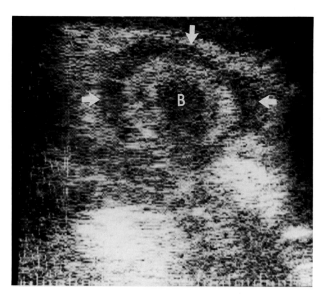

Fig. 14-44. Bladder rupture. Transverse suprapubic sonogram demonstrating the "bladder within the bladder" (arrows) typical of perivesical fluid collection. (*B*, bladder.) (From Kauzlaric and Barmeir,[53] with permission.)

Endometriosis

Endometriosis occurs in 15 to 30 percent of premenopausal women.[56] It commonly involves the ovaries, fallopian tubes, broad and round ligaments, cervix, vagina, peritoneum, and pouch of Douglas.[57] The urinary tract is involved in 2 to 10 percent, with the bladder being the most common urologic site.[56,57] The exact pathogenesis of ectopic endometriosis is unknown. The endometrial element may originate in the uterine wall and reach ectopic positions by direct extension, implantation, or metastasis.[57] Usually the bladder is invaded from without by endometrial tissue penetrating the bladder wall and extending into the bladder lumen.

The symptoms of vesical endometriosis are variable. Most patients experience a sense of pressure in the suprapubic region, which is usually relieved by voiding, with intermittent complaints of urinary urgency, frequency, and burning.[57] Hematuria occurs in 50 percent of cases.[57] The symptoms are cyclic and occur with the menstrual period. A mass is palpable in up to 50 percent of patients depending on its size. At least 50 percent of patients have a history of pelvic surgery.[57]

It is best to time the ultrasound on the day of maximal hormonal stimulation. With vesical endometriosis, a mass along the bladder wall projecting intraluminally may be seen[56,57] (Fig. 14-45). It may be seen as irregular multiple mounds with defined borders. Ultrasound has the advantage of defining the filling defect and its extent.[57]

Neurofibromatosis

Neurofibromatosis is an inherited disorder of the neurilemma cells with characteristic cutaneous, neurologic, and bone lesions. It is an inherited, autosomal dominant, hamartomatous disorder of neural crest origin that affects 1 in 3,000 children with a 3:1 ratio of boys to girls.[58] Classic symptoms include café-au-lait spots and mesodermal tumors of the viscera and nervous system.[58] Visceral involvement is uncommon, but when it occurs the gastrointestinal tract is frequently affected. Urinary tract involvement is rare. Children with urinary tract involvement may have enlarged genitalia.[58] When there is involvement of the bladder, patients often experience frequency, incontinence, urgency, hematuria, or abdominal pain. The patients are treated conservatively as long as urinary function is maintained. If obstruction develops, an ileal or sigmoid conduit may be necessary.[59]

Although these lesions may be confined to the bladder, there may be diffuse involvement of the pelvis, with the distal urethra, prostate, seminal vesicles, spermatic cords, and testes affected. These tumors are derived from the pelvic autonomic plexuses, which form a complex and interrelated meshwork of nerve fibers innervating the distal ureter, base of the bladder, and other pelvic structures.[59] The bladder tumors are closely associated with the trigone, ureters, and urethra and are thought to arise from the vesicoprostatic or vesicovaginal plexus.[58]

Neurofibromatosis may be seen as massive thickening of the bladder wall on ultrasound (Figs. 14-46 and 14-47). There may be focal or diffuse bladder wall thickening with loss of the normal hypoechoic detrusor and extension into the prostate or uterus.[58] There may also be

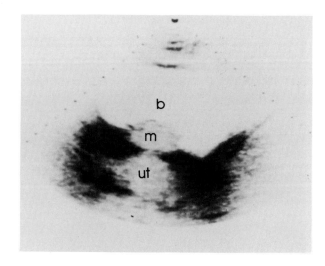

Fig. 14-45. Bladder endometriosis. Transverse scan demonstrating the mass *(m)* situated along the posterior wall of the bladder *(b)*. Note the extent of the mass and its relationship to the uterus *(ut)*. (From Kumar et al,[57] with permission.)

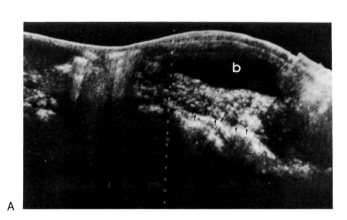

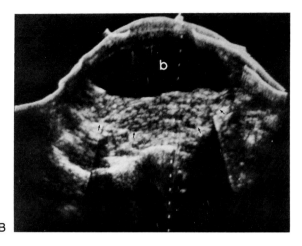

A   B

Fig. 14-46. Bladder neurofibromatosis. **(A)** Longitudinal and **(B)** transverse scans of the bladder *(b)* showing marked thickening of the posterior and superior walls (arrows). (From Miller et al,[59] with permission.)

pelvic tumor. Ultrasound may be helpful in screening such patients for identification of early lesions of the bladder to help prevent the late complications of unresectable disease.[58] The differential diagnosis would have to include embryonal sarcoma or advanced rhabdomyosarcoma, multiple previous operations, neurogenic bladder, and recurrent cystitis/hemorrhagic cystitis/cytoxan cystitis. Since generalized neurofibromatosis is usually present, the diagnosis is not difficult.[59]

Common Primary Bladder Tumors

Ninety-five percent of bladder tumors are epithelial or urothelial. Benign papillomas most commonly occur along the lateral wall; the trigone is the next most common site. These lesions are usually small (0.5 to 2 cm). Malignant tumors of the bladder account for 3 percent of cancer dealths. Ninety percent are transitional cell carcinomas, with 5 percent squamous cell carcinomas; ade-

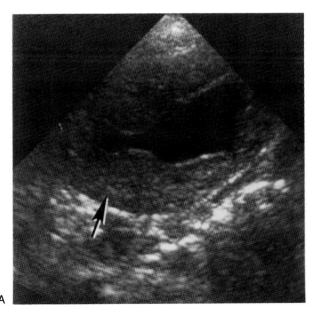

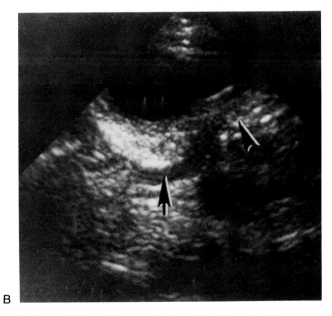

A   B

Fig. 14-47. Bladder neurofibromatosis. Neurofibromatosis of the bladder with extension into the subarachnoid space in a 6-month-old infant girl. **(A)** Transverse sonogram showing the thickened bladder wall (arrow). **(B)** Transverse sonogram showing the dilated distal ureter (arrow) obstructed by the bladder mass extending into the retrovesical region (arrowhead). (From Shapeero and Vordermark,[58] with permission.)

nocarcinomas are rare. Bladder cancer is more common in males, with a 3 : 1 ratio in the fifth and sixth decades.[8] Painless hematuria is the most common presenting symptom in 60 percent of patients.[4,33]

There is a broad spectrum of epithelial bladder tumors from innocuously benign to malignant. Grossly, there may be villous tufts and fronded papillary growths to sessile nodular infiltrating tumors. Local invasion may involve the prostate, seminal vesicles, and retroperitoneum. Forty percent are deeply invasive tumors with metastases to lymph nodes, but hematogeneous spread occurs only late in the disease. The factors affecting curability are depth of infiltration, histologic type, grade of malignancy, and presence of lymphatic or venous permeation of the bladder wall in the region of the tumor.[7,60] The single most important factor is the depth of infiltration, which is defined as the deepest point in the bladder wall to which the tumor has spread.[60] The most important factor in deciding the therapy schedule is the clinically determined stage.[7]

Cystoscopy with biopsy is considered the most accurate method to detect bladder tumors, but it is invasive, causes discomfort, and often requires anesthesia.[4] Ex-

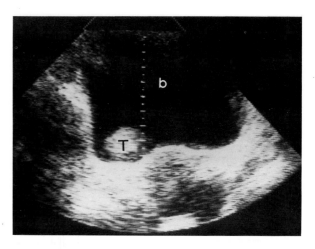

Fig. 14-49. Bladder tumor. Pedunculated. Papillary transitional cell carcinoma. Transverse real-time scan through the bladder *(b)* showing spherical solid mass *(T)* arising from the bladder wall, projecting intraluminally. No acoustic shadowing is seen. (From Bree and Silver,[34] with permission.)

cretory urography, the most common radiologic examination, is relatively insensitive, with an accuracy of 70 percent.[4] Ultrasound is helpful as an initial screen of patients with suspected bladder tumors. Nontechnical factors that affect detection include the size and location of the tumor, bladder distension, obesity of the patient, and the operator's skill.[4]

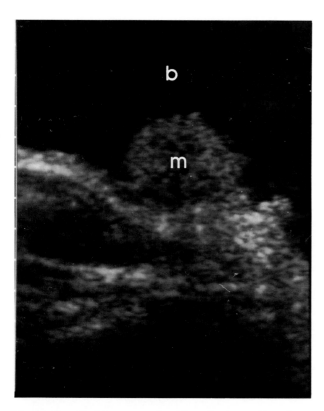

Fig. 14-48. Bladder tumor. On this sagittal magnified view, a large (2.5-cm) broad-based mass *(m)* is seen inseparable from the posterior bladder *(b)* wall. At color Doppler, there was increased flow at the base of the mass. This was found to be a squamous papilloma with severe atypia.

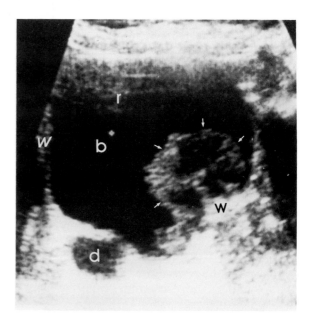

Fig. 14-50. Bladder tumor. Polypoid. Transverse scan of the bladder *(b)* showing a large (3 × 4 cm) polypoid bladder tumor (arrows) with a wide base involving the posterior wall and trigone. The tumor has papillary margins and is of mixed echogenicity. (*d,* diverticulum; *r,* reverberation; *w,* bladder wall.) (From Abu-Yousef et al,[60] with permission.)

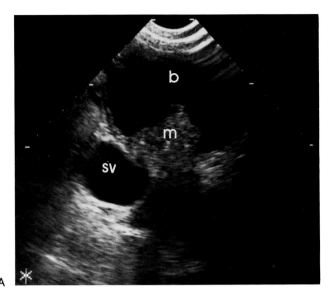
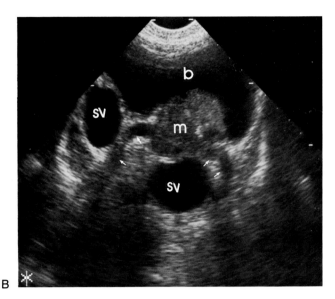

A   B

Fig. 14-51. Bladder tumor. Signet cell (adenocarcinoma) bladder tumor. This patient was noted to have bilateral hydronephrosis. **(A)** Sagittal view of the bladder *(b)* showing a mass *(m)* in the region of the prostate projecting into the bladder. (*sv*, seminal vesicles.) **(B)** Transverse view of the bladder *(b)* showing both obstructed ureters (arrows) as well as cystic dilatation of the seminal vesicles *(sv)* bilaterally. Views of the left ureter are seen in Figs. 14-3E & F. (*m*, mass.)

Ultrasound reveals certain findings in bladder tumors. Accurate detection depends on the size and location of the neoplasm.[61] Villous tufts appear as small projections of the epithelium that, unless numerous, are difficult to define. Small papillomas project from the bladder mucosa and can be pedunculated (Figs. 14-48 and 14-49). If they arise from the bladder base, the pedicle may be obscured. Fronding is seen as a well-defined lesion. A rounded, soft tissue mass 2 to 4 cm in diameter may be seen with polypoid tumors (Figs. 14-50 and 14-51). Massive tumor may be seen obliterating the bladder lumen. The more invasive tumors have a broader base and spongy texture or are solid, returning low-level echoes (Figs. 14-52 and 14-53). The more sessile ones are irregular on the surface because they frequently are necrotic and ulcerated. The intramural lesions are well-defined in outline and are shown to be located within the bladder wall. An infiltrating wall lesion may produce wall thickening with loss of the concave inner border and little intraluminal mass (Fig. 14-53). Infiltrating tumors occasionally show little intraluminal component and are harder to identify. They vary from producing high- to low-level echoes and are usually homogeneous. Exophytic tumors produce focal filling defects of increased or mixed echogenicity arising from the inner surface of the bladder wall. The deeply invasive lesions break through the wall with less definition, and the tumor is seen as a pelvic mass. Extravesical tumor is usually lower in echodensity than perivesical fat and connective tissue.[7]

Ultrasound is an additional diagnostic tool for detection of bladder tumors and is indicated when cystoscopy can not be done or is inconclusive. Bladder tumors appear as echogenic structures protruding into the echofree bladder lumen and are easily seen by ultrasound. The detection accuracy is related to tumor size. Bladder tumors less than 0.5 cm, regardless of location, and those of any size located in the bladder neck or dome areas are

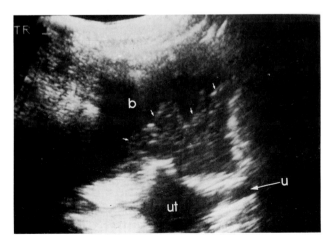

Fig. 14-52. Bladder tumor. Broad-based. Large solid tumor (arrows) obstructing the left ureter *(u)*. The bladder *(b)* wall remains well-defined. The uterus *(ut)* is outlined behind the bladder wall adjacent to the tumor. (From Morley,[7] with permission.)

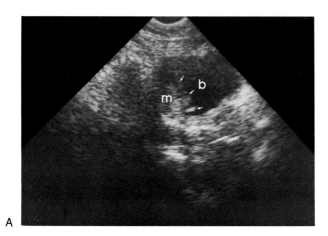 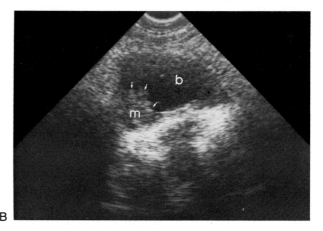

Fig. 14-53. Bladder tumor. Recurrent transitional cell carcinoma. Right **(A)** longitudinal and **(B)** transverse scans of the bladder *(b)* showing echodense mass *(m,* arrows) involving the right lateral wall of the bladder.

difficult to detect.[61] With 1-cm tumors the accuracy is 83.3 percent, and with 2-cm tumors it is 95 percent.[61] The diagnostic accuracy is 95 percent for tumors greater than 0.5 cm in size and situated on the posterior or lateral wall of the bladder.[61]

It is impossible to perform detailed staging of bladder tumors by ultrasound alone. It is usually possible to determine whether the tumor is superficial, whether it has invaded the bladder muscularis, or whether it has spread outside into the pelvic soft tissue. Superficial tumors are usually villous, fronded, or papillary, often with a narrow pedicle (Figs. 14-48 to 14-51). The bladder outline and capacity are normal, as are the pelvic soft tissues. This would correspond to a stage 0 and A in Jewett's classification.

When the tumor invades the bladder wall, the lesion may vary from a broad-based spongy papillary lesion to a solid, sessile, or intramural growth. With involvement of the mucosa and submucosa, stage T1 in the TNM system is reached.[60] It is impossible to separate mucosa from submucosa on ultrasound. The underlying echodense bladder wall appears smooth and interrupted by the less echogenic tumor (Fig. 14-54). No bladder deformity or decreased capacity is seen, and it is not associated with hydronephrosis.

Superficial muscle involvement (stage B1 or T2) causes decreased elasticity of the bladder wall adjacent to the tumor. In stage T2, the superficial invasion of the muscular wall is seen as interruption of the superficial layer of the echogenic wall (Fig. 14-55). There is no associated bladder wall deformity, decreased capacity, or hydronephrosis.

With deeper invasion (stage B2), the bladder wall is rigid and the bladder capacity is decreased, with associated significant residual urine volume. With deep

muscular wall involvement, the stage is T3A. In this stage, the whole thickness of the hyperechoic bladder wall is interrupted by the relatively hypoechoic tumor tissue (Fig. 14-56). There is no associated bladder deformity or decreased capacity, but hydronephrosis is often

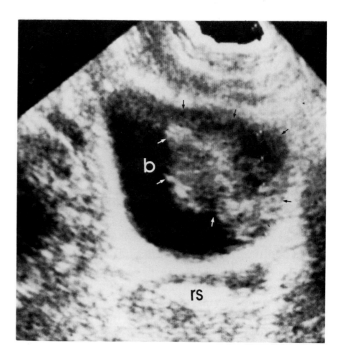

Fig. 14-54. Bladder tumor. Stage T1 transitional cell carcinoma. Transverse scan of the pelvis showing a large polypoid tumor (white arrows) occupying most of the bladder *(b)* lumen and involving a large area of mucosa. Despite the size of the tumor, the muscular wall (black arrows) that underlies the whole extent of the tumor is intact in its entirety, indicating a very superficial tumor. *(rs,* rectosigmoid colon.) (From Abu-Yousef et al,[60] with permission.)

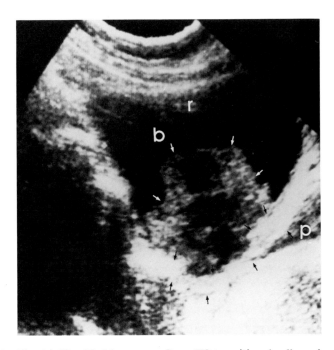

Fig. 14-55. Bladder tumor. Stage T2 transitional cell carcinoma. Parasagittal scan demonstrating a large exophytic mass (white arrows) in the bladder *(b)* trigone. This relatively hypoechoic tumor is seen to infiltrate the superficial layer of the underlying echogenic muscle wall (black arrows). (*p*, prostate; *r*, reverberation.) (From Abu-Yousef et al,[60] with permission.)

is a tendency to overstage the lesion, particularly if the tumor is bulky with a small pedicle. This group can be accurately staged by conventional clinical methods. Tumors confined to the bladder wall (stages B1 and B2) also are overstaged by ultrasound when compared with conventional methods. With the deeply invasive tumors (stages C and D), the accuracy of ultrasound in staging rises and the major errors of understaging are rare. The accuracy is 48 to 55 percent in staging the superficial tumors, 78 percent for involvement of the bladder wall, and 91 to 100 percent for the deeply invasive group.[7,60] The tumors at the base and the posterior and lateral walls are more easily staged than those involving the anterior wall and dome.[7]

Several factors interfere with the ability of ultrasound to accurately stage these bladder tumors.[60] These include obesity, incomplete bladder distension, anterior location of the tumor, and bullous cystitis. Tumors on the anterior wall are usually poorly imaged because they lie outside the focal zone of the transducer. Reverberations in the anterior aspect of the bladder may also hide these tumors. Adequate bladder distinsion is essential but not always possible. Bladder wall edema can obscure the bladder wall.

Investigators have evaluated the accuracy of ultrasound in the detection and staging of bladder carci-

associated. Once the tumor extends beyond the bladder wall in the perivesical fat but without involvement of the other perivesical organs, it is stage T3B.[60] The echogenic bladder wall is deformed, and there is decreased bladder capacity. The perivesical space is involved by the less echogenic tumor (Fig. 14-57). Hydronephrosis is usually present. With deep muscle invasion (stage B2), the ultrasound features are similar to those of tumor that has invaded the perivesical fat (stage C).[7]

Tumors that have invaded the perivesical fat and pelvic soft tissue (stages C and D) are usually sessile, although sometimes solid exophytic growths invade deeply. With a stage T4 tumor, there is extension to the perivesical organs, seminal vesicles, prostate, and rectum.[60] The whole thickness of the underlying bladder wall is interrupted by the less echogenic tumor (Fig. 14-58). Hydronephrosis is present. The tumors are identified as in pelvic soft tissues, either as infiltration areas of low-level echoes or as solid tumor masses. The ureter is commonly involved in the lateral wall. The bladder capacity is nearly always decreased, and there is significant residual volume.[7] With stage TN, there are metastases to nodes, whereas stage TM indicates distant metastases.[60]

What is the accuracy of ultrasound in staging bladder tumors? With superficial tumors (stages 0 and A), there

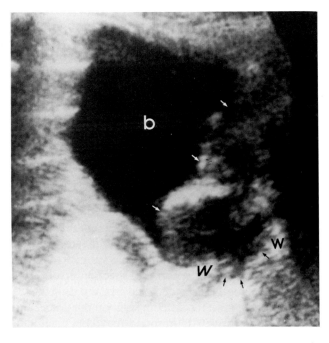

Fig. 14-56. Bladder tumor. Stage T3A transitional cell carcinoma. Longitudinal scan showing an exophytic infiltrating tumor (white arrows) arising from the trigone area. The whole thickness of the underlying muscle wall is infiltrated by the echogenic tumor tissue (black arrows). (*w*, intact muscle wall; *b*, bladder.) (From Abu-Yousef et al,[60] with permission.)

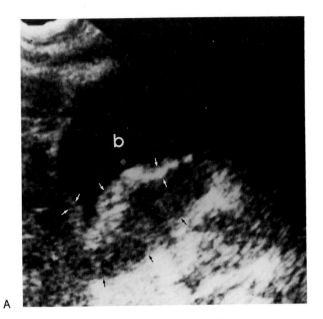
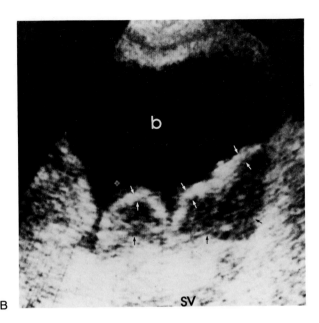

Fig. 14-57. Bladder tumor. Stage T3B transitional cell carcinoma. **(A)** Longitudinal and **(B)** transverse scans showing a large infiltrating mass (black arrows) extending beyond the muscle wall (white arrows) in the perivesical space. The bladder *(b)* itself is markedly deformed. No extension of the tumor to the perivesical organs is seen. (*sv*, seminal vesicles.) (From Abu-Yousef et al,[60] with permission.)

noma.[62] Staging by ultrasound has been accurate in 83 percent of all tumors stages, with the lowest value of 69 percent for T2/T3A tumors.[62] Four lesions smaller than 2 to 3 mm were missed at the bladder dome, the ventral wall, and the side wall.[62] The authors concluded that ultrasound was a reliable noninvasive technique for detecting bladder tumors and for preoperative local staging.[62]

Ultrasound should be the first screening method in patients with macro- or microhematuria.[62] Lesions as small as 2 to 3 mm may be detected if the bladder is well distended.[62]

Other authors have evaluated serial ultrasound in the evaluation of bladder cancer.[63] Close evaluation of patients with bladder tumors is necessary to evaluate the response of the tumor to therapy and recurrence of lesions in patients with a history of successfully treated tumors.[63] The ability of ultrasound to detect the presence or absence of bladder tumors has varied from 58 to 94 percent in various reports.[63] Detection errors have been due to poorly distended bladders and difficulty in detecting lesions on the anterior wall, on the dome, and at the bladder neck.[63] Ultrasound may be a useful adjunct to cystoscopy and may be a dependable means of decreasing the frequency of invasive procedures to evaluate the extent of bladder disease.[63] The use of these two techniques together may improve the accuracy achieved by using cystoscopy alone.[63]

Active Bleeding Associated with Bladder Tumor

Ultrasound demonstration of fluid movement within the bladder has been described previously. The "ureteral jet phenomenon" is said to be visualized because of differences in the specific gravity of the urine entering the bladder and that already present.[64] Urine has a lower specific gravity than plasma, and red blood cells have been shown to be echogenic.[64] As such, blood entering a urine-filled bladder may be hyperechoic and may be visualized by ultrasound.[64] A stream of echoes arising from a bladder mass may represent bleeding, ruling out the possibility that the echoes are caused by urine entering the bladder.[64]

Tumor of a Vesical Diverticulum

A bladder diverticulum represents a cavity formed by herniation of the bladder mucosa through the muscular wall joined by a constricted neck to the bladder cavity proper.[65] These diverticula tend to occur in areas of congenital weakness of the muscular wall; the most common region is around the ureteral meati or in the posterolateral surface of the bladder.[65]

The incidence of carcinoma within a diverticulum ranges from 0.8 to 7 percent.[65] Lower urinary tract obstruction is a causative factor for both diverticula and

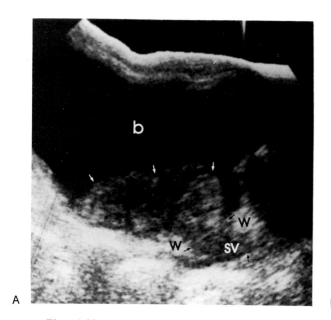

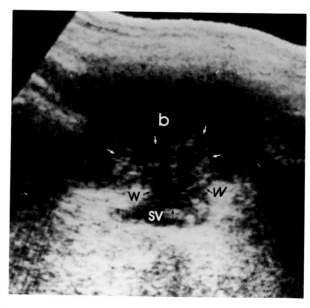

Fig. 14-58. Bladder tumor. Stage T4 transitional cell carcinoma. **(A)** Longitudinal and **(B)** transverse scans at the level of the seminal vesicles *(sv)* showing infiltration of the whole thickness of the muscle wall *(w)* by the relatively less echogenic tumor tissue (arrows), with infiltration into the seminal vesicles. There were only two sections that showed deep infiltration of the tumor, which explains how easy it is to understage bladder tumors by cystoscopy and biopsy. (*b*, bladder.) (From Abu-Yousef et al,[60] with permission.)

carcinoma.[65] Chronic inflammation is associated with diverticula and has been considered a carcinogenic agent.[65] An intradiverticular echogenic mass without acoustic shadowing, in an area in continuity with the bladder, distinguishes the mass from an extravesical mass and limits the differential diagnosis to neoplasia and intradiverticular blood clots or debris.[65]

Urachal Tumors

Urachal tumors are also bladder-related tumors. Eighty percent occur in men from 50 to 60 years old and are associated with vague symptoms.[3] Most are mucinous adenocarcinomas, arising from the intramural (irregularity in dome of bladder) or supravesicular (abdominal mass) portion of the urachus.[3] The supravesicular ones are often cystic and encapsulated, whereas the intramural ones are usually small and solid.

Entities That Mimic Bladder Tumors

Several entities may mimic the ultrasound appearance of tumor. These include blood clots, benign prostatic hypertrophy (BPH), cystitis, and bladder trabeculae.[4] Blood clots usually move with changes in patient posi-

tion (Figs. 14-2 and 14-25). BPH is usually in a central location, and its relation to the prostate may help differentiate it from a bladder tumor (Fig. 14-29). Bladder trabeculae may also mimic bladder lesions. Trabeculations are usually 1 to 3 mm in size; tumors are seldom this size category[4] (Figs. 14-28 and 14-29). In cystitis, there is usually decreased echogenicity, a smoother outline, and lack of involvement of the muscular wall (Figs. 14-30 to 14-38). Because the mucosal involvement is usually more diffuse, the transition from edematous to normal mucosa is usually more gradual. If a focal hyperechoic lesion is seen, it is more likely to be tumor.

Transurethral Evaluation

Transurethral evaluation may be performed under local, spinal, or general anesthesia.[66] Transducers of 5.5, 7, and 10 MHz are interchangeable and are mounted on the end of a long rod, which is rotated through 360 degrees by a motor.[66] The bladder is filled with sterile water, saline, or glycine.[66] Multiple scans are performed during bladder distension, with the position of the transducer altered.

The normal bladder is smooth and symmetric, with a well-defined wall 3 to 6 mm thick.[66] Masses projecting into the lumen of the bladder are echogenic and remain fixed when the patient's position is altered.[66] When tumors infiltrate the deeper layers of the bladder, they produce a decrease in echodensity of the muscle and can result in the loss of wall mobility, depending on the extent of invasion[66] (Fig. 14-59).

This technique of transurethral ultrasound appears to help in the staging of transitional cell tumors of the bladder.[66] On the basis of the depth of invasion, it may be determined whether transurethral resection of the tumors will be adequate or whether segmental resection or cystoprostatectomy is required.[66] The adequacy of transurethral resection may be assessed. Computed tomography (CT) or magnetic resonance imaging (MRI) is needed for assessment of pelvic lymph nodes.[66]

Transvaginal Evaluation

A number of ultrasound methods (transabdominal, transrectal, transvesical) have been described for the evaluation of bladder tumors. Transvaginal or endovaginal ultrasound is a relatively new mode of evaluation of bladder tumors.[67] The image obtained by this technique has high resolution because the transducer is placed very close to the structure being studied (Fig. 14-60). The transvaginal method eliminates the subcutaneous fat, intervening bowel, and bowel gas, which all affect the transabdominal approach. It appears to be superior to the transabdominal approach.[67] It is especially helpful in examining obese patients and those whose tumor is located on the anterior wall or at the bladder neck.[67]

Uncommon Primary Bladder Tumors

Leiomyoma

Benign mesothelial tumors such as leiomyoma of the bladder are rare, with only 0.7 percent of leiomyomas found in the bladder.[68] These tumors represent between 0.1 and 0.5 percent of bladder tumors.[68,69] They are frequently asymptomatic and are found incidentally, although the submucosal form is the most common and most likely to be symptomatic.[69] These lesions are most often located in the trigone and are of variable size.[69] On ultrasound a solid intramural mass with intact mucosa may be visualized.[68] Ultrasound may be able to detect an intact bladder mucosa, its submucosal location, and the relationship of the mass to the cervix, vagina, and urinary bladder[69] (Fig. 14-61). The final diagnosis may not be made on the basis of the ultrasound, but an intact urothelium overlying the submucosal bladder tumor should cause the examiner to consider leiomyoma of the bladder.[68]

Pheochromocytoma

Accounting for fewer than 0.06 percent of bladder tumors, pheochromocytomas are rare bladder neoplasms.[70] Most are located submucosally, often with significant intravesical extension, and demonstrate ulceration of the overlying mucosa.[70] Most patients present with hematuria, and more than half experience signs and symptoms of increased catecholamine secretion.[70] Ultrasound may be helpful in demonstrating a submucosal

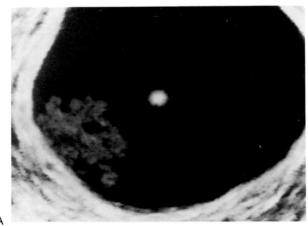

A

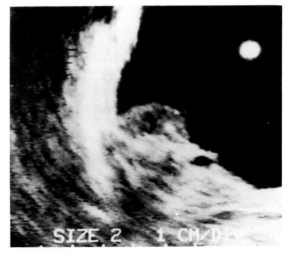

B

Fig. 14-59. Bladder tumor. Transurethral evaluation. **(A)** Transurethral ultrasound scan demonstrating a superficial bladder tumor. **(B)** Transurethral ultrasound scan demonstrating an invasive bladder tumor. (From Wolkoff and Resnick,[66] with permission.)

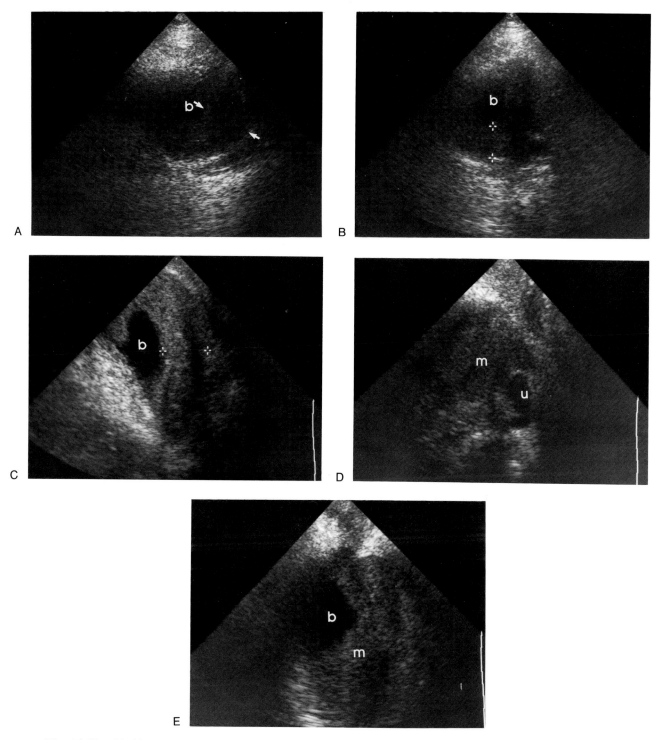

Fig. 14-60. Bladder tumor. Grade III transitional cell carcinoma. Endovaginal evaluation. This patient was noted to have left hydronephrosis. On transabdominal **(A)** sagittal and **(B)** transverse views (which appear similar) of the bladder *(b)*, a poorly defined mass (arrows, calipers) is seen involving the posterior, left, and inferior portions of the bladder wall. On endovaginal **(C & D)** sagittal and **(E)** transverse views, the tumor (calipers, *m*, 20 mm) is seen much more clearly and involves the inferior, posterior, and left bladder *(b)* wall. The dilated left ureter *(u)* is seen in Fig. D.

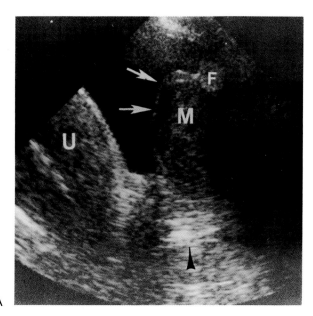
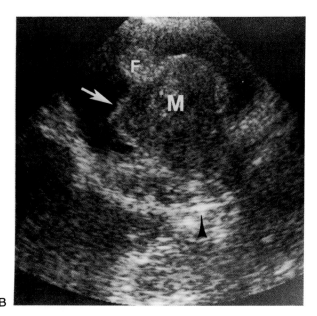

Fig. 14-61. Bladder tumor, leiomyoma. **(A)** Longitudinal and **(B)** transverse sonograms showing a relatively homogeneous submucosal solid mass *(M)* at the bladder base distinct from the uterus *(U)* and vagina (arrowhead, vaginal air). Intact echogenic mucosa (arrows) covers the mass. A Foley balloon *(F)* is located adjacent to the mass. (From Illescas et al,[69] with permission.)

solid mass and determining its relationship to the uterus, cervix, and urinary bladder[70] (Fig. 14-62).

Rhabdomyosarcoma

Mesodermal bladder tumors are uncommon tumors. They tend to be intramural, encapsulated masses. They are more common in adults, although lesions such as

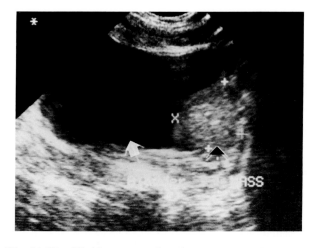

Fig. 14-62. Bladder tumor, pheochromocytoma. Transverse sonogram showing a relatively homogeneous, submucosal solid mass (arrowhead, calipers) in the left posterior and superior aspects of the bladder (arrow) separate from the uterus. (From Puvaneswary and Davoren,[70] with permission.)

angioma are more common in children. The malignant variety of sarcomatous growth is uncommon. They produce a bulky mass that protrudes into the bladder lumen.

As the most common soft tissue sarcoma of childhood, rhabdomyosarcoma, a cancer of embryonic mesenchyme, represents between 5 and 15 percent of all malignant solid tumors in children and is the most common tumor of the lower genitourinary tract in the first two decades of life.[71] There has been an association between rhabdomyosarcoma and systemic neurofibromatosis.[71] Most patients present with symptoms of obstruction or frank urinary retention.[71]

Rhabdomyosarcoma characteristically extends by local invasion and hematogenous spread.[71] It should be suspected when there is a mass of the bladder base or prostate[71] (Fig. 14-63). The urine-filled bladder serves as an anatomic landmark, with mass lesions readily observed protruding into the bladder lumen.[71]

Secondary Bladder Tumors

Metastatic bladder tumors usually develop from direct extension, by implantation from a primary lesion of the upper tract, or by lymphatic or hematogenous spread. Those that occur most commonly from direct extension are from the cervix, uterus, prostate, and rectum, in that order. Carcinoma of the cervix is particu-

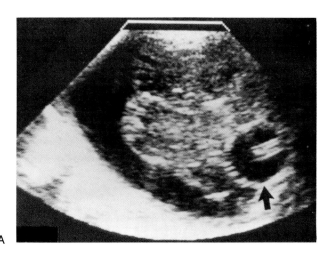
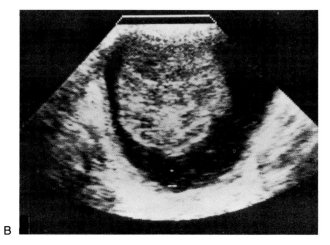

A   B

Fig. 14-63. Bladder tumor, rhabdomyosarcoma. **(A)** Longitudinal ultrasound scan of the bladder showing an intraluminal lobulated mass (arrow, inflated balloon of Foley catheter). **(B)** Transverse section of the intravesical mass. (From Bahnson et al,[71] with permission.)

larly prone to spread into the bladder wall, especially in the region of a ureteric orifice (Fig. 14-64). Endometrial carcinoma less commonly involves the bladder. Advanced prostatic carcinoma can extend into the bladder wall, but it more commonly spreads into the seminal vesicles and perivesical connective tissue.[7]

URETERAL ABNORMALITIES

Congenital

The ureter develops as an outgrowth of the wolffian (mesonephric) duct during the fourth week of embryonic life.[27,72] Later, the ureter and mesonephric duct separate, entering the bladder at different levels. The caudal end of the ureteric bud is eventually incorporated into the urogenital sinus. There is a 2 to 3 percent incidence of congenital anomalies of the ureter at autopsy.[8] Renal duplication can result from either bifurcation of the bud, incomplete duplication or accessory buds from the wolffian duct, or complete duplication.[27] In males, the mesonephric duct empties into the canal of the epididymis, vas deferens, and ejaculatory duct at the lateral aspect of the verumontanum. In females, the mesonephric duct atrophies, becoming the duct of the epoophora or Gartner's duct, which extends to the anterolateral vaginal wall and ends near the orifice of Bartholin's gland.[72] Developmental anomalies of the lower ureter are frequently associated with renal agenesis or dysplasia and may be associated with anomalies of other mesonephric duct derivation.[73] Ureteral ectopia is more common (70 to 90 percent) in females than males, and 10 to 20 per-

cent of cases, regardless of the sex, involve a nonduplicated ureter.[73]

When the ureteric bud originates more cephalad than normal from the mesonephric duct, the ureter may insert into the structures derived from the portion of the mesonephric duct cephalic to the normal origin of the ureteric bud.[73] This includes the posterior urethra, ejaculatory duct, seminal vesicle, and vas deferens. Most of the extravesicle ectopic ureters in males are either single or part of a duplex system, inserting into the posterior urethra (47 to 62 percent) or seminal vesicle (3 to 37 percent). The ejaculatory duct and vas deferens are less frequently involved (40 percent).[73] In females, the ec-

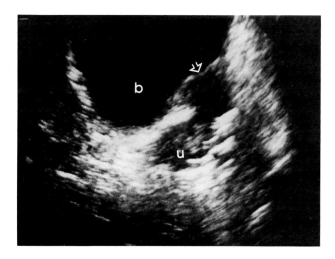

Fig. 14-64. Metastatic bladder tumor. Stage IV carcinoma (arrow) of the cervix, invading the bladder *(b)* and surrounding the dilated ureter *(u)*. (From Morley,[7] with permission.)

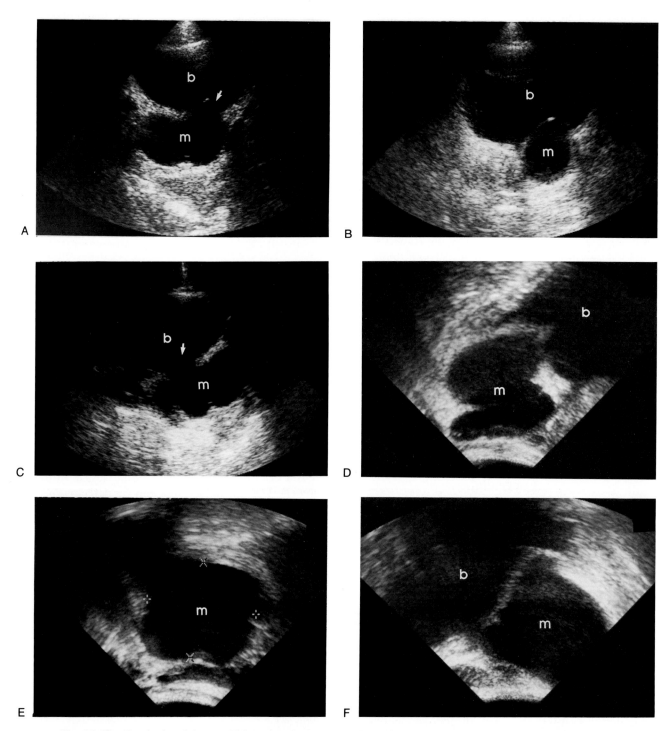

Fig. 14-65.   Seminal vesicle cyst. This patient had only one identifiable kidney (right). On transabdominal left
(A) sagittal and **(B & C)** transverse views of the urinary bladder *(b)*, a cystic mass *(m)* is demonstrated posterior to
and to the left of the bladder. It could not be determined from these views whether the mass was related to the
ureter or the bladder. On several views, it appeared to communicate with the bladder (arrow). On **(D & E)** sagittal
and **(F)** transverse transrectal views, a cystic mass *(m)* is seen in the region of the left seminal vesicle. It is separate
from the bladder *(b)*. The right seminal vesicle appears normal.

topic ureter can implant in the trigone, urethra, perineum, uterus, or vagina.[27]

A more cephalic origin of the ureteric bud from the mesonephric bud also explains the renal dysplasia or agenesis often associated with ureteral ectopia. With the more cephalic origin of the ureteric bud, the elongating ureter may fail to meet the nephrogenic blastema in the proper orientation to stimulate normal renal parenchymal development. The incidence and severity of the renal abnormalities increase as the origin of the ureter becomes more cephalic from its normal origin.[73]

With ipsilateral renal malformation, there may be faulty development of the mesonephric duct, resulting in an internal genital anomaly.[74] Involution of the mesonephros (the provisional kidney) takes place approximately during the seventh week of life, after having given rise to the wolffian ducts (laterally) and the ureteric buds and müllerian ducts (paramedially).[74] Involution of the müllerian ducts in males results in the appendix of the testis and the prostatic utricle in adults, whereas the wolffian ducts differentiate into the internal genital tract (appendix of epididymis, paradidymis, epididymis, ductus deferens, ejaculatory duct, seminal vesicles, and vesical hemitrigone).[74] Involution of the wolffian ducts in females results in remnants (epoophoron, paraophoron, and Gartner's duct), whereas the müllerian ducts develop into the ostium tubae, the uterine tubes, the uterus, and the upper two-thirds of the vagina.[74]

There are ipsilateral internal genital abnormalities in association with renal agenesis in 20 to 70 percent of cases.[74] The main abnormalities in males include hemitrigone asymmetry, agenesis and cysts of the seminal vesicles, wolffian paravesical cyst (due to segmental atresia of the ejaculatory duct), cystic dilatation of the prostatic utricle (considered as a müllerian duct remnant), and ectopic drainage of the ureter into the seminal vesicle.[74] Most frequent are cysts and agenesis of the seminal vesicle.[74]

The main abnormalities in females include bicornuate or unicornuate uterus and vaginal duplication or atresia, leading to hematocolpos and hematometra.[74]

Seminal Vesicle Cyst

Cystic diseases of the seminal vesicle may be either congenital or acquired.[75] The congenital ones are associated with anomalies of the ipsilateral mesonephric duct.[75] Most are associated with ectopic insertion of the ipsilateral ureter into the mesonephric duct derivatives such as the bladder neck, the posterior prostatic urethra, the ejaculatory duct, or the seminal vesicle. Ipsilateral renal dysgenesis is often associated with congenital seminal vesicle cyst.[75] A seminal vesicle cyst may result from incomplete absorption of the mesonephric duct with the ureter attached to the side of the seminal vesicles or from atresia of the ejaculatory duct. Most of these patients (80 percent) have renal dysgenesis or duplication (8 percent) of the collecting system.[75]

In most, the presenting symptom of seminal vesicle cysts is pain, which may be abdominal, flank, pelvic, or

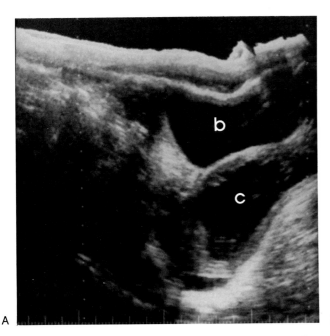 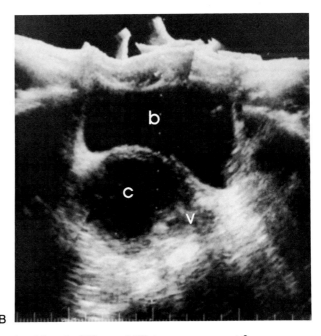

Fig. 14-66. Gartner's duct cyst. **(A)** Sagittal scan 2 cm to the right of midline and **(B)** transverse scan at 2 cm above the symphysis. A relatively cystic mass *(c)* is seen in the lateral vaginal *(v)* wall. (*b*, bladder.)

perineal and may be exacerbated by ejaculation.[75] These lesions are diagnosed in the second and third decades of life with symptoms of dysuria, pelvic pain, and ejaculatory disturbances.[7,72] Transabdominal and transrectal ultrasound can confirm the cystic nature of these masses.[75] On ultrasound, one sees a cystic structure situated within the seminal vesicle just superior to the prostate and posterior to the bladder[7,21] (Fig. 14-65). These lesions may be quite large and are thin-walled.[21] Particularly helpful in defining intraprostatic anatomy is transrectal ultrasound, which confirms the seminal vesicle origin of the cyst.[75]

Gartner's Duct Cyst

Gartner's duct represents incomplete obliteration of the atrophic mesonephric duct in females. Cysts may develop in these ducts, lying along the lateral wall of the vagina (Fig. 14-66). They may be asymptomatic or may cause pain, swelling, and dyspareunia.[7,72]

Double or Bifid Ureter

Double and bifid ureters are relatively common. They are invariably associated with either totally distinct double renal pelves or anomalous development of a very large kidney, with a partially bifid pelvis terminating in separate ureters. They are commonly joined within the bladder wall, producing a single ureteral orifice. Double ureters commonly unite at some point midway to create a Y shape.[8]

Retrocaval Ureter

As a relatively uncommon congenital anomaly that results from anomalous development of the infrarenal segment of the inferior vena cava, retrocaval ureter results in medial deviation of the posteriorly located ureter with resulting hydronephrosis.[76] The incidence of this abnormality in postmortem series is approximately 1 in 1,000, and the right ureter is almost invariably affected.[76]

Symptoms related to this abnormality usually appear in young adulthood. These patients may be asymptomatic or may have symptoms resulting from ureteral obstruction including flank pain, hematuria, recurrent urinary tract infections, and nephrolithiasis.[76] In patients with no or only a few symptoms and absent or mild hydronephrosis, conservative therapy is indicated.[76] Those who have marked hydronephrosis and parenchymal atrophy may be candidates for nephrectomy if the contralateral kidney has good function.[76]

The diagnosis of retrocaval ureter should be suspected when there is ultrasound evidence of hydronephrosis and proximal hydroureter, especially on the right side.[76] An attempt should be made to look for medial deviation of the ureter posterior to the inferior vena cava[76] (Fig. 14-67). This may be best demonstrated in an oblique projection and may be helped if the patient is in the left lateral decubitus position during coronal scans.[76] In this position, the posteromedial course of the ureter may be best demonstrated. When a retrocaval ureter is identified in an asymptomatic patient or if the patient has mild symptoms with minimal hydronephrosis, ultrasound may be used to monitor the patient for evidence of increasing hydronephrosis, parenchymal atrophy, renal infection, and nephrolithiasis.

Miscellaneous Anomalies

Other anomalies involving the ureter include anomalous valves, narrowing or strictures, kinks, and torsion.[8] Diverticula are saccular outpouchings in the ureteral wall. Hydroureter may be congenital or acquired. The congenital type may be related to an innervation defect of the musculature. The acquired type may be associated with some low ureteral obstruction or pregnancy. Megaloureter (i.e., massive enlargement of the ureter) is usually associated with some congenital defect of the kidney, particularly polycystic kidney.[77]

Ureterocele

An ectopic ureterocele is the third most common cause of hydronephrosis in neonates.[78] It causes a palpable mass in 50 percent of children.[78] A ureterocele is a cystic dilatation of the submucosal segment of the intravesical ureter with narrowing of the ureteric orifice.[7,34,78-82] It may cause significant obstruction of the ipsilateral ureter and can obstruct the bladder neck. If it is associated with an upper-pole collecting system, there is often dilatation or hydronephrosis. Most ectopic ureteroceles insert into the lower urinary bladder or urethra. With simple ureteroceles, the ureter inserts into the bladder in its normal location. This entity has been described in adults.[83]

To make the diagnosis with ultrasound, the examiner must carefully scan the fluid-filled bladder. Demonstration of the ureterocele depends on the sonic reflection of the ureterocele wall interposed between the bladder and the ureterocele fluid contents.[82,84] The intravesical dilatation of the ureterocele is composed of both bladder and ureteric wall and is clearly defined on ultrasound.[7] As such, it is seen as an anechoic thin-walled mass of variable size and shape, projecting into the bladder[21] (Figs. 14-68 to 14-73). When the ectopic ureterocele inserts into the lower bladder or urethra, it is seen quite low in the pelvis and one must angle steeply under the symphysis when scanning (Figs. 14-71 to 14-73). With a simple ureterocele, the anechoic mass is seen in the area of the normal ureteral orifice (Figs. 14-68 to 14-70). This can be confirmed by the presence of ureteral jets.

Ectopic Ureterocele Without Ureteral and Calyceal Dilatation.

In some patients with ectopic ureteroceles, the upper moiety is severely dysplastic and does not function.[85] With this situation, the calyces and ureter are not dilated, resulting in the rare entity termed ureterocele disproportion.[85] This is seen with a tiny dysplastic upper pole and a diminutive ureter. The indirect urographic and direct sonographic signs of duplication are ab-

sent or extremely subtle.[85] The presence of the ureterocele in the bladder may be the only clue to the duplication.[85] Duplication with ectopic ureterocele should still be a likely diagnosis when an ectopic ureterocele is defined by ultrasound without other signs of a duplex system.[85]

Variation in Appearance of Ectopic Ureter and Ureterocele.

In some cases of extreme dilatation and tortuosity, ectopic ureters sometimes mimic multiseptated, cystic abdominal masses[85] (Fig. 14-73). The proximal portions of some severely dilated ureters are surprisingly small.[86] Most ectopic ureters are dilated because of obstruction at or near the distal orifice. Most arise from the superior pelvis (upper moiety) of a duplex kidney, with 10 to 20 percent arising from a solitary pelvic kidney.[86] A ureterocele may be simulated by an ectopic

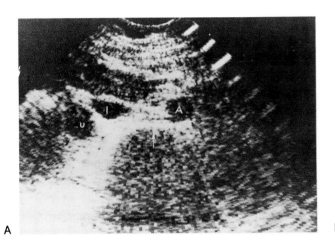

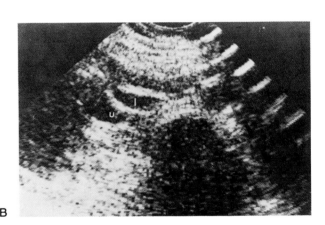

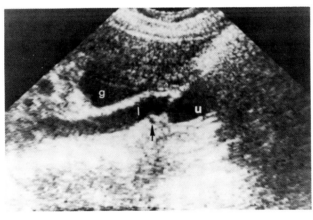

Fig. 14-67. Retrocaval ureter. **(A)** Supine transverse scan showing the dilated proximal ureter *(u)* posterolateral to the inferior vena cava *(I)*. (*A*, aorta; arrow, anterior aspect of the vertebral column with posterior shadowing.) **(B)** Supine transverse scan several centimeters below that in Fig. A, showing that the dilated ureter *(u)* assumes a more posterior position with respect to the inferior vena cava *(I)*, as the former appears to terminate abruptly. **(C)** Right anterior oblique longitudinal scan showing the inferior vena cava *(I)* anterior to the posteriorly located dilated ureter *(u)*. (*g*, gallbladder; arrow, right renal artery.) (From Schaffer et al,[76] with permission.)

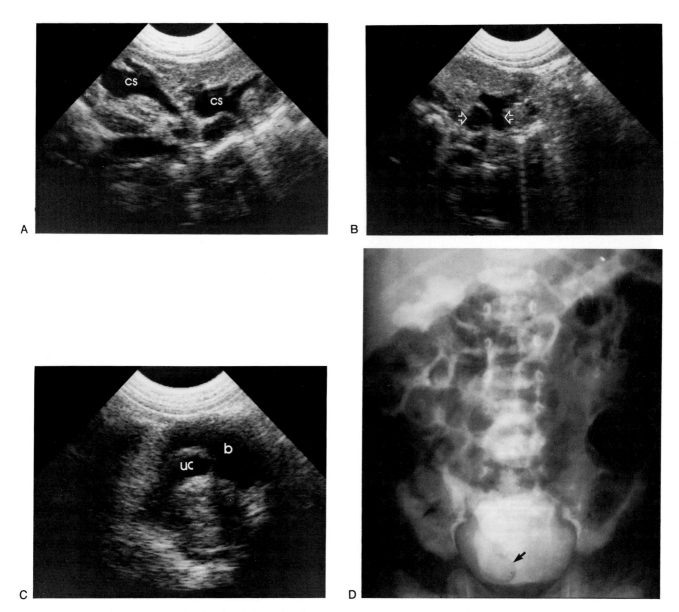

Fig. 14-68.   Ureterocele, simple. **(A)** Longitudinal and **(B)** transverse scans of the right kidney showing dilatation of a bifid collecting system *(cs).* In Fig. B, the two systems (open arrows) are identified. **(C)** Transverse scan of the bladder *(b)* showing a cystic (anechoic) mass *(uc)* in the area of the right ureteral orifice. This represents a simple ureterocele. **(D)** Intravenous pyelogram confirming the diagnosis. (arrow, ureterocele.) (From Seeds et al,[98] with permission.)

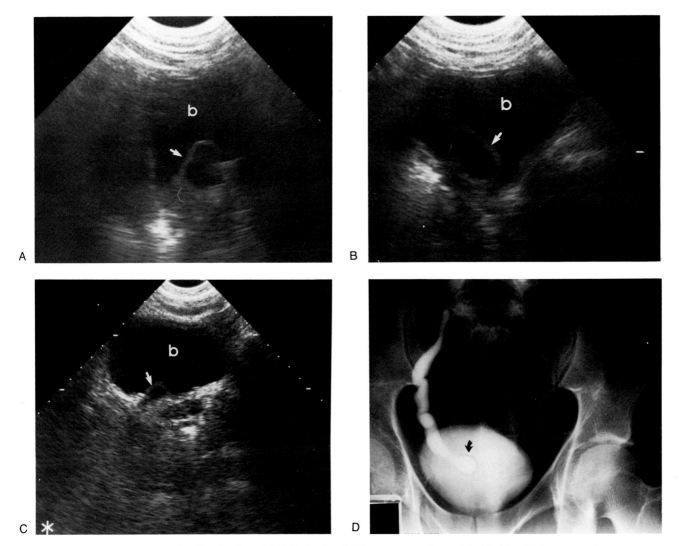

A

B

C ✳

D

Fig. 14-69. Ureterocele, simple. Case 1. **(A)** Sagittal and **(B)** transverse views of the bladder *(b)* demonstrating a cystic mass (arrow) in the region of the right ureteral orifice. There was no associated hydronephrosis or ureteral dilatation. Case 2. **(C)** Transverse view of the bladder *(b)*, showing a small cystic mass (arrow) in the region of the right UVJ. **(D)** This represented a simple ureterocele (arrow) as seen on the IVP. There was no associated hydronephrosis, although there did appear to be some dilatation of the distal ureter on the IVP.

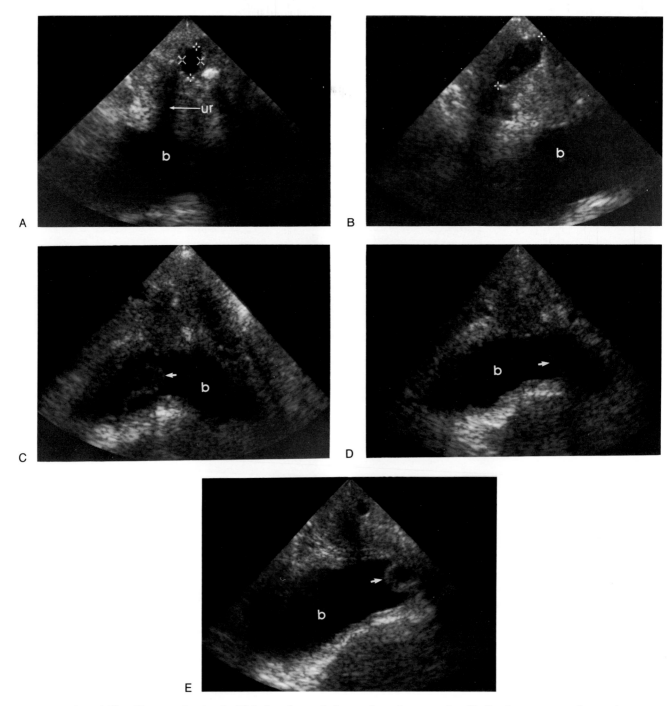

Fig. 14-70.   Ureterocele, simple. This female was being evaluated transperineally for the presence of several urethral diverticuli. Not only was a urethral *(ur)* diverticulum (calipers, 14 mm, 20 mm) demonstrated on **(A)** sagittal and **(B)** coronal views, but also bilateral simple ureteroceles (arrow) were noted on the **(C & D)** postvoid coronal and **(E)** sagittal views. The left one was best seen on the sagittal view (Fig. E). These could not be demonstrated when the urinary bladder *(b)* was distended.

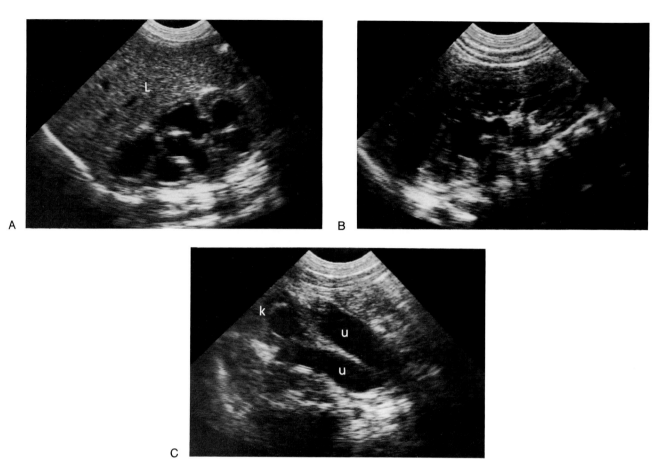

Fig. 14-71. Ureterocele, ectopic. Sagittal scans of the **(A)** right and **(B)** left kidneys demonstrating marked dilatation of the collecting system on the right with moderate hydronephrosis on the left. (*L*, liver.) **(C)** Transverse view of the right kidney *(k)* showing two dilated ureters *(u)*. *(Figure continues.)*

ureter indenting the lower vesical wall.[86] Ectopic ureteroceles are dynamic structures, and therefore change in shape and size with changes in intravesical pressure.[86] It may be difficult to detect the lower pole of a duplex kidney because of displacement by the dilated upper renal pelvis and ureter.[86] It may be equally difficult or impossible to define the renal parenchyma associated with an ectopic ureter because of diminutive dysplasia or, less commonly, acquired atrophy.[86] Dysplasia is diagnosed by seeing highly echogenic parenchyma, lack of corticomedullary differentiation, and occasionally massive enlargement by cysts.[86]

The entities to be differentiated include (1) renal duplication, (2) multiseptated cystic abdominal mass, (3) inability to identify renal parenchyma, (4) ectopic ureter with narrow proximal segment, (5) ectopic ureter simulating ectopic ureterocele, (6) extravesical protrusion of ectopic ureterocele, and (7) renal dysplasia.[86]

Calculi in Ureteroceles. Simple ureteroceles are most commonly encountered in adults, more frequently in females; they are an incidental finding and are usually left alone.[87] They may become symptomatic as a result of urinary tract infections or calculus formation.[87] Operative treatment becomes necessary when calculi occur in ureteroceles, since they cannot pass spontaneously.[87] Calculi within ureteroceles may be tiny and may be radiolucent. The ureterocele and the fluid-filled bladder provides an ideal medium for detecting the lesion. Ultrasound may identify the ureterocele as well as the echogenic stone with its shadow[87] (Fig. 14-74).

Transitional Cell Carcinoma of a Simple Ureterocele. The ultrasound accuracy in diagnosing transitional cell carcinoma of the bladder is directly related to the size and location of the tumor; tumors arising from the posterior or lateral bladder wall are most easily visualized.

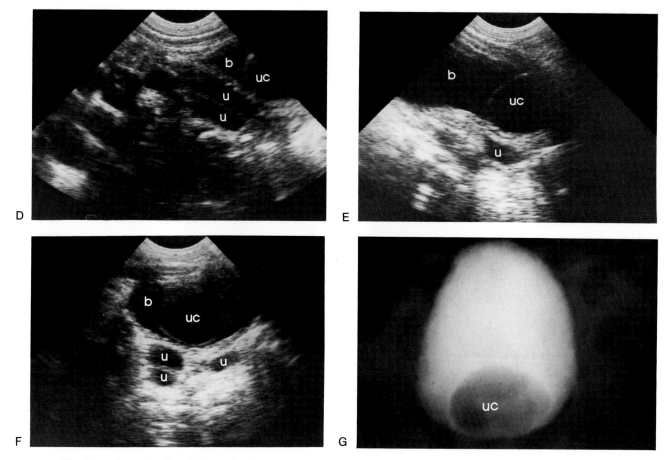

Fig. 14-71 *(Continued).*   **(D)** Longitudinal view of the pelvis also showing two dilated ureters *(u)*. *(b,* bladder; *uc,* ureterocele.) **(E)** Longitudinal and **(F)** transverse views of the bladder *(b)* demonstrating an ectopic ureterocele *(uc)* as a cystic mass in the bladder *(b)* base. In Fig. F, two dilated ureters *(u)* are seen on the right with one on the left. **(G)** Cystogram confirming the diagnosis. *(uc,* ureterocele.)

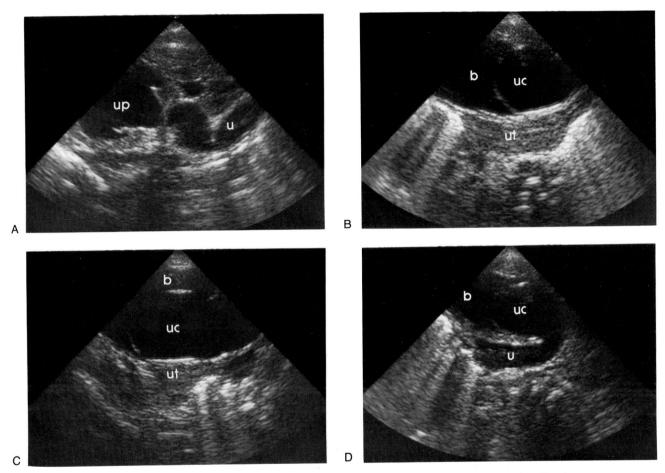

Fig. 14-72. Ureterocele, ectopic. **(A)** Sagittal view of the left kidney with a dilated upper-pole collecting system *(up)* and dilated ureter *(u)*. **(B)** Sagittal and **(C)** transverse views of the bladder *(b)* showing a large cystic mass *(uc)* filling the bladder in its lower extent. *(ut, uterus.)* **(D)** Sagittal view to the left showing the relationship of the ureter *(u)* to the ureterocele *(uc)*. *(b, bladder.)*

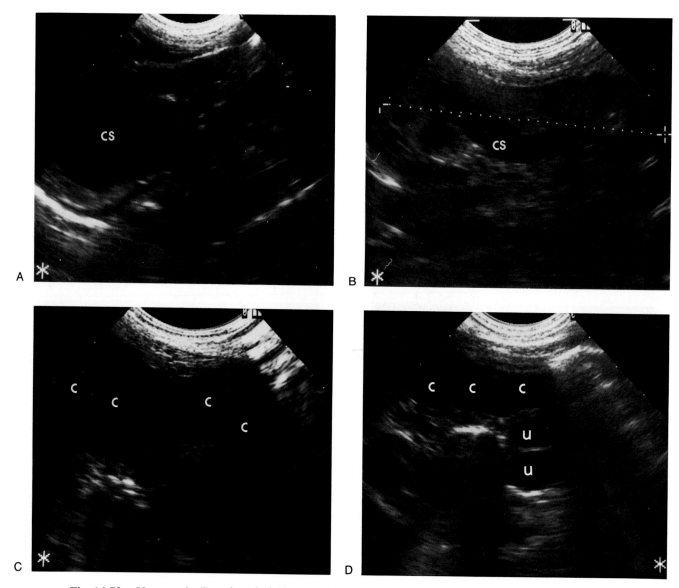

Fig. 14-73. Ureterocele. Ectopic, mimicking multiseptated cystic abdominal mass. Bilateral sagittal views of **(A)** the right and **(B)** left kidneys showing dilatation of both upper-pole collecting systems *(cs)*. (calipers, length of left kidney.) **(C & D)** Transverse views of the pelvis showing multiple cystic masses *(c)* in the region of the bladder. Two dilated ureters *(u)* are seen on the left in Fig. D. *(Figure continues.)*

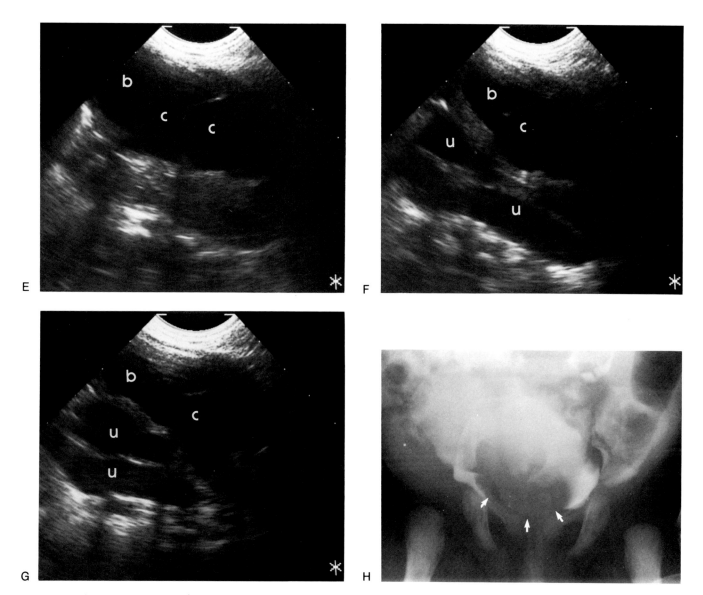

E

F

G

H

Fig. 14-73 *(Continued).* Sagittal views **(E)** in the midline, **(F)** to the right, and **(G)** to the left demonstrating multiple cystic masses *(c)* in the region of the bladder *(b)*. Two dilated ureters *(u)* are seen posteriorly on both sides. This patient had multiple ectopic ureteroceles. **(H)** Contrast image demonstrating the multiple mass effects (arrows).

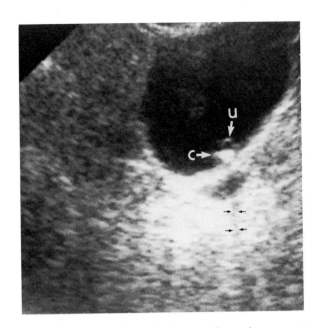

Fig. 14-74. Ureterocele, calculi. An oblique ultrasonogram through the urinary bladder showing the wall of the ureterocele (*u*) and a calculus (*c*) with shadowing (black arrows). (From Khan et al,[87] with permission.)

These lesions appear as irregular echogenic masses that are either polypoid or sessile and project into the bladder lumen with no associated shadow.[88] Transitional cell carcinoma is a rare lesion associated with a simple ureterocele.[88] With this abnormality, a complex cystic mass protruding into the lumen of the bladder may be seen; the mass has an irregular echogenic rim at its periphery and is not gravity dependent.[88]

Ureterovesical Obstruction and Megaloureter

Ureterovesical junction obstruction and megaloureter occur secondary to muscular dysfunction of the distal ureter.[89] Terminal ureteral dysfunction is thought to be secondary to progressive cell deficiency in the cloaking muscular coat of the ureter, terminating in an adynamic, collagenous segment that serves as a functional obstruction.[89]

With ultrasound, there is characteristically dilatation of the lower ureter or dilatation of the entire ureter increasing distally, and there is hyperperistalsis of the dilated ureter, which ends in a curved, nondistensible segment just above the bladder submucosal tunnel.[89] The

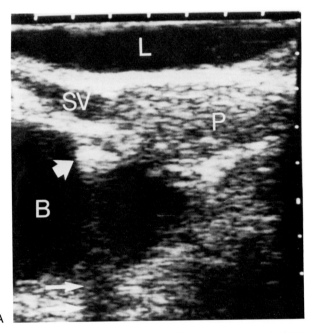

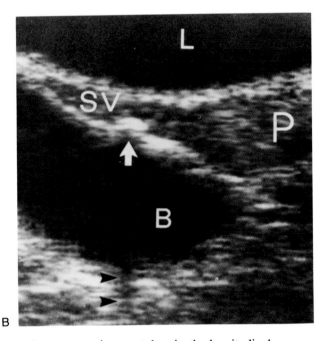

Fig. 14-75. Ureteral calculi, transrectal. **(A & B)** Transrectal sonograms in men taken in the longitudinal projection with the patients prone, heads to left, showing ureteral calculi at the UVJ (thick white arrow). Note the acoustic shadow caused by calculi (long white arrows, Fig. A; arrowheads, Fig. B). (*B*, bladder; *P*, prostate; *SV*, seminal vesicles; *L*, fluid-filled condom containing the transducer.) (From Lerner and Rubens,[90] with permission.)

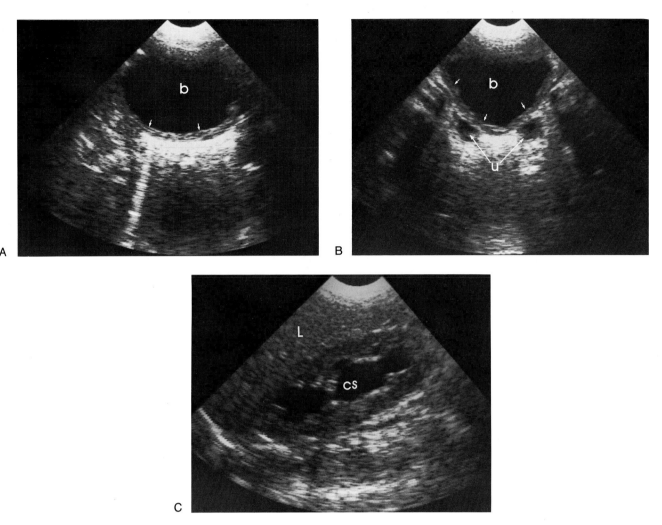

Fig. 14-76. Posterior urethral valves. **(A)** Longitudinal and **(B)** transverse scans of the bladder *(b)* showing a thickened bladder wall (arrows). The dilated ureters *(u)* are seen posterior to the bladder in Fig. B. Additionally, there is bilateral hydronephrosis. **(C)** Longitudinal scan of the right kidney demonstrating dilatation of the collecting system *(cs)*. (*L*, liver.)

dilatation of the distal ureter is often disproportionate to the appearance of the upper collecting system, involving lower ureteral hyperperistalsis and a sharply tapered incurving distal adynamic segment that is 1 to 3 cm long.[89] Real-time ultrasound can facilitate early diagnosis of UVJ obstruction and prevent significant loss of renal function.[89] The characteristic ultrasound features include (1) progressively distal dilatation of the ureter, which ends in a narrow, curved segment 1 to 3 cm long; (2) hyperperistalsis in the lower ureter, often with to-and-fro movement, terminating in a narrowed segment that is adynamic; and (3) disproportionate dilatation of the lower ureter compared with the upper ureter and renal pelvis.[89]

Transrectal Evaluation of Calculi

Transabdominal ultrasound performed through a distended urinary bladder detects only 79 percent of UVJ calculi compared with 68 percent for excretory urography; only 25 percent of calculi are directly observed by ultrasound.[90] The remainder are suggested by findings of moderate hydronephrosis and/or hydroureter on the symptomatic side[90] (Fig. 14-75). Transrectal ultrasound may be helpful in the direct diagnosis of distal ureteral calculi when excretory urography is equivocal or contraindicated.[90] The acoustic shadowing of distal ureteral calculi is reliably detected because the shadow interrupts the bladder.[90] Transrectal ultrasound may be considered

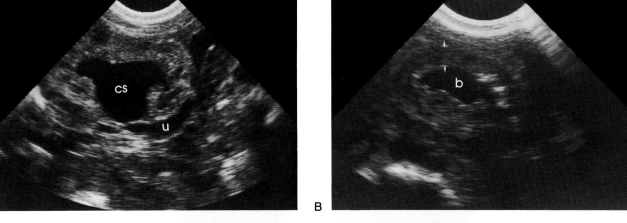

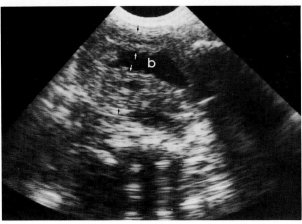

Fig. 14-77. Posterior urethral valves. Case 1. **(A)** Longitudinal left lateral decubitus scan of the right kidney demonstrating dilatation of the collecting system *(cs)* and ureter *(u)*. **(B)** Longitudinal scan of the bladder *(b)* showing a markedly thickened bladder wall (arrows). Case 2. **(C)** Longitudinal scan showing a thickened bladder *(b)* wall (arrows). (Fig. C from Seeds et al,[98] with permission.)

an adjunct to urography in patients presenting with renal colic and distal ureteral obstruction of uncertain cause.[90]

URETHRAL ABNORMALITIES

Congenital

Posterior Urethral Valves

Posterior urethral valves are the most common cause of urinary obstruction in male infants and are the second most common cause of hydronephrosis in neonates. Fifty percent are discovered within the first 3 months of life, with 75 percent identified within the first year of life.[91] The obstruction of urinary outflow produces marked dilatation of the posterior urethra and a thick-

ened, trabeculated bladder. The ureters become dilated, elongated, and tortuous with hydronephrosis. The hydronephrosis is usually bilateral but can be asymmetric, depending on the degree of reflux.[78]

Normally there are mucosal folds in the male urethra. These folds are straight, extending inferiorly from the verumontanum and dividing into two to four folds that then diverge. With posterior urethral valves (type I), a flap of mucosa is seen along the anterior urethral wall, which has a slitlike opening below the verumontanum.[91]

As congenitally occurring thick folds of mucous membrane located in the posterior urethra distal to the verumontanum, posterior urethral valves obstruct the outflow of urine from the bladder, which responds to the increased resistance by detrusor hypertrophy.[92] The bladder walls become thickened with increased trabeculation, sacculation, and diverticulum formation. Proximal to the valves, the urethra undergoes a fusiform dilation while the bladder neck remains relatively narrow.[92]

With hypertrophied detrusor and trigone, there may be involvement of UVJ in two ways: (1) vesicoureteral incompetence with reflux and (2) vesicoureteral obstruction.[92] Massive hydrouretronephrosis may result. Urine may leak into the perirenal space (urinoma), peritoneal cavity (urine ascites), or pleural space (urothorax), with or without a demonstrable tear in the collecting system with back pressure in the pelvicalyceal system.[92] The associated vesicoureteral reflux may occur as a result of a primary abnormality of the UVJ or as a result of the presence of a periureteral (Hutch) diverticulum.[92] Renal dysplasia may result if an early onset of vesicoureteral reflux in fetal life interferes with normal renal development.[92] Following valve ablation with relief of the urethral obstruction, there may be persistence or progression of this dilatation, which may become a serious management problem.[92] With persistent hydroureteronephrosis, whether associated with vesicoureteral reflux or not, there may be progression through renal dysplasia, reflux nephropathy, and chronic pyelonephritis to chronic renal failure.[92]

With posterior urethral valves, a spectrum of ultrasound findings are seen. Whereas the normal bladder has a thin, sharply defined wall, dilatation and thickening of the bladder are seen almost exclusively with an obstructive lesion. The bladder dilates, and there is muscular hypertrophy, which can be identified on ultrasound (Figs. 14-76 to 14-78). The marked hypertrophy of the bladder muscle may simulate a solid echogenic mass.[93] The dilated ureters are seen as lucent tubes medial to the kidney and posterior to the bladder[79] (Fig. 14-76). If a dilated posterior urethra is seen with a distended bladder with a thickened wall, the diagnosis of posterior urethral valves may be made[81,93,94] (Figs. 14-79 and 14-80). Other causes of a dilated posterior urethra include prune-belly syndrome, neurogenic bladder, urethral stricture, and urethral tumor.[94]

Urethral Diverticula

There is an intricate net of paraurethral ducts and glands surrounding the female urethra. Urethral diverticula are thought to result from infection and obstruction of these glands.[1] A diverticulum is formed when rupture of the resultant retention cyst or abscess occurs into the urethra.[1] In other cases, the etiology may be congenital or may be direct trauma from instrumentation, insertion of foreign bodies, or childbirth.[1] Most of the diverticula open into the middle one-third of the urethra; one-third of patients have multiple or compound diverticula.[1]

These diverticula occur in 1 to 6 percent of the general population.[1] They are frequently associated with chronic lower urinary tract symptoms including dysuria, hematuria, dyspareunia, and incontinence, although 20 percent of patients may be asymptomatic.[1] The classic presentation, which is uncommon, includes dribbling after voiding, the presence of a mass, and expression of pus from the urethra on physical examination.[1] Although voiding cystourethrography has been used for screening, its overall accuracy is only 65 percent.[1]

The evaluation of urethral diverticula has been described transabdominally, but the described diverticula

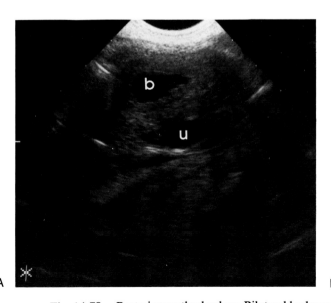
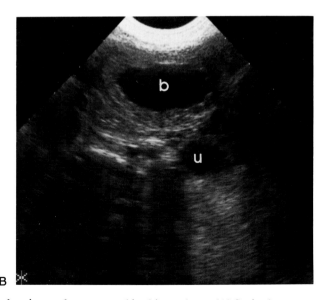

Fig. 14-78. Posterior urethral valves. Bilateral hydronephrosis was demonstrated in this newborn. **(A)** Sagittal and **(B)** transverse views of the bladder *(b)*, showing wall thickening. A dilated ureter *(u)* is seen on the left.

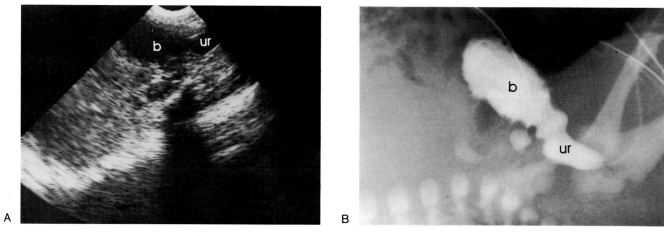

Fig. 14-79. Posterior urethral valves. **(A)** Longitudinal scan of the bladder *(b)* showing a dilated posterior urethra *(ur)*. **(B)** Voiding cystourethrogram demonstrating the dilated posterior urethra *(ur)*. *(b,* bladder.) (From Seeds et al,[98] with permission.)

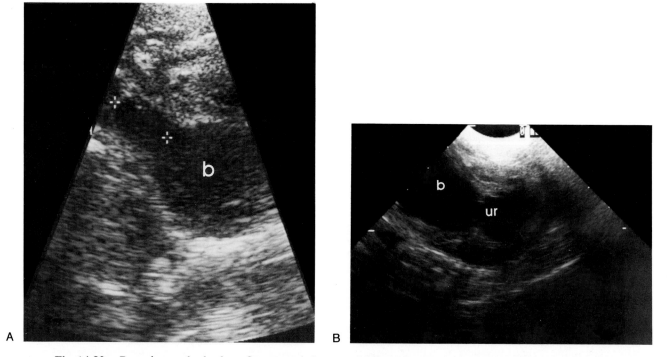

Fig. 14-80. Posterior urethral valves. On prenatal ultrasound, bilateral severe hydronephrosis was seen, as well as a dilated prostatic urethra (calipers) on **(A)** coronal view of the fetal bladder *(b)*. **(B)** On postnatal view of the bladder *(b)*, the dilated urethra *(ur)* was seen.

were 2 to 4.5 cm. By using transperineal (or endovaginal) ultrasound, the identification of small lesions may be possible (Figs. 14-81 and 14-82). With this method, the higher-frequency near-focus endovaginal probes lead to improved visualization. Transperineal ultrasound allows improved three-dimensional visualization of the diverticula in relation to the urethra.[1] In surgical planning, the AP relationship is particularly important and is shown well on sagittal scans.[1] Transperineal ultrasound has the great advantage of being noninvasive, unlike the contrast studies typically used. Although the ultrasound appearance of urethral diverticula is characteristic, it is not pathognomonic of this entity.[1] This technique should be useful in screening for urethral diverticula.

Urodynamics with Ultrasound

As a complex action, micturition involves the following sequence of events: (1) the pelvic floor and urethral sphincter relax; (2) the detrusor muscle contracts until the bladder is empty; (3) the detrusor contraction subsides; (4) the urethral sphincter and pelvic floor contract once more; and (5) a resting position is achieved.[95] This process may be observed by fluoroscopy or ultrasound imaging.

For evaluation of the bladder and/or urethra, ultrasound may be performed by using transvaginal or transrectal imaging of the lower urinary tract. The advantages of ultrasound are the absence of radiation, the ability to provide continuous observation throughout

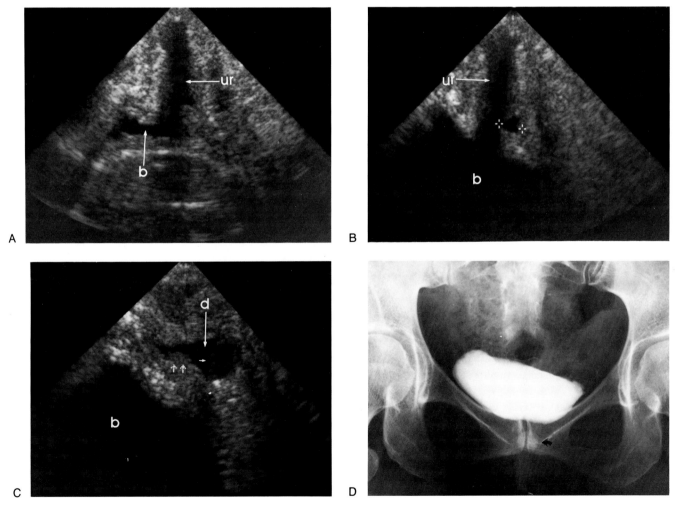

Fig. 14-81. Urethral diverticula. **(A)** Sagittal, magnified view, postvoid, demonstrating the normal urethra *(ur)*. *(b,* bladder.) **(B)** Coronal, prevoid view demonstrating a small cystic area (calipers, diverticulum, 6.2 mm) to the left of the urethra *(ur)*. *(b,* bladder.) **(C)** Sagittal view showing a larger diverticulum *(d,* 14 × 11 mm) containing a fluid-fluid level (small arrow), along with its connection (arrows) to the area of the urethra. *(b,* bladder.) **(D)** Voiding cystogram showing the larger diverticulum (arrow).

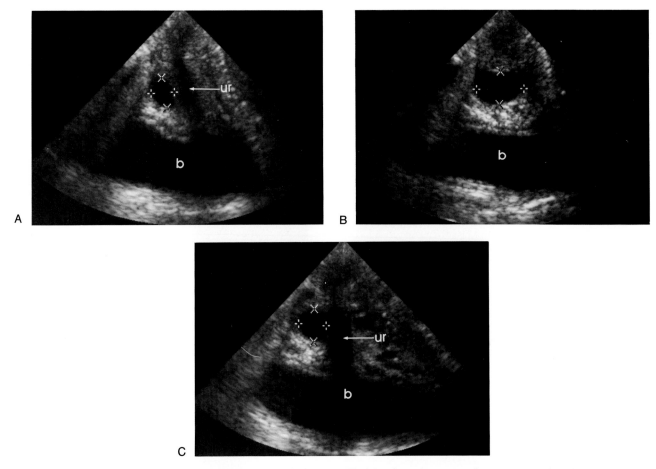

Fig. 14-82. Urethral diverticula. Sagittal **(A)** midline and **(B)** right views demonstrating a urethral diverticulum (calipers) as a lucent structure (11 × 15 mm). (*b*, bladder; *ur*, urethra.) **(C)** Coronal view showing the diverticulum to the right of the urethra *(ur)*. The diverticulum projects to the right of and superior to the urethra. (*b*, bladder.)

the cycle of bladder filling and emptying, and the ability to repeat the evaluation as often as required.[95]

Transrectal ultrasound and urodynamic studies can be valuable in evaluating voiding dysfunction in spinal cord injury patients as well as other patients.[96] With ultrasound, excellent images of the bladder neck, prostatic urethra, prostate, and external sphincter are produced, allowing for accurate diagnosis of detrusor-sphincter dyssynergia, detrusor-bladder neck dyssynergia, prostatic hypertrophy, and bladder neck strictures.[96]

In this technique, the patient is examined in the lithotomy, sitting, or lateral position. The condom-covered probe is inserted into the rectum with lubricant and is positioned so that it is facing the urethra.[96] In normal patients, the bladder neck is closed during the filling phase and the urethra is empty. With voiding, the bladder neck and urethra are clearly visualized. Bladder neck opening and funneling of the prostatic urethra can be evaluated.[96]

Ultrasound Evaluation of Stress Incontinence

Transrectal sagittal ultrasound has been used to image the bladder and urethra in a dynamic fashion. It may be helpful in the evaluation of patients for the diagnosis of urinary stress incontinence.[97] Endovaginal or transperineal ultrasound may also prove helpful (Fig. 14-83). By using the transrectal probe, the posterior urethrovesical angle is measured under both strain and nonstrain conditions.[97] When these results are compared with the radiographic chain cystourethrogram, the ultrasound is shown to be superior.[97] It may estimate the posterior urethrovesical angle accurately and differentiate between patients with and without stress urinary incontinence.[97]

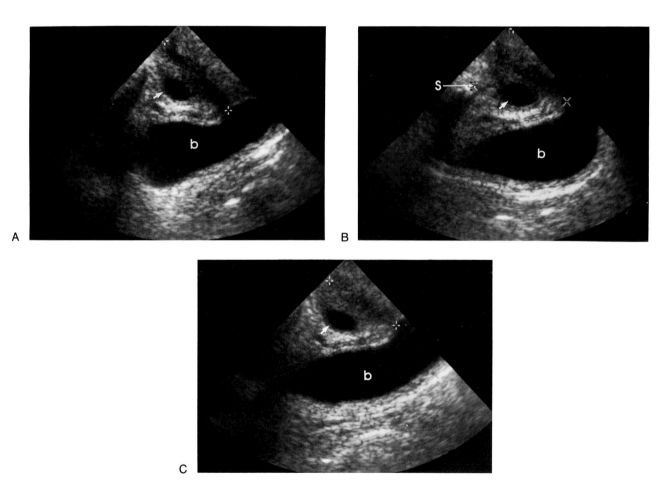

Fig. 14-83. Stress incontinence. (Same patient as in Fig. 14-82.) **(A–C)** Successive sagittal transperineal scans showing how dramatically the angle of the urethra (calipers) changes with straining (Fig. A, patient at rest; Fig. C, patient at maximum strain). In Fig. B, the approximate level of the symphysis *(S)* is marked. Determination of the distance from the symphysis to the bladder neck and from the symphysis to the urethra may be useful in the evaluation of stress incontinence. (arrow, diverticulum; *b*, bladder.)

REFERENCES

1. Keefe B, Warshauer DM, Tucker MS, Mittelstaedt CA: Diverticula of the female urethra: diagnosis by endovaginal and transperineal sonography. AJR 1991;156:1195
2. Richmond DH, Sutherst JR, Brown MC: Screening of the bladder base and urethra using linear array transrectal ultrasound scanning. J Clin Ultrasound 1986;14:647
3. Han SY, Witten DM: Carcinoma of the urachus. AJR 1976;127:351
4. Abu-Yousef MM, Narayana AS, Franken EA Jr, Brown RC: Urinary bladder tumors studied by cystosonography. Part I. Detection. Radiology 1984;153:223
5. Jequier S, Rousseau O: Sonographic measurements of the normal bladder wall in children. AJR 1987;149:563
6. Slovis TL, Perlmutter AD: Recent advances in pediatric urological ultrasound. J Urol 1980;123:613
7. Morley P: The bladder. p. 139. In Rosenfield AT (ed): Clinics in Diagnostic Ultrasound. Genitourinary Ultrasonography. Vol. 2. Churchill Livingstone, New York, 1979
8. Robbins SL, Cotran RJ: The lower urinary tract. p. 1186. In: Pathological Basis of Disease. WB Saunders, Philadelphia, 1979
9. Mirk P, Maresca G, Fileni A, Vincenzoni M: Sonography of normal lower ureters. J Clin Ultrasound 1988;16:635
10. Hennigan HW Jr, DuBose TJ: Sonography of the normal female urethra. AJR 1985;145:839
11. Mchean GK, Edell SL: Determination of bladder volumes by gray scale ultrasonography. Radiology 1978;128:181
12. Erasmie U, Lidefelt KJ: Accuracy of ultrasonic assessment of residual urine in children. Pediatr Radiol 1989;19:388
13. Kremer H, Dobrinski W, Mikyska M et al: Ultrasonic in vivo and in vitro studies on the nature of the ureteral jet phenomenon. Radiology 1982;142:175
14. Elejalde BR, de Elejalde MM: Ureteral ejaculation of urine visualized by ultrasound. J Clin Ultrasound 1983;11:474
15. Dubbins PA, Kurtz AB, Darby J, Goldberg BB: Ureteric jet effect: the echographic appearance of urine entering the bladder. A means of identifying the bladder trigone and assessing ureteral function. Radiology 1981;140:513
16. Burge HJ, Middleton WD, McClennan BL, Hildebolt CF: Ureteral jets in healthy subjects and in patients with unilateral ureteral calculi: comparison with color Doppler US. Radiology 1991;180:437
17. Jequier S, Paltiel H, Lafortune M: Ureterovesical jets in infants and children: duplex and color Doppler US studies. Radiology 1990;175:349
18. Marshall JL, Johnson ND, DeCampo MP: Vesicoureteric reflux in children: prediction with color Doppler imaging. Radiology 1990;175:355
19. Wan YL, Lee TY, Tsai CC et al: The role of sonography in the diagnosis and management of urachal abscesses. J Clin Ultrasound 1991;19:203
20. Bouvier JF, Pascaud E, Maihes F et al: Urachal cyst in the adult: ultrasound diagnosis. J Clin Ultrasound 1984;12:48
21. Rifkin MD, Needleman L, Kurtz AB et al: Sonography of nongynecologic cystic masses of the pelvis. AJR 1984;142:1169
22. Cacciarelli AA, Kass KJ, Yang SS: Urachal remnants: sonographic demonstration in children. Radiology 1990;174:473
23. Richman TS, Taylor KJW: Sonographic demonstration of bladder duplication. AJR 1982;139:604
24. Hayden CK Jr, Swischuk LE: The urinary tract. p. 334. In: Pediatric Ultrasonography. Williams & Wilkins, Baltimore, 1987
25. Pollack HM: Specific disorders of the urinary tract. In: Clinical Urography. WB Saunders, Philadelphia, 1990: 773, 1700
26. Wyly JB, Resende CMC, Teele RL: Ultrasonography of the complicated duplex kidney: further observations. Semin Ultrasound CT MR 1984;5:35
27. Kessler RM, Altman DH: Real-time sonographic detection of vesicoureteral reflux in children. AJR 1982; 138:1033
28. Mann CI, Jequier S, Patriquin H et al: Intramural teflon injection of the ureter for treatment of vesicoureteral reflux: sonographic appearance. AJR 1988;151:543
29. Gore MD, Fernbach SK, Donaldson JS et al: Radiographic evaluation of subureteric injection of teflon to correct vesicoureteral reflux. AJR 1989;152:115
30. Giuliano CT, Cohen HL, Haller JO, Glassberg KI: The sting procedure and its complications: sonographic evaluation. J Clin Ultrasound 1990;18:415
31. Janus C: Sonographic appearance of the abnormally positional Foley catheter. J Ultrasound Med 1985;4:439
32. Lebowitz RL, Vargas B: Stones in the urinary bladder in children and young adults. AJR 1987;148:491
33. Cronan JJ, Simeone JF, Pfister RC et al: Cystosonography in the detection of bladder tumors: a prospective and retrospective study. J Ultrasound Med 1982;1:237
34. Bree RL, Silver TM: Sonography of bladder and prevesical abnormalities. AJR 1981;136:1101
35. Rosenfield AT, Taylor KJW, Weiss RM: Ultrasound evaluation of bladder calculi. J Urol 1979;121:119
36. Abu-Yousef MM, Narayana AS, Brown RC: Catheter-induced cystitis: evaluation by cystosonography. Radiology 1984;151:471
37. Rifkin MD, Kurtz AB, Pasto ME, Goldberg BB: Unusual presentations of cystitis. J Ultrasound Med 1983;2:25
38. Goodling GAW: Varied sonographic manifestations of cystitis. J Ultrasound Med 1986;5:61
39. Manco LG: Cystitis cystica simulating bladder tumor at sonography. J Clin Ultrasound 1985;13:52
40. Kauzlaric D, Barmeir E: Sonography of emphysematous cystitis. J Ultrasound Med 1985;4:319
41. Goodling GAW: Sonography of Candida albicans cystitis. J Ultrasound Med 1989;8:121
42. Suzuki T, Yasumoto M, Shibuya H, Suzuki S: Sonography of cyclophosphamide hemorrhagic cystitis: a report of two cases. J Clin Ultrasound 1988;16:183
43. Boag GS, Nolan RL: Sonographic features of urinary bladder involvement in regional enteritis. J Ultrasound Med 1988;7:125
44. Speirs RT, Raghavendra BN, Rausen A et al: Ultrasound findings in diffuse granulomatous cystitis in chronic granulomatous disease of childhood. Urol Radiol 1990;12:106

45. Duffis AW, Weinberg B, Diakoumakis EE: A case of cystitis glandularis with associated pelvic lipomatosis: ultrasound evaluation. J Clin Ultrasound 1990;18:733

46. Shapeero LG, Friedland GW, Perkash I: Transrectal sonographic voiding cystourethrography: studies in neuromuscular bladder dysfunction. AJR 1983;141:83

47. Brandt TD, Neiman HL, Calenoff L et al: Ultrasound evaluation of the urinary system in spinal-cord-injury patients. Radiology 1981;141:473

48. Perkash I, Friedland GW: Catheter-induced hyperreflexia in spinal cord injury patients: diagnosis by sonographic voiding cystourethrography. Radiology 1986;159:453

49. Amis ES Jr, Newhouse JH, Olsson CA: Continent urinary diversions: review of current surgical procedures and radiologic imaging. Radiology 1988;168:395

50. Hertzberg BS, Bowie JD, King LR, Webster GD: Augmentation and replacement cystoplasty: sonographic findings. Radiology 1987;165:853

51. Mezzacappa PM, Price AP, Kassner EG et al: Cohen ureteral reimplantation: sonographic appearance. Radiology 1987;165:851

52. Carrington BM, Johnson RJ: Vesicovaginal fistula: ultrasound delineation and pathological correlation. J Clin Ultrasound 1990;18:674

53. Kauzlaric D, Barmeir E: Sonography of traumatic rupture of the bladder: "bladder within a bladder" appearance of extraperitoneal extravasion. J Ultrasound Med 1986;5:97

54. Winsett MZ, Fagan CJ, Bedi DG: Sonographic demonstration of bladder-flap hematoma. J Ultrasound Med 1986;5:483

55. Wan YL, Hsieh H, Lee TY, Tsai CC: Wall defect as a sign of urinary bladder rupture in sonography. J Ultrasound Med 1988;7:511

56. Goodman JD, Macchia RJ, Macasaet MA, Schneider M: Endometriosis of the urinary bladder: sonographic findings. AJR 1980;135:625

57. Kumar R, Haque AK, Cohen MS: Endometriosis of the urinary bladder: demonstration by sonography. J Clin Ultrasound 1984;12:363

58. Shapeero LG, Vordermark JS: Bladder neurofibromatosis in childhood: noninvasive imaging. J Ultrasound Med 1990;9:177

59. Miller WB Jr, Boal DK, Teele R: Neurofibromatosis of the bladder: sonographic findings. J Clin Ultrasound 1983;11:460

60. Abu-Yousef MM, Narayana AS, Brown RC et al: Urinary bladder tumors studies by cystosonography. Part II. Staging. Radiology 1984;153:227

61. Itzchak Y, Singer D, Fischelovitch Y: Ultrasonographic assessment of bladder tumors. I. Tumor detection. J Urol 1981;126:31

62. Denkhaus H, Crone-Munzebrock W, Huland H: Noninvasive ultrasound in detecting and staging bladder carcinoma. Urol Radiol 1985;7:121

63. Dershaw DD, Scher HI: Serial transabdominal sonography of bladder cancer. AJR 1988;150:1055

64. Bisset RAL, Khan AN: Detection of active bleeding from a transitional cell carcinoma of the bladder by ultrasonography. J Clin Ultrasound 1987;15:269

65. Saez F, Pena JM, Martinez A et al: Carcinomas in vesical diverticula: the role of ultrasound. J Clin Ultrasound 1985;13:45

66. Wolkoff L, Resnick MI: Transrectal ultrasonography for staging tumors of the urinary bladder. Urol Clin North Am 1989;16:815

67. Tsyb AF, Slesarev VI, Komarevtsev VN: Transvaginal longitudinal ultrasonography in diagnosis of carcinoma of the urinary bladder. J Ultrasound Med 1988;7:179

68. Bornstein I, Charboneau JW, Hartman GW: Leiomyoma of the bladder: sonographic and urographic findings. J Ultrasound Med 1986;5:407

69. Illescas FF, Baker ME, Weinerth JL: Bladder leiomyoma: advantages of sonography over computed tomography. Urol Radiol 1986;8:216

70. Puvaneswary M, Davoren P: Phaechromocytoma of the bladder: ultrasound appearance. J Clin Ultrasound 1991;19:111

71. Bahnson RR, Zaontz MR, Maizels M et al: Ultrasonography and diagnosis of pediatric genitourinary rhabdomyosarcoma. Urology 1989;33:64

72. Arger PH, Zarembok I: Ultrasound efficacy in evaluation of lower genitourinary tract anomalies. J Clin Ultrasound 1977;3:61

73. Weyman PJ, McClennan BL: Computed tomography and ultrasonography in the evaluation of mesonephric duct anomalies. Urol Radiol 1979;1:29

74. Trigaux JP, Van Beers B, Delchambre F: Male genital tract malformations associated with ipsilateral renal agenesis: sonographic findings. J Clin Ultrasound 1991;19:3

75. King BF, Hattery RR, Lieber MM et al: Congenital cystic disease of the seminal vesicle. Radiology 1991;178:207

76. Schaffer RM, Sunshine AG, Becker JA et al: Retrocaval ureter: sonographic appearance. J Ultrasound Med 1985;4:199

77. Gerzof SG, Gale ME: Computed tomography and ultrasonography for diagnosis and treatment of renal and retroperitoneal abscess. Urol Clin North Am 1982;9:185

78. Barth RA, Mindell HJ: Renal masses in the fetus and neonate: Ultrasonographic diagnosis. Semin Ultrasound, CT MR 1984;5:3

79. Mascatello VJ, Smith EH, Carrera GF et al: Ultrasonic evaluation of the obstructed duplex kidney. AJR 1977;129:113

80. Frank JL, Potter BM, Shkolnik A: Neonatal urosonography. p. 159. In Rosenfield AT (ed): Clinics in Diagnostic Ultrasound. Genitourinary Ultrasonography. Vol. 2. Churchill Livingstone, New York, 1979

81. Friedman AP, Haller JO, Schulze G, Schaffer R: Sonography of vesical and perivesical abnormalities in children. J Ultrasound Med 1983;2:385

82. Summer TE, Crowe JE, Resnick MI: Diagnosis of ectopic ureterocele using ultrasound. Urology 1980;15:82

83. Brenner RJ, DeMartini WJ, Goodling GAW, Hedgcock MW: Ultrasonographic demonstration of a simple ureterocele and dilated ureter in an adult. J Clin Ultrasound 1978;6:431

84. Rose JS, McCarthy J, Yeh H-C: Ultrasound diagnosis of ectopic ureterocele. Pediatr Radiol 1979;8:17

85. Share JC, Lebowitz RL: Ectopic ureterocele without ureteral and calyceal dilatation (ureterocele disproportion): findings on urography and sonography. AJR 1989; 152:567

86. Nussbaum AR, Dorst JP, Jeffs RD et al: Ectopic ureter and ureterocele: their varied sonographic manifestations. Radiology 1986;159:227

87. Khan AN, Boggis CM, Ashleigh RJ: Ultrasonography of calculi in ureteroceles. J Clin Ultrasound 1989;17:439

88. Forer LE, Schaffer RM: Transitional cell carcinoma of a simple ureterocele: a specific sonographic appearance. J Ultrasound Med 1990;9:301

89. Wood BP, Ben-Ami T, Teele RL, Rabinowitz R: Ureterovesical obstruction and megaloureter: diagnosis by real-time US. Radiology 1985;156:79

90. Lerner RM, Rubens D: Distal ureteral calculi: diagnosis by transrectal sonography. AJR 1986;147:1189

91. Sty JR, Starshak RJ: Sonography of pediatric urinary tract abnormalities. Ultrasound CT MR 1981;2:71

92. Macpherson RI, Leithiser RE, Gordon L, Turner WR: Posterior urethral valves: an update and review. RadioGraphics 1986;6:753

93. Gilsanz V, Miller JH, Reid BS: Ultrasonic characteristics of posterior urethral valves. Radiology 1982;145:143

94. McAlister WH: Demonstration of the dilated prostatic urethra in posterior urethral valve patients. J Ultrasound Med 1984;3:1989

95. Fellows GJ: Dynamic ultrasonography for voiding dysfunction. Urol Clin North Am 1989;16:809

96. Shabsigh R, Fishman IJ, Krebs M: The use of transrectal longitudinal real-time ultrasonography in urodynamics. J Urol 1987;138:1416

97. Chang HC, Chang SC, Kuo HC, Tsai TC: Transrectal sonographic cystourethrography: studies in stress urinary incontinence. Urology 1990;36(6):488

98. Seeds JW, Mittelstaedt CA, Mandell J: Pre- and postnatal ultrasound diagnosis of congenital obstructive uropathies. Urol Clin North Am 1986;13:131

15

Penis

Carol B. Benson
Peter M. Doubilet

SONOGRAPHY AND SONOURETHROGRAPHY

TECHNIQUE

High resolution ultrasound with transducer frequencies of 5 to 10 MHz is used to image the penis. Linear scanners are optimal because the structures to be imaged are superficial. An alternative, more cumbersome approach is to use a sector scanner with a standoff device.[1,2] For evaluation of the tissues of the three corpora, the penis is scanned directly in longitudinal and transverse planes from either the ventral or dorsal surface. To image the bulbous portion of the corpus spongiosum and the proximal portions of the corpora cavernosa, scanning can be performed through the scrotum and perineum by elevating the testicles.

Sonographic examination of the anterior urethra is performed after antegrade or retrograde distension of the lumen with fluid. The antegrade method of distending the urethra requires the patient to begin voiding. A Zipser clamp is placed on the glans once a full stream is achieved to maintain a filled lumen. Retrograde filling is performed by injection of 10 to 20 ml of lidocaine urologic jelly through a wide-tipped syringe placed in the urethral meatus. A Zipser clamp is applied to maintain distension. The retrograde technique is usually preferable to the antegrade method, especially when the patient is unable to void or achieve a full stream.

All portions of the anterior urethra are assessed in transverse and longitudinal planes. The penile portion of the urethra is scanned from the dorsal aspect of the penis.

When needed, scanning from the ventral surface may provide added information. The distal bulbous urethra is scanned through the scrotum, and the proximal bulbous urethra transperineally.[1-4]

NORMAL ANATOMY

The penis contains three cylindrical columns of spongy tissue, two corpora cavernosa located dorsolaterally, and the corpus spongiosum situated ventrally in the midline. The corpora cavernosa are composed of a sponge-like meshwork of endothelial-lined sinusoids, capable of considerable enlargement when engorged with blood during an erection. The corpus spongiosum is composed of spongy tissue similar to that of the corpora cavernosa and contains the urethra. The enlarged proximal aspect of the corpus spongiosum is the bulbous portion. Distally, the corpus spongiosum expands to form the cone-shaped glans.

The corpora cavernosa are surrounded by a layer of fibrous connective tissue called the tunica albuginea. Between the paired corpora is an incomplete layer of fibrous connective tissue called the septum penis. All three corpora are surrounded by two fascial layers, Buck's fascia (deep) and Colles fascia (superficial).[5,6]

The portion of the urethra lying within the penis and traveling through the corpus spongiosum, is the anterior urethra. Its proximal segment, the bulbous urethra, extends from the urogenital diaphragm to the suspensory ligament of the penis at the penoscrotal junction and is the widest segment of the urethra. The penile or pendulous urethra is that portion lying within the free part of the penis. The fossa navicularis is the distalmost aspect of the penile urethra, lying in the glans.

Normal Sonographic Appearance

In the nonerect state, the corpora cavernosa and spongiosum are homogenous in echotexture and similar in size (Fig. 15-1). The tunica albuginea surrounding each corpus cavernosum appears as a thin echogenic line. Within the corpus cavernosum, the cavernosal artery is seen as a pair of dots on transverse view and a narrow tubular structure on longitudinal view. The normal diameter of the cavernosal artery in the flaccid state ranges from too small to measure (<0.3 mm) to 1.0 mm, with a mean of 0.3 to 0.5 mm.[1,7,8]

When collapsed, the urethra is not visualized sonographically within the corpus spongiosum. After distension of the lumen, the normal urethra is identified as a tubular structure measuring at least 4 mm in diameter (Fig. 15-2). The wall of the urethra appears as a smooth, thin echogenic line between the fluid-filled lumen and the spongy tissue of the corpus spongiosum.[1,2,9]

PATHOLOGY

Fibrosis and Scarring

Scarring or fibrosis may involve the corpora, tunica albuginea, or surrounding tissues. These lesions may cause penile deformity during erection, as the inelastic nature of the fibrosis leads to bending of the penis toward the side of the lesion. In some cases erection is painful, leading to impotence.

Lesions within the corpora cavernosa appear sonographically as irregularly shaped echogenic foci within the usually homogenous spongy tissue (Fig. 15-3). They vary in thickness and may be bilateral.[2]

When the fibrotic plaque involves the tunica albuginea of the corpus cavernosum it is termed Peyronie's disease. These plaques are usually located on the dorsal side of the penis. Noncalcified tunical plaques may resolve spontaneously. Calcified lesions or those that persist and are symptomatic may be surgically corrected by excision and repair.[2,10]

Ultrasound is useful in Peyronie's disease to identify the location and extent of the tunical fibrotic plaque, as well as to detect the presence of calcification. The plaque appears sonographically as an area of echogenic thickening of the tunica albuginea. Calcified lesions are brightly echogenic with acoustic shadowing[1,2,11,12] (Fig. 15-4).

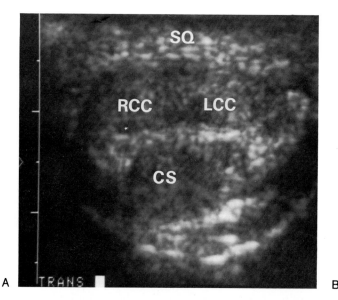
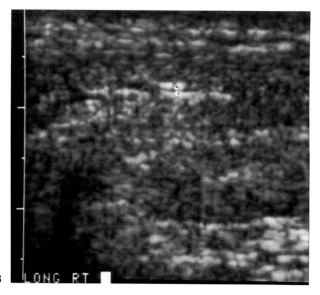

Fig. 15-1.   Normal penis. **(A)** Transverse sonogram of penis showing three corpora (*RCC & LCC,* right and left corpora cavernosa; *CS,* corpus spongiosum) of similar sizes and homogenous echotexture surrounded by subcutaneous tissue and fascial layers *(SQ).* **(B)** Longitudinal image of corpus cavernosum with bright walls of cavernosal artery (calipers) visible within the otherwise homogenous tissue.

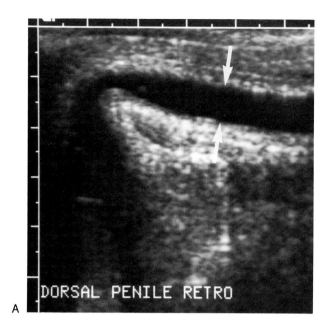

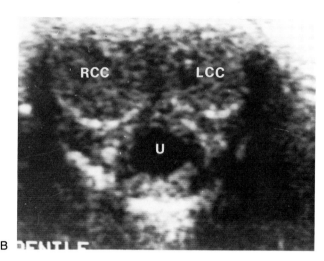

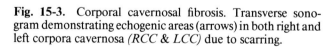

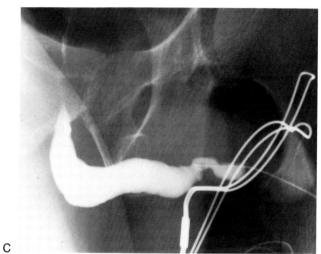

Fig. 15-2. Normal sonourethrogram. **(A)** Distended urethra (arrows) has thin, smooth walls and even caliber lumen. **(B)** Transverse sonogram showing distended urethra *(U)* in corpus spongiosum. *(RCC & LCC,* right and left corpora cavernosa.) **(C)** Radiograph of urethra distended with contrast demonstrating urethral contour and caliber. (Fig. B from Doubilet et al,[2] with permission.)

C

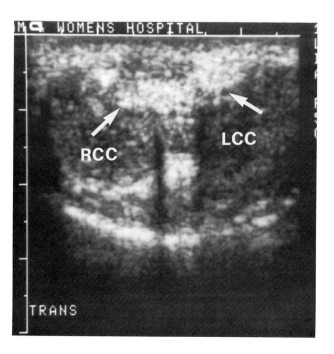

Fig. 15-3. Corporal cavernosal fibrosis. Transverse sonogram demonstrating echogenic areas (arrows) in both right and left corpora cavernosa *(RCC & LCC)* due to scarring.

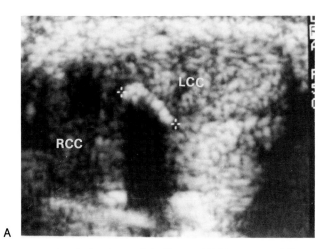

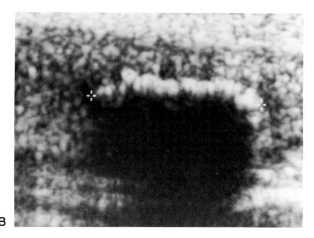

Fig. 15-4. Peyronie's disease. **(A)** Transverse oblique sonogram showing calcified plaque (calipers) along tunica albuginea between the right and left corpora cavernosa *(RCC & LCC)*. **(B)** Longitudinal sonogram demonstrating calcified tunical plaque (calipers). (From Doubilet et al,[2] with permission.)

Masses

A variety of benign and malignant cystic and solid masses may occur in the penis. Cysts may develop from the periurethral, bulbourethral (Cowper's), or anterior urethral (Littre's) glands (Fig. 15-5). Sebaceous gland retention cysts may arise in the skin (Fig. 15-6). Inflammatory masses, including abscesses and granulomata, may involve any of the structures of the penis. Solid tumors may be benign or malignant: the former include angiomas, fibromas, and a variety of dermatologic lesions; the latter include squamous cell carcinomas, melanomas, or soft tissue sarcomas.

Ultrasound serves a number of purposes in the evaluation of penile masses. It can characterize a lesion as a simple cyst, complex cyst, or solid mass. The size of the lesion and extent of corporal involvement can be assessed. Sonourethrography may be useful to define the relationship of the lesion to the urethra[2] (Fig. 15-7).

Trauma

Blunt or penetrating penile trauma may lead to hematomas, disruption of fibrous or fascial layers, or disruption of the anterior urethra. Acute bending of the erect

Fig. 15-5. Periurethral cyst. Longitudinal sonourethrogram showing cyst (arrows) separate from distended urethra (*U*, small arrows). (From Doubilet et al,[2] with permission.)

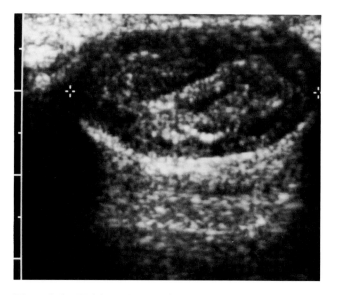

Fig. 15-6. Epidermal retention cyst. Sonogram showing complex mass (calipers) located in subcutaneous tissues of the penis. (From Doubilet et al,[2] with permission.)

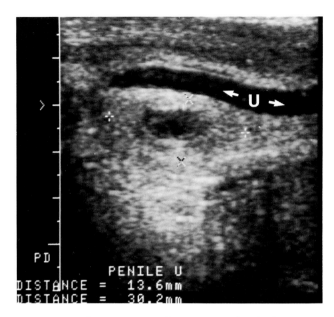

Fig. 15-7. Inflammatory penile mass. Longitudinal sonourethrogram showing complex mass with cystic center (calipers) adjacent to normal urethra (*U*, arrowheads) distended with jelly. (From Benson et al,[1] with permission.)

penis may result in fracture of the corpus cavernosum with rupture of the tunica albuginea.

The location and size of post-traumatic hematomas is easily determined by ultrasound. The sonographic appearance of the hematoma, like hematomas elsewhere, varies with the age of the lesion. Acutely they are complex masses that may be more echogenic than surrounding tissues. With time the hematoma becomes cystic with septations.

With a penile fracture, rupture of the tunica albuginea is diagnosed sonographically by identifying an area of discontinuity in the echogenic line of the tunica albuginea (Fig. 15-8). The length of disruption can be measured by ultrasound and related abnormalities can be identified, such as a hematoma or corporal sinusoidal tissue protruding through the defect.[2]

Priapism

Priapism is persistence of a painful erection in the absence of sexual activity or desire. Priapism is most often idiopathic, but can also occur in patients with sickle cell anemia, chronic granulocytic leukemia, and other hematologic diseases. The persistent erection is thought to result from clot filling all or part of the caver

nosal spongy tissue. Prolonged priapism can lead to sinusoidal disruption and cavernosal fibrosis.[13]

On ultrasound examination, the involved portion of the corpus cavernosum is dilated and filled with homogenous material of increased echogenicity (Fig. 15-9). The echogenic area may have well-defined borders, or poorly defined margins that gradually merge with normal cavernosal tissue.

Urethral Strictures

Narrowing or stricture of the urethra may be a congenital abnormality or may be acquired as a result of urethral infection, Reiter syndrome, Wegener's granulomatosis, trauma, or iatrogenic insult. The most common infectious etiology is gonorrhea. Iatrogenic causes include instrumentation, prolonged indwelling catheters, or surgery. Patients with strictures present with symptoms of impaired urine flow, including hesitancy, nocturia, hematuria, split stream, and postvoid dribbling. Therapeutic options include dilatation, internal urethrotomy, and surgery.[14]

Sonourethrography, performed by scanning the fluid-distended urethra, is used to diagnose, evaluate, and follow urethral strictures. A stricture is identified as a narrowed segment of the urethral lumen typically with irregularity and thickening of the wall (Fig. 15-10). The location, degree of narrowing, and length of the stricture can be determined accurately. Dilatation of the lumen proximal to the stricture may be identified. Sonourethrography is also useful for determining the presence and extent of spongiofibrosis around a stricture. Spongiofibrosis appears as echogenic tissue distorting the surrounding corporal parenchyma[1-4] (Fig. 15-11). Its identification is important in determining whether the stricture can be treated successfully by urethrotomy alone or will require open surgical correction.

Sonourethrographic findings with urethral strictures correlate well with radiologic contrast urethrography with respect to location, length, and diameter of the lesions[1-4] (Fig. 15-10). A disadvantage of sonourethrography as compared with contrast radiologic studies is its inability to evaluate the posterior urethra. This limitation is minor, however, in that most strictures occur in the anterior rather than posterior urethra.[14] Sonourethrography, on the other hand, has several advantages over radiologic techniques. Ultrasound does not use ionizing radiation, so that sonourethrography is ideal for evaluating patients who require repeated studies to follow a stricture over time. In addition, sonography provides information about surrounding spongiofibrosis, which radiologic studies cannot assess.[1-4]

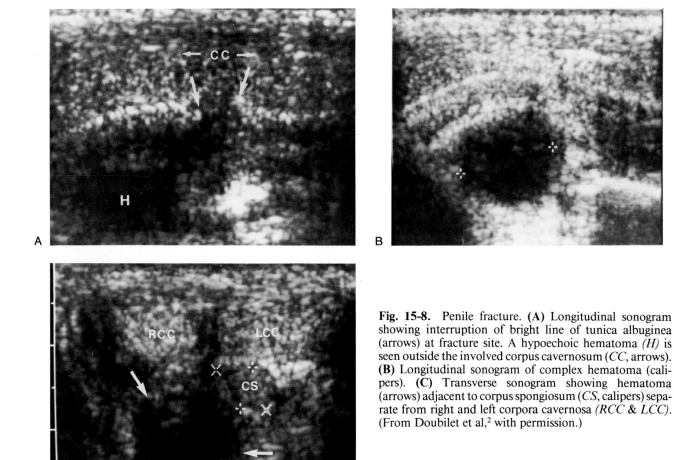

Fig. 15-8. Penile fracture. **(A)** Longitudinal sonogram showing interruption of bright line of tunica albuginea (arrows) at fracture site. A hypoechoic hematoma *(H)* is seen outside the involved corpus cavernosum (*CC*, arrows). **(B)** Longitudinal sonogram of complex hematoma (calipers). **(C)** Transverse sonogram showing hematoma (arrows) adjacent to corpus spongiosum (*CS*, calipers) separate from right and left corpora cavernosa *(RCC & LCC)*. (From Doubilet et al,[2] with permission.)

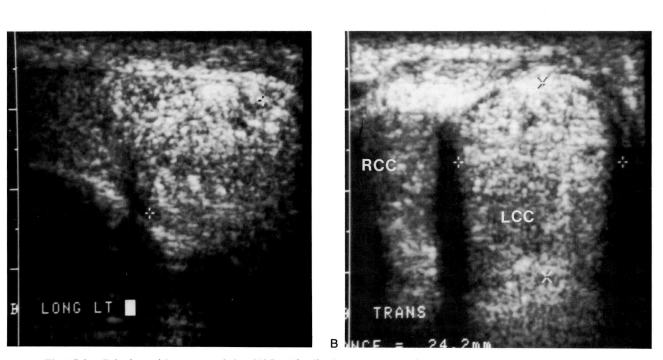

Fig. 15-9. Priapism with cavernosal clot. **(A)** Longitudinal sonogram showing expansion of a segment of corpus cavernosum by echogenic clot (calipers). **(B)** Transverse sonogram showing enlarged left corpus cavernosum (*LCC*, calipers) filled with clot next to small right corpus cavernosum *(RCC)*. (From Benson et al,[34] with permission.)

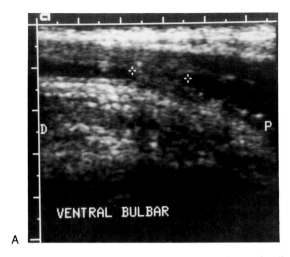 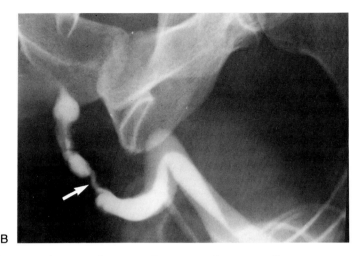

Fig. 15-10. Urethral stricture. **(A)** Longitudinal sonourethrogram demonstrating narrowed segment of lumen (calipers) with irregular wall. (*P*, proximal urethra; *D*, distal urethra.) **(B)** Radiologic urethrogram showing same stricture (arrow).

Urethral Foreign Bodies and Stones

Foreign bodies may be introduced into the urethra through the meatus. Their presence can cause infection, urethral obstruction, or damage to the urethral wall. Solid objects may be identified by ultrasound by scanning longitudinally and transversely until an echogenic object is identified along the course of the urethra. Sonourethrography is used to ascertain whether the foreign body is contained within the urethra or has extended through the urethral wall into the tissue of the corpus spongiosum (Fig. 15-12). After removal of the

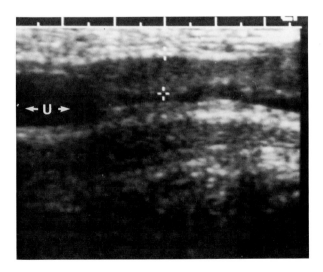

Fig. 15-11. Urethral stricture with spongiofibrosis. Longitudinal sonourethrogram demonstrating fibrosis involving spongiosal tissue (calipers) around a stricture. (*U*, arrowheads, urethra.) (From Doubilet et al,[2] with permission.)

foreign body, continuity of the wall can be assessed by sonourethrography.[1,2]

Calculi may arise primarily in the urethra or may originate in the kidneys or bladder and pass into the urethra. Primary urethral calculi usually occur within a urethral diverticulum or proximal to a stricture. Calculi often cause pain and may occasionally cause urethral obstruction. They may be removed by penile massage, via a urethroscope, or by urethrotomy.

Sonographically, a urethral calculus appears as a brightly echogenic focus with acoustic shadowing located along the course of the urethra (Fig. 15-13). It is important to scan the penis prior to, during, and following distension of the urethra with urologic jelly in order to avoid missing a stone that might be pushed proximally out of the field of view during the injection[1,2] (Fig. 15-14).

Other Urethral Lesions

Urethral diverticula may be congenital or acquired. Patients may present with symptoms of infection, due to urinary stasis, or obstruction, resulting either from compression or from a valve-like flap associated with the lesion. On sonourethrography, diverticula appear as anechoic fluid-filled lesions adjacent to the urethra. They may change in size with distension and emptying of the urethra. Some diverticula may not fill during retrograde urethral distension, but instead may require antegrade radiologic or sonographic studies for diagnosis.[1,2]

Benign and malignant lesions may arise in the urethra. Benign masses include polyps, papillomata, and condylomata acuminata. Malignant urethral tumors are rare,

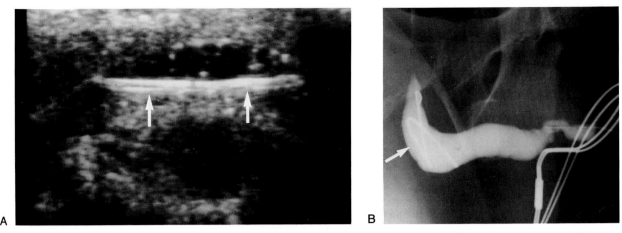

Fig. 15-12. Foreign body in urethra. **(A)** Sonourethrogram showing echogenic linear foreign body within urethra (arrows). **(B)** Contrast radiologic urethrogram showing paper clip (arrow) in bulbous urethra. (From Benson et al,[34] with permission.)

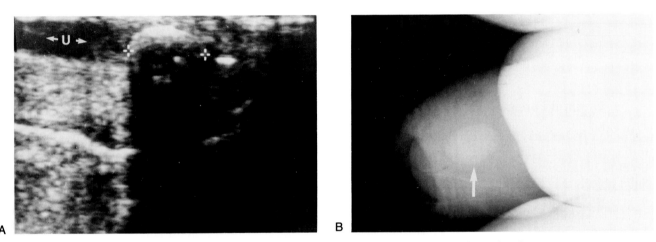

Fig. 15-13. Urethral calculus. **(A)** Sonogram showing oval echogenic stone (calipers) in distal urethra (*U*, arrows). **(B)** Radiograph demonstrating stone (arrow) in penis. (From Doubilet et al,[2] with permission.)

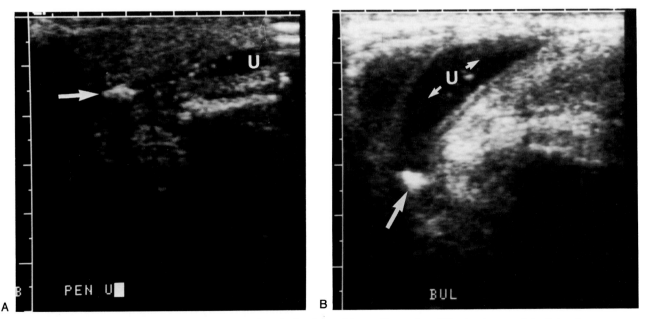

Fig. 15-14. Urethra calculus. **(A)** Echogenic calculus (arrow) in penile urethra *(U)* prior to complete distension. **(B)** Stone (large arrow) dislodged to proximal bulbous urethra (*U*, arrows) after retrograde filling. (From Benson et al,[1] with permission.)

with squamous cell carcinoma being the most common histologic type. Other malignant tumors include transitional cell carcinomas, which may arise in the posterior urethra, and adenocarcinomas, which may arise in the bulbous urethra.[15]

The size of a urethral mass, the extent of involvement of surrounding penile parenchyma, and the presence of proximal dilatation due to obstruction can be assessed by sonography and sonourethrography. Urethral masses may appear as soft tissue lesions of altered echogenicity when compared with the homogenous echotexture of surrounding penile corpora.[2]

DOPPLER ASSESSMENT OF ERECTILE FUNCTION

TECHNIQUE

The hemodynamic function of the penis can be evaluated using high resolution ultrasound in combination with spectral and color Doppler before and after pharmacologic induction of erection with papaverine or prostaglandin E_1 (PGE$_1$).[7,16-22] The examination begins with real-time scanning of the flaccid penis in longitudinal and transverse planes to evaluate the spongy tissue of the corpora cavernosa. The diameters of both cavernosal arteries are measured. Doppler of each cavernosal artery may be performed, although in most patients no flow will be detected in the flaccid state. A tourniquet is then placed at the base of the penis, 45 to 60 mg of papaverine is injected intracorporally, and the tourniquet is removed 2 minutes later. At this time, the diameter of each cavernosal artery is measured (Fig. 15-15). Three to seven minutes after papaverine injection,

each cavernosal arterial Doppler waveform is obtained and peak systolic and end-diastolic velocities are measured[1,7,16,20,22-25] (Fig. 15-16). Color Doppler may permit more rapid acquisition of Doppler waveforms by improving the ability to locate small arteries.[22,25] Seven to ten minutes after injection, color or spectral Doppler is used to look for venous flow in the dorsal or cavernosal veins. Penile tumescence and rigidity are assessed based on penile angle, that is, the angle the penis makes with respect to vertical when the patient is standing.[7]

NORMAL ERECTILE FUNCTION

The blood supply to the penis is via the common penile artery, which arises from the internal pudendal artery, a branch of the internal iliac artery. The common

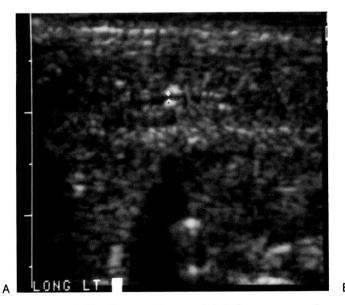
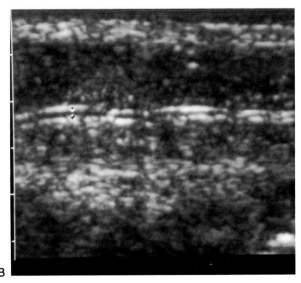

Fig. 15-15. Cavernosal artery. **(A)** Calipers measure diameter of cavernosal artery on longitudinal sonogram of flaccid penis. **(B)** After induction of erection with papaverine, the walls of the cavernosal artery (calipers) appear brighter and the diameter is larger.

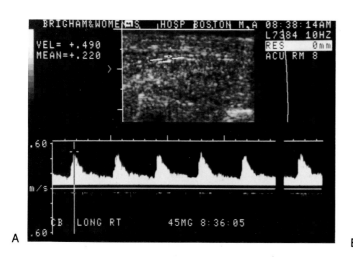 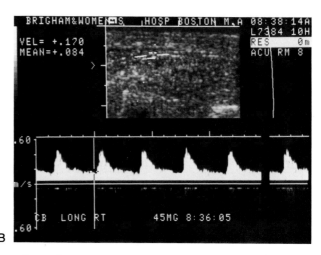

Fig. 15-16. Cavernosal arterial waveform. **(A)** Spectral waveform of cavernosal artery shortly after papaverine injection showing peak systolic velocity of 49 cm/s (caliper, VEL = +.490 m/s) and **(B)** end-diastolic velocity of 17 cm/s (caliper, VEL = +.170 m/s). (From Benson et al,[34] with permission.)

penile artery has three main branches: the artery to the bulbous portion of the corpus spongiosum; the dorsal artery, which supplies the glans and distal corpus spongiosum; and the cavernosal artery, which supplies the corpus cavernosum. The cavernosal artery gives rise to small helicine arteries that extend into the spongy erectile tissue of the corpus cavernosum.[26] Venous drainage of the glans and proximal corpus spongiosum is primarily via the dorsal vein. The corpora cavernosa are drained by small emissary veins that pass through the tunica albuginea to crural and cavernosal veins at the base of the penis.[16]

During erection the cavernosal artery dilates, permitting a large increase in blood flow to the corpora. As the corpora cavernosa become engorged with blood, the small emissary veins are compressed against the tense tunica albuginea, occluding outflow of blood.[10,17,27]

Normal erectile function requires psychological health, normal endocrine balance, an intact nervous system, adequate penile blood supply, and normal cavernosal sinusoidal tissue. Penile erection is initiated and maintained by neurologic activity propagated through the internal pudendal sensory nerves and the parasympathetic cavernosal motor nerves, which arise from sacral nerves two, three, and four.[10] Parasympathetic motor activity stimulates smooth muscle relaxation of the cavernosal arteries and sinusoids, leading to dilatation of the cavernosal arteries, increased blood flow to the penis, and filling of the sinusoidal spaces with blood. The spongy erectile tissue expands until the tunica albuginea is tense. At this stage of erection, the small veins that drain the corpora cavernosa become compressed

against the tunica albuginea and outflow of blood from the distended corpora is occluded. Penile tumescence and rigidity are maintained by continued inflow of blood and minimal venous drainage.[10,17,27]

Normal Findings

In normally potent patients in the nonerect state, the diameter of the cavernosal arteries measures 0.2 to 1.0 mm, with a mean of 0.3 to 0.5 mm. No flow will be detected by Doppler in most cases.[7,8,21,23–25] When flow is identified, peak systolic velocity is typically 10 to 15 cm/s.[22,24]

Three to seven minutes after papaverine injection, the cavernosal artery dilates about 0.5 mm to approximately twice its preinjection diameter.[8,17,20,24] The walls of the artery become prominent because the sinusoids around them are expanded with blood and have decreased echogenicity. The peak systolic velocity in the cavernosal arteries is normally above 30 cm/s, most often greater than 35 cm/s.[7,8]

With the development of an erection, there is a progressive increase in the intracorporal pressure leading to a gradual decrease in end-diastolic flow. When full tumescence is obtained the intracorporal pressure exceeds diastolic arterial pressure, and end-diastolic flow ceases or even reverses[22] (Fig. 15-17).

Seven to ten minutes after papaverine injection, with the development of a normal erection, no flow will be detected in the dorsal or cavernosal veins by color or spectral Doppler.

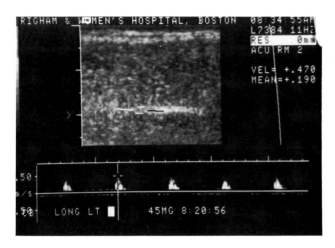

Fig. 15-17. Cavernosal arterial waveform with erection. With development of full erection, waveform demonstrates absence of diastolic flow.

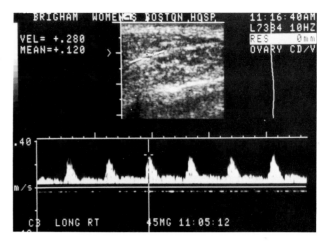

Fig. 15-18. Moderate arterial insufficiency. Peak systolic velocity on cavernosal artery waveform measures 28 cm/s (caliper, VEL = +.280 m/s).

PATHOLOGY

Organic impotence is defined as the inability to generate or maintain an adequate erection for normal sexual activity in the absence of psychological dysfunction. Organic causes can be found in 50 to 90 percent of all cases of impotence.[16,18] In such cases, surgical and medical therapies may be available to treat the specific cause of erectile dysfunction. Before invasive studies are performed, preliminary evaluation should exclude neurologic and endocrinologic causes of impotence, as well as impotence occurring as a side effect of medication or alcohol. Sleep monitoring is used to exclude psychogenic causes.

Arterial Insufficiency

Arterial insufficiency results from occlusion or stenosis of the cavernosal or internal pudendal artery or of any of the feeding arteries, such that the required increase in arterial flow for an erection cannot be generated or maintained. Approximately 30 percent of patients with hemodynamic causes of impotence have isolated arterial insufficiency.[16,23] Patients with mild to moderate arterial insufficiency may be successfully treated with self-injection of vasoactive agents such as papaverine, phentolamine, or PGE_1.[16,23] More severe arterial disease can sometimes be treated successfully with angioplasty or arterial bypass surgery from the inferior epigastric artery to the deep dorsal vein. When pharmacologic and revascularization procedures fail or are inapplicable, prosthetic implantation may be performed.[8,28,29]

The presence and degree of arterial insufficiency can be determined from duplex studies of the cavernosal arteries after papaverine injection. The peak systolic velocity appears to be the single best indicator of arterial function. Peak systolic velocities below 30 cm/s are indicative of arterial insufficiency. Peak velocities between 25 and 30 cm/s suggest moderate arterial disease (Fig. 15-18) and those less than 25 cm/s indicate severe disease[1,7,8,16,17,24,25] (Fig. 15-19). Other measurements related to the cavernosal artery, including increase in diameter during development of an erection, do not correlate well with arterial function.[7,8,18]

Once the diagnosis of arterial insufficiency has been made by Doppler studies and the degree of impairment

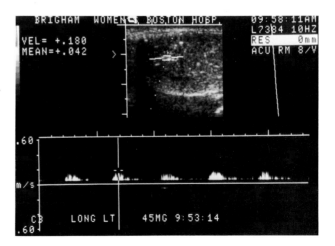

Fig. 15-19. Severe arterial disease. Arterial waveform demonstrates low peak systolic velocity (18 cm/s) (caliper, VEL = +.180 m/s) after induction of erection with papaverine.

has been estimated, angiographic studies should be performed in patients in whom arterial bypass procedures or angioplasty might be considered. This diagnostic procedure accurately delineates vascular anatomy and is necessary for surgical planning.

Venous Incompetence

Erectile dysfunction owing to venous incompetence results from failure of the engorged cavernosal spongy tissues to compress the emissary veins draining the corpora against the tunica albuginea.[16] As a result, blood escapes the corpora rapidly despite increased arterial flow, and full erection is not generated or maintained. Isolated veno-occlusive disease accounts for approximately 15 percent of organic impotence due to hemodynamic abnormalities.[16,23] Patients with this isolated abnormality respond well to venous ligation procedures.[30,31]

Duplex ultrasound diagnosis of venous incompetence can be made only if arterial function is normal. When the venous leak drains through the dorsal vein, the diagnosis can be established with spectral or color Doppler by detecting flow in the dorsal vein 7 to 10 minutes after papaverine injection[7,32] (Fig. 15-20). In many cases, however, venous leakage occurs only through the cavernosal or crural veins, which lie too deep in the pelvis to permit detection of flow by Doppler. In these patients the following observations 7 to 10 minutes after papaverine injection are suggestive of venous incompetence: end-diastolic flow in the cavernosal arteries greater than 5 cm/s[25] (Fig. 15-21) and/or failure to generate and maintain an adequate erection despite normal cavernosal arterial systolic velocities.[7]

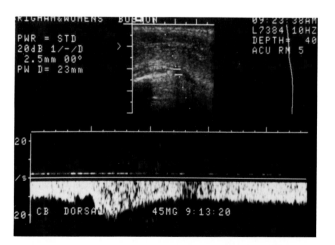

Fig. 15-20. Venous incompetence. Doppler of dorsal vein after induction of erection with papaverine demonstrating significant flow due to venous leakage. (From Benson et al,[34] with permission.)

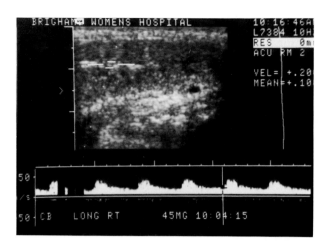

Fig. 15-21. Venous incompetence. Cavernosal arterial waveform demonstrating significant end-diastolic flow (caliper, VEL = +.200 m/s) 12 minutes after papaverine injection, a secondary sign of venous leakage.

Although duplex studies are useful in the diagnosis of venous incompetence, definitive diagnosis often requires dynamic pharmacocavernosometry. This examination involves monitoring intracorporal pressures during controlled infusion of saline into the corpora.[33] Once the diagnosis of venous leakage is established, cavernosography is performed to define sites of venous drainage in order to plan surgical ligation procedures.[8]

Combined Arterial and Venous Disease

In 50 to 70 percent of patients with hemodynamic factors causing impotence, combined arterial insufficiency and venous incompetence are found.[16,23] In these patients therapeutic options are limited. Patients with mild to moderate arterial disease and venous incompetence may have sufficient arterial flow to be treated successfully by surgical venous ligation. If arterial impairment is severe, however, prosthetic implantation may be the only available treatment.[8,32]

The diagnosis of combined arterial and venous disease cannot be made using duplex ultrasound because the sonographic signs of venous incompetence do not apply in the setting of arterial insufficiency. In patients with impaired arterial flow, the cavernosal sinusoids may never fill to the point of occluding the small draining veins of the corpora cavernosa. Persistent diastolic flow will be seen on the cavernosal arterial waveform because the intracavernosal pressure will not reach the level achieved during a normal erection. Even if flow is detected in the dorsal vein, it cannot be determined whether this results from venous incompetence or from cavernosal filling that is insufficient to occlude the draining veins.[8]

Whenever duplex studies indicate arterial insufficiency and surgical repair is considered, cavernosometry should be performed to determine whether there is coexistent venous incompetence. If a venous leak is identified and arterial insufficiency is mild to moderate (peak velocity >25 cm/s) the patient may be a candidate for venous ligation therapy since arterial function may be adequate to generate an erection. If the arterial insufficiency is severe (peak velocity <25 cm/s), neither venous ligation nor arterial revascularization procedures should be considered.[8]

REFERENCES

1. Benson CB, Doubilet PM, Richie JP: Sonography of the male genital tract. AJR 1989;153:705
2. Doubilet PM, Benson CB, Silverman SG, Gluck CD: The penis. Semin Ultrasound CT MR 1991;12:157
3. McAninch JW, Laing FC, Jeffrey RB: Sonourethrography in the evaluation of urethral strictures: a preliminary report. J Urol 1988;139:294
4. Gluck CD, Bundy AL, Fine C et al: Sonographic urethrogram: comparison to roentgenographic techniques in 22 patients. J Urol 1988;140:1404
5. Goss CM: Gray's Anatomy. 37th American Ed. Churchill Livingstone, New York, 1989
6. Tanagho EA: Anatomy of the lower urinary tract. p. 46. In Walsh PC, Gittes RF, Perlmutter AD, Stamey TA (eds): Campbell's Urology. 5th Ed. WB Saunders, Philadelphia, 1986
7. Benson CB, Vickers MA: Sexual impotence caused by vascular disease: diagnosis by duplex sonography. AJR 1989;153:1149
8. Benson CB, Vickers MA, Aruny J: Evaluation of Impotence. Semin Ultrasound CT MR 1991;12:176
9. Ney C, Friedenberg RM: Radiographic Atlas of the Genitourinary System. 2nd Ed. JB Lippincott, Philadelphia, 1981
10. Krane RJ: Sexual function and dysfunction. p. 700. In Walsh PC, Gittes RF, Perlmutter AD, Stamey TA (eds): Campbell's Urology. 5th Ed. WB Saunders, Philadelphia, 1986
11. Chou YH, Tiu CM, Pan HB et al: High-resolution realtime ultrasound in Peyronie's disease. J Ultrasound Med 1987;6:67
12. Hamm B, Friedrich M, Kelami A: Ultrasound imaging in Peyronie disease. Urology 1986;28:540
13. Walsh PC, Wilson JD: Impotence and infertility in men. p. 217. In Braunwald E, Isselbacher KJ, Petersdorf RG et al (eds): Harrison's Principles of Internal Medicine. McGraw-Hill, New York, 1987
14. Devine CJ: Surgery of the urethra. p. 2853. In Walsh RC,

15. Gittes RF, Perlmutter AD, Stamey TA (eds): Campbell's Urology. 5th Ed. WB Saunders, Philadelphia, 1986
15. Hopkins SC, Grabstald H: Benign and malignant tumors of the male and female urethra. p. 1441. In Walsh PC, Gittes RF, Perlmutter AD, Stamey TA (eds): Campbell's Urology. 5th Ed. WB Saunders, Philadelphia, 1986
16. Krysiewicz S, Mellinger BC: The role of imaging in the diagnostic evaluation of impotence. AJR 1989;153:1133
17. Mueller SC, Lue TF: Evaluation of vasculogenic impotence. Urol Clin North Am 1988;15:65
18. Paushter DM: Role of duplex sonography in the evaluation of sexual impotence. AJR 1989;153:1161
19. DuPlessis DJ, Bornman MS, Koch Z, Van der Merwe CA: Penile ultrasonography in impotence. S Afr J Surg 1987;25:69
20. Lue TF, Hricak H, Marich KW, Tanagho EA: Vasculogenic impotence evaluated by high-resolution ultrasonography and pulsed Doppler spectrum analysis. Radiology 1987;59:777
21. Collins JP, Lewandowski BJ: Experience with intracorporal injection of papaverine and duplex ultrasound scanning for assessment of arteriogenic impotence. Br J Urol 1987;59:84
22. Schwartz AN, Wang KY, Mack LA et al: Evaluation of normal erectile function with color flow Doppler sonography. AJR 1989;153:1155
23. Lue TF, Mueller SC, Jow YR, Hwang TIS: Functional evaluation of penile arteries with duplex ultrasound in vasodilator-induced erection. Urol Clin North Am 1989;16:799
24. Shabsigh R, Fishman IJ, Quesada ET et al: Evaluation of vasculogenic erectile impotence using penile duplex ultrasonography. J Urol 1989;142:1469
25. Quam JP, King BF, James EM et al: Duplex and color Doppler sonographic evaluation of vasculogenic impotence. AJR 1989;153:1141
26. Quain R: The vascular anatomy of the human body. Taylor-Walton, London, 1844
27. Melman A: The evaluation of erectile dysfunction. Urol Radiol 1988;10:119
28. Virag R, Zwang G, Dermange H, Legman M: Vasculogenic impotence: a review of 92 cases with 54 surgical operations. Vasc Surg 1981;15:9
29. Goldstein I: Overview of types and results of vascular surgical procedures for impotence. Cardiovasc Intervent Radiol 1988;11:240
30. Abber JC, Lue TF: Surgery for venogenic impotence: early results, abstracted. J Urol 139:297, 1988
31. Garofalo FA, Bennett AH. Surgery for corporovenous leakage, abstracted. J Urol 139:400, 1988
32. Vickers MA, Benson CB, Richie JP: High resolution ultrasonography and pulsed wave doppler for detection of corporovenous incompetence in erectile dysfunction. J Urol 1990;143:1125
33. Padma-Nathan H, Goldstein I, Krane RJ: Evaluation of the impotent patient. Semin Urol 1986;4:225
34. Benson CB, Doubilet PM, Vickers MA: Sonography of the penis. Ultrasound 1991;8:89

16

Scrotum

Carol B. Benson
Peter M. Doubilet

TECHNIQUE

Sonographic examination of the scrotum is best performed by using a linear transducer with frequencies in the range of 5 to 10 MHz. The transducer is applied directly to the scrotum with aqueous coupling gel. Both testicles should be scanned in their entirety in transverse and longitudinal planes, and the echogenicities of the two testicles should be compared. The epididymal head and, when visible, the body and tail should be imaged. The spermatic cord should be scanned from the inguinal canal to the scrotum.[1]

Spectral and color Doppler can be used to assess blood flow in the scrotum. Pulsed or spectral Doppler is performed by placing the sample gate over the artery or region from which flow velocity waveforms are to be obtained. This permits quantitative assessment of blood flow. The spermatic cord can be examined to evaluate flow to the scrotum, and the capsular arteries of the testicle can be interrogated to assess flow within the testicle. Color Doppler is performed in the same manner as two-dimensional ultrasound and provides a qualitative anatomic assessment of blood flow. For optimal results, the Doppler settings should be adjusted for low velocities to visualize the small testicular arteries. Flow in the testicle, epididymis, and scrotal wall should be compared in the two hemiscrota to examine for asymmetry.[2,3] Color Doppler may be useful in locating vessels for further evaluation by pulsed Doppler.

Normal Ultrasound Appearance

The wall of the scrotum is normally 2 to 5 mm thick. The testicles are ovoid structures with homogeneous echogenicity of medium intensity (Fig. 16-1). The two testicles should be symmetric in size and echogenicity. The tunica albuginea encapsulating the testicle appears as a thin bright line around its margins. At the mediastinum testis, where the tunica albuginea invaginates and ducts and vessels enter the parenchyma, a bright circular region on transverse view or a bright band on longitudinal view is seen at the periphery of the testicle.[1]

The head of the epididymis, situated over the superolateral aspect of the testicle, has homogeneous echotexture similar to that of the testicle and is up to 10 mm thick (Fig. 16-2). The epididymal body is not usually seen, but occasionally is visible as a thin band coursing along the posterolateral side of the testicle with lower echogenicity than the epididymal head or testicular parenchyma (Fig. 16-2). The epididymal tail is sometimes seen at the inferior pole of the testicle. A small amount of anechoic fluid is normally seen between the layers of the tunica vaginalis surrounding the testicles.[1]

Spectral Doppler studies of the capsular and centripetal arteries of a normal testicle demonstrate low flow with a low-resistance pattern. On color Doppler the capsular arteries are visualized surrounding the testicle and the centripetal arteries are seen within the testicle (Fig. 16-3 and Plate 16-1). The arteries to the epididymis are

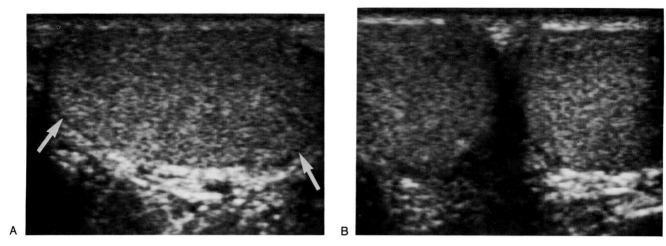

Fig. 16-1. Normal testicle. **(A)** Longitudinal sonogram of ovoid testicle with homogeneous echotexture (arrows). **(B)** Transverse sonogram of both testicles showing symmetry in size and echotexture.

more difficult to identify and, when seen, demonstrate higher resistance.[2]

NORMAL ANATOMY

The scrotum is a cutaneous pouch divided into two lateral compartments. Each compartment contains a testicle, epididymis, vas deferens, and spermatic cord, all of which carry blood vessels, nerves, and lymphatics. The median raphe separates the two compartments. The scrotal wall is composed of several layers of tissue. From outside in, these are the skin, dartos fascia, external spermatic fascia, cremaster muscle, internal spermatic fascia, and a thin layer of fatty tissue.

The scrotal sac is lined internally by the parietal layer of the tunica vaginalis. The visceral layer of the tunica vaginalis is reflected over and surrounds most of the testicle, the epididymis, and the proximal portion of the spermatic cord. A small area of the posterior surface of the testicle is not covered by the tunica vaginalis. At this site, termed the *bare area,* the testicle is anchored against the scrotal wall, preventing torsion. Blood vessels, lymphatics, nerves, and spermatic ducts travel through the bare area.

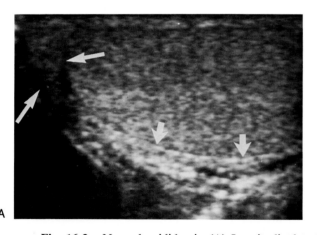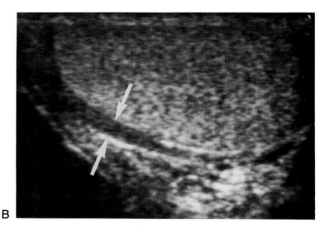

Fig. 16-2. Normal epididymis. **(A)** Longitudinal testicular sonogram showing the epididymal head (long arrows) superior to the upper pole of the testicle. The tunica albuginea surrounding the testicle is visible as a thin bright line (short arrows) posteriorly. **(B)** The epididymal body (arrows) is visible as a thin hypoechoic band coursing behind the testicle.

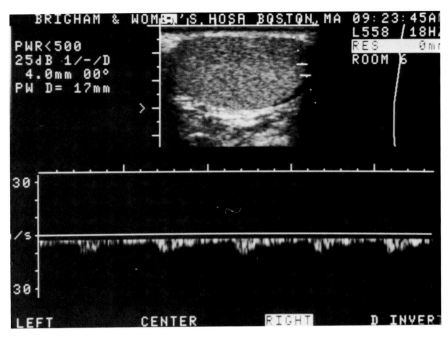

Fig. 16-3. Testicular Doppler. The Doppler gate is placed over the capsular artery at the periphery of the testicle with the arterial waveform displayed below the image. (See also Plate 16-1.)

The testicle is an ovoid structure measuring approximately 2 to 3 cm in diameter and 3 to 5 cm long. It is composed of multiple small lobules containing seminiferous tubules radiating toward the rete testis in the posterior testicle, and is encapsulated by a dense fibrous connective tissue layer called the tunica albuginea. The tunica albuginea invaginates into the posterior aspect of the testicle, where the efferent ductules and blood vessels enter to form a vertical septum called the mediastinum testis. Sperm are produced in the lobules of the testicle and are carried by the seminiferous tubules to the rete testis in the mediastinum and thence into 8 to 20 efferent ductules in the head of the epididymis.

The epididymis is a tortuous, elongated structure situated along the posterolateral aspect of the testicle. The head of the epididymis is located over the upper pole of the testicle. The body courses along the posterolateral surface of the testicle to the tail, located inferior to the lower pole of the testicle. The efferent ductules, carrying sperm produced in the testicle, converge to a single larger duct in the body and tail of the epididymis; this duct becomes the vas deferens in the spermatic cord.

Remnants of developmental structures may be present as appendages. The appendix testis, a remnant of the müllerian ducts, is commonly found on the testicle near the epididymal head. The appendix epididymis, located on the head of the epididymis, is a remnant of the mesonephron. Two other embryonic remnants, the paradidymis and the vas aberrans, may be seen associated with the spermatic cord and epididymis.[4,5]

Arterial blood is supplied to the scrotum wall by branches of the pudendal arteries and to the scrotal contents by the testicular, deferential, and cremasteric arteries through the spermatic cord. The testicular (or internal spermatic) artery arises directly from the aorta; the deferential artery is a branch of the vesical artery; and the cremasteric (or external spermatic) artery arises from the inferior epigastric artery. Both the deferential and cremasteric arteries anastomose with the testicular artery. The testicle is supplied primarily by the testicular artery via capsular branches around the periphery of the testicle and their small centripetal arteries that course into the testicular parenchyma. The epididymis is also supplied primarily by the testicular artery. The vas deferens receives its blood flow from the deferential artery.[5]

The pampiniform plexus is a network of veins that arise in the mediastinum and travel in the spermatic cord. The venous network converges into three veins: the testicular (or internal spermatic) vein, which drains into the inferior vena cava on the right and into the left renal vein on the left; the deferential vein; and the cremasteric (or external spermatic) vein.[4]

MALIGNANT TESTICULAR TUMORS

Primary Testicular Cancer

Primary testicular cancer usually occurs in men aged 20 to 35 years. Most patients present with a palpable mass or painless testicular enlargement, although up to 15 percent present with symptoms related to metastatic spread. Another 10 percent of patients present with symptoms of epididymitis that may not resolve on antibiotic therapy, and 15 percent of cases are first detected following trauma.[6]

The incidence of testicular cancer in cryptorchid testicles is 48 times that in normally descended testicles. There is also an increased incidence of carcinoma in cryptorchid testicles treated by orchiopexy, although it is not as high as in untreated undescended testicles. The contralateral, normally descended testicle is at slightly increased risk for developing cancer than in a patient with bilaterally normally positioned testicles.[7] For this reason, sonography is useful for screening patients at increased risk for cancer to detect early nonpalpable cancers.[6]

Ninety-five percent of primary testicular cancers are of germ cell origin. These tumors include seminomas (40 to 50 percent), embryonal cell carcinomas (15 to 20 percent), teratocarcinomas (5 to 10 percent), and chorio-

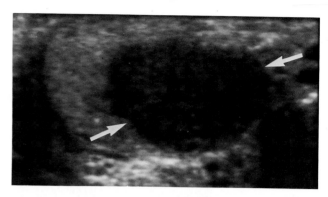

Fig. 16-5. Seminoma. Sonogram of the testicle containing a well-defined, homogeneous tumor (arrows) with markedly decreased echogenicity.

carcinomas (rare). Forty percent of germ cell tumors are mixed, comprising two or more of the above cell types. Non-germ cell tumors, the remaining 5 percent of malignant neoplasms, may arise from the Sertoli cells, Leydig cells, or mesenchymal tissues.[7]

Sonography plays a major role in detecting and characterizing intrascrotal masses. It is extremely sensitive for detecting testicular masses and highly accurate at distinguishing cystic from solid lesions.[1] Sonography can accurately differentiate intratesticular from extratesticular masses. This distinction is critical to patient manage-

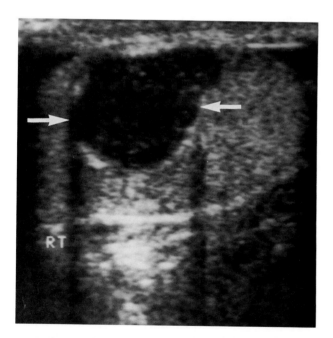

Fig. 16-4. Primary testicular tumor. Longitudinal sonogram of the right testicle demonstrating a well-defined mass (arrows) with decreased echogenicity except for some calcification at the periphery of the tumor.

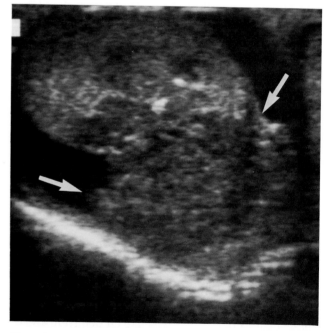

Fig. 16-6. Aggressive germ cell tumor. Longitudinal sonogram demonstrating tumor (arrows) growing outside the testicle into the scrotal wall.

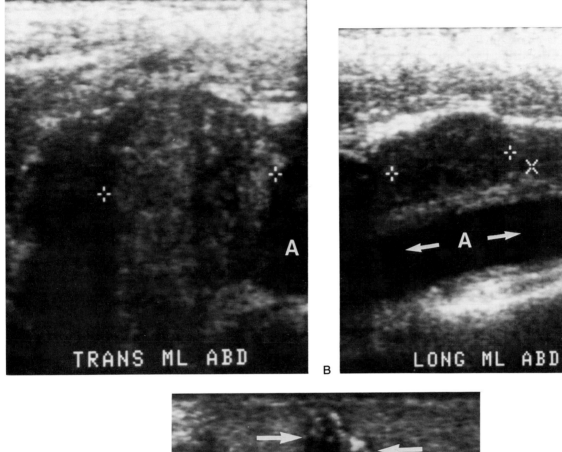

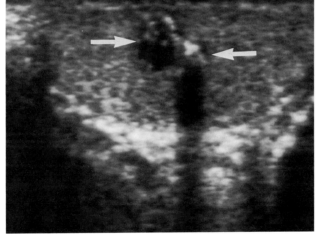

Fig. 16-7. Retroperitoneal germ cell tumor with "burned-out" testicular primary. **(A)** Transverse sonogram of the upper abdomen demonstrating a large tumor mass (calipers) in the retroperitoneum adjacent to the aorta *(A)*. **(B)** Longitudinal sonogram of the mid-abdominal aorta (*A*, arrows) demonstrating preaortic lymphadenopathy (calipers). **(C)** Longitudinal sonogram of the right testicle demonstrating a small tumor mass (arrows) with calcification.

ment because most intratesticular masses are malignant and most extratesticular tumors are benign.[1,8-10] Although ultrasound is very sensitive for detecting testicular masses, it cannot be used to distinguish different types of malignant tumors. The sonographic features of a mass may be suggestive of a particular type of tumor

(e.g., seminoma) but there is too much overlap to establish a histologic diagnosis with certainty.

On ultrasound, malignant tumors are usually well-defined intratesticular masses surrounded by normal testicular parenchyma (Fig. 16-4). The lesions are most often hypoechoic or heterogeneous with areas of decreased echogenicity. Occasionally a testicular tumor is predominantly hyperechoic. Seminomas tend to be more homogeneous and hypoechoic than other germ cell tumors (Fig. 16-5), and they may be multifocal. Cystic areas and calcifications are rare in pure seminomas but are common in nonseminomatous tumors. Embryonal cell carcinomas, the most aggressive of the germ cell cancers, may be very large by the time of ultrasound examination, and there may be sonographic evidence of local invasion through the tunica albuginea and into the epididymis (Fig. 16-6). Distant metastases may be seen. Pure choriocarcinomas are also quite aggressive and metastasize early; they may have cystic areas that are due to hemorrhage and necrosis.[6,11]

Some patients with extragonadal germ cell tumors are found to have regressed or "burned-out" tumors in the testicle. The extragonadal tumor most probably represents viable metastases from a primary testicular neoplasm that has undergone necrosis and fibrosis by the time of detection. On ultrasound, the regressed tumor may appear as an echogenic focus or a solitary small mass of increased or decreased echogenicity within the testicle (Fig. 16-7). No viable tumor cells are found on pathologic examination.[6,8,12–14]

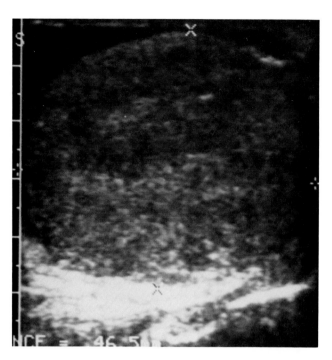

Fig. 16-8. Metastatic oat cell carcinoma. Longitudinal sonogram demonstrating enlarged testicle (calipers) filled with poorly defined areas of decreased echogenicity due to metastatic cancer.

Other Testicular Cancers

Testicular metastases may arise from a variety of primary cancers, most commonly from the genitourinary tract and less often from the lungs or gastrointestinal tract. The testicle is also a common site of leukemia and lymphoma. In some cases, the testicle is the only site of recurrence of lymphoma or leukemia because the blood-gonadal barrier may lead to inadequate treatment of testicular tissue.[6] Sonography is a useful screening tool in these patients because it is highly sensitive for detecting early recurrent disease.[15]

Metastatic disease, lymphoma, or leukemia in the testicle usually has one of two sonographic appearances. In some cases, one or more intratesticular masses are identified. In others, the involved testicle is enlarged and there are ill-defined areas of decreased echogenicity that gradually blend into normal testicular parenchyma[6] (Fig. 16-8).

BENIGN TESTICULAR TUMORS

Sertoli cells, Leydig cells, and mesenchymal tissues of the testicle may give rise to benign as well as malignant tumors. Ultrasound is unable to distinguish benign from malignant testicular tumors, because both types appear as solid intratesticular masses. In most cases, surgical

resection and histopathologic examination is required to prove that a tumor is benign.[1,6]

TESTICULAR CYSTS AND CALCIFICATIONS

Simple testicular cysts are benign lesions that increase in frequency with advancing age. They may be single or multiple and are usually nonpalpable and asymptomatic. On ultrasound they are similar in appearance to cysts elsewhere in the body: anechoic, with thin, smooth walls and distal acoustic enhancement (Fig. 16-9). Most are located close to the mediastinum.[1,16–18]

Small calcifications are occasionally seen in the testicle as tiny echogenic foci. In most cases only two or three such foci are seen, but occasionally there are many tiny echogenic foci throughout both testicles in a diffuse process that has been called testicular microlithiasis (Fig. 16-10). Microlithiasis may be seen in normal patients, but it is sometimes associated with pathologic conditions such as cryptorchidism, Kleinfelter syndrome, sterility, and tumors.[19] Large intratesticular calcifications may be seen as isolated foci in regressed germ cell tumors or associated with a mass in active germ cell tumors.[11]

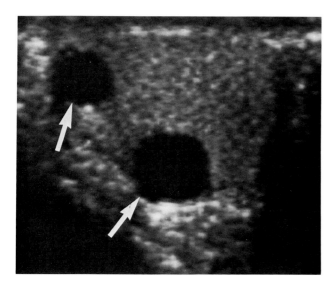

Fig. 16-9. Testicular cysts. Transverse image of the testicle showing two cysts (arrows), which are round and anechoic with thin smooth walls.

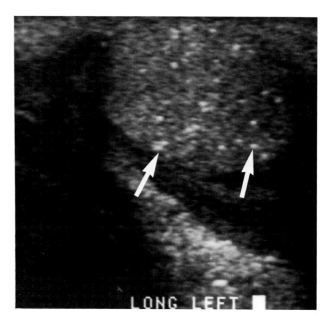

Fig. 16-10. Microlithiasis. Sonogram of the testicle (arrows) containing multiple scattered, very bright echoes due to tiny calcifications.

INFECTIONS

Infectious processes involving the scrotal contents are most often bacterial in origin. Retrograde spread of the organism from the urinary tract is the most common mechanism, although hematogenous seeding of bacteria may occur. Patients present with fever, pain, and swelling.

The infection usually begins in the epididymis and may spread to involve the adjacent testicle or spermatic cord. Severe cases may result in abscess formation in the epididymis or testicle. Scrotal infections usually respond to an antibiotic regimen, although surgery may be required if an abscess is present.

The sonographic findings in acute epididymitis include thickening of the epididymis and, in some cases, alteration of its echotexture. A reactive hydrocele may be present. Increased blood flow in and around the epididymis may be identified by color Doppler (Fig. 16-11 and Plate 16-2). If an abscess is present, complex cystic areas may be seen in the enlarged epididymis[1] (Fig. 16-12).

Spread of infection to the testicle leads to a diffuse decrease in the echogenicity of the testicle or a focal hypoechoic area that is usually located at the periphery of the testicle near the involved portion of the epididymis (Fig. 16-13). Occasionally, focal orchitis appears as an intratesticular mass indistinguishable from a tumor. Clinical symptoms may strongly suggest an infectious process, but these lesions should still be monitored to resolution after antibiotic therapy to ensure that a neoplasm is not present.[20]

TESTICULAR TORSION

The testicle is anchored to the scrotal wall at its bare area. In some cases this bare area is small, leaving a thin stalk of reflected tunica vaginalis surrounding testicular vessels and ducts. This anomaly, the "bell-clapper" de-

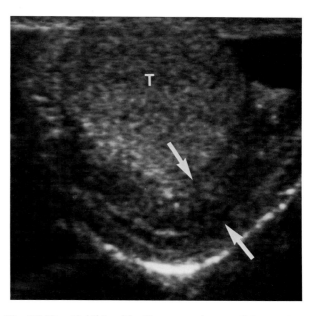

Fig. 16-11. Epididymitis. Transverse image of the scrotum showing a markedly thickened epididymis (arrows) surrounding the testicle *(T)*. (See also Plate 16-2.)

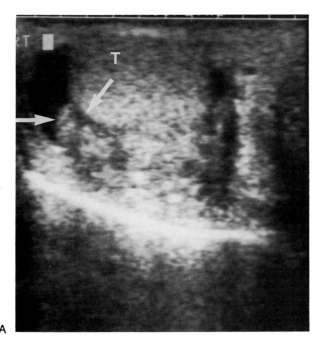 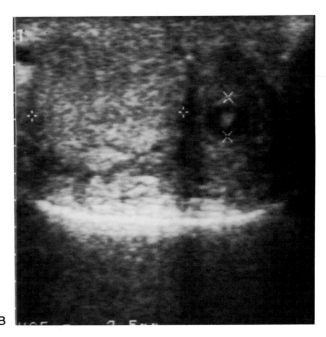

A B

Fig. 16-12. Epididymitis with epididymal abscess. **(A)** Transverse sonogram showing marked thickening of the epididymal body (arrows) behind testicle *(T)*. **(B)** Longitudinal image of the thickened epididymal tail inferior to the testicle ('+' calipers), which contains a hypoechoic collection ('X' calipers) due to abscess.

formity, is bilateral in 40 percent of cases.[21,22] It results in an excessively mobile testicle that is at risk for twisting on its narrow stalk. Torsion occurs when the testicle turns one or more times on this short mesenteric stalk, obstructing blood flow and leading to severe pain.[23] Initially, the veins in the twisted cord are compressed, lead-

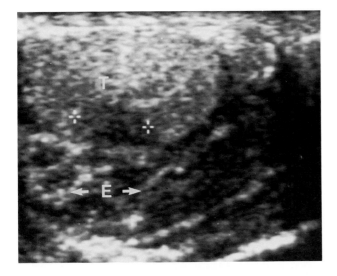

Fig. 16-13. Focal orchitis. Scrotal sonogram demonstrating a poorly defined hypoechoic area (calipers) in the testicle *(T)* adjacent to thickened epididymis *(E*, arrows).

ing to congestion and edema in the testicle and along the spermatic cord. Eventually, pressure within the testicle rises to the point of arterial obstruction, which in turn leads to testicular ischemia and sometimes hemorrhage. The later the diagnosis is made, the greater the likelihood of testicular necrosis. In particular, the testicle is virtually always unsalvageable if diagnosis is delayed beyond 24 hours.[22]

The ultrasound image is normal in the early stages of torsion, up to approximately 4 hours after the cord has twisted. Spectral and color Doppler, on the other hand, are abnormal during this period, demonstrating absence of flow within the testicle and epididymis.[3,23] It is important to compare Doppler signals from the affected and unaffected sides to ensure that the Doppler settings are appropriate for detecting normal testicular flow. In some cases, color Doppler may identify twisted blood vessels that terminate abruptly in the spermatic cord.[24]

The ultrasound image becomes abnormal after about 4 hours, demonstrating an enlarged, hypoechoic testicle (Fig. 16-14). Heterogeneous areas of increased and decreased echogenicity may be seen within the testicle if hemorrhage has occurred. Other findings include enlargement of the epididymis, reactive hydrocele, and scrotal wall thickening.[3,10,25] As in the early phase of torsion, Doppler demonstrates absence of flow within the testicle and epididymis. In this latter phase, increased

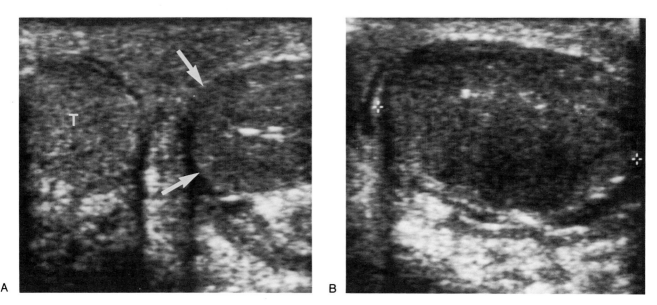

Fig. 16-14. Testicular torsion. **(A)** Transverse image of the left testicle (arrows), which is enlarged and diffusely hypoechoic compared with the normal right testicle *(T)*. **(B)** Sagittal image of the enlarged, diffusely hypoechoic left testicle (calipers).

flow may be identified in the scrotal wall as a result of reactive hyperemia.

If the condition is left untreated, the swelling resolves and the testicle ultimately atrophies. At this stage, ultrasound demonstrates a small, hypoechoic testicle.

Clinically, it may be difficult to distinguish torsion from epididymitis/orchitis. Prior to the introduction of duplex ultrasound (combining imaging and Doppler), radionuclide scanning was the only accepted method for distinguishing between these two pathologic entities. Duplex ultrasound now provides an alternative method with similar accuracy and greater convenience.[24,26,27]

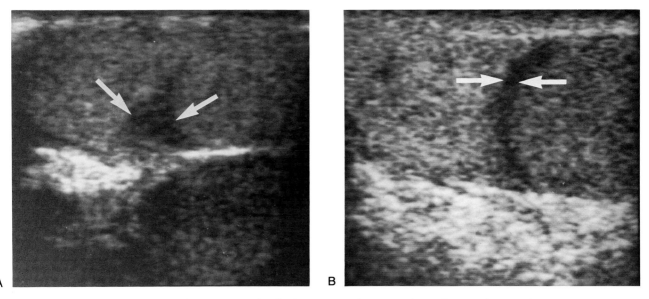

Fig. 16-15. Wedge infarction. **(A)** Longitudinal sonogram demonstrating a focal testicular infarct (arrows), which is wedge-shaped and extends to the periphery of the testicle. **(B)** Follow-up sonogram 5 months later demonstrating narrowing of the wedge infarction to a thinner hypoechoic band (arrows) in the testicle.

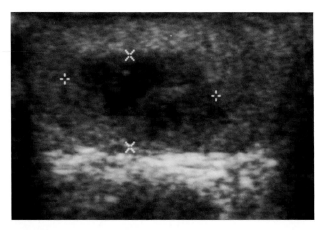

Fig. 16-16. Focal infarction. Testicular sonogram demonstrating a complex mass (calipers) in the testicle due to infarction. This mass is indistinguishable from a tumor sonographically.

INFARCTS

Patients with focal infarction of testicular parenchyma commonly present with pain. The typical sonographic appearance of an acute infarct is a wedge-shaped hypoechoic lesion extending to the periphery of the tes-

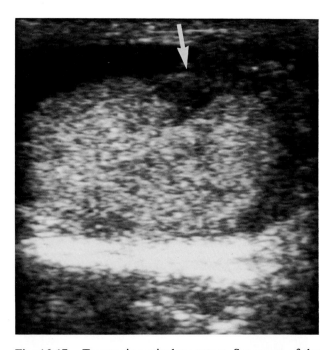

Fig. 16-17. Traumatic testicular rupture. Sonogram of the right scrotum demonstrating abrupt interruption of the oval contour of the testicle (arrow) due to rupture of the tunica albuginea. Hypoechoic extruded testicular parenchyma and blood are seen surrounding the testicular remains. Echoes in fluid surrounding the testicle represent a hematocele.

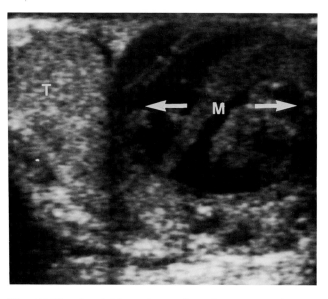

Fig. 16-18. Scrotal hematoma. Scrotal sonogram demonstrating a complex mass (*M*, arrows) of resolving hematoma adjacent to and compressing the testicle *(T)*.

ticle (Fig. 16-15). Cystic areas may develop within the lesion as a result of hemorrhage and necrosis. With time, the wedge becomes thinner and may eventually resolve to a linear hypoechoic scar[11] (Fig. 16-15).

Occasionally, an infarct will not extend to the tunica albuginea, but instead will appear as a hypoechoic intratesticular mass surrounded by normal parenchyma (Fig. 16-16). This appearance may be indistinguishable from that of a malignant tumor.

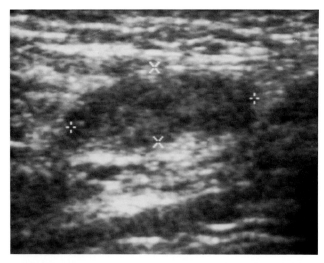

Fig. 16-19. Undescended testicle. Sonogram of the left groin demonstrating an ovoid mass (calipers) attributable to the atrophic cryptorchid testicle. The testicle is smaller and less echogenic than a normal testicle.

TRAUMA

Trauma to the scrotum may lead to disruption or contusion of the testicular parenchyma, rupture of the tunica albuginea, and hematomas involving the testicle, epididymis, tunica vaginalis (hematocele), or scrotal wall. Surgical intervention is usually required only when the tunica albuginea is ruptured.

Ultrasound is useful for management of patients with testicular trauma because it can accurately delineate the extent of injury. Testicular parenchymal injury or hemorrhage appears as alteration of the normally homogeneous echotexture. Rupture of the tunica albuginea is diagnosed on the basis of loss of the smooth testicular contour and discontinuity of the echogenic line representing the tunica albuginea (Fig. 16-17). Hematomas in the epididymis or scrotal wall have a variable sonographic appearance. Like hematomas elsewhere in the body, their echocharacteristics depend in large part on their age (Fig. 16-18). Hematoceles appear as complex fluid collections surrounding the testicle.[1]

CRYPTORCHIDISM

Undescended testes are usually located at or below the inguinal ring.[8,28,29] If orchiopexy is not performed at an early age, they become atrophic and are at high risk for cancer. Ultrasound is useful for locating these testes if orchidectomy is planned. Sonographically, they are ovoid structures that are smaller and more hypoechoic than normal testicles (Fig. 16-19). As mentioned above, ultrasound is also useful to screen for cancer in patients with surgically corrected cryptorchidism, as these testicles are at an intermediate risk for cancer.

EXTRATESTICULAR ABNORMALITIES

Epididymal Cysts

Spermatoceles are benign cysts arising from the ducts in the epididymis. They often occur as a result of a previous inflammatory process. The cysts are located most often in the head of the epididymis, but also may be seen in the epididymal body or tail. They may be single or multiple, and their frequency increases with age.

Sonographically, they appear as extratesticular lesions that are round and anechoic with thin smooth walls and distal acoustic enhancement (Fig. 16-20). Their size is variable, up to several centimeters in diameter.

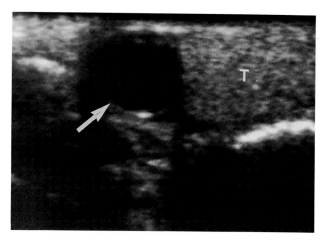

Fig. 16-20. Spermatocele. Longitudinal scrotal image demonstrating a cyst (arrow) in the epididymal head above the testicle *(T)*.

Masses

Extratesticular solid masses are usually benign tumors arising from the epididymis, tunica albuginea, or spermatic cord. Those arising from the spermatic cord are most often of mesenchymal origin, whereas those arising from the tunica or epididymis are often benign adenomatoid tumors.[6,11]

A major role of ultrasound in evaluating an extratesticular mass is in determining its location, and, in particular, verifying that it lies outside the testicle (Fig. 16-21). Ultrasound can also accurately differentiate cystic lesions, especially spermatoceles, from solid masses. Mesenchymal tumors of the spermatic cord, including fibromas, lipomas, and angiomas, are located along the

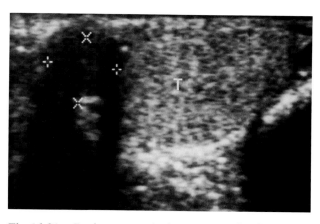

Fig. 16-21. Benign extratesticular mass. Longitudinal scan of the right scrotum showing a well-defined hypoechoic mass (calipers) superior to and separate from the testicle *(T)*.

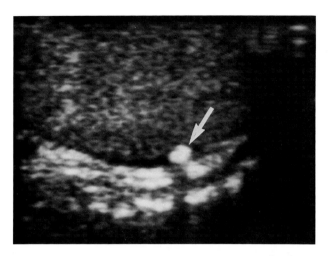

Fig. 16-22. Scrotal calculus. Sonogram demonstrating freely mobile calculus (arrow) in the scrotum between the layers of the tunica vaginalis.

Varicoceles

A varicocele is dilatation of the veins in the pampiniform plexus of the spermatic cord. It is usually unilateral, occurring more commonly on the left than the right, but may be bilateral. Varicoceles may cause infertility because they are associated with low sperm counts and decreased motility. This may be the result of increased intrascrotal temperature. Surgical repair of a varicocele frequently results in improved fertility.[30]

On ultrasound, a varicocele appears as an extratesticular collection of serpiginous structures measuring at least 2 mm in diameter (Fig. 16-23 and Plate 16-3). Having the patient perform the Valsalva maneuver or stand may increase venous diameter, making the varicocele more obvious. Blood flow may be identifiable by Doppler, especially during the Valsalva maneuver (Fig. 16-23 and Plate 16-3). This occasionally helps to confirm the diagnosis of varicocele, but failure to detect flow does not exclude this diagnosis since the velocity may be too low to detect.[1]

Hydrocele

A hydrocele is a collection of fluid in the scrotum between the visceral and parietal layers of the tunica vaginalis. Hydroceles may be congenital or acquired. Acquired hydroceles are often idiopathic but may be the result of intrascrotal inflammation or, rarely, a tumor.

course of the spermatic cord and usually are homogeneous in echotexture with clearly defined margins. Adenomatoid tumors are usually small, less than 1 cm in diameter, with homogeneous echogenicity similar to or slightly more echogenic than that of testicular parenchyma.[6] Scrotal calculi are freely mobile calcifications located between the layers of the tunica vaginalis. They are brightly echogenic and cast an acoustic shadow (Fig. 16-22).

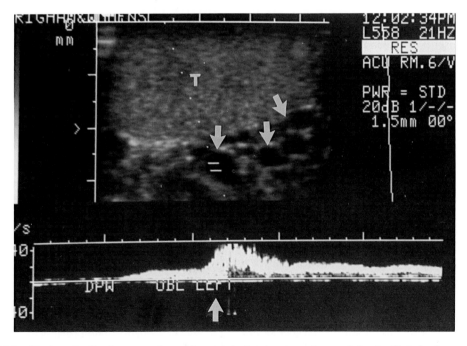

Fig. 16-23. Varicocele. Duplex scan of serpiginous tubular structures (arrows) due to dilated veins are identified around the testicle *(T)*. Doppler interrogation demonstrates venous flow on the waveform below the image. The flow was augmented (arrowhead) by performing the Valsalva maneuver. (See also Plate 16-3.)

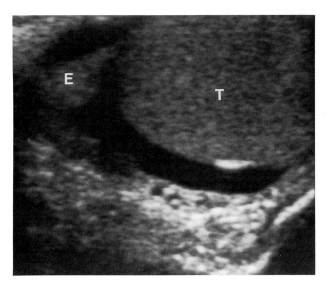

Fig. 16-24. Hydrocele. Longitudinal sonogram demonstrating increased fluid around the testicle *(T)* and epididymis *(E)* between the layer of the tunica vaginalis.

On ultrasound, anechoic fluid is seen in the scrotum surrounding the testicle and epididymis (Fig. 16-24), except where the testicle is anchored to the scrotal wall at the bare area. In some cases, small particles or septations are seen in the fluid. Sonography can be helpful in deter-

mining the etiology of acquired hydroceles, especially when evaluating the testicle for cancer when scrotal distension limits the reliability of the physical examination.

Hernia

In an inguinal hernia a section of the bowel can herniate through a patent processus vaginalis into the scrotum. The patient may present with scrotal enlargement of unknown etiology. Ultrasound is helpful for excluding other causes of scrotal enlargement such as a mass, cyst, or hydrocele. In some cases, ultrasound will make the definitive diagnosis of hernia by demonstrating peristalsing loops of bowel in the scrotum[11] (Fig. 16-25).

REFERENCES

1. Benson CB, Doubilet PM, Richie JP: Sonography of the male genital tract. AJR 1989;153:705
2. Middleton WD, Thorne D, Melson GL: Color Doppler ultrasound of the normal testes. AJR 1989;152:293
3. Tumeh SS, Benson CB, Richie JP: Acute disease of the scrotum. Semin Ultrasound CT MR 1991;12:115
4. Tanagho EA: Anatomy and surgical approach to the urogenital tract. p. 46. In Walsh PC, Gittes RF, Perlmutter AD, Stamey TA (eds): Campbell's Urology, 5th Ed. WB Saunders, Philadelphia, 1986
5. Gray H, Goss CM: Anatomy of the human body, 29th Ed. Lea & Febiger, Philadelphia, 1973
6. Benson CB: The role of ultrasound in diagnosis and staging of testicular cancer. Semin Urol 1988;6:189
7. Garnick MB, Prout GR, Canellos GP: Germinal tumors of the testis. p. 1937. In Holland JF, Frei E (eds): Cancer Medicine. Lea & Febiger, Philadelphia, 1982
8. Krone KD, Carroll BA: Scrotal ultrasound. Radiol Clin North Am 1985;23:121
9. Paulson DF, Einhorn L, Peckham M, Williams SD: Cancer of the testis. p. 786. In DeVita VT, Hellman S, Rosenberg SA (eds): Cancer—Principles and Practice of Oncology. JB Lippincott, Philadelphia, 1982
10. Hill MC, Sanders RC: Sonography of benign disease of the scrotum. Ultrasound Annu 1986;197
11. Doherty FJ: Ultrasound of the nonacute scrotum. Semin Ultrasound CT MR 1991;12:131
12. Shawker TH, Javadpour N, O'Leary T et al: Ultrasonographic detection of "burned-out" primary testicular germ cell tumors in clinical normal testes. J Ultrasound Med 1983;2:477
13. Grantham JG, Charboneau JW, James EM et al: Testicular neoplasms: 29 tumors studied by high-resolution US. Radiology 1985;157:775
14. Bohle A, Studer UE, Sonntag RW et al: Primary or secondary extragonadal germ cell tumors? J Urol 1986; 135:939

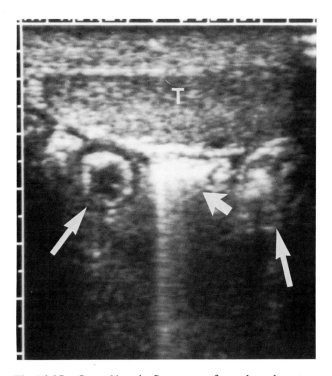

Fig. 16-25. Scrotal hernia. Sonogram of an enlarged scrotum demonstrating multiple loops of peristalsing bowel (arrows) including air in some loops (short arrow). The herniated bowel is compressing the testicle *(T)*.

15. Phillips G, Kumari-Subaiva S, Sawitsky A: Ultrasonic evaluation of the scrotum in lymphoproliferative disease. J Ultrasound Med 1987;6:169

16. Hamm B, Fobbe F, Loy V: Testicular cysts: differentiation with ultrasound and clinical findings. Radiology 1988; 168:19

17. Rifkin MD, Jacobs JA: Simple testicular cyst diagnosed preoperatively by ultrasound. J Urol 1983;129:982

18. Gooding GAW, Leonhardt W, Stein R: Testicular cysts: US findings. Radiology 1987;163:537

19. Doherty FJ, Mullins TL, Sant GR et al: Testicular microlithiasis: a unique sonographic appearance. J Ultrasound Med 1987;6:389

20. Lentini JF, Benson CB, Richie JP: Sonographic features of focal orchitis. J Ultrasound Med 1989;8:361

21. Kogan SJ: Acute and chronic scrotal swellings. p. 1947. In Gullenwater JY, Grayhack JT, Howards SS et al (eds): Adult and Pediatric Urology. Year Book Medical Publishers, New York, 1987

22. Rajfer J: Testicular torsion. p. 1962. In Walsh PC, Gittes RF, Perlmutter AD, Stamey TA (eds): Cambell's Urology. 5th Ed. Vol. 2. WB Saunders, Philadelphia, 1986

23. Middleton WD, Siegel BA, Melson GL et al: Acute scrotal disorders: prospective comparison of color Doppler US and testicular scintigraphy. Radiology 1990;177:177

24. Ralls PW, Larsen D, Johnson MB, Lee KP: Color Doppler sonography of the scrotum. Semin Ultrasound CT MR 1991;12:109

25. Fowler RC, Chennells PM, Ewing R: Scrotal ultrasonography: a clinical evaluation. Br J Radiol 1987;60:649

26. Jenson MC, Lac KP, Halls JM, Rall PW: Color Doppler sonography in testicular torsion. J Clin Ultrasound 1990;18:446

27. Ralls PW, Jenson MC, Lac KP et al: Color Doppler sonography in acute epididymitis and orchitis. J Clin Ultrasound 1990;18:383

28. Weiss RM, Carter AR, Rosenfield AT: High resolution real-time ultrasonography in the localization of the undescended testis. J Urol 1986;135:936

29. Friedland GW, Chang P: The role of imaging in the management of the impalpable undescended testis. AJR 1988;151:1107

30. Sherins RJ, Howards SS: Male infertility. p. 640. In Walsh PC, Gittes RF, Perlmutter AD, Stamey TA (eds): Campbell's Urology. 5th Ed. WB Saunders, Philadelphia, 1986

17

Prostate

David Thickman
Steve H. Parker

Until recently, the primary method for the evaluation of the prostate gland was digital rectal examination (DRE). While this simple, inexpensive technique remains valuable, the imaging modalities of ultrasound, computed tomography (CT), and magnetic resonance imaging (MRI) play a significant role in the diagnosis and assessment of prostate disease. Transabdominal and transperineal ultrasound techniques visualize the prostate, but lack sufficient anatomic definition to be useful in identifying prostate cancer.[1-3] In 1974, Watanabe et al[4] developed a special chair for transrectal ultrasound (TRUS) of the prostate. The development of handheld gray-scale transrectal sonography in the 1980s made examination of the internal architecture and anatomy possible, as well as the detection of abnormalities. These developments have placed TRUS in the first line in the diagnosis of prostate disease. This chapter reviews the anatomy of the prostate and surrounding tissues, the sonographic appearance of the normal prostate and seminal vesicles, the technique of endorectal sonography, biopsy techniques, diseases affecting the prostate, and the position of transrectal ultrasound in the diagnostic armamentarium including its potential future contributions.

TECHNIQUE

Most top-of-the-line ultrasound equipment manufacturers offer state-of-the-art endoluminal probes for the examination of the prostate gland. While early transduc-

ers used the 3.5-MHz crystals, newer transducers are using higher frequencies, up to 7 or 10 MHz. These provide improved anatomic detail and contrast resolution. A variety of transducer types have been used: mechanical sector, phased array, linear, and curved linear transducers. Some of these are side-fire and others are end-fire. Furthermore, some have been combined into single probes, thus permitting examination in transverse or longitudinal planes with a single endorectal insertion. Unfortunately, this advantage of the biplane probes is lost sometimes when sonographically guided biopsy of the prostate is considered since transrectal biopsy using these probes can be difficult. Most probes for biopsy have been designed with the transducer oriented to give a longitudinal view of the prostate gland.

The linear and curved linear transducers give a rectangular field of view. Most phased array and sector scanners produce a pie-shaped sector with fields of view between 90 and 110 degrees. Some mechanical sector equipment provides rotational modes yielding a 360 degree field of view in the transverse plane.

The ease of performing the examination has improved considerably in the last decade from the time the patient was asked to insert into his rectum a rigid transducer fixed to a chair. The surfaces of the probes currently in use are coated with a coupling agent before insertion. A condom or two affixed to the transducer with rubber bands is used to cover the transducer and assure cleanliness. Some transducers have a built-in separate channel through which water can be instilled to create a water path or standoff. This permits placement of the prostate in the focal zone of the transducer, removes the prostate from near-field artifact, and places the prostate within the larger field of view of the sector image. Some transducers, particularly the linear array and curved linear array varieties, do not require a water path.

It is typical to have patients prepare for the examination by administration of an enema 2 hours before the study. This removes fecal material that may interfere with the quality of the examination. Additionally, having the patient arrive with a full bladder provides the opportunity to determine the amount of residual urine in the bladder following voiding.

It is easiest to place the patient in a decubitus position on a standard stretcher or examining table. Prior to insertion of the transducer, a digital rectal examination is performed. The probe should be well lubricated and inserted with the transducer facing anteriorly toward the prostate. Initial posterior direction of the tip will aid insertion and conform to the anatomic structure of the rectum. The probe should be well situated within the rectum at the level of the prostate prior to insufflation of the water path.

The prostate should be fully examined in the transverse and longitudinal planes. The examination should extend from the most superior extent of the seminal vesicles and bladder base to the apex of the prostate and membranous urethra. Longitudinal examination extends from the most right lateral extent of the seminal vesicle and border of the prostate to the similar area on the opposite side. All areas must be seen in two planes. In addition to the seminal vesicles, prostate, and bladder base, attention must be paid to the periprostatic tissues and rectal wall. All of these structures should be well documented in both planes. Following the examination the transducer is cleaned and should be placed in a sterilizing and disinfecting solution.

Biopsy

Although interventional techniques using ultrasound are covered in Chapter 19, some aspects of biopsy of the prostate using ultrasound guidance are covered briefly here. Transperineal and transrectal biopsy are the most common routes of obtaining prostate tissue using ultrasound guidance. Transrectal biopsy is performed at most centers because it is fast, easy to perform, and is very well tolerated by the patient. Most biopsies of the prostate are performed using a core needle, between 18 and 14 gauge. The Biopty gun (Radiplast, Uppsala, Sweden) and its disposable analogs have made obtaining excellent tissue material routine (Fig. 17-1). Serious bleeding complications from prostate biopsy are extremely rare. Hematuria or hematospermia occur in up to two-thirds of cases, but generally resolve without medical treatment.[5] Infection is likely to be the most devastating complication and occurs in approximately 16 percent of patients without antibiotic prophylaxis.[5] It is now standard practice to begin a course of appropriate antibiotics the day before the performance of transrectal biopsy. This reduces the complication rate to 2.4 to 5.8 percent.[6,7]

Using a longitudinally oriented transducer and a biopsy guide, the core needle can be inserted into suspicious areas within the prostate gland under direct sonographic visualization. This permits biopsies to be performed on suspicious areas identified by sonography and DRE. The accuracy of a prostatic biopsy approaches 100 percent[8]; this is likely an overestimation since 30 percent of cancers have been discovered by random performance of prostate biopsy of regions believed to be normal by transrectal ultrasound.[6,9] Ultrasound-guided biopsies are better than digitally guided biopsies. Studies

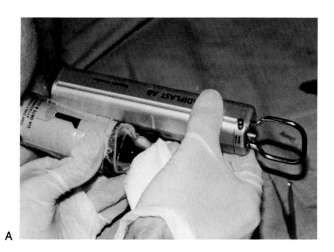
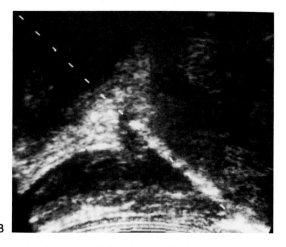

A

B

Fig. 17-1. (A) This photograph shows the endorectal transducer in the operator's left hand with the transrectal biopsy device inserted in tandem with the right hand. (B) The echogenic needle is seen along the biopsy tract projected as dashed lines. The ultrasound biopsy guide permits accurate and predictable placement of the needle.

have shown that ultrasound-guided biopsies are positive in nearly all cases of positive DRE-guided biopsies and detect cancer in 53 percent of patients with negative DRE-guided biopsy.[6] However, it should be noted that the histologic tumor grade from radical prostatectomy specimens is higher than the grade obtained from biopsy specimens in 26 percent of cases.[10] In approximately 69 percent there will be agreement between biopsy and prostate specimen histologic grade, and in 5 percent the grade of the tumor found in the radical prostatectomy specimen will be lower than that found in the biopsy specimen.

In addition to ultrasound visualization of palpable lesions and of suspicious areas in the prostate gland, ultrasound-guided prostate biopsy can be used to locally stage prostate cancers. Biopsies of areas of extraprostatic abnormality can be performed, including bladder, rectum, and seminal vesicle (Fig. 17-2). Furthermore, by proper placement of the biopsy device, specimens that include the extraprostatic tissue, the prostate capsule, and the gland or tumor can be obtained. This approach can provide histologic confirmation of local staging of prostate cancer.

EMBRYOLOGY

At the end of the first trimester of fetal life, androgenic hormones from the fetal testes cause the epithelium of the cranial portion of the urethra, the urogenital sinus, to proliferate into the surrounding mesenchyme and form prostatic buds. Prior to this the bladder, urethra, and mesenchyme have developed. At this stage, the ejacula-

tory ducts can be identified penetrating a small, flattened verumontanun. The prostate arises from the proximal urethra, which already shows the anterior angulation of the adult configuration. Early outgrowths, 14 to 20 in number, arise from the endoderm of the urogenital sinus that surrounds the urethra; some of these regress. Initially these outgrowths, which are the glandular epithelium of the prostate, are solid. As they invest the acinus, they begin to branch, become tubular, and invade the surrounding mesenchyme, which is differentiating into muscular tissue. As the prostate grows, it incorporates striated muscle from the urethral sphincter. Most of the growth is along the lateral aspects, which gives rise to the outer glandular zone. Outgrowth from the dorsal wall produces the internal zone of glandular tissue.[11,12]

The male urethra contains the prostatic urethra and the portions derived from the urogenital sinus. The prostatic urethra is derived from the vesicourethral portion of the cloaca, and the incorporated ends of the mesospheric ducts. The remainder of the prostatic urethra is formed from the urogenital sinus. The verumontanum and the utricle lie in the midportion of the prostatic urethra. The fused caudal tip of the müllerian ducts is believed to induce formation of the midline müllerian tubercle by contact with the urogenital sinus. The müllerian tubercle gives rise to the prostatic utricle.

The epididymis, vas deferens, and ejaculatory ducts are formed from the mesonephric duct (wolffian duct). At the beginning of the second trimester, a swelling at the termination of the mesonephric duct begins formation of the seminal vesicle. The seminal vesicle elongates. Diverticula bud from the wall of the duct producing numerous convoluted channels. During the third trimester, the enlargement of the seminal vesicles causes them to move from posterior to the trigone of the bladder to their normal anatomic position at the side of the trigone beneath the bladder base.[3,11-13]

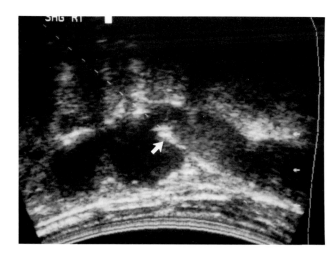

Fig. 17-2. Biopsy of seminal vesicle. Ultrasound can be used to accurately guide transrectal biopsy of tissues adjacent to the prostate, in this case, the seminal vesicle. The needle generates a linear echogenic focus (arrow) along the predicted biopsy path.

NORMAL ANATOMY

The prostate is a firm conical structure located behind the inferior border of the symphysis pubis, anterior to the rectum, directly inferior to the urinary bladder, and superior to the superficial transverse perineal muscle and perineal body. It completely surrounds the proximal urethra and is composed of glandular and fibromuscular tissue. It sits in the low pelvis like an inverted pyramid with the larger base superior and the smaller apex inferior. The prostate is surrounded by a capsule composed of an inner layer of smooth muscle and an outer layer of collagen. There is marked variability in the amounts of these tissues and the prostatic capsule should not be regarded as a well-defined structure. There are several breaches of the capsule: bladder neck, entrance of ejaculatory ducts and neurovascular bundle, and the anterior apex.

The prostate measures approximately 5 cm transversely at the base, by 2 cm from anterior to posterior, and by 3 cm longitudinally. It weighs approximately 20 g. The prostate can be described using two anatomic systems. The classic method divides the prostate into five lobes.[11] The anterior lobe is situated between the anterior border of the prostate and the urethra. The median lobe is the area of the prostate between the ejaculatory ducts and the urethra. The posterior lobe is bounded by the ejaculatory ducts anteriorly and by the posterior border of the prostate. The remaining two lobes of the prostate are the right and left lateral lobes, which make up the mass of the gland. They are contiguous with the posterior lobe and the urethra. Anteriorly they are joined by the isthmus, a band of fibromuscular tissue.

While this anatomic description of the prostate is useful in respect to physical examination and staging of prostate cancer, a second system based on internal histologic architecture is more commonly used in the description of imaging studies and is helpful in using location to identify probable disease. This schema divides the prostate into zones based on differences in histologic composition first popularized by McNeal.[13] An advantage of this system is that certain disease processes, such as benign prostatic hyperplasia, originate in the inner area of the gland, whereas other diseases, such as prostate cancer, have a tendency to arise in the outer portion of the gland. Furthermore, these zones can be distinguished by TRUS and MRI.

The zonal anatomy of the prostate is somewhat like peeling an onion. The central landmark of this model is the urethra, which makes a 35-degree bend in the middle of the prostate (Figs. 17-3 and 17-4). The apex of the angle divides the urethra into proximal and distal portions of nearly equal size. Periurethral glands are scattered the length of the proximal urethra. About 90 percent of the ducts of the prostate gland and the ejaculatory ducts empty into the distal prostatic urethra. The verumontanum and utricle are part of the distal urethra. The entire length of the prostatic urethra is surrounded by sphincteric muscle and comprises the periurethral zone.

The peripheral zone of the prostate is the most posterior portion and comprises the largest portion of the prostate gland. It is composed of small acini with smooth walls lined by simple columnar epithelium. It makes up 70 percent of the normal gland. Just deep to the peripheral zone is the central zone, which makes up about 20 percent of the prostate gland. The anterior border of the central zone is formed by the urethra, the small periurethral zone, and the lateral lobes of the transition zones. The central zone is composed of large irregular spaces of acinar tissue whose ducts enter the convexity of the verumontanum adjacent to the openings of the ejaculatory ducts. Multiple ridges and septi project into the lumen of the gland, which is composed of crowded epithelial cells with large nuclei. The central zone surrounds the ejaculatory ducts, the orifices of which empty at the apex of the verumontanum. The ejaculatory ducts are sur-

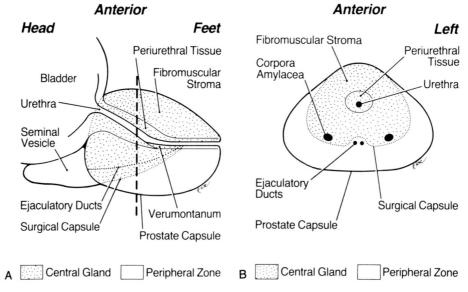

Fig. 17-3. Diagrams of zonal anatomy of the prostate. **(A)** Sagittal diagram shows relationships of urethra to fibromuscular stroma, central gland, and peripheral zone. Note ejaculatory ducts travel in central gland. **(B)** Transverse diagram shows surgical capsule demarcating separation of central gland from peripheral zone. (From Lee et al,[116] with permission.)

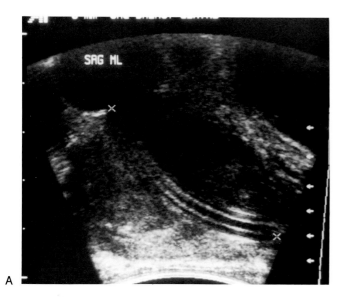 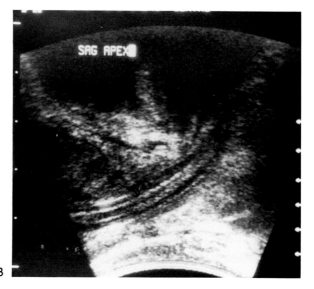

A   B

Fig. 17-4. Sagittal ultrasound of the prostate with Foley catheter in urethra. **(A)** The urethra, which is demarcated by the echogenic borders of the catheter, is seen coursing posteriorly from the bladder within the prostate. **(B)** The urethra makes a gentle angulation at its midportion and then courses anteriorly to the apex of the prostate.

rounded by the thin invaginated extraprostatic space. Thus, the central zone is a cone-shaped area of tissue extending from the base of the prostate to the verumontanum. The boundary between the peripheral zone and the central zone is the surgical capsule (it is not a true capsule). It is formed by the difference in histologic composition of the central and peripheral zones and is so named because it is the level to which the adenomatous gland is removed by transurethral resection.

Just deep to this is the urethra surrounded by the periurethral region containing multiple tiny ducts, acini, and muscle. Posterolateral and slightly superior to the verumontanum are two small lobules of glandular tissue, the transition zone. This accounts for approximately 5 percent of the glandular prostate and is composed of tissue histologically identical to that of the peripheral zone. Finally, the anterior fibromuscular stroma or band extends from the anterior portion of the urethra to the anterior margin of the prostate and from the bladder neck to the apex of the prostate. It is composed mainly of smooth muscle and is a nonglandular portion of the prostate.

In summary, the zonal anatomy of the prostate is based on histologic consideration. This is of consequence in that 70 to 80 percent of cancers arise in the peripheral zone with the remaining portions distributed in the transition zone and central zone. Benign prostatic hyperplasia arises primarily in the central and transition zones.

The complex zonal anatomy is not entirely distingui-

shable by ultrasound. The peripheral zone is generally distinguishable from the central zone, but the central and transition zones have a similar echotexture. Because of its location, the anterior fibromuscular band generally does not produce confusion. This, with transrectal ultrasound, the prostate is generally described as having a peripheral or outer zone and a central or inner zone.

Periprostatic Tissues and Relationships

The prostate sits superior to the urogenital diaphragm. Posteriorly, Denonvilliers fascia and areolar tissue separate the prostate from the rectum. Anterolaterally, the prostate is separated from adjacent structures by fat, lymphatic vessels, nerves, and fascial tissues. The arterial supply branches from the internal iliac artery with major supply entering the prostate at the bladder neck and arborizing over the capsule. The periprostatic venous plexus (Santorini's plexus) courses along the lateral borders of the prostate. It moves anteriorly as it courses inferiorly along the prostate. This venous plexus separates the prostate from the levator ani and obturator interni muscles. The neurovascular bundles enter the posterolateral portion near the base of the prostate on either side. They are composed of the urethral branch off of the inferior vesical artery and nerve branches off of the prostatic plexus, that accompany the vessels. Near the apex of the prostate is an extraprostatic space called the trapezoid area (Fig. 17-5). It is bordered by the mem-

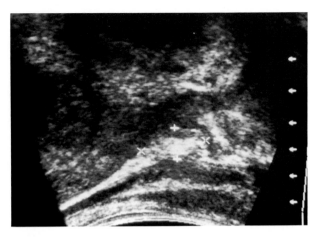

Fig. 17-5. Sagittal ultrasound of the prostate apex shows the normal echogenic trapezoid area (white markers).

branous urethra anteriorly, rectum posteriorly, prostate superiorly, and rectourethralis muscle inferiorly. This area is important because it is contiguous with an area of weakness in the apical prostatic capsule from which tumors can easily invade[8] (Fig. 17-6).

The prostatic portion of the urethra runs approximately 3 cm from the base of the bladder to the end of the prostate. The verumontanum arises near the apex of the slight anterior angulation formed by the superior portion of the prostatic urethra with the inferior portion. The seminal vesicles are two sacs composed of cylindrical tubes between the posterior surface of the bladder and the rectum. They are superior to the prostate. Each is about 3 to 5 cm long and 1 to 2 cm in width. The size of the seminal vesicles decreases insignificantly following

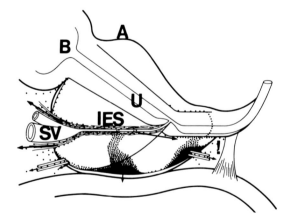

Fig. 17-6. Sagittal diagram of patterns of spread of outer gland tumors including extension into trapezoid area. The arrows and dots show routes of tumor spread. (*A*, anterior; *B*, bladder; *U*, urethra; *SV*, seminal vesicle, *IES,* invaginated extraprostatic space.) (From Lee et al,[8] with permission.)

ejaculation.[14] This convoluted tube ends in a narrow straight duct, which with the ipsilateral vas deferens forms the ejaculatory duct. The ejaculatory ducts enter the base of the prostate in the central zone and run for 2 cm to end in slit-like orifices of the prostatic utricle.

PHYSIOLOGY

The prostate, seminal vesicles, and Cowper's glands produce the seminal fluid that serves as a medium for the transportation of sperm. The vas deferens, which conducts the sperm from the testes, joins with the seminal vesicle to form the ejaculatory duct. The prostate produces a complex fluid with a slightly acid pH, which comprises the major portion of the ejaculation fluid. The seminal vesicles contribute fluid high in sugar (fructose), in addition to amino acids, prostaglandins, and fibrinogen. These fluids are considered to be important in the maintenance and activation of spermatozoa.

NORMAL ULTRASOUND APPEARANCE

A variety of sonographic appearances of the normal prostate gland have been described. All agree that the sonographic appearance is symmetric from side to side. The region of the anterior fibromuscular stroma is hypoechoic and may be anechoic. The periurethral tissues are hypoechoic.[15] At times the opposed borders of the urethra may cause a central area of echogenicity within this zone. The remainder of the prostate has been described as homogeneous hypoechoic or isoechoic tissue and in many cases the zonal anatomy is not distinguished.[16,17] However, with newer higher frequency transducers the peripheral and central zones can be identified (Fig. 17-7). The echogenicity of the central zone has been described as greater than that of the peripheral zone[18] and the central zone has been described as hypoechoic compared with the peripheral zone.[19] It has been our experience that the echotexture of these zones can vary, but typically the homogeneous peripheral zone is somewhat more echogenic than the central zone. The peripheral zone also produces tighter, more compact echoes, whereas the sonographic appearance of the inner zone is one of loose, more heterogeneous echoes. The inner zone appears to become more inhomogeneous and less echogenic with increasing age. In any event, these two zones are generally separated by a thin, curvilinear hypoechoic border that corresponds to the surgical capsule of the prostate[17] (Fig. 17-8). The true prostatic capsule

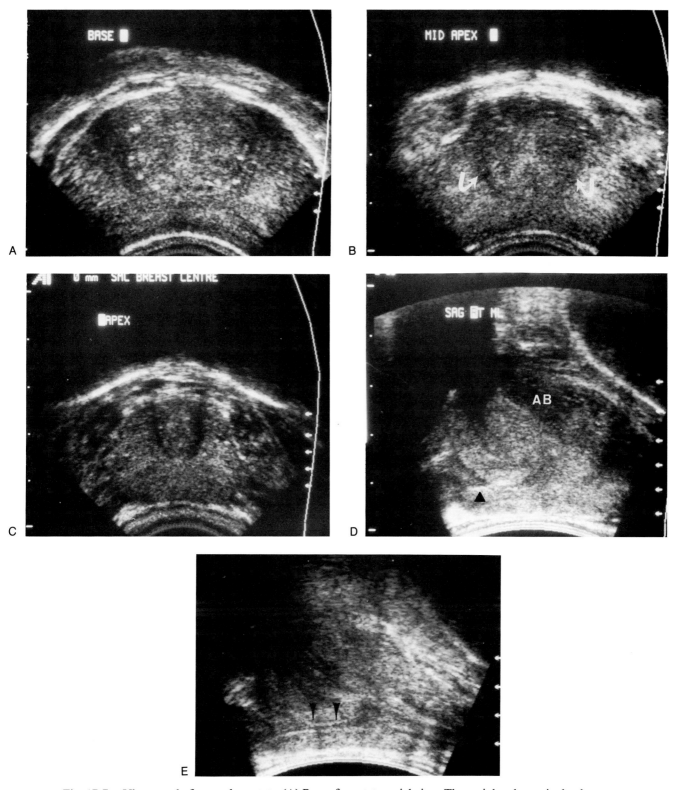

Fig. 17-7. Ultrasound of normal prostate. **(A)** Base of prostate, axial view. The peripheral zone is clearly seen slightly more echogenic than the central gland. The peripheral zone surrounds the posterior and lateral borders of the central gland. **(B)** Middle of the prostate, axial view. The peripheral zone is homogeneous and composed of small tight echoes. It is separated from the central gland by the surgical capsule (arrows). Note the course echotexture of the more hypoechoic central gland. The anterior fibromuscular band is relatively echopenic. **(C)** Apex of prostate, axial view. Most of the gland is composed of peripheral zone at this level. **(D)** Parasagittal view of normal prostate. The entrance of the ejaculatory duct into the prostate produces the beak sign (arrowhead). The anterior fibromuscular band *(AB)* is a broad echopenic area. The peripheral zone is a large homogeneous echogenic area posteriorly. **(E)** Sagittal view of prostate. The ejaculatory ducts (arrowheads) are seen coursing to the verumontanum in the middle of the gland.

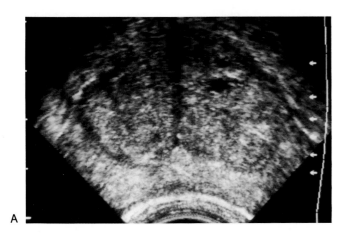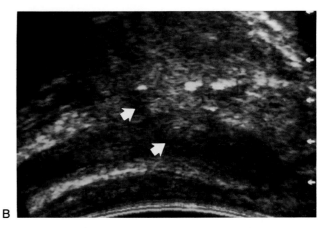

Fig. 17-8. Surgical capsule. **(A)** Axial projections demonstrate the curvilinear appearance of the fairly well-defined hypoechoic surgical capsule. **(B)** Sagittal projection demonstrates well-defined surgical capsule (arrows).

may be seen as a thin echogenic band surrounding the prostate. Many times exact sonographic definition of the capsule is not seen, which is not surprising given its limited histologic delimitation.

The seminal vesicles are typically symmetric structures that are generally more hypoechoic than the prostate.[18-20] They are elongated cones that project like ears from the posterosuperior border of the prostate. Their central portion is hypoechoic with areas of increased echogenicity from the walls of the excretory epithelium. They are surrounded by echogenic fat. The seminal vesicles can be followed inferiorly where they join the ampullary portion of the vas deferens to form the ejaculatory ducts (Fig. 17-9). The angles of the seminal vesicle, which are formed by the entrance of the ejaculatory ducts into the prostate, should be symmetric bilaterally. The area where the duct enters the prostate has been described as having a beak appearance (Fig. 17-7D). The ejaculatory ducts may be traced through the prostate to the slightly echogenic verumontanum (Fig. 17-7E).

Following transurethral prostatectomy, the sonographic appearance of the prostate is altered and varies with the amount of tissue removed, the passage of time since the procedure, and physiologic state such as bladder pressure and micturition (Fig. 17-10). Generally, the post-transurethral resection prostate is thin with a preserved peripheral zone and a scant or absent inner zone. The urethra is widened with a funnel shape, the widest portion at the bladder base.

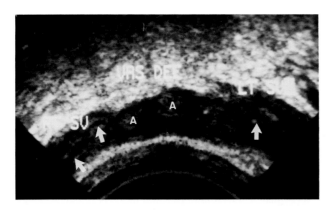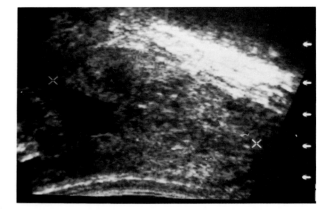

Fig. 17-9. Transverse view of seminal vesicles. The seminal vesicles are cylindrical hypoechoic lobulated structures. Ducts (arrows) are seen as relatively anechoic tubes within the seminal vesicle. The ampullary *(A)* portion of the vas deferens is seen.

Fig. 17-10. Sagittal view of prostate following transurethral resection. The proximal urethra is dilated, portions of the central zone have been removed, and the peripheral zone is preserved.

PROSTATE DISEASE

Adenocarcinoma

Prostate cancer is a pervasive disease and a significant health problem. It is estimated that there will be over 120,000 new cases of prostate cancer in 1991. It is the most common malignancy and the second leading cause of cancer-related death among men in the United States.[21] Interestingly, the age-adjusted cancer death rate from prostate cancer has remained stable for the last 50 years. The age-adjusted mortality for blacks, however, is higher than for whites with the overall 5-year survival being 75 percent for white men and 62 percent for black men. Thirty-four percent of prostate cancers are no longer localized at the time of diagnosis. It seldomly affects men under 45 years of age. Autopsy studies show that prostate cancer may occur in 30 to 40 percent of men over age 60, in half of those over 70, and in up to 80 percent of men 90 years and older.[22]

In addition to age, several factors have been related to the development of prostate cancer. There has been no definite linkage of prostate cancer with benign prostatic hyperplasia, sexual activity, or venereal disease, but it is related to a positive family history. Also, it is related to endogenous hormonal factors and appears to be related to environmental factors, as illustrated by the increased incidence in oriental men in the United States as compared with those in Japan.[3] Preliminary data suggest that there is an increased incidence of lymphoma in patients with prostate cancer.[23]

Adenocarcinoma is by far the most common malignant neoplasm of the prostate. Approximately 70 percent of prostate cancer arises in the peripheral zone. Of the remaining 30 percent, approximately one-third arise in the central zone and two-thirds originate in the transition zone. Localization of a lesion to a particular zone in the prostate is only a guideline as to the likelihood that it is malignant. Malignancies can arise anywhere in the prostate. Furthermore, prostate cancer can be multifocal. In addition to multifocality, the histology of multiple cancers can be heterogeneous (e.g., areas of well-differentiated carcinoma can be found adjacent to areas of poorly differentiated carcinoma in the same specimen).[22] Some authors have noted a relationship between histologic dedifferentiation of tumor and tumor volume.[13,24] It is hypothesized that as the tumor grows, it also becomes less differentiated. Others believe that tumors retain their degree of malignancy and, therefore, poorly differentiated tumors are large because they grow rapidly not because the tumors change their degree of malignancy with growth.[25]

Patients with carcinoma of the prostate often present with symptoms and signs of prostatism, including frequency of micturition, urgency, and hesitancy usually associated with a weak stream. Occasionally, hematuria will be present. Less common presentations include bone pain due to bone metastasis with or without pathologic fracture, obstruction, uremia due to ureteral compression, and change in bowel habits due to compression by the enlarged prostate tumor. Some prostate cancers are found on incidental physical examination or during transurethral resection for benign prostatic hyperplasia.

An elevation of acid phosphatase is highly suggestive of prostate cancer, but is not specific since elevations may be caused by recent invasive procedures, prostate infarction, prostatitis, and biopsy.[26] Furthermore, elevations have been identified following DRE in normal patients. On rare occasions, other nonprostatic malignancies have produced elevations of prostatic acid phosphatase. Acid phosphatase is limited as a screening technique since it is frequently normal in early, limited prostate cancer. Also, up to 22 percent of patients with bone metastasis from prostate cancer have normal serum acid phosphatase levels.[27] Therefore, if the acid phosphatase is normal, prostate cancer is not excluded.

Prostate-specific antigen (PSA) was identified in 1979. It is produced solely by normal and neoplastic ductal tissue of the prostate, and is a well-established monitor of patients who have had radical prostatectomy.[28] In these patients, the PSA should return to normal or female levels. Postoperative elevations in PSA are extremely sensitive in identifying recurrent disease. However, its role as a screening test for prostate cancer is more controversial. Its sensitivity ranges from 73 to 96 percent, but its specificity is limited since PSA elevations can be found in 55 to 85 percent of patients with benign prostatic hyperplasia (BPH) and enlarged glands.[29,30] Furthermore, elevations in PSA can be found following invasive procedures such as digital rectal examination, cytoscopy, and biopsy. The latter can produce up to a 57-fold increase above normal levels.

Histologic grading of prostate cancer is used as a prognostic tool. It is dependent on the degree of cellular differentiation. A multitude of systems have been used including Gleason sums, Gleason grades, M.D. Anderson grades, Mayo Clinic grades, Mostofi grades, and Gaeta grades.[3,31] This proliferation of grading systems is a reflection of disappointment in predicting clinical outcome, complexity of the grading systems, and reproducibility. Since capsular invasion and penetration are highly correlated with tumor volume, and since tumor volume is somewhat correlated with histologic grade, histologic grade of a prostate cancer may predict local invasion.

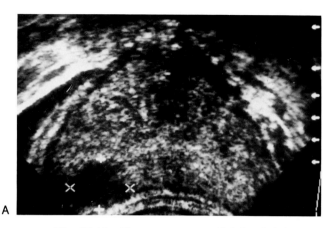

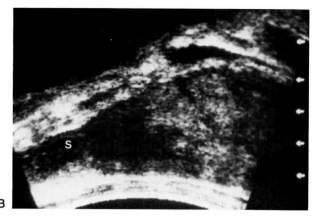

Fig. 17-11. Prostate cancer, well defined. **(A)** Transverse view shows a well-defined hypoechoic lesion in the right peripheral zone (crosshatches). **(B)** The cancer is also seen in the sagittal view. Note the normal seminal vesicle *(S)* junction with the prostate.

Ultrasound Appearance

The historical description of prostate cancer on ultrasound is varied, but it is now generally accepted that early prostate cancer appears as a hypoechoic or echopenic area within the homogeneous prostate gland. Early studies with B-mode and initial gray scale scanners reported prostate cancers to be hyperechoic.[32-35] With improvement in technique and higher frequency transducers, it was recognized that the appearance of most prostate carcinomas, particularly small prostate carcinomas, was hypoechoic (Fig. 17-11). In a review of 221 patients with histologically proven prostate cancer, 96 percent of the cancers were identified as ill-defined hypoechoic areas[36] (Figs. 17-12 and 17-13). This point of view has been further strengthened by comparison with

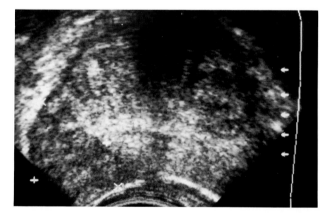

Fig. 17-12. Prostate cancer. Transverse view shows a less well-defined hypoechoic tumor (crosshatches) in the right peripheral zone and extending along the right lateral border.

the gold standard of whole or hemisectioned histologic mounts of prostate specimens. In these studies, the ultrasound appearance of areas of prostate cancer was hypoechoic or slightly hypoechoic in 29.7 to 76 percent, isoechoic in 24 to 56.5 percent, and hyperechoic or mixed in 15 percent.[37-40]

The causes of the varied echographic appearance of prostate cancers remain incompletely understood. In part, the ultrasonographic appearance is related to the variety of histopathologic appearances and cellular compositions of the tumor (Fig. 17-14). There is an association between sonographic appearance and Gleason grade in which the most well-differentiated carcinomas (pattern 1) and intermediate grade tumors (pattern 3) are the most hypoechoic. Tumors that invade and admix with stroma (pattern 2) tend to be isoechoic. Tumors that contain hyperechoic regions correspond to pattern 5.[22] The sonographic appearance has also been related to the degree of stromal fibrosis. With minimal stromal fibrosis, cancers are hypoechoic. With increasing degrees of fibrosis, the sonographic appearance shows increasing echogenicity.[41] Furthermore, the degree of stromal fibrosis is inversely related to the differentiation of the cancer; however, considerable overlap in histologic grade is apparent. On the other hand, in another study the echopenic appearance of prostate cancer was directly related to the amount of gland involved. Isoechoic tumors were less than 0.5 cm and hyperechoic tumors were less than 1 cm, whereas hypoechoic tumors covered the full range with a mean of 3 cm.[38] A unique sonographic appearance of small stippled echogenicity within a hypoechoic lesion has been associated with Gleason pattern 5, comedocarcinoma[40,42] (Fig. 17-15). The regions of increased echogenicity correspond to

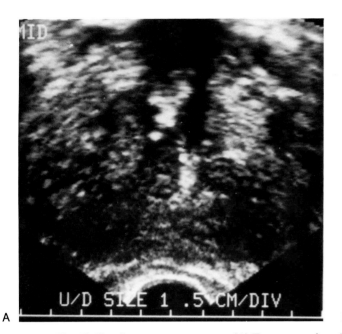

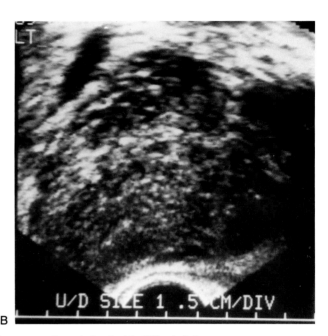

A

B

Fig. 17-13. Large prostate cancer. **(A)** Transverse view shows an enlarged gland with diffusely inhomogeneous echoes, which is confirmed in **(B)** the sagittal view. No well-defined focus is seen. This cancer, which involves the entire gland, can be easily overlooked sonographically.

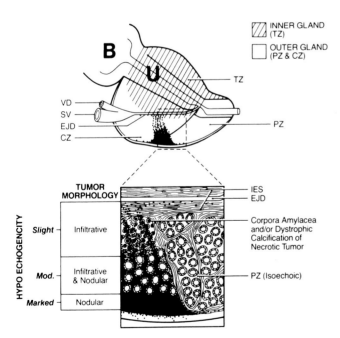

Fig. 17-14. Relationship of echographic appearance to tumor morphology. Tumors become less hypoechoic with increasing tumor infiltration. (*B*, bladder; *U*, urethra; *CZ*, central zone; *PZ*, peripheral zone; *TZ*, transition zone; *EJD,* ejaculatory duct; *SV,* seminal vesicle; *VD,* vas deferens; *IES,* invaginated extraprostatic space.) (From Lee et al,[8] with permission.)

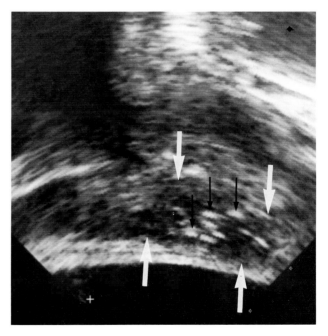

Fig. 17-15. Comedocarcinoma, sagittal view. Within the hypoechoic tumor (white arrows), there are multiple nonshading echogenic structures (black arrows) corresponding to necrotic debris within the acini and ducts of the prostate. (From Lile et al,[42] with permission.)

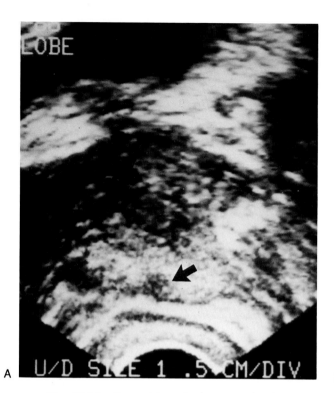

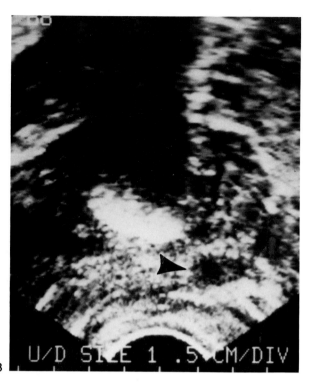

Fig. 17-16. Prostatitis and prostate cancer in same patient. **(A)** Sagittal view of left prostate shows a small hypoechoic area (arrow) in the peripheral zone. Biopsy result showed prostatitis. **(B)** Sagittal view of right prostate shows a small hypoechoic area (arrowhead) in the peripheral zone. The sonographic appearance of this lesion resembles that in Fig. A, but biopsy result showed prostate cancer.

areas of central necrosis and microcalcification within the tumor.

In summary, early prostate cancer is typically recognized as a hypoechoic lesion. Biopsies of areas of asymmetry in gland contour, heterogeneous echotexture, or regions of decreased, increased, or mixed echotexture are likely warranted in the appropriate clinical setting.[43] Biopsies are performed because many benign entities, such as prostatitis, BPH, and infarction may mimic the sonographic appearance of prostate cancer (Figs. 17-16 to 17-18).

The ability of TRUS to detect prostate cancer is better than DRE[28,44,45]; its sensitivity appears to be nearly twice that of DRE. However, the issue of detection of prostate cancer by TRUS remains complex and unsettled. The sensitivity of TRUS in the detection of prostate cancer ranges from 70 to 96 percent, the specificity from 54 to 88 percent, and the predictive value of a positive ultrasound from 47 to 56 percent.[45-48] A better estimation of the accuracy of TRUS for the detection of prostate cancer can be obtained by comparison of sonographic findings with full-mount histopathology. In two studies the sensitivity of TRUS was 52 to 59 percent.[49,50] Our results in 35 patients who underwent radical prostatectomy with comparison of preoperative TRUS with full-

mount histology showed similar results: sensitivity 55 percent and specificity 70 percent for the identification of prostate cancer.[51] Although these studies show a limited sensitivity of TRUS for the identification of individual prostate cancers within the prostate gland, we identified a prostate cancer in 76 percent of patients with prostate cancer.

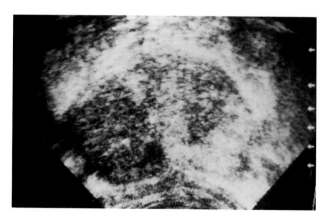

Fig. 17-17. Prostatic infarction, transverse view. The large hypoechoic area in the right prostate resembles carcinoma (see Fig. 17-12). Biopsy result of this nonspecific finding showed bland infarction.

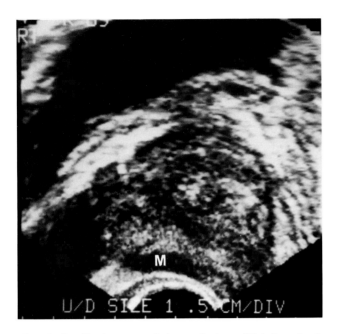

Fig. 17-18. Benign prostatic hyperplasic, sagittal view. A relatively well-defined hypoechoic mass *(M)* is seen in the peripheral zone. It has the classic appearance and location of prostate cancer, but this lesion proved to be prostatic hyperplasia. This is not the typical location for this entity.

Several regimens have been proposed to improve detection by combining TRUS with other means of identifying prostate cancer, such as DRE, PSA, and assessments of prostate volume. In 225 patients with negative DREs, TRUS identified suspicious areas in 96 patients of whom 28 (29 percent) had cancer. PSA levels greater than 4 ng/ml identified 71 percent of the cancers. Examination of the group of patients in whom a biopsy was performed because a suspicious lesion was identified on TRUS, shows that the percent of negative biopsy results is reduced by half when the ultrasound findings are combined with a PSA level greater than 4 ng/ml (50 to 21 percent).[52] Furthermore, the chance of a positive biopsy result is triple for an abnormality identified on sonography when associated with a PSA level greater 4 ng/ml (7 to 22 percent). Others have identified improvement in the positive predictive value for the identification of prostate cancer from 41 percent using TRUS alone to 61 percent using TRUS combined with positive DRE. Additionally, results showed an increase in detection to 52 percent when TRUS was combined with abnormal PSA levels greater than 2.6 ng/ml, and finally, an increase to 71 percent when TRUS was combined with positive DRE and positive PSA.[53] Others have developed an index based on calculations of prostate volume from transverse, longitudinal, and anteroposterior diameters of the prostate gland. Using a ratio of PSA level divided by calculated prostate volume (V), subjects could be grouped into normal, benign disease, and malignant disease categories. Patients with prostate cancer had mean PSA/V ratios of 1.73 (range 0.26 to 5.8) whereas the mean PSA/V ratios for patients with benign disease and normal subjects were all less than 0.2 and had a maximum range value of 0.25.[54] All these regimens may eventually become valuable in improving both the detection of prostate cancer and the specificity of transrectal ultrasound. Ultimately, though, it remains necessary to obtain tissue.

Screening

By far, the most controversial use of TRUS, however, is screening. Supporters of screening point out that TRUS is noninvasive, well tolerated, and detects twice as many cancers as DRE. Thus, supporters believe that DRE should be viewed as an adjunct to TRUS rather than vice versa.[44] Skeptics argue that since only a small percentage of prostate cancers are lethal, early detection of possibly nonlethal cancers is unlikely to change overall mortality rates.[55] Owing to the inherent morbidity and mortality of prostatectomy, skeptics further contend that ultrasound screening could harm more patients, rather than help.

Theoretically, however, TRUS detects only the significant, lethal cancers. Nonlethal cancers, which are present in 30 percent of autopsy specimens in men older than 50 years of age, are quite small with a volume of less than 0.5 cm^3.[44] On the other hand, nonpalpable cancers detected by TRUS tend to be larger,[44] lethal cancers, but they are still less than 1.5 cm and, therefore, potentially curable.[44] In addition, it has been shown that nonpalpable cancers detected by TRUS are just as clinically significant (i.e., by Gleason grade) as palpable tumors when controlled for size and location.[56]

Skeptics cite the substantial cost involved in screening with TRUS because of its low specificity. There is some evidence, however, that the cost of detecting a prostate cancer with TRUS screening is not significantly different than the cost of detecting a breast cancer with mammography screening.[57]

Unlike cervical cancer screening in which one test (Pap smear) serves as the screening tool, any screening program for prostate cancer would likely involve a combination of two or three tests: DRE, TRUS, and PSA. The latter used in a screening manner (PSA > 4.0 ng/ml) detects cancers not suspected on DRE alone.[58] This combination of tests would be similar to breast cancer screening in which clinical examination, mammography, and breast ultrasound combine to elevate the sensitivity of the overall screening.

In light of accumulated TRUS and PSA data, it is apparent that DRE alone should no longer be considered the sole or most useful means of detecting prostate cancer. Eventual screening regimens may well reserve TRUS for those patients with elevated PSA, abnormal DRE or both. Alternatively, TRUS may be used as a "front-line" screening tool in conjunction with DRE and PSA.

Staging

Accurate staging of prostate cancer is critically important because it directly affects therapeutic options and management and alters prognosis. Several staging systems have been proposed, but the two most common are the Whitmore-Jewett and the TNM systems. The Whitmore-Jewett system classifies prostate cancer into four categories: A through D. Stage A tumors which are not palpable and not suspected clinically, are typically diagnosed by transurethral resection of the prostate for BPH or bladder outlet obstruction. Stage A is subdivided into A1 (focal disease) and A2 (diffuse disease). Stage B tumors are confined to the prostate and are palpable on DRE. These tumors, which have not extended beyond the capsule, are subdivided into B1 (focal tumors < 2 cm in size) and B2 (diffuse involvement). Palpable prostate cancers that extend beyond the prostatic capsule but have no evidence of distant metastases are stage C. When there is minimal extracapsular involvement, the cancer may be subclassified stage C1. With more extensive extracapsular extension including bladder outlet obstruction and involvement of the seminal vesicles it is subclassified C2. Prostate cancer that has metastasized to distant areas is stage D. Stage D0 tumors have elevated serum acid phosphatase levels, but normal bone scans. D1 tumors have metastatic pelvic lymph node involvement, and D2 tumors show clinical evidence of metastases to bone, lymph node, or other distant sites. The TNM staging system and the American Urologic Association system are summarized in Table 17-1.

DNA flow cytometry, a technique for quantitating the amount of DNA in tumor cells, has been used preliminarily to yield prognostic information in prostate cancers of advanced stage. It is well recognized that an alteration in the nuclear cytoplasmic ratio is an indicator of cancer. In many cases these alterations are the result of chromosomal changes that are reflected in abnormal DNA content. Using a flow cytometer, the DNA content in tumor cells is measured by a fluorescent technique and displayed as a histogram. Thus, the ploidy of the tumor cells can be determined. One report shows that 15 percent of DNA diploid (normal) tumors and 75 percent of abnormal DNA ploidy patterns (tetraploid or aneuploid) progressed. Furthermore, at 5 years, 21 percent of patients with diploid tumors died, whereas 57 percent of patients with nondiploid prostate cancer died.[59]

Although the choice of the most appropriate treatment for prostate cancer is controversial, it remains essential to accurately stage the disease, because which treatment is chosen (of the multitude that exist) is based on this staging. A radical prostatectomy, an operative procedure designed to cure carcinoma of the prostate, is usually performed only on tumors that are confined to the prostate. Thus it is crucial for an imaging study to distinguish stage B from stage C disease[60] (Fig. 17-19). Differentiation of stage B1 from stage B2 disease may be of prognostic significance in patients undergoing radiation therapy. However, appropriate therapeutic management regarding treatment of patients with stage B or

TABLE 17-1. Comparison of Two Staging Systems for Prostate Cancer

American Urologic Association	TNM
A: no palpable lesion A1: focal A2: diffuse	T0: no evidence of primary tumor T1a: ≤ 3 microscopic foci T1b: > 3 microscopic foci
B: limited to prostate B1: discrete small nodule B2: diffuse	T2: clinical tumor confined to gland T2a: tumor ≤ 1.5 cm greatest diameter T2b: Tumor ≥ 1.5 cm diameter, or more than one lobe
C: local extension C1: < 70 g; no seminal vesicle spread C2: > 70 g; seminal vesicle involved	T3: invades apex, beyond capsule bladder neck, seminal vesicle without fixation T4: fixed or invades adjacent structures other than T3
D: metastatic disease D1: pelvic lymphadenopathy, hydronephrosis D2: bone, distant lymph node, organ or soft tissue metastases	N1: single lymph node ≤ 2 cm N2: single node 2 to ≤ 5 cm, or multiple nodes < 5 cm diameter N3: lymph node metastasis > 5 cm diameter M1: distant metastasis

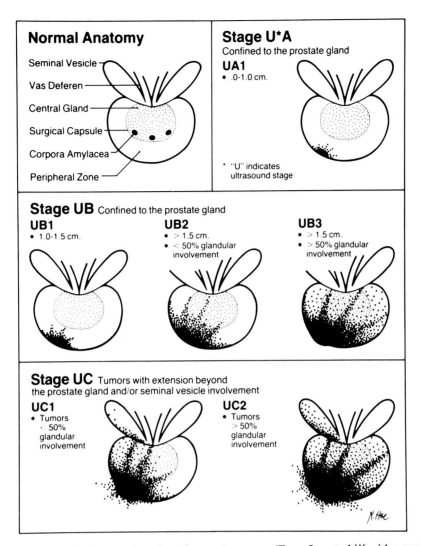

Fig. 17-19. Diagram of ultrasound staging of prostate cancer. (From Lee et al,[116] with permission.)

less prostate cancer remains controversial. In addition, although it is recognized that traditional radical prostatectomy can provide up to 15 years of disease-free survival, there is no firm evidence to support radical prostatectomy rather than radiation therapy.[61-63]

It is well recognized that patients with clinical stage B or less disease will have evidence of capsular penetration or seminal vesicle involvement in 8 to 70 percent of cases. Also, clinical stage B cancers demonstrate more advanced disease at operation around 40 percent of the time or greater.[17,60] It is therefore critical that TRUS identify extracapsular extension and seminal vesicle involvement. Results of numerous studies are disappointing in this regard. The ability of TRUS to differentiate stage B from stage D disease in respect to extracapsular penetration ranges from a sensitivity of 50 to 89 percent, specificity 50 to 91 percent, and a predictive value of a

positive result from 55 to 92 percent.[46,47,64-67] In regard to seminal vesicle involvement, most studies show low sensitivity (20 to 60 percent) and high specificity (89 to 100 percent).[64,66,67] Sensitivities as high as 92 percent with specificities of 99 percent have been reported, but the predictive value of a positive result in this study was only 40 percent.[68] These results are further confirmed by a large multi-institutional trial evaluating TRUS in the staging of prostate cancer. Of 219 patients with preoperative transrectal ultrasonography prior to radical prostatectomy, the sensitivity of transrectal ultrasound for identifying patients with stage C disease was only 66 percent and the specificity for confirming stage B disease was only 46 percent.[50] These data indicate that the value of TRUS in accurate staging of prostate cancer and in distinguishing stage B from stage C disease is limited. However, it must be recognized that TRUS is more accurate than DRE in both the detection and staging of prostate cancer (Figs. 17-20 and 17-21). The ability of TRUS to stage cancer may be improved by using staging-directed transrectal biopsies. Biopsy of the prostate to include the capsule, seminal vesicles, and bladder wall may prove to be effective in more accurately staging this disease, although this awaits confirmation.

There is no well-defined method for a workup of the patient with prostate cancer. For the lesion identified by TRUS, biopsy of suspicious areas, particularly regions that would affect staging, can be performed at the time of prostate biopsy. Patients with elevated alkaline phosphatase and very high PSA levels should have a bone scan. CT evaluation of the abdomen, pelvis, and retroperitoneum is of limited value in early prostate cancer. In those patients clinically believed to have stage C or greater disease, CT can identify and measure sites of involvement for monitoring therapeutic outcome. The role of MRI is unsettled. It holds a great promise in identifying extracapsular extension of prostate cancer. Furthermore, it may detect lymph node involvement and show disease that has metastasized to the bone.

Transrectal ultrasound has been used to monitor patients following operative therapy and chemotherapy (Fig. 17-22). In 20 patients who underwent radical prostatectomy or radical cystoprostatectomy, TRUS identified recurrence in 19 (95 percent).[69] Nearly three-fourths of the recurrences were hypoechoic and the remainder were isoechoic. TRUS was useful in performing biopsies of suspicious areas. However, a potential pitfall was the inability of TRUS to differentiate tumor recurrence from postoperative change and fibrosis.

Ultrasound has also been used to monitor changes in prostate volume in patients undergoing gonadotropin

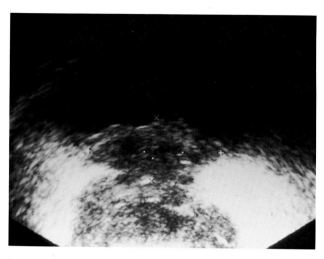

Fig. 17-21. Prostate carcinoma involving the bladder. Axial projection of the base of the prostate demonstrates a hypoechoic lesion (crosshatches) involving the trigone region of the bladder.

releasing hormone (GnRH) analog treatment for prostate cancer.[70] In a small series of 13 patients, TRUS measurement of prostate volume showed a decrease in 12 patients, but an increase in 1. However, clinical responsiveness of disease showed that only eight improved, whereas five progressed. Therefore, measurement of prostate volume by TRUS is of limited value in these patients. The exact role of TRUS of the prostate in monitoring and followup of treated patients remains undetermined. Its place, along with other potential methods such as PSA and MRI, remains to be investigated.

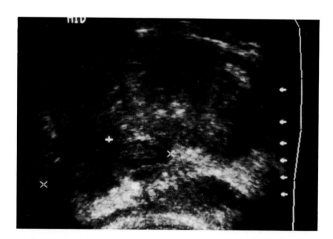

Fig. 17-20. Prostate carcinoma involving the rectum. Axial projection of the midgland of the prostate demonstrates a hypoechoic lesion (crosshatches) involving the peripheral zone of the right lobe extending into the rectum.

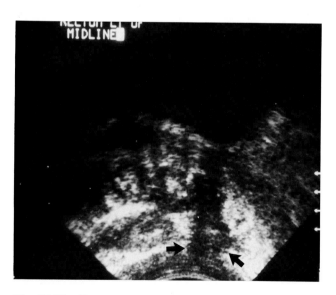

Fig. 17-22. Recurrent prostate carcinoma. Columnar hypoechoic region (arrows) extending from the bladder to the rectum is biopsy-proven recurrent prostate carcinoma 3 years after prostatectomy.

Lymphoma

Lymphoma involvement of the prostate is rare. Primary lymphoma of the prostate makes up less than 0.2 percent of extranodal non-Hodgkins' lymphoma. Secondary involvement of the prostate is estimated to occur more frequently, generally less than 10 percent of cases (range 8 to 20 percent of cases).[71,72] Lymphoma of the prostate occurs in a wide-ranged age group with a mean of about 60 years. Patients present with obstructive symptoms, abdominal mass, hematuria, or sepsis. The median survival of patients with lymphoma of the prostate is 13 months.[73]

Enlargement of the gland may be identified by TRUS. Focal and diffuse hypoechoic areas within the prostate are seen with lymphomatous involvement.[72]

Sarcomas

Adenocarcinoma of the prostate is by far the most common malignancy of this gland. Sarcomas are rare lesions that may affect the prostate[74] (Fig. 17-23).

Rhabdomyosarcoma

These tumors are composed of sheets of round to spindle-shaped cells with relatively uniform hyperchromatic nuclei and occur primarily in the first decade of life. Of rhabdomyosarcomas, approximately 20 percent arise in the prostate and genitourinary system. At the time of diagnosis, the tumors are relatively large measuring on average 5 to 20 cm.[75] They may produce obstructive uropathy and may involve the rectum producing

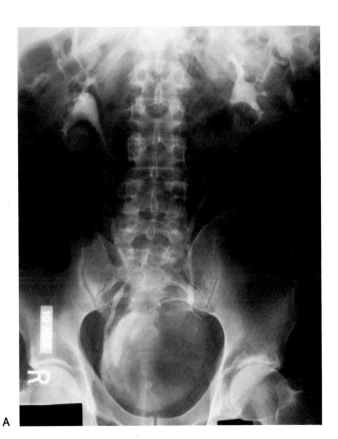

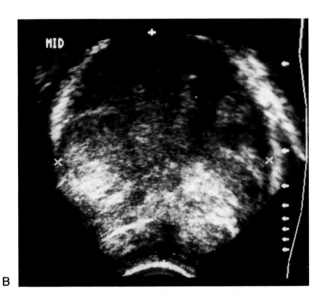

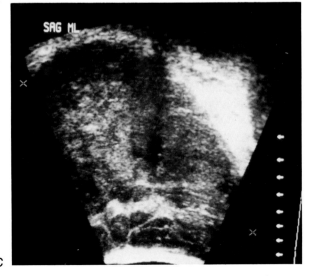

Fig. 17-23. Undifferentiated sarcoma of the prostate. **(A)** Excretory urogram demonstrates marked deviation of the distal left ureter to the right of midline secondary to large mass in pelvis. The bladder is considerably effaced. **(B)** Axial ultrasound demonstrates marked enlargement of the heterogeneous gland. **(C)** Sagittal projection shows enlargement of the gland with multiple septated hypoechoic regions occupying the peripheral zone corresponding to tumor infiltration. There is diffuse hypoechoic heterogeneity of the central gland.

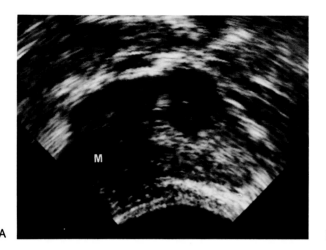

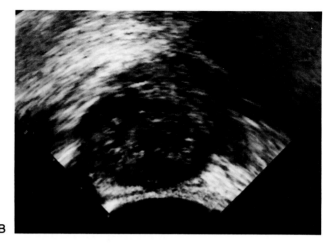

Fig. 17-24. Leiomyosarcoma of the prostate. **(A)** Axial projection demonstrating hypoechoic mass *(M)* extending from the right peripheral zone and beyond the true prostatic capsule. **(B)** Sagittal projection demonstrating the fairly well-defined hypoechoic lesion, again extending beyond the true prostatic capsule.

bloody stools, constipation, and inability to empty the rectum.[76] Rhabdomyosarcomas can grow rapidly and invade adjacent structures. These tumors are of two types: embryonal (65 percent) and alveolar (35 percent). The alveolar type tends to occur in the second and third decades and the embryonal in the first and second decades.[75] The 3-year survival is about 50 percent, though some patients are completely cured with current multidrug and multimodality therapy.

Leiomyosarcoma

Leiomyosarcoma is the second most common type of sarcoma to involve the prostate (Fig. 17-24). It usually occurs between 40 and 70 years of age,[75] and presents as a large bulky tumor (2 to 24 cm long) with diffuse infiltration of surrounding tissue. It typically produces frequent, urgent, and difficult urination. It metastasizes to the lung, liver, and the genitourinary tract. The 3-year survival is approximately 22 percent with less than 10 percent surviving at 5 years.

Leiomyosarcoma and other sarcomas can be mimicked histopathologically by a postoperative spindle cell nodule.[77] This is a recently described benign tissue reaction that occurs weeks to months following an operative procedure, such as transurethral resection. Awareness that this benign entity may mimic sarcomas is important in preventing inappropriate radical therapy.

Other Sarcomas

The sonographic appearance of other sarcomas has been described in case reports. An extraskeletal Ewing sarcoma and an extraosseous osseogenic sarcoma have

been recognized as hypoechoic infiltrative lesions.[75] Other rare sarcomas have been reported, including mixed tumors, malignant schwannoma, granulocytic sarcoma, and radiation-induced sarcoma.[75,78,79]

Metastasis

Metastatic tumors of the prostate from distant sites are uncommon, with an incidence of less than 1 percent. When metastatic disease is recognized in the prostate,

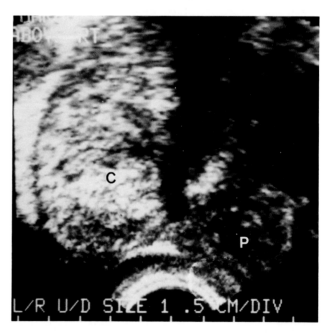

Fig. 17-25. Adenocarcinoma of the rectosigmoid involving the base of the prostate. Axial projection reveals a large, relatively hyperechoic rectosigmoid carcinoma *(C)* extending to the relatively hypoechoic right base of the prostate *(P)*.

the prognosis is dismal. Direct invasion of the prostate by local tumors is more common (Fig. 17-25). Transitional cell carcinoma of the bladder is associated with transitional cell carcinoma of the prostate. Involvement of the prostate has been seen in 12 to 43 percent of radical cystoprostatectomy specimens for bladder cancer. In a recent study of 58 men with transitional cell cancer of the bladder, prostate involvement was found in 34 percent. Of those, 50 percent had urethral invasion, 35 percent stromal invasion, 20 percent ejaculatory duct and seminal vesicle invasion, and 15 percent involved periprostatic tissues. All lesions were hypoechoic on TRUS.[80]

A small cell, bronchial cell carcinoma has been identified as a hypoechoic lesion metastatic to the prostate.[81] While metastatic lesions to the prostate mimic primary prostate cancer, two cases of prostate cancer mimicking primary rectal tumor have been identified. TRUS of the prostate in these cases was normal, but focal thickening of the rectum was identified. Biopsy results showed prostate cancer.[82]

Prostatic Intraepithelial Neoplasia

Prostatic intraepithelial neoplasia (PIN) is used to describe atypical lesions of prostatic epithelium. This lesion is noncancerous, but is considered by some to be premalignant. It is differentiated from prostatic cancer by the preservation of the basal cell layer at the periphery of the prostatic acinus, which rests on an intact basement membrane. The atypical cells can be found in the duct or acinus portion of the gland.[83] PIN appears to be related to increasing age. Furthermore, its extent and grade are more advanced when associated spatially with invasive carcinoma. Prostate cancers have been observed to arise

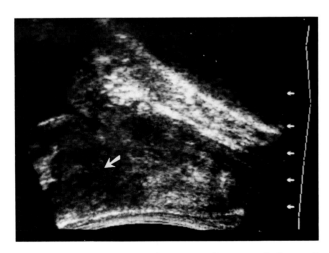

Fig. 17-26. Sagittal scan of prostate with prostatic intraepithelial neoplasia. This hypoechoic lesion (arrow) in peripheral zone is a sonographic mimic of prostate cancer.

directly from PIN and this entity occurs more commonly in prostates with adenocarcinomas.

Sonographically, PIN mimics the appearance of prostate cancer (Fig. 17-26). It is recognized as a hypoechoic lesion within the prostate gland,[84,85] and will be found in approximately 10 percent of biopsies of hypoechoic lesions identified by TRUS.[85,86] The size of this lesion is intermediate between the size of noncancerous lesions and cancer. Furthermore, the PSA is elevated in PIN above that found in benign conditions, but lower than that found in cancers.[86]

Benign Prostatic Hyperplasia

Benign prostatic hyperplasia or nodular hyperplasia is the most common disease to affect the prostate. Microscopic changes can be seen as early as the fourth decade. Autopsy studies show that 90 percent of men older than 80 years of age have BPH. This disease arises exclusively in the transitional and periurethral zones. The nodular hyperplasia that becomes clinically significant generally arises in the transition zone, which has a higher volume in men over 40 years of age compared with younger men.[87] The BPH involving the transition zone is glandular whereas that involving the periurethral zone is stromal.

The etiology of BPH is uncertain but a pathogenetic model has been proposed. In this model, stromal cells revert to an embryonic state. This causes induction of branches, budding, and growth of prostatic ducts. Of note, the presence of testosterone is necessary for the development of BPH.

Clinically, patients with BPH present with symptoms of bladder outlet obstruction and increased resistance to urine flow. Hesitancy, dribbling, and urinary retention are seen. Urinary tract infections, prostatic calculi, and bladder and urethral diverticula may develop. The bladder outlet obstruction may lead to dilatation of the renal collecting system and ureters. Prolonged obstruction by prostatic hyperplasia may lead to renal failure. The urinalysis is not specific. Hematuria, for which BPH is one of the most common causes, proteinuria, glycosuria, crystalluria, and bacteriuria can be seen.

The classic sonographic description of prostatic hyperplasia is an enlarged gland composed of homogeneous echoes (Fig. 17-27). It is symmetric and has a regular continuous border. However, echogenic· structures have been seen in one-third of BPH cases. Discrete nodules may be seen in the inner gland.[43] An inhomogeneous pattern within the gland has been reported in about one-fourth of the cases[88] (Fig. 17-28). Small cysts correlating with cystic dilatation of the acini can be seen associated with BPH (Fig. 17-29). These are retention cysts of the prostate, and may be indistinguishable from

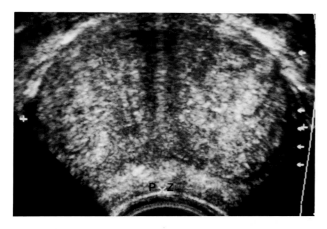

Fig. 17-27. Benign prostatic hyperplasia. Note markedly enlarged central gland, which is effacing the peripheral zone *(PZ)*. In an enlarged gland such as this, the transducer may need to be rocked to the right and left in order to visualize the entire gland.

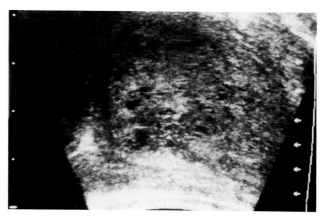

Fig. 17-29. Benign prostatic hyperplasia. Sagittal view demonstrates cystic changes within the hyperplastic central gland.

cystic atrophy changes within prostatic hyperplasia.[89] Both of these cysts are generally in the central gland and increase in number with increasing degree of benign hyperplasia. These are the most common cysts seen in the prostate, and may contain corpora amylacea or calculi[90] (Fig. 17-30). An inhomogeneous pattern within the gland has been reported in about one-fourth of the cases.[88]

Treatment of BPH can be pharmacologic, mechanical, or operative. With androgenic deprivation, symptoms will improve in approximately 60 percent of patients. Transurethral balloon dilation of the urethra and prostate has met with limited success, although it is a simple, safe, and easily repeated procedure. Simple prostatectomy, which involves removal of the hyperplastic gland to the surgical capsule, can be performed from the

transurethral or open routes. Neither operative method involves resection of tissue in the peripheral zone of the prostate.

Prostatitis

Prostatitis encompasses a variety of benign inflammatory disorders of the prostate including acute and chronic prostatitis, bacterial and nonbacterial prostatitis, and granulomatous prostatitis.[91]

Acute

Acute suppurative prostatitis presents with sudden fever, chills, discomfort with voiding, low back pain, and pain in the perineum and rectum. Acute prostatitis is

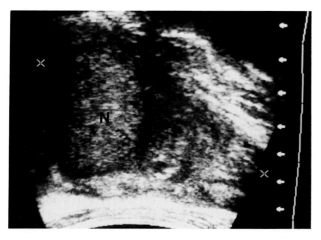

Fig. 17-28. Benign prostatic hyperplasia. Sagittal view shows a discrete, large hyperplastic nodule *(N)* occupying the majority of the cephalic portion of the central gland.

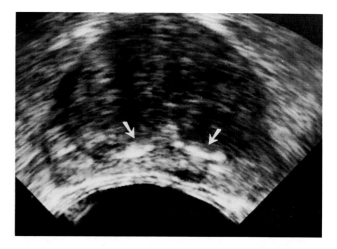

Fig. 17-30. Benign prostatic hyperplasia with corpora amylacea. Enlarged central gland is noted with echogenic regions (arrows) along the surgical capsule corresponding to corpora amylacea.

frequently accompanied by acute cystitis and is caused by the same bacteria that cause urinary tract infections. Diagnosis of acute prostatitis is made in the presence of appropriate history and positive urine culture or a culture of prostatic secretions. DRE typically defines a prostate that is enlarged, tender, warm, and indurated. Acute bacterial prostatitis generally responds to antibiotic treatment.

On rare occasion, acute bacterial prostatitis can lead to prostatic abscess. Most prostatic abscesses occur in the elderly and in immunocompromised patients, including those with acquired immunodeficiency syndrome (AIDS) and patients positive for human immunodeficiency virus (HIV) infection. There is generally a history of recent instrumentation of the lower urinary tract. These patients present with fever and symptoms due to prostate enlargement, including urinary retention. In addition to the bacterial organisms that cause acute prostatitis, prostate abscesses are also caused by anaerobic bacteria and, rarely, yeast. Abscess of the prostate can be diagnosed by CT and ultrasound. Sonography shows a hypoechoic or anechoic mass within the prostate and may even mimic a cyst[89] (Fig. 17-31). It may have thick walls and septations.[92-94] TRUS can be helpful in guiding needle aspiration of the mass to obtain diagnosis and material for culture. Furthermore, ultrasound can be used for guidance of drainage of the abscess.

Chronic

Chronic prostatitis may present with frequency, dysuria, urgency, hematospermia, low back pain, and perineal and scrotal pain. The prostate may be normal to tender and boggy on DRE. Microscopic examination of prostatic secretions shows increased numbers of white blood cells (> 10 per high power field). Histologically,

chronic prostatitis is recognized by aggregates of lymphocytes, plasma cells, and macrophages within the prostatic stroma.

Chronic bacterial prostatitis is the most common cause of relapsing urinary tract infections in men with normal excretory urograms. It is a condition difficult to diagnose and to treat. *Escherichia coli* is the most common cause of chronic bacterial prostatitis. Calcification within the prostate may serve as a nidus for infection. This condition is difficult to treat because it results in an alkalinization of the tissues produced by the chronically inflamed prostate. Antibiotics do not penetrate the prostate well in the alkaline environment.

Chronic nonbacterial prostatitis is more common than the bacterial form. In addition to the symptoms described above, patients may also complain of painful ejaculation. The cause of nonbacterial prostatitis is unknown. A variety of organisms including *Chlamydia trachomatis, Trichomonas vaginalis,* and *Ureaplasma urealyticum* have been proffered as etiologic agents, but conclusive evidence has been illusive. Others think the cause is autoimmune or related to intraprostatic urinary reflux with subsequent chemical irritation. Intraprostatic urinary reflux may be a major cause of prostatic calculi. The course of chronic nonbacterial prostatitis is one of relapses and remissions.

Chronic prostatitis produces a heterogeneous echopattern in the prostate on TRUS (Fig. 17-32). Areas of increased echogenicity and acoustic shadowing from prostatic calculi are common. The periprostatic venous plexus is commonly engorged and dilated. Additionally, the seminal vesicles may be enlarged and contain dilated ducts with thickened septae. These changes may be asymmetric. Thickening of the bladder neck has also been recognized.[95]

Granulomatous prostatitis is a unique form of prostatitis that may be secondary to a variety of infectious

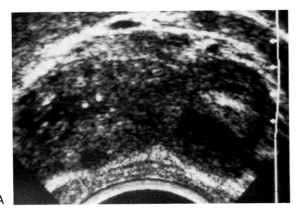
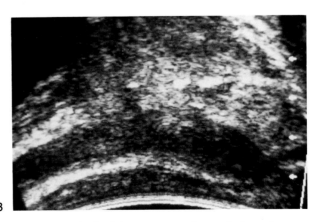

A   B

Fig. 17-31. Acute prostatitis. **(A)** Axial projection demonstrates markedly inhomogeneous hypoechoic and irregular gland diffusely enlarged with prostatitis. **(B)** Sagittal projection demonstrates the peripheral zone to be extremely hypoechoic and extending to the seminal vesicles suggesting stage C prostate carcinoma.

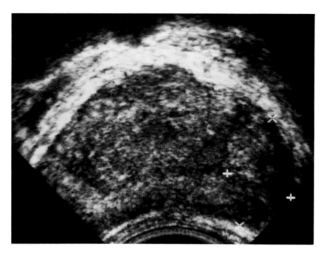

Fig. 17-32. Prostatitis. Axial projection demonstrates an inhomogeneous peripheral zone in the left lobe (crosshatches) representing chronic prostatitis.

agents, secondary to inflammatory processes, a result from biopsy, and systemic granulomatous diseases.[96] Approximately 10 percent are asymptomatic, but more common symptoms include voiding with irritation, fever, chills, urinary retention, and hematuria. It affects men from the second to ninth decade. Most patients report a relatively recent history of urinary tract infection. On DRE, a diffusely indurated gland (80 percent) or hard focal nodules (20 percent) may be felt. The appearance on physical examination raises the clinical suspicion of malignancy. Increased red blood cells and white blood cells are found on urinalysis. Pathologically a granulomatous reaction with lipid-laden macrophages, plasma cells, giant cells is identified. Sonographically a hypoechoic area in the prostate is seen.

Malakoplakia

Malakoplakia has traditionally been reported to be extremely rare in the prostate. It is a granulomatous disorder that most commonly affects the bladder, followed in frequency by the kidney, ureter, testis, and then prostate.[97] With increasing use of prostate ultrasound and transrectal biopsy, however, malakoplakia of the prostate appears to be more prevalent than previously reported.[98]

The lack of familiarity with malakoplakia of the prostate may have contributed to its misdiagnosis in the past. Cases of malakoplakia have been misdiagnosed as granulomatous prostatitis or chronic inflammation.[99,100] There has been one reported case in which a patient with prostatic malakoplakia underwent prostatectomy because the initial biopsy specimens were misdiagnosed as carcinoma.[101] Since malakoplakia can be treated medically rather than surgically, it is important that the physicians involved in the diagnosis of prostate disease be familiar with this condition.

The etiology of malakoplakia has not been definitely established, although there seems to be a close relationship with urinary tract infection, specifically with *E. coli* infection.[101,102] Grossly, malakoplakia manifests as multiple soft plaques, thus giving rise to the term *malakoplakia* (malakos, soft and plakos, plaque). Microscopically the characteristic feature is the presence of Michaelis-Guttman bodies, which are macrophages with an intracellular, concentrically laminated, basophilic, intracytoplasmic body. Ultrasonographically, malakoplakia of the prostate reveals hypoechoic regions sometimes indistinguishable from carcinoma of the prostate (Fig. 17-33). In addition, the true prostatic capsule can be quite irregular and actually suggest stage C prostate carci-

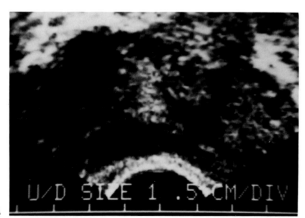
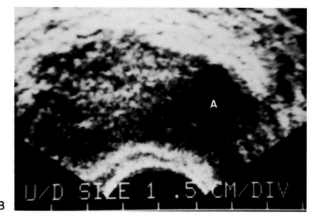

Fig. 17-33. Malakoplakia of the prostate. **(A)** Diffuse, irregular hypoechoic lesion of the right lobe of the prostate, axial projection. **(B)** Sagittal projection shows diffusely hypoechoic peripheral zone with the apex *(A)* markedly involved. (From Chantelois et al,[98] with permission.)

noma. Therefore, transrectal biopsy is essential to establish an accurate diagnosis.

Prostate Cysts

Utricle cysts are believed currently to be a midline cystic dilation of the prostatic utricle. Müllerian duct cysts are also midline cysts resulting from remnants of incompletely regressed müllerian ducts. These are extremely difficult to differentiate sonographically, clinically, and embryologically. Müllerian duct cysts may arise anywhere along the ductal remnants. Therefore, they generally extend cephalad and are slightly lateral from midline. They may extend beyond the prostate and may present as a pelvic mass. They usually occur in the third and fourth decade and produce a variety of symptoms including pain, dribbling, and obstructive and irritative urinary tract symptoms. Prostatic utricle cysts always arise at the verumontanum and are always in the midline. They are generally small (1 to 10 mm) and occur earlier, usually before the age of 20 years. Unlike müllerian cysts, utricle cysts are associated with genitourinary abnormalities (hypospadias, renal agenesis, intersex).[103] Neither cyst contains sperm. They may be complicated by pus or hemorrhage and carcinoma has been associated with both types of cyst in up to 3 percent.[89,90,20] TRUS guidance can be used for drainage.[104]

SEMINAL VESICLE DISEASE

Congenital Anomalies

A variety of congenital anomalies may affect the seminal vesicles from agenesis to the implantation of an ectopic ureter.[105] The latter is often associated with ipsilateral renal agenesis. Absence of the seminal vesicle or vas deferens has been associated with cystic fibrosis and cryptorchidism.

Benign Lesions

Cysts are usually encountered as early as the third decade. Symptoms include prostatism, painful ejaculation, frequency, and dysuria. Seminal vesicle cysts have been associated with infertility.[106] They are thought to be the result of obstruction at the confluence of the seminal vesicles and ejaculatory ducts. This obstruction may be congenital or acquired secondary to prostatitis. Cysts of the seminal vesicle may become large. Aspiration may show the presence of sperm. Cysts of the seminal vesicle have been associated with abnormalities of the upper

urinary tract including renal agenesis and multicystic dysplasia.[106]

Calcification within the seminal vesicle may be seen in patients with diabetes mellitus, granulomatous infection or chronic suppurative infection, and with chronic renal failure. Chronic infection may cause small seminal vesicles, in turn causing low ejaculatory volume.[20] Calcifications will be recognized sonographically as echogenic material with posterior acoustic shadowing. Sonography of acute infection or abscess may show a complex or hypoechoic fluid collection. TRUS can be used to guide aspiration or drainage.[105,107,108]

Neoplasm

Primary

Primary neoplasms of the seminal vesicles are rare. Cystadenoma and cystadenosarcoma may occur. Other rare benign neoplasms such as mesenchymoma and mesonephric hamartoma have been reported.[109,110] However, when cystadenosarcoma occurs in the seminal vesicles, it is especially difficult to confirm the seminal vesicles as the primary site. These tumors are usually papillary or anaplastic. They tend to invade adjacent structures early. The prognosis is poor and radiotherapy tends to produce better results than radical surgery.

Secondary

Metastatic involvement of the seminal vesicles is more common than involvement by a primary tumor. Direct extension from prostate cancer is the most common metastatic tumor. Seminal vesicle involvement occurs in approximately 10 percent of presumed early prostate cancer. Additionally, involvement of the seminal vesicles can occur with bladder cancer and anorectal cancers. Metastatic involvement of the seminal vesicles from distant sites is extremely rare.

EJACULATORY DUCTS

Cysts

Ejaculatory duct cysts are relatively common findings on TRUS. Most small cysts are asymptomatic, but larger cysts may present with perineal pain, dysuria, hematospermia, and ejaculatory pain. They are caused by obstruction of the ejaculatory ducts that is either secondary or congenital. Small anechoic masses are seen along the course of the ejaculatory ducts (Fig. 17-34). Small cysts

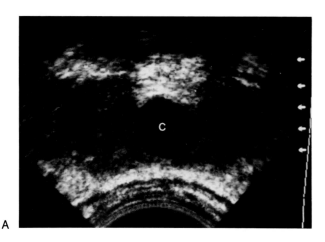

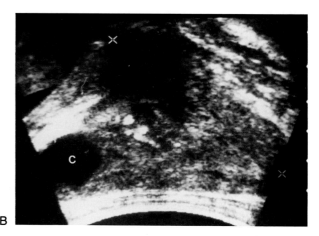

Fig. 17-34. Ejaculatory duct cyst. **(A)** Axial projection; **(B)** sagittal projection. (*C*, cyst.)

are confined to the central zone whereas larger ejaculatory duct cysts may extend cephalad to the prostate and may mimic müllerian duct cysts. Ejaculatory duct cysts are lateral to midline at the base of the prostate and in the midline when they occur at the verumontanum. Cystic dilatation of the ipsilateral seminal vesicle may occur. Aspiration of the cysts may show sperm.[90]

FUTURE DIRECTIONS

As the accuracy of prostate ultrasound improves and the controversy over its utilization for screening is resolved, other uses for prostate ultrasound will emerge. These future applications will include not only expansion of diagnostic capabilities, but the introduction of treatment modalities as well.

In the diagnostic realm, color Doppler and duplex ultrasound performed with the endorectal transducer may be helpful both in locating and in distinguishing between benign and malignant lesions (Fig. 17-35 and Plate 17-1). Color Doppler may be helpful in detecting subtle, small, or isoechoic lesions by identifying the increased vascularity in the borders of tumors. One would presume, as in malignancies in other tissues, that the arteriovenous shunting within a prostate neoplasm would create a low resistance, high velocity pattern on spectral Doppler. Thus, the low resistivity index produced by malignancies should be differentiable from other less vascular entities like benign prostatic hyperplasia and infarction. Preliminary experience, however, has not substantiated this supposition (McLeary, personal communication, May 1991).

Needle-directed treatments such as alcohol ablation and localized chemotherapy are becoming commonplace in other regions of the body. Instillation of absolute alcohol into liver metastases, parathyroid adenomas, and renal cysts has been successfully reported.[111,112]

Theoretical problems with needle-directed treatment of prostate carcinoma include bacterial contamination of the treatment-induced necrotic tissue secondary to the transrectal approach. Coverage with oral antibiotics may not be sufficient to suppress infection in this instance. In addition, prostate ultrasound is known to underestimate the size and number of neoplastic lesions in the prostate.[51] The success of ablation would therefore need to be confirmed with followup biopsy.

Another possible application of ultrasound in the diagnosis and treatment of prostate disease would be tagging an ultrasound contrast agent to monoclonal antibodies, which would seek and attach only to involved

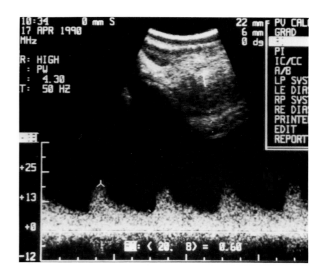

Fig. 17-35. Doppler ultrasound of prostate. Duplex ultrasound of prostatic nodule in the peripheral zone. This nodule has a low resistance pattern with high diastolic flow. The resistivity index is 0.6 (see also Plate 17-1).

regions of prostate cancer. This technique would not only facilitate determination of the number and size of prostate lesions, but could also be used to identify residual tumor after treatment.

Other ultrasound-guided treatment modalities currently under investigation include hyperthermia[113] and cryosurgery.[114,115] Hyperthermia involves heating the inner gland of the prostate to temperatures that cause necrosis and eventual dissolution of the majority of the inner gland. Results equivalent to TURP (transurethral resection, prostate) might be achieved with this procedure. Cryosurgery is being investigated as an alternative to prostatectomy. This treatment consists of freezing the prostate with an ultrasound-guided probe to necrose the entire gland. With concomitant ultrasound visualization, necrosis of the prostate can be continuously monitored during both procedures.

The debate over using prostate ultrasound for screening for prostate cancer should not obscure its potential for extension beyond its present horizons. Expanded diagnostic capabilities as well as treatment possibilities are already being investigated and will certainly become a part of the diagnostic and therapeutic regimens for prostate disease in the near future.

REFERENCES

1. Greenberg M, Neiman HL, Brandt TD et al: Ultrasound of the prostate: analysis of tissue texture and abnormalities. Radiology 1981;141:757
2. Henneberry M, Carter MF, Neiman HL: Estimation of prostatic size by suprapubic ultrasonography. J Urol 1979;121:615
3. Rifkin MD: Ultrasound of the Prostate. Raven Press, New York, 1988
4. Watanabe H, Igari D, Tanahasi Y et al: Development and application of new equipment for transrectal ultrasonography. J Clin Ultrasound 1974;2:91
5. Gustafsson O, Norming U, Nyman CR, Oshtrom M: Complications following combined transrectal aspiration and core biopsy of the prostate. Scand J Urol Nephrol 1990;24:249
6. Hodge KK, McNeal JE, Stamey TA: Ultrasound guided transrectal core biopsies of the palpably abnormal prostate. J Urol 1989;142:66
7. Weaver RP, Noble MJ, Weigel JW: Correlation of ultrasound guided and digitally directed transrectal biopsies of palpable prostatic abnormalities. J Urol 1991;145:516
8. Lee F, Siders DB, Torp-Pedersen ST et al: Prostate cancer: transrectal ultrasound and pathology comparison. Cancer 1991;67:1132
9. Palken M, Cobb OE, Simons CE et al: Prostate cancer: comparison of digital rectal examination and transrectal ultrasound for screening. J Urol 1991;145:86
10. Rannikko S, Salo JO: Radical prostatectomy as treatment of localized prostatic cancer. Scand J Urol Nephrol 1990;24:103
11. Williams PL, Warwick R, Dyson M, Bannister LH: Gray's Anatomy. 37th Ed. Churchill Livingstone, New York, 1989
12. Tarragho EA: Anatomy of the lower urinary tract. p. 46. In Walsh PC, Gittes RF, Perlmutten AD, Stamey TA (eds): Campbell's Urology. 5th Ed. WB Saunders, Philadelphia, 1986
13. McNeal JE: The prostate gland: morphology and pathobiology. Monogr Urol 1983;4:3
14. Hernandez AD, Urry RL, Smith JA Jr: Ultrasonographic characteristics of the seminal vesicles after ejaculation. J Urol 1990;144:1380
15. Hardt NS, Kaude JV, Li KC et al: Sonography of the prostate: in vitro correlation of sonographic and anatomic findings in normal glands. AJR 1988;151:955
16. Rifkin MD: Endorectal sonography of the prostate: clinical implications. AJR 1987;148:1137
17. Hernandez AD, Smith JA Jr: Transrectal ultrasonography for the early detection and staging of prostate cancer. Urol Clin North Am 1990;17:745
18. Waterhouse RL, Resnik MI: Applications of prostate ultrasonography. Suppl Urol 1990;36:18
19. Fornage BD: Normal US anatomy of the prostate. Ultrasound Med Biol 1986;12:1011
20. Carter SSC, Shinohara K, Lipshultz LI: Transrectal ultrasonography in disorders of the seminal vesicles and ejaculatory ducts. Urol Clin North Am 1989;16:773
21. Boring CC, Squires TS, Tong T: Cancer statistics, 1991. CA 1991;41:19
22. Miller GJ: Histopathology of prostate cancer: prediction of malignant behavior and correlation with ultrasonography. Suppl Urol 1989;33:18
23. Liskow AS, Neugunt AI, Benson M et al: Multiple primary neoplasms in association with prostate cancer in black and white patients. Cancer 1987;59:380
24. Lee F, Torp-Pedersen ST, Siders DB: The role of transrectal ultrasound in the early detection of prostate cancer. CA 1989;39:337
25. Gleason DF: Histologic grading of prostatic carcinoma. p. 83. In Bostwick DG (ed): Pathology of the Prostate. Churchill Livingstone, New York 1990
26. Ordonez NG, Ro JY, Ayala AG: Application of immunocytochemistry in the pathology of the prostate. p. 137. In Bostwick DG (ed): Pathology of the Prostate. Churchill Livingstone, New York 1990
27. Sy FA, Gursel EO, Veeneja RJ: Positive random iliac bone biopsy in advanced prostatic cancer. Urology 1973;2:125
28. Drago JR: The role of new modalities in the early detection and diagnosis of prostate cancer. CA 1989;39:326
29. Stamey TA, Yang N, Hay AR et al: Prostate specific antigen as a serum marker for adenocarcinoma of the prostate. N Engl J Med 1987;317:909
30. Seamonds B, Yang N, Anderson K et al: Evaluation of prostate-specific antigen and prostatic acid phosphatase as prostate cancer markers. Urology 1986;28:472

31. Miller GJ: Pathologic aspects of prostate cancer: prediction of malignant potential. Suppl Urol 1989;34:5

32. Harada K, Tanahashi Y, Igari D et al: Clinical evaluation of inside echo patterns in gray scale prostatic echography. J Urol 1980;124:216

33. Greenberg M, Neimen HL, Vogelzang R, Falkowski W: Ultrasonographic features of prostatic carcinoma. J Clin Ultrasound 1982;10:307

34. Rifkin MD, Kurtz AB, Choi HY, Goldberg BB: Endoscopic ultrasonic evaluation of the prostate using a transrectal probe: prospective evaluation and acoustic characterization. Radiology 1983;149:265

35. Resnik MI, Willard JW, Boyse WH: Transrectal ultrasonography in the evaluation of patients with prostatic carcinoma. J Urol 1980;124:482

36. Griffiths GJ, Clements R, Jones DR et al: The ultrasound appearances of prostatic cancer with histologic correlation. Clin Radiol 1987;38:219

37. Salo JO, Rannikko S, Makinen J, Lehtonen T: Echogenic structure of prostatic cancer image on radical prostatectomy specimens. Prostate 1987;10:1

38. Jones DR, Griffiths GJ, Parkinson MC et al: The correlation of histopathological, microradiographic and ultrasonographic features in disease of the prostate gland. Br J Radiol 1989;62:1059

39. Dahnert WF, Hamper UM, Eggleston JC et al: Prostatic evaluation by transrectal sonography with histopathologic correlation: the echopenic appearance of early carcinoma. Radiology 1986;158:97

40. Hamper UM, Seth S, Walsh PC, Epstein JI: Bright echogenic foci in early prostatic carcinoma: sonographic and pathologic correlation. Radiology 1990;176:339

41. Rifkin MD, McGlynn ET, Choi H: Echogenicity of prostate cancer correlated with histologic grade and stromal fibrosis: endorectal US studies. Radiology 1989;170:549.

42. Lile R, Thickman D, Miller GJ, Crawford E: Prostatic comedocarcinoma: correlation of sonograms with pathologic specimens in three cases. AJR 1990;155:303

43. Burks DD, Drolshagen LF, Fleischer AC et al: Transrectal sonography of benign and malignant prostatic lesions. AJR 1986;146:1187

44. Lee F, Littrup PJ, Torp-Pedersen ST et al: Prostate cancer: comparison of transrectal US and digital rectal examination for screening. Radiology 1988;168:389

45. Jansen H, Gallee MP, Schroder FH: Analysis of sonographic pattern in prostatic cancer: comparison of longitudinal and transversal transrectal ultrasound with subsequent radical prostatectomy specimens. Eur Urol 1990;18:174

46. Hauzeur C, Corbusier A, Bossche MV, Schulman CC: Transrectal ultrasound in the diagnosis and staging of prostatic carcinoma. Eur Urol 1990;18:107

47. Hamper UM, Seth S, Walch PC et al: Capsular transgression of prostatic carcinoma: evaluation with transrectal US with pathologic correlation. Radiology 1991;178:791

48. Clements R, Griffiths GJ, Peeling WB, Ryan PG: Experience with ultrasound guided transperineal prostatic needle biopsy: 1985–1988. Br J Urol 1990;65:362

49. Carter HB, Hamper UM, Sheth S et al: Evaluation of transrectal ultrasound in the early detection of prostate cancer. J Urol 1989;142:1008

50. Rifkin MD, Zerhouni EA, Gatsonis CA et al: Comparison of magnetic resonance imaging and ultrasonography in staging early prostate cancer: results of a multi-institution cooperative trial. N Engl J Med 1990;323:621

51. Thickman D, Parker SH, Hopper KD et al: Comparison of transrectal ultrasound of the prostate with whole-mount histologic specimen: accuracy of detection. Radiology 1989;173:143

52. Cooner WH, Mosley BR, Rutherford CL Jr et al: Clinical application of transrectal ultrasonography and prostate specific antigen in the search for prostate cancer. J Urol 1988;139:758

53. Lee F, Torp-Pedersen S, Littrup PJ et al: Hypoechoic lesions of the prostate: clinical relevance of tumor size, digital rectal examination, and prostate-specific antigen. Radiology 1989;170:29

54. Veneziano S, Pavlica V, Querze R et al: Correlation between prostate-specific antigen and prostate volume, evaluated by transrectal ultrasonography: usefulness in diagnosis of prostate cancer. Eur Urol 1990;18:112

55. Chodak GW: Screening for prostate cancer. Role of ultrasonography. Urol Clin North Am 1989;16:657

56. Lee F Jr, Bronson JP, Lee F et al: Nonpalpable cancer of the prostate: assessment with transrectal ultrasound. Radiology 1991;178:197

57. Torp-Pederson ST, Littrup PJ, Lee F, Mettlin C: Early prostate cancer: diagnostic costs of screening transrectal ultrasound and digital rectal examination. Radiology 1988;169:351

58. Catalona WJ, Smith DS, Ratliff TL et al: Measurement of prostate-specific antigen in serum as a screening test for prostate cancer. N Engl J Med 1991;324:1156

59. Winkler HZ, Rainwater LM, Myers RP et al: Stage D1 prostatic adenocarcinoma: significance of nuclear DNA ploidy patterns studied by flow cytometry. Mayo Clin Proc 1988;63:103

60. Walsh PC, Lepor H: The role of radical prostatectomy in the management of prostatic cancer. Cancer 1987;60:526

61. Prostate Cancer Consensus Conference: The management of clinically localized prostate cancer. JAMA 1987;258:2727

62. Bagshaw MA: Current conflicts in the management of prostatic cancer. Int J Radiat Oncol Biol Phys 1986;12:1721

63. Pilepich MV, Bagshaw MA, Asbell SO et al: Radical prostatectomy or radiotherapy in carcinoma of prostate. Urology 1987;30:18

64. Enlund A, Pedersen K, Boeryd B, Varenhorst E: Transrectal ultrasonography compared to histopathological assessment for local staging of prostatic carcinoma. Acta Radiol 1990;31:579

65. Pontes JE, Eisenkraft S, Watanabe H et al: Preoperative evaluation of localized prostatic carcinoma by transrectal ultrasonography. J Urol 1985;134:289

66. Andriole GL, Coplen DE, Mikkeleson DJ, Katalona

WJ: Sonographic and pathological staging of patients with clinically localized prostate cancer. J Urol 1989;142:1259

67. Hardeman SW, Causey JQ, Hickey DP, Soloway MS: Transrectal ultrasound for staging prior to radical prostatectomy. Urology 1989;34:175

68. Terris MK, McNeal JE, Stamey TA: Invasion of the seminal vesicles by prostatic cancer: detection with transrectal sonography. AJR 1990;155:811

69. Parra RO, Wolf RM, Huben RP: The use of transrectal ultrasound in the detection and evaluation of local pelvic recurrences after a radical urologic pelvic operation. J Urol 1990;144:707

70. Matzkin H, Greenstein A, Braf Z: Clinical importance of prostatic measurements in follow-up of GnRH analog-treated prostatic carcinoma patients. Urology 1990;36:214

71. Rainwater LM, Barrett DM: Primary lymphoma of prostate: transrectal ultrasonic appearance. Urology 1990;36:522

72. Patel DR, Gomez GA, Henderson ES, Gamarra M: Primary prostatic involvement in non-Hodgkin lymphoma. Urology 1988;32:96

73. Lewi HJE, Stewart ID, Seywright M et al: Urinary tract lymphoma. Br J Urol 1986;58:16

74. Tetu B, Singley JR, Bostwick DG: Soft tissue tumors. p. 117. In Bostwick DG (ed): Pathology of the Prostate. Churchill Livingstone, New York, 1990

75. Smith BH, Dechner LP: Sarcoma of the prostate gland. Am J Clin Pathol 1972;58:43

76. Tannenbaum M: Sarcomas of the prostate gland. Urology 1975;5:810

77. Huang W, Ro JY, Grignon DJ et al: Postoperative spindle cell nodule of the prostate and bladder. J Urol 1990;143:824

78. Frame R, Head D, Lee R et al: Granulocystic sarcoma of the prostate: two cases causing urinary obstruction. Cancer 1987;59:142

79. Scully JM, Uno JM, McIntyre M, Mosely S: Radiation-induced prostatic sarcoma: a case report. J Urol 1990;144:746

80. Terris MA, Villers A, Freiha FS: Transrectal ultrasound appearance of transitional cell carcinoma involving the prostate. J Urol 1990;143:953

81. Kromann-Andersen B, Sommer P, Glenthoj A: Non-prostatic malignant disease mimicking prostatic cancer. Int Urol Nephrol 1990;22:133

82. Lorentzen T, Torp-Pedersen S, Nolsoe C: Transrectal ultrasound findings of prostate cancer mimicking primary rectal tumor. Acta Radiol 1990;31:625

83. Garnett J: Editorial comment. J Urol 1989;142:1512

84. Brawer MK, Rennels MA, Nagle RB et al: Prostatic intraepithelial neoplasia: a lesion that may be confused with cancer on prostatic ultrasound. J Urol 1989;142:1510

85. Devonec MM, Fendler JP, Monsallier M et al: The significance of the prostatic hypoechoic area: results in 226 ultrasonically guided prostatic biopsies. J Urol 1990;143:316

86. Lee F, Torp-Pedersen ST, Carroll JT et al: Use of transrectal ultrasound and prostate-specific antigen in diagnosis of prostatic intraepithelial neoplasia. Urology Suppl. 1989;34:4

87. Greene DR, Egawa S, Hellerstein DK, Scardino PT: Sonographic measurements of transition zone of prostate in men with and without benign prostatic hyperplasia. Urology 1990;36:293

88. Hendrikx AJM, Doesburs WH, Reintjes AGM et al: Effectiveness of ultrasound in the preoperative evaluation of patients with prostatism. Prostate 1988;13:199

89. Hamper UM, Epstein JI, Sheth S et al: Cystic lesions of the prostate gland: a sonographic-pathologic correlation. J Ultrasound Med 1990;9:395

90. Ngheim HT, Kellman GM, Sandberg SA, Craig BM: Cystic lesions of the prostate. Radiographics 1990;10:635

91. Meares EM Jr: Prostatitis—acute and chronic. p. 71. In Paulson DF (ed): Prostatic Disorders. Lea & Febiger, Philadelphia, 1989

92. Papanicolaou N, Pfister RC, Stafford SA, Parkhurst EC: Prostate abscess: imaging with transrectal sonography and MR. AJR 1987;149:981

93. Thornhill BA, Morehouse HT, Coleman P, Hoffman-Tretin JC: Prostatic abscess CT and sonographic findings. AJR 1987;148:899

94. Rorvik J, Daehlin L: Prostatic abscess: imaging with transrectal ultrasound. Scand J Urol Nephrol 1989;23:307

95. Di Trapani D, Pavone C, Serretta V et al: Chronic prostatitis and prostatodynia: ultrasonographic alterations of the prostate, bladder neck, seminal vesicle and periprostatic venous plexas. Eur Urol 1988;15:230

96. Bude R, Bree RL, Adler RS, Jafri SZ: Transrectal ultrasound appearance of granulomatous prostatitis. J Ultrasound Med 1990;9:677

97. Stanton MJ, Maxted W: Malakoplakia: a study of the literature and current concepts of pathogenesis, diagnosis and treatment. J Urol 1981;125:139

98. Chantelois AE, Parker SH, Sims JE, Horne DW: Malacoplakia of the prostate sonographically mimicking carcinoma. Radiology 1990;177:193

99. Anderson T, Kristiansen W, Ruge S, Hansen JPH: Malakoplakia of the prostate causing fatal fistula to rectum. Scand J Urol Nephrol 1986;20:153

100. Lou TY, Teplitz C: Malakoplakia: pathogenesis and ultrastructural morphogenesis: a problem of altered macrophase (phagolysosomal) response. Hum Pathol 1974;5:191

101. Koga S, Arakaki Y, Matsuoka M, Ohyama C: Malakoplakia of the prostate. Eur Urol 1985;11:137

102. McClure J: Malakoplakia of the prostate: a report of two cases and a review of the literature. J Clin Pathol 1979;32:629

103. Shabsigh R, Lerner S, Fishman IJ, Kadmon D: The role of transrectal ultrasonography in the diagnosis and management of prostatic and seminal vesicle cysts. J Urol 1989;141:1206

104. Migleari R, Scarpa RM, Campus G, Usai E: Percutane-

ous drainage of utricular cyst under ultrasound guidance. Br J Urol 1988;62:385

105. King BF, Hattery RR, Lieber MM et al: Seminal vesicle imaging. Radiographics 1989;9:653

106. Roehrborn CG, Schneider H, Rugendorff EW, Hamann W: Embryological and diagnostic aspects of seminal vesicle cysts associated with upper urinary tract malformation. J Urol 1986;135:1029

107. Fox CW, Vaccaro JA, Kiesling VJ Jr, Belville WD: Seminal vesicle abscess: the use of computerized coaxial tomography for diagnosis and therapy. J Urol 1988;139:384

108. Asch MR, Toi A: Seminal vesicles: imaging and intervention using transrectal ultrasound. J Ultrasound Med 1991;10:19

109. Islam M: Denign mesenchymoma of seminal vesicles. Urology 1979;13:202

110. Kinas H, Kuhn MJ: Mesonephriz hamartoma of the seminal vesicle: a rate cause of a retrovesical mass. NY State J Med 1987;87:48

111. Livraghi T, Vettori C, Lazzaroni S: Liver metastases: results of percutaneous ethanol injection in 14 patients. Radiology 1991;179:709

112. Tanaka K, Okazaki H, Nakamura S et al: Hepatocellular carcinoma: treatment with a combination therapy of transcatheter arterial embolization and percutaneous ethanol injection. Radiology 1991;179:713

113. Caastaneda F, Landas S, Babbs C et al: Transurethral thermic debulking of the prostate for BPH: a preliminary animal study. (Abstract) 16th Annual Meeting Interventional Radiology, Society of Cardiovascular and Interventional Radiology, San Francisco, California, February 16–21, 1991, p. 166

114. Onik GM, Cohen J, Rubinsky B: Percutaneous transperineal cryoprostatectomy using transrectal ultrasound guidance. (Abstract) 16th Annual Meeting Interventional Radiology, Society of Cardiovascular and Interventional Radiology, San Francisco, California, February 16–21, 1991, p. 162

115. Onik G, Porterfield B, Rubinsky B, Cohen J: Perataneous transperineal prostate cryosurgery using transrectal ultrasound guidance: animal model. Urology 1991;37:277

116. Lee F, Littrup PJ, Kumasaka GH et al: The use of transrectal ultrasound in the diagnosis, guided biopsy, staging and screening of prostate cancer. Radiographics 1987;7:627

18

Peripheral Vascular System

Susan A. Mulligan
D. Bradley Koslin

Evaluation of the peripheral vascular system by duplex sonography requires knowledge of vascular anatomy and flow patterns in both normal and diseased vessels. High resolution sonographic equipment is required to provide detailed evaluation of the vascular structures and to assess their flow characteristics.

This chapter provides a framework for interpretation of vascular anatomy and flow phenomena by sonography. Discussion of the venous system, both lower and

upper, is followed by discussion of the arterial system. Each section begins with a discussion of the technique used followed by the anatomy and specific pathology, including venous thrombosis, venous insufficiency, arteriovenous fistula, arterial stenosis and occlusion, and others. Also, the diagnostic performance of sonography is compared with other methods, outlining pitfalls in examination, technique, and interpretation.

LOWER EXTREMITY VENOUS EVALUATION

TECHNIQUE

Compression Ultrasound

The main diagnostic procedure in venous ultrasound evaluation is the assessment of vein compressibility.[1-10] The thin venous wall should completely collapse, with coaptation of the walls when minimal pressure is applied by the transducer on the skin overlying the venous segment.[2-10] The importance of assessing venous compressibility cannot be overemphasized; the detection rates for diagnosis of deep venous thrombosis (DVT) are not significantly altered when compression ultrasound is compared with compression ultrasound plus either pulsed or color Doppler examination.[11]

Compressibility is assessed primarily with the transducer oriented transversely to the venous segment (Fig. 18-1). Transverse orientation minimizes the possibility that the vein will be oblique to the scan plane, and thus maximizes sensitivity to thrombus that is located asymmetrically within the lumen. A normal vein without thrombus will compress completely with only a small amount of pressure applied to the overlying skin surface. Increased pressure may be necessary when surrounding edema is present. The contour of the accompanying artery should not be altered by the amount of pressure necessary to compress the normal vein.

Incomplete compressibility may result from intrinsic obstruction, either acute thrombus (Fig. 18-2) or thickened venous walls from prior DVT, or extrinsic obstruc-

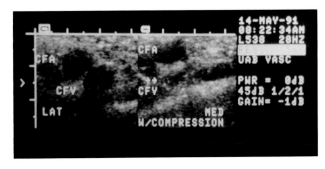

Fig. 18-1. Dual transverse gray-scale images show the common femoral vein *(CFV)* medial to the common femoral vein *(CFA)*. In this normal volunteer, compression view demonstrates complete coaptation of the CFV walls.

tion more proximally. The sonographic distinction between acute versus chronic thrombus can be difficult, and is discussed below. However, Murphy and Cronan[12] have demonstrated that acute thrombus can be diagnosed if the vein is distended. They report that comparison of the venous diameter with that of the accompanying artery can aid in this distinction; if the vein diameter is more than 50 percent greater than its companion artery, the presence of an acute DVT is strongly suggested.[12]

The following is a brief summary of sonographic technique of the lower extremities:

1. The legs should be scanned with slight external rotation, preferably with the head elevated 20 to 30 degrees for better venous filling.

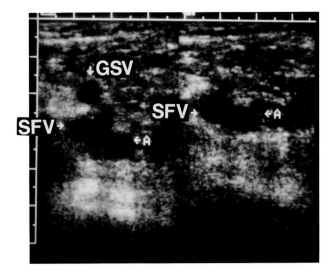

Fig. 18-2. Dual transverse gray-scale images in this patient show full compressibility of the greater saphenous vein *(GSV)* located anterior to the proximal superficial femoral vein. However, the superficial femoral vein *(SFV)*, medial to the superficial femoral artery *(A)*, does not compress, which is consistent with thrombus at this level.

2. Each venous segment is scanned in both transverse and longitudinal planes. Transverse scanning provides optimal evaluation of compressibility, because the transducer may slide off the vein obliquely and mural thrombus may be overlooked. Venous flow patterns are assessed, evaluating phasicity and change of flow with Valsalva maneuver and/or augmentation (see below).

3. A high frequency (5- to 7-MHz) transducer is commonly used, although a 3-MHz transducer may sometimes be necessary for adequate penetration of a markedly enlarged leg.

4. The extraluminal soft tissues are examined carefully to detect ancillary findings; namely, Baker's cyst, abscess, node enlargement, pseudoaneurysm, and arteriovenous fistula.[11,13]

5. Flow analysis with color and spectral Doppler requires that scale settings, sample volume placement, and Doppler angle are chosen to optimize sensitivity to slow flow.

6. Scanning begins transversely at the inguinal crease, identifying the common femoral–greater saphenous junction.

7. The common femoral vein is followed as far superiorly as it can be visualized; bowel gas may obscure visualization above the inguinal ligament.

8. The common femoral vein is evaluated caudally into the thigh, and its bifurcation is visualized, with the origin of the deep femoral vein seen posterolaterally. The superficial femoral vein is then followed caudally; if visualization is lost, the report should state the extent to which the vein was visualized.

9. Evaluation of the popliteal vein is usually performed with the patient in the lateral decubitus position.

10. The proximal portions of the deep calf veins are evaluated, and if focal symptoms are present in the calf, the underlying veins are assessed for compressibility.

11. In patients with thrombus, mapping of its extent is very important, particularly in patients who will undergo percutaneous placement of an inferior vena cava filter.[14] The ipsilateral common femoral vein may be used for filter placement access if thrombus is limited to the superficial femoral vein.[14,15]

12. If thrombus is identified that is believed to be "free-floating" or loosely adherent, no further compression or distal augmentation maneuvers should be utilized. The patient should not be allowed to ambulate after the procedure, and the radiologist should notify the referring physician immediately.[16]

Provocative Maneuvers

Venous disease in the legs may be diagnosed by documentation of intraluminal thrombus and/or alteration in flow patterns. Several provocative maneuvers may be used to assess venous flow patterns including the Valsalva maneuver, the inspiration/expiration maneuver, and the augmentation maneuver, which is performed distal or proximal to the region scanned.

Valsalva Maneuver

To implement the Valsalva maneuver, the patient is asked to bear down to increase abdominal pressure. During the Valsalva, increased pressure within the abdomen results in decreased venous return, and venous flow decreases or ceases within the lower extremity veins being examined. The diameter of the leg veins also increases during the Valsalva maneuver.[2,17–19] After release of the abdominal muscular contraction, the venous flow returns, often with increased flow for the first several seconds after Valsalva release (Plate 18-1).

Patient cooperation is necessary for the proper performance and interpretation of the Valsalva maneuver. Infirm and/or elderly patients may not be able to comply with such commands, which limits its utility.[2]

Inspiration/Expiration Maneuver

The changes of venous flow pattern with inspiration and expiration are helpful in assessing leg veins for thrombus. The patient is asked to inspire deeply, with diaphragmatic excursion downward resulting in increased abdominal pressure. Thus, during inspiration, a normal response is decreased venous flow in the legs; upon expiration, abdominal pressure decreases and venous flow increases. If there is continuous flow, without the expected change in flow with respiration, venous compression and/or occlusion should be suspected.[6,17]

Both the Valsalva and inspiration/expiration maneuvers allow assessment of venous patency upstream from the site being directly assessed. However, nonocclusive thrombus may not be detectable with such indirect evaluation. Isolated iliac venous occlusive thrombus may be missed, since collateral venous pathways may develop in patients with this disorder, and the collateral channels may result in normal physiologic response in the veins distal to the occluding thrombus.

Despite these limitations, the inspiration/expiration and Valsalva maneuvers are useful for evaluating venous flow patterns. Abnormal responses to these provocative tests may result from intrinsic or extrinsic venous obstruction.

Augmentation Maneuver

External compression of the calf and thigh is used to augment venous flow routinely in our laboratory. The examiner's hand grasps the calf or thigh muscles, and applies a slow, gentle squeeze distal to the venous segment being evaluated; the normal response is a subsequent increase in venous flow, which returns to baseline in several seconds (Plate 18-2).[6,17]

An abnormal response to augmentation is failure to demonstrate increase in venous flow; this implies obstruction of the venous segment between the site being squeezed and the vein being directly imaged. Collateral veins may serve as conduits between these two locations, and result in false-negative augmentation evaluation.

NORMAL ANATOMY

The lower extremities are drained by the deep and superficial systems, which are connected by perforating veins (Fig. 18-3). The deep veins provide most of the venous return from the legs, accompany the principal arteries, and share the same names.[20,21]

The deep calf veins are usually paired and lie on either side of the single anterior tibial, posterior tibial, and peroneal arteries. The popliteal vein is formed by the confluence of the anterior and posterior tibial veins, and is located posteromedial to the popliteal artery in the more caudal portion of the popliteal fossa. The popliteal vein courses posterior to the popliteal artery as it passes between the two heads of the gastrocnemius muscle, and then lies posterolateral to the popliteal artery in the more superior portion of the popliteal fossa[20] (Plate 18-3).

The superficial femoral vein is a continuation of the popliteal vein, beginning at the adductor hiatus, accompanying its artery throughout the thigh, while the deep femoral vein takes a more posterolateral course, draining into the superficial femoral vein posteriorly from 4 to 10 cm below the level of the inguinal ligament.[20] The superficial femoral vein lies posterolateral to the superficial femoral artery in the distal thigh, the vein posterior to the artery in the mid-thigh, and medial to the artery in the proximal thigh.

The common femoral vein is formed by the superficial femoral and deep femoral veins and continues as the external iliac vein above the level of the inguinal ligament.

The greater saphenous vein, the longest vein in the superficial system, originates at the level of the medial malleolus. It courses superiorly just deep to the skin surface of the medial calf and thigh and drains into the anteromedial aspect of the common femoral vein. It is not accompanied by an artery. The lesser saphenous vein originates behind the lateral malleolus, and ascends over the posterior calf, passing between the two heads of the gastrocnemius muscle, and usually joins the popliteal vein[20] (Plate 18-4).

Normal variants in the venous system are common;

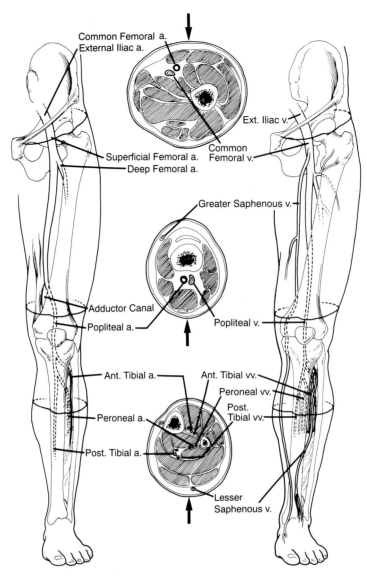

Fig. 18-3.   Illustration of the left leg arterial and venous anatomy; cross sections of the proximal thigh (arrow, anterior), knee and mid-calf regions (arrow, posterior) demonstrate pertinent vascular anatomy.

the superficial femoral and popliteal veins are duplicated or bifid in approximately 25 percent of individuals.[20]

DEEP VENOUS THROMBOSIS

Deep venous thrombosis of the lower extremity is a common disorder, which may lead to life-threatening pulmonary embolism and/or disabling venous insufficiency if not promptly diagnosed and adequately treated.[22-29] Clinical diagnosis is difficult, because patients with DVT have nonspecific complaints and may

be asymptomatic.[21,30-32] A reliable, reproducible method for noninvasive evaluation of patients who may have DVT of the legs is therefore highly desirable.[33-35] Sonographic evaluation of the venous system has become the mainstay for diagnosis of DVT of the lower extremities.[1,11,17,21,36-39] Ultrasound examinations consist of B-mode imaging, compression, and Doppler assessment, the latter employing continuous-wave, pulsed Doppler, and color Doppler. Because a variety of sonographic criteria and instrumentation are employed for detection of leg thrombus, it is crucial to define the ultrasound technique that has been utilized when reviewing reported rates of detection.[11]

Detection Rates

Several groups of investigators have examined the detection rate of DVT by compression sonography, duplex ultrasound, and color Doppler.[2-5,9,10,40,41] Detection of thrombus above the popliteal trifurcation by venous compression ultrasound has a proved sensitivity of 93 percent and a specificity of 99 percent when compared with contrast venography, as validated in several laboratories.[2-5,10,41] Statistical evaluations of previously published data have analyzed the sensitivity and specificity of compression and duplex ultrasound for lower extremity venous thrombosis.[7,36] These studies demonstrate that compression ultrasound is highly sensitive and specific for detection of thrombus at and above the knee, time- and cost-effective, and reproducible.

The addition of Doppler methods to compression ultrasound has not been shown to dramatically change the already high sensitivity and specificity figures for thrombus detection.[11] However, venous flow assessment may help determine thrombus extent and venous occlusion. Color Doppler often expedites the detection of veins in swollen, edematous extremities and within the calf.[42,43]

Rose et al[43] have reported a prospective study of 75 lower limbs of 69 consecutive patients, whose color Doppler study was performed within 24 hours of the contrast venogram. Color Doppler for detection of DVT had 96 percent sensitivity and 100 percent specificity above the knee; these values fell to 73 percent and 86 percent for the infrapopliteal deep veins. In 30 extremities (40 percent), technical factors caused limited ability to visualize and evaluate the calf veins; compromised visibility resulted from multiple factors, including prominent calf swelling, obscuration by adjacent veins, obesity, and local pain.[43]

Color Doppler also aids in identifying blood vessels, evaluating the perivascular soft tissues, and distinguishing nonocclusive from occlusive thrombus. In areas where compressibility is suboptimal, color Doppler demonstration of normal flow patterns can confirm venous patency.[11]

Below-Knee Thrombosis

Poor detection rates have been reported for the detection of DVT of the calf by compression ultrasound,[7,36] but Yucel et al[44] have recently reported a sensitivity of 88 percent and specificity of 96 percent using compression ultrasound to detect isolated calf DVT. The addition of color Doppler to compression ultrasound aids in detection and evaluation of the calf veins, but the examination time remains increased.[14,42-44] Without proximal extension, calf vein thrombus is believed to have little role in embolic phenomenon, but several investigators

argue the contrary.[42,45-48] The role of calf vein thrombus in the development of the postphlebitic syndrome is unknown.[49]

Our laboratory does not routinely evaluate calf veins for thrombus, but performs serial examinations to assess for propagation of thrombus into the popliteal vein in patients with continued symptoms and/or clinical suspicion who have had prior negative sonographic examinations. The appropriate interval for reexamination has yet to be proven; however, we typically reassess these patients in 3 to 5 days to determine whether thrombus can be detected.[49] If the referring physician believes that therapy of calf DVT is warranted and color Doppler is negative, then contrast venography is obtained.

Pitfalls

Iliac Veins

Isolated external and common iliac venous thrombosis may be difficult to diagnose with duplex sonographic evaluation, because these vessels are often obscured by overlying bowel gas and cannot be directly imaged. Even if the vessels are visualized, compression maneuvers may be suboptimal because of the increased depth of the iliac veins.[50,51]

Partial obstruction of the iliac veins and/or chronic iliac vein thrombosis with subsequent collateral venous pathways are especially difficult to detect with duplex sonographic techniques. In both instances, venous flow characteristics may be normal. Isolated iliac thrombosis is relatively uncommon, but can be missed by duplex evaluation even with careful technique.[51]

Femoral Veins

Evaluation of the common and superficial femoral vein is relatively straightforward in most patients, unless there is marked swelling and/or obesity, which may make evaluation of compressibility more difficult. Poorly echogenic thrombi may be missed, particularly if attention is not paid to the choice of Doppler gain settings and flow assessment.

Compressibility may be difficult to assess in two regions: in the proximal thigh at the level of the inguinal ligament, and more distally within the adductor canal. Within these regions, mild resistance to compression may be within normal limits, and comparison with the other leg at these levels is helpful.[11,50] If resistance to compression is mild, symmetrical, and the vein does fully compress, these findings are likely related to the patient's body habitus and are within normal limits. However, if the vein does not fully compress, or the resistance to compression is unilateral only, thrombus is suspected. Evaluation of augmentation and flow characteristics are valuable for assessment of these regions in question, particularly with color Doppler.[11]

The superficial femoral vein is commonly duplicated, and full compressibility should be established in both segments of the duplicated vein.[52]

Popliteal Veins

The more proximal portions of the popliteal vein within the adductor canal may also be slightly more difficult to compress than those more caudally. Comparison with the opposite leg is important to determine if thrombus is responsible.

Calf Veins

Within the calf, color Doppler assists in identifying the deep veins, but their course may be too deep to allow evaluation of compressibility. Their small size, paired distribution, and overlap with collateral veins make detection of small thrombi difficult. Several investigators have employed compression ultrasound and color Doppler to evaluate for calf vein thrombus, as described above. However, at our institution, symptomatic regions within the calf are examined. If no thrombus is detected, then serial examinations may be helpful to detect propagation of thrombus into the popliteal or femoral veins.

Acute versus Chronic Deep Venous Thrombosis

The venous segments involved by prior episodes of DVT can have a variety of appearances.[12,53-56] Sonographic findings at follow-up examination depend on the time interval since the initial diagnosis, and the course of thrombus resolution or progression. Murphy and Cronan[12] have evaluated patients with documented DVT by serial duplex ultrasound more than 6 months from the time of initial diagnosis; 50 percent of the veins involved had returned to a normal appearance. Persistent abnormalities after 6 months included:

> Persistent occlusion
> Intimal thickening with thickened, stiff walls
> Recanalization of the original lumen, with incompetent valves

In those patients with persistent occlusion, recurrent acute thrombus may be suspected if the vein diameter is increased and the thrombus slightly compressible. If the thrombus does not compress at all, and if the vein diameter is normal or contracted, then chronic venous

thrombus may be suspected. Recanalized veins with intimal thickening may not fully compress; color Doppler examination may be helpful to distinguish flowing blood within the lumen from the peripheral thickened intima[12] (Plate 18-5).

Echogenicity has not proved to be a reliable indicator of thrombus age; although acute thrombus may be minimally echogenic, and chronic thrombus more echogenic, marked variability in thrombus echogenicity has been demonstrated.[12]

Ideally, a new baseline for comparison should be established in patients with documented DVT, performed within 6 months to 2 years after the initial diagnosis.[12,49] Two groups of investigators have demonstrated that the majority of change in acutely thrombosed veins occurs within 6 months of the initial diagnosis of acute DVT.[12,53] Serial compression sonography may prove useful in the evaluation of thrombus progression, tendency for embolization, and effectiveness of therapy.[49]

Venous Compression Ultrasound in Patients with Suspected Pulmonary Embolism

The use of compression ultrasound as a *primary* method of diagnosing pulmonary embolism is *strongly discouraged.*[49] In one prospective study, 29 percent of patients with angiographically proven pulmonary emboli had normal bilateral contrast venograms of the legs at the time of the pulmonary angiogram.[57] Conversely, demonstration of thrombus in either or both lower extremities does not prove or exclude pulmonary embolism. Therefore, compression sonography is not appropriate as a primary method for the detection of pulmonary embolism. Several investigators recommend noninvasive evaluation for lower extremity thrombosis as a secondary method in evaluating patients who have an indeterminate ventilation-perfusion scan; however, this strategy requires further confirmation with appropriately designed clinical trials.[57-59]

VENOUS INSUFFICIENCY

The chronic venous stasis syndrome has been referred to by many names, including the *postphlebitic syndrome,* which implicates thrombophlebitis as its etiology.[60] In patients who do not have a history of DVT, the venous valve cusps become incompetent without a recognizable cause, and this is termed *primary venous incompetence.*[61] Patients with venous insufficiency suffer from a variety of complaints, including pain, skin discoloration, induration, edema, and ulceration.[60,61]

Chronic venous stasis syndrome is caused by valvular incompetence in the deep or superficial veins, which results in retrograde flow of blood (reflux) and an increased ambulatory venous pressure.[62]

Many methods are currently available for the evaluation of patients with venous insufficiency; these include ambulatory venous pressure measurements, descending venography, photoplethysmography, and duplex ultrasound.[63] Flow reversal within the venous system may be detected by duplex sonography.[62,64] Several provocative maneuvers may induce venous reflux, including the utilization of Valsalva maneuver or thigh compression to provoke retrograde venous flow. Some investigators propose that the patient should be scanned in the standing position, evaluating the influence of gravity on venous reflux.[62,64] With the patient standing, the calf is compressed externally, often by application of a pressure cuff. Superficial and deep venous flow is observed with duplex ultrasound during and after application of calf compression; reversed venous flow after release of calf compression indicates venous reflux.[64]

Duplex scanning has been investigated to determine its efficacy in the detection of venous incompetence.[62,64,65] In a study by Szendro et al[64] duplex ultrasound examinations were evaluated in 23 patients and 6 volunteers. The examinations were performed with the subject standing to assess flow reversal induced by gravity. Comparison with venous pressure measurements showed that duplex scanning had a sensitivity of 84 percent and a specificity of 88 percent for the detection of venous insufficiency.[64]

A prospective study by Rosfors et al[65] compared duplex scanning with descending phlebography for the detection of venous incompetence, showing agreement in 15 of 23 lower extremities. Disagreements resulted primarily in patients with minor degrees of reflux; these were underestimated by ultrasonographic examinations. In four patients, duplex scanning diagnosed isolated calf valvular insufficiency, which is impossible to demonstrate with descending phlebography if the proximal valve segment is competent.[65]

The final role of duplex ultrasound in the evaluation of venous valvular insufficiency remains to be defined. These initial studies are encouraging; color Doppler may improve detection rates and aid in the determination of site and severity of venous reflux.[66]

UPPER EXTREMITY VENOUS EVALUATION

Indications for upper extremity venous sonography include central venous catheter complications[67-71]; dialysis access arteriovenous fistulas[14,72-74]; and arm edema from other etiologies[67,68,75] (including effort, mastectomy, node enlargement, neoplasm, intravenous drug abuse).

TECHNIQUE

The following is a summary of the sonographic technique of the upper extremities.[67]

1. Use a 7-MHz transducer for the arm and neck examination and a 5-MHz transducer for the infraclavicular transpectoral approach.
2. Begin the ultrasound examination at the elbow, and follow the basilic and brachial veins along the medial aspect of the upper arm.
3. Assess compression in the transverse plane, and follow the course of the veins with both the transverse and longitudinal views.
4. Evaluate the distal axillary vein under the arm; then utilize the infraclavicular approach to image the proximal axillary vein and distal subclavian vein.

5. Examine the proximal subclavian vein and distal innominate vein with a supraclavicular approach.
6. Utilize spectral/color Doppler settings and a Doppler angle of less than 60 degrees to optimize detection of slow flow.

The diagnosis of venous thrombosis is indicated by noncompressibility, direct visualization of mural thrombus with luminal narrowing, or absence of color flow within the lumen.[67-70,76] Visualization of venous collaterals may be confirmatory evidence, implying a more chronic obstruction.[67]

NORMAL ANATOMY

In contrast to the leg, the dominant venous drainage route of the upper extremity is via the superficial venous system (Fig. 18-4). The deep veins of the arm are small, paired, and accompany the arteries. The principal superficial veins are the cephalic, basilic, and median veins. The cephalic vein drains the radial aspect of the hand, coursing over the anterolateral forearm and upper arm to join the axillary vein immediately inferior to the

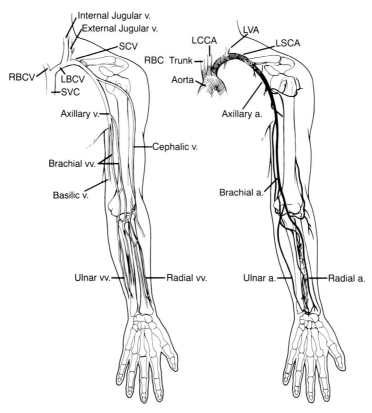

Fig. 18-4.   Illustration of the left arm arterial and venous anatomy. (*RBCV & LBCV,* right and left brachiocephalic veins; *SCV,* subclavian vein; *LCCA,* left common carotid artery; *LVA,* left vertebral artery; *LSCA,* left subclavian artery; *RBC Trunk,* right brachiocephalic trunk; *SVC,* superior vena cava.)

clavicle. The basilic vein originates over the ulnar aspect of the distal forearm, continuing along the anteromedial surface of the forearm, and continues as the axillary vein; its contributaries include the brachial veins. The median vein of the forearm is located anteriorly, joining the basilic or medial cubital vein.

The axillary vein continues as the subclavian vein as it passes the lateral border of the first rib, and is then joined by the internal jugular vein at the medial border of the anterior scalene muscle to form the brachiocephalic vein.[77]

VENOUS THROMBOSIS/CENTRAL VENOUS CATHETER EVALUATION

Although upper extremity venous thrombosis is less common than DVT of the legs, the incidence of arm thrombosis has increased, likely resulting from the increased utilization of central venous catheters and transvenous cardiac pacemakers.[69,70] Local infection and distant embolization can result from upper extremity thrombus. The actual incidence of pulmonary embolism resulting from arm thrombus is difficult to quantitate, because most reports of arm venous thrombosis are retrospective studies or case reports.[78] Monreal et al[78] performed a prospective study of 30 patients with venographic evidence of arm thrombus who were also evaluated with ventilation-perfusion scans. Their results show that 4 of 20 patients with catheter-related thrombus had lung scans highly suggestive of pulmonary embolism, while the 10 patients without catheters had no high probability lung scans.[78] Pulmonary embolism appears to be more common in reported series with a larger proportion of patients with catheter-related arm thrombosis; arm thrombus may lead to pulmonary embolism, particularly in patients with central venous catheters.[78]

DIALYSIS ACCESS ARTERIOVENOUS FISTULA

Upper extremity vascular access grafts for hemodialysis may be either end-to-side or end-to-end venoarterial shunts from the radial or brachial artery.[74] A prosthetic loop graft may sometimes be employed in the antecubital fossa of the proximal forearm, connecting the basilic vein to the brachial artery[72,74] (Plate 18-6). Knowledge of the patient's surgical anastomotic procedure is helpful in the sonographic evaluation of the arteriovenous communication.

Complications that may occur are venous stenosis, either proximal to or at the anastomotic site; pseudoaneurysm at the fistula site; and distal arterial steal, caused by arterial obstruction proximal to the fistula. Color Doppler evaluation is difficult to utilize in the diagnosis of localized stenosis at the fistula site or proximal venous stenosis.[14,72,73] Patients whose flow precludes satisfactory dialysis are best evaluated by a fistulogram.[72] However, analysis of a pulsatile mass or distal ischemia can be evaluated with color Doppler, because duplex evaluation can detect pseudoaneurysm or proximal arterial obstruction with distal arterial steal.[14,72]

LOWER AND UPPER EXTREMITY ARTERIAL EVALUATION

Sonographic evaluation of arterial disease involves a targeted examination to answer the pertinent clinical question. If aortoiliac evaluation is necessary, the patient should fast for at least 4 to 6 hours prior to the procedure.

Currently, duplex imaging of upper and lower extremity arteries is performed for the following indications:

1. Evaluation of suspected pseudoaneurysm, arteriovenous fistula
2. Analysis of perivascular soft tissues for detection of hematoma, abscess
3. Serial examination after surgical and/or percutaneous interventions

Although some have proposed the use of duplex arterial evaluation for screening of patients with claudication,[14] appropriate clinical trials have not yet proved the validity of this approach.

Typically lower and upper extremity arteries will be best evaluated with either a 5- or 7-MHz transducer; more proximally within the body the 3-MHz transducer may be necessary.
3. Color Doppler is routinely utilized to examine regions of suspected arterial stenosis; gain settings are adjusted to increase sensitivity to slow flow in regions of decreased flow. Doppler sample volume is increased if no flow is detected initially.
4. Measurements of peak velocity are performed with Doppler angle of less than or equal to 60 degrees to avoid significant errors in velocity determination; comparison with baseline peak velocity established more proximally is used to grade stenosis severity (Table 18-1).[79]
5. The perivascular soft tissues and adjacent venous structures are also examined for possible hematoma, pseudoaneurysm, and arteriovenous fistula. Color Doppler techniques aid in this analysis, because with optimal settings, abnormal flow patterns and extraluminal flow may be readily detected.

TECHNIQUE

High resolution sonographic equipment is essential for the diagnosis of extremity arterial disease. The following steps are performed in the evaluation of patients with suspected arterial abnormalities in our laboratory.

1. With the patient supine, the extremity is examined in both transverse and longitudinal planes contiguously.
2. The choice of transducer depends on the depth of the vessel under investigation; the highest frequency transducer that allows visualization of the vessel is selected.

TABLE 18-1. Grading of Arterial Lesion Severity with Color Doppler[a]

Peak Velocity	Interpretation
No increase	Normal diameter
Increase of 30–100%	1–49% diameter reduction
Increase of >100%	50–99% diameter reduction
No flow	Occlusion

[a] Grade of stenosis severity is based on angle-corrected peak velocity at the stenosis, compared with baseline measurement established in the arterial segment proximal to the stenosis. Occlusions are diagnosed when no flow is demonstrated despite attempts at maximizing sensitivity to slow flow.
(Data from Jager et al[79] and Mulligan et al.[80])

NORMAL ANATOMY

Lower Extremity

Caudal to the inguinal ligament, the external iliac artery continues as the common femoral artery. The common femoral artery is located lateral to the common femoral vein (Fig. 18-3). The common femoral artery bifurcates into the deep femoral artery (profunda femoris) and superficial femoral artery approximately 4 cm caudal to the inguinal ligament. The deep femoral artery often lies posterior to the superficial femoral artery. The superficial femoral artery courses along the anteromedial aspect of the thigh, supplying several unnamed muscular branches and the descending geniculate artery before entering the adductor canal. The proximal superficial femoral artery rarely bifurcates, and when it does, it reunites at the adductor canal.[81] The superficial femoral artery continues as the popliteal artery distal to the adductor canal, coursing between the heads of the gastrocnemius muscle behind the knee. The popliteal artery usually bifurcates at its termination into the anterior and posterior tibial arteries. The anterior tibial artery courses through the interosseous membrane, lying medial to the fibular neck, and descends anterior to this membrane along the medial border of the fibula. In the foot, it passes toward the midline of the dorsum of the foot as the dorsalis pedis artery. The posterior tibial artery courses medially through the calf, giving off the peroneal artery approximately 2 to 3 cm distal to the popliteal bifurcation. The posterior tibial artery continues toward the foot, passing just behind the medial malleolus. The peroneal artery occasionally arises from the popliteal artery; it courses posteriorly in the calf, terminating at the ankle.

Upper Extremity

The subclavian artery is located below the clavicle, and continues as the axillary artery as it passes the lateral aspect of the first rib, distal to the origin of the costocervical trunk (Fig. 18-4). As it courses past the level of the anatomic neck of the humerus, the axillary artery continues as the brachial artery, located in the medial bicipital groove, and is easily palpable. Below the elbow, the brachial artery bifurcates into an ulnar and radial artery, the latter is usually a smaller, more direct continuation of the brachial artery.[82]

ARTERIAL STENOSIS AND OCCLUSION

Evaluation of arterial obstruction can be performed noninvasively by a variety of methods, including sonographic duplex techniques.[79,83-85] Although the contrast angiogram remains the mainstay of diagnosis for peripheral arterial obstruction, particularly in patients in whom surgery is contemplated, duplex sonography may be utilized to evaluate postsurgical patients and may detect arterial disease prior to surgery.[80,85-95]

Diagnostic criteria for the evaluation of arterial stenosis and occlusion are based on waveform analysis; specifically, elevations of peak systolic velocity from baseline established more proximally within the artery, and estimation of spectral broadening.[79,83,96-99] Peak systolic velocity determinations are more reproducible, suffer less from technical factors in their interpretation, and are used exclusively in our laboratory to determine stenosis severity.

Peak systolic arterial velocity must be determined with a Doppler angle of less than 60 degrees. The use of an appropriate Doppler angle will avoid the great errors in measurement of velocity if larger angles are utilized. Color Doppler techniques aid in identifying regions of increased brightness in areas of increased mean flow velocity; however, spectral evaluation is required to determine the peak velocity.

Four diagnostic categories are utilized to grade arterial lesions: 0 percent, 1–49 percent, 50–99 percent diameter reduction, and occlusion (Table 18-1).[79] The grade of stenosis is based on angle-corrected determinations of peak systolic velocity at the stenosis compared with peak systolic velocity in the arterial segment proximal to the stenosis. If the peak velocity more than doubles from the baseline established proximally, 50 to 99 percent diameter reduction is diagnosed (Plate 18-7). Arterial occlusion is diagnosed when no flow is demonstrated despite maximizing sensitivity to slow flow by increasing Doppler gain, decreasing scale, and increasing sample volume.[80]

Color Doppler and Grading of Arterial Lesions

Careful attention to color Doppler technique is necessary for optimal results. Nonvisualization of iliac arterial segments remains an obstacle for the evaluation of arterial disease extent, particularly in preoperative patients. However, at and below the level of the inguinal ligament, detection and grading of arterial lesions by color Doppler is much improved.[80]

Underestimation of the severity of arterial disease can result despite optimal color Doppler technique. Mapping of arterial disease requires diligence and familiarity with normal and postoperative arterial anatomy. Stenosis severity may be difficult to assess in regions obscured by calcified plaque. Arterial segments with calcified plaque remain difficult to analyze with color Doppler, and should be regarded as indeterminate when grading stenosis.[14,80]

ARTERIOVENOUS FISTULA AND PSEUDOANEURYSM

Duplex ultrasound and color Doppler are particularly adept at detecting complications of femoral artery catheterizations, particularly arteriovenous fistulae and pseudoaneurysms. In addition to detecting these complications, duplex ultrasound and color Doppler are able to differentiate them from hematomas. While these complications are uncommon, their incidence increases in patients undergoing percutaneous transluminal coronary angioplasty (particularly in the setting of thrombolytic therapy), percutaneous aortic valvulotomy, and electrophysiologic testing.[100] Other factors that increase the risk of developing a complication include multiple arterial punctures, arterial and venous cannulation, hypertension, and improper technique.[100,101]

Arteriovenous Fistula

An arteriovenous fistula is an abnormal communication between the arterial and venous systems. These lesions shunt blood from the high pressure arterial system into the low pressure (and low resistance) venous system. An arteriovenous fistula, when symptomatic, can have systemic and local effects. Systemic symptoms include high-output congestive heart failure and angina. Local effects include claudication resulting from decreased arterial flow and venous stasis due to increased venous pressure.[102,103]

Duplex ultrasound and color Doppler are complementary methods for the detection of arteriovenous fistula, which cannot be detected with the use of B-mode scanning alone. Duplex ultrasound findings include the following:

1. Abnormal arterial waveform proximal to the fistula with the loss of the normal triphasic wave form that is replaced by continuous forward flow during diastole.
2. Distal to the fistula, arterial flow may be decreased with respect to the opposite leg. Sometimes, the triphasic waveform is not seen.
3. In the vein at and immediately proximal to the fistula, continuous high velocity venous flow is present. This flow will lack respiratory variation and will often exhibit arterial pulsations.

Color Doppler findings of arteriovenous fistula include the following:

1. Direct visualization of an arteriovenous communication (high-velocity jet of blood) (Plate 18-8).
2. A colorful "speckled" mass at the level of the fistula and/or adjacent vein with extremely turbulent flow demonstrated on waveforms taken from the site of these "speckles."
3. "Spreading" of color pixels in the soft tissues adjacent to the fistula at scanner settings in which color pixels were not seen in soft tissues elsewhere.[102]

The forward continuous diastolic arterial flow seen proximal to the fistula is due to the decreased peripheral resistance of the receiving venous system. The turbulent flow at the site of the arteriovenous fistula that results in the "speckled" mass is due to the large pressure gradient between the arterial and venous systems.[100] In our experience, the perivascular "spread" of color may disappear when firm pressure is applied with a transducer. When an apparent connection between the artery and vein is seen in the absence of the other findings described above, the diagnosis of an arteriovenous fistula should be made with caution since this finding can be mimicked by vessels that cross or are located immediately adjacent to each other.[102]

Pseudoaneurysm

A pseudoaneurysm is a pulsatile hematoma that results from the leakage of blood into the soft tissues abutting the punctured artery, with subsequent fibrous encapsulation and failure of the vessel wall defect to heal.[104] Pseudoaneurysms may require prompt surgical repair because they can be a source of emboli, a site of infection, and a cause of local pressure effects. They can also rupture, which may result in exsanguination.[105,106]

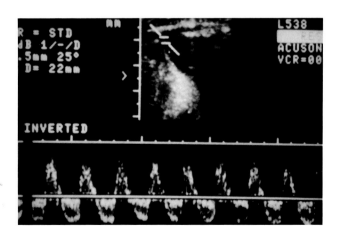

Fig. 18-5. To-and-fro pattern within the neck of this pseudoaneurysm of the superficial femoral artery, the characteristic spectral waveform.

During B-mode scanning, a pseudoaneurysm may appear as an anechoic or complex cystic mass, and may on occasion mimic a hematoma. The echogenic material within the pseudoaneurysm represents thrombus. Duplex ultrasound and color Doppler are both able to identify pseudoaneurysm. Doppler of the pseudoaneurysm demonstrates arterial flow that may or may not be turbulent but is continuous throughout the cardiac cycle. With color Doppler, swirls of color are seen within the pseudoaneurysm[107] (Plate 18-9). A characteristic spectral waveform of the blood flow has been reported in the neck of the pseudoaneurysm, called *to-and-fro*[104,105] (Fig. 18-5). During systole, blood flows from the artery into the pseudoaneurysm, and during diastole, blood returns to the artery from the pseudoaneurysm, resulting in the to-and-fro pattern. This flow reversal is caused by the drop in arterial pressure during diastole. Flow velocity is lower in diastole than in systole because the pressure gradient between the pseudoaneurysm and the artery is smaller in diastole than in systole.[105]

ACKNOWLEDGMENTS

We would like to thank Lincoln L. Berland, M.D., Mitzi D. Fields, R.T., R.D.M.S., R.V.T., Michael Clements, R.T., R.D.M.S., Pamela McEachern, R.T., R.D.M.S., Curtis E. Cagle, R.T., R.D.M.S., and David Fisher for their assistance in this effort.

REFERENCES

1. Hobson RW, Mintz BL, Jamil Z et al: Diagnosis of acute deep venous thrombosis. Surg Clin North Am 1990;70:143
2. Raghavendra BN, Horii SC, Hilton S et al: Deep venous thrombosis: detection by probe compression of veins. J Ultrasound Med 1986;5:89
3. Appleman PT, De Jong TE, Lampmann LE: Deep venous thrombosis of the leg: US findings. Radiology 1987;163:743
4. Dauzat MM, Laroche J-P, Charras C et al: Real-time B-mode ultrasonography for better specificity in the noninvasive diagnosis of deep venous thrombosis. J Ultrasound Med 1986;5:625
5. Vogel P, Laing FC, Jeffrey RB Jr et al: Deep venous thrombosis of the lower extremity: US evaluation. Radiology 1987;163:747
6. Talbot SR: B-Mode evaluation of peripheral veins. Semin Ultrasound CT MR 1988;9:295
7. White RH, McGahan JP, Daschback MM et al: Diagnosis of deep-vein thrombosis using duplex ultrasound. Ann Intern Med 1989;111:297
8. Rosner NH, Doris PE: Diagnosis of femoropopliteal venous thrombosis: comparison of duplex sonography and plethysmography. AJR 1988;150:623
9. Cronan JJ, Dorfman GS, Scola FH et al: Deep venous thrombosis: US assessment using vein compression. Radiology 1987;162:191
10. O'Leary DH, Kane RA, Chase BM: A prospective study of the efficacy of B-scan sonography in the detection of deep venous thrombosis in the lower extremities. J Clin Ultrasound 1988;16:1
11. Cronan JJ: Evaluation of the femoral popliteal venous system. p. 65. Color Doppler Ultrasonography Course. AIUM syllabus. American Institute of Ultrasound in Medicine, Atlanta, 1991
12. Murphy TP, Cronan JJ: Evolution of deep venous thrombosis: a prospective evaluation with US. Radiology 1990;177:543
13. Chaudhuri R, Salari R: Baker's cyst simulating deep vein thrombosis. Clin Radiol 1990;41:400
14. Foley WD, Erickson SJ: Color Doppler flow imaging. AJR 1991;156:3
15. Mewissen MW, Erickson SJ, Foley WD et al: Thrombosis at venous insertion sites after inferior vena caval filter placement. Radiology 1989;173:155
16. Yedlicka JW, Hunter DW, Letourneau JG: Pulmonary embolism after femoral vein compression during sonography: case report. Semin Intervent Rad 1990;7:24
17. Zwiebel WJ: Anatomy and duplex characteristics of the normal deep veins. Semin Ultrasound CT MR 1988;9:269
18. Raghavendra BN, Rosen RJ, Lam S et al: Deep venous thrombosis: detection by high-resolution real-time ultrasonography. Radiology 1984;152:789
19. Effeney DJ, Friedman MB, Gooding GAW: Iliofemoral venous thrombosis: real-time ultrasound diagnosis, normal criteria, and clinical application. Radiology 1984;150:787
20. Kadir S: Venography. p. 536. In Kadir S (ed): Diagnostic Angiography. WB Saunders, Philadelphia, 1986
21. O'Leary DH, Kane RA: Venous ultrasonography of the lower extremities. p. 304. In Taylor KJW, Burns PN, Wells PNT (eds): Clinical Applications of Doppler Ultrasound. Raven Press, New York, 1988
22. Kakkar VV: Deep vein thrombosis: detection and prevention. Circulation 1975;51:8
23. Lindner DJ, Edwards JM, Phinney ES et al: Long-term hemodynamic and clinical sequelae of lower extremity deep vein thrombosis. J Vasc Surg 1986;4:436
24. Strandness DE Jr, Langlois Y, Cramer M et al: Long-term sequelae of acute venous thrombosis. JAMA 1983;250:1289
25. Rollins DL, Lloyd WE, Buchbinder D: Venous thrombosis: the clinical problem. Semin Ultrasound CT MR 1988;9:277
26. Mudge M, Hughes LE: The long term sequelae of deep vein thrombosis. Br J Surg 1978;65:692
27. Hufnagel CA: Deep venous thrombosis: an overview. Angiology 1990;41:337
28. Otoya J, Nemcek AA Jr, Green D: Venous thromboembolism. Chest 1989;96:1169

29. Moser KM: Venous thromboembolism. Am Rev Respir Dis 1990;141:235

30. Harmon B: Deep vein thrombosis: a perspective on anatomy and venographic analysis. J Thorac Imaging 1989;4:15

31. Froehlich JA, Dorfman GS, Cronan JJ et al: Compression ultrasonography for the detection of deep venous thrombosis in patients who have a fracture of the hip. J Bone Joint Surg (Am) 1989;71:249

32. Dorfman GS, Froehlich JA, Cronan JJ et al: Lower-extremity venous thrombosis in patients with acute hip fractures: determination of anatomic location and time of onset with compression sonography. AJR 1990;154:851

33. Whitehouse GH: Venous thrombosis and thromboembolism. Clin Radiol 1990;41:77

34. Redman HC: Deep venous thrombosis: is contrast venography still the diagnostic "gold standard"? Radiology 1988;168:277

35. Barnes RW, Nix ML: Clinical and noninvasive assessment of venous disease as related to pulmonary embolism. J Thorac Imaging 1989;4:8

36. Becker DM, Philbrick JT, Abbitt PL: Real-time ultrasonography for the diagnosis of lower extremity deep venous thrombosis. Arch Intern Med 1989;149:1731

37. Comerota AJ, Katz ML, Greenwald LL et al: Venous duplex imaging: should it replace hemodynamic tests for deep venous thrombosis? J Vasc Surg 1990;11:53

38. Knighton RA, Priest DL, Zwiebel WJ et al: Techniques for color flow sonography of the lower extremity. RadioGraphics 1990;10:775

39. Mantoni M: Diagnosis of deep venous thrombosis by duplex sonography. Acta Radiol 1989;30:575

40. Foley WD, Middleton WD, Lawson TL et al: Color Doppler ultrasound imaging of lower-extremity venous disease. AJR 1989;152:371

41. Lensing AWA, Prandoni P, Brandjes D et al: Detection of deep-vein thrombosis by real-time B-mode ultrasonography. N Engl J Med 1989;320:342

42. Polak JF, Culter SS, O'Leary DH: Deep veins of the calf: assessment with color Doppler flow imaging. Radiology 1989;171:481

43. Rose SC, Zwiebel WJ, Nelson BD et al: Symptomatic lower extremity deep venous thrombosis: accuracy, limitations, and role of color duplex flow imaging in diagnosis. Radiology 1990;175:639

44. Yucel EK, Fisher JS, Egglin TK et al: Isolated calf venous thrombosis: diagnosis with compression US. Radiology 1991;179:443

45. Bartter T, Hollingsworth HM, Irwin RS et al: Pulmonary embolism from a venous thrombus located below the knee. Arch Intern Med 1987;147:373

46. Philbrick JT, Becker DM: Calf deep venous thrombosis: a wolf in sheep's clothing? Arch Intern Med 1988;148:2131

47. Moreno-Cabral R, Kistner RL, Nordyke RA: Importance of calf vein thrombophlebitis. Surgery 1976;80:735

48. Kakkar VV, Howe CT, Flanc C et al: Natural history of postoperative deep-vein thrombosis. Lancet 1969;2:230

49. Dorfman GS, Cronan JJ: Sonographic diagnosis of

thrombosis of the lower extremity veins. Semin Interven Radiol 1990;7:9

50. Wright DJ, Shepard AD, McPharline M et al: Pitfalls in lower extremity venous duplex scanning. J Vasc Surg 1990;11:675

51. Zwiebel WJ: Sources of error in duplex venography and an algorithmic approach to the diagnosis of deep venous thrombosis. Semin Ultrasound CT MR 1988;9:286

52. Quinn KL, Vandeman FN: Thrombosis of a duplicated superficial femoral vein. J Ultrasound Med 1990;9:235

53. Cronan JJ, Leen V: Recurrent deep venous thrombosis: limitations of US. Radiology 1989;170:739

54. Krupski WC, Bass A, Dilley RB et al: Propagation of deep venous thrombosis identified by duplex ultrasonography. J Vasc Surg 1990;12:467

55. Mantoni M: Deep venous thrombosis: longitudinal study with duplex US. Radiology 1991;179:271

56. Thomas ML, McAllister V: The radiological progression of deep venous thrombus. Radiology 1971;99:37

57. Hull RD, Hirsh J, Carter CJ et al: Pulmonary angiography, ventilation lung scanning, and venography for clinically suspected pulmonary embolism with abnormal perfusion lung scan. Ann Intern Med 1983;98:891

58. Kelley MA, Carson JL, Palevsky HI et al: Diagnosing pulmonary embolism: new facts and strategies. Ann Intern Med 1991;114:300

59. Hull RD, Raskob GE, Coates G et al: A new noninvasive management strategy for patients with suspected pulmonary embolism. Arch Intern Med 1989;149:2549

60. Train JS, Schanzer H, Peirce EC II et al: Radiological evaluation of the chronic venous stasis syndrome. JAMA 1987;258:941

61. Kistner RL: Primary venous valve incompetence of the leg. Am J Surg 1980;140:218

62. Vasdekis SN, Clarke GH, Nicolaides AN: Quantification of venous reflux by means of duplex scanning. J Vasc Surg 1989;10:670

63. Raju S, Fredericks R: Evaluation of methods for detecting venous reflux: perspectives in venous insufficiency. Arch Surg 1990;125:1463

64. Szendro G, Nicolaides AN, Zukowski AJ et al: Duplex scanning in the assessment of deep venous incompetence. J Vasc Surg 1986;4:237

65. Rosfors S, Bygdeman S, Nordstrom E: Assessment of deep venous incompetence: a prospective study comparing duplex scanning with descending phlebography. Angiology 1990;43:463

66. Athanasoulis CA, Yucel EK: Venous reflux: assessing the level of incompetence. Radiology 1990;174:326

67. Knudson GJ, Wiedemeyer DA, Erickson SJ et al: Color Doppler sonographic imaging in the assessment of upper-extremity deep venous thrombosis. AJR 1990;154:399

68. Grassi CJ, Polak JF: Axillary and subclavian venous thrombosis: follow-up evaluation with color Doppler flow US and venography. Radiology 1990;175:651

69. Hubsch PJS, Stiglbauer RL, Schwaighofer BWAM et al: Internal jugular and subclavian vein thrombosis caused by central venous catheters: evaluations using Doppler blood flow imaging. J Ultrasound Med 1988;7:629

70. Gaitini D, Kaftori JK, Pery M et al: High-resolution real-time ultrasonography: diagnosis and follow-up of jugular and subclavian vein thrombosis. J Ultrasound Med 1988;7:621

71. Weissleder R, Elizondo G, Stark DD: Sonographic diagnosis of subclavian and internal jugular vein thrombosis. J Ultrasound Med 1987;6:577

72. Middleton WD, Picus DD, Marx MV et al: Color Doppler sonography of hemodialysis vascular access: comparison with angiography. AJR 1989;152:633

73. Surratt RS, Picus D, Hicks ME et al: The importance of preoperative evaluation of the subclavian vein in dialysis access planning. AJR 1991;156:623

74. Hunter DW, So SK: Dialysis access: radiographic evaluation and management. Radiol Clin North Am 1987;25:249

75. Nemmers DW, Thorpe PE, Knibbe MA et al: Upper extremity venous thrombosis; case report and literature review. Orthop Rev 1990;19:164

76. Kerr TM, Lutter KS, Moeller DM et al: Upper extremity venous thrombosis diagnosed by duplex scanning. Am J Surg 1990;160:202

77. Lundell C, Kadir S: Upper extremity veins. p. 177. In Kadir S (ed): Atlas of Normal and Variant Angiographic Anatomy. WB Saunders, Philadelphia, 1991

78. Monreal M, Lafoz E, Ruiz J et al: Upper-extremity deep venous thrombosis and pulmonary embolism: a prospective study. Chest 1991;99:280

79. Jager KA, Phillips DJ, Martin RL et al: Noninvasive mapping of lower limb arterial lesions. Ultrasound Med Biol 1985;11:515

80. Mulligan SA, Matsuda T, Lanzer P et al: Peripheral arterial occlusive disease: prospective comparison of MR angiography and color duplex US with conventional angiography. Radiology 1991;178:695

81. Kadir S: Arteriography of the lower extremity vessels. p. 254. In Kadir S (ed): Diagnostic Angiography. WB Saunders, Philadelphia, 1986

82. Kadir S: Arteriography of the upper extremities. p. 172. In Kadir S (ed): Diagnostic Angiography. WB Saunders, Philadelphia, 1986

83. Moneta GL, Strandness DE Jr: Peripheral arterial duplex scanning. J Clin Ultrasound 1987;15:645

84. Kohler TR, Nance DR, Cramer MM et al: Duplex scanning of aortoiliac and femoropopliteal disease: a prospective study. Circulation 1987;76:1074

85. Strandness DE Jr: Noninvasive evaluation of arteriosclerosis: comparison of methods. Arteriosclerosis 1983;3:103

86. Bandyk DF, Cato RF, Towne JB: A low flow velocity predicts failure of femoropopliteal and femorotibial bypass grafts. Surgery 1985;98:799

87. Bandyk DF: Postoperative surveillance of infrainguinal Bypass. Surg Clin North Am 1990;70:71

88. Barnes RW: Noninvasive evaluation of peripheral vascular disease. S Med J 1986;79:55

89. Bandyk DF, Kaebnick HW, Bergamini TM et al: Hemodynamics of in situ saphenous vein arterial bypass. Arch Surg 1988;123:477

90. Bandyk DF, Seabrook GR, Moldenhauer P et al: Hemodynamics of vein graft stenosis. J Vasc Surg 1988;8:688

91. Barnes RW, Thompson BW, MacDonald CM et al: Serial noninvasive studies do not herald postoperative failure of femoropopliteal or femorotibial bypass grafts. Ann Surg 1989;210:486

92. Cohen JR, Mannick JA, Couch NP et al: Recognition and management of impending vein-graft failure. Arch Surg 1986;121:758

93. Polak JF, Donaldson MC, Dobkin GR et al: Early detection of saphenous vein arterial bypass graft stenosis by color-assisted duplex sonography: a prospective study. AJR 1990;154:857

94. Leopold PW, Shandall AA, Kay C et al: Duplex ultrasound: its role in the non-invasive follow up of the in situ saphenous vein bypass. J Vasc Surg Technol 1987;11:183

95. Polak JF, Karmel MI, Mannick JA et al: Determination of the extent of lower-extremity peripheral arterial disease with color-assisted duplex sonography: comparison with angiography. AJR 1990;155:1085

96. Campbell WB: Doppler waveform analysis in the management of lower limb arterial disease. Ann R Coll Surg Engl 1986;68:103

97. Campbell WB, Fletcher EL, Hands LJ: Assessment of the distal lower limb arteries: a comparison of arteriography and Doppler ultrasound. Ann R Coll Surg Engl 1986;68:37

98. Capper WL, Amoore JN, Clifford PC et al: Non-invasive assessment of lower limb ischaemia by blood velocity wave-form analysis. S Afr Med J 1987;71:695

99. Field JP, Musson AM, Zwolak RM et al: Duplex arterial flow measurements in normal lower extremities. J Vasc Technol 1989;13:13

100. Sheikh KH, Adams DB, McCann R et al: Utility of Doppler color flow imaging for identification of femoral arterial complications of cardiac catheterization. Am Heart J 1988;117:623

101. Liu J, Merton DA, Mitchell DG et al: Color Doppler imaging of the iliofemoral region. RadioGraphics 1990;10:403

102. Roubidoux MA, Hertzberg BS, Carroll BA et al: Color flow and image-directed Doppler ultrasound evaluation of iatrogenic arteriovenous fistulas in the groin. J Clin Ultrasound 1990;18:463

103. Igidbashian VN, Mitchell DG, Middleton WD et al: Iatrogenic femoral arteriovenous fistula: diagnosis with color Doppler imaging. Radiology 1989;170:749

104. Mitchell DG, Needleman L, Bezzi M et al: Femoral artery pseudoaneurysm: diagnosis with conventional duplex and color Doppler US. Radiology 1987;165:687

105. Abu-Yousef MM, Wiese JA, Shamma AR: The "to-and-fro" sign: duplex Doppler evidence of femoral artery pseudoaneurysm. AJR 1988;150:632

106. Helvie MA, Rubin JM, Silver TM et al: The distinction between femoral artery pseudoaneurysms and other causes of groin masses: value of duplex Doppler sonography. Am Heart J 1988;150:1177

107. Polak JF, Donaldson MC, Whittemore AD et al: Pulsatile masses surrounding vascular prostheses: real-time US color flow imaging. Radiology 1989;170:363

19

Interventional Abdominal Ultrasound

John P. McGahan

Percutaneous aspiration drainage procedures have become a vital portion of day-to-day clinical practice because of their safety, simplicity, and effectiveness. While needle puncture and aspiration were first described in 1930,[1] it was not until the early 1970s that both Holm[2] and Goldberg[3] independently devised ultrasound transducers that could be utilized for aspiration or biopsy techniques. Since that time, advances in ultrasound instrumentation and refinement of aspiration/biopsy techniques have dramatically increased intervention ultrasound applications within the abdomen. This chapter reviews some of these applications and procedures.

ULTRASOUND ADVANTAGES

Probably one of the most important considerations when selecting a technique for guidance of aspiration or drainage in the abdomen is the accuracy and safety provided by the guidance system (Table 19-1). The inherent accuracy and safety of the procedure outweighs most other considerations, such as expediency or the cost of imaging technology. Recent technologic advances include development of ultrasound guidance systems and specially designed ultrasound needles, which allow for needle placement into a target lesion under real-time control. A previous publication[4] has demonstrated that ultrasound can precisely guide needle biopsies in lesions

as small as 1 cm in critical anatomic areas (Fig. 19-1). This precision is necessary for a successful procedure and often makes sonography the first choice in guiding interventional procedures. Ultrasound may be used to not only confirm needle placement, but redirect needle position under real-time control.

Other advantages of ultrasound include development of compact portable units that may be transported throughout the hospital to guide interventional procedures.[5,6] A review of over 100 ultrasound-guided aspiration or drainage procedures performed at our institution revealed that approximately one-third of these were performed within the hospital intensive care units.[6] While it is inconvenient for a radiologist to leave the radiology department, bedside guidance of aspiration or drainage procedures avoids the risk and inconvenience of transporting a critically ill patient (Fig. 19-2). Bedside ultrasound guidance for performance of invasive procedures will probably increase in the future.

Ultrasound guidance of invasive procedures has other advantages in that the procedure can be performed quite expediently, and that ultrasound equipment is relatively inexpensive compared with other imaging procedures. Ultrasound may also be used to confirm drainage of a fluid collection and check for complications such as a postaspiration hematoma.

Recent reports demonstrate the utility of pulsed Doppler or color Doppler as an aid in avoiding complications of aspiration or biopsy. Duplex sonography, and, more recently, color Doppler have been shown to be

TABLE 19-1. Ultrasound Advantages

Accurate
Needle visualization
Real-time control
Portable
Expedient
Inexpensive
Confirm drainage
Check for complications
Doppler/color flow to avoid vascular structures

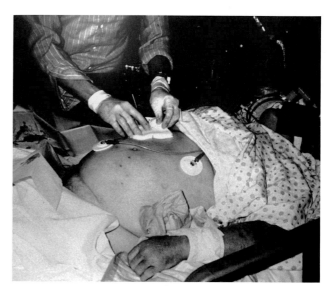

helpful in identifying the vascular nature of a mass and avoiding vascular structures within the needle path. Selective use of duplex sonography or color Doppler (Fig. 19-3 and Plate 19-1) before abdominal aspiration procedures provides information that should serve to minimize the further risk of hemorrhage associated with modern biopsy techniques. Either color flow or Doppler may be used to identify potential vascular areas to help to avoid the complications associated with needle or catheter insertion.[7]

A major disadvantage of ultrasound is its limitation by overlying patient drains and/or dressings, abdominal bowel gas, and rib artifacts.

Fig. 19-2. Portable ultrasound. An advantage of ultrasound is that it can be used at the patient's bedside. In this example, the catheter has been inserted into the gallbladder of a patient in the intensive care unit and sterile dressings are being placed around the catheter.

PATIENT PREPARATION

Proper patient consent must be obtained before performing any aspiration biopsy or drainage procedure. The procedure must be explained in detail, including the risks, benefits, and alternatives. A historical review of the patient must be obtained concerning easy bruising, abnormal bleeding during surgery or tooth extraction, and any medication that may prolong bleeding.[8] Coagulation studies and hemoglobin and/or hematocrit counts are obtained when indicated based on patient history and the site and nature of invasive procedure.

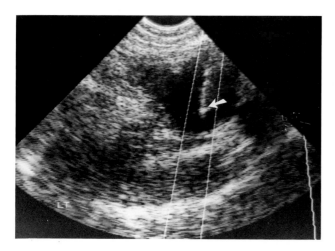

Fig. 19-1. Percutaneous biopsy. Using biopsy guidance attachments, a 22-gauge needle (arrow) is placed between precalibrated grids into a node. Cytology revealed recurrent cervical carcinoma.

ANESTHESIA

The use of analgesia and premedication for ultrasound-guided abdominal aspiration, biopsy, or drainage procedures is determined individually depending on the difficulty of the procedure and the wishes of the patient. For instance, if a simple paracentesis is performed, usually only local anesthesia is necessary. However, patients are often apprehensive and uncomfortable and may experience some pain during other procedures. My preference is to place an intravenous catheter prior to the procedure in those who are elderly, have multiple medical problems or in whom a difficult procedure is anticipated. An intravenous catheter is used for administration of analgesia prior to abdominal percutaneous procedures.

The choice of medication for patient comfort, relief of anxiety, and to control pain is dependent on the procedure, the patient, and the attending physician. Interven-

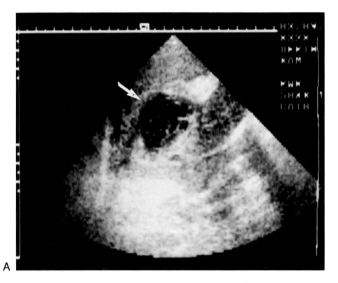
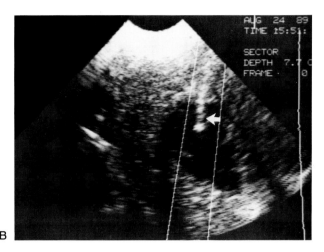

Fig. 19-3. Infected biloma. **(A)** Fluid collection (arrow) in the liver. **(B)** A 22-gauge needle (arrow) is placed transhepatically into the fluid collection avoiding the vascular region identified with color Doppler (see also Plate 19-1). (From McGahan[48] with permission.)

tionalists should only administer medications with which they are thoroughly familiar. Closely reading package inserts for dosages and potential side effects is mandatory and consultation with other health care professionals should be obtained before administering any unfamiliar medications. My preference for medication is intravenous premedication with a combination of narcotics and tranquilizers. These medications may be gradually titrated via the intravenous route. Typical narcotics used to produce analgesia and sedation include fentanyl, morphine sulfate, or meperidine. The main side effect of these narcotics is dose-dependent respiratory depression. For this reason, resuscitation equipment and naloxone (Narcan) must be available.

Typical tranquilizers that may be administered by the intravenous route include use of diazepam (Valium) and a more potent benzodiazepine derivative, midazolam hydrochloride (Versed). When using either of these medications, especially the more potent medication Versed, patients should be continuously monitored for early signs of underventilation or apnea, which could lead to hypoxia or cardiac arrest.[9,10]

For more complicated interventional procedures in the abdomen, other methods of anesthesia may be necessary. For instance in performing biliary drainage, with combined ultrasound and fluoroscopic guidance, pain may be controlled with epidural anesthesia.[11] Anesthesia standby or general anesthesia may be occasionally needed for complicated interventional procedures, or when performing interventional techniques in the pediatric patient.

GUIDANCE METHODS

Most commonly, ultrasound guidance of abdominal aspiration procedures such as simple paracentesis uses *indirect ultrasound guidance.* Using this technique, the ultrasound probe is used to select the site on the patient's skin for puncture. The transducer is removed and the site is marked with pressure from the hub of the needle. The angle and depth of the puncture are preselected from the ultrasound image and aspiration or drainage procedures are then performed. This method is used to perform biopsy or drainage of large abdominal masses or fluid collections.

When biopsy or aspiration of very small lesions or fluid collections within the abdomen is performed, direct needle guidance is often helpful; either a *freehand method* or a *needle guidance system* is used.

Freehand Method

Using the freehand method, scanning is performed to optimize visualization of both the lesion and the needle. The position may be either adjacent to the transducer and parallel to the scan plane or more remote from the transducer and perpendicular to the scan plane (Fig. 19-4). The freehand method with a linear array probe is highly accurate in aspiration or biopsy of small lesions (1 to 2 cm) in critical anatomic areas.[4] A sector probe may also be used to guide aspiration biopsy of deeper lesions within the abdomen. My preference is to place the needle

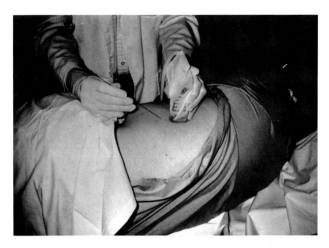

Fig. 19-4. Freehand technique. The needle is inserted to the side of the transducer and advanced under ultrasound observation. The transducer need not have sterile coverings when the needle is inserted in a location remote from the transducer. (From McGahan and Brant,[9] with permission.)

parallel rather than perpendicular to the scan plane to try to visualize not only the needle tip but the shaft of the needle.

Another option when using the freehand method is to place the transducer in sterile coverings. If no coverings are used, the probe is cleansed and placed to the side of the sterile field. A disadvantage of placing the scanhead in a sterile sheath is decreased depth penetration and some loss of resolution. However, I often find it necessary to reposition the probe when performing an invasive procedure and therefore I often place the ultrasound probe in sterile coverings. Sterile gel or povodine iodine (Betadine) is used as the acoustic coupling agent.

Needle Guidance Systems

There have been a number of needle guidance systems that are currently available. These include a dedicated biopsy transducer with holes or grooves built into the

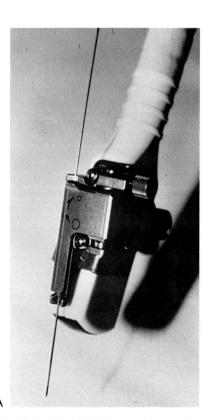

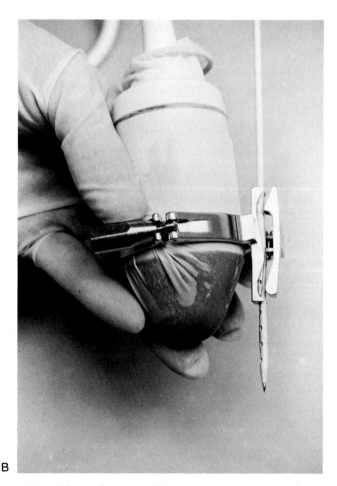

A   B

Fig. 19-5. (A & B) Biopsy guidance attachments. Two different fixed metal biopsy guidance attachments that allow a variety of different needles sizes or catheters to be utilized for either aspiration, biopsy, or drainage procedures. (From McGahan and Brant,[9] with permission.)

transducer face. More commonly, biopsy guides are now attached to the transducer. Attachable needle guides that fasten to the transducers are available from all manufacturers. These guidance systems are designed with slots or grooves sized to the different needle sizes or small catheters (Fig. 19-5). The angle, direction, and depth of the needle can be continuously monitored with real-time. The guidance system holds the needle firmly along a predetermined course displayed as a calibrated line on the video monitor of the ultrasound unit (Fig. 19-6). All needle guides allow placement of small needles (22-gauge), with some guides allowing placement of larger needles or small trocar catheters.

Other Systems

Guidance systems have also been developed for specially designed endoluminal ultrasound probes. These transrectal transducers are commonly used for transrectal biopsy of the prostate. Transvaginal transducers are commonly used for oocyte retrieval. Occasionally, the only potential drainable fluid collection or mass for biopsy may be deep within the pelvis and is best approached with a transvaginal or transrectal transducer (Figs. 19-7 and 19-8). Therefore, those performing aspiration, biopsy, or drainage procedures in the abdomen should be familiar with these types of newer endoluminal scanners that may be used to guide interventional procedures within the pelvis.

NEEDLE SELECTION

There are a number of different needles that may be used for percutaneous aspiration/biopsy. All needles differ in length, inside and outside diameter, wall thickness, flexibility, needle tip and stylet design, sonographic detectability, and suitability for cytology or for tissue cores for histology (Fig. 19-9). Most commonly, aspiration of a simple cyst can be performed with a 22- or 23-gauge needle while aspiration of abscesses with thick purulent debris will require a larger needle or catheter.

CYTOLOGY

Tissue diagnosis may be performed with either cytologic or histologic techniques. The "skinny" needle has become popular for cytologic diagnosis. Using fine needle aspiration (FNA), cytologic diagnosis is usually possible with a very thin needle (22 or 23 gauge). In general, thinner needles yield smaller specimens for diagnosis, but are associated with lower incidence of complications.[12,13]

Beveled edge needles such as the Chiba, Menghini, or Turner needles have been shown by experimental data to yield more suitable specimens for cytologic diagnosis than nonbeveled needles with circumferential sharpened tips like the Greene or Madayag needles. There are

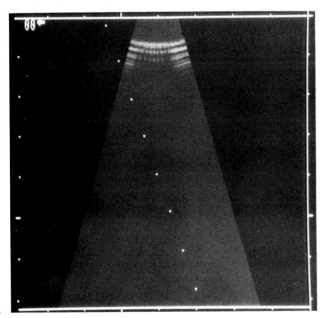

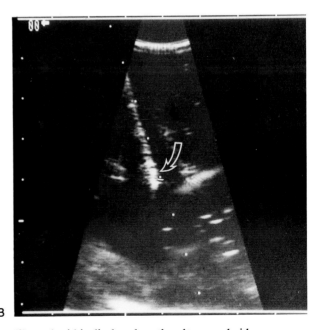

A   B

Fig. 19-6. Biopsy guidance needle attachment. **(A)** A precalibrated grid is displayed on the ultrasound video output monitor demonstrating the proposed trajectory of the needle before placement. **(B)** Needle is placed into a water path and the needle (curved arrow) follows the proposed trajectory.

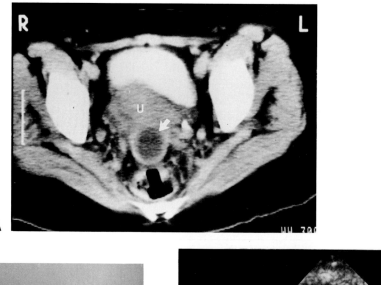

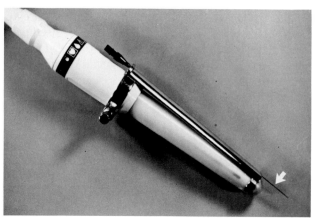

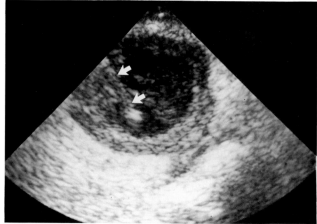

Fig. 19-7.   Transvaginal aspiration. **(A)** Well-demarcated and localized fluid collection (arrow) is noted posterior to the uterus (*U*). **(B)** In these situations, a transvaginal guidance may be used for needle (arrow) placement into the fluid collection. **(C)** Echogenic needle (arrows) is placed into the fluid collection utilizing the transvaginal route.

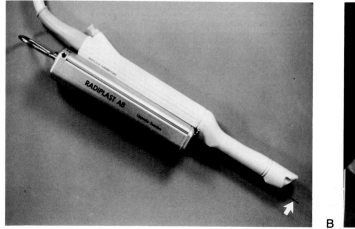

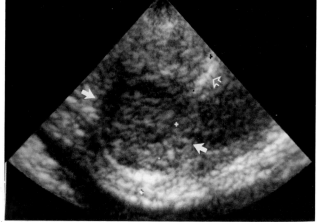

Fig. 19-8.   Prostate biopsy. **(A)** The Biopty gun was originally intended for use for prostate biopsies. As such, the Biopty-type gun is fitted to a transrectal transducer for prostate biopsy, with distal needle tip (arrow). (Fig. A from McGahan and Gerscovich,[49] with permission.) **(B)** Using the transrectal route, an echogenic tip of the biopsy needle (open arrow) is positioned within the path of a prostate nodule (arrows), before firing the automated gun.

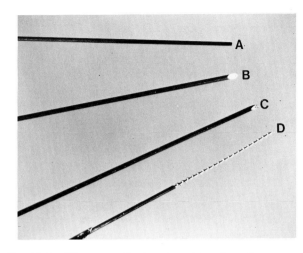

Fig. 19-9. Biopsy needle tips. A variety of needles are available for percutaneous biopsy, including **(A)** the Greene needle with the stylet removed showing the nonbeveled tip; **(B)** the Chiba needle with a sharpened beveled tip; **(C)** the Franseen needle with a cutting edge; and **(D)** the Rotex needle with the screw inner stylet. (From McGahan and Brant,[9] with permission.)

a variety of other needles and tips including the Franseen, which has three cutting serrations at the needle tip. The Rotex needle has a screw inner stylet, which is excellent for sonographic visibility, but tissue specimens may prove to be difficult to remove or become macerated with removal from the stylet[4,12] (Fig. 19-9). There are other specially designed needles such as the Surecut (Meadox Surgimed, Oakland, NJ) or the PercuCut self-aspiration needles (E-Z-EM, Inc., Westbury, NJ), which are designed for core tissue specimens.

A number of manufacturers have designed needles that are scored, abraded, or have surface roughenings to increase sonographic visibility.[14] Alternatively, before performing an aspiration/biopsy under ultrasound guidance, scoring the needle (placing circumferential markings) with a scalpel may improve needle detection.

When performing FNA for cytology, once the needle is properly positioned, the inner stylet is removed and a syringe is attached to the needle and approximately 10 ml of negative suction is applied with a hand-held syringe. Simultaneously, several up-and-down movements are made within the lesions. A rotatory motion of the needle may be helpful to increase tissue retrieval.[15] Release of negative suction is needed as the needle is removed from the lesion so as not to aspirate more proximal contents into the syringe. Some authors use a technique in which they preload the syringe with 2 ml of saline to flush the specimen from the needle shaft into the test tube if a cytologist is not available. Our preference is to have a cytologist in the room who does an

immediate cytologic staining to evaluate adequacy of tissue specimen.

A recent report advocated a *nonaspiration technique* for performance of cytology. A 22-gauge spinal needle is inserted into the lesion. Once the needle tip is confirmed in the lesion, the stylet is removed. Without attaching a syringe, several gentle, rapid in-and-out movements of the needle are performed for 10 seconds or until fluid is seen in the needle hub. Cytology retrieval is reported to be excellent.[16]

HISTOLOGY

Histologic diagnosis to demonstrate tissue architecture requires a core specimen, obtained from a large cutting needle (14 to 20 gauge). An automated Biopty gun was introduced for performance of ultrasound-guided prostate biopsies (Figs. 19-8, 19-10, and 19-11). The BARD/Radiplast Biopty gun (BARD Urological Divisions, Covington, GA; Radiplast, Uppsala, Sweden) is used with a large gauge biopsy-cut needle. These Biopty-cut needles consist of an inner trocar with a 1.7-cm sample notch. The inner trocar is placed into an outer cannula of the needle. The Biopty gun consists of a handheld device that automatically triggers a two-stage rapid firing of the Biopty-cut needle. The spring loaded Biopty gun accepts two separate hubs of the needle trocar and the cannula, which can be placed within the gun either before or after the mechanism is cocked. The gun is fired, and the inner trocar and its sample notch are thrust forward 2.3 cm (Fig. 19-12). This is followed almost instantaneously by a forward thrust of the outer cannula, which shears off the tissue sample. Needles that have a shorter thrust have also been developed.

Recently, percutaneous biopsies of abdominal organs have been successfully performed with the automated Biopty gun system.[17,18] The Biopty gun needle may be placed under ultrasound guidance. After the needle is placed to the desired location by ultrasound, allowance is made for the 2.3-cm needle excursion before the gun is fired. This specimen is placed in formalin for pathologic review. There are several manufacturers that now have disposable automated Tru-cut type needles, which are available in sample sizes from 14 to 20 gauge (Fig. 19-10). Advantages of these automated needles are the elimination of the "crush" artifact and obscuration by blood that are common problems associated with thin needle biopsy techniques. Patient discomfort is minimal with the rapid firing of these needles and the procedure time is reduced.

Several recent articles have attested to the safety and increased accuracy of these new automated biopsy-type

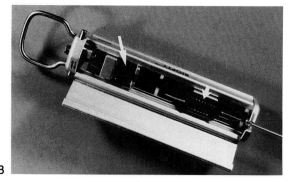

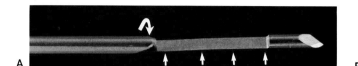

A   B

Fig. 19-10. Biopty-cut needle. **(A)** The inner 1.7-cm sample notch (arrows), which is thrust forward approximately 2.3 cm followed almost instantaneously by forward thrust of the outer cannula (curved arrow) with firing of the Biopty gun. (Fig. A from McGahan and Gerscovich,[49] with permission.) **(B)** The Biopty gun in which the proximal portion of the inner trocar (long arrow) and outer sheath (short arrow) is placed into the automated device before use.

devices.[19] These articles have demonstrated the efficacy of automated biopsy guns and excellent tissue retrieval compared with conventional biopsy needles.[20] For instance, Poster et al[21] demonstrated the accuracy of this technique by providing core biopsy specimens for definitive histologic diagnosis of renal parenchymal disease in biopsy of native pediatric kidneys. They utilized an 18-gauge automated biopsy needle and now exclusively use these automated biopsy needles in performance of percutaneous ultrasound-guided biopsy of native pediatric kidneys. We have found utilization of these automated guns, for ultrasound-guided percutaneous biopsy, to be

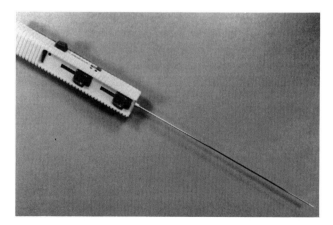

Fig. 19-11. Disposable cutting needle. A number of manufacturers have automated disposable needles that are used to obtain a core biopsy. This one is manufactured by Medi-Tech, Boston Scientific Corporation, Watertown, MA. This is very similar to the BARD Biopty gun except that the complete system is disposable.

quite helpful in obtaining histologic specimens of solid organs within the abdomen. We have often used both cytologic techniques and automated biopsy guns and have had several cases in which cytology was indeterminate and histology specimens with an automated biopsy device were definitive for carcinoma. A potential disadvantage of using the larger needles is increased hemorrhagic complications as compared with the skinny biopsy needles. In general, hemorrhagic complications are increased with the use of large bore needles.[12,13] However, to date complications have not been a major problem in our experience or for others using the automated biopsy devices.[19–21]

These automated cutting needles have been used with a high success rate elsewhere in the abdomen, such as in the performance of pancreatic biopsies.[22] Using this technique, Elvin et al[22] did not hesitate to pass an 18-gauge needle through the colon as long as this was the shortest available path that avoided any major vessels. In 47 of their patients, there were no cases of biopsy-induced pancreatitis and no cases of adverse sequelae of needle passage through the colon. Complications included only two cases of vasovagal reaction and two cases of mild pain. They believe that their results show that a cut biopsy of the pancreas is a useful, reliable, and nontraumatic method in the diagnosis of pancreatic malignancy. These authors also believe that the results of their study support the impression that diagnostic yield and complication rate of cutting-needle biopsy techniques compare well with that of FNA for pancreatic tumor biopsy. Thus, it seems that the use of these automated biopsy-type needles will be utilized further in performance of biopsies in the abdomen.

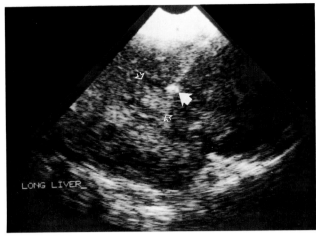
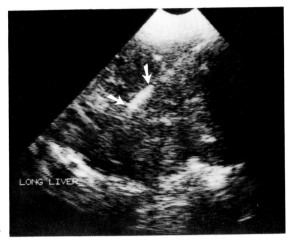

A   B

Fig. 19-12. Specimen of liver metastases taken with a BARD Biopty gun. **(A)** The 18-gauge Biopty-type needle is placed into a liver with the tip (arrow) visualized at the edge of a circumscribed liver lesion (open arrows). **(B)** The needle is then fired approximately 2.3 cm through the liver taking a core specimen (arrows) from the liver. Histology demonstrated metastatic colon carcinoma.

ABSCESS DRAINAGE

Percutaneous catheter drainage of abdominal abscesses has been shown to be a safe and effective alternative to operative drainage. Percutaneous drainage avoids the morbidity associated with operation and the necessity for general anesthesia. Percutaneous abscess drainage has proven to be an effective alternative to surgical techniques. In general, there are only a few contraindications to percutaneous drainage of abdominal abscesses. These include (1) poorly defined abscesses such as pancreatic phlegmons that are not amenable to catheter drainage; (2) extensive abdominal abscesses with either multicompartment involvement or in multiple locations within the abdomen; (3) infected necrotic materials, such as pancreatic necrosis, which require surgical debridement; (4) lack of a safe access route due to overlying bowel or overlying vascular structures; and (5) major bleeding problems including coagulopathies.[23]

Computed Tomographic Guidance

In general, my preference is to use computed tomography (CT) rather than ultrasound when possible for draining abscesses in the mid-abdomen. CT better defines the extent of the abdominal abscess and more importantly visualizes the overlying bowel, which could be inadvertently transgressed during catheter placement. Simple aspiration procedures such as paracentesis are usually performed under ultrasound guidance. Abdominal abscesses in solid organs, such as the liver, are easily drained with ultrasound.

Ultrasound/Fluoroscopic Control

Combined ultrasound/fluoroscopic guidance may be used to drain liver abscesses, the gallbladder, biliary tract or a renal collecting system. Initial needle puncture is guided by ultrasound while guide wire exchange/catheter manipulation is monitored by fluoroscopy. Combined use of ultrasound for initial needle placement and fluoroscopy for catheter placement via the guide wire exchange technique optimizes the advantage of both guidance systems in performing abdominal drainage procedures.[24]

Ultrasound Guidance

In some situations, patients may be so desperately ill that they cannot be moved to the radiology department. Recently developed techniques, such as emergency percutaneous cholecystostomy for acute cholecystitis, are routinely performed under ultrasound guidance at the patient's bedside.[25,26]

Technique

When performing catheter drainage, a safe access route must be determined. The cavity is first aspirated and purulent material is obtained. The catheter is usually inserted via the guidewire exchange technique. Most patients are on a broad spectrum of antibiotics for underlying sepsis prior to drainage. Various catheters may be utilized for drainage. Nonviscus fluid collections are probably adequately drained with size 8 to 10 French catheters. More viscus fluids are best evacuated with a double lumen sump-type catheter. Recent research has demonstrated the small size of the catheter stopcock may be a limiting factor in fluid egress.[27]

After the abscess cavity has been drained, the patient is rescanned with ultrasound or CT to check for adequacy of catheter drainage. The patient is then followed closely for catheter output, decreased pain, normalization of temperature, and laboratory parameters. The patient's antibiotics are adjusted for appropriate culture and sensitivity. A follow-up fluoroscopic abscessogram is helpful to identify the size and configuration of the abscess cavity and to note fistulous communications.[28] Most low output enteric fistulas with outputs less than 50 ml/d were generally resolved with a combination of percutaneous drainage and antibiotic therapy. However, higher output fistulas of over 200 ml/d may not close with catheter drainage alone.[29,30]

SPECIFIC ANATOMIC AREAS

Abdomen

The diagnostic accuracy of retroperitoneal and pelvic lymph node biopsy varies from 65 to 90 percent.[31] This wide variation is due to the need to obtain a large tissue sample required to accurately diagnose cell patterns in lymphoma.[32] Ultrasound may be used to guide FNA

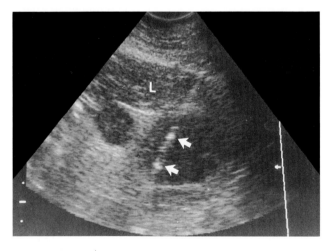

Fig. 19-13. Liver biopsy. Using freehand ultrasound guidance, a 22-gauge needle (arrows) is placed into a focal hypoechoic hepatic nodule. Cytology revealed undifferentiated adenocarcinoma. (*L*, liver.)

when adenopathy is sonographically visualized (Fig. 19-1). Biopsy techniques are similar to those previously described and perhaps use of automated core cutting biopsy-type needles will improve retrieval rates.

Either diagnostic or therapeutic paracentesis is easily performed under ultrasound guidance. The fluid is localized and the needle or catheter is inserted into a fluid collection usually with ultrasound guidance. When performing aspiration of fluid collections within the abdomen, inadvertent placement of the catheter through a loop of bowel must be avoided. Even insertion of a small gauge needle through the colon, then subsequent passage into a fluid collection may potentially contaminate a noninfected fluid collection, thus creating an abscess.

Liver

Fine needle aspiration is a safe and accurate method for cytologic diagnosis of malignancy (Fig. 19-13). FNA techniques have shown an accuracy rate in cytologic diagnosis of hepatic malignancy as high as 95 percent in a large series.[33,34] It is likely that with the use of automated Tru-cut biopsy needles of moderate size (18 to 20 gauge), the diagnostic yield for malignancy may increase without significant increase in morbidity (Fig. 19-12).

Ultrasound may also decrease complication rates and increase diagnostic yield when performing histologic biopsy of the liver for hepatic architecture. Greiner and Franken[35] compared liver biopsy techniques using a "blind" biopsy and ultrasound-guided biopsy using a 14-gauge cutting needle. Ultrasound knowledge of liver topography reduced the complication rate in this series from 1.4 to 0.2 percent and the need for analgesia from 4.5 to 1.1 percent in performance of core liver biopsies. In cases of Calides syndrome, the bowel may be interposed between the liver and the abdominal wall, a situation that could be disastrous if the "blind" biopsy is performed using a very large bore biopsy needle. Use of ultrasound before performance of biopsy may be helpful to prevent this complication.

Ultrasound may be used in the future to guide percutaneous ablation of liver lesions. Figure 19-14 demonstrates ultrasound-guided destruction of normal liver in the animal model, using radiofrequency electrocautery. Ultrasound may be used to guide other methods of percutaneous ablation of tumors within the liver or other organs.[36]

Gallbladder

Gallbladder biopsy is performed similarly to other aspiration/biopsy techniques. Preoperative knowledge of the gallbladder carcinoma may change the surgical man-

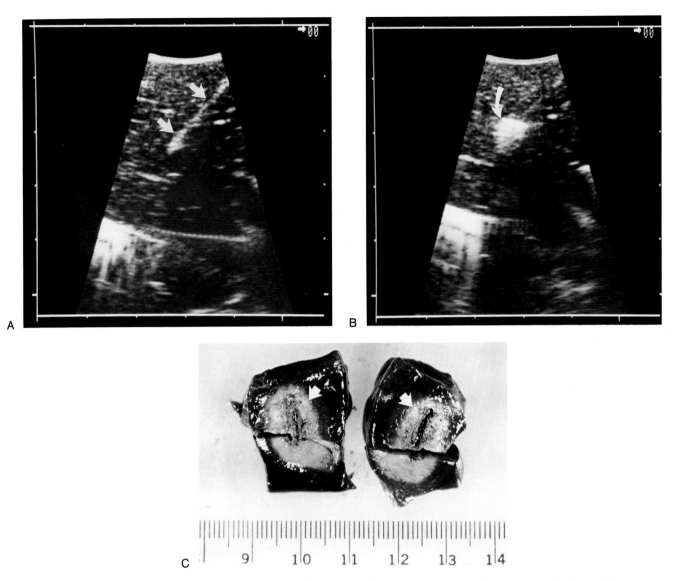

Fig. 19-14. Hepatic ablation. **(A)** A specially designed needle (arrows) is inserted into the hepatic tissue. **(B)** Using radiofrequency electrocautery, a well-demonstrated echogenic region (curved arrow) is noted about the needle tip. (Figs. A & B from McGahan et al,[36] with permission.) **(C)** A pathologic specimen demonstrates an area of central scar with surround area of coagulation (arrows) in this deep hepatic ablation.

agement of the patient from a simple cholecystectomy to a cholecystectomy with a wedge resection of the liver in an area of possible hepatic invasion.[37]

Emergency cholecystectomy is associated with higher mortality rates than is elective cholecystectomy. A number of recent reports have shown that percutaneous cholecystostomy may be helpful in management of hospitalized patients with suspected acute cholecystitis.[25,26] Ultrasound is frequently used to guide percutaneous cholecystostomy. As the ultrasound unit is portable, the entire procedure is performed at the patient's bedside. The catheter system may be placed transhepatically

under ultrasound guidance into the gallbladder using the trocar/Seldinger technique. It is best that the catheter used for performance of percutaneous cholecystostomy has a securing device such as a Cope loop to prevent catheter dislodgment from the gallbladder[25] (Figs. 19-15 and 19-16).

In most circumstances, percutaneous cholecystostomy is a temporizing procedure for patients with acute cholecystitis before more definitive treatments such as cholecystectomy can be performed. However, in a number of patients, percutaneous cholecystostomy has been proven to be a definitive treatment for acute acalculous

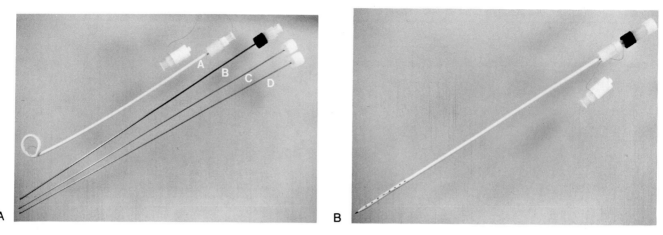

Fig. 19-15. Drainage catheter. **(A)** The McGahan drainage catheter is composed of four components including a 25-cm long pigtail catheter with a Cope loop *(A)*, a cannula *(B)*, and a blunted obturator *(D)* used to straighten the catheter. Once the catheter and the cannula are assembled together, the inner blunted obturator is removed and replaced with a sharp inner stylet *(C)*, so that the catheter may be inserted via the trocar method. **(B)** The catheter is loaded on the cannula and the sharp inner stylet for placement via the trocar method. (From McGahan,[25] with permission.)

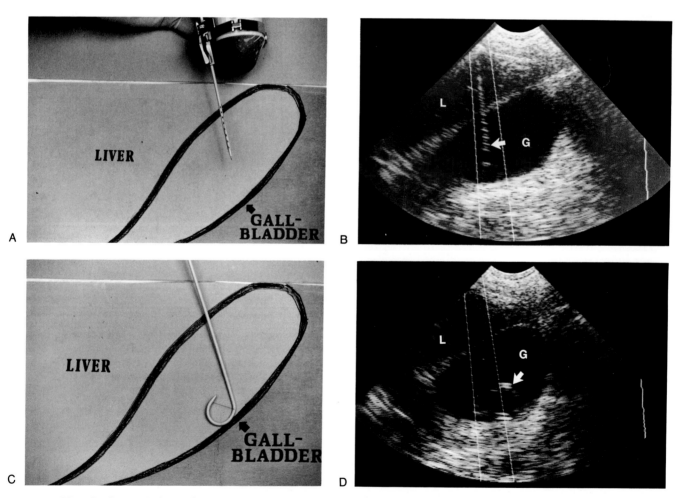

Fig. 19-16. Technique of percutaneous cholecystostomy—trocar method. **(A & B)** With sonographic guidance, a cholecystostomy catheter (arrow) is placed transhepatically via the trocar method into the gallbladder *(G)*. *(L,* liver.) **(C & D)** Once in the gallbladder, the stylet and the cannula are removed while the catheter is simultaneously advanced into the gallbladder *(G)* and the distal loop of the catheter (arrow) is reformed. *(L,* liver.) (From McGahan,[50] with permission.)

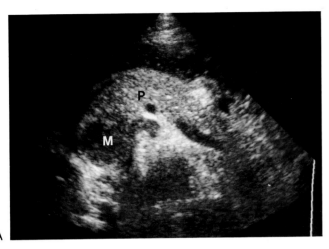

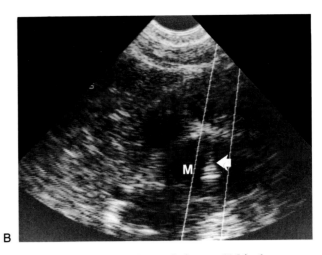

A

B

Fig. 19-17. Pancreatic biopsy. **(A)** Transverse real-time ultrasound demonstrated a hypoechoic mass (*M*) in the head of the pancreas (*P*). **(B)** Using sonographic guidance, a needle (arrow) is placed into the mass (*M*). Cytology revealed pancreatic carcinoma.

cholecystitis, thus avoiding cholecystectomy.[26] Recently, percutaneous cholecystostomy has been shown to be useful as an alternative to transhepatic drainage of the biliary drainage.[38]

Biliary Tract

Percutaneous transhepatic cholangiography and drainage are usually performed under ultrasound guidance. However, combined ultrasound/fluoroscopic guidance has been shown to be helpful to optimize the benefits of both procedures.[24] Using the combined ultrasound and fluoroscopic approach, selected ducts may be punctured under ultrasound guidance for either percutaneous transhepatic cholangiography or as the site of definitive catheter placement. Some authors have advocated the use of ultrasound alone for percutaneous transhepatic biliary drainage.[39] My preference is to use ultrasound for initial needle puncture with catheter manipulation by the guidewire exchange technique using fluoroscopic control. Ultrasound is used to identify the exact site of ductal dilatation for initial needle puncture.[24]

Pancreas

Percutaneous ultrasound-guided FNA/biopsy for diagnosis of malignancy in the pancreas has been shown to have an accuracy rate slightly less than that for cytologic diagnosis in the liver[40] (Fig. 19-17). Most recently, the use of ultrasound-guided 18-gauge automated biopsy gun has been proven to be highly accurate in diagnosis of pancreatic malignancy.[22]

Peripancreatic fluid collections may develop during an episode of acute pancreatitis. Many of these fluid collections disappear spontaneously. Ultrasound needle aspiration may be used to determine if these fluid collections are infected (Fig. 19-18). Later, mature fibrotic walls develop around fluid collections, and are termed *pancreatic pseudocysts.* The pseudocysts may in fact be either infected or noninfected and may be treated with percutaneous drainage.

Needle aspiration may be used to determine if a pancreatic pseudocyst is sterile or infected. There is a high reoccurrence rate with simple aspiration of pancreatic pseudocysts. Alternatively, recent published series of re-

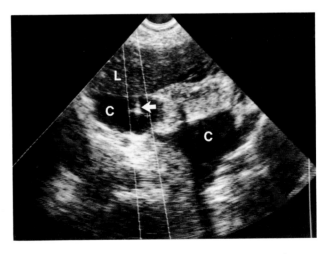

Fig. 19-18. Pancreatic aspiration. Transverse scan demonstrating a 22-gauge needle (arrow) being passed transhepatically into a peripancreatic fluid collection. This and a second fluid collection (*C*) were aspirated with ultrasound guidance. (*L*, liver.) (From McGahan et al,[6] with permission.)

sults of percutaneous drainage of either infected or non-infected pseudocysts are excellent. The overall cure rate by catheter drainage alone was greater than 90 percent.[41] In most cases, CT rather than sonography is the primary method of drainage.

Ultrasound-guided percutaneous fine needle puncture of the pancreatic duct may be followed by cholangiography.[42] Using this technique, pancreatic fluid can be aspirated for cytologic diagnosis. Under fluoroscopic control, the duct may be opacified. This technique is not widely used and more experience should be gained before considering this a routine procedure.

Kidney

Renal biopsies are performed either for cases of suspected malignancy or for histologic diagnosis of renal architecture. Whatever needle is used, ultrasound is helpful in marking the site and depth of the renal cortex. Using ultrasound-guided core needle techniques, renal tissue is recovered in greater than 95 percent of cases[43] (Fig. 19-19). Also promising is a recent report about the use of automated Biopty guns in performance of renal biopsies.[21]

Most renal cysts can be characterized by ultrasound. Indications for percutaneous aspiration of a simple cyst include (1) thick or irregular walls; (2) wall calcifications; (3) internal echoes or presence of septations; (4) presence of a solid mass arising from the wall; and (5) discrepancy in imaging results as to cystic or solid nature of a mass.[44]

Ultrasound-guided FNA of a cyst is similar to other previously explained techniques. A 22-gauge thin wall needle is passed directly into the cyst under ultrasound

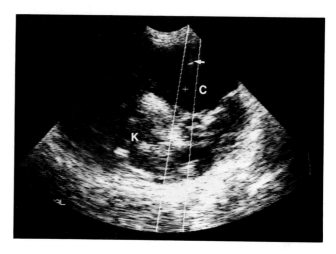

Fig. 19-20. Renal cyst aspiration. Renal cyst puncture was performed on this symptomatic patient using a biopsy guidance attachment. The echogenic needle (arrow) is noted between the precalibrated grid lines as it passes into the renal cyst (*C*). (*K*, kidney.) (From Lindsay et al,[44] with permission.)

guidance (Fig. 19-20). Investigation of the cyst fluid includes culture and sensitivity, lipids (Sudan stain), lactate dehydrogenase (LDH), protein, and glucose. A small amount of protein (<2.5 g/dl), and LDH (<25.5 μ/L) may be obtained from a simple cyst.[45] Increased LDH is associated with malignancy.[46]

Ultrasound has gained wide acceptance as the imaging modality for initial needle placement for percutaneous nephrostomy.[47] Most commonly, ultrasound is used to access the dilated renal collecting system and the catheter is placed via the Seldinger technique under fluoroscopic control.

Pelvis

There are few descriptions of FNA of the pelvis under ultrasound guidance. Any pelvic abnormality well visualized with ultrasound can be aided by sonographic needle guidance. These include abnormalities of the ovaries and uterus. FNA of ovarian masses presents certain problems. Ovarian malignancies often have a complex echostructure. If an ovarian malignancy coexists with a benign cyst, the biopsy may sample the cyst and not the malignancy. Spillage of cyst contents from a mucinous cystadenocarcinoma may lead to pseudomucinous peritonei—a potentially devasting complication.

More recently, endoluminal transducers that may be placed in close proximity to pelvic contents have been developed. Special biopsy guidance systems have been developed and allow for transvaginal aspiration and biopsy of the pelvis. Most commonly, this is used for

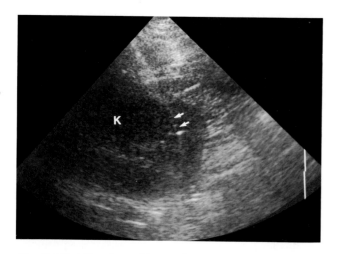

Fig. 19-19. Renal core biopsy. Sixteen-gauge needle (arrows) was placed percutaneous under freehand ultrasound guidance into the lower pole of the kidney (*K*). (From Lindsay et al,[44] with permission.)

transvaginal biopsy of ovarian follicles for oocytes retrieval for in vitro fertilization programs. However, this technique may also be used for other applications such as aspiration/biopsy of pelvic masses. Transvaginal ultrasound may also be used for aspiration or drainage of pelvic fluid collections when other routes are inaccessible (Fig. 19-7).

Specialized transducer probes are routinely utilized for either transrectal or tranperitoneal biopsy of the male prostate. The transrectal technique is most commonly used with an automated Biopty-type gun in performance of prostate biopsy (Fig. 19-10).

SUMMARY

Ultrasound may be used to guide aspiration, biopsy, or drainage procedures in the abdomen. Ultrasound has several advantages as compared with other imaging modalities because it is very precise and allows for direct needle visualization under real-time control. Most ultrasound units are portable and therefore many emergency procedures may be performed at the patient's bedside. It is certain that with refinement of aspiration, biopsy, and drainage techniques and further advances in ultrasound instrumentation, there will be a future increase in the use of ultrasound guidance for abdominal interventional procedures.

ACKNOWLEDGMENTS

Special thanks to Karen Anderson for preparation of this chapter.

REFERENCES

1. Blady JV: Aspiration biopsy of tumors in obscure or difficult locations under roentgenoscopic guidance. AJR 1939;42:515
2. Holm HH, Kristensen JK, Rasmussen SN et al: Ultrasound as a guide in percutaneous puncture technique. Ultrasonics 1972;10:83
3. Goldberg BB, Pollack HM: Ultrasonic aspiration transducer. Radiology 1972;102:187
4. Reading CC, Charboneau JW, James EM, Hurt MR: Sonographically guided percutaneous biopsy of small (3 cm or less) masses. AJR 1988;151:189
5. McGahan JP: Aspiration and drainage procedures in the intensive care unit: percutaneous sonographic guidance. Radiology 1985;154:531
6. McGahan JP, Anderson MW, Walter JP: Portable real-time sonographic and needle guidance systems for aspiration and drainage. AJR 1986;147:1241
7. McGahan JP, Anderson MW: Pulse Doppler sonography as an aid in ultrasound-guided aspiration biopsy. Gastrointest Radiol 1987;12:279
8. Rapaport SI: Preoperative hemostatic evaluation: which tests, if any? Blood 1983;61:229
9. McGahan JP, Brant WE: Principles, instrumentation, and guidance systems. p. 1. In McGahan JP (ed): Interventional Ultrasound. Williams & Wilkins, Baltimore, 1990
10. Neff CC: Analgesia for abdominal interventional procedures. p. 12. In Ferrucci JT Jr, Wittenberg J, Mueller PR, Simeone JF (eds): Interventional Radiology of the Abdomen. 2nd Ed. Williams & Wilkins, Baltimore, 1985
11. Teplick SK, Harshfield DL, Brandon J, Rosenberg H: Pain management for major percutaneous biliary procedures. Radiology 1990;177:(P):175
12. Andriole JG, Haaga JR, Adams RB, Nunez C: Biopsy needle characteristics assessed in the laboratory. Radiology 1983;148:659
13. Haaga JR, LiPuma JP, Bryan PJ et al: Clinical comparison of small- and large-caliber cutting needles for biopsy. Radiology 1983;146:665
14. McGahan JP: Laboratory assessment of ultrasonic needle and catheter visualization. J Ultrasound Med 1986; 5:373
15. Wittenberg J, Mueller PR, Ferrucci JT Jr et al: Percutaneous core biopsy of abdominal tumor using 22 gauge needles: further observations. AJR 1982;139:75
16. Fagelman D, Chess Q: Nonaspiration fine-needle cytology of the liver: a new technique for obtaining diagnostic samples. AJR 1990;155:1217
17. Ragde H, Aldape HC, Blasko JC: Biopty: an automatic needle biopsy device—its use with an 18-gauge Tru-cut needle (Biopty-cut) in 174 consecutive prostate core biopsies. Endosonographique 1987;3:5
18. Parker SH, Hopper KD, Yakes WF et al: Image-directed percutaneous biopsies with a biopsy gun. Radiology 1989;171:663
19. Bernardino ME: Automated biopsy devices: significance and safety. Radiology 1990;176:615
20. Hopper KD, Baird DE, Reddy VV et al: Efficacy of automated biopsy guns versus conventional biopsy needles in the pygmy pig. Radiology 1990;176:671
21. Poster RB, Jones DB, Spirt BA: Percutaneous pediatric renal biopsy: use of the biopsy gun. Radiology 1990;176:725
22. Elvin A, Andersson T, Scheibenpflug L, Lindgren PG: Biopsy of the pancreas with a biopsy gun. Radiology 1990;176:677
23. Jeffrey RB Jr: Abdominal abscesses: the role of CT and sonography. p. 129. McGahan JP (ed): Interventional ultrasound. Williams & Wilkins, Baltimore, 1990
24. McGahan JP, Raduns K: Biliary drainage using combined ultrasound fluoroscopic guidance. J Interventional Radiol 1990;5:33
25. McGahan JP: A new catheter design for percutaneous cholecystostomy. Radiology 1988;166:49
26. McGahan JP, Lindfors KK: Percutaneous cholecystos-

tomy: an alternative to surgical cholecystostomy for acute cholecystitis? Radiology 1989;173:481

27. D'Agostino H, Park Y, Moyers P et al: Influence of the stopcock connection in the performance of percutaneous drainage catheters. Radiology 1990;177(P):276

28. Kerlan RJ Jr, Pogany AC, Jeffrey RB et al: Radiologic management of abdominal abscesses. AJR 1985;144:145

29. Kerlan RK Jr, Jeffrey RB Jr, Pogany AC, Ring EJ: Abdominal abscess with low output fistula: successful percutaneous drainage. Radiology 1985;155:73

30. Jeffrey RB Jr, Tolentino CS, Federle MP, Laing FC: Percutaneous drainage of periappendiceal abscesses: review of 20 patients. AJR 1987;149:59

31. Bernardino ME: Percutaneous biopsy. AJR 1984;142:41

32. Zornoza J, Cabanillas J, Altoff TM et al: Percutaneous needle biopsy in abdominal lymphoma. AJR 1981;136:97

33. Grant EG, Richardson JD, Smirniotopoulos JG, Jacobs NM: Fine-needle biopsy directed by real-time sonography: technique and accuracy. AJR 1983;141:29

34. Schwerk WB, Durr HK, Schmitz-Moormann P: Ultrasound guided fine-needle biopsies in pancreatic and hepatic neoplasms. Gastrointest Radiol 1983;8:219

35. Greiner L, Franken FH: Sonographically assisted liver biopsy—replacement for blind needle biopsy? Dtsch Med Wochenschr 1983;11:108, 368

36. McGahan JP, Browning PD, Brock JM, Tesluk H: Hepatic ablation using radiofrequency electrocautery. Invest Radiol 1990;25:267

37. McGahan JP, Gerscovich E, Lindfors KK: Gallbladder disease: perspectives in diagnosis and treatment. Radiol 1989;1:171

38. vanSonnenberg E, D'Agostino HB, Casola G et al: The benefits of percutaneous cholecystostomy for decompression of selected cases of obstructive jaundice. Radiology 1990;176:15

39. Lameris JS, Obertop H, Jeekel J: biliary drainage by ultrasound-guided puncture of the left hepatic duct. Clin Radiol 1985;36:269

40. Porter B, Karp W, Forsberg L: Percutaneous cytodiagnosis of abdominal masses by ultrasound guided fine-needle aspiration biopsy. Acta Radiol [Diagn] 1981;22:663

41. vanSonnenberg E, Wittich GR, Casola G et al: Percutaneous drainage of infected and noninfected pancreatic pseudocysts: experience in 101 cases. Radiology 1989;170:757

42. Ohto M, Karasawa E, Tsuchiya Y et al: Ultrasonically guided percutaneous contrast medium injection and aspiration biopsy using a real-time puncture transducer. Radiology 1980;136:171

43. Afschrift M, Mets T, Matthijs E, Lameire N: A 2 year experience with percutaneous renal biopsy under ultrasonic guidance. Acta Clin Belg 1981;36:237

44. Lindsay DJ, Lyons EA, Levi CS: Urinary tract. p. 199. In McGahan JP (ed): Interventional Ultrasound. Williams & Wilkins, Baltimore, 1990

45. Clayman RV, Williams RD, Fraley EE: The pursuit of the renal mass. N Engl J Med 1979;300:72

46. Phillips GN, Kumari-Subaiya S: Renal cyst puncture: LDH as a tumor marker. Presented at the annual meeting of the Radiological Society of North America, Chicago, 1986

47. Pedersen H, Juul N: Ultrasound-guided percutaneous nephrostomy in the treatment of advanced gynecologic malignancy. Acta Obstet Gynecol Scand 1988;67:199

48. McGahan JP: Ultrasound-guided abdominal aspiration/drainage procedures. p. 443. In Rumack CM, Wilson SR, Charboneau JW (eds): Diagnostic Ultrasound. Mosby-Year Book, St. Louis, 1991

49. McGahan JP, Gerscovich GO: Interventional ultrasound update. Appl Radiol 1991;20:10

50. McGahan JP: Gallbladder. p. 159. In McGahan JP (ed): Interventional Ultrasound. Williams & Wilkins, Baltimore, 1990

Index

Page numbers followed by f *denote figures; those followed by* t *denote tables.*

A